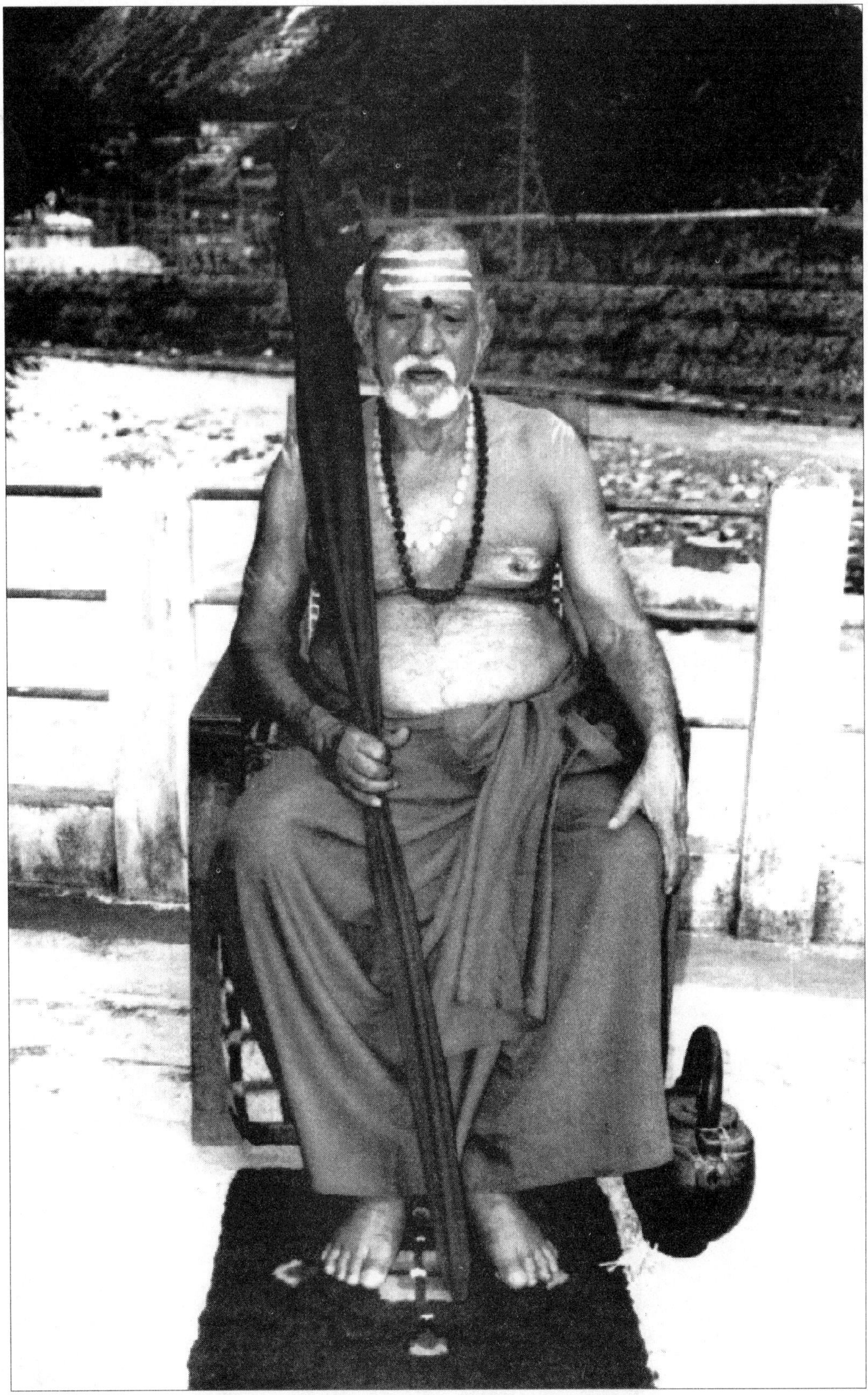

Dedicated to His Holiness 1008 Sri Sri Srimat Swami Narayan Tirthaji Maharaj

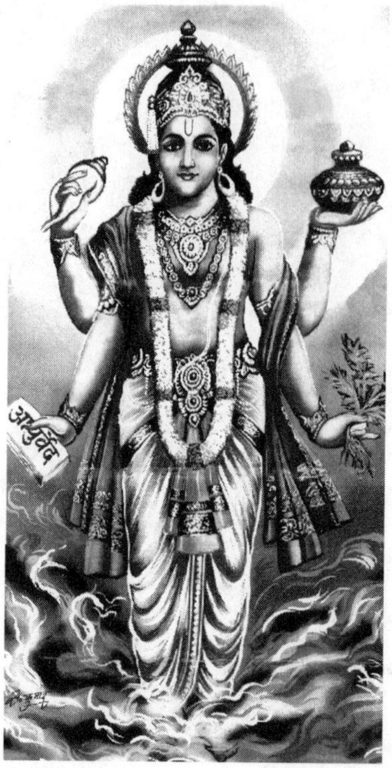

Dhanwantari: Divine father of Āyurvedic Medicine

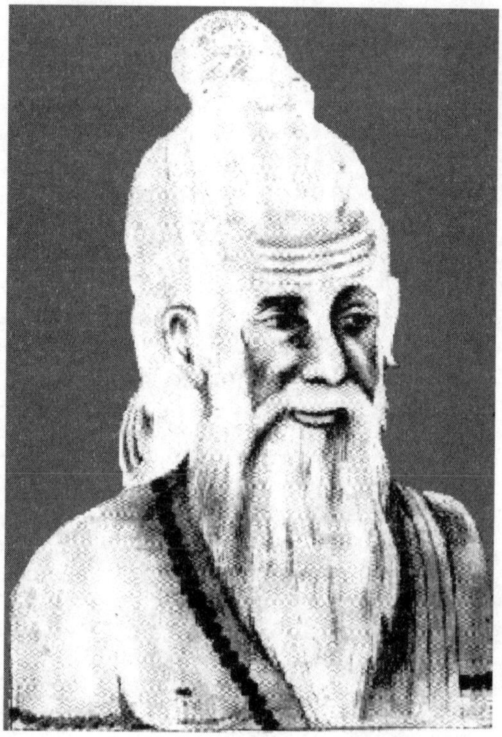

Māhāriṣhi Bharadwaj:Human father of Āyurvedic Medicine

The Ayurveda Encyclopedia

Natural Secrets to Healing, Prevention, & Longevity

Swami Sada Shiva Tirtha

Technical Editor
Dr. R. C. Uniyal

Contributing Editors
Dr. S. Sandhu, Dr. J.K. Chandhok

Second Edition

Publisher
Ayurveda Holistic Center Press
82A Bayville Ave
Bayville, NY 11709 USA
http://ayurvedahc.com/press.htm

ISBN 0-9658042-2-4
Library of Congress Catalog Card Number 97-077845

Edited by Guru Amrit Kaur Khalsa and Rob Paton of Caduceus Press, NJ
Book cover design by Linda Parks; Boulder, Colorado

This book is a reference manual, and is not intended to treat, diagnose, or prescribe. The information in this book is in no way intended to substitute for health consultations with licensed practitioners.

Some of the medical pictures appear courtesy of the Software Marketing Corporation's Bodyworks 3.0 CD-ROM program.
Some of the Indian clipart appears courtesy of Prium Graphics' KalashKala 1.0 program (617) 444-4103. All Hindi words used in KalashKala ver. 1.0 were created using Saralfonts, a product of SaralSoft, located in California.

Printed in Canada

Table of Contents

Dedication

Dedicated to my beloved baba, His Holiness 1008, Sri Sri Srimat Swami Narayan Tirthaji Maharaj, without whose Divine silence and blessings, this book could never have been written or published.

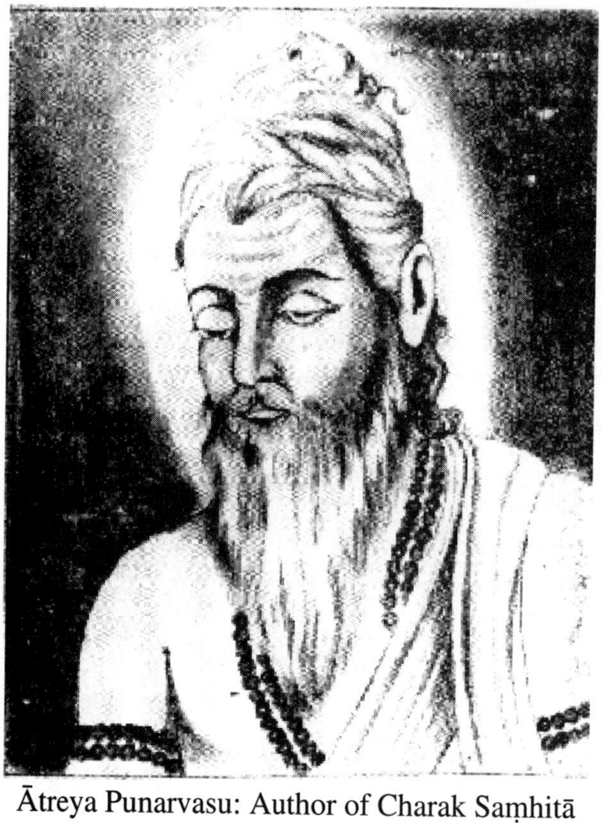

Ātreya Punarvasu: Author of Charak Saṃhitā

A Psalm of Dedication

(In memory of the Christmas in Montreal, 1952)

Who are Thou, Magnum Marvel
Hanging in the cross-bar of cruelty?
Veneration to Thee!
Does the soul of Eternal Pathos-
Stalled in the body of man
Role Defiance to Death?
A man never Thou art.
The petty strip of a loin-cloth
shies to bring Thy body bare to all eyes
But is forced to slip off Thy slim waist;
Thy arms wide apart,
Thy bellowing feet locked together,
For Thy palm and Thy soles to get
Teethed in canine hooks.
Thy sores drain Thy red hot blood.
And, what eyes are Thine!
Wide and Large azure pools,
Half-lid but flowing
The tears of mercy sublime
That roll down Thy sturdy cheeks
To mix up with Thy blood
And drench the arid bosom of Earth-
with the elixir of graceful piety.
And, here Thou art lofty- alone
Ignoring ignorance of Soul.
Thy golden curly locks
Spray the Spree of love sincere;
The crown of thorn about Thy head-
Meant to mean the message of Envy-
Beams luster of halo to clouds
As also to gloom and the glum;
And Thou stickest fast
As the scare-craft of Sin and the Devil.

✞ ✞ ✞

Memory hits at the glimpses old.
I get to have seen Thee before-
sometime and somewhere else.
Pray wait till I may gather up.
Well perhaps Thou are the One
That on the beginning of the world
Cupped Thy palm to hold all the venom
And drenched Thy throat blue
To deliver the gods in heaven
As also all the beings of earth
Against the puff of poison.
It is Thine to keep everything
And every being playing pure-
Pure in form and in spirit.
Certainly yes I cognize Thee.
Thou art Civa the Benevolence.

ॐ ॐ ॐ

And,
Did I not meet Thee once more yet
on the foot of a mighty oak
In the dense of a wood-Land hilly?
can it be a miss? Oh no.
These broad and big eyes
Shedding compassion of love
For all beings pining in penance
This pose of unstirring fortitude
of forbearing Forgiveness,
This untold agony of loving sacrifice
These cherry lips inviting
A thousand kisses of gratitude
And still tending a resolute vow-
All these were then and there-in.
There Thou satest stalled
To a humble seat of dried stalk,
As fixed as a doll divine,
And Thy lips muttering a stout oath-
- I don't fail to recollect it-
This sitting be mine Last
To soak me dry if
Knowledge unbound fling not its door
Open unto me and let me find
The means to free the soul
out of all coverings and bondage
Those eyes like the brightest stars
Glowed in the wild forlorn
Becoming the go to pilgrims fair.
Nothing can con nor whiff my ken
to find in Thee that one indeed-
Buddha Idol of Love Enlightened

☯☯☯

It's all the grace of Thy blessings
That my memory blooms to brighten

Thy vision in full splendor of glory.
I met Thee, to be sure,
Amidst the havoc of bloody Kuruxetra.
Hero of all heroes, Thou wert
In the driver's box of a chariot-
The chariot of mighty Arjuna
Drawn by four stallions white,
All brave, bold and proud-
To drive Thy faithful through the killing spree
To Eternal Security.
The reins of the shooting chargers
Were in Thy fists fixed;
Sanguinity roared and danced
Before Thy graceful eyes
But could by no means disturb
Thy serene, care-free comfort;
The same unbridled locks
Dangled in the wind by Thy shoulders;
The same rosy resolute lips bore
The assurance of faith unvexed.
And how much blood Thou hadest
The selfish monsters to shed to turn
The yellow sandy breast of Kuruxetra
Into a wild stretch of a ruddy mud!
The pangs of the dying ones,
The tears of widows and mothers,
The loud roars of enmity
The deep sighs of the destitute
And all these violence
Thou hadst to nook in Thy breast.
Was that, the task, too much for Thee
And, is it why Thou shiftest Thyself
To this far and far distance,
To ride the cross, and
To drain Thy noble blood in drops
In atonement for what Thou hadst to course?
Thou winst Thy Self
And dost wean the children of God
To savour truth, purity and faith.
Certainly Yes, O Magnum Marvel,
Thou art He that buggied Arjuna,
Thy brother and Thy Lamb as well,
From the foul hell to Proud Paradise

ॐ ॐ ॐ

Ah! Thy Supreme Holy Excellency!
Eternal Existence
Paramount Life-Intelligence-Bliss!
Amalgam of total Beauty- Harmony- Music!
Thou art Sole Energy to spring motion forth.
And Nature is Thy modus operandi.
Salutations to Thee.
Blow the blind off the sockets of sight
And jut Thy revelation
more solemn and profound.
I, the most petty and low of Thy Lambs
Beg to pray for riddance
From the dismal abyss of falsehood-
- Boastful and selfish Ignorance.
Holdst me up.
Heedest my passion's groan,
Bathest me in faith divine
Brushest all scars of violation off
With Thy breath and Thy glance.
And foundst in my heart my soul
Long forgotten to feel.
Be it Thou pleasure to accept
- My ovation to Civa in Thee
- My tributes to Buddha in Thee
- My homage to Krishna in Thee
And be it Thy kindness superb
To turn this dolt in me
Into a fair forehead Arya,
The holy and ever progressive friar
To the goal of self-immolation-
Clear, complete and perfect-
Against the slips of whom
Fore-and-aft standst Thou
Ever and for-ever.

Bhikshu Suddev
May 20, 1994; Shankar Math
Uttarkashi, India

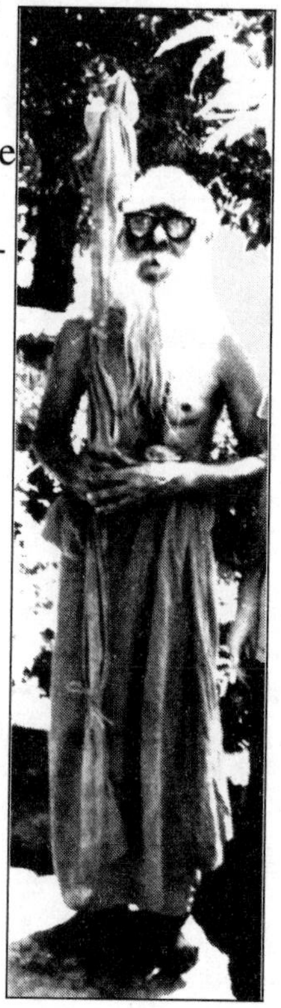

Foreword

I am happy to write these few words by way of introduction to, and appreciation of Shri Swami Sada Shivaji's book entitled, *The Āyurveda Encyclopedia: Taking Control of Your Health; Natural Secrets To Healing, Prevention, & Longevity for Families and Practitioners*.

Āyurveda is a science of life that deals with the problems of longevity, and suggests a safe, gentle, and effective way to rid diseases afflicting our health. Āyurveda is regarded as the fifth *Veda*—by its virtue—and has been practiced in India for thousands of years. Medicinal plants and their utility are widely described in the *Vedas*; especially in *Atharva Veda.* To understand Āyurveda, it is necessary that we should have a good knowledge of its basic principals. Swamiji has clearly described these basic principals in his book, *The Āyurveda Encyclopedia.* This book covers approximately two years worth of study at India government-recognized Āyurveda colleges and universities. I congratulate Swamiji for writing this magnificent work.

Dr. S.N. Srivastava
B.A.M.S. (K.U.)
U.G.T.T. (I.M.S., B.H.U)
Head of Department, Kayachikitsa
Government Āyurvedic College
Gurukul Kangri
Hardwar, India

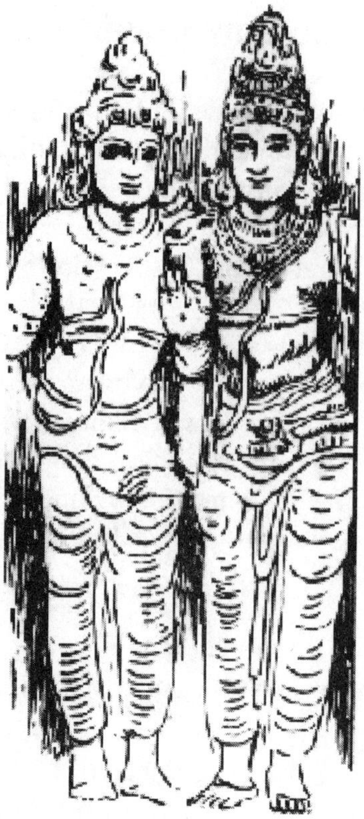

Aṣhwin Twins: The Celestial Physicians

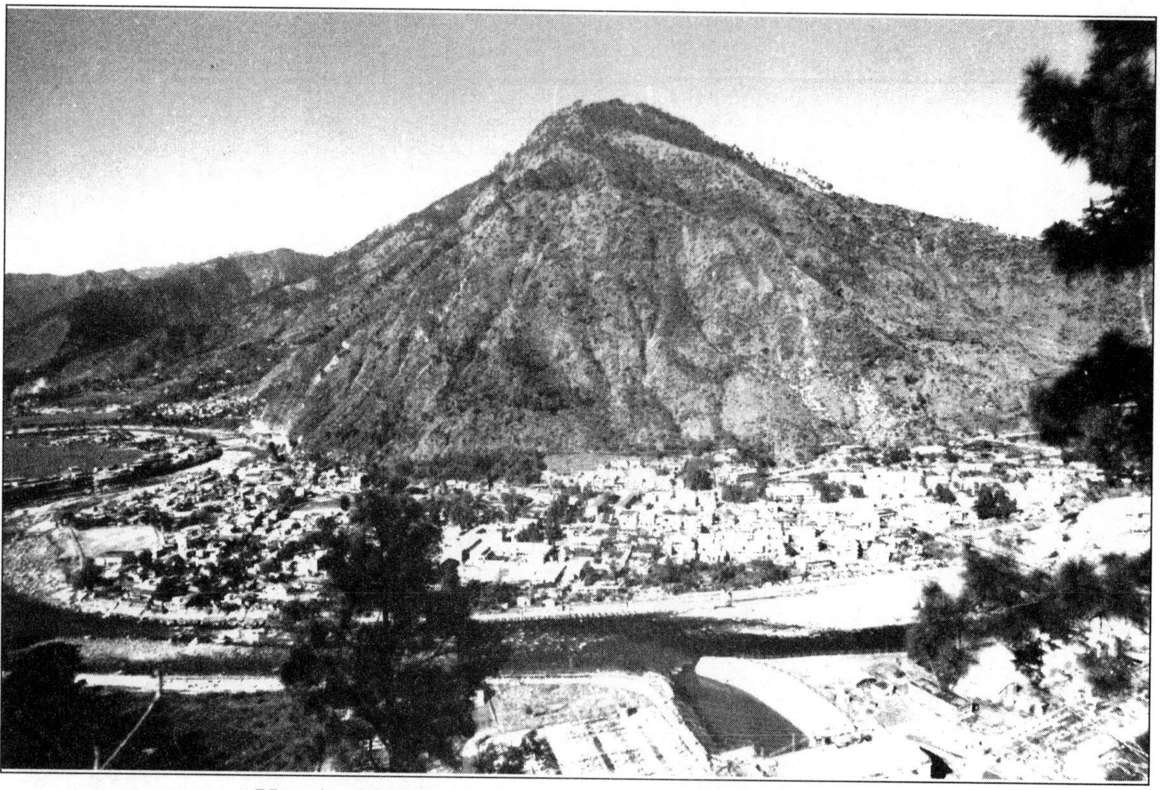

Uttarkaṣhi: Himalayan Mountains and Ganges River

Acknowledgments

My first two teachers, Dr. Vasant Lad and Dr. David Frawley, were the first authors in the U.S. to present Āyurveda in a simple, thorough, and clear manner. Deeper studies with Dr. Frawley provided me with an excellent foundation for practicing the subject; his teachings have formed my initial groundwork of the subject. Personally, he reflects the teachings through his generous nature. I am grateful for his early influences.

As I progressed further into the study of Āyurveda, Dr. R. H. Singh, professor and head of the department of *Kayachikitsa*, Institute of Medicinal Sciences at Benares Hindu University (BHU) and Dr. I. P. Singh, professor of Āyurveda at BHU, generously shared some of their time to personally tutor and allow me to tour the BHU Āyurveda clinic with their students. Dr. I.P. Singh spent many days privately tutoring me on herbology and the spiritual foundations of the subject. BHU is among the most respected Āyurvedic universities in India, and it was a great blessing to have such esteemed teachers share their time, knowledge, and experience.

Following my Guruji in India to the Himalayan town of *Uttarkaṣhi*, I was fortunate enough to be introduced to Dr. Ram Chandra Uniyal, with whom I have studied for many years. He kindly allowed me to sit in on his consultations and gain greater practical experience of pulse analysis and treatment of disease. Dr. Uniyal, a recognized expert on Himalayan mountain herbs, took the photographs of the herbs in this book and reviewed the book for technical accuracy. Without his input on the herbal therapies in Section 4, it would have been impossible to complete this work.

Another peer review member, Dr. Satnam S. Sandhu, provided several insights on the tradition of Āyurveda, as well as some reflections in the realm of Western medicine. His assistance, technical and otherwise, has been crucial to the accuracy and authenticity of this book.

The third peer review member was Dr. J. Kishan Chandhok who has gone through many chapters with a fine tooth comb, helping to clarify many important points.

The author of the poem, A Psalm of Dedication (page ix), is Swami Suddev Tirtha, my elder *guru* brother, was an extremely learned man, yet simple and humble. I am honored to accept and print his wonderful poem about the universality of religion. The underlying theme of this book is the universality of Āyurveda as a healing science and how it integrates simply with all other forms of healing, including modern medicine. He expired several months before the publication of this book, and is dearly remembered.

Dr. Anil Kumar Darji also deserves recognition for providing some modern explanations for Āyurvedic pathologies, as well as some of the herbal energetics in the materia medica.

Special thanks to the *haṭha yoga* models who generously donated their time and talents: Jeff Caughey, certified Āyurvedic Practitioner/certified *haṭha yoga* instructor; Ray Pesonen, *yoga* teacher; Dr. Baldev Anand, *Pañcha karma* specialist; and Chris Deutsch, *yoga* student.

Countless thanks are also due to Guru Amrit Kaur Khalsa and Rob Paton of Caduceus Press, who edited this book. They worked above and beyond the call of duty, taking a personal interest in this project.

Finally, I am most grateful to my Guruji, His Holiness 1008 Sri Sri Srimat Swami Narayan Tirthaji Maharaj, without whose blessings and grace this task could never have been achieved.

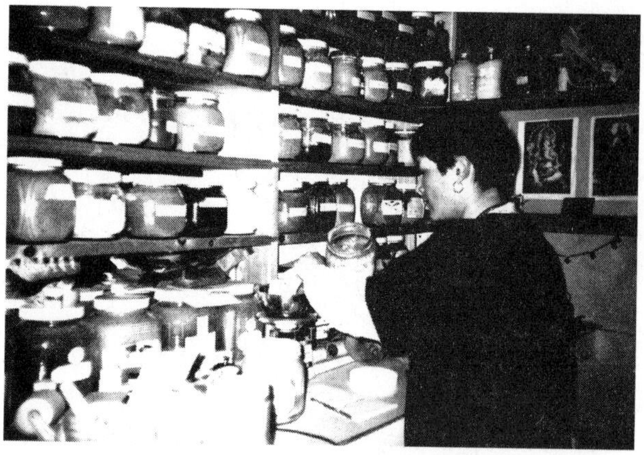

Certification student practicing herb mixing
Ayurveda Holistic Center, Bayville, NY, USA

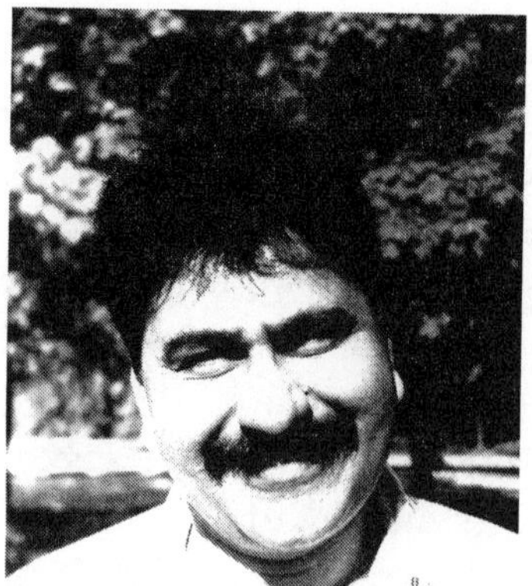

Dr. Satnam Sandhu

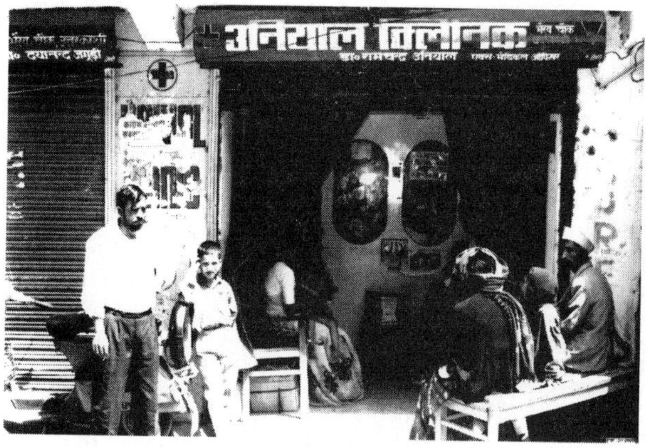

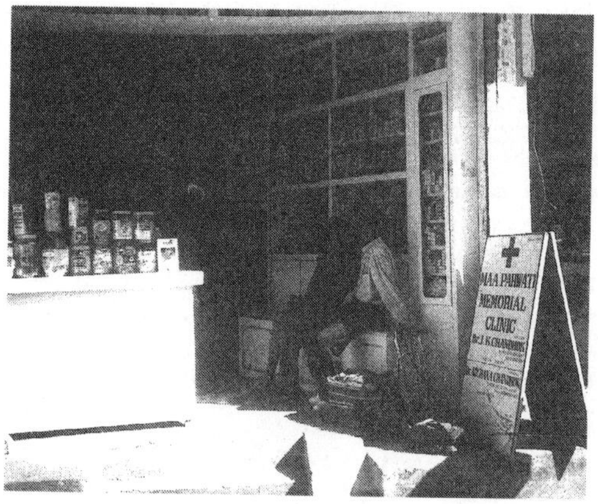

Two Ayurveda Holistic Center branches in Uttarkashi (Himalayas), India

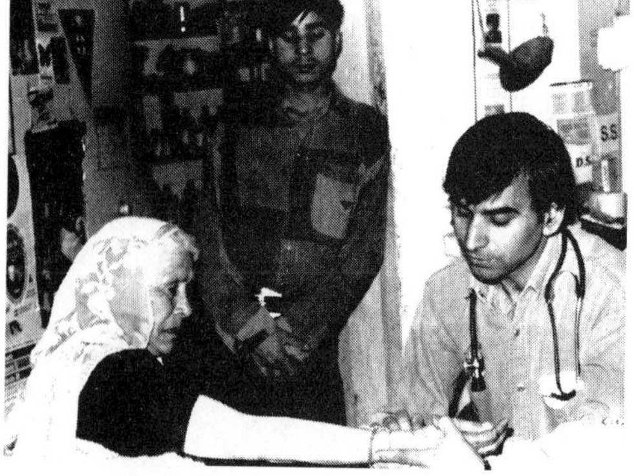

Dr. Ram Chandra Uniyal taking
patient's pulse at the Uttarkashi center

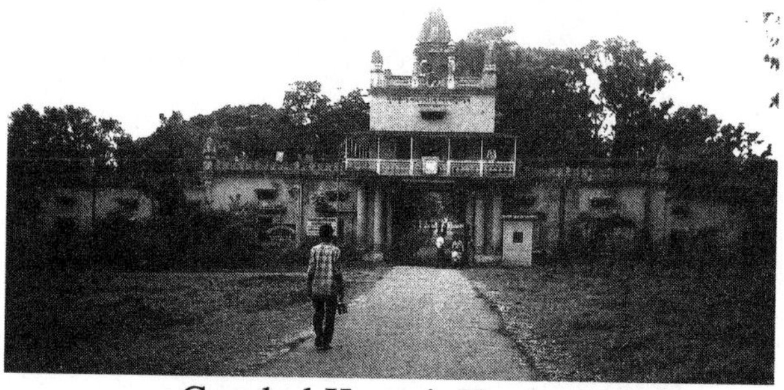

Gurukul Kangri; Hardwar India
Ayurveda Government College

Introduction

The knowledge of Āyurveda was handed down from Brahmā to Dakṣha Prajāpati, onto the Aṣhwin twins (the divine doctors), then passed to Indra. Sage Bharadvāja volunteered to go to heaven to receive this wisdom from Indra, and so became the first human to receive the knowledge of Āyurveda. He passed it to Ātreya, then onto Punarnavasu and finally Agniveṣha.

This book was written at the request of my students, who sought a deeper understanding of the Āyurvedic process. To that end I have endeavored to provide the following: a deeper insight into the spiritual foundation of Āyurveda; a complete analysis of how diseases are caused and how they progress—information not previously available in English-language books on the subject; photographs of the Āyurvedic herbs; a more comprehensive materia medica; diacritical marks to facilitate pronunciation of Sanskrit (original Āyurvedic language) words; an expanded discussion of the Āyurvedic use of *haṭha yoga* and *prāṇāyāma* with photographs; an expanded *pañcha karma* chapter; a discussion of current research on many of the Āyurvedic herbs; a discussion of the complimentary relationship between Western and Āyurvedic methods; and discussions based not only on traditional Āyurvedic thought, but also on the practical results of my experiences and those of other Āyurvedic doctors and practitioners.

To achieve these ends, the ancient Āyurvedic texts were consulted along with books by contemporary authors. The purpose was to synthesize ancient tradition with modern use. Authentic *Vedic* spiritual books have also been researched to better incorporate the spiritual dimension of Āyurveda.

An attempt has been made to present the material in a simple and instructive manner, accessible even to those with little prior knowledge of Āyurveda. We hope it will unite Western and Āyurvedic traditions.

This book is composed of four sections:

1. Āyurvedic Theory/Fundamentals
2. Constitution (*Doṣha*) and Illness Diagnosis
3. Therapeutic Modalities
4. Specific Illnesses and Diseases (Diagnosis, pathology, and therapies)

Āyurveda, when practiced correctly, allows for intuition and individual differences. One of the main points of this book is that the information presented here is only a starting point in education—it is not to be followed blindly. Too often readers treat what is written in books as gospel, even if such suggestions may be harmful to their particular conditions. The Āyurvedic practitioner and the patient must examine many elements before choosing an appropriate therapy (e.g., age, strength, *doṣha,* geography, climate, culture, etc.). Further, the patient is encouraged to rely on common sense and intuition. Slavishly following the words of a book, verbatim, can be dangerous. Please, dear readers, accept this information as educational—not dictatorial.

This book is offered in devotional service. It is my hope that it will be read with devotion; knowledge without devotion is like driving a car without oil, or like growing a beautiful flower without a scent.

Bayville, NY, USA
January, 1998

The first printing of 5,000 copies sold out in less than 1 year - September 1999

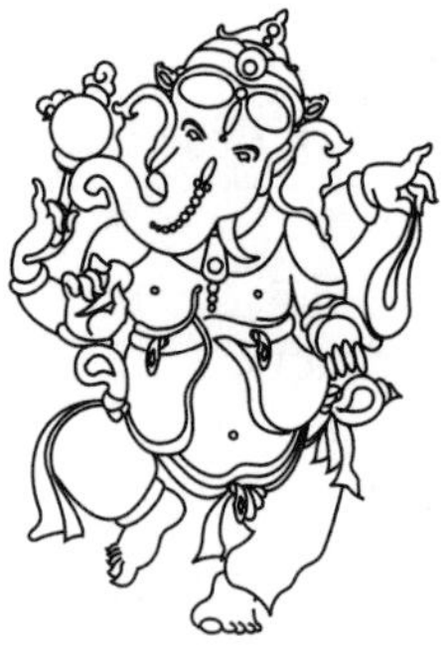

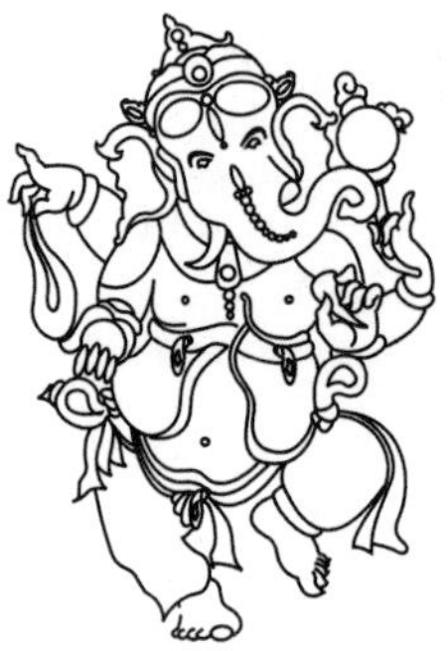

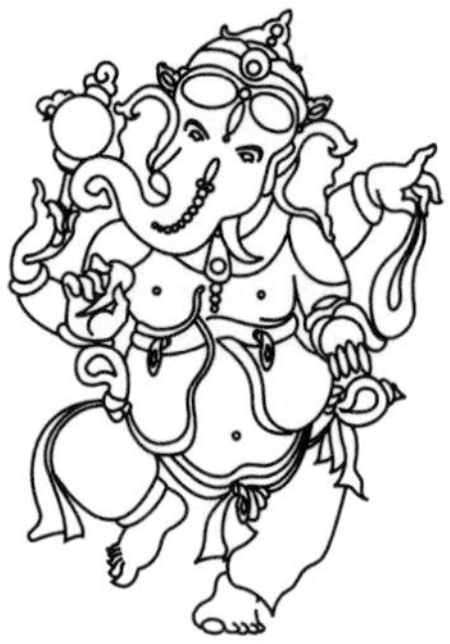

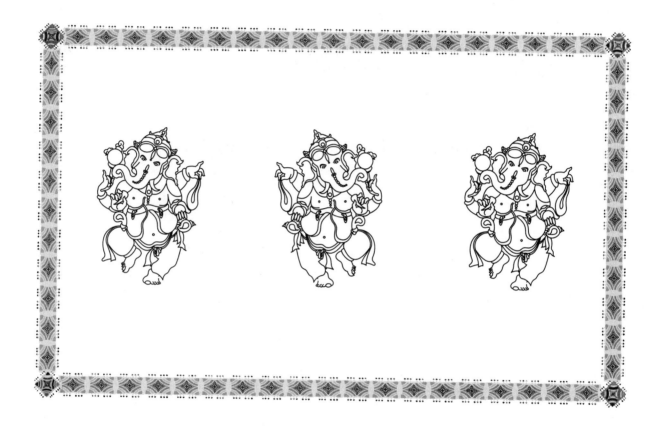

Section 1

Āyurvedic Fundamentals

आयुर्वेद सूत्रस्थान

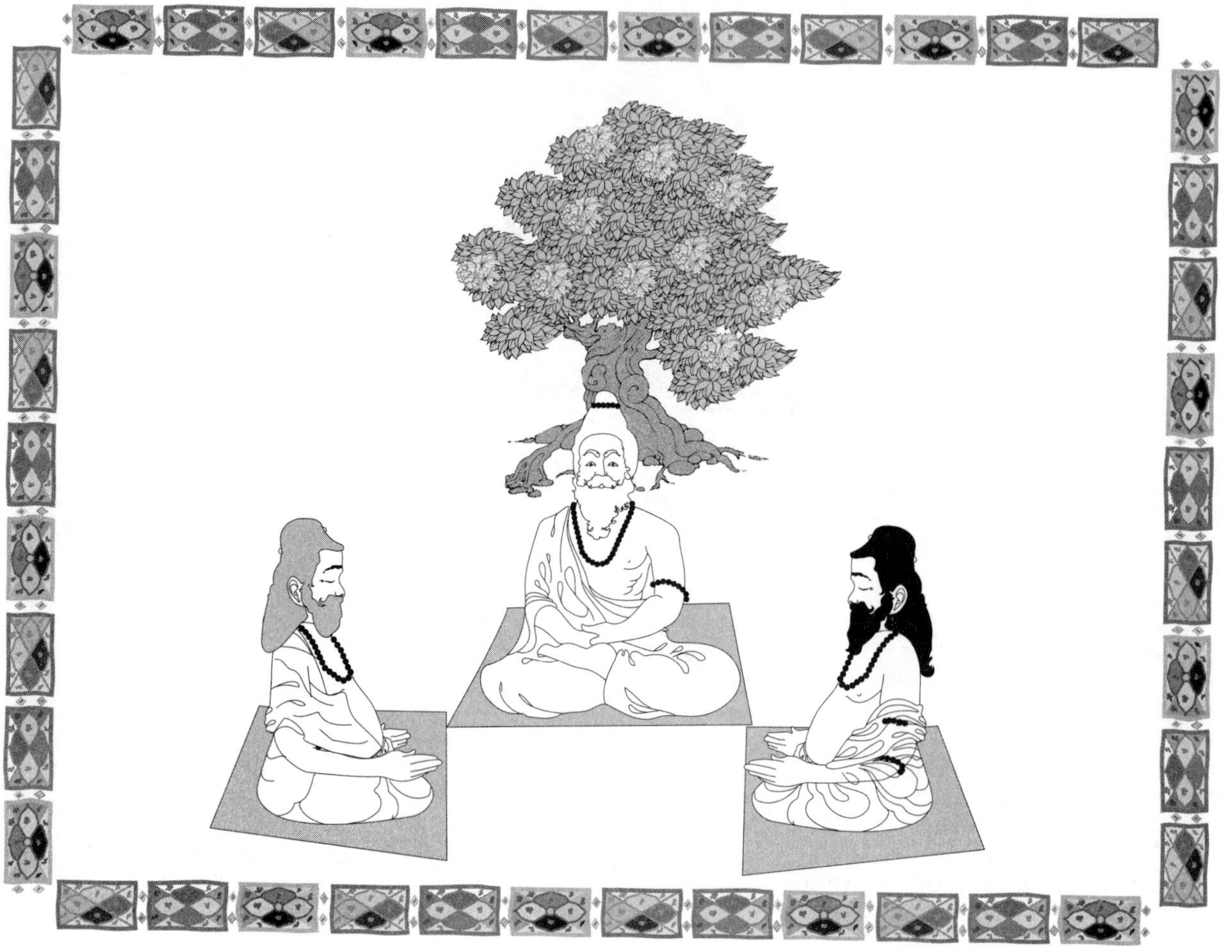

Like an oasis is a mirage of the desert,
this world is an illusion of Brahman.
Upanishadic wisdom

Chapter 1
Overview of Āyurveda

Āyurveda, the "science of life," or longevity, is the holistic alternative science from India, and is more than 5,000 years old. It is believed to be the oldest healing science in existence, forming the foundation of all others. Buddhism, Taoism, Tibetan, and other cultural medicines have many similar parallels to Āyurveda. The secret of Āyurveda's individualized healing method was preserved in India, whereas it has been lost or superseded in other cultures.

The First World Medicine

Āyurveda (pronounced Aa-yer-vay-da), said to be a world medicine, is the most holistic or comprehensive medical system available. Before the arrival of writing, the ancient wisdom of healing, prevention, and longevity was a part of the spiritual tradition of a universal religion. Healers gathered from the world over, bringing their medical knowledge to India. *Veda Vyasa*, the famous sage, preserved the complete knowledge of Āyurveda in writing, along with the more spiritual insights of ethics, virtue, and Self-Realization. Others say Āyurveda was passed down from God to his angels, and finally to humans.

The methods used to find this knowledge of herbs, foods, aromas, gems, colors, *yoga*, *mantras*, lifestyle, and surgery are fascinating and varied. The sage, physicians/surgeons of the time were the same sages or seers, deeply devoted holy people, who saw health as an integral part of spiritual life. It is said that they received their training of Āyurveda through direct cognition during meditation. That is, the knowledge of the use of the various methods of healing, prevention, longevity, and surgery came through Divine revelation; guessing, or animal testing was unnecessary. These revelations were transcribed from oral tradition into written form, interspersed with aspects of mortal life and spirituality.

Originally four main books of *Vedic* spirituality existed. Topics included health, astrology, spiritual business, government, military, poetry, and ethical living. These are known as the *Vedas*: *Ṛik, Sama, Yajur,* and *Atharva*. Āyurveda was used along with *Vedic* astrology (called *Jyotiṣh*, that is, one's "inner light"). Eventually, Āyurveda was organized into its own compact system of health and considered a branch of *Atharva Veda*. This *upaveda*/branch dealt with the healing aspects of spirituality; although, it did not directly treat spiritual development. Passages related to Āyurveda from the various *Vedas* were combined into separate books dealing only with Āyurveda. Among the *Ṛik Veda's* 10,572 hymns are discussions of the three constitutions (*doṣhas*): air (Vāyu), fire (Pitta), and water (Kapha). Topics comprised organ transplants, artificial limbs, and the use of herbs to heal diseases of the mind and body and to foster longevity. Within the *Atharva Veda's* 5,977 hymns are discussions of anatomy, physiology, and surgery.

There were two schools of Āyurveda at the time of *Ātreya*, the school of physicians and the school of surgeons. These two schools transformed Āyurveda into a scientifically verifiable and classifiable medical system. Through research and testing, they dispelled the doubts of the more practical and scientific minded, removing the aura of mystery that surrounded Divine

History of Āyurveda

Brahma

Dakṣha Prājapatī

Aṣhwini Kumar
(celestial physicians)

Indra
(Sat Yuga)

Divodasa Dhanwantari
(Treta Yuga)
(develops school of surgery
9-6th century BC.)

Kaṣhyap
(Dwapar Yuga)
(children/gynecological)

Bharadwaj
(Dwapar Yuga)
(human father of
Āyurvedic medicine)

Sushrut
(Sushrut Samhitā
written 5-4th century BC)

Ātreya Punarvasu

(Ātrea develops school of
physicians 8-6th century BC)

(Ātrea writes Charak
Saṃhitā 1st century AD

Aṣhṭhāñga Hṛidayam written
(8th century AD)

Mādhava Nidan written
(treatise on diagnosis -9th century AD)

Mercury first used - 14th century AD

Śhārṅgadhara Saṃhitā written
(Āyurvedic recipes- 13th century AD

revelation. Consequently, Āyurveda grew in respect and became a widely used system of healing in India. People from many countries came to Indian Āyurvedic schools to learn about this medicine in its entirety. Chinese, Tibetans, Greeks, Romans, Egyptians, Afghanis, Persians, and others traveled to absorb the wisdom and bring it back to their own countries. India's Silk Road, an established trade route between Asia (China, Tibet, etc.), the Middle East (Afghanistan, Persia, etc.), and Europe (Rome, Greece, etc.), provided a link between cultures. On this route travelers first discovered Āyurveda.

Charak and *Suṣhrut* are two reorganizers of Āyurveda whose works are still extant. The third major treatise is called the *Aṣhṭāñga Hṛidayam*, a concise version of the works of *Charak* and *Suṣhrut*. Thus, the three main ancient Āyurvedic texts still in use are the *Charak Saṃhitā* (compilation), *Suṣhrut Saṃhitā,* and the *Aṣhṭāñga Hṛidaya Saṃhitā*. These books are believed to be over 1,200 years old and contain the original and complete knowledge of this Āyurvedic world medicine. Consequently, Āyurveda is the only complete ancient medical system in existence.

Charak represents the *Ātreya* school of physicians, discussing physiology, anatomy, etiology, pathogenesis, symptoms and signs of disease, methodology of diagnosis, treatment and prescription for patients, prevention, and longevity. Internal and external causes of illness are also considered. *Charak* maintains that the first cause of illness is the loss of faith in the Divine. In other words, when people do not recognize that God dwells within all things, including themselves, this separation of vision creates a gap. This gap causes a longing or suffering for oneness of vision. This suffering then manifests itself as the beginning of spiritual, mental, and physical disease. External influences on health include time of day, the seasons, diet, and lifestyle. An entire section is devoted to discussions of the medicinal aspects of herbs, diet, and reversal of aging.

Suṣhruta comes from the *Dhanvantari* school of surgeons. In America, a society of surgeons named themselves the *Suṣhruta Society* in remembrance of the Āyurvedic father of surgery. This text presents sophisticated accounts of surgical equipment, classification of abscesses, burns, fractures, and wounds, amputation, plastic surgery, and anal/rectal surgery. Human anatomy is described in great detail, including descriptions of the bones, joints, nerves, heart, blood vessels, circulatory system, etc., again, corroborated by today's methods of mechanical investigation. From the *Suṣhrut Saṃhitā*, the first science of massage is described using *marma* points or vital body points, later adapted into Chinese acupuncture. Even the popular Polarity Massage Therapy in America was developed after advocates studied massage in India.

Eight Branches of Āyurveda

The ancient Āyurvedic system was astoundingly complete. In the colleges of ancient India, students could choose a specialty from eight branches of medicine.

1. Internal Medicine (*Kāyachikitsā*). This is related to the soul, mind, and body. Psychosomatic theory recognizes that the mind can create illness in the body and vice versa. The seven body constitutions and seven mental constitutions were delineated here: Vāyu (air/energy), Pitta (fire), Kapha (water), Vāyu/Pitta, Vāyu/Kapha, Pitta/ Kapha, and a combination of all three (tridoṣha). Although finding the cause of an illness is still a mystery to modern science, it was the main goal of Āyurveda. Six stages of the development of disease were known, including aggravation, accumulation, overflow, relocation, a buildup in a new site, and manifestation into a recognizable disease. Modern equipment and diagnosis can only detect a disease during the fifth and sixth stages of illness. Āyurvedic physicians can recognize an illness in the making before it creates more serious imbalance in the body. Health is seen as a balance of the biological humors, whereas disease is an imbalance of the humors. Āyurveda creates balance by supplying deficient humors and reducing the excess ones. Surgery is seen as

a last resort. Modern medicine is just beginning to realize the need to supply rather than to remove, but still does not know how or what to supply.

Additionally, there are over 2,000 medicinal plants classified in India's materia medica. A unique therapy, known as *pañcha karma* (five actions), completely removes toxins from the body. This method reverses the disease path from its manifestation stage, back into the blood stream, and eventually into the gastrointestinal tract (the original site of the disease). It is achieved through special diets, oil massage, and steam therapy. At the completion of these therapies, special forms of emesis, purgation, and enema remove excesses from their sites of origin. Finally, Āyurveda rejuvenates–rebuilding the body's cells and tissues after toxins are removed.

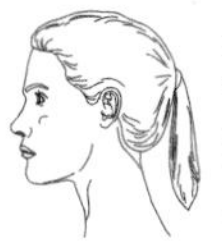

2. Ears, Nose, and Throat (*Śhālākya Tantra*). *Suṣhruta* reveals approximately 72 eye diseases, surgical procedures for all eye disorders (e.g., cataracts, eyelid diseases), and for diseases of the ears, nose, and throat.

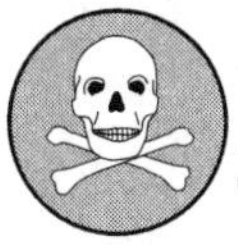

3. Toxicology (*Viṣhagara-vairodh Tantra*). Topics include air and water pollution, toxins in animals, minerals, vegetables, and epidemics; as well as keys for recognizing these anomalies and their antidotes.

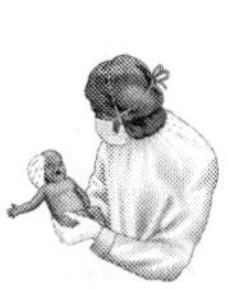

4. Pediatrics (*Kaumāra bhritya*). In this branch prenatal and postnatal care of the baby and mother are discussed. Topics include methods of conception; choosing the child's gender, intelligence, and constitution; and childhood diseases and midwifery.

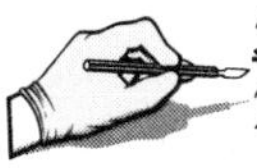

5. Surgery (*Śhalyā Tantra*). More than 2,000 years ago, sophisticated methods of surgery were known. This information spread to Egypt, Greece, Rome, and eventually throughout the world. In China, treatment of intestinal obstructions, bladder stones, and the use of dead bodies for dissection and learning were taught and practiced.

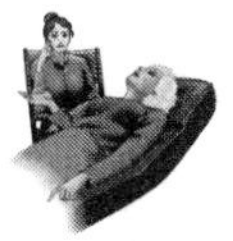

6. Psychiatry (*Bhūta Vidyā*). A whole branch of Āyurveda specifically deals with diseases of the mind (including demonic possession). Besides herbs and diet, *yogic* therapies (breathing, *mantras*, etc.) are employed.

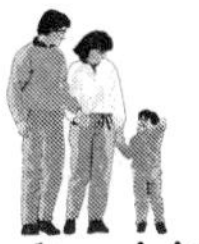

7. Aphrodisiacs (*Vājikarana*). This section deals with two aspects: infertility (for those hoping to conceive) and spiritual development (for those eager to transmute sexual energy into spiritual energy).

8. Rejuvenation (*Rasāyana*). Prevention and longevity are discussed in this branch of Āyurveda. *Charak* says that in order to develop longevity, ethics and virtuous living must be embraced.

The Decline of Āyurveda

The alert person may now ask why, if Āyurveda is so exceptional, is it not widely practiced in India today. This is a valid question, which has an equally valid answer. Āyurveda, like all of *Vedic* philosophy, adheres to the belief in *Sanātana dharma*, or accepting everything in its appropriate time and place, and rejecting nothing. All aspects of medicine may be useful, but the appropriate treatment must be used when required. This is why Āyurveda does not reject modern medicine. The Indian temperament allows all religions to express themselves freely in India. Buddhism, Jainism, and other religions grew in India and influenced the thinking of many people. Eventually, a time came when all religions lost some degree of their spiritual link, and egos vied for first place. Gentle spiritual medicine lost ground. Divisiveness was followed by foreign conquest. Āyurvedic colleges were closed and books destroyed. One nation forced Āyurvedic doctors to add information on meat to the translations of the Āyurvedic texts. Another religion did not believe in harming the body in any manner and destroyed the books on Āyurvedic surgery. *Nalanda*, at *Patna*, India, a famous Āyurvedic university, was the main university at the center of the Silk Road, where students from China, Tibet, the Middle East, and Europe came to study. This institution was among those destroyed by various conquerors. During the nineteenth and early twentieth centuries, the British ruled India and closed the remaining Āyurvedic universities (although Āyurveda continued to be practiced in secret). The knowledge was preserved by the *guru-śhishya* relationship (teacher-student) and passed from one generation to the next by word of mouth as it had centuries before. Finally, in 1920 Āyurveda reemerged and, with the help of the Indian government's assistance, universities were rebuilt. Now more than 150 Āyurvedic universities and 100 Āyurvedic colleges are flourishing in India, with plans for more educational facilities in development. Thus, Āyurveda, without resisting or rejecting other systems, is slowly returning to recognition and reestablishing its true value. Keep in mind that just as some unethical western medical practices exist, unethical Āyurvedic pharmacies and doctors can also be found in India today.

The oldest medicine, Āyurveda, is now the last to be rediscovered. This world medicine may not only unite healing practices, but also peoples, cultures, and religions. The impact of its reawakening is astounding, as we see its effectiveness and demand in the United States growing in leaps and bounds. Among the respected teachers of Āyurveda, many include the original spiritual integration, reestablishing ancient Āyurveda, intact in modern society. Spiritual Āyurveda, the original world medicine, will soon find validation and universal acceptance in all areas of society and the world.

What may surprise some people is the degree of insight these ancient, mystical doctors, or *ṛiṣhis* (seers) had. Without the aid of modern technological x-ray machines or CT-scans, they knew of the inner workings of the human body. One can read in the ancient Āyurvedic texts of the development of the fetus, month by month. It is astonishing how these ancient descriptions are validated by today's technologies. Even the distance from the planets and the duration of their orbits were nearly identical to today's technological measurements. It is enough to make even the most skeptical of us sit up and consider Āyurvedic insights.

So we see the foundation for the integration of Āyurveda and modern medicine. Too many people on both sides of the holistic-vs-allopathic (modern) medicine debate want to deny the need for the other science. Because of Āyurveda's all-embracing philosophy, we see how all types of healing are compatible. No one will be put out of a job.

Spiritual Āyurveda

We have discussed Āyurveda, the "science of life" as the original world medicine. Yet Āyurveda is more than this; it is a spiritual science. This is the most important aspect of Āyurveda.

Around 1500 B.C. the book, the *Charak Saṃhitā* discussed these spiritual principles. It said that even if Āyurvedic doctors had a complete knowledge of Āyurveda but could not reach the inner Self or soul of the patient, they would not be effective healers. Furthermore, if the practitioner were more concerned with fame and fortune, and not with spiritual development (Self-Realization), they would not be effective healers.

To understand the spiritual nature of Āyurveda, we must know something about the *Vedic* roots of philosophy, spirituality, and universal religion. According to the ancient *Vedic* scriptures of India there is a goal to life. We are not simply born, to live, and then to die without some meaning or purpose. Albert Einstein reflected this idea when he said *God does not play dice with the universe*. Order and reason exist in life. According to *Vedic* philosophy life is Divine and the goal of life is to realize our inner Divine nature. Āyurvedically speaking the more a person realizes their Divine nature the healthier they are. Thus it is the responsibility of the Āyurvedic doctor to inspire or help awaken the patient to their own inner Divine nature. Positive thinking or love is the best medicine. When patients are taught they have this Divinity within themselves, they feel a connection to life and God (however each patient defines God). For atheists, we speak of the greater mystical power, which is synonymous to God. This connection allows patients to feel they have a handle on life and an ability to develop their own inner nature. After this, secondary therapies of herbs, diet, meditation, etc. are offered.

Even modern medical doctors are finding a link between their healthy patients and the patient's degree of spiritual faith. Spirituality changes the definition of health, giving it added dimension. Two types of health can now be seen-diagnosed health and true health. Often when a patient is diagnosed as healthy, they still may not feel healthy or alive. This is due to psychosomatic conditions where a troubled mind affects the health of the body. The deepest level of mental agitation is the longing for a deeper spiritual connection.

Āyurveda suggests true health is based on the healthy functioning of four areas of life; physical/mental health, career or life purpose, spiritual relationships, and spirituality. First one needs to be physically and mentally able to do work and play. Then persons need to work to support themselves and afford a social life. Work however is defined as making a living doing something meaningful or purposeful. To do this type of work one needs to use their innate or God-given talents; they need to work at something they love to do. It is this love that cultures spirituality.

All too often we find people working at jobs that they dislike. Often people are forced into a "practical" career by parents or societal beliefs. Other persons lack the self-worth and confidence to challenge themselves to find and live their dreams. Working in meaningless, unfulfilling jobs can create mental and physical disorders.

The most extreme example of illness caused by lack of purpose is cancer. Āyurveda considers cancer an emotionally caused disease. By not having a purpose in life (i.e., suppressing life) people create life within their body—cancer. When seriously ill people discuss what they would love to do (instead of what they are told to do) life returns to their eyes. As they begin to follow up on these ideas, some remarkable recoveries are seen. Purposeful career is then an aspect of this new definition of health.

The third realm of health is spiritual relationships. When persons are healthy and purposefully working, they can now begin to truly enjoy their social life. These days we have become acutely aware of the emotional and physical abuses that exist in many people's relationships. Co-dependency and enabling are often used terms to describe relationship diseases. From the spiritual standpoint if one is dependent on anything other than God, co-dependency exists. People look for something lasting or permanent; only God is eternal and everlasting. Spiritual development directs one to focus inwardly to discover their eternal nature instead of the ever-changing outer realm of life. For relationships to be healthy all people must continue to develop their individual inner spiritual lives. Then they are able to share their growing spiritual fullness with their spouse and others.

Too often individuals are attracted to one another because they see a quality that they think they do not have. In reality each person has all the human qualities within themselves because inner eternal Divinity, by definition, contains everything. Further, if one can see a quality in another they must have it within themselves in order to recognize it. When the main focus in people's lives is the Divine, then troubles that seemed like mountains are seen as molehills. Thus the third dimension of health involves healthy spiritual relationships.

Once people are sound in body and mind, work in a purposeful career and have fulfilling spiritual relationships, life develops a state of grace. People then become eager to devote more time to spiritual development, the final dimension of health. Personal spiritual development is seen on many levels. The body becomes more relaxed, the mind more calm and alert; and one becomes more personable in relationships. Yet the most profound developments take place inwardly; Divinity grows within. Gradually one also begins to see the Divinity in others and all of life.

This is the multi-dimensional definition of health according to Āyurveda. Life is composed of many elements; it is not seen as independent parts. If one aspect of life becomes imbalanced all the other aspects are affected. Rather than merely treating a symptom, Āyurveda looks to the root cause or underlying reasons of illness. The body may be sick because of mental or career stress. Rather than instruct the patient to merely take a drug or an herb to heal the physical condition, the practitioner of Āyurvedic medicine looks to restore balance within the patient (e.g., calming the mind or finding a more purposeful job). The deepest root level is spiritual development. Thus, all four areas of life must be cultivated; mind/body, career, spiritual relationships, and inner spiritual development.

The Development of Allopathic Medicine

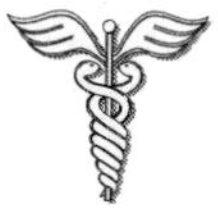

Not long ago in America herbal and naturopathic medicines were the common healing modalities. Grandmothers and mothers gave family members natural or herbal remedies when they were sick.

Parallel to the onset of the industrial revolution came the rise in allopathic medicine; not because it was better, but because more money was available for its propagation. A chief developer of allopathic medicine was Andrew Carnegie, who saw a better financial future for himself in investing large sums of money to develop allopathic research and diagnostic machinery instead of encouraging natural medicine research. Thus allopathy had the backing to develop and surpass natural medicine.

This statement is not meant to discredit the effectiveness and usefulness of modern medicine, but merely intended to underline the point that herbal medicine was also an effective healing method, but it was swept under the rug in the name of progress and was viewed less enthusiastically. Now, due to difficult economic times, the high cost of medical care, and hazardous side effects from drugs, people have been forced to return to alternative measures for relief. As with any groundswell at the grassroots, when something works the word gets out. People are returning to alternative or complimentary healthcare in droves.

Self-Healing & Self-Realization

The main theme of Āyurveda is that people can adequately educate themselves to take control of their own health. This is achieved by monitoring and balancing one's nutritional and lifestyle habits to heal, prevent illness, and develop longevity. Āyurveda teaches that people are their own best healers. One's intuition is better at discerning subtle health imbalances than relying on another person. All that is needed is some basic guidelines offered by the Āyurvedic practitioner.

The ability to take control of one's health inspires self-worth and self-empowerment. Faith in one's intuitive abilities is further engendered when persons actually see the positive results from their efforts. Realizing one has the ability to take control of one's own health is itself a key factor in healing.

Self-reliance is also the most important component in spiritual development. Individuals can learn to rely on their own intuition [along with guidelines laid out by one's spiritual mentor or *guru* and from the scriptures]. As one begins to see positive results developing in their spiritual

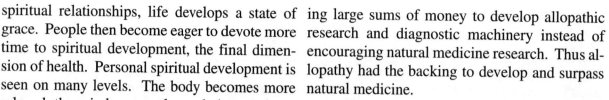

life, doubts begin to vanish: clarity, confidence, and mental peace begin to dawn.

The mental peace of Self-Realization is said to be the true state of life because it is eternal, non-changing. *Vedic śhastras* (scriptures) speak of the three legs of truth; what the scriptures say, what the *guru* or spiritual guide says, and what one experiences for oneself. Only when all three sources are found to be saying the same thing is something accepted as truth. But it is personal experience that must also be known; it is not enough to follow something dogmatically with blind faith.

Doubts are mental agitation. When doubts are dispelled the mind gains a state of peace. In Self-Realization one knows truth in its eternal nature; they cannot be swayed or agitated. The first step towards Self-Realization is developing the ability to not be swayed by others if you experience things differently. The American poet Thoreau, after reading the *Vedic* scriptures, expressed it this way:

If a man cannot keep pace with his companions,
perhaps it is because he hears the beat of a different drummer.
Let him step to the beat he hears,
no matter how measured or far away.

The Āyurvedic practitioner instills this philosophy in the patient, who then experiences and respects inner intuition and Divinity. When patients see that the practitioner believes they have such Divine qualities, they usually respond in kind.

A psychological study highlights the value of expectation. Two teachers were given classes of students with average abilities. One teacher was told their class was above average while the other teacher was told they had an average class. The first teacher went to class expecting exceptional work from the students and treated them accordingly. The other teacher just taught the average curriculum. The supposed above average class performed above average. Thus, when the Āyurvedic practitioner treats a patients with respect, recognizing their inner intuitive abilities, the patients automatically develop a greater sense of self-worth and faith that they can take control of their health.

As self-worth develops, people are not as easily swayed by peer pressure, whether pressed to take drugs or lead an unethical life. Low self-esteem causes people to abuse themselves. Having someone recognize one's inner Divinity and self-healing abilities develops confidence. Experiencing positive results from self-healing and spiritual development further generates confidence, health, mental peace, and Divinity.

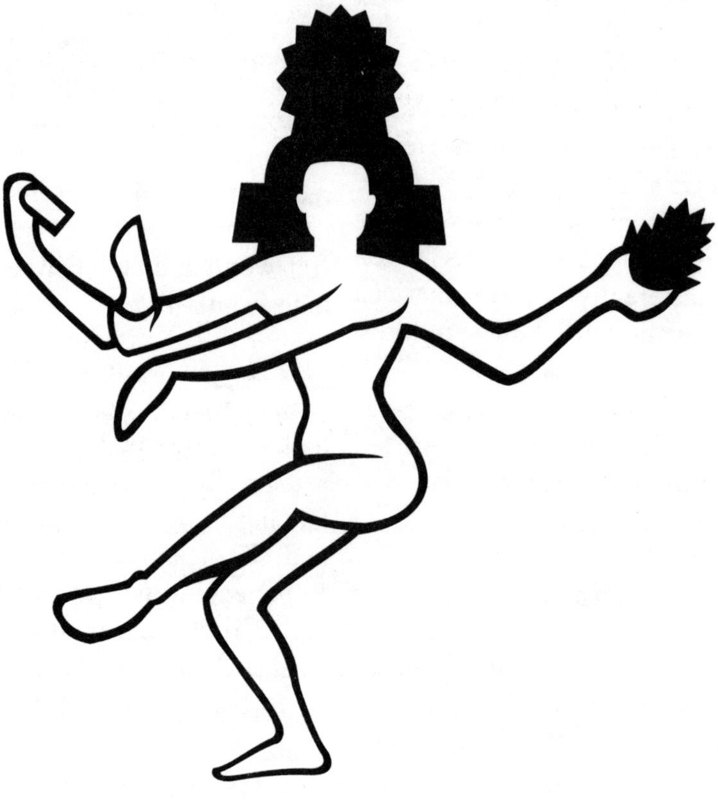

A plate, a cup and a bowl
are all made from the same clay.
Like this, all creation is made from
the same eternal Brahman.
Upanishadic wisdom

Chapter 2
The Human Universe

The *Vedic* scriptures say that there is an inextricable link between humans and the universe. The very elements of human life exist outside in the cosmos as well. As the poet Walt Whitman said, "I believe a blade of grass is no less than the journeywork of the stars." In order to understand the universe and environmental situations, and to understand human health concerns, one needs to appreciate the common link between them: the elements of creation.

The *Vedas* discuss the process of creation. First, there was the eternal, Divine, unmanifest existence: ever present. It is said that life was created from within the eternal, like a thread that comes from within a spider to be woven into a web. Creation eventually dissolves back into the eternal like the spider returning the web into itself.

One may ask how the nonmoving eternal can appear to move or create something. Here, the *Vedic* literature, known as the *Upaniṣhads*, offers a metaphor: Just as the desert appears to create an oasis without moving to create it, so does the nonmoving eternity appear to produce this illusory creation. The creation is called illusory because it is not lasting; only eternity is real because it is everlasting.

There is not enough space in this book to justly discuss this topic. This is a mere offering into the insight of the origin of creation as explained by the ancient *Vedic ṛishis* (seers).

As creation developed, it formed three underlying principles that uphold all life: the laws of creation, maintenance, and dissolution. Everything in life is born or created, it lives, and then it dies. These principles are known as *sattwa, rajas,* and *tamas*, respectfully, and are called the three *guṇas* or tendencies. All of life, human and celestial, obey these laws.

The Elements: Building Blocks of Life

The creation principle developed five essential elements—or building blocks that all life forms contain: ether, air, fire, water, and earth. We can easily see how life was created from the subtlest to the grossest matter. From eternity, the subtlest form of matter is ether. Ether mixing with eternity creates air, a more observable or experiential element. As air moves, it eventually creates friction, which creates heat or fire. Heat produces moisture, thus creating water, the densest element yet: if one tries to walk through water, one is slowed by its density. Finally, water produces the densest form of matter, earth. The *Vedas* say that all of the creation, including humans, are made up of combinations of all five essential elements. These elements are the subtlest aspects of human life, finer than the molecular, atomic, or subatomic levels.

This is the level that Āyurvedic healing works on. Focusing on the cause of the grosser levels of life, the denser aspects will be taken care of since they are made up of these five elements. Just as a strong foundation supports a strong building, when the five elements (the foundation of all matter) are strong and balanced in a person, they will automatically balance the more material levels.

Thus, Āyurveda does not need to look at isolated parts of the human anatomy, or at the vitamin, chemical, or nutritional level of health. It simply balances the elements, and this balances the more physical levels.

A person diagnosed with a duodenal ulcer is an example of this balancing. Rather than create a name for a symptom, Āyurveda identifies the illness as an excess of the fire element. Acid is a byproduct of heat. Āyurveda will look to see in what part of the patient's life overheating occurs. It may be due to eating excessive fiery foods and spices like tomatoes and peppers. One's career may be causing undue anger (i.e., hot temper). Perhaps the person drinks alcohol (firewater).

Once the cause is learned, suggestions for reducing a person's excessive intake of fire are discussed. Simultaneously, the patient is advised to use more of the air and water elements to balance the heat with coolness (air cools heat, water puts out the fire).

Thus, the holistic approach of Āyurveda seeks the cause of an illness and restores balance, using the insight of the elemental creation of the universe.

The Āyurvedic Body

Personalizing the healing process is a uniqueness that Āyurveda brings to the holistic field of health. From the insights of the *Vedic* sages, we learn that people are different and need to be individually treated.

Expanding upon this elemental view, the Āyurvedic practitioner understands that people are made up of various combinations of the elements. Some people have more air in their system, some people have a more fiery constitution. Others are predominantly made up of water. Still others are combinations of fire and air, fire and water, or air and water. Some people have an equal amount of all three elements (ether is combined in air and earth within water).

Thus a more air-predominant individual needs to take in less air and more fire and water. A water person already has an excess of water, so there is a need to reduce the intake of water and to increase the fire and air elements in the diet and lifestyle.

Personalized Healing

The general Āyurvedic approach is threefold.

1. Determining one's elemental constitution (*doṣha* or *prakṛiti*),
2. Learning the elemental cause of illness (*vikṛiti*), and
3. Applying therapeutic recommendations to balance elements causing the illness, without causing an imbalance to the *doṣha* (constitution).

This unique, personalized approach not only makes healing effective, but gentle as well. Other holistic measures may work, yet still aggravate the person's *doṣha*. Āyurveda is the only holistic science that needn't warn people that they may feel worse while the diseases or toxins are being removed before they will feel better. Because of its balancing approach, gentleness marks the entire healing process.

Qualities of the Three Doṣhas

Parallel to the three *guṇas* (*sattwa, rajas,* and *tamas*) in creation are the three *doṣhas*, or constitutions, in the human body: Vāyu (or Vāta), Pitta, and Kapha. Vāyu may be understood as nerve force, electro-motor, physical activity or that which is responsible for motion. It is commonly called air. The root, 'va' means to spread. In Western terms, it is the electricity setting the organism into motion, maintaining the equilibrium between Pitta and Kapha (inerts).

Vāyu relates to the nerve-force.
It is responsible for all movement
in the mind and body.
The movement of Vāyu even regulates the
balance of Pitta and Kapha.

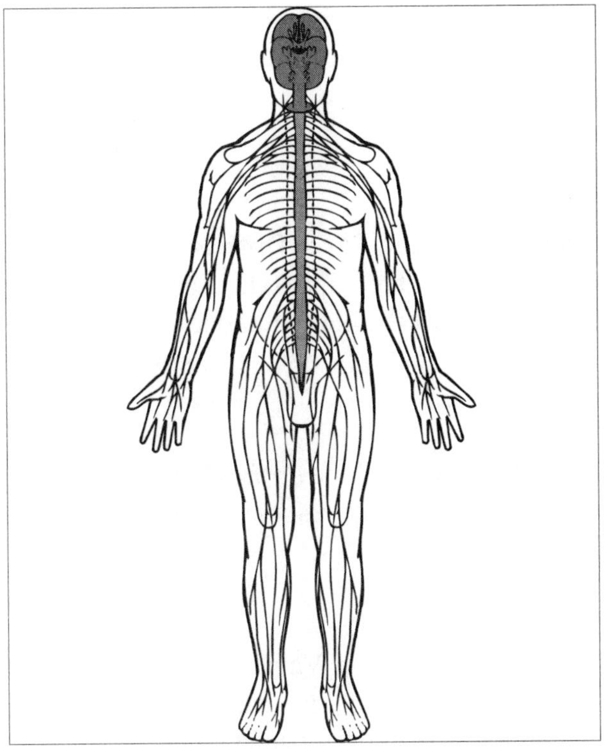

The nerve network of the mind and body.

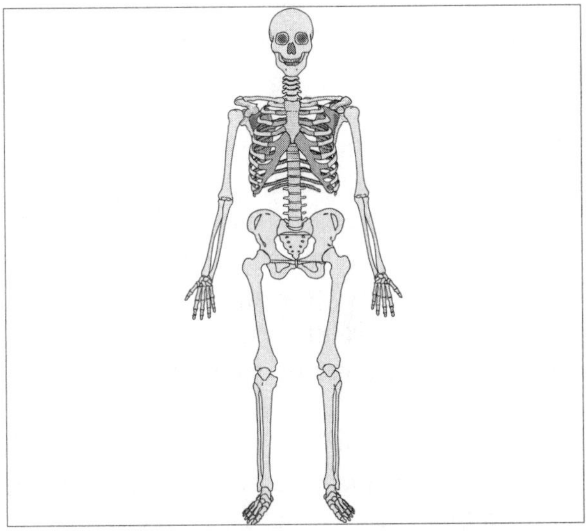

The bones are primarily affected by Vāyu

Pitta relates to internal fire, bile, body heat, digestive enzymes, physio-chemical, biological, metabolic and endocrine systems. It is responsible for digesting the chyle into a protoplasmic substance like sperm and ovum.

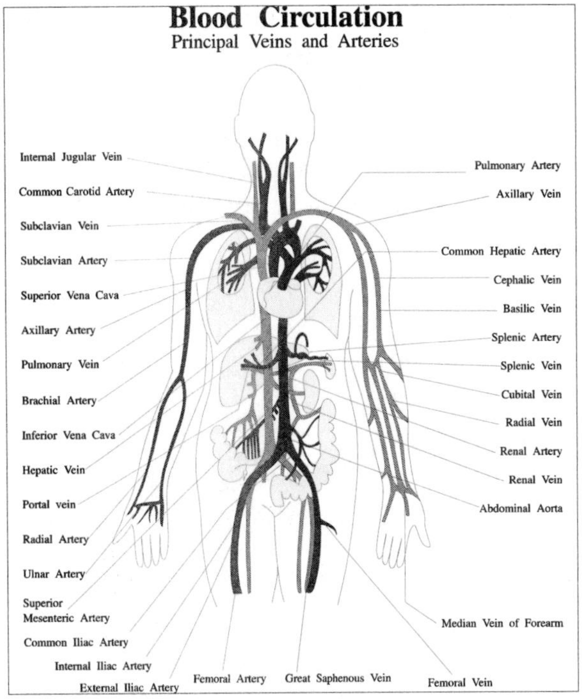

Pitta relates to the endocrine system...

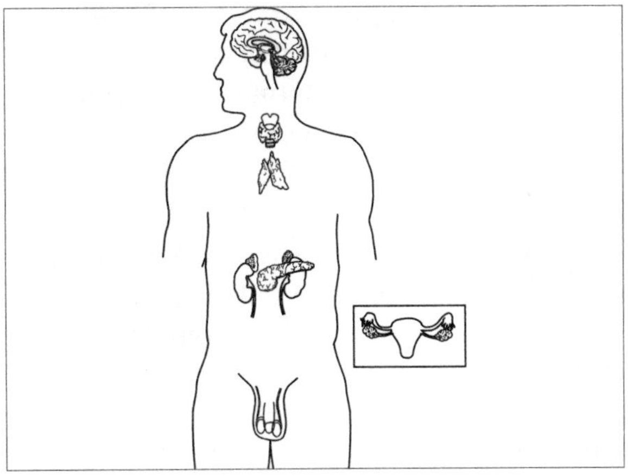

and digestive system.

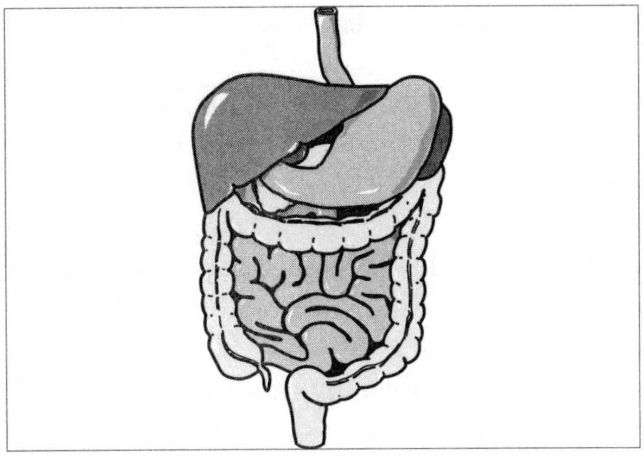

Kapha fills the intercellular spaces of the body as connective tissue. Examples of these tissues include mucus, synovial fluid, and tendons. Kapha is responsible for the gross structure of the body (solid and liquid/phlegm-plasma). Each person is made up of a combination of these elements.

The knee bones are examples of areas that are lubricated by Kapha.

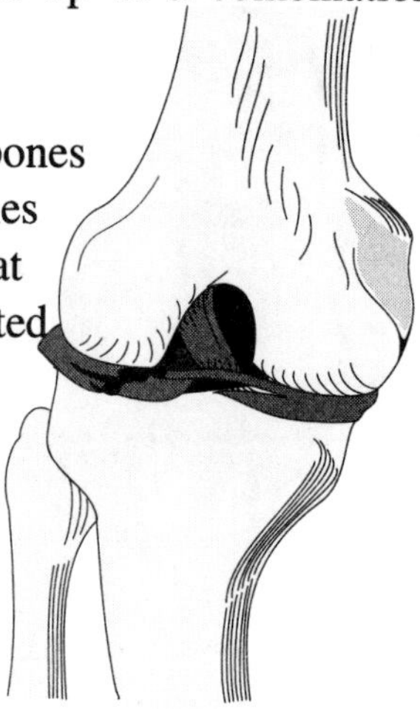

Together, the *doṣhas* are responsible for catabolic and anabolic metabolism. Catabolism breaks down complex internal bodies, and Vāyu (air energy) sets this energy free into simpler waste. Anabolism takes food and builds it into more complex bodies. The summit of the metabolic process is protoplasm or essential matter [proteins, carbohydrates, lipids, inorganic salts]. Lifeless food becomes living protoplasm and is set free as useful energy or excess heat or motion that is emitted from the body. Thus, the purpose of the three *doṣhas* is to move the lymph chyle (the byproduct of digested foods) throughout the body. This nourishes and builds the body tissues. When any or all of the *doṣhas* develop imbalance, the body ceases to be nourished, and disease develops.

The three *doṣhas* (Vāyu, Pitta, Kapha) exist throughout the entire body, in every cell, yet are predominant (their sites of origin) in the colon, small intestine, and stomach, respectively. Some authorities say that Vāyu primarily resides below the navel, Pitta from the navel to the heart, and Kapha, above the heart.

Vāyu is also found in (governing) the waist, thighs, ear, bones, and skin. Pitta also governs the navel, sweat, lymph, blood, eye, and skin. Kapha additionally controls the chest, throat, head, bone joints, small intestine, plasma, fat, nose, and tongue.

Properties of the Three Doṣhas

Vāyu: Dry, light, cold, rough, subtle, moving
Pitta: Slightly oily, hot, light, odorous, liquid
Kapha: Oily, cold, heavy, slow, smooth, slimy, static.

Each of the three *doṣhas* have five divisions or responsibilities.

5 Vāyus

Each of the five Vāyus is responsible for various physical and mental functions of the cerebral-spinal and sympathetic nerves.

Prāṇ is located in the head and governs the chest, throat, mind, heart, sense organs, intelligence, expectorating, sneezing, belching, inspiration, and swallowing of food—outward movement.

Udān resides in the chest and controls the nose, navel, and throat, and is responsible for initiating speech, effort, enthusiasm, the capacity to work, complexion, and memory—upward movement.

Vyān is found in the heart and rapidly moves throughout the body. It regulates all body movements, including walking, raising and lowering of the body parts, and opening and closing the eyes.

Samān is located near the digestive fire. It works in the alimentary tract (absorbing nutrients and excreting wastes), and other abdominal organs. It holds food in the alimentary tract, helps digest it, separates nutrients from waste, and eliminates the waste—equalized movement.

Apān is seated in the colon, and controls the waist, bladder, genitals, and thighs. Its main function is downward movement of wastes (feces, urine), reproductive fluid, menstrual fluid, and it also controls the downward movement of the fetus.

5 Pittas

Pāchaka exists in the small intestine, stomach, and colon as non-liquid heat, bile, or digestive fire. The fire digests and transforms food, emulsifying food fats and separating absorbable nutrients from waste, so they may be passed to lacteals by absorption. [Food becoming partially digested in the stomach is known as chyme. This chyme passes into the small intestine where it becomes digested by the pancreatic juice and bile. The usable byproduct is lymph and fatty matter, or chyle. The chyle moves through lacteals, or lymphatic vessels which carry chyle from the small intestine to the thoracic duct. From the thoracic duct, the chyle is sent into the blood.] *Pāchaka* (digestive enzymes), through digestion, automatically nourishes the other four Pittas.

Rañjaka is located in the stomach, liver, and spleen, and gives color to lymph chyle when it is transformed into blood as it passes through the liver and spleen.

Sādhaka is found in the heart. It helps in performing mental functions such as knowledge, intelligence, and consciousness by maintaining rhythmic cardiac contractions.

Ālochaka resides in the retina of the eyes and governs sight.

Bhrājaka resides in the skin. It regulates complexion by keeping secretions from the sweat and sebaceous glands of the skin active.

5 Kaphas

Avalaṃbaka is found in the chest and creates cohesion, softness, moistness, and liquidity, which results in maintaining body strength.

Kledaka is in the stomach, liquefying hard food masses.

Bodhaka is found in the tongue and is responsible for taste.

Tarpaka exists in the head and nourishes the sense organs.

Śhleṣhaka is located in the bone joints and lubricates them.

People who are predominantly an air (Vāyu) *prakṛiti* will have different experiences depending on whether their *doṣha* is balanced or in excess. Balanced Vāyu-*prakṛiti* individuals will be adaptable, cheerful, have natural healing tendencies, be thin-framed, and very tall or very short. If there is excess Vāyu in their bodies, they may be very thin, have dry skin, gas, constipation, bone problems, or arthritis. They may talk very fast or become easily tired. Mentally, they may quickly grasp concepts but soon forget them; be anxious, worried, fearful, or nervous.

Pitta-dominant individuals, when healthy and balanced, will be warm, and have clear, penetrating thoughts. They will tend to be leaders and/or athletic. They will be of moderate, muscular build, and will be passionate. When they overheat, they may find themselves impatient, hot-tempered, or too critical. Physically, they will develop heat-related problems like ulcers, infections, rashes or acne, eye problems, or high blood pressure.

The Kapha-paramount individuals, when balanced, are loyal and calm. Physically, they are big boned and strong, with deep-toned voices. When Kapha is excessive, they tend toward water excesses like water retention, being overweight, or having bronchitis. Mentally, they will find themselves lethargic, too attached, and sentimental.

As we discussed earlier, each person is made up of a combination of these elements, yet each usually has a combination predominantly of two or all three of these elements. These elements in turn, form three physiological principles, Vāyu (ether and air), Pitta (fire), and Kapha (water and earth). Like the elements, people are predominantly made up of one or more or these *doṣhas*.

People fall into seven *prakṛiti* categories:

1. Vāyu 5. Pitta/Kapha
2. Pitta 6. Kapha/Vāyu
3. Kapha 7. Tridoṣhic (equal amounts).
4. Vāyu/Pitta (combination)

These constitutions may be further subdivided, 8, 9. Vāyu/Pitta (with Vāyu or Pitta being

predominant)
10, 11. Vāyu/Kapha (with Vāyu or Kapha being predominant)
12, 13. Pitta/Kapha (with Pitta or Kapha being predominant)
14-19. Tridoṣhic (six additional constitutions, with one or two *doṣhas* being more predominant: e.g., Vāyu predominance, Pitta and Kapha predominance, etc.)

Three external reasons cause *doṣhas* to become increased (imbalanced):
1. Time of day or season (e.g., around noontime is ruled by Pitta; Fall is predominantly a Vāyu time)
2. From inadequate, excessive or untimely sensory experiences (e.g., excessive loud music, overeating)
3. Actions. (e.g., excessive speaking, inadequate exercise, etc.)

Agnis: Digestive Fire (Enzymes)

Most diseases are due to poor digestion. *Agni* (enzyme) is found in the alimentary canal and digests food. *Samāgni* is produced by the normal digestion of the three *doṣhas*. Digestive activity (healthy, deficient or excessive) is governed by the *doṣhas* becoming aggravated. The three *doṣhas* produce three *agnis* (*viṣhamāgni, tīkṣhnāgni* and *mandāgni* respectively). Excess Vāyu in the body produces weak, irregular digestion, and causes gas.

Excess Pitta creates a situation like an overheated furnace. Food burns up quickly, and persons experience burning sensations, thirst, acid indigestion, etc. In some cases the *agni* fire even burns up nutrients, causing malnutrition.

When excess Kapha is in the digestive tract, the digestive fire is low, making it difficult to digest any foods. As a result, a person feels dull, poor, inadequate, and lethargic; the stomach is heavy, or the person may experience constipation. Vāyu disorders produce hard stools from the dryness caused by gas. Pitta stools are soft or liquid due to excess heat. Kapha stools are moderate. A healthy stool is also moderate and easily eliminated once or twice a day.

Thirteen *agnis* reside in the body and are responsible for digestion,

Jatharagni: Works at the gastrointestinal level, governing basic digestion and the 12 other *agnis*.

5 *Bhutagnis*: Metabolize the five elements that are present in the body's tissues. They are a form of heat that is always present in all the tissues that are responsible for proper function and development of the tissues.

7 *Dhatagnis*: Metabolize in the seven tissues (*dhātus*). This is a biochemical process beyond food digestion. It includes anabolic and catabolic activity.

Body Tissues and Wastes (The 7 Dhātus and 3 Malas)

Tissue Layers (Dhātus)

The Āyurvedic view of the body has many similarities to modern beliefs. Seven tissue systems (*dhātus*) are in the body. Each tissue is primarily governed by one of the three elements. Each *dhātu* is developed or transformed out of the previous tissue layer, starting with *rasa* (plasma). If plasma is not healthy, then all the other layers will also be affected.

Tissue Layer (*Dhātus*)	Governing *Doṣha*
1. plasma (*rasa*)	Kapha/water
2. blood (*rakta*)	Pitta/fire
3. muscle (*māṃsa*)	Kapha/water
4. fat (*medas*)	Kapha/water
5. bone (*asthi*)	Vāyu/air
6. nerves fluid/marrow (*majjā*)	Kapha/water
7. reproductive tissues (*śhukra*)	Kapha/water

With insight into the governing *doṣha*, the cause of a diseased *dhātu* is accurately determined. For example, if a person has cancer in the blood, we know that excess Pitta (heat, toxins) exists in the blood. If a person has osteoporosis, then too much Vāyu is in the bones. Muscular Dystrophy would be an example of a muscular or Kapha problem.

Once the elemental cause of the illness is known, therapies are used to balance the system through reducing the excess elements(s) and increasing the deficient one(s). Therapies include the use of herbs, foods, and lifestyle variations.

Signs and Symptoms of Vitiated Tissues (Dhātus)

Tissues (*Dhātus*)	Signs and Symptoms
Plasma (*rasa*)	restlessness, palpitation, cardiac pain, exhaustion without cause, irritated by loud noises
Hemoglobin Blood (*rakta*)	roughness, dryness, skin cracks, loss of luster
Muscle (*māṃsa*)	emaciation (especially of buttocks, neck, and abdomen)
Fat (medas)	cracking joints, eye lassitude, overly thin, exhaustion,
Bone (*asthi*)	falling hair, nails, teeth, loose joints
Marrow (*majjā*)	thinness, weakness, bone lightness, Vāyu bone diseases
Reproductive Essence (*śhukra*)	weakness, dry mouth, pallor, lassitude, exertion, impotence, non-ejaculation of semen

Body Wastes (Malas)

Another important factor in health is the proper elimination of waste: feces, urine, and sweat (miscellaneous waste includes tears (eye), spit (tongue), oily secretions (skin), mucoid secretions (mucus membrane), and smegma (genitalia excreta). *Malas* (bodily wastes) help maintain the functioning of our organs.

Feces (*purīṣha*) provide support and tone, as well as maintaining the temperature of the colon. Improper functioning can lead to Vāyu illness like worry, fear, ungroundedness, nervousness, headaches, gas, distention, and constipation. Functioning of the feces is damaged by excessive use of purgatives, colonics, worry, and fear (fear can both create improper functioning or be a byproduct of this dysfunction). It is also damaged by excessive travel, the wrong foods (such as "junk food," or those foods that are too light or too heavy), oversleeping, coffee, drugs, antibiotics, insufficient exercise, and prolonged diarrhea. In Āyurvedic literature it has been clearly stated that debilitated persons suffering from tuberculosis should not be given any kind of purgatives, as it is the feces that preserve the temperature of such persons.

Urine (*mūtra*) expels water and other solid wastes from the body. Poor urine elimination results in bladder pain or infection, difficult urination, fever, thirst, dry mouth, or dehydration. It is damaged by diuretic drugs, alcohol, excessive sex, trauma, fright, or too few liquids.

Sweat (*sweda*) controls the body temperature by way of expelling excess water and toxins, cools the body, moistens the skin and hair, carries excess fat from the body, and purifies the blood. Excess sweating can cause skin diseases (usually Pitta related) like eczema, boils, fungus, burning skin, dehydration, fatigue, or convulsions (Vāyu-caused). Deficient sweating can result in stiff hair, skin fissures, dry skin, dandruff, wrinkles, or susceptibility to colds and flu (i.e., peripheral circulation). Sweating is damaged by too much dry food, lack of salt, excess or deficient exercise, excessive use of diaphoretic herbs or excess sweating.

Life Sap (Ojas)

Ojas (the life sap) is the essence of all the tissues (*dhātus*). It pervades every part of the body. (Some authorities believe *ojas* is a combination of eight different drops *(aṣhtabindu)* of liquid, secreted from the pineal gland.) *Ojas* is depleted by excessive sex, drugs, talking, loud music, insufficient rest or burnout, and high technology. Signs of diminished *ojas* are fear, worry, sensory organ pain, poor complexion, cheerlessness, roughness, emaciation, immune system disorders, and easily contracting diseases.

Tastes (Rasas)

Āyurveda says there is a total of six tastes. Each taste is governed by a *doṣha*. These tastes may either aggravate or pacify the *doṣhas, dhātus*, and *malas*.

Taste (*Rasa*)	*Doṣha* Aggravated	*Doṣha* Balanced
sweet/*swādu*	Kapha	Vāyu/Pitta
sour/*amla*	Pitta/Kapha	Vāyu
salty/lavaṇa	Pitta/Kapha	Vāyu
pungent/*katu*	Pitta, Vāyu (in excess)	Kapha
bitter/*tikta*	Vāyu	Pitta/Kapha
astringent/*kaṣhaya*	Vāyu	Pitta/Kapha

Tastes provide varying degrees of nourishing strength. Sweet taste is the most nourishing, and as each taste becomes less nourishing, it becomes more bitter, until it is astringent—and the least nourishing.

This is also the order of tastes that get digested (so eating sweets first is better, and astringent foods last). Some authorities state that if one were to eat sweets last, the body would digest this taste first, letting the other tastes pass undigested through the system. By the time the sweets are digested, the other foods have passed through the system without being digested. Other authorities believe that a little sweet taste at the end of the meal stimulates digestion.

Every substance, including some foods, may have more than one taste (i.e., primary and secondary tastes). Substances alleviate *doṣhas*, aggravate *doṣhas*, or maintain health. When health is at least slightly in balance, persons are advised to have a little of each taste daily. *Rasa* is discussed in a Chapter 6, the chapter on nutrition.

Potency: (Vīrya)/After Taste: (Vipāka)

The qualities of substances are either hot (*ūṣhnā*) or cold (*sīta*). Hot tastes generally aggravate Pitta and mitigate Vāyu and Kapha. Cold tastes mitigate Pitta and aggravate the rest.

After digestion, one experiences an aftertaste, which is either sweet, sour, or pungent. Again, this is important in balancing or imbalancing the *doṣhas*. These aspects will also be discussed in the chapter on nutrition.

20 Qualities (Guṇas)

Each substance has qualities associated with one *doṣha*. Again, like increases like and opposites reduce *doṣhas, dhātus,* and *malas*. Āyurveda has developed a remarkably detailed and precise analysis of the qualities. These attributes are used in finding which qualities will heal or aggravate the *doṣhas*. For example, substances that are heavy and cold are not suggested for those with weak digestion, such as Vāyu and Kapha *doṣhas*. Foods that are hot and oily heal the Vāyu *doṣha*.

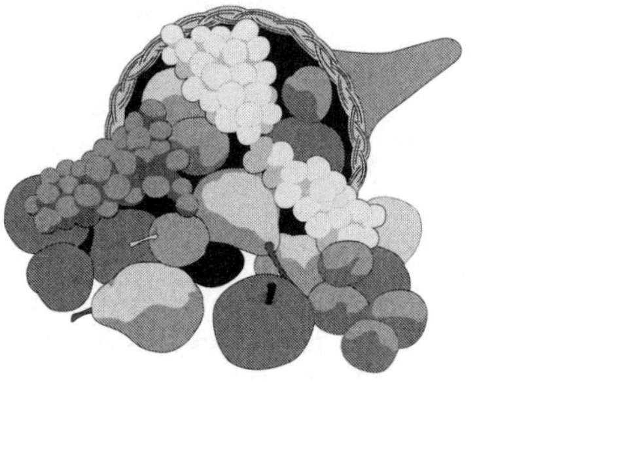

In the table below the 20 *guṇas* or qualities are listed.

1. heavy/*guru*	11. light/*laghu*
2. slow/*manda*	12. quick/*tekṣhna*
3. cold/*hima*	13. hot/*ūṣhnā*
4. oily/*snighda*	14. dry/*rūṣha*
5. smooth/*śhlakṣhna*	15. rough/*khara*
6. solid/*sāndra*	16. liquid/*drava*
7. soft/*mridu*	17. hard/*kathina*
8. stable/*sthira*	18. moving/*cala*
9. subtle/*sūkṣhma*	19. large/*sthūla*
10. non-slimy/ *viṣhada*	20. slimy/*picchila*

Disease (*roga*) is caused by deficient, improper, or excess contact with 1) seasons (e.g., excess cold in winter), 2) sensory objects (e.g., overeating), and 3) activities (e.g., over exercise). Health (*arogya*) is achieved through proper contact with the three.

Disease is caused by imbalancing the *doṣhas*. For example, if a Pitta *doṣha* (fiery person) eats much ginger, they will create excess fire in the body. This results in Pitta disorders like acid indigestion. Diseases occur due to internal or external factors, and reside in the body or mind. Disease is caused by *rajas* (overactivity) and *tamas* (lethargy) psychological/ spiritual factors.

Three Mental Qualities: Sattwa, Rajas, Tamas

The three *guṇas, sattwa, rajas,* and *tamas* are found in nature and in the mind, paralleling the three *doṣhas* of the body. *Sattwa*, or purity, is the preferred mental state because a person with this quality is calm, alert, kind, and thoughtful. A person whose mind is predominantly *rajasic* (too active) is always seeking diversions (incessant activity). The *tamasic*-predominant mind is a dull, lethargic mind.

Just as combinations of Vāyu, Pitta, and Kapha exist for the body, the mind has combinations of *sattwa*, *rajas*, and *tamas*. Individuals whose minds are *sattwic* and *rajasic* are those who enthusiastically study spiritual and holistic measures to improve themselves. *Rajasic/tam-asic* minded people will actively work and exercise to overcome their lethargy.

Mental balance and the development of purity and peace develop the mind towards a *sattwic* mind. This is the first stage of *samādhi* or spiritual realization.

To decide the cause of illness, the practitioner observes, questions, and takes the pulse of the patient. Illness can be understood by learning its cause, or seeing it in its incubatory, beginning, developmental, or advanced stages.

The Vāyu Mind

When Vāyu doṣha persons are balanced, they are cheerful, creative, and adaptable. When Vāyu doṣhas are imbalanced, they are worried, nervous, fearful, and giddy.

The mental constitution of Vāyu individuals tends towards fear, anxiety, and insecurity. They can easily be deceived with threats or promises. They do not have much courage, are of solitary nature, and possess few intimate friends (although they form friends with those in other social circles). Vāyu people do not make good leaders or followers and are not materialistic (as they spend and earn freely).

Sattwic influence creates comprehension, the need for unity and healing, and creates a positive mental outlook.

Rajasic influence creates indecisiveness, unreliability, hyperactivity, and anxiety.

Tamasic influence creates fear, a servile attitude, dishonesty, depression, self-destructiveness, addictive behavior, sexual perversions, animal instincts, or suicidal thoughts.

The Pitta Mind

When Pitta doṣha individuals are healthy or balanced, they are

goal-oriented, powerful, warm, athletic.
When Pitta doṣhas are imbalanced, they are burnt out, angry, impatient, irritable, critical.

Mental Pitta individuals possess fiery emotions like irritability, anger, and hate. Mentally, they have abilities of penetration, yet can be aggressive and seldom sentimental. They are determined, articulate, convincing, and yet may try to dominate others with their will and ideas. They are self-righteous and may become fanatical. Pitta people are good leaders, ambitious, and work hard to achieve great goals. They help their families and friends, but are cruel and unforgiving to enemies. Also, they are bold, adventurous, daring and enjoy challenges. Although they have much clarity, they lack compassion.

Sattwic influence creates clarity, intelligence, leadership, warmth, and independence.

Rajasic influence creates willfulness, ambition, anger, manipulation, vanity, impulsiveness, and aggressiveness.

Tamasic influence creates vindictiveness, violence, hate, criminality, and psychopathic behavior.

The Kapha Mind

These people are the emotional ones, full of love, desire, romance, and sentiment. However, they also have the negative emotions of lust and greed. Kapha *doṣhas* find it hard to adapt to new situations, yet they are very loyal. They have many friends and are close to their families, communities, religions, and countries. They are more comfortable with practical knowledge than with abstract ideas.

When Kapha doṣha persons are healthy they love to cook for others, are strong, and loyal.
Imbalanced Kapha doṣhas become lethargic, hoarding, overly materialistic

Sattwic influence creates calmness, peace, love, compassion, faith, nurturing, and forgiveness.

Rajasic influence creates greed for money, material luxuries, and comfort. They are too sentimental, controlling, attached, and lustful.

Tamasic influences create dullness, sloth, lethargy, depression, lack of care and a tendency to steal.

Developing Samādhi: Divine Peace

Some patients have one type of physical constitution combined with another type of mental constitution (i.e., a heavy and nervous person has a Kapha body and Vāyu mind). Consequently, when suggesting healing measures for the Kapha body illness, the practitioner takes care not to aggravate the Vāyu mental constitution. In this example, fire-increasing measures are recommended, including herbs, foods, and aromas, but not air-increasing ones. Mental disease is related to *rajas* and *tamas*, the activity and lethargy principles of the three *guṇas* (qualities). The *guṇas* also reflect the level of the soul's development. If the mind is *sattwic,* or pure, then clarity exists. *A sattwic*-minded person perceives the knowledge of Divinity. A *sattwic* mind is also the first stage of *samādhi.* Poor mental discrimination is the cause of all illness, making one dishonest, self-destructive, and hurtful to others. One would overindulge in "junk food," entertainment, etc. The best way to heal is by following a *sattwic* lifestyle. This includes meditation, compassionate actions, ethical and virtuous behavior, healthy, organic foods, and living within the rhythms of nature. People in whom *sattwa* predominates, see the good in all things (including the value an illness may offer), and they are the healthiest people as well.

Tamas creates lethargy, dullness, and a cloudy perception. This is caused by fear and ignorance, and plays on one's animal nature. A person with this frame of mind would choose not to do much of anything. When this mental quality is predominant, such persons will suppress their emotions. Emotional suppression is a major cause of severe illness, like cancer. Stagnancy describes their emotional makeup. Negative mindedness and self-destruction define their personality.

Rajas causes a turbulent, or distracted, mind. It makes one look outside for comfort and fulfillment. It causes one to seek external validation. *Rajas* makes one think love is derived from an external relationship, not from within. It makes one willful, egoistic, and manipulative.

When *rajas* and *tamas* exist in the mind simultaneously, activity is devoted to greedy purposes. These persons also overextend themselves for those ends. They blame others for their condition and expect others to cure them.

When *rajas* is free from a trace of *tamas*, it then can develop purer activities, like studying or learning about health and spirituality. Yet the *rajasic*-minded person may still burn out during the learning process.

Often, just as people have some qualities of all three *doṣhas*, that mind has some of each *guṇa*. Seven mental *guṇa* types exist: *sattwa, rajas, tamas, sattwa-rajas, sattwa-tamas, rajas-tamas,* and *triguṇa* (equal amounts of the three *guṇas*). Just as external factors may cause *doṣha* derangement, the *rajasic* nature of our modern technological society may cause mental *rajasic* derangements.

Mental Qualities: Prāṇa, Tejas & Ojas

The mind has three governing agents similar to Vāyu, Pitta, and Kapha. They are called *prāṇa* (air), *tejas* (fire), and *ojas* (life sap). Again, it is the balance of these three elements that decide mental balance and clarity. Too much *prāṇa* will create anxiety, worry, insomnia, and loss of memory and concentration. (This *prāṇa* is different from the air we think of as respiration. Here, *prāṇa* means life-force, soul, or *kuṇḍalinī śhakti*). Excess *prāṇa* dries up *ojas*, the sap that creates one's spiritual life sap. Through meditation, *ojas* becomes transmuted into life energy, or "*kuṇḍalinī śhakti*," which develops one's Self-realization. Spiritually speaking, an undetectable tube runs up the middle of our spine called the "*suṣhumṇā*" in which the *kuṇḍalinī* energy travels. Without this *śhakti* energy, not only is our physical and mental health used up, but so is our spiritual development. Excess *tejas* also depletes *ojas* by burning it up, whereas excess *ojas* can create a lethargic person.

Doṣhas and the Organs

Each organ is primarily governed by one *doṣha*. By knowing which *doṣha* controls which organs, one achieves the health of the appropriate organ, through balancing the elements (*doṣhas*)

Vāyu	Pitta	Kapha
colon*	small intestine*	stomach*
brain	liver	lungs
thighs	spleen	pericardium
bones	gall bladder	triple warmer
kidney	kidney	
urinary bladder	heart	urinary bladder
pancreas	pancreas	pancreas
	uterus	testes

** Origin Sites of the doṣhas*

By merely knowing which *doṣha* is related to which tissue layer and body system, Āyurveda can identify and bring balance to health problems. For example, diabetes is a condition of the water (glucose) metabolism *srota.* Kapha *doṣha* causes this condition (from sweet tastes). By removing water-increasing foods and herbs from one's diet, and eating fire and air increasing foods (bitter and pungent tastes), diabetes is controlled. Certain herbs like *śhilājit* and *guḍmar*, and special Āyurvedic *abhyañgas* (massage-like) are also used specifically for healing the pancreas and kidneys.

Health, Excess & Deficiencies of the Dhātus

Plasma/Rasa

Excess: Saliva, phlegm, blocked channels, loss of appetite, nausea, Kapha is increased throughout body.

Deficient: Rough skin, dry lips, dehydration, weariness and exhaustion after slight activity, intolerance to sound, tremors, palpitations, heart pain, a sense of emptiness, poor nutrition.

Healthy: Good complexion, healthy hair, vitality, compassionate, and happy.

Blood/ Rakta

Excess: Skin disease, abscesses, liver, and spleen enlargement, hypertension, tumors, delirium, poor digestion, jaundice, burning sensation, bleeding, redness in skin, eyes, and urine.

Deficient: Low blood pressure, pallor, low skin luster, blood vessel collapse, shock, desiring sour and cold foods, loose and dry hair, dry, rough, cracked skin.

Healthy: Good color in cheeks, hands, feet, lips, tongue lustrous eyes, warm skin, vital yet sensitive to sun and heat, passion.

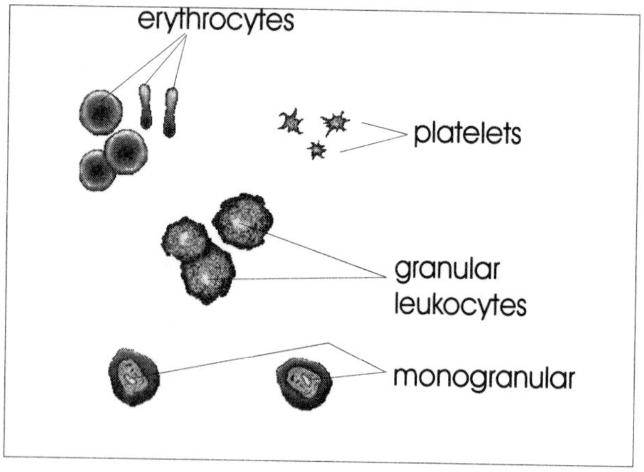

Muscle/Māṃsa

Excess: Enlarged liver, swelling, tumors in muscle sites, heaviness or swelling of glands, overweight or obesity, irritability, aggression, fibroids, miscarriage, low sexual vitality.

Deficient: Weariness, loose limbs, lack of coordination, emaciation of hips, back of neck and abdomen, fear, unhappiness, insecurity.

Healthy: Able to exercise, strong, adaptable. Well developed neck, shoulder and thigh muscles. Courageous, integrity, fortitude and a strong character.

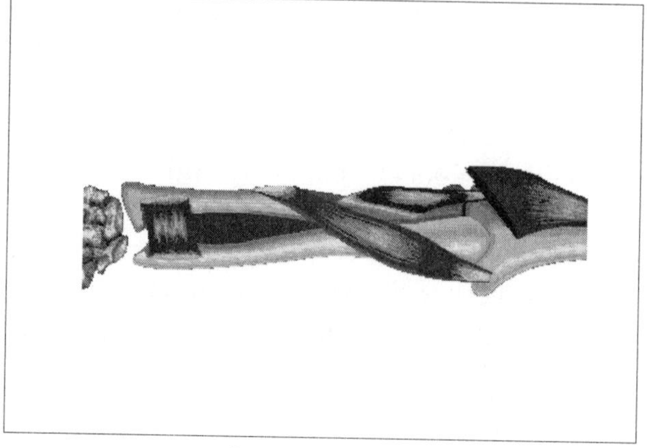

Rotator Muscles

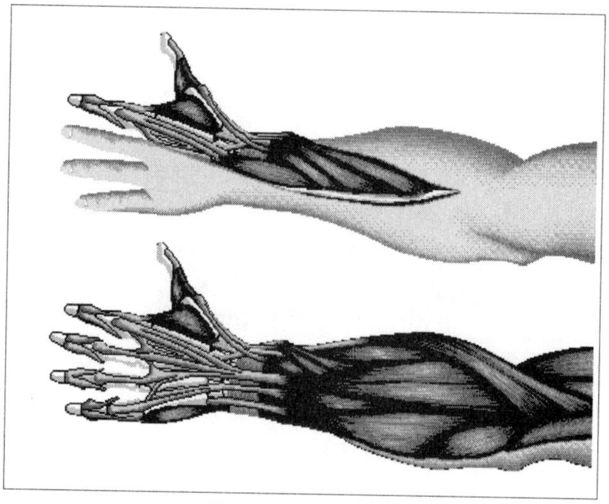

Extensor Muscles

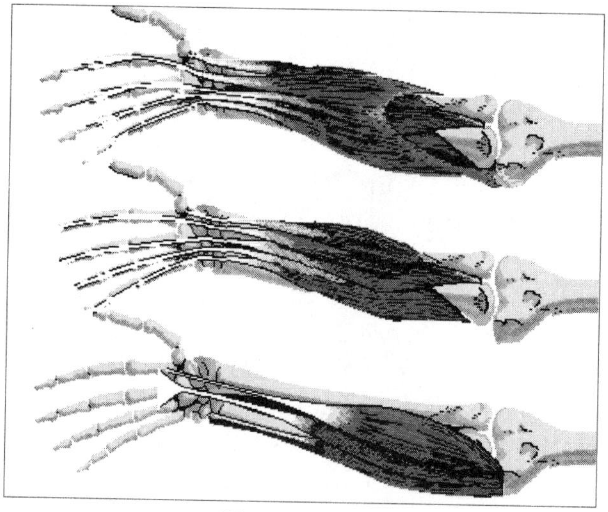

Flexor Muscles

Fat/Medas

Excess: Overweight and obesity, lacking mobility, asthma, fatigue, sexual debility, thirst, diabetes, shortened life span, hypertension, breast, sagging belly and thighs, emotional fear and attachment.

Deficient: Weary eyes, fatigue, cracking joints, enlarged spleen, limb emaciation, thin abdomen, brittle or weak hair, bones, nails, teeth.

Healthy: Lubricated tissues, oily hair, eyes, feces. Ample body fat (not excessive). Melodious voice, loving, joyful, humorous, affectionate.

Bone/Asthi

Excess: Spurs, extra bones and teeth, extra large frame, joint pain, low stamina, anxiety, arthritis, bone cancer, or gigantism in extreme cases.

Deficient: Pain or loose joints, falling of teeth, hair and nails, poor bone and tooth formation, fatigue, dwarfism in extreme cases.

Healthy: Large joints, and prominent bones, flexibility, long, feet, large, strong, white teeth, patient, consistent, stable, hard working.

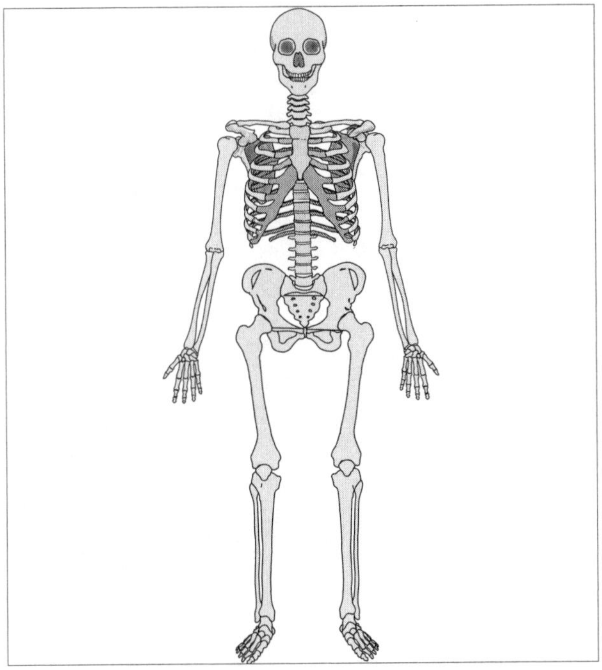

Marrow/ Majjā

Excess: Limbs, eyes and joint (origin) heaviness, deep non-healing sores, cloudy eyes, and infections.

Deficient: Weak and porous bones, small joint pain, seeing spots or darkness before the eyes, dizzy, low sexual vitality, feeling emptiness, and fear. Vāyu becomes imbalanced from low nerve tissue supply.

Healthy: Strong joints, clear eyes, good speech, able to withstand pain, sharp, clear, sensitive mind with good memory, open, feeling, compassionate, receptive.

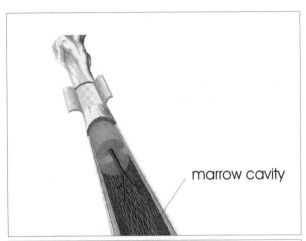

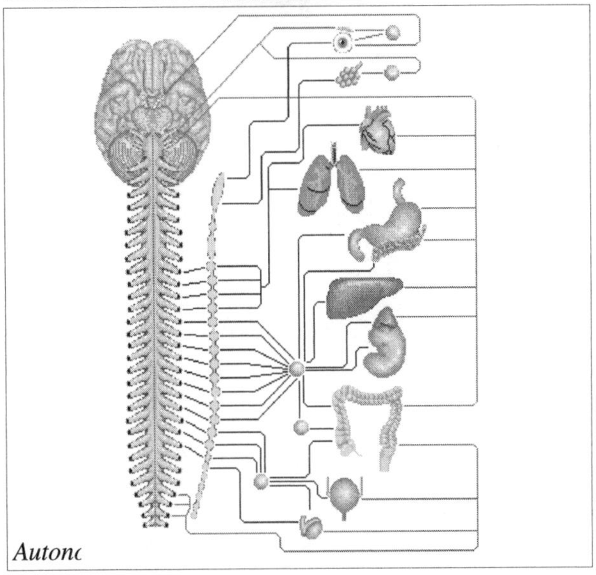

Semen/ Śhukra

Excess: Excess sexual desire that leads to anger, excess semen, semen stones, and a swollen prostate.

Deficient: Low vitality and sexual desire, impotence, sterility, difficult and slow ejaculation, bloody semen. One may experience lassitude, weariness, a dry mouth, lower back pain, fear, anxiety, lack of love.

Healthy: Attractive body, lustrous eyes, good hair growth, well formed sexual organs, charm, loving, compassionate, empathic.

Excess produces Kapha. Deficiencies produce Vāyu.

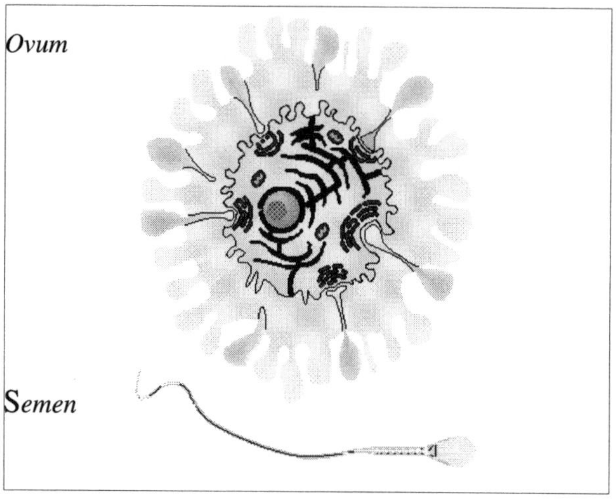

Srotas: Body Channel Systems

Other parallels exist between East and West concerning *srotas*. *Srotas* are the channels, pores, or systems that carry or circulate the *doṣhas* and tissues (*dhātus*) or their elements to the various organs. During this process of circulation the *dhātus* are transformed from the first to the last tissue layer (*rasa* through *śhukra*). Each *dhātu* has two aspects: nutrition for its own tissue layer, and sustenance for the next developing *dhātu*.

Āyurveda notes 16 systems, several more than those that are currently considered. The origin sites which carry each *dhātu* are listed on the next page.

Systems (*Srotas*)	Main Organ Site: Related *Doṣha*	Signs of Excess
Respiratory (Vital Breath) *Prāṇavaha Srotas*	heart, colon; nose, trachea, lungs alimentary tract, plurae: Vāyu	hyperventilation
Digestive *Ānnavaha Srotas*	digestive/small intestine: Pitta	hyperacidity, diarrhea
Metabolism (water) *Udakavaha Srotas*	palate and pancreas: Kapha	hunger, hypoglycemia
Lymphatic/Plasma *Rasavaha Srotas*	heart and blood vessels: Kapha	edema, swollen glands, lymphatics
Circulatory/Blood (Hemoglobin) *Raktavaha Srotas*	liver and spleen: Pitta	hypertension, disorders of skin, spleen, or bleeding; abscesses, jaundice, inflammations
Muscular *Māṃsavaha Srotas*	ligaments and skin: Kapha	tremors
Fat/Adipose *Medavaha Srotas*	kidney and organ coverings: Kapha	edema, obesity
Skeletal *Asthivaha Srotas*	adipose tissue, hips: Vāyu	extra bone tissue
Marrow *Majjāvaha Srotas*	bones and joints: Vāyu	insomnia, pain, tremors, hypersensitivity, overly perceptive
Reproductive *Śhukravaha Srotas*	external genitals: Kapha	premature ejaculation, leukorrhea, spermatorrhea, nocternal emission
Sebaceous/Sweat *Swedavaha Srotas*	fat and hair follicles: Kapha	excessive oily sweat
Excretory *Purīṣhavaha Srotas*	rectum and colon: Vāyu	diarrhea
Urinary *Mūtravaha Srotas*	kidney and urinary bladder: Kapha	excess or frequent urination
Female Reproductive *Artavaha Srotas*	uterus (menstruation, hormones): Pitta	menorrhagia (excess menstruation)

From this chart we see that a Vāyu excess will create problems in the colon, rectum, skeleton, or nervous system. Pitta derangement occurs in the female reproductive, digestive, and circulatory systems. Kapha rules the remaining channels: metabolic, lymphatic, muscular, adipose, reproductive, sebaceous, and female reproductive subsystem (breast milk system). When these *srotas* are depleted, specific symptoms develop:

Systems (*Srotas*)	**Signs of Deficiency**
Vital Breath *Prāṇavaha*	breathing abnormalities (e.g., shortness of breath) with sound or pain
Digestion *Annavaha*	dry tongue, palate, lips, throat, pancreas, excessive thirst, low appetite
Water *Udakavaha*	loss of hunger, anorexia, indigestion, nausea, vomiting, hyperglycemia
Plasma *Rasavaha*	loss of hunger, anorexia, nausea, heaviness, drowsiness, fever and fainting, anemia, circulatory blocks, impotence, emaciation, poor digestion, early gray hair and wrinkles, dehydration
Hemoglobin *Raktavaha*	rough skin, fissures, cracks, loss of lustre, dryness, collapsed veins and areteries, desire for cold & sour things, anemia, digestive disorders, purpura
Muscle *Māṃsavaha*	vitiation of muscle tissue, inflamed uvula or cervix, tonsillitis, boils, goiter, inflamed epiglottis, hemorrhoids (dilated blood vessels in the anal region or rectal tumors of the mucous membranes), muscle tumors, granular tumors, peeling skin, muscle spasms, poor muscle tone
Fat *Medavaha*	incubatory signs and symptoms of urinary disorders including diabetes mellitus, matted hair, emaciation, dry skin
Bone *Asthivaha*	weak bones and teeth, deficient bone and tooth tissue; cracking sensation in teeth, bone pain, discoloration and loss of hair and nails, osteoporosis
Marrow *Majjāvaha*	joint pain, giddiness, fainting, joint abscesses, nerve numbness, Parkinson's (nerves not firing to muscles)
Reproductive *Śhukravaha*	impotency, sterility, or sick progeny
Feces *Purīṣhavaha*	constipation (may occur with pain and sound)
Urine *Mūtravaha*	scanty, difficult, or painful urination
Sweat *Swedavaha*	lack of or deficient sweat, rough skin, burning sensation, hair standing on end
Uterus *Artavaha*	scanty or delayed menses, hormone deficiencies
Breast Milk *Stanyavaha*	lack of breast milk

Channels (*Srotas*)	**Causes of *Srota* Vitiation**
Vital Breath *Prāṇavaha*	Suppressing natural urges, oils, when hungry, exercising
Water-Metabolism *Udakavaha*	heat, indigestion, alcohol, dry foods, excessive thirst
Digestion *Annavaha*	unwholesome/indigestible food
Plasma *Rasavaha*	excess heavy, cold, oily foods, over worry
Hemoglobin *Raktavaha*	hot, oily, irritating foods and drinks, sun and fire exposure
Muscle *Māṃsavaha*	heavy foods, sleeping right after meals
Fat *Medovaha*	no exercise, day naps, fatty food
Bone *Asthivaha*	exercise that irritates and rubs bones, Vāyu increasing foods
Marrow *Majjāvaha*	crushing, excess liquids, injury and compression of bone marrow, dry foods
Repro-ductive *Śhukravaha*	untimely intercourse, suppression of sexual urge, excessive sexual indulgence
Urine *Mūtravaha*	suppressing urine urge, eating, drinking, and intercourse when there is an urge to urinate
Feces; *Purīshavaha*	suppressing the urge to defecate, eating overly large meals, eating before digesting the last meal
Sweat/ Swedavaha	excess exercise, heat, anger, grief, fear, untimely eating of hot and cold things

Channels (*Srotas*)	**Symptoms of Blocks**	**Symptoms of Overflow**
Vital Breath *Prāṇavaha*	cough, asthma, hiatal hernia	perforated lungs
Water-Metabolism *Udakavaha*	diabetes, pancreatic cancer, dry tongue, palate, lips, and throat	anorexia, watery vomiting
Digestion *Annavaha*	tumors	vomiting, perforated stomach or intestines (i.e., ulcer)
Plasma *Rasavaha*	severe swollen glands, lymph obstruction, lymph cancer	bleeding with cough
Hemoglobin *Raktavaha*	arrhythmia, liver or spleen enlargement	bleeding
Muscle *Māṃsavaha*	chronic inflammations, muscle tumors	tearing of muscle tissue
Fat *Medovaha*	fat tumors (subcutaneous and usually benign), arteriosclerosis	tearing of adipose tissue
Bone *Asthivaha*	calcification, spurs, cancer	bones breaking
Marrow *Majjāvaha*	convulsions, coma, MS	damage
Repro-ductive *Śhukravaha*	impotentency, swollen testes, prostate stones, uterine tumors	sperm in bladder
Urine *Mūtravaha*	difficult or painful urination, obstructions or stones	bladder bursting
Feces; *Purīshavaha*	tumors, intestinal blocks, diverticulitis, constipation or scanty stool, pain, sound	colon perforation
Sweat/ Swedavaha	no sweating	sweat in plasma
Uterus *Artavaha*	pain, dysmenorrhea, amenorrhea, chlorosis, tumors	menses or urine in stool
Breast Milk *Stanyavaha*	No milk, pain, swelling, mastitis, cysts, tumors, cancer	breast injury

Using cross-referencing, by knowing a symptom, Āyurveda finds the imbalanced *srota*.

Srotas include, veins (*śhirā*), arteries (*dhamanī*), capillaries (*rasavahini*), ducts (*nāḍī*), passages (*pantha*), tracts (*marga*), spaces inside the body (*śharīrachidra*), ducts [open at one end and closed at the other] (*samvṛitāsamvṛita*), residence (*sthāna*), containers (*āśhaya*), and abodes (*niketa*). They are the visible and invisible areas in the body's tissue elements. Affliction of these *srotas* creates vitiation of the tissues that reside there or pass through them (i.e., vitiation of one, leads to depletion of the other). Vāyu and Kapha *doṣhas* cause vitiation of the *srotas* and tissue elements (*Charak Saṃhitā - Vimānasthāna* Ch. 5 verse 9).

The 13 Natural Urges

Āyurveda, we have already said, emphasizes gentle and natural methods. To highlight this, Āyurveda notes that certain bodily urges are natural and necessary for proper health and functioning of the mind, emotions, and body. The result of suppressing these natural urges creates serious health problems.

13 Natural Urges and the Results of Suppressing Them

1. Sleep: Insomnia, fatigue, headache, deranges the vital force.

2. Cry: Eye disease, allergies, light-headedness, heart disease (suppressed emotions).

3. Sneeze: Headache, facial nerve pain, numbness, weak senses, lung disorders, respiratory allergies.

4. Breathe: Coughing, asthma, shallow breath, low vitality, heart disease.

5. Belch: Cough, hiccups, anorexia, difficult breathing, palpitations.

6. Yawn: Tremors, numbness, convulsions, insomnia, harms nervous system, deranges Vāyu.

7. Vomit: Nausea, anorexia, edema, anemia, fever, skin diseases, damages Kapha.

8. Eat: Low appetite and digestion, malabsorption, light-headedness, deranges the whole body and mind, suppresses the *agni* fire and Pitta.

9. Drink: Dryness, deafness, fatigue, heart pain, bladder pain, lower backache, headache, damages Kapha and Vāyu.

10. Urinate: Kidney and urinary system derangement, difficult or painful urination, bladder pain, lower backache, headache, deranges Vāyu and Kapha.

11. Ejaculate: Weakens the reproductive and urinary systems, penis and testes pain, swollen prostate, difficult urination, cardiac pain, insomnia, malaise, Vāyu derangement.

12. Defecate: Weakens the colon, excretory and digestive *srotas*, causes constipation, abdominal weakness, abdominal distention, headaches, muscle cramps, deranges Vāyu.

13. Flatulate: Causes constipation, difficult urination, abdominal pain, distention, weakens Vāyu, air wastes are absorbed into the bones and marrow, aggravating arthritis and nerves.

It is for these reasons that Āyurveda advises that people follow nature's call, living naturally and gently, without straining or forcing.

Four Disease Conditions

All diseases are said to fall into one of four categories: those that are easily healed, those that are difficult to heal, those that are controllable but cannot be healed, and those that cannot be healed. Each form of disease has specific features.

Easily Healed: People able to receive all therapies, adults, self-controlled persons, not having the vital organs affected, having mild or few causes, or are currently in the first three of the six stages of development (see second section following this). Other indications include no secondary complications or diseases; or the disease is different from the *doṣha*, *dhātu*, region, season and constitution. Further signs include, favorable planetary influence, having a proper practitioner and therapy, or disease arising from only one *doṣha*. Other signs include diseases that manifest themselves in only one disease pathway (i.e., inner, outer, central), or those that have recently begun to develop.

Difficult But Able to be Healed: Diseases requiring surgery, dual *doṣha* illness, or tridoṣhic illness (some believe tridoṣha belongs in the next category).

Controllable But Not Able to be Healed: Illness remaining throughout life, which have symptoms of easily healed description, are controllable through using appropriate foods, herbs, nutrition, and lifestyle regimens.

Unable to be Healed: Symptoms that are the opposite of diseases that can be healed (described above), long lasting (and involving all seven *dhātus* and important vital organs), causing anxiety, delusion and restlessness, showing fatal signs, and causing loss of sensory organs.

Requirements of the Practitioner & Patient

Practitioners are required to have both proper education and experience learned from a qualified teacher, to be ethical and virtuous, and to follow their own Āyurvedic lifestyle and spirituality—in actions, words, and thoughts.

Patients should want to be healed, and should be able and willing to take responsibility to heal themselves or to be open to the therapies administered.

The practitioner should be honest and tell patients when they are unable to suggest healing measures, and recognize a patient who does not really want to be healed. The practitioner is not advised to attempt healing persons who cannot be healed. They will gain a reputation as an unscrupulous pretenders, just out to make money.

Effects on Doṣhas:
Time, Geography and Age

The environment also plays a role in the balance of the *doṣhas*. Each humor has certain times of the day when it is predominant. It is sometimes necessary to avoid imbalancing one's *doṣha* by considering these effects.

Prevailing *Doṣha* times of the Day		
Kapha	7-9 A.M.	7-9 P.M.
Kapha/Pitta.	9-11 A.M.	9-11 P.M.
Pitta	11 A.M.-3 P.M.	11 PM-3 AM
Vāyu	3-5 P.M.	3-5 A.M.
Vāyu/Kapha	5-7 P.M.	5-7 A.M.

Thus, a Pitta *doṣha* person would not be advised to spend much time in the sun between 11:00 and 3:00 P.M. They should avoid working at this time as well, since they will be more susceptible to overheating their systems during this time of day.

Geography

Geography affects a person in the same manner as the seasons. Hotter climates will aggravate Pitta *doṣhas*. Cold and damp northwest regions will bother the Kapha person. Dry and cold climates will aggravate the Vāyu *doṣha*. Consider this example of geographical therapy: If a person has a Kapha condition, he or she may be advised to visit the mountains or desert where it is drier. This climate causes the person to heal properly and quickly. (See Chapter 12 for a detailed discussion of seasons).

Age

Although a person's *doṣha* generally does not change during their life, five stages need to be considered due to age.

The 5 *Doṣha* Stages of Life

Age	Main *Doṣha*
Birth-15 years	Kapha
15-27 years	Kapha/Pitta
27-42 years	Pitta
42-56 years	Pitta/Vāyu
56+ years	Vāyu

Generally, we see a tendency for children to get colds and congestion, a Kapha condition, whatever their *doṣha*. During a person's mid-years, more Pitta illness occurs. In the later years, we see Vāyu attacking the bones and memory of the elderly. Simply by considering age factors, a person can stay healthy and balanced, avoiding the problems that come with age.

Humor-Imbalancing Priorities

We have discussed the situations that imbalance the humors: internal (foods, mind, emotions, and body) and external (i.e., environmental and the lifestyle). When two of these factors simultaneously affect an individual, one component will have more of an effect on one's *doṣha* than the other.

1. Constitution outweighs environment

If the constitution is kept balanced, environmental factors will not aggravate a condition. For example, if children maintain a balanced constitution, they will be less susceptible to Kapha-type colds and flu in the winter. Environmental factors include spiritual (*karmic*) situations such as past life influences.

2. Lifestyle outweighs environment

Following a lifestyle that balances their *doṣha* protects people from environmental aggravations (i.e., cold weather will not seriously affect Vāyu persons if they take measures to keep warm).

3. Internal intake (of foods and drinks) outweighs external exposure

Seasonal temperatures cannot cause any imbalance if a person eats herbs and foods that balance one's *doṣha*.

4. Mind and emotions outweigh physical factors

A calm, peaceful mind and cheerful disposition will keep away physical imbalances. (Worry will cause physical illness. A clear, calm mind will prevent bodily disease).

5. Degree of factors is most significant

An excess of any one cause of an imbalance will create an illness. Too hot a summer day, too much worry, too much junk food, etc., will override any other balancing measures.

6. Combinations of factors outweigh individuals

Two or more agents acting on a person, will be more problematic than just one component.

Three Desires

Intelligent persons are advised to pursue good health, wealth, and Self-Realization. Health is the basis of life, so living a healthy lifestyle (i.e., wholesome diet and lifestyle, and adequate rest,) is essential. Living a long life without adequate financial resources is sure to promote troubles. The goal of life, according to Āyurvedic precepts, is Self-Realization. By living a healthy life and not being troubled by financial matters, persons have the time to focus on the prime goal of life. Thus Āyurveda suggests people live lives of charity, compassion, nonviolence, celibacy, devotion to Divinity and *sādhanā* (meditation) or prayer (see the discussion on *Yama* and *Niyama* in Chapter 13). These measures help to develop one's Self-Realization. By ignoring these principles, people are forced to be reborn repeatedly until they follow these measures and gain Self-Realization.

Management of the Doṣhas

Vāyu is reduced through heat and moistness.

Pitta is reduced through leisure and cold.

Kapha is reduced through heat, dry, and lightness.

Vāyu (*Apān* Vāyu) gathers and becomes excessive while food is in the large intestine (originating site). Western medicine has a parallel view. Carbohydrates become fermented and proteins become putrefied. This produces gas in the colon. Vāyu is alleviated when food is in the stomach. This is why it is suggested that Vāyu individuals have a meal every 3-4 hours. In this way, putting food in the stomach reduces the Vāyu accumulated since the last meal. Because the colon is the organ that is the main site of Vāyu and mostly affects air, Āyurveda recommends enemas (*bastis*) to cleanse the excess Vāyu from the colon.

Pitta gathers and becomes excessive when food is in the duodenum and small intestine (originating site). It is reduced when the food reaches the colon. Thus, an excess of Pitta may create heartburn about two hours after meals. Because the small intestine is the main site of Pitta, purgation (*virechana*) is recommended. From the western point of view, the Pitta (*Pachak* Pitta) is parallel to the digestive enzymes secreted by the pancreas, liver, etc. that are active in the duodenum and small intestine.

Kapha gathers and becomes excessive in the stomach just after eating (*Kledaka* Kapha). Kapha moistens the food and passes it on to the small intestine for the action of Pitta. It is the sluggishness of Kapha that causes one to feel sleepy after eating a meal. If an excess of Kapha develops, one may feel nauseous or want to vomit just after eating. Kapha is relieved when food is in the small intestine. The parallels to Kapha in western medicine are mucoid secretions and saliva. When food is eaten, secretions from the mucus membranes (in the intestines) moisten the food. These secretions from the lungs rise into the trachea (from the ciliary action) and move to the throat. Then the secretions are swallowed and move down the esophagus and finally, into the stomach. Āyurveda calls these excess secretions water, or Kapha.

In Western medicine expectorants are used to remove the excess secretions. These expectorants have minor emetic properties. In large doses, these expectorants cause vomiting (emesis). Likewise, Kapha *doṣha* is balanced by *vaman* (emesis). [See diagram below]

The Path of Food Moistening Secretions

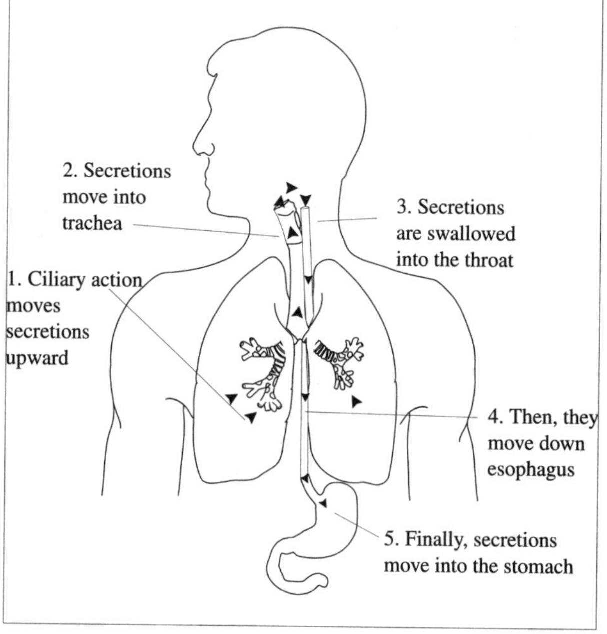
2. Secretions move into trachea
3. Secretions are swallowed into the throat
1. Ciliary action moves secretions upward
4. Then, they move down esophagus
5. Finally, secretions move into the stomach

Underlying Causes of Health: Agni, Āma and Ojas

The main cause of illness is a poor digestive system. If the digestive fire (*agni*) does not burn strongly enough, foods do not get digested. If food is not digested, nutrients cannot be absorbed. When foods do not get digested, they sit and accumulate in the colon, becoming a breeding ground for yeast infections, toxins, gas, and constipation. Undigested foods are called *āma*. *Āma* is the root cause of most problems in the body, resulting from excess Vāyu or Kapha (or both). If the *agni* burns too much, heat and acid build up in the system, creating Pitta problems.

Digestion begins in the mouth and stomach as

saliva acts upon the food to digests it. The food is moved from the mouth to the stomach (*āmāṣhaya*) by *Prāṇa* Vāyu. Once in the stomach the food takes on a predominantly sweet (*madhura*) taste. Food mixes with the digestive enzymes (*Pāchaka* Pitta). *Samāna* Vāyu moves the food to the duodenum (*grahanī*) where digestion continues due to the digestive fire or *agni* (*koṣṭhāgni*), assuming a pungent taste. The liver and pancreas are involved in the digestive process. Finally, the large intestine (Vāyu) absorbs the air and ether elements. Here, undigested foods become feces, and water is absorbed, transferred, and eliminated through the urine.

Properly digested food creates nutritional essence, chyle, or plasma (*rasa*). Improperly digested food becomes undigested food toxins (*āma*) that are the cause of most diseases.

Earth foods build protein bulk, such as muscles. Watery foods build vital fluids and fat. Fiery foods build enzymes and hemoglobin. Air foods build bone and nerve plexuses, and ether foods build the mind.

The health of the immune system determines whether diseases are warded off. Āyurveda notes that there is a sap-like material called *ojas* (perhaps analogous to pineal gland secretion) that coats the immune system and protects it from disease. If the *agni* fire is too low or too high, this life sap will be diminished. Just like the tree that creates a sap over the bruise in the bark to protect and heal the bruise, our life sap (*ojas*) protects and heals us from illness.

Too much dryness or too much heat and fire eats away the life sap. A weak immune system is the cause of all illness, from colds to multiple sclerosis to AIDS. To heal the immune system, one needs adequate rest and pure (*sattwic*) foods and herbs that specifically rebuild the *ojas* (life sap). Examples include blanched almonds or tahini, and *ojas* building herbs like *śhatāvarī* and *aśhwagandhā*, respectively.

Summary

So, we have seen that by knowing the constitution and elemental cause of one's illness (*vikṛiti*), by knowing which tissue layers (*dhātus*), systems, and organs are governed by which *doṣha*, and by knowing how to balance the *agni* fire and build the *ojas*, Āyurveda offers an individualized, simple, gentle, and effective form of healing.

All diseases can be caused by any of the humors, depending on which sites they relocate to, so the patient is examined completely, using all possible methods. Since disease development (pathogenesis) is the same for all *doṣhas*, only the humors, stages, sites, and directional movement of the humors are examined. Humors have to return to their origin sites to be eliminated.

Āyurveda emphasizes promoting health, preventing disease, and enhancing longevity (rejuvenation or age reversal). By using *rasāyana*- (rejuvenation) promoting herbs and diet, good conduct, daily routine, and seasonal living longevity is developed.

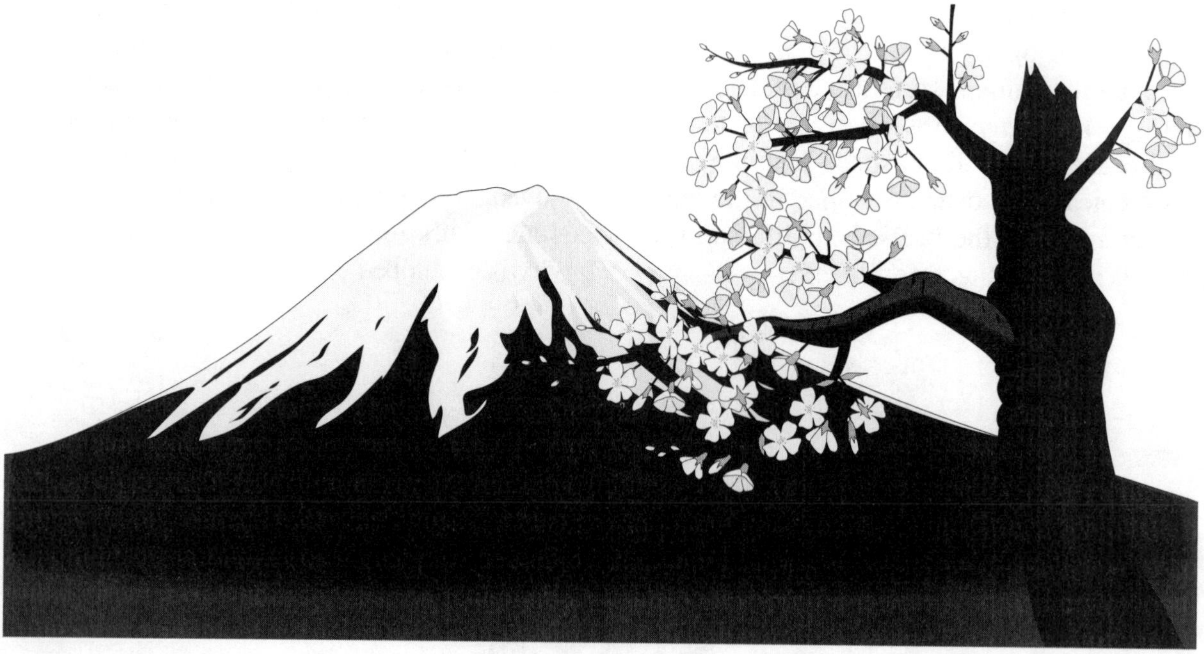

Section 2

Āyurvedic Analysis

आयुर्वेद निदानस्थान

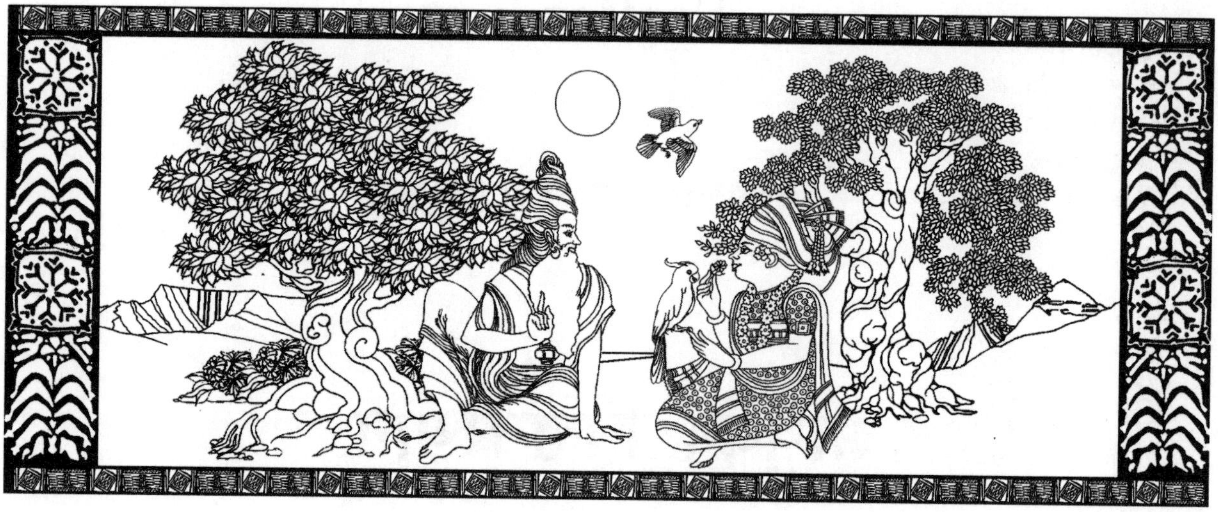

The physician should examine the disease first,
then the drug and finally the management.
They should always proceed
with prior knowledge.
Charak Saṃhitā

Chapter 3
Analyzing
Constitutions and Diseases

Overview

Ayurveda, according to *Charak Saṃhitā,* was a scientific and logical interpretation, in which tridoṣha theory was enumerated along with management of Vāyu, Pitta, and Kapha. Nature was seen as uniform, and rational knowledge was emphasized over the supernatural. Symposia were held for practitioners to express opinions and to arrive at an accepted view of truth. Lord *Ātreya* presided over the talks.

Rather than analyze and name millions of body parts and diseases, *Charak Saṃhitā* holds that it is happiness and unhappiness that result in health and disease respectively. The healthy or holistic person is termed *Puruṣha,* or eternal Divinity. The causes of illness are *deha-manasa,* or psychosomatic reasons; mind affects body and body affects mind. Thus, the 'partial' view has no place and *Sattwavajaya,* or holistic psychotherapy, has its origins in the Āyurvedic science. Āyurveda then, is seen as a highly accurate and personalized method of analyzing people's constitutions and illnesses; it recommends and provides gentle, natural and effective therapies.

Āyurveda relies totally on nature to heal, while Āyurvedic therapies only help in the healing process. *Swabhavoparama* (recession by nature) is the method of using herbs, diet, lifestyle, and other therapies (discussed in the next section) to return the mind and body back to its natural state of balance.

The nature of an illness is learned through five methods.

1. Cause (*nidāna)*
2. Premonitory or incubatory signs (*pūrvarupa*)
3. Signs and symptoms (*rupa*)
4. Diagnostic tests (*upaṣhaya*)
5. Pathology or stages of manifestation (*samprapti*)

1. *Nidāna* or etiology (cause)—All diseases are caused by the aggravation of the *doṣhas*.

2. *Pūrvarupa* (hidden or incubatory signs)—Signs and symptoms cannot be attributed to any specific *doṣha* due to their mild nature. Two forms exist;

a) Symptoms may occur due to one or more of the aggravated *doṣhas* and disappear when the disease manifests, or

b) Symptoms that develop into the specific disease.

3. *Rupa* (signs and symptoms)—Manifestations of the disease are clearly observed.

4. *Upaṣhaya* (diagnostic tests)—When practitioners cannot determine the cause of the illness through the other methods they test with herbs, food, or habits. These therapies show whether they heal or aggravate the illness.

5. *Samprapti* or pathogenesis (disease development)—Not merely symptoms or signs, this is the actual manifestation of disease. Five kinds of development exist:

a) The varieties of a disease.

b) The different aspects of the *doṣhas* causing the illness.

c) Whether a disease is of primary or secondary nature.

d) The severity of the illness, strong or weak (e.g., due to age, general health, etc.).

e) Time of digestion, day, or season when the *doṣha* is predominant.

Etiology: Cause of All Disease

All diseases are caused by aggravation of the *doṣhas*. This aggravation of different *doṣhas* is caused by the intake of improper diet and the leading of an improper lifestyle (*Mithya Āhar Vihar*). The three causes of illness are excessive, insufficient, or improper use of,

1. The senses
2. Actions
3. Seasonal factors

1. Unsuitable use of the senses: Unwholesome contact of the senses (taste, touch, sight, sound, and smell) with objects. For example, sound (hearing loud voices, noise pollution cause serious mind and health problems). Touch (contact of the skin with chemicals, hot objects, or overly cold objects). Sight (exposure to too much light, such as staring at the sun).

2. Actions: Relate to body, speech, and mind. These include, conduct, urge, posture, concern, and emotions. Thoughts and decisions leading to harmful or unhealthy situations are said to be errors of the intellect. Spiritually speaking, the first intellectual error is to believe that anyone or anything is separate from oneself. The Āyurvedic texts say that this is the first cause of all diseases, the loss of faith in the Divine.

3. Seasonal factors: Vāyu accumulates during the dry or dehydrating heat of the summer (*Grīṣhma*: mid-May to mid-July). It becomes aggravated during the rainy season (*Varṣha*: mid-July to mid-September), which causes weakened digestion, acidic atmospheric conditions, and gas produced from the earth.

Pitta accumulates during the rainy season due to the acidic conditions of the atmosphere and a weakened digestion. It is aggravated during autumn (*Śharat*: mid-September to mid-November) when the heat returns (perhaps equivalent to Indian Summer). This occurs after the cooling spell of the rainy season.

Kapha accumulates during the cold season (*Śhiśhira*: mid-January to mid-March) due to the cold and damp caused by the winds, clouds, and rain. It gets aggravated during the spring (*Vasant*: mid-March to mid-May) when the warm weather liquefies the accumulating Kapha (from the cold season).

Seasonal Increases of the Doṣhas

Doṣha	Accumulate	Aggravate	Normalize
Vāyu	Summer/ *Grīṣhma*	Rainy/ *Varṣhā*	Autumn/ *Śharat*
	mid-May - mid-July	mid-July - mid-Sept.	mid-Sept.- mid-Nov.
	heat is dry, dehydrating	weak digestion, acidic rain, earth gas	sun and warmth
Pitta	Rainy/ *Varṣhā*	Autumn/ *Śharat*	Winter/ *Hemanta*
	mid-July - mid-Sept.	mid-Sept.- mid-Nov.	mid-Nov. - mid-Jan.
	weak digestion, acidic rain	sun and heat returns	cold, moist
Kapha	Cold/ *Śhirśha*	Spring/ *Vasant*	Summer/ *Grīṣhma*
	mid-Jan. - mid-March	mid-March - mid-May	mid-May - mid-July
	cold, damp	warmth, liquefies	warm, dry

Vāyu Increasing Causes: Bitter, salty, and astringent tastes, dry, light, cold foods, fasting, waiting longer than three or four hours between meals, suppression or premature initiation of the 13 natural urges, staying awake late at night, prolonged high pitched speaking, excess emesis and purgation, sudden grief, fear, worry, or anxiety; excessive exercise or sexual intercourse; the end of the digestive process.

Pitta Increasing Causes: Pungent, sour, and salty tastes, foods causing heat and burning sensations, anger, autumn, the middle of digestion, sun or heat exposure, exhaustion, eating with indigestion.

Kapha Increasing Causes: Sweet, sour, and salty tastes, oils, heavy or indigestible foods, overeating, cold foods, lack of exercise, excess sleeping, naps, inadequate emesis and purgation, eating before hungry, in the spring, before noon and early night, the first stage of digestion.

Factors Increasing All *Doṣhas*: Eating excessively, improper diet, uncooked, contaminated or incompatible foods; spoiled food and drinks; dried vegetables, raw root vegetables. Other factors include eating fried sesame seeds and molasses, mud, barley beer, foul and dry meat, eating food out of season; direct breeze, negative thoughts, living in mountain slopes. Malefic positioning of the planets and constellations, improper administration of therapies, illegal actions, and being too inactive also increase all the *doṣhas*.

Food Intake and Doṣha Illness

Improper quantity of food results in impairing strength, complexion, weight, distention, longevity, virility, and *ojas*. It afflicts the body, mind, intellect, and senses, causing harm to the *dhātus* (tissues)—especially Vāyu. Food taken in excess aggravates all three *doṣhas*. Obstructions are produced in the stomach and move through the upper and lower tracts, producing diseases according to one's *doṣha*.

Vāyu: Colic pain, constipation, malaise, dry mouth, fainting, giddiness, irregular digestive power, rigidity, hardening and contracting of vessels.

Pitta: Fever, diarrhea, internal burning sensation, thirst, intoxication, giddiness, and delirium.

Kapha: Vomiting, anorexia, indigestion, cold fever, laziness, and heaviness.

Disease Development: Six Stages

Earlier, it was briefly mentioned that six stages of disease development exist. However, modern medical technology can only see the last two stages of any illness. Āyurveda offers insight into the earlier stages and enables those monitoring their health to take care of any small imbalances well before developing any serious illness. The six stages of disease development are:

1. Accumulation: Illness begins in one of the three main *doṣha* sites: stomach (Kapha), small intestine (Pitta), or the colon (Vāyu). Excess Kapha in the stomach creates a blockage in the system that leads to lassitude, heaviness, pallor, bloating, and indigestion. Pitta accumulation creates burning sensations, fever, hyperacidity, bitter taste in the mouth, and anger. The collecting of Vāyu creates gas, distention, constipation, dryness, fear, fatigue, insomnia, and the desire for warm things.

The value of monitoring these experiences within one's body and mind leads to the earliest detection of an imbalance, while it is still in its hidden or incubatory stages.

2. Aggravation: As the imbalanced elements (humors) continue to increase, the symptoms mentioned above become more aggravated and will be noticed in other parts of the body as well. Kapha aggravation causes a loss of appetite, indigestion, nausea, excess saliva, heaviness in the heart and head, and oversleeping. The aggravated Pitta experience is one of increased acidity, burning sensations in the abdomen, lowered vitality, or insomnia. Vāyu aggravation results in pain and spasm in the abdomen, gas and rum-

bling in the bowels, and light-headedness.

3. Overflow: Once the origin site is full with the excess humor (element), it will begin to overflow into the rest of the body using different channels of transportation. The *doṣhas* begin to overflow into the GI tract, then join with the circulating plasma and blood. During circulation the humors then begin to seep into the organs, *dhātus* (tissues), and *malas* (waste). Simultaneously, symptoms at the origin site continue to grow worse.

4. Moving and localization at a distant site: The humors will move to wherever a weak site exists in the body. This is where and when specific diseases begin to develop. For example, a Vāyu illness could move to the bones and begin to create arthritis. If the duodenum is weak, humors deposit themselves there and create an ulcer (usually a Pitta condition). Kapha moves to organs like the lungs when weakened. Healing is still simple, even at this fourth stage of illness.

5. Manifestation: This is the first stage of the development of illness for which Western science can detect signs of disease. Here, diseases become fully developed, showing signs of clinical features. Names are given to imbalances of the humors, such as cancer, bronchitis, arthritis, etc.

6. Distinction/Chronic Complications: In this last stage, the symptoms become clear enough so that the elemental cause may be determined. For example, Vāyu asthma will cause dry skin, constipation, anxiety, attacks at dawn, and the desiring of warmth. Pitta asthma will show yellow phlegm, fever, sweating, and attacks at noon and midnight. Asthma brought on by Kapha will create white phlegm, water in the lungs, and attacks during the morning and evening.

Some practitioners describe this stage as the chronic phase of development. For example, if one develops an inflammation or abscess in stage five, in stage six, complications set in, and the abscess may burst and become a chronic ulcer.

Three Disease Pathways

In our consideration of the Āyurvedic view of the body, we also learn of the classification of illness and the healing process through the three paths that disease travels.

Inner: This is the digestive tract involving diseases of the GI tract. These diseases are easy to heal because toxins are expelled through the tract. Diseases of the inner path include fever, cough, hiccups, enlarged abdomen or spleen, internal edema, vomiting, and hard stools.

Outer: This path refers to the plasma/skin, blood, and superficial tissues. Toxic blood and skin diseases are harder to heal because removing an illness from the tissue is more difficult. Symptoms include abdominal and other malignant tumors, edema, and hemorrhoids.

Central: This path refers to muscle, fat, bone, marrow, and deeper nerve tissues. This is the most delicate area of the body, affecting the heart, head, bone joints, and urinary bladder. The most difficult diseases develop here, such as cancer or arthritis. These diseases develop between the inner and outer paths.

Signs and Symptoms of Disease, by Doṣha

Excess Vāyu: Drooping, dilation, loss of sensation, and weakness; continuous, cutting, pricking, crushing, or splitting pain; obstruction, contraction, or constriction; twisting, tingling, thirst, tremors, roughness, dryness, throbbing, curvatures, gas, winding, stiffness, or rigidity; astringent taste in mouth, blue/crimson discoloration, partial vacuums in bodily liquids.

Excess Pitta: Burning sensation, reddish discoloration, heat, high digestive fire, pus, ulcers, perspiration, moistness, debility, fainting, toxicity, bitter and sour tastes in the mouth, oozing, fungus.

Excess Kapha: Oiliness, hardness, itching irritations, cold, heaviness, obstructions, toxic or mucus coatings inside the *srotas* (channels), loss of movement, swelling, edema, indigestion, excessive sleep, whitish complexion, sweet and salty tastes in the mouth.

Three Kinds of Diseases

All diseases arise from bad actions occurring in one's

1. Present life (finding a specific cause of the illness). These are healed with therapies of the opposite nature.

2. Past lives (no apparent cause for an illness). These are healed after the action has worked itself out.

3. A combination of both (diseases that suddenly manifest as terrible, profound and severe). These require a combination of therapies and the cessation of harmful activities.

Diseases are either primary (initial symptoms) or secondary (complications arising later). If the secondary complications of the *doṣhas* do not subside when the primary causes are healed, additional therapies must be administered.

Analysis of Factors

For healing to occur, the practitioner carefully studies and decides the condition of the vitiated tissues (*dhātus*) and wastes (*malas*), patient's habitat, strength, and digestive power. He needs to learn the constitution, age, mind, lifestyle, diet, the stage of the disease, and the season, before recommending the appropriate therapy. (Symptoms may appear mild or severe, depending upon the patient's total strength (mental and physical). Thus, the practitioner needs to make a careful and complete analysis).

After determining individual body type and the elemental cause and development of illness, the next step is to analyze the patient's constitution and illness (*prakṛiti* and *vikṛiti* respectively).

The Doṣhas - Deciding the Cause of Disease: General Approach

The practitioner has several methods of learning the *prakṛiti* (constitution) and the *vikṛiti* (illness) of patients:

1. Authoritative Instruction
2. Direct Observation
3. Inference

1. Authoritative Instruction comes from a teacher who has had much experience in determining the cause and nature of constitutions and illness.

2. Observation includes visual analysis of the face, finger nails, eyes, tongue, urine, stool, complexion, and shape; it also includes auditory observations of the tone of voice, listening for intestinal gurgling, cracking sounds of bones and fingers, coughing or hiccups, as well as by palpation, most notably the evaluation of the pulse. By noticing certain characteristics, the practitioner begins to learn the *doṣha* or *prakṛiti* (constitution), and the *doṣha* imbalance that may be causing the illness (*vikṛiti*).

Āyurvedic observation is a threefold approach: questioning, observing, and palpating (touch). To gain information that is not readily observable, the practitioner addresses questions directly to the patient and also asks the patient to complete a questionnaire or self-test (see appendix 2).

Discussion with the patient helps reveal the *prakṛiti* and *vikṛiti*. Discussing one's family and personal health history, and learning of the patient's symptoms round out the consultation.

Questionnaires are self-tests which ask a series of mental and physical questions that help the practitioner decide a person's mental and physical *doṣha* and illness.

3. Inference Through reasoning the practitioner gains indirect knowledge about the state of various health conditions. The situations learned through inference are summarized in the follow-

ing table:

Patient Knowledge Through Inference

Condition	Inferred From
agni (digestive fire)	digestive power
strength	exercise capacity
sensory abilities	capacity to correctly perceive
mental abilities	understands instructions
mental *guṇa (sattwa, rajas, tamas)*	expression (e.g., gentle, harsh, angry)
anger	revengeful
grief	sorrowful
fear	apprehension
joy	happy mood
pleasure	satisfied face & eyes
courage	resolute mind
mental stability	expressing balance, lack of mistakes
desire	amount of requests the patient makes
intelligence	comprehension of spiritual discussion
deception	subsequent actions

Only after a careful analysis of all three areas—that is, considering the cumulative information,—does a practitioner determine the *prakṛiti* (constitution) and *vikṛiti* (illness). The practitioner would not make quick judgments based on only one or two signs. Often people have characteristics of all three *doṣhas,* so the practitioner finds the one or two *doṣhas* that predominate. Sometimes a patient is tridoṣhic, or having equal parts of all three *doṣhas*. [It is not important what *doṣha* a person is (i.e., there is no preferred constitution). What is important is that one's constitution is balanced.]

By observing, listening, and questioning, the practitioner learns of one's constitution and illness. Below are general guidelines that show which *doṣha* is in excess. Sometimes the patient may use words like "dry," "hot," or "lazy," which alerts the practitioner to the *doṣha* being deranged.

Observation

Face: The face offers various clues to help the practitioner determine the disorder. A thin facial structure is an indication of a Vāyu *prakṛiti*. A wide structure is more of a Kapha constitution. Strong muscular, or moderate facial structure suggests Pitta *doṣha*.

The picture of a face (below) shows which organs may be imbalanced or diseased.

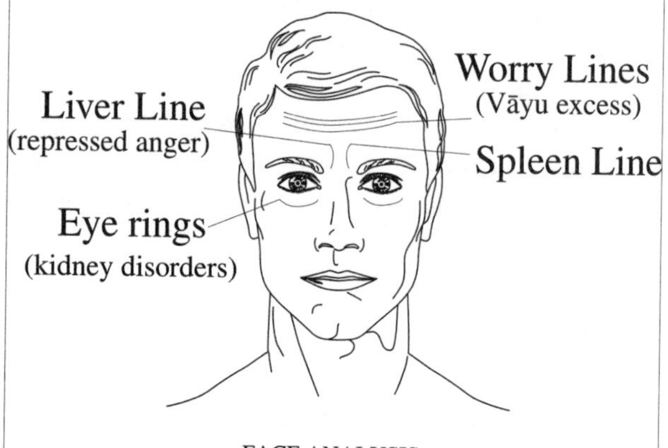

FACE ANALYSIS

Mouth: Vāyu excess—foul and smelly, Pitta excess—bitter, Kapha excess —sweet, Tridoṣhic excess—all symptoms.

Tongue: The tongue also offers many signs about health. Its size, shape, and coating help the practitioner decide the humor causing the illness.

Coating: Suggests *āma* or toxin in the system. When only a little coating is on the tongue, the person is generally healthy. A thick, white coating indicates *āma* (Kapha). Thick, greasy, yellow, or inflamed tongues suggest *āma* fermentation (Pitta).

If a coating is on the front third of the tongue, this indicates Kapha toxins (*āma*), the middle third shows Pitta *āma,* and the back third suggests Vāyu *āma.* Should the coating be on two thirds of the tongue, or on the entire tongue, then there is a dual *doṣha* or tridosha *āma* excess.

Color: A blackish brown color shows Vāyu disorders. Yellow, green or reddish suggests Pitta problems in the liver or gall bladder. Kapha problems are revealed by a whitish color. Blue may suggest heart problems, blue or purple would indicate stagnation or liver disorders. Vāyu problems yield a dull or pale color. Kapha conditions are pale colored.

Size: Vāyu *doṣhas* have a small, long, thin, or trembling tongue. Pitta *doṣhas* have a medium tongue with a sharp tip. Kapha people have large, thick, round tongues with thick lips.

Marks:Teeth-like marks around the front arc/edge of the tongue means that nutrients are not being absorbed.

A line down the middle of the tongue suggests immune problems. Cracks in the tongue shows Vāyu imbalances.

By brushing or scraping the tongue with a toothbrush or spoon, excess mucus is removed. This process releases repressed emotions as well. Below is a diagram of a tongue, with the corresponding areas from which organ health can be detected.

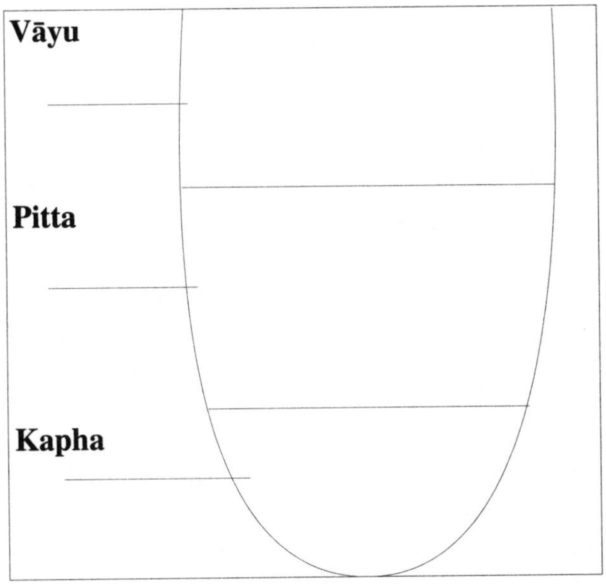

The diagram below shows where on the tongue the *doṣhas* are reflected.

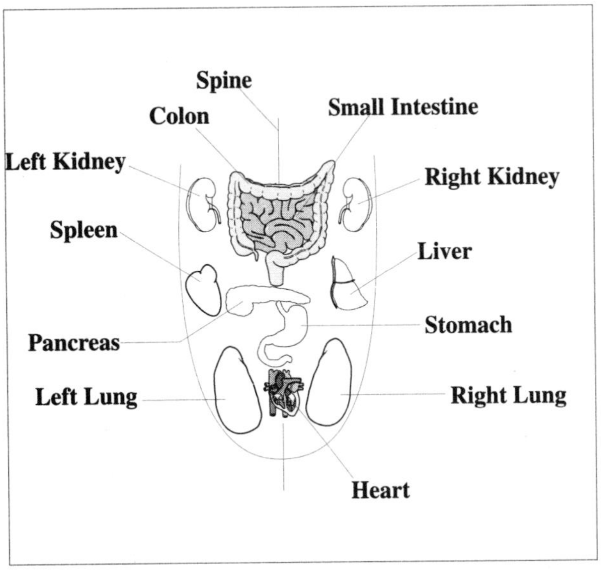

ORGANS AND THE TONGUE

<u>Eyes</u>: The eyes also help show an individual's *doṣha*. Generally, Vāyu eyes are small and unsteady. Pitta eyes are sharp and piercing, and reddish or bloodshot. Large, wide and white eyes suggest Kapha *doṣha*. Healthy eyes are serene, cheerful, and beautiful.

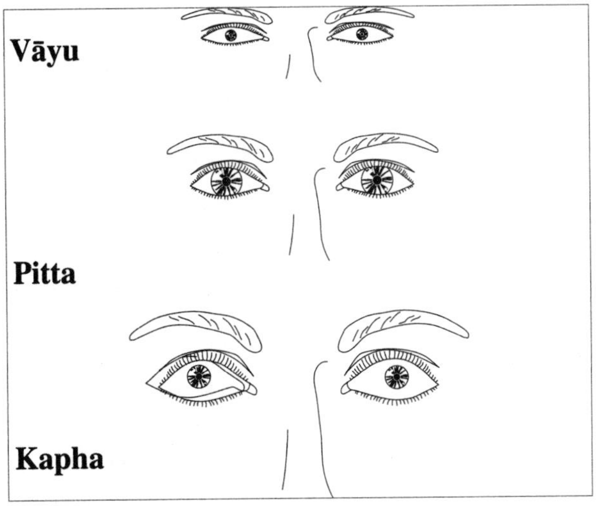

<u>Nails</u>: The nails also help reveal one's *doṣha* and illness. Vāyu nails are thin, brittle, and cracking.

Biting the nails shows Vāyu nervousness. Lines in the nail show malabsorption. Pitta nails are medium in size and pinkish in color. Wide, strong, white colored nails suggest Kapha *doṣha*.

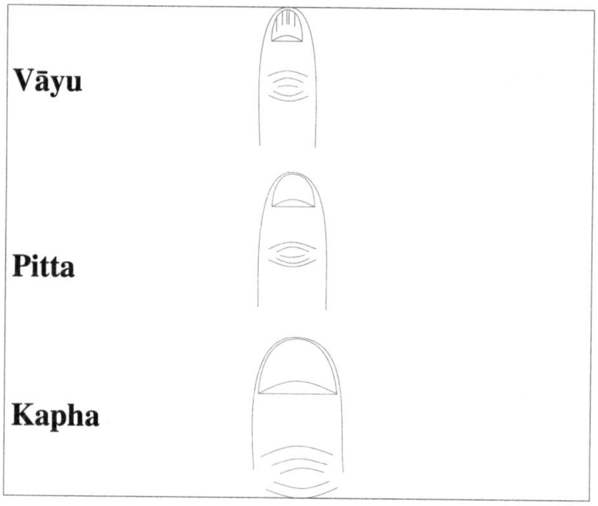

Small white spots on the nails, reveal calcium or zinc deficiencies, or calcium deposits in certain organs. Spots on the ring finger suggest calcium deposit in the kidney. If the spots are on the middle finger nail the deposit is in the small intestine. When spots are on the index finger, the deposits are in the lungs. See the diagram below.

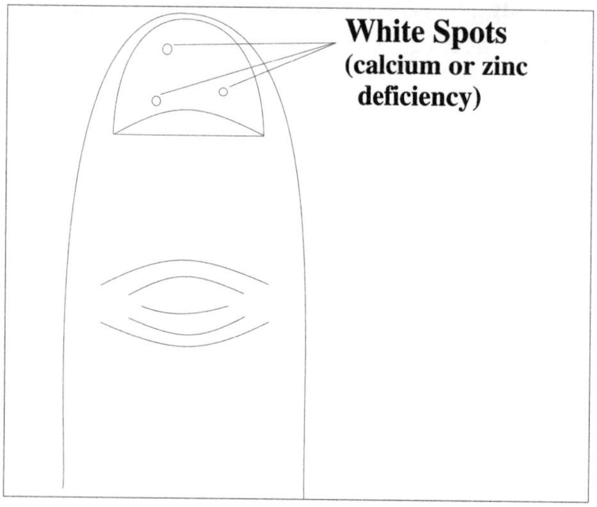

Lips: Thin, dry, or cracked lips are signs of Vāyu excesses. Medium sized lips reveal a Pitta *doṣha*. Wide, thick lips suggest a Kapha *doṣha*.
Voice: Deep tonal voices are characteristic of Kaphas. A moderate speaker, with a tendency towards arguing, suggests a Pitta person. A person with a low, weak voice indicates a Vāyu individual.

Pulse Analysis

A healthy pulse is thick and strong
A sick pulse is thick and dull, or sluggish
- Nāḍīprakasam: Ch. 2 verse 4

Pulse Analysis: This is a science in itself. Although it takes many years to become proficient in this practice, pulse reading offers many insights, including *doṣha* knowledge, general health, and organ health. Since pulse reading requires much skill, one may decide the *prakṝiti* (constitution) and *vikṛiti* (illness) without even using pulse analysis.

Two Āyurvedic texts deal exclusively with the intricacies of pulse analysis: *Nāḍīvijñānam* (meaning the science or knowledge of pulse diagnosis), by *Māhāriṣhi Kanada* (circa 7th century B.C.), and *Nāḍīprakaṣham* by *Śhaṅkar Sen* (19th-20th Century AD). The basic belief is that the pulse reveals different qualities, rates, and temperatures, and appears stronger in different positions for each *doṣha*.

Pulse analysis takes a long time to master, and many factors may cause inaccurate readings, so it is advised not to take pulses under certain conditions.

Time of Taking Pulse: The pulse is read or analyzed when the patient and practitioner are at rest. *Nāḍīprakaṣham* suggests taking the pulse in the morning, when the pulse is cool (afternoon pulse is hot; evening pulse is fast). The ideal constitution (*doṣha*) pulse is read upon waking in the morning (before 10:00 a.m.), after expelling stool and urine, and before eating.

Constitution Pulse: 6:00-10:00 a.m.
Illness (Imbalance) Pulse: 10:00 a.m. on.

Finding the Pulse

Two schools of thought exist on this subject. The author of *Nāḍīvijñānam* suggests that the index finger be placed on the radial pulse of the wrist, just under the thumb (see the diagram below). The middle finger is placed just under the index finger (but not resting on the bony protrusion [radial tubercle]), and the ring finger is placed closest to the elbow.

श्रङ्गुष्ठामूले करयोः पादयोर्गल्फदशतः

कपालपार्श्वयोः षड्भ्यो नाडीभ्यो व्याधिनिर्णयः ॥१॥

Śhraṅguṣhṭhāmūle karayoḥ
pādayorgalphadaśhataḥ |
kapālapārśhvayoḥ ṣhaḍbhyo nāḍībhyo
vyādhinirṇayaḥ || *verse 1*||
Nāḍīvijñānam

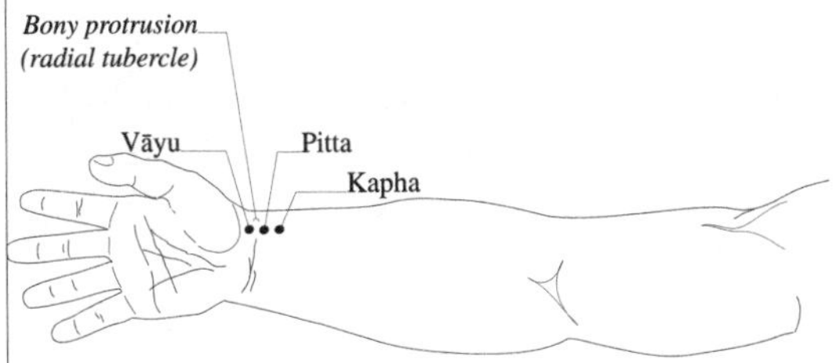

A second school suggests the index finger should be placed on the radial pulse below the flex in the wrist (i.e., two finger widths below the thumb root). As before, the other two fingers are positioned below it. In both cases, finger pressure on the wrist is applied lightly.

Some suggest taking the pulse of the right hand for men, and the left hand for women (except when they have a fever). Others suggest checking both pulses. When taking one's own pulse, males use their left hand and take the right pulse. Females take the left hand pulse with their right hand.

The practitioner's left palm supports the patient's elbow, with the right hand fingers pressing the artery. The patient's elbow and wrist are slightly bent. Finger pad tops are soft and can easily read the pulses. Fingers are placed between the wide bone below the thumb and the thin bones (in the middle of the wrist).

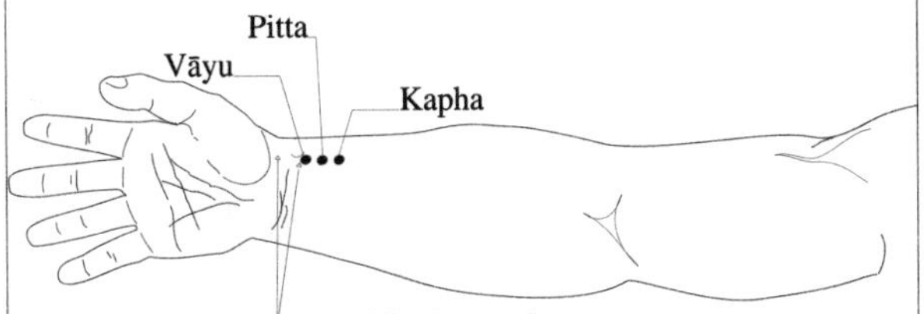

The second positioning option.
Vāyu pulse now begins just below the radial tubercle

Many factors may cause inaccurate readings, so it is advised not to take pulses under certain conditions.

Accurate Pulse Taking	
Take Pulse	**Do Not Take Pulse**
between meals	after meals
when rested	after exercise or strenuous work
after bathroom	when nature calls
	with fever
	during or after bath
	after sunbathing
	after sex
	after massage
	while sitting near fire

Finding the pulse of Vāyu persons may be hard due to the weakness of their pulse. Kapha pulses may also be difficult to find or read because of excess fat or thick skin. The pulse under the ring finger may also be difficult to find because the pulse moves deeper into the arm as it gets farther away from the wrist. [Other positions to find the pulse include at the lower ankles and at the temples.]

Although the pulse becomes slower as one gets older, the general rule in deciding *doṣhas* is:

Pulse Rate

Doṣhas	Pulses
Vāyu	80-100
Pitta	70-80
Kapha	60-70

Pulse Quality

A most interesting and unusual method to learn the constitution (*prakṛiti*) or present imbalance (*vikṛiti*) is the quality of the pulse. When the *doṣhas* are aggravated, the pulse expresses itself in various ways.

Vāyu pulses have the personality or quality of a snake, feeling quick, thin, thready, irregular, and crooked, with symptoms of nervousness, indigestion, Vāyu fevers.

Pitta pulses feel like a frog: bounding or jumpy, regular (or if irregular, it has a consistent pattern), with symptoms of heat, insomnia, diarrhea, vertigo, hypertension, eye, or skin problems. When the pulse is also felt as wiry, hard, stiff, and fast, there are corresponding symptoms of Pitta asthma, rheumatism, gout, chronic headaches, and bleeding disorders.

Kapha pulses are swan-like: regal, slow, and constant. Some people say it is a warm pulse, while others say it is cold. Related symptoms are coughing, melancholy, constipation, bronchial disorders, and overweight.

Vāyu/Pitta pulses alternate between snake and frog qualities. The pulse feels knotty, restless, intermittent, imperceptible, thick, and thin. Health issues include thirst, vertigo, headaches, suppressed urine, extremity pain, and heat.

Pitta/Vāyu pulses feel jumpy and hard, with heat and blood related symptoms being predominant.

Vāyu/Kapha pulses alternate between snake and swan qualities, weak and forceful, vanishing, hollow, slippery, and irregular qualities. Symptoms include chills, extremity pain, frequent urination, cough, insomnia, drowsiness, feeling slow and fast, soft and expanded. Sometimes chronic complaints arise around the new and full moon.

Kapha/Vāyu pulses feel soft and slow.

Pitta/Kapha pulses alternate between frog and swan qualities, with symptoms of both fire and water excesses. Pitta concerns are more aggravated.

Kapha/Pitta pulses alternate between swan and frog qualities, with predominantly Kapha symptoms, and secondary Pitta complaints.

Tridoshic (all three doṣhas) pulses will show all three qualities: snake, frog, and swan. Pulse movements are periodic, quick, jumpy, and slow.

Healthy pulse has no signs of dullness. In the morning the pulse feels cool and steady, at noon it feels warm. The pulse moves quickly in the evening. These three pulses indicate the person has been healthy for a long while and will continue to be healthy for some time to come.

Pulse-Doṣha Detection

One method is to lightly place fingers on the pulse positions until a pulse is first felt under one finger. If the pulse if first noticed under the index finger, this shows a Vāyu *doṣha* (before 10 a.m.) or Vāyu imbalance (after 10 a.m.). The middle finger suggests a Pitta *doṣha* or Pitta imbalance. A Kapha *doṣha* pulse is first felt under the ring finger. Sometimes this method is inaccurate because of the pulse being more easily felt closer to the wrist.

Some practitioners believe that whichever finger the pulse is first felt (i.e., index/Vāyu, middle/Pitta, ring/Kapha) will tell whether an illness is located in a Vāyu, Pitta, or Kapha organ (or the *prakṛiti* before 10 a.m.). Should the pulse be felt under two fingers simultaneously, then both *doṣhas* are imbalanced (or a dual-*doṣha prakṛiti* before 10 a.m.). Sometimes one may feel the pulse under one or two fingers strongly and yet feel a mild pulse under the second or third finger. The fainter pulses suggest a slight imbalance of the corresponding *doṣha*.

For example, a pulse is first felt under the index finger and then a milder pulse is felt under the middle finger. This shows a main Vāyu imbalance, with a secondary Pitta disorder. If the pulse is felt under all three fingers (either strongly or mildly), then all the *doṣhas* are imbalanced.

Pulse quality, position, and rate are the three best pulse methods to decide one's *doṣha*.

> After 10:00 a.m. one only learns the *vikṛiti* (current imbalance or disease) from both the quality and position of the pulse.

The practitioner takes the pulse from the thumb side of the client (radial side), not reaching across from the pinky side (ulnar side).

Pulse Qualities Signs for Health and Disease

Abscess- agitated, fiery
Acidity- crooked, shaky, wide, slippery, slow
Anemia- faint, felt at intervals
Anger- accelerated
Appetite (loss of)- steady, slow, hard, mild
Asthma- thin, steady, accelerated, hard, speedy, intense, felt under all three fingers, hollow
Bile- hot
Boils- (hard) bilious
Colic- (pulse according to the *doṣhas*)
(with abdominal worms)- expanded
Convulsions- wide and rapid
(hysterical)- crooked and rapid
Constipation- frog, strong
Cough- trembling, thin, restless, slow, hot, swan
Deafness- quick and spreading
Diabetes- knotty
(mellitus)- thin
(insipidus)- Vāyu: Crooked, thin.
Pitta: Fast.
Kapha: Slow
Diarrhea (chronic)- [after evacuations] gentle, weak.
Vāyu: Crooked.
Pitta: Fast.
Kapha: mild
Dysentery-
(Vāyu)- crooked
(Pitta)- restless
(Kapha)- cold, slow, swan-like
(with mucus)- wide, inert, dull
(two *doṣhas*) both pulses, respectively
(caused by three *doṣhas*) disappears, or is imperceptible
(after bowel evacuation) energy-less
Dysmenorrhea- steady, quick
Edema- sometimes weak, thin, cold, stopping
Eye Diseases- hard, slow, slippery, crooked
Fainting- lightning-like
Fear- weak
Healthy/Nourished- rises or jumps upward, pure, stays in place, steady, not slow,
Feces (suppression)- hard, heavy, or frog
Fever- heated
Full-blooded- slightly hot and heavy
Fistula-in-ano- dull Kapha pulse
Gonorrhea- thin, knotty, inert; pulse at joint
Good Digestion- soft, mild, quick, not dull
Gout (acute)- slow, crooked, hard, mild
Headaches- weak, changeable
Heart diseases- swan
Hemorrhage- hard, slow
Hemorrhoids- (differs according to the *doṣha* deranged)
Hernia- rises and jumps
Hiccup- much trembling and fast
Hoarse/loss of voice- thready, grave, twisting,

tricky, thin, hard, inert
Hungry- restless, unsteady, wavering
Hysteria- weak, fast
Indigestion- slow, hard, or inert; cool, swan-like
(Chronic)- under nourished, slow
Insanity- speedy and turning, crooked
Jaundice- weak, splitting, and expanded
Mucus- wide, hot
Negative Thoughts (evil spirits)- hot, curved
Nose Diseases- agitated, slowed
Obesity- thick, slow
Parasites- sometimes disappears, is slow, or fast
Phlegm- thick and slow
Pregnant- weak, slow
Rheumatism- thin, fast
Satiated- steady and slow
Sciatica- wide, crooked, slow
Sex (afterwards)- weak and accelerated
(passion)- deranged
Sinus- agitated, fiery
Spleen enlargement- trembling, restless, and becoming speedy
Suppression of urges (repeatedly)- hard, heavy
Thirst- leech-like
Thyroid (enlarged)- wide, slow
(hypo)- slow
Toxic blood (bile)- slow, hard, and mild
Tumor (abdominal)- restless, gyrates, quick
(throat)- wide, slow, trembling
Urine (suppressing or discharge pain)- heavy, hard, urgent
stones- frog, low, crooked
inability (obstruction)- frog
other diseases- thin, knotty, inert
Vāyu disorders- thin and fast
Vomiting- thick, slowed, disappears (elephant and swan-like)
Wasting- weak or differing movements

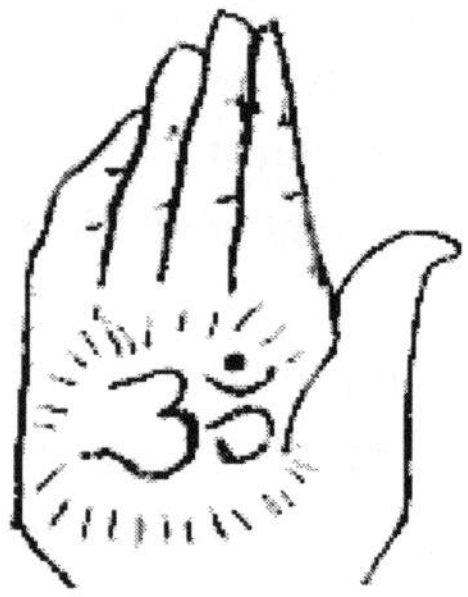

Nature of Pulse Depending Upon Diet Intake
Foods and Qualities

Food	Pulse
Oils	thick, wide
Sweets	wide, frog-like
Banana	snake/frog
Fried Foods	snake/frog
Fasting	weak, accelerated
Meat	wide, hard, jumps up
Milk	slow
Molasses	snake/frog
Liquids	hard
Dry Foods	snake/frog
Hard Foods	flowing (liquid or soft)
Small Foods	knotty, separate
Nourishing	developed

6 Tastes	Pulse
Sweet	swan
Sour	bird
Salty	speedy, straight
Hot/Acidic	frog, warm, light
Bitter	worm
Astringents	hard, weak
Multiple tastes	several pulses

Onset of Fevers

Depending upon the time and *doṣha* causing fever, the pulse yields different readings.

Vāyu- generally a slow, weak pulse, especially when beginning during times of
(accumulation)- slow, weak [occurring during digestion, in the summer, and at noon, and mid-night].
(excess)- heavy, hard, quick [after digestion,

in the afternoon, end of night, and in the rainy season].

Pitta- (accumulating)- clearly felt under all three fingers, and quickens its pace [after meals, morning, evening, and during the rainy season].

(excess)- hard, quick, bursting pulse [occurs while digesting, at noon and midnight, and in autumn].

Kapha- (accumulating or in excess)- weak, thin, thready, cold [during digestion, evening, the end of night, in autumn and in winter].

Vāyu/Pitta Fever- thick, hard, undulating.
Vāyu/Kapha Fever- slow and hot.
Vāyu/Kapha Fever- dry and quick.
Pitta/Kapha- slow, thready, weak, sometimes cool, sometimes cold and slow.
Tridoṣhic Fever- the symptoms described above appear during their respective periods of excess.
Pulse Before Fever- a short period that exhibits a frog-like pulse.
Intermittent Fever- the pulse is felt at the root of the thumb or at its side, on alternating days. When fevers appear every three or four days, the pulse is hot, gyrating, and receding.
Fever with Hot and Sour Foods- raises the pulse rate.

Pulses That Determine Causal Doṣha

Vāyu Fever with Air Accumulation: Soft, thin, steady, slow, and faint.
Vāyu Fever with Air Excess: Large, hard, and rapid.
Pitta Fever with Fire Accumulation: Full, straight, felt under all three fingers, and quick.
Pitta Fever with Fire Excess: Hard, fast, piercing, and pulsing upwards.
Kapha Fever with Kapha Accumulation: Hard, slow, and cool
Kapha Fever with Kapha Excess: Thread-like, slow, and cool.
Vāyu=Pitta Fever: Unsteady, wavy, thick, and hard.
Vāyu/Kapha Fever: Slightly warm, and slow.
Kapha/Vāyu Fever: Hard and rough.
Pitta=Kapha Fever: Thin, cool, and steady.
Fever Caused by Negative Thoughts (Spirits): Speedy, flowing, and hot.

If a person's pulse is continuously
cool and slow in the morning,
hot at noon, and fast in the evening,
It is a healthy pulse.

Organ Pulses

Pulses at the three wrist positions also reveal the health of 12 different body organs. This information can be found by taking the pulse at a light and deep level. This is possible because certain "meridian" or energy lines connect the organ energy currents to corresponding wrist positions. Superficial or light pulses generally relate to the hollow organs, while the deep positions mostly reveal the solid organs.

The same three fingers and wrist positions are used as before, except the organ pulses are taken on both wrists. [Of the two finger placement systems described earlier, i.e., just under the thumb joint and under the bone, the latter positioning is used for taking the organ pulse.] The practitioner first get a feel for the general pulse by using all three fingers. Then, they press one finger to an organ pulse site. The two pulses (general and specific) are then compared for strength (i.e., deciding if the organ pulse is stronger or weaker than the general pulse). Practitioners can even determine conditions such as noting smoke in the lungs. This may reveal that the person is a cigarette smoker. Fire organ positions, like the liver, spleen, and gall bladder can feel hot or electric when Pitta is excessive in these organs. The urinary bladder pulse may reflect an urgency or fullness if the bladder is full. This would suggest the need for persons to attend to nature's call.

Some practitioners, use the right hand at superficial and deep positions to gain spiritual insights about the patient. (An approach used by some practitioners is mentally to ask the "pulse" what it is that the patient needs to hear right now. The first thought entering their head thereafter is the answer.) It is said that the various pulse methods take 10-15 years to master.

Again, no one indication is used by itself when deciding the health of an organ. Only after assessing the total person does the practitioner reach a decision as to the patient's *prakṛiti* and *vikṛiti*. The practitioner looks at all the mental and physical traits found through observation, questionnaire, and discussion.

Organ Pulse Positions

Left Hand		
Position	Light	Deep
1st	small intestine	heart
2nd	stomach	spleen
3rd	urinary bladder	kidney
Right Hand		
Position	Light	Deep
1st	colon	lungs
2nd	gall bladder	liver
3rd	pericardium	spiritual pulse

A more advanced determination of the organ pulse analysis also exists. The index, middle, and ring fingers relate to Vāyu, Pitta, and Kapha *doṣhas* respectively. The upper, middle, and lower areas of each finger tip show which *doṣha* is imbalancing which organ.

The index finger pressing at the superficial position of the right hand (colon) is such an example. If the pulse is felt in the middle of the index finger, a Pitta imbalance exists in the colon. If the pulse is felt on the upper portion of the index finger, Vāyu is causing the disorder. Colon disorders caused by Kapha are noted by the pulse being felt at the lower portion of the index finger. Should the pulse be felt at two areas (e.g., the upper and middle of the finger tip), then two *doṣhas* are causing the excess.

Questionnaire

Another Āyurvedic *doṣha* analysis tool is a self-test filled out by the patient. The self-test questions reflect the patient's total life span (not just the new or current symptoms caused that day, week, or year). Some practitioners offer two different questionnaires, one to learn the *prakṛiti* and one to learn about the cause of the illness (*vikṛiti*). (During consultation discussions the current illness (*vikṛiti*) is discussed.)

To find out one's *doṣha*, questions are asked about the patient's mind, body, and emotional well being. Below is a sample of the questions that offer insight into the patient's *prakṛiti* (nature).

[Note: V stands for Vāyu, P stands for Pitta, and K stands for Kapha.] After checking the category that best describes one's total life experiences, the practitioner totals the number for each category V, P, K. The result will decide the *doṣha*. For example, if there are 10-V, 20- P, and 30- K, the person is a Kapha *doṣha*. If the sum is 25-V, 25-P and 10-K, the person is Vāyu/Pitta *doṣha*. If the sum is 20-V, 20-P, and 20-K, the person is Tridoṣhic. Separate totals for the mental and physical questions reveal any differences between the *doṣhas* of the mind and body.

Outer Conditions

Frame:

V- tall or short, thin, bony
P- medium, average development
K- wide, stocky, stout, big, well-developed body

Weight:

V- low, protruding veins and bones, can't keep weight on; may be heavy but with fluctuating weight and spongy tissues.
P- moderate, muscular; excess red meat and greasy foods add excess weight.
K- heavy, hard to keep weight off, obesity

Head:

V- thin, long, small, unsteady, stiff necks
P- moderate
K- stocky, large, square-ish, steady

Hair:
V- curly, brown, dry, coarse, sparse, full bodied
P- straight, blond or reddish, early gray or bald, soft, fine
K- oily, thick, very wavy, dark brown or black, lustrous, abundant

Forehead:
V- small, wrinkles
P- moderate with folds
K- large and broad

Face:
V- long, thin, wrinkled, small, dull
P- moderate, sharply contoured
K- large, round, fat, pale, softly contoured

Skin:
V- thin, cold, rough, cracked, dry, prominent veins
P- warm, pink, freckles, acne, moles, moist, rashes, easy sunburn, delicate, sensitive
K- thick, cold, smooth, white, soft, moist, oily, edema, fatty

Complexion:
V- dull, darkish brown, lackluster
P- flushed, reddish, freckled, glowing, discolor tion
K- pale, whitish

Eyes, Lashes, and Brows:
V- small, dry, brown, unsteady
P- medium, red, thin, green, piercing, light sensitive
K- wide, oily, white, attractive, prominent, cry easily, discharge in eyes, steady but dull focus

Nose:
V- thin, long, and pointed, small, dry, crooked
P- average, sharp, and pointed
K- thick, firm, big, oily

* Nose, eyes, and complexion will vary depending on racial/cultural characteristics.

Lips:
V- thin, small, dry, unsteady, darkish, biting
P- medium, soft, red
K- large, thick, oily, smooth, firm, attractive

Teeth/Gums: (varies according to hygiene)
V- thin, small, dry, rough, crooked, spaces, buck teeth, receding gums
P- medium, soft pink, gums bleed easily
K- large, white, attractive, thick, soft pink, oily

Neck:
V- thin, long, loose tendons
P- moderate
K- large, thick, square

Shoulders:
V- small, thin, flat, hunched
P- medium
K- broad, thick, firm

Frame:
V- small, thin bones
P- average
K-large bones

Upper Torso:
V- small, thin, narrow, underdeveloped, doesn't gain weight easily
P- moderate, wiry
K- large, broad, well developed, overdeveloped, gain weight easily

Arms:
V- small, thin, long, low development, bony elbows
P- moderate, wiry
K- large, thick, round, well developed, fleshy

Hands:
V- small, narrow, dry, rough, cold, unsteady, fissured, lines, bony knuckles
P- moderate, warm, pink
K- large, thick, cool, firm, oily, square, unlined

Legs:
V- very short or long legs, thin, bony knees, runs and walks a lot, walking coordination is unsteady
P- average
K- large, stocky, can stand for long periods

Thighs:
V- thin, narrow
P- moderate
K- fat, round, well developed, cellulitis
Calves:
V- small, tight, hard
P- soft, loose
K- firm, shapely

Feet:
V- small, thin, rough, long, dry, unsteady, fissured, need to be oiled daily
P- moderate, soft pink, good circulation and complexion
K- large, thick, firm

Joints:
V- small, thin, dry, unsteady, cracking, prominent
P- moderate, loose, soft
K- large, thick, well built

Nails: (mineral absorption)
V- small, thin, dry, rough, cracked, fissured, dark
P- medium, soft, pink
K- large, thick, white, smooth, oily, firm

Sweat/Odor: (vegetarians sweat less than meat eaters)
V- odorless, scanty
P- strong smell, profuse, hot
K- pleasant smell, moderate when exercising, cold

Feces:
V- scanty, dry, hard, painful, or difficult, gas, constipation
P- abundant, loose, yellowish, burning diarrhea
K- moderate, solid, pale, mucus in stool

* Pitta persons with fevers get constipation. Kaphas may get constipation but stool is not hard.

Urine:
V- scanty, colorless, bubbly, difficult
P- profuse, yellow, red, burning
K- moderate, whitish, milky

<u>Inner Conditions</u>
Appetite/Food:
V- erratic, variable, eats quickly, likes warm, oily food
P- sharp, strong, eats moderately fast, likes cold food
K- low, constant, eats slowly, likes warm, dry food

Taste:
V- sweet, sour, salty, oily, spicy foods
P- sweet, bitter, astringent, raw or steamed, bland foods
K- pungent, bitter astringent, spicy, non oily foods

* *Āma* (toxins) in the system causes one not to follow the above natural inclinations.

Circulation:
V- low, variable, palpitations, aggravated by wind, cold, and dryness
P- excellent, warm, aggravated by heat, fire, and sun
K- slow, steady, aggravated by cold and dampness

Life Pace:
V- fast, unsteady, erratic, hyperactive
P- moderate, purposeful, goal-oriented
K- slow, steady, regal

Endurance:
V- low or fluctuating
P- moderate to high, heat intolerance, pushes until one burns out

K- strong, steady, slow starters, moderate performance

Disease Tendency:
V- nervous and immune system diseases, pain, arthritis, mental, bones
P- infections, febrile, blood, inflammatory diseases, yellow or green mucus
K- respiratory diseases, clear or white mucus, edema, obesity

Disease Resistance:
V- poor, weak immune systems
P- moderate, infections, bleeding
K- good, strong immune system, consistent

<u>**Medicinal Healing Tendency:**</u>
V- quick, low dosages, nervous reactions
P- moderate
K- slow, higher dosages

Pulse: (quality is the most important thing)
V- 80-100, irregular, rapid, snake-like quality
P- 70-80, wiry, frog-like quality
K- 60-70, slow, warm, steady, wide, swan-like quality

Sexual Nature:
V- variable, strong desire but low energy, few children
P- moderate, passionate, domineering, quarrelsome
K- constant, low, devoted, many children

Pain: (blocked or wrong movements in the *srotas* cause the severest pain)
V- severe - sharp, shocking, disruptive, churning, beating, throbbing, tearing, variable, colic, migratory, intermittent
P- moderate - burning, steaming, swelling, bleeding
K- mild - heavy, dull, constant, congestion

Fever:
V- moderate heat, variable, irregular, thirst, anxious, restless
P- highest heat, burning, thirst, sweating, irritable, delirious
K- lowest heat, dull, heavy, constant

Discharges:
V- noises (joint cracking, moaning, sighing), gas
P- blood, bile, yellow or green pus
K- mucus, clear or white pus, salivation, water

Mouth:
V- dry, astringent taste
P- bitter, pungent taste, salivation
K- sweet, salty tastes, excess salivation, discharge of mucus

Throat:
V- dry, rough pain, constricted esophagus
P- sore, inflamed, burning
K- swollen, dilated, edema

Stomach:
V- frequent belching, and/or hiccuping, feeling a sense of constriction, variable appetite, less secretions
P- cancer, ulcers, burning, sour or pungent (eructations) belches or hiccups, excess appetite, heart burns
K- slow digestion, sweet or mucoid belching, nausea, vomiting

Liver/ Gall Bladder:
V- dry, rough, irregular activity, scanty secretions
P- soft, inflamed, abscesses, increased activity, excess bile, gall stones (most liver and gall bladder problems are Pitta related)
K- enlarged, heavy, firm, little bile, lower activity

Intestines:
V- dry, distention, gas, constipation, disorders of peristalsis
P- excess secretions, inflamed, ulcers, abscesses, tumors, cancer, bleeding, perforation, rapid peristalsis

K- coated with mucus, obstructed, edema, tumors, distention, slow peristalsis

Initial Signs of Disease:
V- variable, irregular rapid onset
P- high fevers, moderate onset
K- constant, slow onset from congestion

Mental Traits

Sensitivities:
V- noise
P- bright lights
K- strong odors

Voice/Speaking:
V- low, weak, whining, monotone, quick, talkative, rambling, imaginative
P- high, sharp, clear, precise, organized, detailed, orators, moderate, argumentative
K- deep, tonal, singers, slow, silent

Dreams/Sleep:
V- flying, running, fearful, light sleep
P- fighting, in color, moderately deep
K- romantic, water, few, heavy, deep sleep

Mind/Senses:
V- fear, anxiety, apathy, sorrow, delusion, unconsciousness, insomnia, needing heat, strongly dislikes cold things, loss of coordination indecisive
P- violent, delirious, dizzy, fainting, needing cold, poor senses, intoxicated, restlessness, heated head, impatient, hot tempered, critical
K- calm, lethargic, stupor, excessive sleep, slow perception, desires heat, dull, inert

Memory/Learning:
V- quick to learn ideas but also forgets quickly, likes to study many things but becomes unfocused, learns by listening
P- focused, penetrating, discriminating, goal-oriented, learns best by reading and with visuals
K- slow to learn but never forgets, learns by association

Nature:
V- adaptable, quick, indecisive
P- penetrating, critical, intelligent
K- slow, steady, dull

Memory:
V- understands ideas quickly, then forgets quickly
P- clear, sharp
K- slow to learn, but once learns, never forgets

Faith:
V- erratic, rebellious, changeable
P- leader, goals, fanatical
K- loyal, constant, conservative

Emotions:
V- anxious, nervous, fearful
P- angry, irritable, argumentative
K- content, calm, sentimental

Habits:
V- travel, culture, humor, eccentric
P- politics, sports, dance, competitive
K- water sports, flowers, cosmetics, business, lazy

Mental Disorders:
V- anxiety attacks, hysteria, trembling
P- rage, tantrums, excess temper
K- depression, sorrow, lethargic

Discussion

Once the *doṣha* has been determined, the present illness or health concern (*vikṛiti*) is discussed. Through a series of questions regarding the degree of air, fire, and water affecting the condition, the *vikṛiti* will become clear.

It is more crucial to learn what the patient experiences than merely naming the illness. Another way of cross-referencing disease is finding the site of the condition. For example, dryness, or general weakness in the colon, bones, and thighs; anxieties, and worry are symptoms of Vāyu. Heat, infection or acid of the liver, spleen, heart, blood, gall bladder; yellow or green mucus, anger, impatience, and irritability are symptoms of Pitta. With dampness, water (e.g., in the lungs), white or clear, abundant mucus, overweight, and lethargy, Kapha is the cause. If symptoms include more than one *doṣha*, then it is possible that both *doṣhas* are the cause.

Different physical and mental imbalances may exist. The practitioner investigates "the cause of the cause." For example, if a person wants to lose weight, therapy can begin in one of three ways. First, one may address the symptom with allopathic weight loss pills. Obviously, this is the most superficial method. Second, one may realize that the cause of the weight is a Kapha tendency and follow appropriate Kapha-reduction therapies. Yet, a deeper level still exists. What is the cause of the overeating? Perhaps it is a Vāyu-imbalanced mind, producing worry or anxiety. Kapha imbalances create a need for love and contentment. These factors may cause a person to eat more. Therapies include herbs and foods to reduce weight, calm the mind, and culture the heart. *Sādhanā* (meditation) is also advised to develop inner calm and Self-love.

When viewing weight gain from another vantage point, finding out what causes anxiety in the person may uncover *dharmic* (life-purpose), *kamic* (spiritual relationship), or spiritual situations, that are making the person unhappy.

The *dharmic* reasons are easily discovered when asking patients if they love the career in which they are presently working. They specifically need to say they love it. When they acknowledge that they do, the practitioner can focus more deeply into *kama* and *mokṣha* (Self-Realization) questioning.

If they admit they are unhappy with their careers, a deeper question is asked; "What is it you would love to do if you could, regardless whether it seems possible or practical?" Often patients realize that once, before they stopped doing something they loved, they did not have a weight problem; only after they stopped doing what they love (e.g., teaching dancing) did the weight gain occur. Thus, the practitioner uncovers the ultimate cause of the weight problem. People doing what they love to do find their lives are transformed in a very short time.

Spiritual lacking is yet another dimension that may cause overeating and overweight. It is the cause of all causes of diseases. An inner lack of fulfillment may exist in one's career, relationship or in their self worth. These persons are urged to begin taking small steps towards involving themselves in whatever they need for inner nourishment. These three topics will be discussed in detail later in the book.

So we see that the discussion portion of the consultation covers mind, body, career, relationships, and spirituality. This makes for a truly holistic investigation.

Nutrition

We have briefly touched upon the topic of tastes, as they are related to the seasons. This may seem quite an unusual way to look at the seasons, but nonetheless, a useful one when considering health. To better understand the idea of taste from the Āyurvedic viewpoint, it needs to be examined more deeply. These insights offer an explanation of the role of tastes in healing. Unique to Āyurveda is a scientific breakdown of tastes, discussed according to energies or energetics. Āyurveda classifies herbs, foods, and drinks into five categories. Each has its own therapeutic effects:

1. Taste
2. Element (property)
3. Heating or cooling effect
4. Post-digestion effect (final taste after digestion)
5. Special properties

Taste: Is considered therapeutic for several reasons. The *Sanskrit* word for taste is *"Rasa"*. It means delight or essence, both of which are healing. A nerve channel extends from the mouth into the head, that brings the essence (one definition of taste) to the brain. This essence stimulates *prāṇa*, which in turn stimulates the *agni* or digestive fires. If the taste of the food is not pleasing, the gastric fires may not digest the food and one will not receive proper nutrition. That is why Āyurvedic cooking is a science unto itself, blending the right amount of herbs for the right taste. In our society, we have mixed our sense of taste with unwholesome (artificial) objects of food (one of the two fundamental causes of disease).

Element: Six tastes originate from the five elements, transmitting their properties: sweet, sour, salty, pungent, bitter, astringent. All tastes essentially belong to the water element, having their origin here. No food consists only of one taste; all five elements are contained in all substances. So when it is said that a food has a certain taste (e.g., sweet), it means predominantly that taste. Similarly, no illness is caused purely by one *doṣha*. However, when a *doṣha* predominates, it is said that an illness is caused by that specific *doṣha*.

Taste	Element	Food
sweet	earth/water	sugar, starches
sour	earth/fire	fermented, acids
salty	water/fire	salt, alkaline
pungent	fire/air	spicy, acrid, aromatic
bitter	ether/air	herbs
astringent	earth/air*	constricting quality with tannin

**Astringents can either aggravate or pacify Kapha due to its earth and air elements, respectively.*

All persons need some of each of the six tastes in their daily diet. However, depending on one's constitution, health condition, and the season, they will take varying amounts of the tastes to balance their *doṣha*. The key is to have a moderate amount of each taste.

The benefits listed on the next page result from ingesting foods that develop these healing measures. However, they relate primarily to the *doṣha*(s) listed. If used by a *doṣha* not listed, they will create excess.

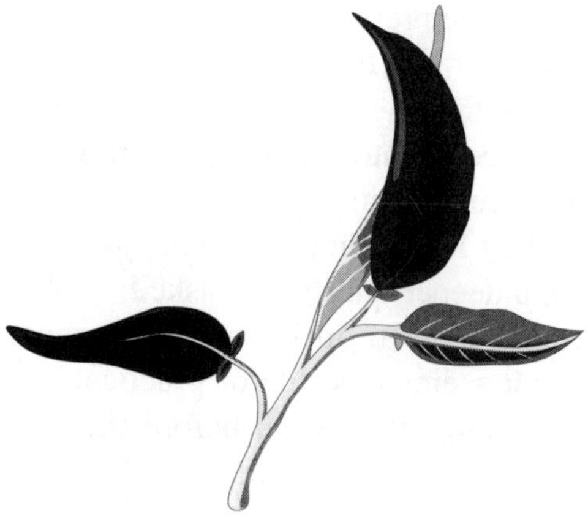

Taste *(Rasa)*	Physical Effect	Mental Effect
sweet VP-	builds & strengthens tissues, life sap *(ojas)*, bones complexion	contentment, pleasure
sour VK-	digestive aid, dispels gas, nourishes, relieves thirst, satiates, helps circulation and elimination, strengthens heart, aids all tissues but reproductive, maintains acidity	wakens mind & senses
salty V-	softening, lubricates tissues, laxative, sedative, digestive aid, promotes sweating, purgative, emetic, softens hard tumors, decongests hard phlegm, maintains mineral balance, holds water, improves taste	calms nerves, stops anxiety
pungent VK-	heals throat diseases and VK allergic rashes, skin diseases, counters water, grease, and fat; digestive aid, dispels gas, removes edema, improves taste, promotes sweat, improves metabolism and organic functions, breaks up stagnant blood or clots and other hard masses, clears channels, relieves nerve pain and muscle tension	opens mind and senses
bitter PK-	heals anorexia, thirst, skin diseases, fever, nausea, burning, parasites, and bacteria; blood purifier, cleanses, detoxifies, reduces fat, tissue, and water excesses; antibiotic, antiseptic, digestive aid, cleanses breast milk, digests sugar and fat	clears senses and emotions
astringent PK-	stops bleeding and cleanses blood, sweat, diarrhea, heals skin and mucus membranes, prolapse, and ulcers; expectorant, diuretic, tightens tissues, dries moisture and fat	cools fiery minds and removes lethargy

V = Vāyu, P = Pitta, K = Kapha, '-' means reduces that *doṣha*

Negative Effects Due To Excess

In the table below are the diseases that result from ingesting foods that create excesses in the *doṣhas*. In excess, eventually any *doṣha* will develop these ailments.

Taste (*Rasa*)	Physical Effect	Mental Effect
sweet K+	excess fat diseases; obesity, diabetes indigestion, malignant tumors, neck gland enlargement	Kapha: lethargy, Vāyu: anxiety
sour P+	flabbiness, loss of strength, fever, thirst, blindness, itching, pallor, Pitta anemia, herpes, small pox	giddiness, anger, impatience, hot temper
salty PK+	hypertension, baldness, gray hair, skin diseases, wrinkles, thirst, herpes, loss of strength, abscesses	anger, impatience, lethargy
pungent P+	thirst, depletion of reproductive fluid and strength, fainting, tremors, waist/back pain	anger, impatience
bitter V+	tissue depletion, Vāyu diseases	anxiety, fear, insomnia
astringent V+	undigested foods, heart pain, thirst, emaciation, virility loss, constipation, blocked channels	anxiety, worry, fear, insomnia

It is interesting that Āyurveda is not concerned with naming diseases. It determines illness according to the excesses and deficiencies of the elements or *doṣhas* (air, fire, and water). When *doṣhas* are balanced, illness does not exist. From this point of view, one can see that by understanding the effects of the six tastes upon the *doṣhas*, nutrition becomes an elemental and effective measure in maintaining the balance of health. The charts shown above also reveal how various diseases are seen to be directly related to tastes and *doṣhas*. Thus, by following an appropriate food plan for one's constitution, a person may maintain health and prevent future illness.

Energy (Vīrya)

This energy causes the activation of tastes. Foods and drinks possess either cool or hot energy (in the body). Each taste has an associated energy.

Taste	Energy	Foods
sweet	cool	sugar
sour	acidic*/hot	yogurt, wine, pickles
salty	hot	table salt, seaweed
pungent	hot	hot peppers, chilies, wine
bitter	cold	alum, goldenseal, gentian
astringent	constricting	alum, oak bark

** Yogurt is sour, sweet, and heavy. Pure forms of the tastes will aggravate one's doṣha more easily than complex versions and thus should be used with care.*

Aggravating	Pacifying
sugar	complex carbohydrates
table salt	sea weed
hot peppers (e.g., cayenne)	mild spices (e.g., cardamom)
alcohol	yogurt, sour fruit
pure bitters (e.g., goldenseal)	mild bitters (aloe gel)
pure astringents (strong tannins)	mild astringents (e.g., red raspberry)

Post Digestive (Vipāka)

Tastes may change at the end of the digestive process. This is due to the digestive *agni* fire juices in the alimentary tract (metabolism). For example, foods or liquids, initially sweet, develop an aftertaste. This taste may be any of the six tastes. These aftertastes also affect a person's constitution.

6 Tastes	Post-digestive Taste
sweet, salty	becomes sweet
sour	remains sour
pungent, bitter, astringent	becomes pungent

[Throughout this text, the following abbreviations will occur; 'V' 'P' 'K' stands for Vāyu, Pitta, Kapha respectively. '-' stands for reducing a doṣha and '+' means increasing a doṣha]

Sweet VP- K+ (moist) promotes secretion of Kapha, semen, easy and comfortable gas, and helps the discharge of urine and feces. Produces saliva.

Sour P+ increases the tissues (except the reproductive *dhātu*, which is reduced). It produces bile, acid.

Salty P+ produces saliva.

Pungent P+ (in time) causes gas, constipation, painful urine, reduces semen with difficult discharge.

Bitter PK- V+ produces dryness and gas in the colon.

Astringent PK- V+ constricts, bothers Vāyu.

Emotions and Taste

Each of the six tastes produces or enhances a certain emotion when eaten. Thus, emotional disorders may be balanced by eating and avoiding foods according to their tastes.

Taste	Emotions	Excesses
sweet	desire	Kapha
sour	envy	Pitta
salty	greed	Kapha/Pitta
pungent	anger	Pitta
bitter	grief	Vāyu
astringent	fear	Vāyu

Doṣhas, Nutrition, and the 6 Tastes

Vāyu is balanced by supplementing with moist tastes, sweet, sour, and salty (balancing dryness), and some warm tastes as well. Pitta is balanced by using sweet (moist), and bitter and astringent (cooling) tastes. This helps counter heat-related illness (e.g., infection, rash, anger, impatience). Kapha diseases are removed by using sour and pungent tastes (i.e., they heat and burn up water). Bitter tastes, by causing a drying action, also reduce Kapha.

Sweet: Generally, food is sweet in taste, neutral in energy, and sweet in its post-digestive effect. It decreases Vāyu and Pitta, and increases Kapha. It nourishes and maintains humors, *dhātus* (tissues), and *malas* (wastes).

Sour: Examples of sour tastes include sour fruit, tomatoes, and pickled vegetables. All tissues are nourished by sour tastes—except reproductive tissue (of the sour tastes, only yogurt nourishes all tissues).

Salty: Sea food or condiment. In moderation, salt strengthens all tissues. When used in excess, it depletes tissues.

Pungent: Spices and spicy vegetables do not offer much nutrition, but they stimulate digestion.

Bitter: Such vegetables offer little nourishment. They are useful in clearing and cleansing digestive organs, and in aiding digestion, especially if taken before meals (for Pitta and Kapha *doṣhas*).

Astringent: This is mainly a secondary taste. Astringent foods, like green vegetables or unripe apples, provide minerals but do not build tissue.

Energy: Most foods are neutral in heating and cooling effects. To apply hot or cold therapeutics, appropriate spices and foods are eaten cooked or raw.

Heavy/Light: Most foods tend to be heavy, though many light foods also exist. Spices can make foods lighter. Oils can make them heavier.

Dry/Moist: Foods are also dry or moist. Dryness can be increased by eating dry foods or toast. Moistness can be increased by frying foods or adding liquids.

Special Properties: (Prabhāva)

Herbs also have some subtler, more specific qualities, beyond their traditional rules and definitions. For example, basil, although a heating herb, reduces fever. Herbs with similar energies will have different special properties.

Certain external actions affect the herbs' *prabhāva*; *mantras*, gems, or just the intention or love imparted by the practitioner alters the herbs beyond the general classifications. For example, *āmalakī* (embellica officinalis) and *barhal* (a variety of ficus bengalensis, linn.) both have the same taste, property, energy, and post-digestive taste. Yet *āmalakī* alleviates the *doṣhas* and *barhal* aggravates the *doṣhas*. Also *til* (sesame seeds) and *madan* (randia dumetorum, lamk.) have predominantly sweet, astringent, and bitter tastes. Both are oily and sticky. Yet, *madan* is an emetic, while sesame is not. Similarly, wearing specific stones like topaz, ruby, sapphire, etc., can heal different diseases.

Dual Doṣhas

It is simply a matter of balance. When *doṣhas* are not in a balanced state, one has to increase the depleted *doṣha* and/or decrease the aggravated *doṣha*. When a person has a dual *doṣha* (e.g., Vāyu/Pitta) they are advised to ingest foods and herbs that increase the third or deficient element (e.g., Kapha). Simultaneously, one reduces the intake of foods and herbs that increase the two excessive *doṣhas* (e.g., Vāyu and Pitta).

Foods affect the surface nutrition, while herbs aid the subtle nutrition. There also may be instances when one *doṣha* is greatly excessive, and a second is mildly aggravated. Thus, proper consideration of the degree of derangement is necessary as well.

Tastes and Organs

Each of the six tastes also produces effects on each of the internal organs as well. Again, through ingesting the proper tastes, the health of the organs may be maintained.

Physiology of the 6 Tastes

Āyurveda says that each taste, when found in excess in the body will adversely affect certain organs in the body. This information is used as a cross reference to the five-element view of health and balance, stated earlier.

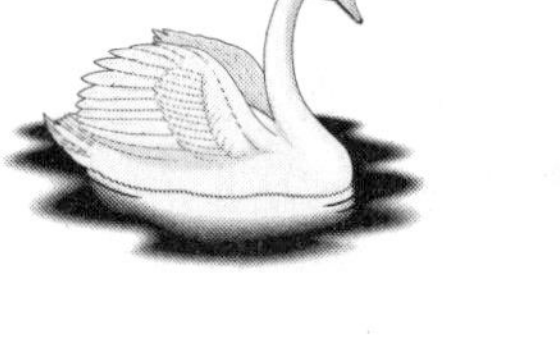

Taste	Organ
sweet	spleen (pancreas)
sour	liver
salty	kidneys
pungent	lungs
bitter	heart
astringent	colon

Thus, Āyurveda offers a unique view of the energetics of taste: six tastes (the initial taste, its hot or cold energy, and its after taste), how tastes are related to the *doṣhas*, organs, diseases, and emotions and their special properties. It is a complete science of the mechanics and energies of nutrition. Further, it reveals a causal relationship between food and health; how one feels is greatly decided by what one eats.

As discussed earlier, Āyurveda aims to remove the cause of an illness. Rather than 'curing' a specific disease, this science addresses the balance of the whole individual. It always considers the three levels of health: body, mind, and external causes. This chapter has examined the Āyurvedic view of how the tastes and energies of foods play a direct role in creating health or illness.

Life habits (external) are considered another essential Āyurvedic healing measure when life style changes are gradually adapted. In the original Āyurvedic texts, people are cautioned to gradually change their habits. Starting or stopping habits (even healthy ones) too suddenly, causes shock to the system. In the chapter on the seasons, a subtle seven-day transition period between seasons is noted and utilized to help people avoid disease during the shift. In the spiritual texts, we find similar wisdom about the transition points at sunrise, noon, sunset, and midnight. It is suggested that these are points of weakness and that the person is better advised to spend these transitional times in *sādhanā* (meditation). [Astrologically, the 1st, 8th, 15th, and 16th days, starting with the new and full moon cycle, are also transitional days best suited for *sādhanā*—or at least reduced activity.]

Even for a healing science that suggests vegetarianism to those who are healthy, Āyurveda does not advise giving up meat "cold-turkey " (no pun intended). Even if a food is bad for one's constitution (e.g., one's favorite vegetables or desserts), or good for their *doṣha*, gradual stopping and starting of any life habit is advised. Gentleness is the key. Similarly, if one too radically undertakes a detoxification program, one may experience uncomfortable cleansing, like diarrhea or excess toxins aggravating the body as they come out. Āyurveda has the unique position of offering a healing process that does not have to make one feel bad before feeling better; one needn't feel punished for changing to a healthier way of life. Thus, healing becomes enjoyable. It makes life better, simpler, more natural, and it enhances spiritual growth as well. It may take some months before a healing effect is felt. Making one or two changes for health, and consistently following them, is better than experimenting here and there without a foundation for growth and healing. The Āyurvedic motto is, "no pain - no pain."

Also, people often look for quick healing—magic medicine that allows them to continue with their bad habits. In fact, illness is a sign (i.e., a teacher) that life is not being lived in balance. Herbs are a food supplement, not magic pills that instantly remove discomfort. Some people may be impatient with this 'gradual' lifestyle development, but it is enhanced lifestyle and not a quick, topical cure that Āyurveda achieves.

Chronic indigestion also needs a slow change. One week of *kicharī* (rice and beans) may be needed for those with severe conditions. Again, some people may be disinclined to make changes, but the alternatives (i.e., illnesses) are less pleasant. Eventually one finds a food plan that feels comfortable.

As discussed earlier, food essence rises through the channel to the brain, so it is crucial that wholesome foods are taken for its *sattwic* (pure) essence. Organic is also very good. *Sattwic* essence positively affects the mind. A completely *Sattwic* mind is the first stage of *samādhi* (*Saibikalpa*).

Suggested Reading

Amber, B.B. *Pulse Diagnosis*. Santa Fe, NM: Aurora Press; 1993.

Lad, V. *Āyurveda; The Science of Self Healing*. Santa Fe, NM: Lotus Press; 1984.

Murthy, K.R. Srikantha. (transl.) *Aṣhṭāñga Hṛidayam*. Varanasi, India: Krishnadas Academy; 1991.

Frawley, D. *Āyurveda Certification Course*. Santa Fe, NM: American Institute of Vedic Studies; 1992.

Frawley, D. *Āyurvedic Healing*. Salt Lake City, UT. Passage Press; 1989.

Frawley, D., Lad, V. *The Yoga of Herbs*. Santa Fe, NM: Lotus Press; 1986.

Gupta, K.R.L. *Science of Sphygmica or Sage Kanad on Pulse*. Delhi, India: Sri Satguru Publications; 1987.

Sharma, P.V. (transl.) *Charaka Saṃhitā*. Varanasi, India: Chaukhambha Orientalia; 1981.

Sharma, R.K., Dash, B. (transl.) *Charaka Saṃhitā*. Varanasi, India: Chowkhamba Sanskrit Series Office; 1992.

Sikdar, J.C. (editor/transl.) *Nāḍīvijñanam and Nāḍīprakaṣham*. Prakrit Bharti Academy: Jaipur, India; 1988.

Singh, Dr. R.H. *Pañcha Karma Therapy*. Chowkhamba Sanskrit Series: Varanasi, India; 1992.

Tirtha, S.S.S. *Spiritual Āyurveda Certification Course*. Bayville, NY: Āyurveda Holistic Center Press; 1992.

Kerala lamp

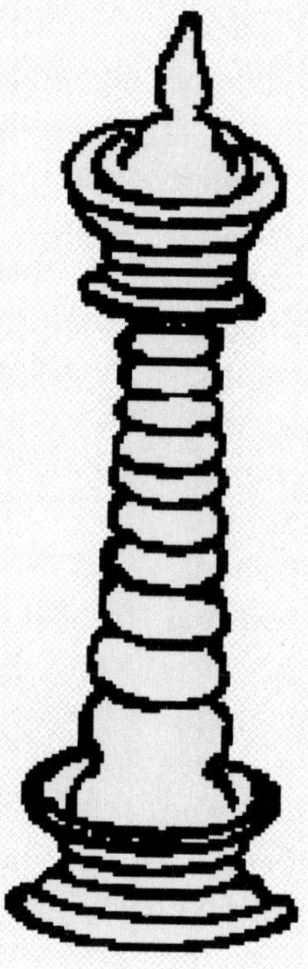

Section 3

Āyurveda Therapies

आयुर्वेद चिकित्सास्थानम

Each therapy discussed in this section reveals Āyurveda's unique "personalized" approach, in the same way the fundamentals and analysis sections revealed individualization according to the three *doṣhas*. Once learned, all other healing therapies from all other cultures may be integrated into this Āyurvedic framework, and can be made more personalized.

This section will cover the following topics :

1. Herbology
2. Nutrition
3. *Pañcha karma*
4. *Abhyañga*
5. Aromatherapy
6. *Haṭha yoga* therapy
5. Sound Therapy: *Mantras, Chakras*, Music
6. Color, Gem, and Ash Therapies
7. Lifestyle counseling and Exercise
8. Psychology, Ethics, and Spiritual Counseling

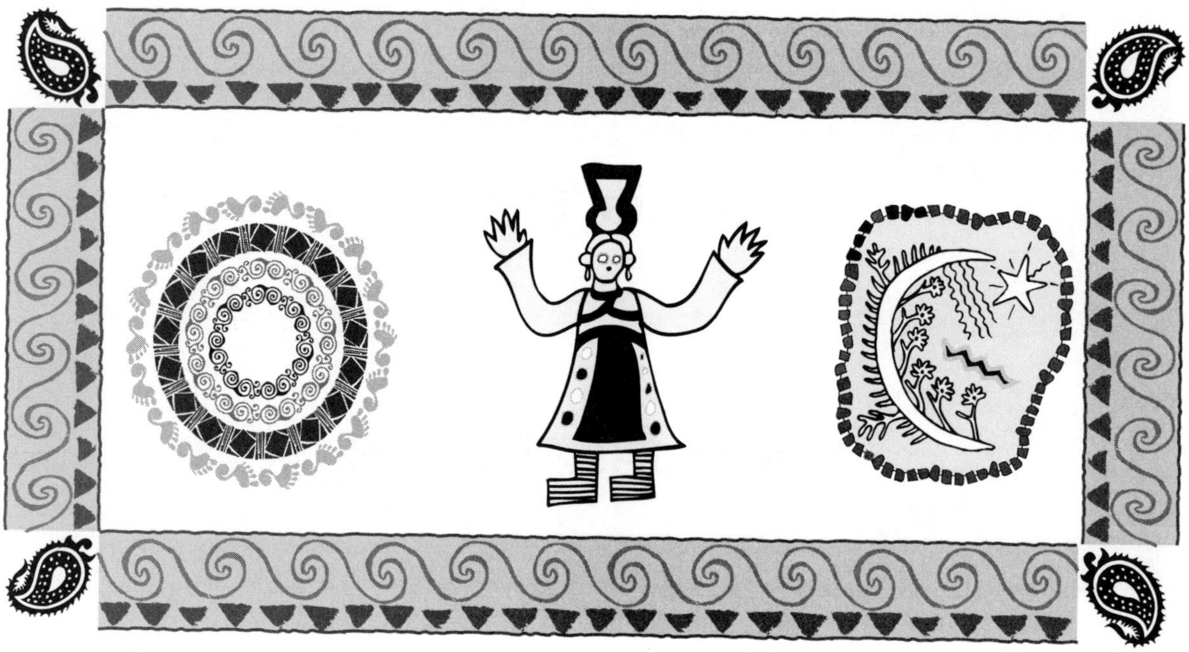

All our sorrows arise because we do not love or establish friendship with the One with whom we should. We Place our love and friendship in people instead of God.
-Swami Shankar Purushottam Tirtha

Chapter 4
Herbology

Herbology

Herbs represent the most effective Āyurvedic approach to healing illness. Their action is strongest when they are fresh, but they may also be used as decoctions, infusions, teas, powders, and pills. Pills have the least power, but retain their potency the longest. Below are some of the most commonly used Āyurvedic herbs available in America today.

Herbs are classified according to which *doṣha* they decrease and increase. Decreasing a *doṣha* is useful for a person of that body type, while an herb that increases one's *doṣha* will aggravate it. For example, a Vāyu person will be helped by ginger, a warm herb, but be irritated by goldenseal, a dry, bitter herb. This is yet another reason the Āyurvedic paradigm is so extraordinary. This personalizing aspect of Āyurveda can be integrated into all other healing systems. Here we will see an example of this by classifying some Western herbs according to the Āyurvedic framework.

Āyurveda uses herbs according to their energies or "energetics." The same five unique classifications discussed under nutrition in the last chapter also apply to herbs. Each herb has its own therapeutic effects.

1. Initial taste
2. Element
3. Heating or cooling effect
4. Post digestion effect
5. Special properties

Taste is considered therapeutic for several reasons. The *Sanskrit* word for taste is *rasa*. It means delight or essence, both of which are healing. If the taste of the food is not pleasing, the gastric fires may not digest the food, and thus proper nutrition is not received. That is why Āyurvedic cooking is a science unto itself, blending the right amount of herbs for the right taste. In our society, we have confused our sense of taste with unwholesome (artificial) objects of food, thereby creating disease.

The Six Tastes

According to Āyurveda, all foods and liquids contain six tastes: sweet, salty, sour, pungent, bitter, astringent, or combinations. As discussed in the previous chapter, each of the six tastes either increase, or decrease, each *doṣha*. To review;

Sweet: Reduces Vāyu and Pitta and increases Kapha
Sour: Reduces Vāyu and increases Pitta and Kapha
Salty: Reduces Vāyu and increases Pitta and Kapha
Pungent: Reduces Kapha and increases Pitta and Vāyu
Bitter: Reduces Pitta and Kapha and increases Vāyu
Astringent: Reduces Pitta and Kapha and increases Vāyu

Everyone needs some of each of the six tastes every day. Depending on one's constitution, however, persons mostly eat from the tastes that balance their *doṣha*. The key is moderation. In fact, a general rule of thumb in life is

Everything in moderation,
including moderation.

Physical and Mental Properties of the Six Tastes

The symbols V, P, K stand for Vāyu, Pitta, and Kapha. For example, VP- K+ is read the following way: Vāyu and Pitta are reduced; Kapha is increased.

Sweet VP- K+

Physical: Strengthens tissues, good for complexion, hair, throat, sense organs, *ojas*, children, and the elderly. It heals broken bones, effects longevity, is an emollient, expectorant, and a mild laxative. Sweet tastes build the body, increase breast milk, and are difficult to digest.

Mental: Provides contentment and is harmonizing.

In Excess: Causes overweight, indigestion, diabetes, fainting, enlarged glands, and cancer.

Salty V- PK+ (V+ in excess)

Physical: Clears channels and pores, improves digestion, produces sweat, enhances taste, penetrates tissues, causes lacerations, and bursting of tissues and abscesses.

Mental: Sedative, calms nerves, stops anxiety

In Excess: Increases blood, causes balding, gray hair, wrinkles, thirst, skin diseases, herpes, weakens body strength.

Sour V- PK+

Physical: Good for the heart, digestion, relieves burning sensations, satiating, moistens, is easily digested, oily, dispels gas, nourishes, relieves thirst, aids circulation, aids all tissues except reproductive, maintains acidity.

Mental: Awakens the mind and senses.

In Excess: Flabbiness, loss of strength, blindness, giddiness, itching irritation, pallor, herpes, swellings, smallpox, thirst, fevers.

Pungent K- P+ (V+ in excess)

Physical: Heals throat diseases, allergic rashes, skin disorders, edema, ulcer swelling; dries oiliness, fat, and water; promotes hunger, taste, and digestion; eliminates *doṣha* excesses, breaks up hard masses, expands body channels.

Mental: Opens the mind and senses.

In Excess: Causes thirst, fainting, tremors and pains, depletes reproductive fluid and strength.

Bitter PK- V+

Physical: Heals anorexia, parasites, thirst, skin disorders, fever, nausea, burning sensations, cleanses breast milk and throat, is easily digested, promotes intelligence, and is drying.

Mental: Clears the senses the emotions.

In Excess: Depletes tissues.

Astringent PK- V+

Physical: Cleanses blood, stops bleeding, sweat, diarrhea, heals ulcers, is drying, difficult to digest, causes indigestion, tightens tissues, heals prolapse.

In Excess: Causes gas, thirst, emaciation, loss of virility; obstructs channels, causes constipation and pain in the heart area, inhibits digestion.

Tastes, Energy and Properties

Hot	**Hotter**	**Hottest**
salty	sour	pungent
Cold	**Colder**	**Coldest**
sweet	astringent	bitter
Dry	**Drier**	**Driest**
astringent	bitter	pungent
Causes Constipation		
Oily	**Oilier**	**Oiliest**
sour	salty	sweet
Promotes elimination of feces, urine, and gas		
Digestibility Difficult	**More Difficult**	**Most Difficult**
salty	astringent	sweet
Digestible Easy	**Easier**	**Easiest**
sour	pungent	bitter

With this information in mind, let us look at the various therapies, beginning with herbs. For each herb, the energetic description offers the triform effect of 'taste—energy—post-digestive taste.' Below are 85 Āyurvedic herbs with uses.

85 Important Āyurvedic Herbs

1. Akarkarā
2. Ādrak (Fresh Ginger) & Śhuṇṭhī (Dry Ginger)
3. Āmalakī
4. Amlavetasa (Rhubarb)
5. Apāmārga
6. Arjuna
7. Arka
8. Aśhoka
9. Aśhwagandhā
10. Ativiṣhā
11. Bākuchī
12. Bhṛiṅgarāj
13. Balā (Indian Country Mallow)
14. Bhūtṛina (Lemon Grass)
15. Bhūāmalakī
16. Bibhītakī
17. Bilwa
18. Bola
19. Brāhmī (Gotu Kola)
20. Bṛihatī
21. Chakra Marada
22. Chāṇgerī, Amlikā
23. Chirāyatā
24. Chitrak
25. Dāruharidrā (Barberry)
26. Devadaru
27. Dhānyak (Coriander/Cilantro)
28. Dhātakī
19. Elā (Cardamom)
30. Eraṇḍa
31. Gauriphal (Red Raspberry)
32. Gokṣhura (Caltrops)
33. Guḍmār
34. Guḍūchī
35. Guggul (Indian Bedellium)
36. Haridra (Turmeric)
37. Harītakī
38. Īśhabgol (Ispaghula or Spogel Seeds)
39. Jaṭāmāṇśhī
40. Kākamāchī
41. Kākanāśhā
42. Kañchanar
43. Kaṇṭkārī
44. Kapikachhū (Ātmaguptā)
45. Kaṭukā
46. Kumari (Aloe Vera)
47. Kumkum (Saffron)
48. Kuśhā (Durba)
49. Kuṣhtha (Kūt)
50. Laghu Patha (Jal Jamnī)
51. Mamīrā (Gold Thread)
52. Mañjiṣhṭhā (Indian madder)
53. Maricha (Black Pepper)
54. Musta (Nutgrass)
55. Nāgkeśhar
56. Nimba (Neem)
57. Nirguṇḍī
58. Paṣhana Bheda
59. Pippalī (Long Pepper)
60. Pravāl (mineral)
61. Punarnavā
62. Rasonam (garlic)
63. Rechanaka (Raktam)
64. Sālam-Miśhrī
65. Sārivā
66. Sarpagandha
67. Śhaṅkh Puṣhpī
68. Śhatāvarī
69. Śhilājit (mineral)
70. Śhwetamusali (White Musali)
71. Snuhi (Vajra)
72. Tagara
73. Tejbal (Tumburu)
74. Tila
75. Trāymān
76. Tulsī (Holy Basil)
77. Twak (Cinnamon)
78. Vachā (Calamus)
79. Vaṃśha Lochana (Bamboo Manna)
80. Vārāhīkand
81. Vāsāka (Vāsāk)
82. Vatsnābh
83. Viḍaṅga
84. Vidārī Kanda
85. Yaṣhṭīmadhu (Licorice)

Ten Traditional Herb Mixtures

1. Triphalā- VPK=, for all tridoṣhic diseases, constipation, diarrhea, eyes, cleansing or detoxing the colon, good for Kapha conditions, gas, distention, diabetes, parasites.
2. Trikatu- VK- P+, for colds, flu, fevers, stimulates appetite, cough, congestion, for low *agni* and *āma*, detoxification.
3. Chyavan Prāśh- VPK=, general tonic, cough, strengthening lungs from asthma etc., long-term healing migraines, good for pregnant mothers, post partum strength, and for babies; anemia, debility, T.B.
4. Sitopaladi- VPK=, colds, flu, fevers, increases appetite, reduces burning sensations in the extremities.
5. Lavaṇ Bhaskar- VK- P+, stimulates appetite, malabsorption, constipation, abdominal pain, tumors.
6. Mahāsudarṣhan- P- VK+, for Pitta fevers, nausea, enlarged liver and spleen.
7. Daśhmūl- VPK = V-, arthritis, strengthens tissues, debility, postpartum condition of females, cold, flu, body pain, and stiffness.
8. Āvipattikar Chūrṇa- P- VPK=, used for hyperacidity, heartburn, ulcers, colitis, stomach pains, indigestion, chronic constipation.
9. Hiṅgwastāk- VPK= mainly V-, indigestion, bloating (upward-moving *apāna*).
10. Yogaraj Guggul- VK- P+ (in excess), arthritis, joint pains, stiffness, cholesterol, arteriosclerosis, rheumatism, gout, lumbago, back pain, hernia, goiter, sciatica, acts on the pituitary gland and hormone swelling, immune system, all Vāyu disorders including nerve disorders, depression, and insomnia; heals bone fractures . Good for circulation, blood purifying, reduces masses, breaks up stagnation, cardiac tonic (reduces mycocardial necrosis), antiseptic, respiratory conditions, pulmonary TB, enlarged and inflamed lymph glands, urinary disorders, endometritis, hemorrhoids, inflamed colon, hepatitis, ulcerated mouth, throat, tooth, and gum problems (gargle), skin conditions, increases white blood cell count. Do not use with acute kidney infections or acute stages of rashes. (*Kaiṣhore Guggul* for Pitta-gout, burning joints, herpes, and all blood diseases; Pure *Guggul* for Kapha. They have similar actions).

[VPK= means good for all *doṣhas*]

Empowering Herbs

When herbs are mixed or prepared, a *bīj* (seed) *mantra* is often recited to empower the herb's properties by enlivening all five elements: ether, air, fire, water, and earth. *Bīj* are the essence of all other *mantras.* Thus of all the *mantras* they have the most power. One such *mantra* is

Om Īng Hrīng Śhrīng
Klīng Sanga Śhamboah Namah

This *mantra* can be repeated once, seven, 31, or 108 times. It may also be repeated in intervals of 108 times. The number 108 is a mystical number in the *Vedic* sciences. Thus, chanting 108 times further empowers the herbs.

An Āyurvedic Story

Two brothers came to their guru. "Baba," said one brother, "our Pitta is excessive in our mouths. Thus, we always argue with each other. Please give us some Āyurvedic medicine to relieve our aggravated Pitta."

Their guruji responded, "Whenever you feel the Pitta rising, each of you are to take a mouthful of water. Neither swallow nor spit it out, as water calms fire and the fire is in the mouth. So long as you keep the water in the mouth, you will not be plagued by arguing."

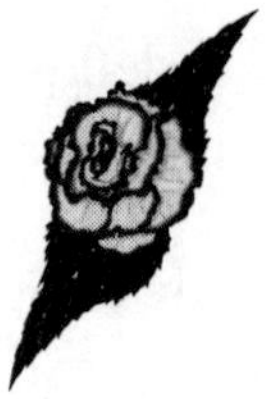

Āyurvedic Materia Medica

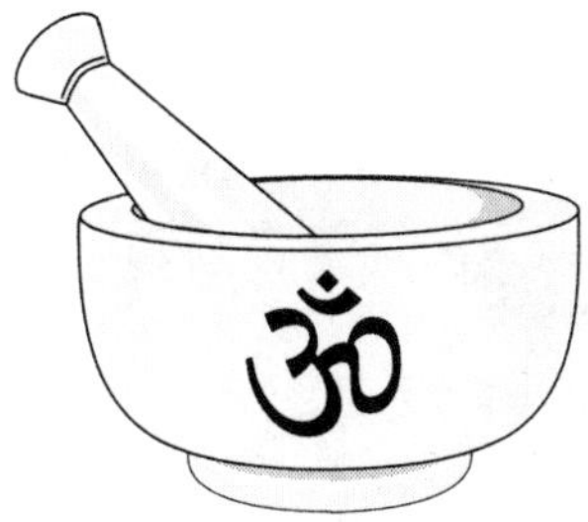

Under the energetics category, the symbols V, P, K stand for *Vāyu*, *Pitta* and *Kapha* respectively. A '+' means an herb increases the *doṣha*, a '-' means the herb reduces the *doṣha*. '=' means it is good for all three *doṣhas*.

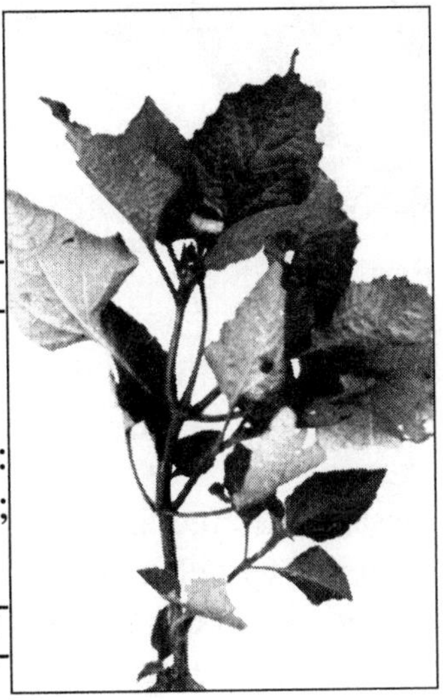

Sanskrit: **Akarkarā**

अकरकरा

Hindi: Akarakara
English: Pellitory
Latin: Anacyclus pyrethrum DC. (Pyrethrum radix)
Part Used: Root
Habitat: Himalayas: 3,000-12,000 feet; Bengal, Arabia
Energetics: pungent/hot/pungent VK- P+
Tissues: Nerves, bones
Systems: Nervous, excretory, reproductive
Action: Stimulant, sialagogue, nerve tonic
Uses: Nerve disorders, bowel conditions, seminal debility, gargle for tooth problems (e.g., toothache), sore throat and tonsils; paralysis, hemiplegia, epilepsy, rheumatism, promotes talking in retarded children, with honey for epilepsy (internal and as snuff), diabetes. Promotes saliva.
Preparation: Powders, pills, paste

Sanskrit: **Ārdrakam/Śhuṇṭha (Śhuṇṭhī)**

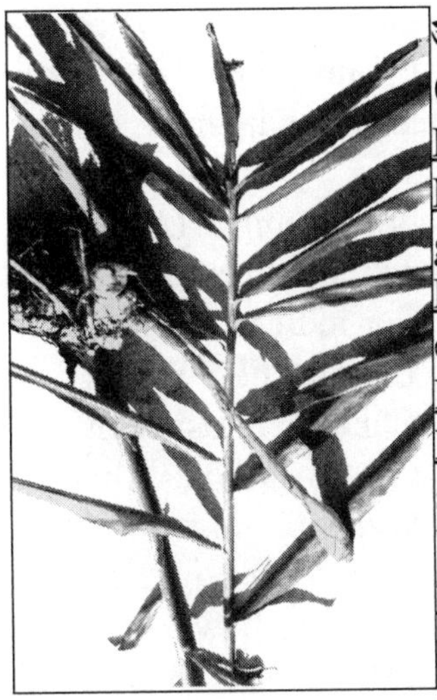

आद्रकम ॥ शुण्ठ (शुण्ठी)

Hindi: Ādrak/Suṇṭh
English: Fresh Ginger/dry Ginger
Latin: Zingiberis officinale roscoe.
Part Used: Rhizomes
Energetics: Pungent, sweet-hot-sweet VK- P+
Tissues: All
Systems: Digestive, respiratory
Action: Analgesic, anti-emetic, aromatic, aphrodisiac, carminative, diaphoretic, digestive, expectorant, nervine, sialagogue, stimulant.
Uses: Ginger is truly a wonder drug, having so many healing properties. It was called the universal medicine. Taken with rock salt it reduces Vāyu; with rock candy it reduces Pitta; with honey it reduces Kapha.

Fresh: Mixed juice with water and cane sugar, boiled to a syrup—add saffron and powders of cardamom, nutmeg, and clove and preserve well. This ginger-jam, called *Allaepauk*, is useful indigestion, flatulence, colic, vomiting, spasms, stomach and bowel pains with fever, colds, cough, asthma, and increasing *Pachaka Agni* (responsible for digestion).

For indigestion, mix equal parts juice with lemon juice and rock salt (found in Indian groceries), and take just before meals. Taking the juice with rock salt, before meals, cleanses the throat and tongue, and increases the appetite. For bile and delirium due to biliousness, take ginger juice with cow's milk (2:7 ratio), boil to half volume and add rock-candy powder, and take before bed. Or mix juice with mango juice, cane sugar, and cow *ghee*; mix and melt to half the quantity and take mornings and evenings.

For sore throats, hoarseness, and laryngitis, sometimes chewing a piece of fresh ginger produces saliva and soothes these conditions. Juice rubbed on navel relieves diarrhea. Ginger and onion juice relieve nausea, vomiting, and retching. Juice with rock candy (twice daily) remedies diabetes (mellitus and insipidus), For nervous headache, mix ginger juice with milk, let dry, and use as snuff.

Dry: With black and long peppers (*trikatu*) it is a carminative. Added to purgatives, it prevents nausea and the gripe. For indigestion and low appetite, mix with *ghee* or hot water. With painful bowels or stomach make an infusion of dry ginger, and mix with 1-2 tbs. castor oil. Alternatively, mix some *asafoetida* with ginger powder. For chronic rheumatic pain (Vāyu or Kapha), colds, excess mucus, take ginger powder tea before bed, and cover up with blankets to promote sweating. In cases of headaches, make a paste of ginger and aloe gel or water, and apply to the head and take a nap or before evening sleep. The same paste may be applied to the face for tooth or face aches. For headaches caused by nerves, mix a paste of ginger, cinnamon, castor root, and cloves (equal parts); and apply to the head.

For fainting, apply a thin paste of ginger and water to the eyelids, or place a mix of *sunṭh*, black pepper and *pippalī* under the nostrils in small pinches. This will also help stupor, delirium and senselessness caused by brain fever.

Other uses: Arthritis, belching, heart disease, laryngitis (use as a tea and an external paste on throat), vomiting, constipation, strengthens memory, removes obstructions in the vessels, incontinence, flatulence, colic, spasms, fever, eye diseases, and asthma. Juice is better for colds, cough, vomiting, deranged Vāyu, and as a diaphoretic. Dry ginger is better for increasing *agni* and reducing Kapha.

Spiritual Uses: Most *sattwic* (spiritually pure) spice

Precautions: Aggravates Pitta (i.e., inflamed skin diseases, fever, bleeding, ulcers, etc.)

Preparation: Fresh juice, infusion, decoction, powder, pill, paste

Sanskrit: **Āmalakī** (meaning: the nurse)

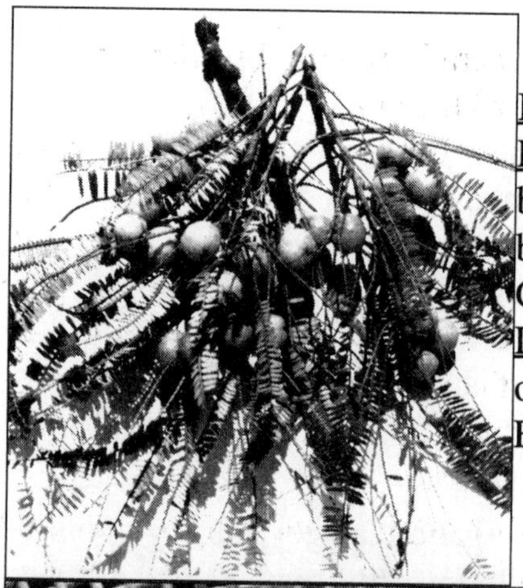

आमलकी

Hindi: Āmla

English: Emblic myrobalan; Indian Gooseberry

Latin: Emblica officinalis Euphorbiaceae

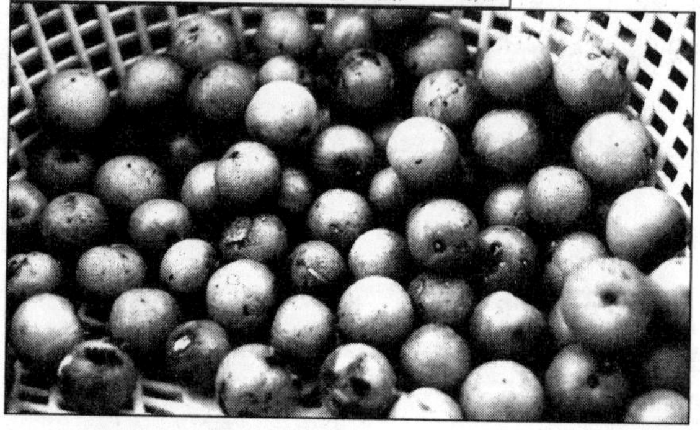

Part Used: Fruit

Habitat: Himalayas, sea coasts, Kashmir, Deccan

Energetics: Mostly sour, but include all tastes (except salty)-cold-sweet VP- (K+ and *āma* in excess)

Tissues: All; increases *ojas*

Systems: Circulatory, digestive, excretory

Action: Aphrodisiac, astringent, hemostatic, laxative, nutritive tonic, refrigerant, rejuvenative (for Pitta), stomachic

Uses: All Pitta diseases, all obstinate urinary conditions, anemia, biliousness, bleeding, colitis, constipation, convalescence from fever, diabetes, gastritis, gout, hair (premature gray/balding), hepatitis, hemorrhoids, liver weakness, mental disorders, osteoporosis, palpitation, spleen weakness, tissue deficiency, vertigo; rebuilds blood, bones, cells, and tissues. It increases red blood cell count and regulates blood sugar; heart tonic, cleanses mouth, stops gum bleeding, stops stomach and colon inflammation; cleanses intestines, strengthens teeth, aids eyesight, highest natural source of vitamin C (3,000 mg per fruit), worms, acidity, eye and lung in-

flammations, ulcerations, G.I. disorders, painful urination, internal bleeding.
Spiritual benefits: It is *sattwic* (pure) in quality, gives love, longevity, and good fortune. For mothers who behave angrily towards their children, it calms and balances their emotions. For children who have lost their mother, it fills them with the sense that their mother is there. Thus, *āmalakī* has another name, *dhatri,* meaning "mother" in *Sanskrit*
Precautions: May cause acute diarrhea in Pitta *doṣhas.* Pregnancy
Prepared: Decoction, powder (1/4-3 tsp.), sweets

Sanskrit: **Amla-vetasa**, Aml Parni
अम्ल वेतस

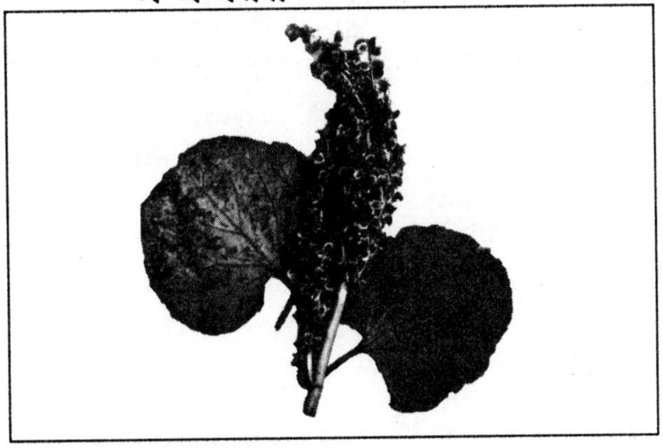

Hindi: Revand-chini, Archu
English: Rhubarb
Latin: Rheum emodi Wall., (R. officinale, R. acuminatum, R. speciforme, R. webbianum, R. moorcroftianum, R australe).
Part Used: Root (dried rhizomes)
Habitat: Himalayas: 8,000-13,000 feet; Kashmir, Nepal, Sikkim, Bhutan, China, Tibet, Russia, Turkey, and many other countries
Energetics: Bitter-cold-pungent PK- V+
Tissues: Plasma, blood, fat
Systems: Excretory, digestive
Action: Purgative, alterative, hemostatic, antipyretic, anthelmintic, stomachic, bitter tonic, cathartic, laxative, atonic indigestion
Uses: Constipation (with fevers, ulcers, infections), diarrhea, Pitta dysentery, jaundice, liver disorders. One of the best purgatives (milder than senna), protects colon tone, used with licorice and psyllium in older and dryer persons (ginger or fennel is added to remove griping action—4 parts rhubarb:1 part ginger or fennel); purges bile, *āma*, stagnant food and blood; reduces weight and fat; is safe for children (also for teething and nutritional balancing), atonic dyspepsia, or indigestion; duodenal catarrh. It is stronger when used with epsom salt.
Preparation: Infusion, powder (1 gm.—laxative; 3 gms.—purgative), pill
Precaution: Pregnancy, chronic diarrhea, chills, not for Vāyu hemorrhoids; not used with gout, rheumatism, epilepsy, or uric acid diseases. It turns the urine yellow but there is no cause for concern

Sanskrit: **Apāmārga**
अपामार्ग

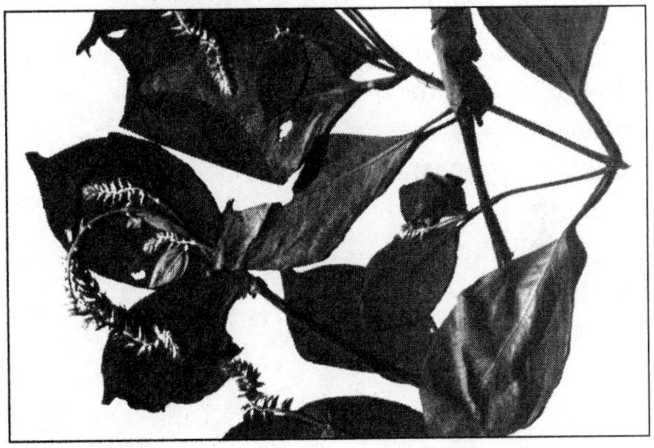

Hindi: Apamara
English: Rough Chaff Tree, Prickly Chaff Flower
Latin: Achyranthes aspera Linn.
Part Used: Herb, leaves, seeds, root flower (whole plant)
Habitat: Small herb throughout India under 4,000 feet
Energetics:
Tissues: Plasma, blood, fat, nerves
Systems: Circulation, digestion, nervous
Action: Diuretic, expectorant, antibilious
Uses: Decoction; diuretic for renal edema, stomach ache, hemorrhoids, boils, skin eruptions;

with honey or rock candy for early stages of diarrhea and dysentery; leaves mixed with *jaggery* or black pepper into a paste as pills for fevers, cough, insect bites, and bee stings. Leaf juice applied to skin for overexposure to the sun. Leaves or seeds are used for poisonous animal bites. Seeds are used as an expectorant, or mixed with rice water for bleeding hemorrhoids. *Khīr* or *Pāyasam* with seeds in milk for brain diseases. Seeds soaked in yogurt/water overnight and ground into an emulsion the next morning heals bilious complaints.
Preparation: Decoction, powder, paste, oil, infusion
Precaution: Do not use while pregnant

Sanskrit: **Arjuna**
अर्जुन

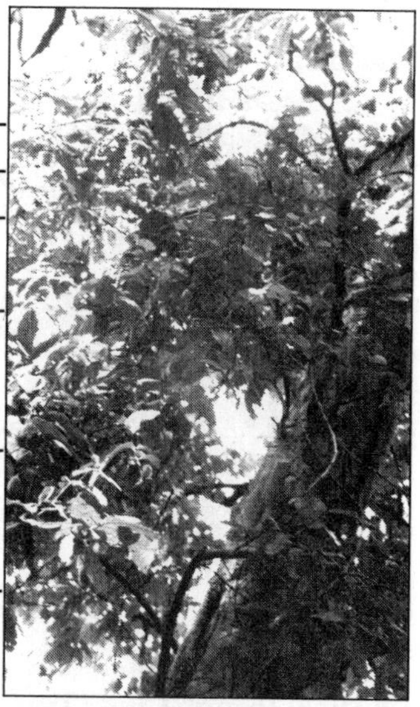

Hindi: Arjun
Latin: Terminalia arjuna W. & A., Pentaptera glabra; P. angustifolia
English: Arjuna Myrobalan
Part Used: Bark
Energetics: Astringent-cold-sweet VPK=
Tissues: Reproductive, plasma, blood
Systems: Digestive, circulatory, reproductive
Action: Cardiac stimulant, rejuvenative, astringent, hemostatic, alterative
Uses: Best herb for heart disease (prevents and helps in the recovery of), angina, heals heart tissue scars after surgery, bile, edema, fractures, contusions, broken bones, diarrhea, malabsorption, venereal disease, heals tissues. Externally—ulcers, acne, skin disorders.
Spiritual Uses: May help the spiritual heart
Preparation: Decoction, herbal wine, powder (1/4-3 tsp.)

Sanskrit: **Arka**
अर्क

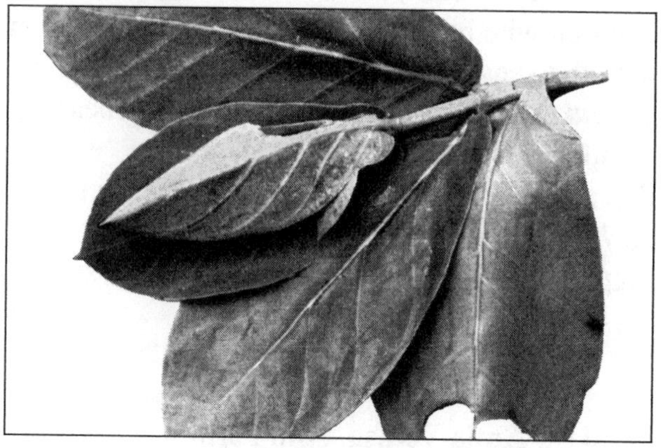

Hindi: Aka
English: Gigantic Swallowort
Latin: Caltropis gigantea R. Br.
Part Used: Root, root bark, leaves, juice, and flowers [two varieties; purple/red flowered or white flowered (C. procera)]
Habitat: Shrub is mainly found in wastelands in lower Bengal, Himalayas, Punjab, Assam, Madras, South India, Sri Lanka, Singapore, Malay Islands, South China
Energetics: Bitter
Tissues: Plasma, muscles, fat, nerves
Systems: Digestion, circulation, nervous, urinary, water metabolism
Action: Special care is taken while using this herb, as it is poisonous. Mucilaginous, digestive, stomachic, tonic, antispasmodic, emetic (large doses), diaphoretic, (root bark—alterative), purgative, expectorant, anthelmintic, acrid, antiparasitical
Uses: Promotes secretion (especially of bile), intestinal muscle sedative, heart (used like digitalis), phlegm purge, depilatory, parasitic infection, reduces pain, difficult/painful urination, skin diseases, abdominal disorders, dysentery, syphilis, fevers with enlarged liver and cough; intermittent fevers, hemorrhoids, edema. Leaves are for paralysis, anesthesia, and toxic asthma. Flowers—digestive tonic and stomachic, small

doses stimulate capillaries, skin (including elephantiasis, leprosy), asthma. Milky juice—violent purgative, G.I. irritant.
Preparation: Paste, powder, pill
Precaution: Special care is to be taken while using this herb, as it is poisonous. Do not use while pregnant. Use only with the advice of an Āyurvedic specialist

Sanskrit: **Aśhoka**
अशोक

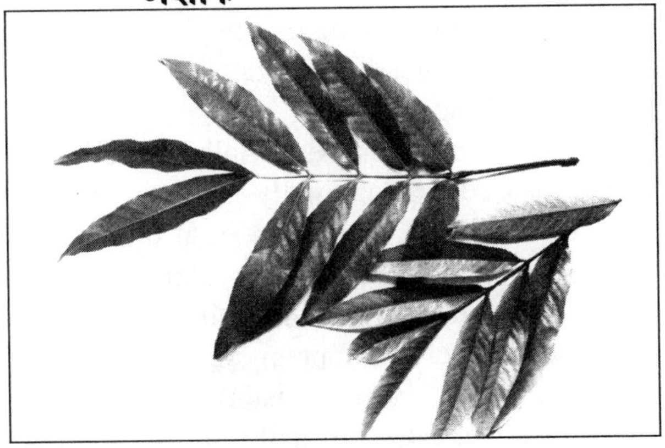

Hindi: Aśhoka, Anganapriya
English: Ashoka Tree
Latin: Saraca indica Linn.
Part Used: Bark
Habitat: Found throughout India; cultivated in gardens for its beautiful flowers
Energetics: pungent, astringent-cold-sweet
Tissues: Blood, fat, reproductive
Systems: Reproductive
Action: Astringent
Uses: A major herb for the uterus; sedative; uterine/ovarian fibroid and tumors, menorrhagia, bleeding hemorrhoids, bleeding dysentery.
Preparation: Decoction, powder, pill, *ghee*, paste, herbal wine
Precaution: May aggravate arrhythmia

Sanskrit: **Aśhwagandhā** (vitality of the horse)
अश्वगन्धा
Hindi: Aśhgandh
Latin: Withania somnifera dunal (Physalis flexu-

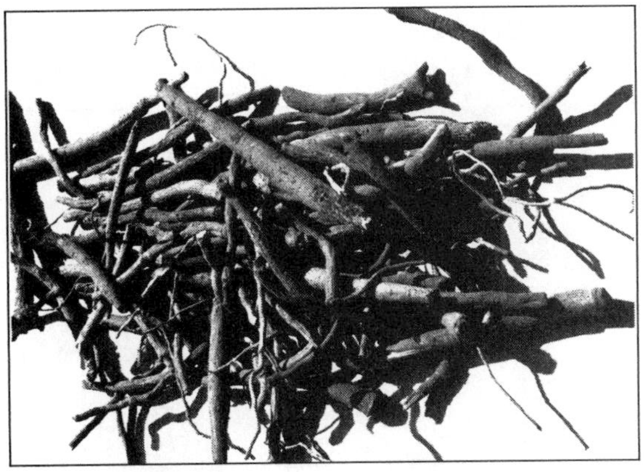

osa); Solanaceae
English: Winter cherry
Part Used: Root
Habitat: This shrub is in Himalayas, 6,000 feet; common in Bombay, Western India, sometimes in Bengal
Energetics: Astringent, bitter, sweet-hot-sweet VK- (P and *āma* + in excess)
Tissues: Muscle, fat, bone, marrow/nerves, reproductive
Systems: Nervous, reproductive, respiratory
Action: Aphrodisiac, astringent, nervine, rejuvenative, sedative, tonic
Uses: AIDS, general debility, nerve exhaustion, convalescence, problems of the elderly, sexual debility, emaciation, memory loss, muscle energy loss, marrow, overwork, tissue deficiency (and promotes tissue healing), insomnia, paralysis, MS, weak eyes, rheumatism, skin afflictions, cough, difficult breathing, anemia, fatigue, infertility, swollen glands, immune system problems, alcoholism, lumbago. Known as Indian ginseng, builds marrow and semen; inhibits aging; one of the best herbs for the mind (clarity, nurturing). Externally—skin diseases, obstinate ulcers, carbuncles, rheumatic swellings. For women, it stabilizes fetus, regenerates hormones, cancer—strengthens one from and for chemotherapy.
Spiritual Uses: *Sattwic*, produces *ojas*
Precautions: Do not take if congested. For cancer and other serious illness, use one or more ounces daily
Preparation: Decoctions, *ghee*, oil, powder (1/4-3 tsp.) herbal wine

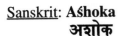

Sanskrit: **Ativiṣhā**

अतिविषा

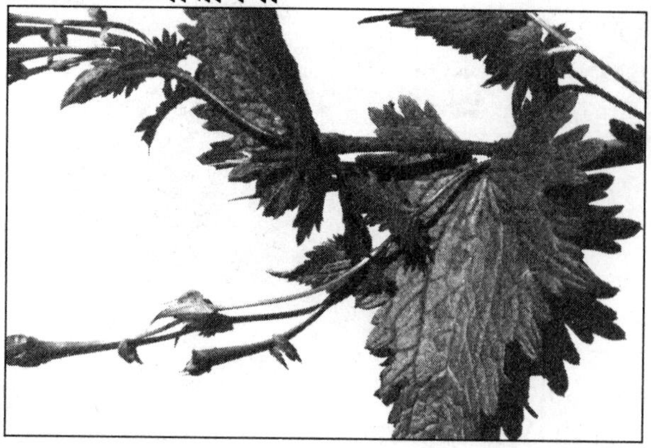

Hindi: Atīs; Atis
English: Indian Atees
Latin: Aconitum hetrophyleum Wall. (A. Cordatum.)
Part Used: Dried tuberous roots
Habitat: Sub-alpine and alpine regions; Himalayas from Indus to Kumaon
Energetics: Bitter, astringent VPK=
Tissues: Plasma, blood
Systems: Digestive, immune, respiratory
Action: Tonic, stomachic, antiperiodic, aphrodisiac, carminative
Uses: Hemorrhoids, vomiting, edema, liver disorders, Kapha and Pitta diseases; convalescing after fever, debility, diarrhea, dysentery, acute inflammations, cough, indigestion, chronic fevers, with honey for coryza.
Preparation: Tincture, decoction, powder

Sanskrit: **Bākuchī**

बाकुची

Hindi: Babchi
English: Babchi Seeds
Latin: Psoralea corylifolia Linn.
Part Used: Seeds
Habitat: Common herbaceous weed found in Bengal, Bombay, throughout the Indian plains
Energetics: Pungent, bitter-hot (or cold)-pungent, bitter VKP= (P+ in excess)
Tissues: Muscles, plasma, blood

Systems: Respiratory, circulatory, muscular, lymphatic
Action: Aromatic, anthelmintic, antibacterial, antifungal, diuretic, diaphoretic, laxative, stimulant, aphrodisiac
Uses: Skin conditions—especially leukoderma, psoriasis (used both internally and as an external paste or ointment), fevers, internal ulcers, bile conditions, improves the color of skin (including removing white spots), hair, nails; tones liver, spleen, and pancreas; impotency, frequent or involuntary urine, cold or painful extremities, joints, or lower back; difficulty breathing, diarrhea, abdominal pain.
Precautions: May increase Pitta when taken alone; do not take with low body fluids; do not use with licorice root
Preparation: Five grams powder twice daily before meals with some coriander and honey (to taste); as an external paste

Sanskrit: **Balā** (meaning: strength giving)

बला

Hindi: Bariar
English: Country Mallow
Latin: Sida cordifolia Linn. (S. herbacea, S. rotundifolia, S. althaeitolia.)
Part Used: Root
Habitat: Grows wild along roadsides throughout the tropical and sub-tropical plains of India and Sri Lanka
Energetics: Sweet-cold-sweetVPK=(K and *āma*

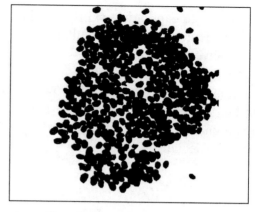

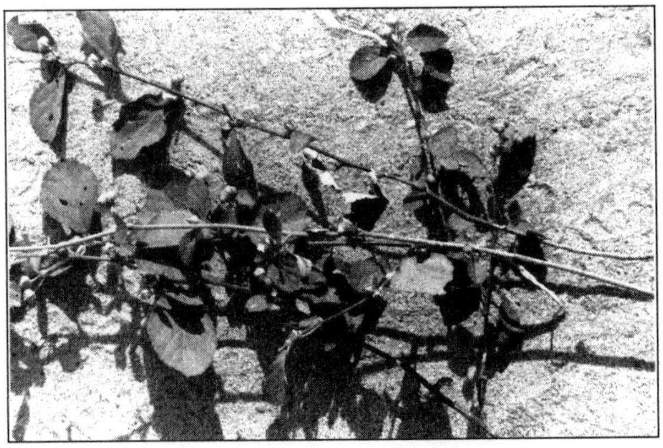

+ in excess)
Tissues: All—especially marrow/nerves
Systems: Circulatory, nervous, reproductive, urinary, respiratory
Action: Analgesic, aphrodisiac, demulcent, diuretic, nervine, rejuvenative, stimulant, tonic, vulnerary
Uses: Heart disease and stimulant; facial paralysis, heals tissues of chronic inflammation, sciatica, insanity, neuralgia and nerve inflammation; removes deep seated and intermittent fevers (with ginger), chronic rheumatism, asthma, bronchitis, emaciation, exhaustion, sexual debility, cystitis, dysentery, leukorrhea, chronic fevers, convalescence, arthritis. Externally it is good for numbness, nerve pain, muscle cramps, skin disorders, tumors, joint diseases, wounds, and ulcers. For cancer, it strengthens persons before and after chemotherapy.
Precautions: Do not take in excess if congested
Preparation: Decoction, powder, medicated oil. For serious illness like cancer, use one or more ounces daily

Sanskrit: **Bhṛiṅgarāj** (or Keśharāja)
भृंगराज
Hindi: Bhangra (meaning, "ruler the hair")
English: None
Latin: Eclipta alba Hassk. or Eclipta erecta Linn.
Parts used: Herb, roots, leaves
Habitat: Throughout India and the southwestern U.S.
Energetics: Bitter, astringent, sweet/cold/ sweet
VPK=

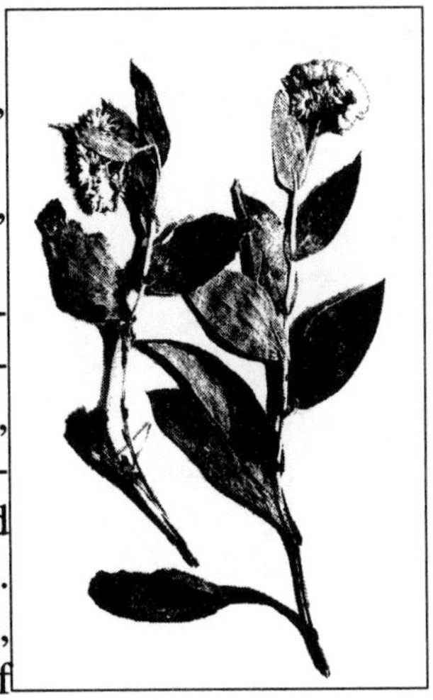

Tissues: Blood, bone, marrow, plasma
Systems: Circulatory, digestive, nervous
Actions: Herbs—alterative, antipyretic, hemostatic, laxative, nervine, rejuvenative, tonic, vulnerary. Roots and leaves are cholagogues. Root—tonic, alterative, emetic, purgative. Leaf juice—hepatic tonic and deobstruent
Uses: This is the main herb for the hair and cirrhosis. It prevents aging, maintains and rejuvenates hair, teeth, bones, memory, sight, and hearing. It is a rejuvenative for Pitta, kidneys, and liver. As an oil, it removes graying, balding, makes the hair darker, and promotes deep sleep. Externally, it draws out poisons and reduces inflammations and swollen glands. It also improves complexion.

The root powder is used for hepatitis, enlarged spleen, and skin disorders. Mixed with salt, it relieves burning urine. Mixed with a little oil and applied to the head, it relieves headache.

Two drops of expressed juice is mixed with eight drops raw honey and given to newborn children with colds and excess mucus. Mixed with castor oil, it removes worms. Juice placed in the ears removes earaches. A leaf decoction is useful for uterine hemorrhaging (two to four ounces twice daily). Leaf paste applied to swollen glands and skin conditions helps them to heal. Leaf juice boiled in coconut oil makes a hair oil to remove gray hair and balding.

For pitariasis, alopecia, and other skin diseases: *Bhṛiṅgarāj* (16 parts), *triphalā, arka,* and *sārivā* (all equal parts) are all mixed with four times as much sesame oil and boiled into a medicated oil.
Preparations: Infusions, decoction, powder, medicated oil and *ghee*
Precautions: Can cause severe chills

Sanskrit: **Bhūtṛiṇ**

भूतृण

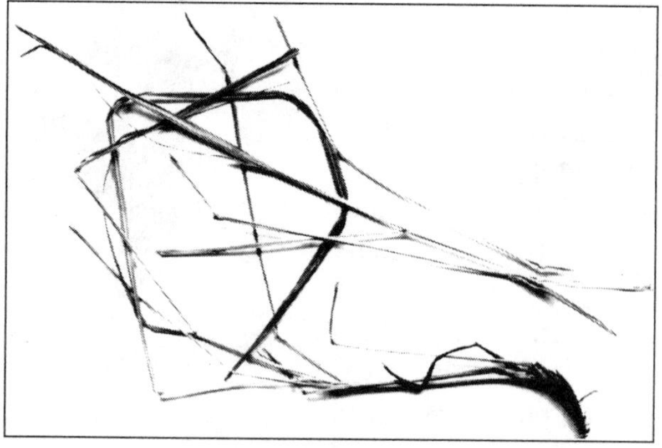

Hindi: Gandhatrana, Harī-chaha
English: Lemon grass
Latin: Andropogon citratus DC. (A. Shoenanthus)
Part Used: Essential oil, herb
Habitat: Grows wild in gardens in India, Sri Lanka and other tropics, in cultivated areas
Energetics: Pungent, bitter-cold-pungent PK- (V+ excess)
Tissues: Fat, nerves
Systems: Nervous, metabolic
Action: Antispasmodic, diaphoretic, diuretic, emmenagogue, stimulant; oil— carminative, refrigerant, stomachic, tonic
Uses: Bowel spasms, colic, diarrhea, dysmenorrhea (neuralgic), fever, gas, colds, G.I. spasms, intestinal mucus membrane tonic and stimulant; vomiting. Oil/external—bath, perfume, and hair oils; with coconut for lumbago, rheumatism, neuralgia, sprains, pains, ringworm; excellent tea for Pitta and kidneys.
Precautions: None
Preparation: Infusion or decoction of leaves, powder

Sanskrit: **Bhūāmalakī**

भूआमलकी

Hindi: Bhūy āmalakī; Niruri
English: None
Latin: Phyllanthus niruri Linn. (P. urinaria)

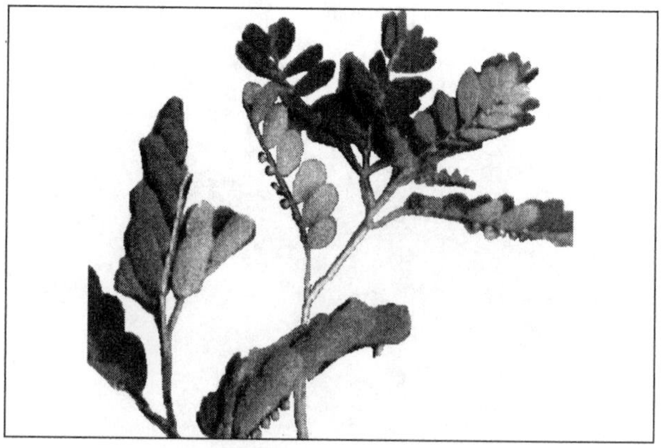

Part Used: Leaves, root, whole plant
Habitat: A perennial herb in Central and Southern India, to Sri Lanka
Energetics: PK- V+
Tissues: Semen, plasma, blood, fat
Systems: Digestive, reproductive, urinary
Action: Bitter, astringent, de-obstruent, stomachic
Uses: The main herb for the liver; colitis, certain edema, gonorrhea, menorrhagia, urogenital diseases, dysentery, diabetes, dyspepsia; jaundice. Externally—poultice for ulcers, inflammations, sores, swellings, itch and other skin diseases; spongy and bleeding gums; uvulitis, tonsillitis.
Preparation: Infusion, juice, poultice, powder, pill

Sanskrit: **Bibhītakī**

बिब्हीतकी

Hindi: Bhaira
English: Beleric Myrobalan
Latin: Terminalia belerica Roxb.
Part Used: Fruit
Habitat: A tree found throughout the Indian forests and plains
Energetics: Astringent-hot-sweet KP-(V+ in excess)
Tissues: Plasma, mus-

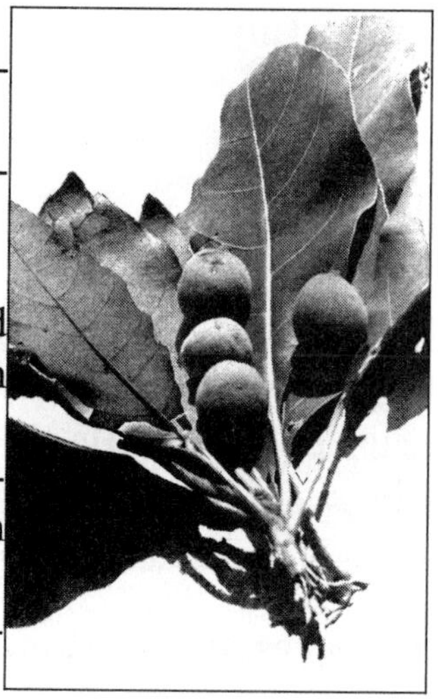

cle, bone
Systems: Digestive, excretory, nervous, respiratory
Action: Anthelmintic, antiseptic, astringent, expectorant, laxative, lithotriptic, rejuvenative, tonic
Uses: Nausea, cold, vomiting, cough, bronchitis, catarrh, chronic diarrhea, dysentery, eye disorders, laryngitis, headache, hemorrhoids, parasites, stones, Kapha digestive disorders, urinary tract stones, stomach, liver disorders, G.I. tract diseases, increases appetite; mixed with honey it is good for sore throats and voice (or used as a gargle). Brain and stomach tonic, Part of the *triphalā* formula. Externally—as an antiseptic lotion; paste for Pitta swellings, eye diseases; dried ripe fruit—edema; with honey for ophthalmia.
Preparation: Infusion, decoction, powder, paste
Precaution: High Vāyu

Sanskrit: **Bilwa** बिल्व

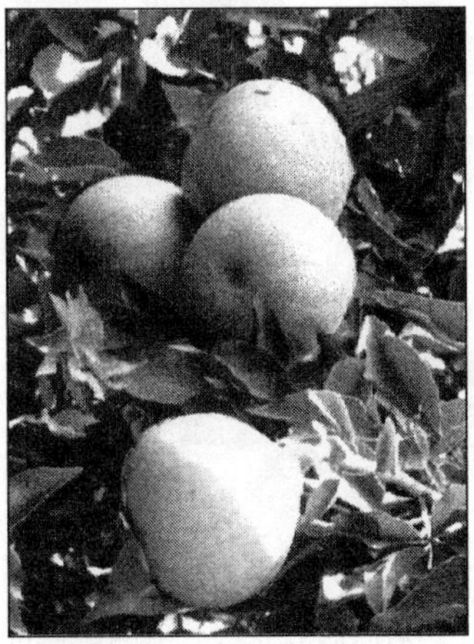

Hindi: Belaphal
English: Bael Fruit
Latin: Aegle marmelos Corr.
Part Used: Fruit, root-bark, leaves, rind, flowers
Habitat: Throughout India from the sub-Himalayan forests to Burma (Myanmar)
Energetics: Sweet/cooling; bitter/pungent (fresh juice) VPK=
Tissues: Plasma, blood, nerves, semen
Systems: Circulatory, digestive, reproductive, nervous
Action: Aromatic, alterative, nutritive, astringent; hemostatic, tonic, laxative, digestive stimulant, stomachic, stimulant, antipyretic, aphrodisiac, antibilious, febrifuge, antiparasitical
Uses: Unripe is better than ripe; heart, stomach, Kapha disorders, intestinal tonic, chronic constipation and dysentery; some forms of indigestion; mucus membrane, chronic, obstinate mucus and catarrhal diarrhea; early stages of sprue and consumption; typhoid, debility, intestinal disorders, prevents cholera and hemorrhoids; intermittent fever (stem bark); hypochondria, melancholia, heart palpitation. Leaf poultice is applied to inflammations; with black pepper for edema, constipation, and jaundice; with water or honey it is good for catarrh and fever. Rind is used for acute and amoebic dysentery, griping pain in the loins and constipation, gas, and colic; sprue, scurvy. Pulp heals Vāyu, Kapha, *āma*, and colic, is constipative.

Sanskrit: **Bola** बोल

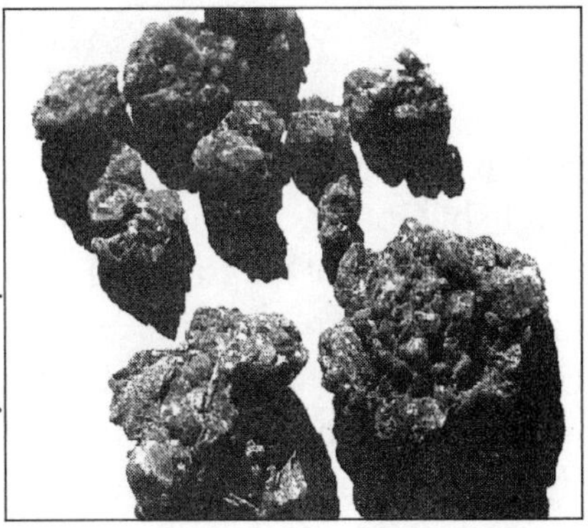

Hindi: Bol
English: Myrrh
Latin: Balasmodendron myrrha Nees. (Commiphora Myrrha)
Part Used: Resin
Habitat: Indigenous to North-East Africa, collected in Southern Arabia and Iran
Energetics: Bitter, astringent, pungent, sweet-heating-pungent KV- (P+ in excess)
Tissues: All
Systems: Circulatory, lymphatic, nervous, reproductive, respiratory
Action: Alterative, analgesic, antiseptic, antispasmodic, emmenagogue, expectorant, stimulant, rejuvenative

Uses: Amenorrhea, anemia, arthritis, asthma, bronchitis, cough, dysmenorrhea, menopause, rheumatism, traumatic injuries, ulcerated surfaces, as an infusion with rose petals (50 parts) used as a mouthwash, mouth inflammations, as a gargle for spongy gums, used in tooth powder, indigestion, wasting diseases, prevents loss of hair, menstrual disorders, and chlorosis problems of young girls.
Precautions: Can create excess Pitta
Preparation: Infusion, powder, pill, paste

Sanskrit: **Brāhmī**- best type: *Than Kuni* (meaning: Divine creative energy)

ब्राह्मी

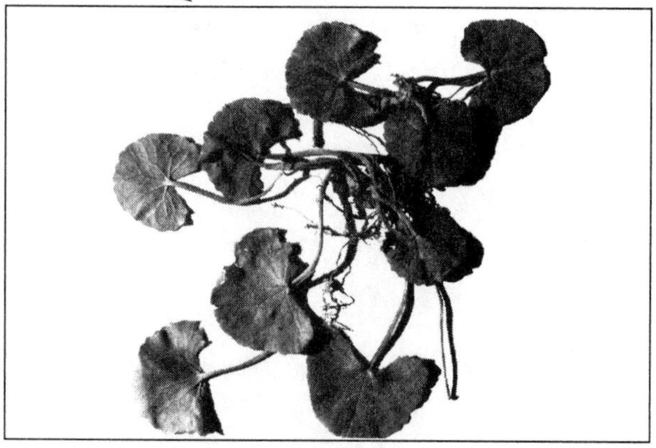

Hindi: Brahma-manduki
English: Gotu Kola, Indian Pennywort
Latin: Hydrocotyle asiatica Linn. Umbelliferae
Part Used: Herb
Habitat: Common throughout India and the world, in shaded, watery places.
Energetics: Bitter-cold-sweet VPK=
Tissues: All except reproductive; mainly blood, marrow, nerve
Systems: Circulatory, digestive, nervous, respiratory, reproductive, excretory
Action: Alterative, diuretic, febrifuge, nervine, rejuvenative
Uses: Adrenal purifier, AIDS, blood purifier, eczema, epilepsy, insanity, hypochondria, fevers (intermittent), hair loss, immune system boost (cleansing and nourishing), liver, longevity, memory, nervous disorders, psoriasis, senility, skin conditions (chronic and obstinate), venereal diseases, tetanus, convulsions, rheumatism, elephantiasis, bowel disorders. Best rejuvenative herb for brain cells and nerves, intelligence.
Spiritual Uses: The most *sattwic* herb
Precautions: Large doses may cause headaches, spaciness, or itching
Preparation: Infusion, decoction, powder, *ghee*, oil

Sanskrit: **Bṛihatī**

बृहती

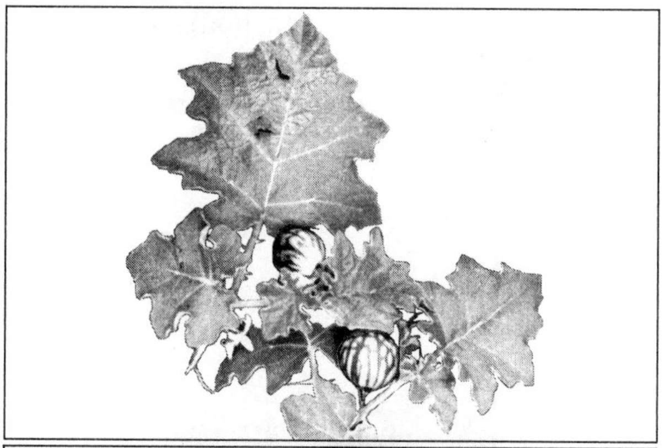

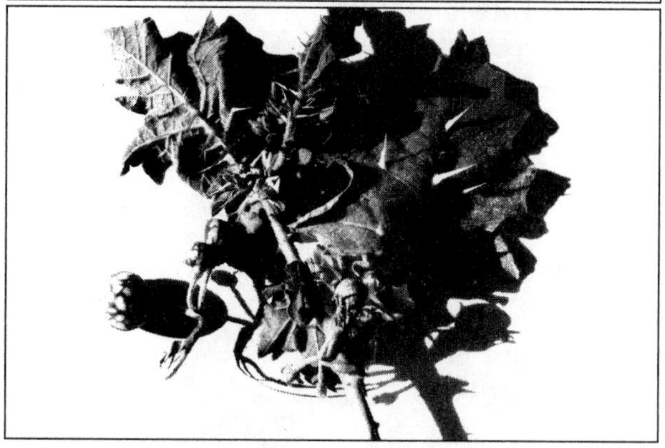

Hindi: Kaṇṭakārī, Birhatta
English: Indian Nightshade
Latin: Solanum indicum Linn.
Part Used: Fruit, root, plant, seeds
Habitat: Common throughout India
Energetics: Astringent
Tissues: Plasma, blood, reproductive
Systems: Respiratory, reproductive, urinary, circulatory
Action: Plant—cordial, aphrodisiac, astringent, carminative, cardiac tonic, resolvent; root—diu-

retic, expectorant, stimulant, diaphoretic.
Uses: Asthma, dry and spasmodic cough; difficult childbirth, chronic fevers, chest pains, colic, gas, worms, scorpion stings, difficult urination, edema, enlarged and spleen; catarrh. Burning seed smoke is used for toothache (it is usually used along with other herbs). The root is one of the *daśhmūl* ingredients, and is usually mixed with other roots. It is good for edema, cough, mucus. Decoctions help dysuria.
Preparation: Decoction, powder

Sanskrit: **Chakra Marda** (ringworm destroyer)
चक्र मर्द

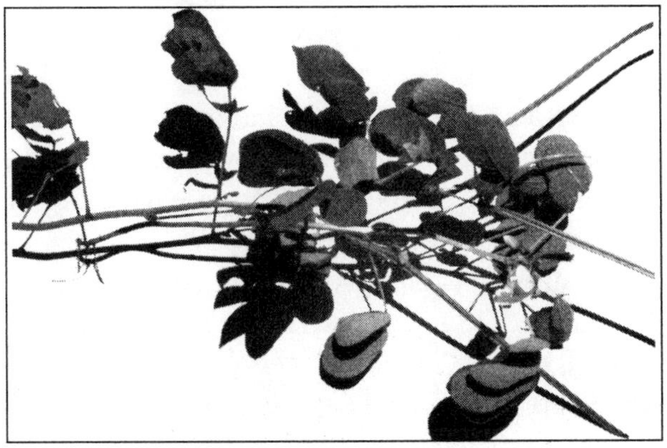

Hindi: Chakunda
English: Cassia
Latin: Cassia tora Linn.
Part Used: Leaves, seeds, roots
Habitat: This small plant grows in dry soil in tropical India and in Bengal.
Energetics: Plasma
Systems: Circulatory
Action: Externally—germicide, antiparasitical; Internally—gentle laxative
Uses: Seeds and leaves are used for skin diseases. Mixed with lime juice, eases skin itch and eruptions; ringworm (used externally). Leaf decoctions (1 part leaves : 10 parts water) given in two ounce doses to children, removes fevers during teething. Leaves boiled in castor oil are applied to foul ulcers and inflammations. As a poultice, leaves hasten suppuration. Warmed they reduce gout, sciatica, and joint pains. Seeds are used as a substitute for tea and coffee.
Preparation: Decoction, paste, poultice, oil

Sanskrit: **Chāṇgerī, Amlikā**
चांगेरी, अमलिक

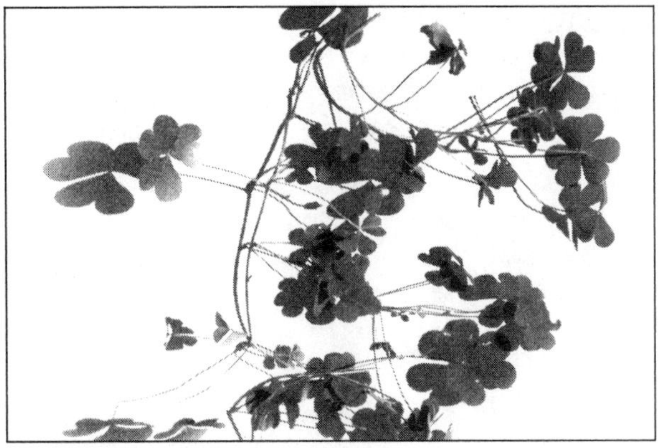

Hindi: Amrul
English: Sorrel
Latin: Oxalis corniculata Linn.
Part Used: Leaves
Habitat: Common weed throughout India
Energetics: Astringent-cold-pungent
Tissues: Plasma, blood
Systems: Digestive, excretory, circulatory
Action: Cooling, refrigerant, antiscorbutic, appetizing, astringent
Uses: Leaves—fever, inflammations, pain, appetite, scurvy, digestion, dyspepsia, intoxication, poisoning, difficult urination, bilious headaches, removes fibers over cornea or opacities of the cornea; Leaves boiled in yogurt/water (*lassi*), or mixed with honey or cane sugar for chronic dysentery, rectum prolapse, thirst and enteritis (small intestine inflammation), hemorrhoids; as a soup for convalescence from diarrhea. Juice—made into sherbet with honey or cane sugar for dysentery, rectum prolapse, thirst. Externally—removes warts, corns, etc.; applied locally as a poultice to inflamed areas and pain. Leaf juice with pepper and *ghee* are applied externally to red spots or other skin eruptions due

to bile, removes warts. Mixed with onions and applied to the head for bilious headaches.
Precautions: Not taken with gout
Preparation: Juice, powder, paste, poultice, pill, soup, confection

Sanskrit: **Chirāyatā** (Kirata-tikta)
चिरायता

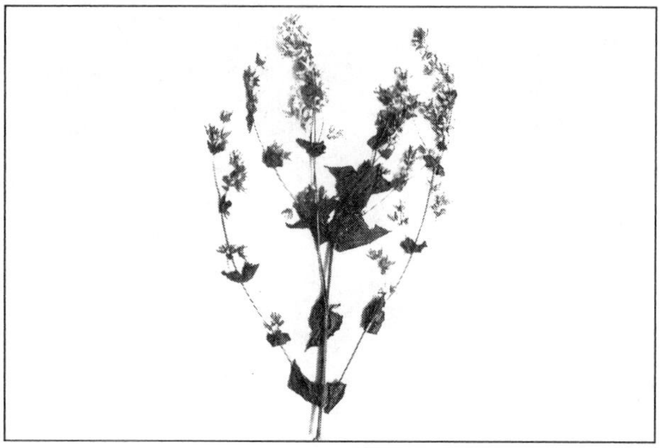

Hindi: Kiryat-charayatah
English: None
Latin: Swertia chirata Ham.
Part Used: Leaves and whole plant
Habitat: Himalayas; over 4,000 feet
Energetics: PK- V+ (King of the Bitters)
Tissues: Plasma, blood, muscle, fat
Systems: Circulatory, respiratory
Action: Anthelmintic, astringent, bitter tonic, febrifuge, stomachic, antidiarrhetic, antispasmodic
Uses: Excellent for fever, skin diseases, blood purifier, worms, wounds, malaria; tonic for heart, liver, and eyes, cough, scanty urine, sciatica, a gentian substitute, toxic blood, enlarged spleen and liver, catarrh, intestinal spasms, anemia, indigestion, obstinate urinary disorders (some say diabetes also), cleanse ulcers; the best form is (*Tinnevelly Nilavembu*).
Precautions: High Vāyu
Preparation: Powder

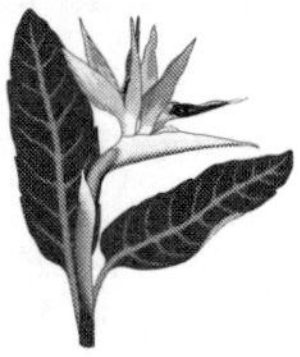

Sanskrit: **Chitrak**
चित्रक

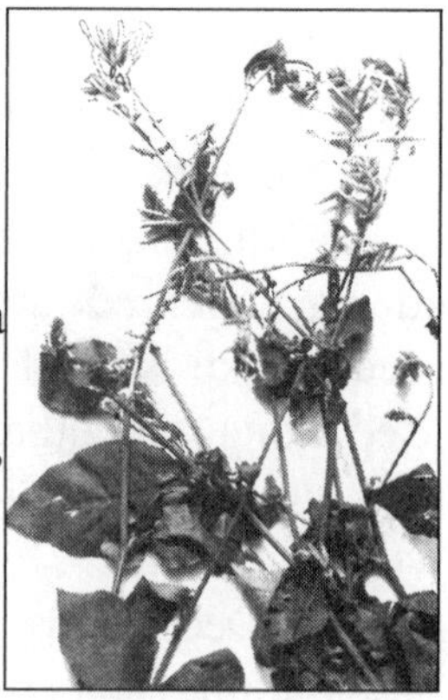

Hindi: Chitra
English: White Leadwort
Latin: Plumbago zeylanica Linn.
Part Used: Root, root bark, seeds
Habitat: Throughout India
Energetics: VK- P, *agni* +
Tissues: Bones, plasma, blood, reproductive
Systems: Nervous, female reproductive
Action: Stimulant, caustic; digestion, antiseptic, antiparasitical
Uses: Sprue, worms, dysmenorrhea, small doses stimulate the central nervous system, externally used as paste it opens abscesses and used for skin diseases and ulcers; colitis, indigestion, hemorrhoids, anasarca, diarrhea, gas, rheumatism, and all joint pains, promotes sweating. Tincture of root bark- intermittent fevers.
Preparation: Paste, powders, pills, tincture
Precaution: Do not use when pregnant; use only in small doses. Due to its very hot nature, it can cause abortion

Sanskrit: **Dāruharidrā, Dāruhaldī**
दारुहरिद्रा, दारुहल्दी

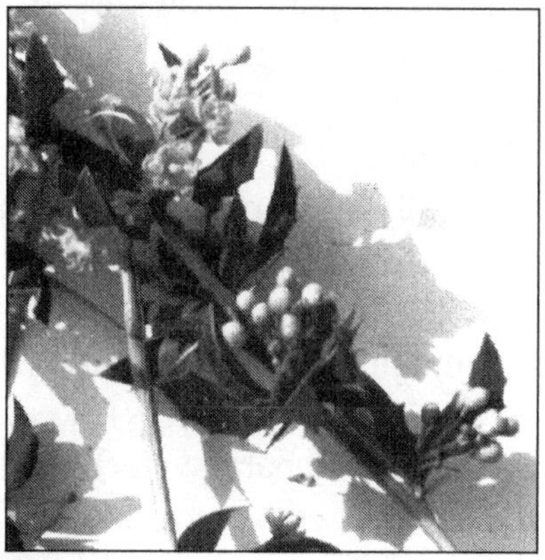

Hindi: Kingor
English: Barberry
Latin: Berberis vulgaris Linn.
Part Used: Berries

Habitat: Found throughout the Himalayas, Nepal, Tibet, Afghanistan
Energetics: Bitter, astringent-heating-pungent PK- V+
Tissues: Blood, fat, plasma
Systems: Circulatory, digestive
Action: Diuretic, antibilious, refrigerant, stomachic, bitter tonic, antiperiodic, alterative, antipyretic
Uses: For bile and urinary conditions, Pitta detoxification, and congestion of abdomen and pelvic cavities; rheumatism, scarlet fever, brain disorders, heat, thirst, nausea; small amounts—tonic; large doses—purgative; excellent herb for jaundice, during pregnancy, mild laxative, periodic neuralgia, fevers, skin diseases, vomiting in pregnancy; fruit—mild laxative/purgative for children, fevers, blood purifier, malaria, gastric and duodenal ulcers; sores, jaundice, enlarged liver and spleen, and regulates liver functioning, diabetes, and toxins/*āma* (with twice as much turmeric); destroys toxins, reduces body fat (with turmeric); renal calculi, abdominal and pelvic congestion; G.I. stimulant, reduces blood pressure.
Precautions: High Vāyu, tissue deficiency
Preparation: Decoction, powder, eye wash, medicated *ghee*, paste

Sanskrit: **Devadaru**
देवदरु

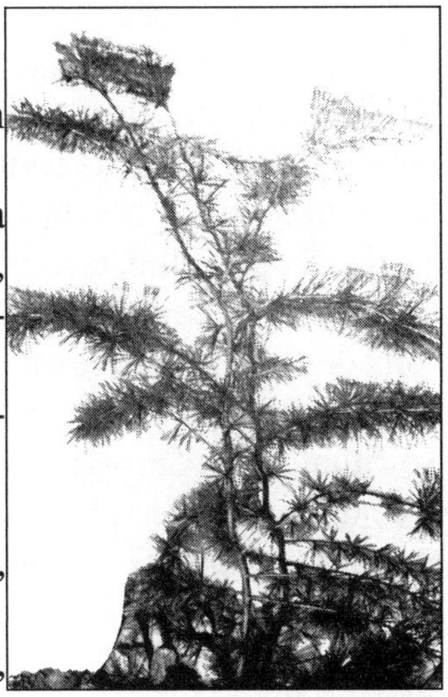

Hindi: Deodar; Tūna
English: Himalayan Cedar
Latin: Cedrus deodara
Part Used: Leaves, wood, bark, turpentine
Habitat: Northern Himalayas
Energetics: PK- V+
Tissues: Plasma, blood, muscle, fat
Systems: Circulatory, respiratory
Action: Wood—carminative; bark—astringent, febrifuge; Leaves—mild turpentine properties
Uses: Inflammation, antispasmodic, anti-poison, paralysis, kidney stones, fevers, external injuries. Bark—bilious, remittent and intermittent fevers, diarrhea, dysentery. In powder form it is applied to ulcers. The dark oil, or tar from the leaves (turpentine), is applied to skin ulcers and other skin diseases. (It is also used for mange on horses and on cattle with sore feet).
Preparation: Oleoresin (oil or tar), powder

Sanskrit: **Dhānyak**
धान्यक

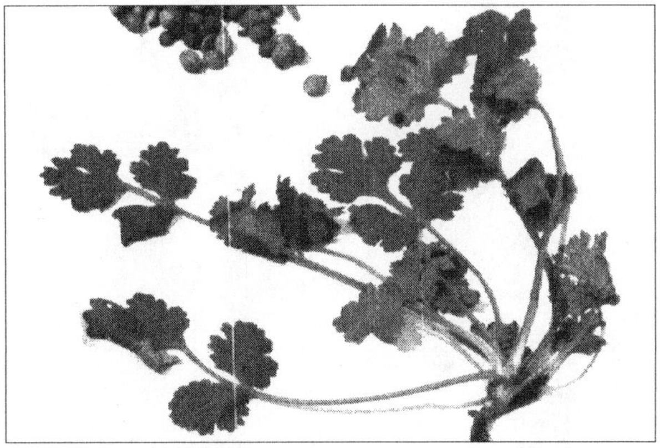

Hindi: Dhania
English: Coriander/Cilantro
Latin: Coriandrum sativum Linn.
Part Used: Seeds, leaves
Habitat: Common throughout India
Energetics: Bitter, pungent-cooling-pungent VPK=
Tissues: Blood, muscle, plasma
Systems: Digestive, respiratory, urinary
Action: Alterative, antibilious, aphrodisiac, aromatic, carminative, diaphoretic, diuretic, stimulant, stomachic, tonic
Uses: Griping, flatulent colic, rheumatism, neuralgia, indigestion, vomiting, intestinal disorders, removes excess Kapha, eyewash, conjunctivitis, relieves internal heat and thirst, skin/rash problems, urogenital system (burning urethra, cystitis, infections, etc.), sore throat, allergies,

hay fever, for all Pitta disorders, burning, juice for allergies, hay fever, and skin rashes (and externally as well); antidotes hot pungent foods, bleeding hemorrhoids. Externally—eye disorders.
Preparation: Cilantro juice, infusions (hot and cold), powder
Precautions: Not to be used in extreme Vāyu nerve tissue deficiency

Sanskrit: **Dhātakī**
धातकी

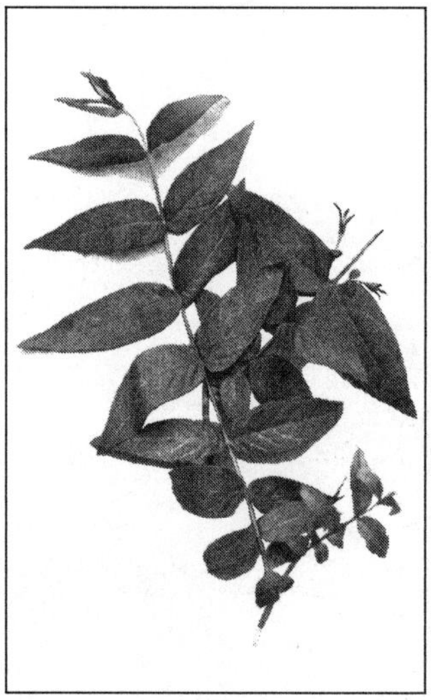
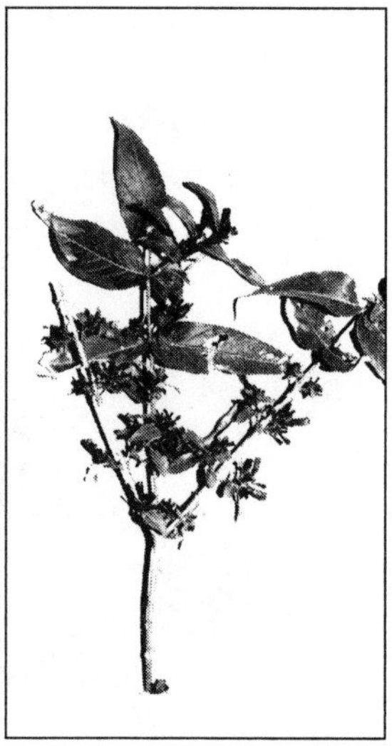

Hindi: Dhai-phul
English: None
Latin: Woodfordia floribunda Salisb. (W. frut icosa; kurz; Lythrum fruticosum Linn.)
Part Used: Flowers, leaves
Habitat: Large shrub found throughout India
Energetics: Astringent, slightly pungent-cold-sweet PK- V+
Tissues: Plasma, blood, reproductive
Systems: Reproductive, excretory
Action: Stimulant, astringent, tonic
Uses: Herpes, flowers in milk—dysentery, diarrhea, etc. Flower powder—mucus membrane disorders, hemorrhoids, liver disorders, internal hemorrhage; leukorrhea, menorrhagia. Leaves—biliousness, headache, fever. Externally, flower powder—ulcers, wounds; decoction as a lotion.
Preparation: Infusion, powder

Sanskrit: **Elā**
एला

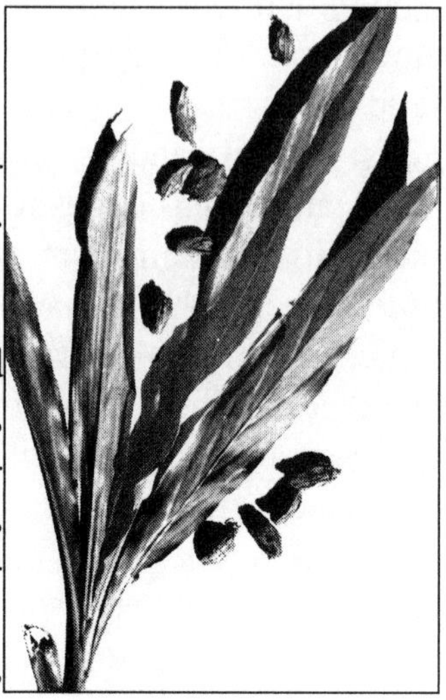

Hindi: Elachi
English: Cardamom
Latin: Elatarria cardamomum Maton (E. repens)
Part Used: Seeds
Habitat: Found throughout Northern, Western, and Southern India, Sri Lanka, and Burma (Myanmar).
Energetics: Pungent, sweet-heating-pungent VK- (P+ in excess - Large *elā*) In the U.S. only the small or *choti elā* is available. *Choti elā* is slightly cooling and better for Pitta than for Vāyu and Kapha).
Tissues: Blood, marrow, nerve, plasma
Systems: Circulatory, digestive, nervous, respiratory
Action: Carminative, diaphoretic, expectorant, digestive stimulant, stomachic
Uses: Absorption of nutrients, asthma, bronchitis, colds, cough, excellent for stomach complaints, hoarseness, indigestion, loss of taste, helps the spleen and pancreas, reduces Kapha in lungs and stomach, stimulates the mind, with milk it reduces mucus formation, detoxifies caffeine in coffee, nervous digestion, vomiting, headache, belching, acid indigestion, nausea, expels Vāyu in colon and digests foods in colon, convalescing from diarrhea, biliousness, respiratory disorders, involuntary urination.
Spiritual Uses: *Sattwic*, gives clarity and joy
Precautions: Ulcers, high Pitta
Preparation: Infusion (don't boil seeds), powder, milk decoction

Sanskrit: **Eraṇḍa, Vātāri**
एरण्ड, वातारि

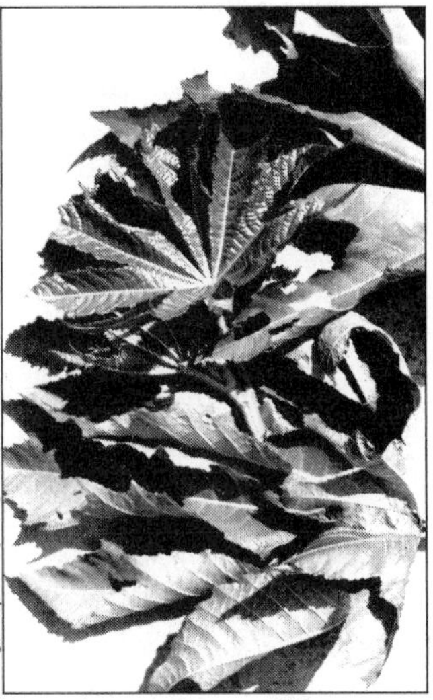

Hindi: Rendi
English: Castor Oil Plant
Latin: Ricinus communis Linn. (R. dicoccus)
Part Used: [two varieties—perennial bushy plant with large fruits and red seeds—yields more oil; smaller annual shrub with small gray or white seeds with brown spots] oil, leaves, roots, seeds, fruit.
Habitat: Common throughout India
Energetics: Pungent, sweet-heating-pungent V-PK+
Tissues: All
Systems: Excretory, urinary, nervous, female reproductive, digestive
Action: Cathartic, demulcent, analgesic, nervine, purgative (in the duodenum); root bark—purgative
Uses: Colic, headache, abdominal disorders, coagulates blood; fruit—enlarged liver and spleen; bark—nervous diseases, rheumatism, lumbago, sciatica; dried root—fevers; leaves—warmed and applied to nursing mother's breasts acts as a galactagogue. When applied to the stomach, promotes menstrual discharge. Applied to painful joints, relieves pain; leaves internally—purgative. Seed decoction—lumbago, sciatica. Seed poultice is applied to mature boils to promote bursting and to reduce gouty and rheumatic swellings. Oil—the "king of the purgatives", "king of Vāyu disorders", inflamed bowels, infantile diarrhea, irritable conditions in debilitated adults and children; to facilitate delivery of baby; after childbirth to mother; in operations for urinary stones; peritonitis, jaundice, dysentery, urinary organ inflammation, articular rheumatism.
For rectum disorders and hemorrhoids, it is given in small doses to soften feces and lubricate the passage. Also helps with ingested glass. As a purgative, it is taken with ginger or *dashmūl* teas. Externally used for sore nipples during breast feeding. In constipation it is used as an enema (2 oz.: 1 pint water). Dropped into the eyes for conjunctivitis and irritations. It increases cow's milk when they eat the leaves. Externally—oil mixed with rice water for leg swelling; oil mixed with coconut oil and water (1:2:6) for itching skin.
Preparation: Oil doses: children- 1 tsp.; adults—2 tsp. - 3 tbs. in tea or boiled milk. Decoction, infusion, poultice, leaf, paste
Precaution: Oil not used for kidney, bladder, bile duct, or intestine infections; jaundice, dysuria

Sanskrit: **Gauriphal**
गौरिफल

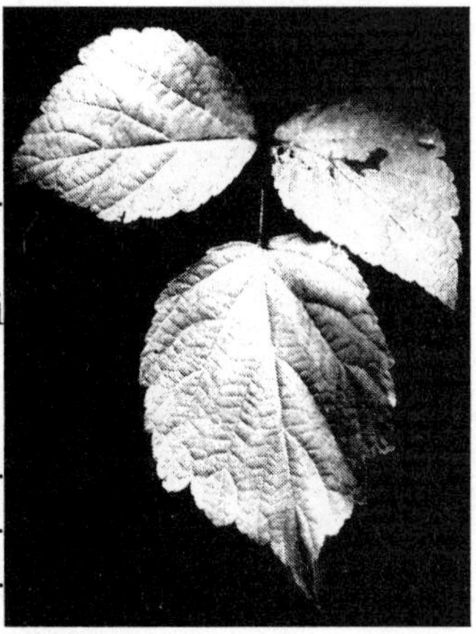

Hindi: None
English: Red Raspberry
Latin: Rubus wallichii
Part Used: Leaves
Habitat:
Energetics: Astringent, sweet-cool-sweet PK- (V+ in excess)
Tissues: Blood, muscles, plasma
Systems: Circulatory, digestive, female reproductive
Actions: Alterative, anti-emetic, astringent, hemostatic, tonic
Uses: Diarrhea, dysentery, female reproductive organs, heartburn, thirst, cholera, hemorrhoids, hemorrhage in stomach, inflamed mucus membranes, intestinal flu, menstruation (irregular or excess), kidneys, liver, nausea, Pitta disorders, pre-childbirth toning, prolapse of uterus or anus, sores, spleen, vomiting, tones lower abdomen muscles, uterine bleeding, sore throats, wounds, ulcers, passive stomach hemorrhage, summer heat.
Precautions: Most varieties promote abortion ex-

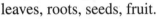

cept American red raspberry; Vāyu constipation
Preparation: Hot or cold infusion, powder, paste

Sanskrit: **Gokṣhura** *(emphasize 'go'. Meaning: shape of the cow's-hoof)*

गोक्षुर

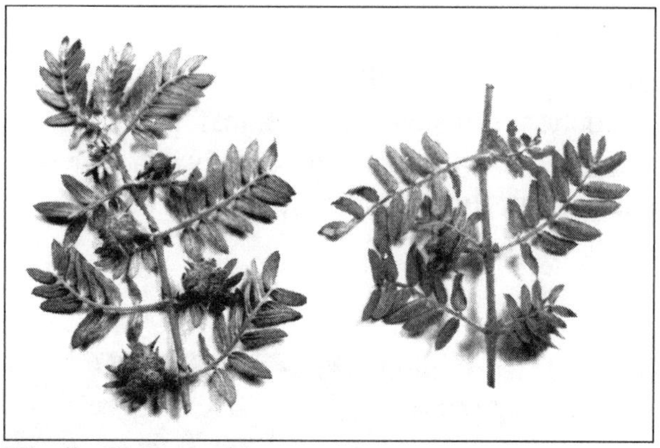

Hindi: Chota-gokhru
English: Small Caltrops, Goats head, Puncture Vine
Latin: Tribulis terrestris Linn. (T. lenuginosus, T. aeylanicus)
Part Used: Fruit
Habitat: Trailing plant common in sandy soil throughout India, Sri Lanka, Madras.
Energetics: Sweet, bitter-cool-sweet VPK=
Tissues: Plasma, blood, marrow/nerve, reproductive
Systems: Nervous, reproductive, respiratory, urinary
Action: Analgesic, aphrodisiac, diuretic, lithotriptic, nervine, rejuvenative, tonic
Uses: Back pain, cough, cystitis (chronic), diabetes, difficult breathing, urourogenital conditions including difficult or painful urination, stones, bloody or burning urine, etc.; Vāyu edema, gout, uterine disorders, hemorrhoids, impotence, infertility, kidney disease (acute inflammation), lumbago, nerve pain, Bright's disease with edema, rheumatism, sciatica, seminal debility, kidney stones, venereal diseases. Strengthens the postpartum woman. Can be used with *punarnavā* (boerhavia diffusa; nyctagineae) for kidney health.
Spiritual Uses: *Sattwic*, promotes clarity, opens crown *chakra* (energy center)
Precautions: Do not use if dehydrated
Preparation: Decoction, powder

Sanskrit: Sarpa-daruṣhtrika
Hindi: **Guḍmār** (meaning: sugar destroying)
गुडमार (common name)

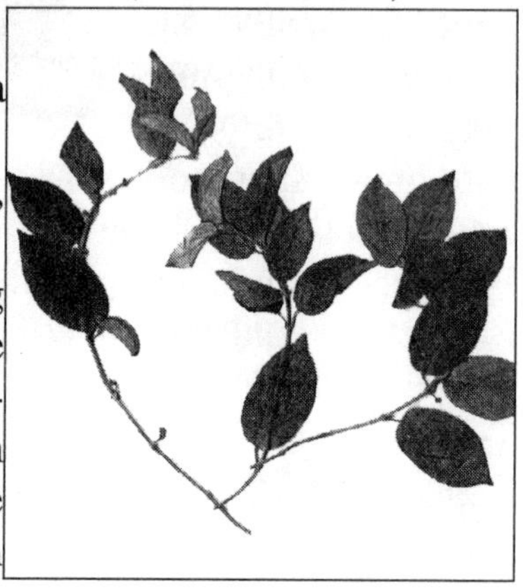

English: None
Latin: Gymnema sylvestre
Part Used: Roots, leaves
Habitat: Climbing plant found in the Himalayas, Central and Southern India, and on the Western *Ghats* in Goa
Energetics: Astringent, refrigerant, tonic PK- V+
Tissues: Plasma, blood, fat, reproductive
Systems: Circulatory, urinary, reproductive
Action: Antiperiodic, diuretic, stomachic,
Uses: One of the main herbs used for healing diabetes mellitus; removes sugar from pancreas, restores pancreatic function; leaves stimulate the circulatory system, increases urine secretion, activates the uterus, swollen glands, cough, fever.
Precautions: Leaves stimulate the heart
Preparation: Decoction, powder

Sanskrit: **Guḍūchī**
गुडूची
Hindi: Amṛitā, Giloy
English: None
Latin: Tinosporia cordifolia Miers; (Menisper mum cordifolium, Cocculuc cordifolia, E. Tinospora)

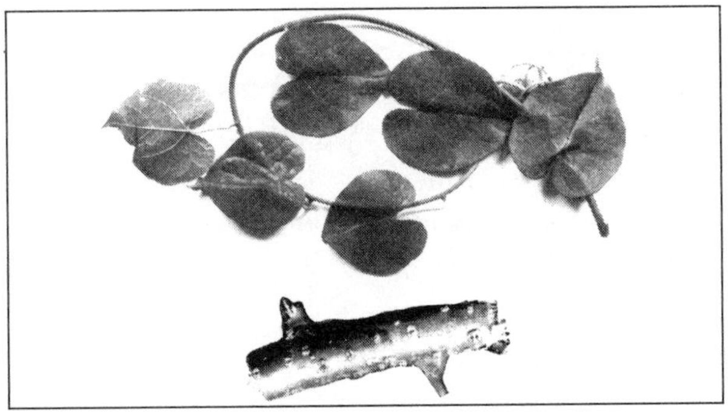

Part Used: Roots, stems
Habitat: Himalayas, throughout Madras Presidency districts
Energetics: Bitter, sweet-hot-sweet VPK=
Systems: Circulatory, digestive
Action: Alterative, antiperiodic, bitter tonic, diuretic, febrifuge
Uses: AIDS and other immune diseases, Pitta diseases, blood purifier, fever and convalescence from fevers, jaundice, digestion, gout, chronic rheumatism, constipation, hemorrhoids, dysentery, Kapha jaundice, skin disease, chronic malarial fevers, tuberculosis, cancer (strengthens persons before and after chemotherapy).
Spiritual Uses: Produces *ojas*
Preparation: Extract, powder, for serious illnesses like cancer, use one or more ounces daily

Sanskrit: **Guggula**
गुग्गुल

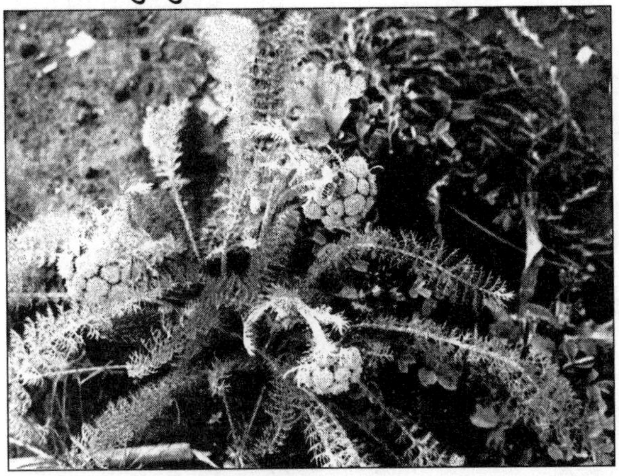

Hindi: Gugal
English: Indian Bedellium
Latin: Balsamodendron mukul Hook. (B. agallocha., Commiphora mukul; C. africana)
Part Used: Resin
Habitat: Eastern Bengal, Mysore, Rajputan, Sind, Assam, Berars, Khandesh
Energetics: All but sour and salty-hot-pungent KV- (P+ in excess)
Tissues: All
Systems: Circulatory, digestive, nervous, respiratory
Action: Alterative, analgesic, antispasmodic, astringent, expectorant, nervine, rejuvenative, stimulant
Uses: The best herb for arthritis, hypercholesterol, bronchitis, cystitis, debility, diabetes, disinfects secretions (e.g., mucus, sweat, urination), endometritis, fat reducing, gout, heals skin and mucus membranes; hemorrhoids, increases white blood cell count, indigestion, leukorrhea, lumbago, menstrual regulator, nervous disorders, neurosis, obesity, plaster for gums and throat ulcers, pus discharges, skin diseases, sores, tissue regenerating catalyst, heals bone fractures, toxin reducing, tumors, ulcers, whooping cough, edema, enlarged cervical glands, parasitic infection, abscesses, rheumatic disorders.
Precautions: Acute kidney infections and rashes; avoid eating sour, sharp indigestible things; exhaustion, sex, sun exposure, alcohol, and anger when taking this herb
Preparation: Powder, pill

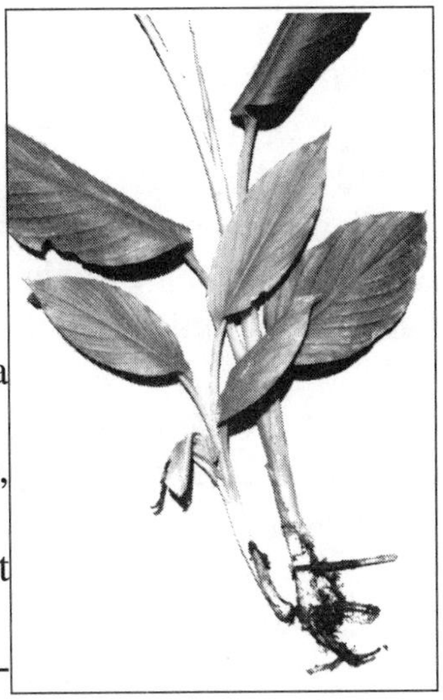

Sanskrit: **Haridrā, Gauri**
हरिद्रा, गौरि
Hindi: Haldi
English: Turmeric
Latin: Curcuma longa Linn.
Part Used: Rhizome, tubers
Habitat: Throughout India
Energetics: Bitter, as-

tringent, pungent-heating-pungent K- (VP+ in excess)
Tissues: All
Systems: Circulatory, digestive, respiratory, urinary
Action: Alterative, anthelmintic, antibacterial/antibiotic, aromatic, carminative, stimulant, tonic, vulnerary
Uses: Amenorrhea, anemia, arthritis, blood purifier, blood tissue formation, circulation, cooking spice, cough, diabetes, worms, jaundice, eye problems, fevers, gas, hemorrhoids, edema, indigestion, ligament stretching, metabolism regulator; mucus relief, and hysteria (from inhaling fumes); pharyngitis, protein digesting, skin disorders, abscess, urinary diseases, wound and bruise healer; a natural antibiotic which also improves intestinal flora; inflammatory bowel syndrome (e.g., ulcerative colitis), Chron's Disease, chronic hepatitis, chronic bronchial asthma, psoriasis, all inflammatory conditions. External—acne, insect bites, sore eyes, with honey or aloe gel for bruises or sprains.
Spiritual Uses: Gives one the Divine Goddess's energy and prosperity; *chakra* and subtle body cleanser; limbers for *yoga āsana* practice
Precautions: Do not use if pregnant, with excess Pitta, with acute jaundice or hepatitis.
Preparation: Infusion, decoction, milk decoction, powder, external paste (with sandalwood).

Sanskrit: **Harītakī**
हरीतकी
Hindi: Hardh, Har
English: Myrobalan, Indian Gall Nut
Latin: Terminalia chebula Retz., (T. reticulata)
Part Used: Fruit
Habitat: Tree grows wild in the forests of Northern India, central provinces, Bengal, Madras, Mysore, southern Bombay presidency
Energetics: All except salty-heating-sweet VPK=
Tissues: All
Systems: Digestive, excretory, nervous, respiratory, female reproductive

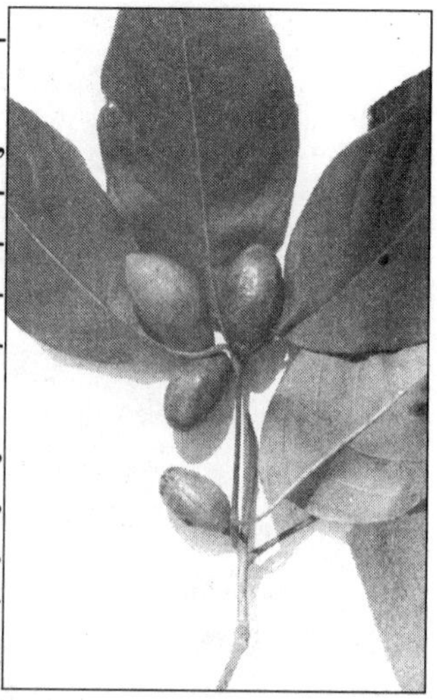

Action: Rejuvenative, tonic, astringent, laxative, nervine, expectorant, anthelmintic, alterative (unripe—laxative/ripe—astringent)
Uses: Jaundice, colic, anemia, cough, asthma, hoarse voice, hiccup, vomiting, hemorrhoids, diarrhea, malabsorption, abdominal distention, gas, fevers, urinary diseases, parasitic infection, tumors, blood purifier, spleen and liver disorders; gargle for sore throat, mouth, or spongy, ulcerated gums; muscular rheumatism, with sugar water for ophthalmia; heart, skin, itching, edema, nervous disorders, rejuvenative, feeds the brain and nerves; small doses—good for both diarrhea and constipation (also chronic); digestion, atonic indigestion, bleeding hemorrhoids, longevity, paralysis, headache, epilepsy, melancholy, memory, wisdom, intelligence, organ prolapse, excessive discharges (cough, sweat, sperm, menorrhagia, leukorrhea); one of the three herbs in *triphalā*. Externally for Vāyu swellings, burns, scalds, skin disorders.
Spiritual Uses: Gives pure awareness (*Śhiva* energy)
Preparation: Decoction, powder, paste, gargle
Precaution: Pregnancy, dehydration, severe exhaustion, emaciation, Pitta if taken in excess

Sanskrit: **Īśhabgol, Snigdhajīrā**
ईशब्गोल, स्निग्धजीरा
Hindi: Isapghul
English: Ispaghula or Spogel Seeds
Latin: Plantago ispagula; P. ovata Forsk.
Part Used: Seeds
Habitat: Throughout India
Energetics: Cool, astringent VPK=

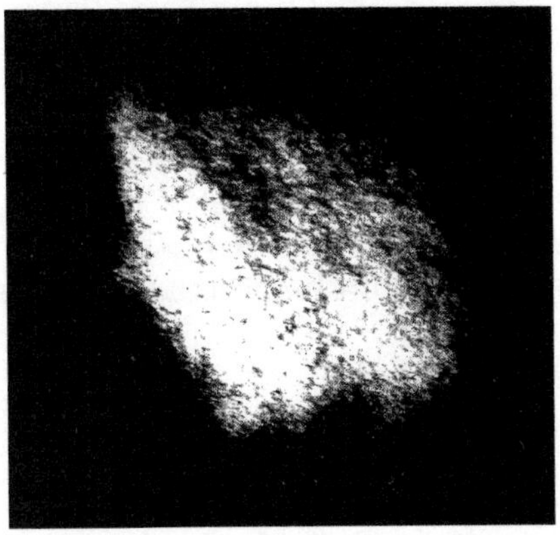

Systems: Digestive/Excretory
Action: Demulcent, emollient, laxative, diuretic
Uses: Excellent for constipation (with warm water) and diarrhea (with cool water). Seeds swell and thicken (mucilage) when soaked in water. It passes through the small intestine undigested, lining the mucus membrane (demulcifying and lubricating). May inhibit intestinal organism growth. The thickened jelly absorbs toxins (*āma*) and bacteria. It is useful for catarrh, chronic dysentery, intestinal problems, bladder, kidney and urethra problems (including inflammations and burning), digestive disorders, and fevers. Further uses include gonorrhea, gastritis, gastric and duodenal ulcers, cystitis, a demulcent for coughs and colds (especially for children).
Preparation: 1-2 tbs. in warm or cool water, stirred until it thickens into a gel

Sanskrit: **Jaṭāmāṇśhī**
जटामांशी

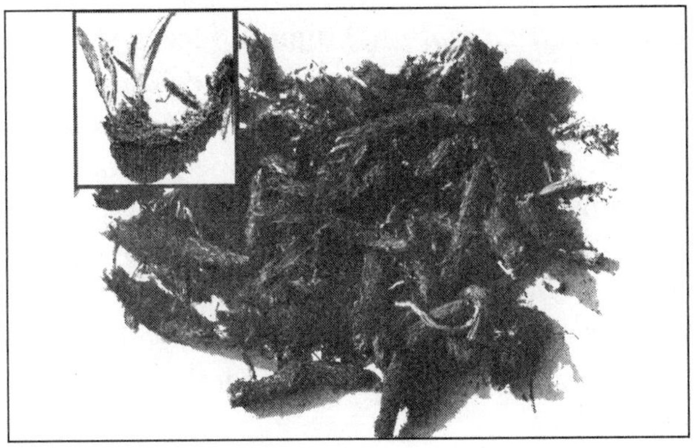

Hindi: Jatamashi, Balchar
English: Muskroot; Indian Spikenard
Latin: Nardostachys jatamansi DC.
Part Used: Rhizome, rhizome oil
Habitat: Himalayas: 9,000-17,000 feet; India, Nepal, Bhutan, Sikkim
Energetics: Bitter, sweet, astringent-cool-pungent VPK=
Tissues: Blood, marrow/nerve
Systems: Circulatory, nervous, digestive, respiratory, reproductive
Action: Aromatic, antispasmodic, diuretic, emmenagogue, nervine, tonic, carminative, deobstruent, digestive stimulant, reproductive
Uses: Complexion, strength, kidney stones, jaundice, removes blood impurities, spasmodic hysteria and other nervous convulsive ailments; heart palpitations, nervous headache, flatulence, epilepsy, convulsions, respiratory and digestive diseases, skin conditions, typhoid, gastric disorders, seminal debility.
Spiritual Uses: Increases awareness
Precautions: None; its sedative properties increase awareness, whereas its cousin, valerian, dulls the mind
Preparation: Infusion, powder

Sanskrit: **Kākamāchī**
काकमाची

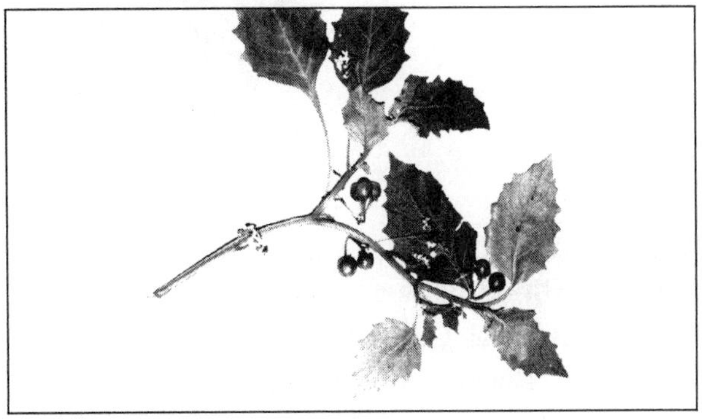

Hindi: Makoy
English: Garden nightshade
Latin: Solanum nigrum Linn. (S. rubrum, S. incertum)
Part Used: Fruit, leaf

Habitat: Throughout India
Energetics
Tissues: Plasma, blood, bones, fat, reproductive
Systems: Circulatory, reproductive
Action: Leaf—alterative, sedative, diaphoretic, diuretic, hydragogue, expectorant; fruit—alterative, tonic, diuretic
Uses: Heart disease (with leg and foot swelling), skin diseases, fruit for edema, hemorrhoids, gonorrhea, inflammatory swellings, enlarged spleen and liver, fevers, promotes perspiration, cough. External—painful, swollen testicles; poultice for rheumatic and gouty joints.
Precaution: Berries may be poisonous for some people
Preparation: Powder, extract, leaves, poultice, syrup, decoction

Sanskrit: **Kāknāśhā** **काकनाशा**

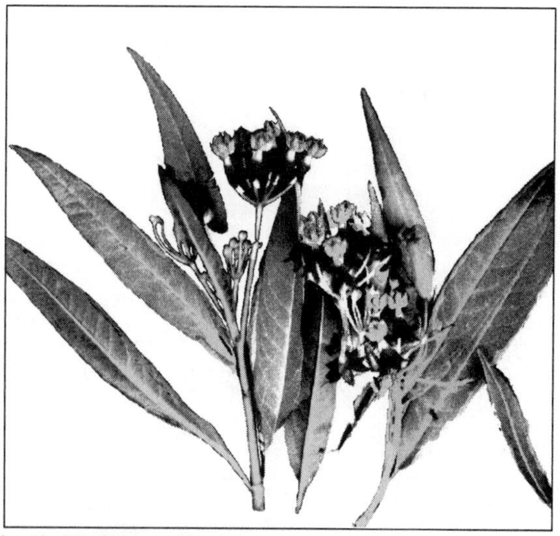

Hindi: Kakatundi
English: Blood Flower
Latin: Asclepias Curassavica, Linn.
Part Used: Leaves, root, flowers
Habitat: Bengal and throughout South India; West Indies, Jamaica
Energetics: Astringent
Tissues: Plasma, blood, muscle, reproductive
Systems: Circulatory, respiratory, excretory, reproductive
Action: Root—purgative, emetic, styptic
Uses: Organic muscular system (especially heart and blood vessels), dysentery, hemorrhoids, gonorrhea.
Preparation: Juice, powder
Precaution: Difficult breathing, vomiting

Sanskrit: **Kañchanar** **काञ्चनर**

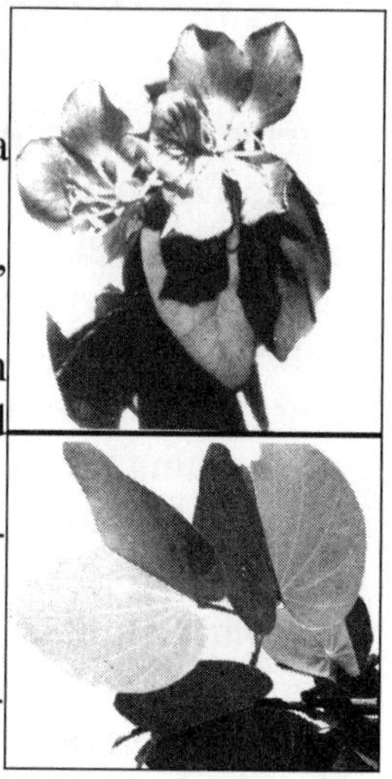

Hindi: Kanchnar
English: Mountain Ebony
Latin: Bauhinia variegata Linn. (B. racemosa)
Part Used: Bark, root, bud, gum, leaves, seed, flowers
Habitat: Sub-Himalayan tract, forests of India and Burma (Myanmar)
Energetics: Sweet, bitter, astringent PK- V+
Tissues: Plasma, blood,
Systems: Digestive, reproductive
Action: Bark—alterative, tonic, astringent; root—carminative; flowers—laxative.
Uses: Worms, gargle with bark liquid for sore throat; bud decoction for cough, bleeding hemorrhoids, hematuria, menorrhagia. Bark emulsified with rice water and ginger for TB, enlargement of neck glands. Bark and ginger paste for TB tumors. Bark decoction for ulcer wash, skin diseases, diarrhea. Buds—diarrhea, worms, hemorrhoids, dysentery. Root decoction—indigestion, heartburn, gas, malaria, weight loss (anti-fat); flowers with sugar—gentle laxative; *Kañchanar guggul*—TB tumors, ulcers, skin diseases, gonorrhea, edema, increase white blood cells. [Ingredients; *kañchanar* bark (10 parts): ginger, black pepper, long pepper, cardamom, cinnamon, *tejpatra* leaves (cassia cinnamon), *triphalā* (1 part of each of the above herbs)]. This is taken every morning with *triphalā* or *khadira* (catechu/ acacia catechu, willd.) decoction.
Preparation: Emulsion, paste, gargle, decoction

Sanskrit: **Kāṇṭkārī**
कांटकारी

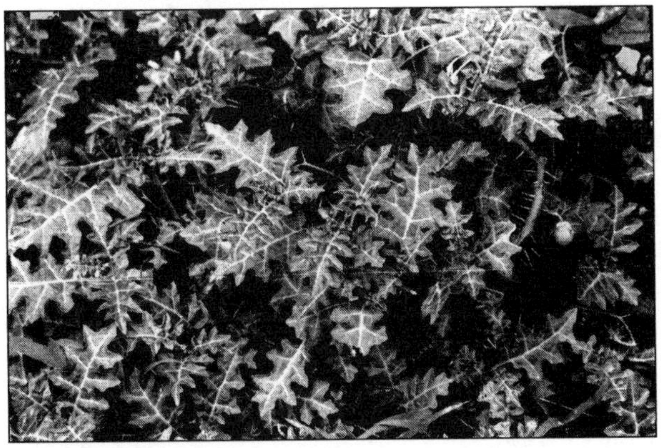

Hindi: Choti Katheri
English: None
Latin: Solanum xanthocarpum Schrad and Wendil
Part Used: Stems, roots, flowers, fruit
Habitat: Grows abundantly throughout India
Energetics: Pungent, bitter VP- K+
Tissues: Plasma, blood, marrow, reproductive
Systems: Respiratory, reproductive
Action: Aperient, digestive, alterative, astringent; stems, fruits, flowers—bitter, carminative; root—diuretic, expectorant, febrifuge.
Uses: One of the *daśhamūl* roots; fever, asthma, TB and other lung diseases; kidney disorders, cough, constipation, fumigation for toothache; juice with whey for diuretic; root with *chirāyatā* and ginger as a febrifuge, berry juice for sore throat, juice with black pepper for rheumatism; decoction for gonorrhea, conception; fruit powder with honey for chronic coughs in children; root decoction with *guḍūchī* for cough and fever.
Preparation: Decoction, powder, juice, fumes

Sanskrit: **Kapikachhū, Ātmaguptā**
कपिकच्छू , आत्मगुप्ता
Hindi: Kavach
English: Cowitch or Cowhage Plant
Latin: Mucuna pruriens Bak. M. prutita (Carpopogon pruiens; Dolichos pruiens)
Part Used: Seeds, root, legumes
Habitat: Annual climbing shrub common in the tropics of India; legumes are eaten as a vegetable

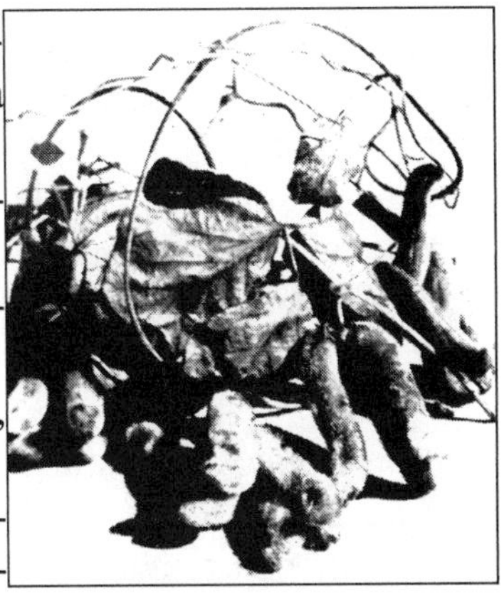

Energetics: Sweet-cool-sweet VP- K+
Tissues: Reproductive
Systems: Nervous, reproductive
Action: Anthelmintic, aphrodisiac, astringent, nervine, tonic, rejuvenative, (root is nervine/tonic)
Uses: Seeds—one of the best tonics and aphrodisiacs for the reproductive system. Indigestion, colic, debility, edema, impotence, infertility, leukorrhea, menorrhagia, roundworm, spermatorrhea, Parkinson's; Generally, it is used with *āmalakī*, *aśhwagandhā*, *śhatāvarī*, *gokṣhura*, white and black musali to make pills and jellies. Roots—fevers, edema, elephantiasis (externally), nervous disorders, including facial paralysis.
Precautions: Do not use when congested
Preparation: Decoction, powder, confections

Sanskrit: **Kaṭukā**
कटुका

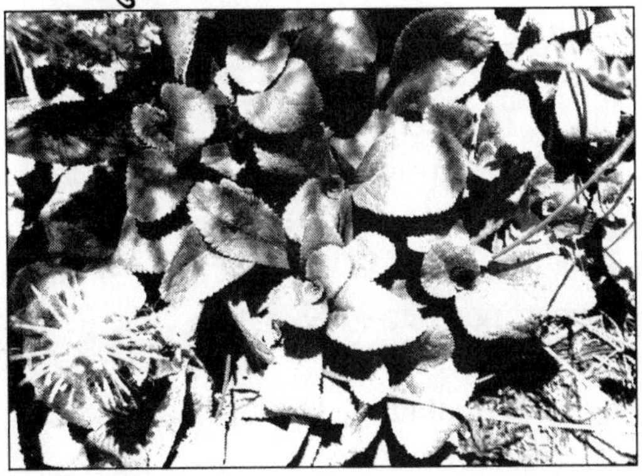

Hindi: Kuṭki, Kaṭki
English: None
Latin: Picrorrhiza kurroa Benth.
Part Used: Dried rhizome
Habitat: North - Western Himalayas, from Kashmir to Sikkim

Energetics: Bitter PK- V+
Tissues: Plasma, blood, marrow/nerves, female reproductive
Systems: Excretory, female reproductive, digestive, circulatory, nervous.
Action: Small doses—bitter stomachic and laxative; large doses—cathartic; anti-periodic, cholagogue
Uses: Epilepsy, paralysis, emmenagogue, emetic, abortifacient, skin diseases, improves eye sight, constipation due to small intestine secretion; with equal parts licorice, raisins, neem bark; for bilious fever; with aromatics for worms in children, fever, malaria.
Preparation: Tincture, extract, powder, pills

Sanskrit: **Kumārī (Ghirita)**
कुमारी

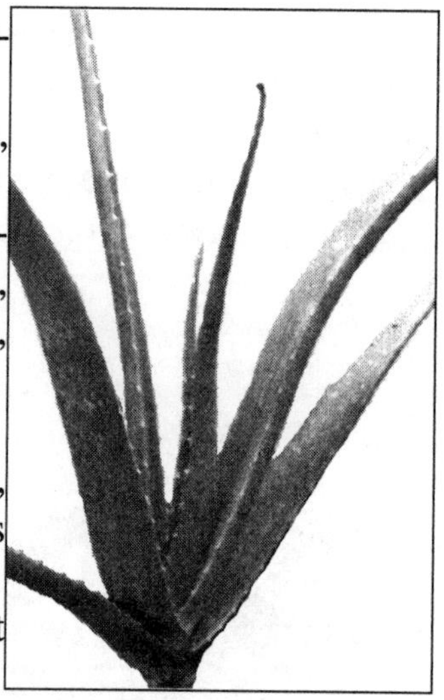

Hindi: Kumari, Gawarpaltra
English: Indian Alces, Aloe Vera
Latin: Aloe barbadensis Mill., Aloe Indica, A. Barbados, A. Vera, Varieties: Officinalis (Liliaceae)
Part Used: Extract, dried juice of leaves and pulp root
Habitat: Throughout India and the world
Energetics: Bitter, astringent, pungent, sweet/cold/sweet VPK= (gel and small doses of powder; powder—PK- V+
Tissues: All
Systems: Circulatory, female reproductive, digestive, nervous, excretory
Action: In small doses—stomachic tonic; large doses—purgative, emmenagogue, anthelmintic; laxative, refrigerant, bitter tonic, alterative, vulnerary, rejuvenative. Aperient, digestive, alterative, astringent; stems, fruits, flowers—bitter, carminative; root—diuretic, expectorant, febrifuge.
Uses: Intestinal worms, hair dye and growth; eye problems, colds, hemorrhoids (confection of leaf pulp); pulp with honey and turmeric—coughs and colds; juice with *asafoetida* gum—colic, infant pneumonia; external leaf juice for skin inflammations and chronic ulcers, brain tonic, Anti-Vāyu rib pain, heart pain, swellings from injury, enlarged spleen (internal and external paste); tender leaves with cumin and rock candy—dysentery with bloody stools; juice and ginger oil—hair oil for insomnia; leaf pulp—conjunctivitis; with small amounts of rock candy and cooked alum (in frying pan)—ophthalmia; with butter—applied to skin ulcers to relieve burning sensation; with turmeric—spleen disorders and enlarged glands; tuber paste with turmeric paste—externally applied to inflamed or diseased breasts; fever, constipation, bursitis, jaundice, hepatitis, enlarged liver, venereal diseases, herpes, amenorrhea, dysmenorrhea, menopause, vaginitis, tumors, regulates fat and sugar metabolism; blood tonic, tones digestive enzymes, kidney disorders, asthma, TB and other lung diseases, ear infections, obesity, Pitta reducing, wasting diseases. Externally for burns, skin rashes, sores. One of the *daśhamūl* roots. Fumigation for toothache; juice with whey for diuretic; root with *chirāyatā* and ginger as a febrifuge, berry juice for sore throat, juice with black pepper for rheumatism; decoction for gonorrhea, conception; fruit powder with honey for chronic coughs in children; root decoction with *guḍūchī* for cough and fever.
Precaution: Do not use when pregnant
Preparation: Confection, tincture, lotion, juice (gel), powder, decoction, paste, pulp, herbal wine, fumes

Sanskrit: **Kum Kuma**
कुम्कुम
Hindi: Zaffran, Kesar
English: Saffron
Latin: Crocus sativus Linn. (C. saffron)

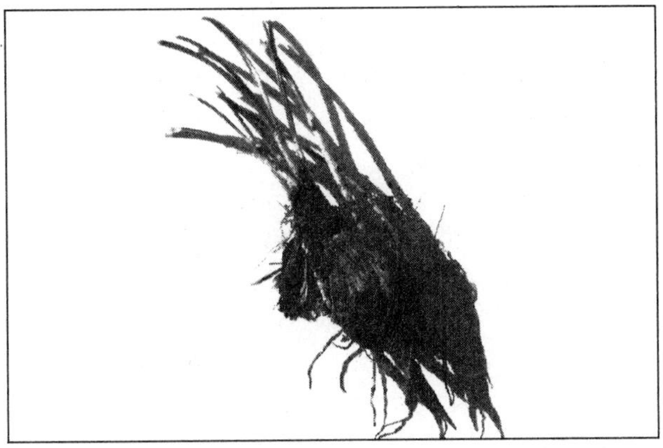

Part Used: Dried stigmas
Habitat: Common wild dwarf-flower in India, U.S. and elsewhere
Energetics: Pungent, bitter, sweet-cool-sweet VPK=
Tissues: All, especially the blood
Systems: Circulatory, digestive, female reproductive, nervous
Action: Alterative, antispasmodic, aphrodisiac, carminative, emmenagogue, rejuvenative, stimulant, stomachic
Uses: Amenorrhea, anemia, asthma, cold, cough, depression, diarrhea, dysmenorrhea, hysteria, female reproductive blood circulator, food assimilation, impotence, infertility, headache, G.I. disorders, leukorrhea, menstrual pain and irregularity; liver enlargement/regulator, lumbago, menopause, neuralgia, Pitta reducer, rheumatism; seminal weakness, spleen regulator, tissue growth stimulator of the reproductive systems, uterus toner.
Spiritual Uses: *Sattwic*, develops love, compassion, and devotion
Precautions: Do not use when pregnant; large doses is narcotic
Preparation: Infusion, milk decoction, powder

Sanskrit: **Kuśhā**
कुशा

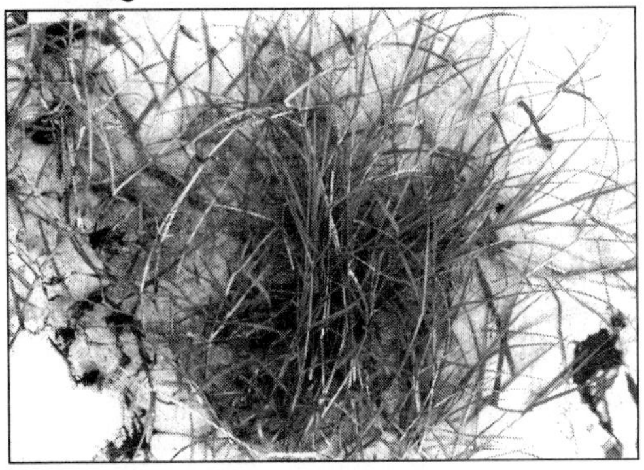

Hindi: Dūrba
English: Sacred Creeping Grass
Latin: Eragrostis cynosuriodes Beauv.
Part Used: Grass, root
Habitat: Grows wild throughout the Himalayas
Energetics: Astringent
Tissues: Plasma, reproductive
Systems: Reproductive, urinary
Action: Grass—hemostatic, coagulant, diuretic; [note: even local grasses (without chemicals sprayed on them) are useful]
Uses: Root—dysentery, menorrhagia, other bleeding disorders like hemorrhoids, purpura, etc.
Preparation: Infusion

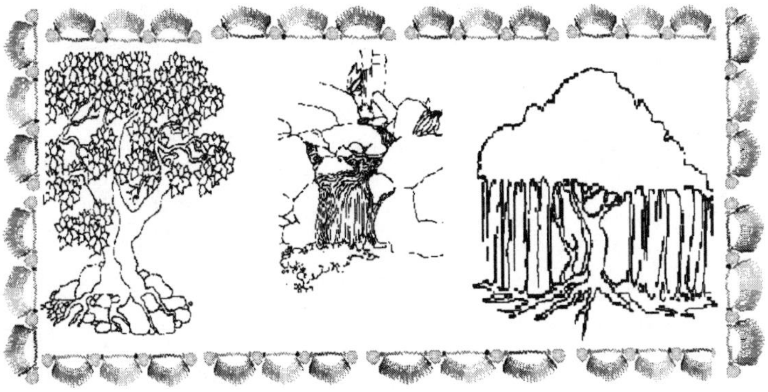

<u>Sanskrit</u>: **Kushtha**
कुष्थ

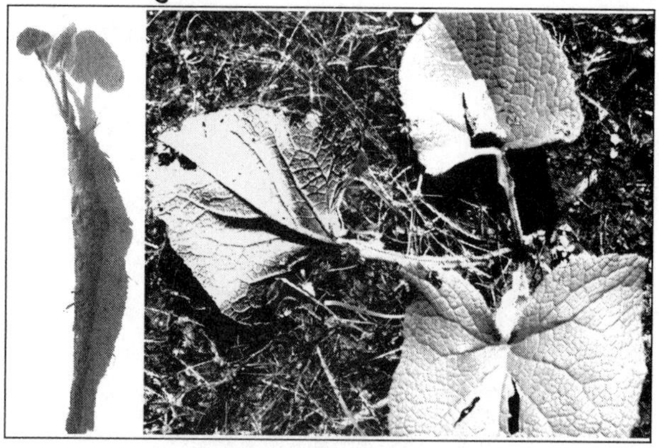

<u>Hindi</u>: Kūt
<u>English</u>: Costus, Kut Root
<u>Latin</u>: Saussurea lappa Clarke.
<u>Part Used</u>: Root
<u>Habitat</u>: Himalayas, Kashmir Valley
<u>Energetics</u>: Pungent, Bitter-hot-rasāyana VPK=
<u>Tissues</u>: Plasma, Blood, Bone
<u>Systems</u>: Circulatory, respiratory
<u>Action</u>: Anthelmintic, antiseptic, aphrodisiac, astringent, antispasmodic, alterative, aromatic, carminative, diuretic, expectorant, insecticidal, prophylactic, stimulant, tonic
<u>Uses</u>: Bronchial asthma (especially vagotonic), gas, phlegm, wasting, cough, loss of hunger (dyspepsia), rib pain, edema, skin diseases, jaundice, all diseases due to Vāyu and Kapha, and asthma; rheumatism (with *choti elā*), cholera, quartan malaria, leprosy, persistent hiccup, blackens gray hair; with musk for toothache, hair wash. As an ointment it is applied externally to wounds, severe ulcerations, skin diseases, tumors, angina.
<u>Preparation</u>: Powder, paste
<u>Precaution</u>: Narcotic effects when smoked. Use only under supervision of a qualified practitioner

<u>Sanskrit</u>: **Laghu Pāṭā, Jal Jamnī**
लघु पाटा, जल जमनी
<u>Hindi</u>: Patha, Harjori
<u>English</u>: Velvet Leaf
<u>Latin</u>: Cissampelos pareira Linn.
<u>Part Used</u>: Root, bark, leaves

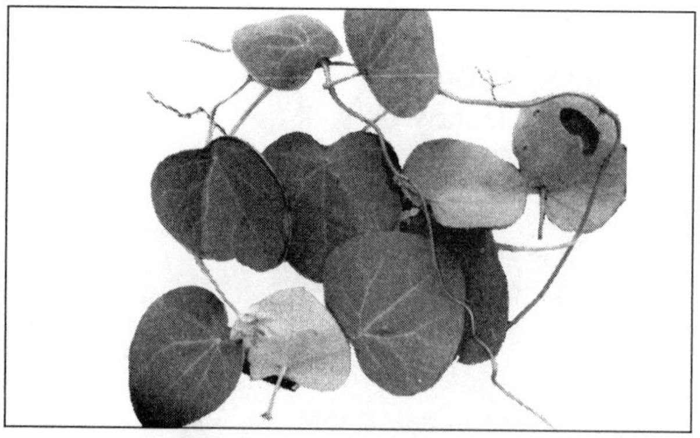

<u>Habitat</u>: Tropical and subtropical India (From Sind and Punjab to South India and Sri Lanka)
<u>Energetics</u>: Very pungent, astringent-hoVK- P+t
<u>Tissues</u>: Plasma, fat, reproductive
<u>Systems</u>: Urinary, digestive, excretory, female reproductive
<u>Action</u>: Mild stomachic, bitter tonic, diuretic, lithotriptic
<u>Uses</u>: Fever, diarrhea, dysentery, acid indigestion, edema, kidney inflammation, Bright's Disease, chronic cystitis, urethral discharge, urinary and bladder diseases, later stages of bowel complaints (taken with aromatics like cardamom); leaves and root paste with bland oil—topically for sores, sinuses, and itches. Recipe for colic; 4 parts *laghu pāṭā*: 5 parts pepper: 3 parts *asafoedita*: 6 parts ginger; mix and add honey to make into a pill. The dose is three to five grains.
<u>Preparation</u>: Decoction, powder, extract

<u>Sanskrit</u>: **Mamīrā, Mishamitita**
ममीरा, मिष्हमितित

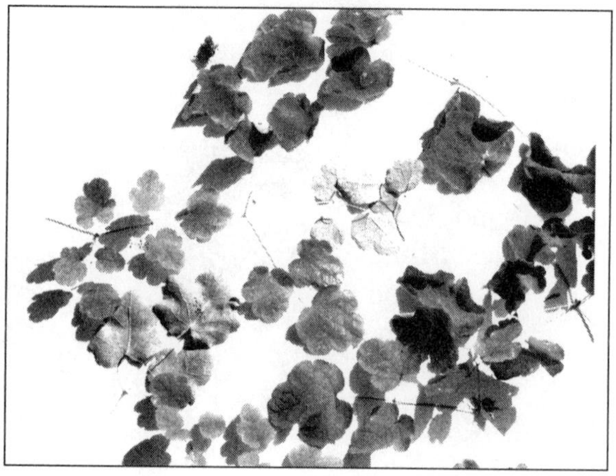

Hindi: Mamira
English: Gold Thread
Latin: Coptis teeta Wall.
Part Used: Dried root
Habitat: Himalayas, Mishmi mountains east of Upper Assam
Energetics: Bitter-cooling-pungent PK- V+
Tissues: Plasma, blood, fat
Systems: Digestive, circulatory
Action: Bitter tonic, antipyretic, alterative
Uses: Improves appetite, restores digestion, gas, visceral obstructions, jaundice, improves bile flow, chronic gall bladder inflammation, debility, convalescence after fevers, debilitating diseases, atonic indigestion, mild forms of intermittent fevers, catarrhal and rheumatic conjunctivitis, dries excessive body moisture (e.g., water retention), all Pitta disorders, anal fissure, ulcerative colitis, vaginal infections, tumors, boils, carbuncles, inflammatory skin conditions; externally applied to sores (including mouth sores).
Preparation: Paste, eye salve, powder, infusion, extract
Precaution: Drying; do not use with nausea or vomiting caused by a stomach hypoactivity or diarrhea due to spleen or kidney deficiency. Long term use aggravates the spleen and stomach

Sanskrit: **Mañjiṣhṭhā** मञ्जिष्ठा
Hindi: Mañjiṭ

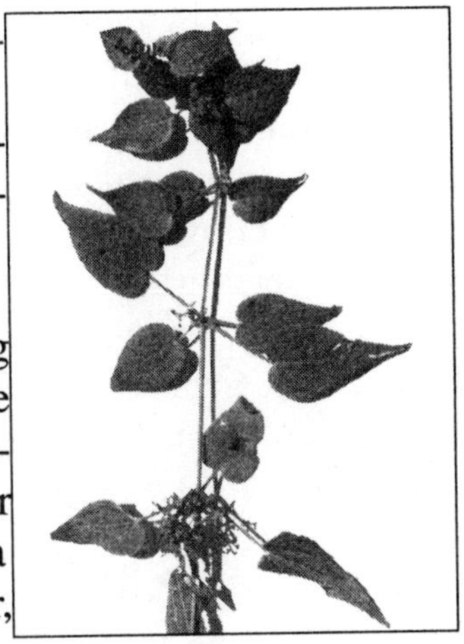

English: Indian Madder
Latin: Rubia cordifolia Linn. (R. manjishta, R. secunda)
Part Used: Root
Habitat: A climbing plant found in the North- West Himalayas, Nilgiris and other hilly districts of India
Energetics: Bitter, sweet-cooling-pungent PK- V+
Tissues: Plasma, blood, muscles
Systems: Circulatory, female reproductive
Action: Alterative, anti-tumor, astringent, diuretic, emmenagogue, hemostatic, lithotriptic
Uses: The best herb for blood purification; blood circulation, controls bleeding, mends broken bones, amenorrhea, cancer, cleanses and regulates liver, spleen, pancreas, and kidneys; diarrhea, dysentery, dysmenorrhea, edema, destroys kidney and gall stones, heart disease, hepatitis, herpes, jaundice, menopause, menorrhagia, painful menstruation, post partum uterus stimulation, paralysis, skin problems, tissue healing, traumatic injuries, skeletal disease, Kapha disorders, joint pain, rheumatoid arthritis, improves complexion and voice, helps destroy benign and malignant tumors.
Precautions: Severe chills, aggravates Vāyu
Preparation: Decoction, powder, paste, *ghee*

Sanskrit: **Maricha** (meaning: sun due to its large amounts of solar energy)

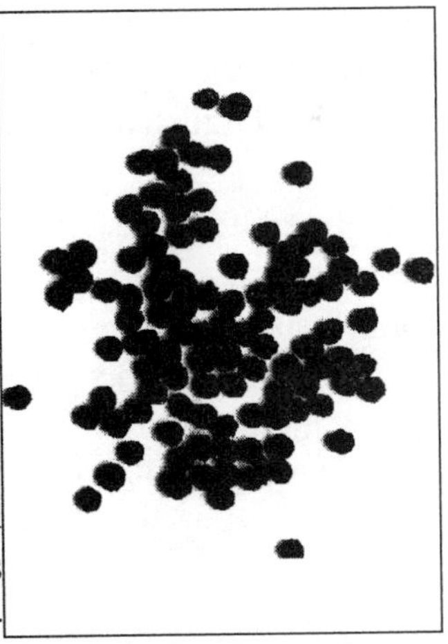

मरिच
Hindi: Gulmirch
English: Black Pepper
Latin: Piper nigrum Linn.
Part Used: Dried unripe fruit
Habitat: Perennial climbing shrub is found throughout India
Energetics: Pungent-heating-pungent VK- P+
Tissues: Plasma, blood, fat, marrow, nerve
Systems: Digestive, circulatory, respiratory
Action: Stimulant, expectorant, carminative, antipyretic, anthelmintic, antiperiodic; externally—rubefacient, stimulant, resolvent
Uses: Asthma, chronic indigestion, colon toxins, obesity, sinus congestion, fever, intermittent fe-

ver, cold extremities, colic, cooking spice, cholera, gastric ailments, gas, diarrhea, hemorrhoids, worms, sore throat; externally—applied as a paste to boils, skin diseases.
Preparation: Infusion, powder, milk decoction, medicated *ghee*
Precaution: Digestive inflammations, high Pitta

Sanskrit: **Musta, Mustaka**
मुस्त, मुस्तक

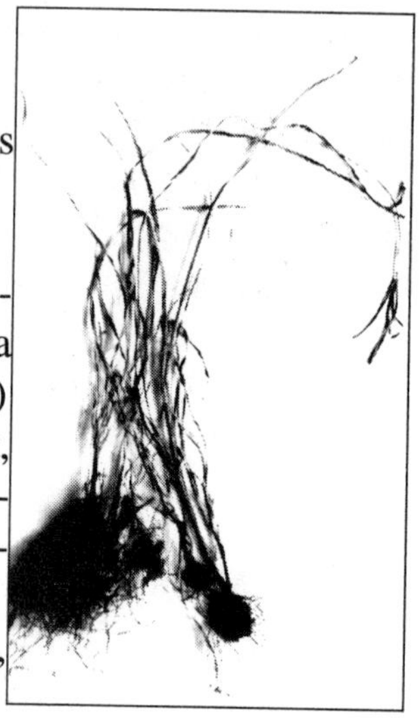

Hindi: Mutha
English: Nutgrass
Latin: Cyperus rotundus Linn.
Part Used: Rhizome
Habitat: Found throughout the plains of India (especially South India)
Energetics: Pungent, bitter, astringent-cool-pungent PK- (V+ in excess)
Tissues: Plasma, blood, muscle, marrow/nerve
Systems: Digestive, circulatory, female reproductive
Action: Alterative, anthelmintic, anti-fungal, anti-parasitic, anti-rheumatic, antispasmodic, aphrodisiac, astringent, carminative, demulcent, diaphoretic, diuretic, emmenagogue, stimulant, stomachic
Uses: Appetite (increases), yeast, candida, diarrhea, dysentery, dysmenorrhea, fevers, gastritis, indigestion, liver (sluggish), harmonizes the liver, spleen, and pancreas; malabsorption, colic, bloody stool, urine, and vomiting blood, promotes memory, convulsions, moodiness, and depression, menstrual disorders (including pain and cramps), PMS, menopause, palpitation, parasites, vomiting, colds, flu, mucus, lowers blood pressure, reduces breast tumors.
Precautions: Constipation and excess Vāyu
Preparation: Decoction, powder

Sanskrit: Nāgkeśhar नागकेशर

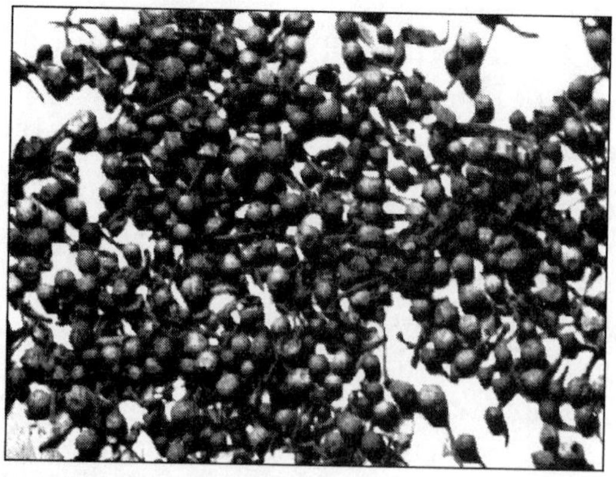

Hindi: Nagakesara
English: Cobra's Saffron
Latin: Mesua ferrea Linn. (M. Roxburghii, M. coromandalina
Part Used: Flower buds, flowers, fruit, seed, root, bark, oil
Habitat: Throughout India
Energetics: dried blossoms, root and bark—bitter; bark—mild astringent; dried flowers and blossoms—astringent; fruit skin—astringent
Tissues: Plasma
Systems: Respiratory, digestive, excretory
Action: Root—aromatic, sudorific
Bark—aromatic, sudorific,
Bark oleo-resin—aromatic, demulcent
Unripe fruit—aromatic, acrid, purgative
Fresh blossoms —stomachic, bitter, aromatic, sudorific
Dried flowers—stomachic, stimulant, carminative
Uses: Leaves—poultice for head colds. Bark and root—decoction, infusion, or tincture for gastritis and bronchitis. Seed Oil—externally for skin conditions (e.g., wounds, sore, etc.), and rheumatism. Dried flowers—oil or decoction fragrance; as a powdered paste or with *ghee,* they are used for bleeding hemorrhoids and dysentery with mucus. Flowers are also used for thirst, excessive perspiration, expectorating cough, indigestion.

Sanskrit: **Nimba**

निम्ब

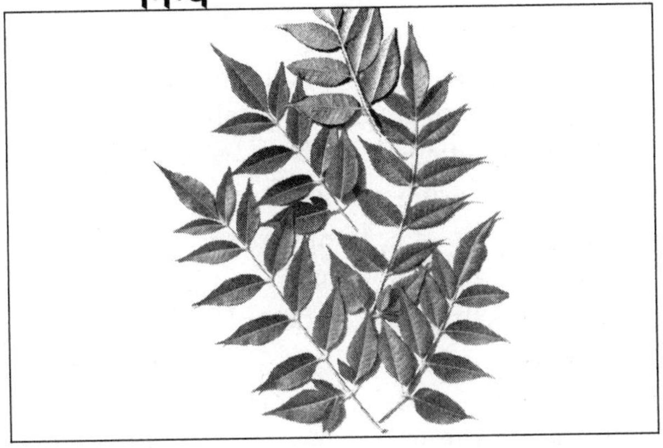

Hindi: Nimb
English: Neem
Latin: Melia azadirachta Linn. (Azadiracta Indica)
Part Used: All
Habitat: This tree grows wild in Iran, the Western Himalayas of India, and is cultivated in other parts of India
Energetics: Bitter-cool-pungent PK- V+
Tissues: Plasma, blood, fat
Systems: Circulatory, digestive, respiratory, urinary
Action:
Root bark—astringent, antiperiodic (prevent recurrence of diseases), tonic
Bark—astringent, antiperiodic, bitter, tonic, vermifuge, antiviral
Fruit—purgative, emollient, anthelmintic
Leaves—discutient, emmenagogue, antiviral
Juice—anthelmintic
Nut Oil—local stimulant, insecticide, antiseptic
Flowers—stimulant, tonic, stomachic
Uses: Arthritis, blood purifier and detoxifier, convalescence after fever, cough, diabetes, eczema, fever (used with black pepper and gentian), inflammation of muscles and joints, jaundice, leukorrhea, malaria, mucus membrane ulcerations, nausea, obesity, parasites, rheumatism, skin diseases/inflammations, cleanses liver, syphilis, thirst, tissue excess, tumors, vomiting, worms, drowsiness. Leaves—heal ulcers in urinary passage, emmenagogue, skin diseases. Fruit—skin diseases, bronchitis. Kernel powder—washing hair.
Precautions: Not used for people on spiritual paths or with emaciation
Preparation: Infusion, decoction, powder, medicated *ghee,* or oil

Sanskrit: **Nirguṇḍī**

निर्गुण्डी

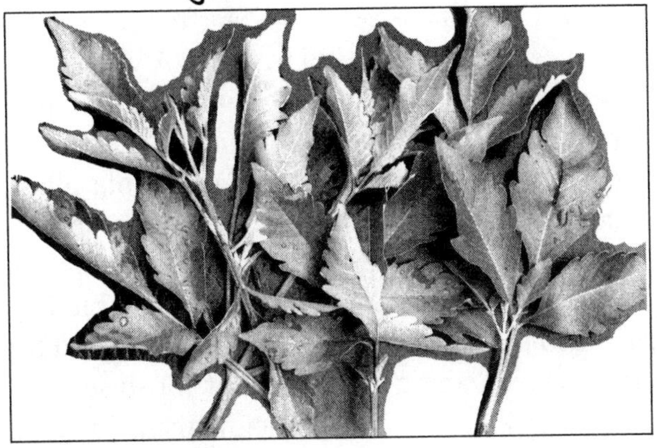

Hindi: Sambhalu
English: Five Leafed Chaste Tree
Latin: Vitex negundo Linn.
Part Used: Roots, root, flowers, leaves, bark
Habitat: Bengal, Southern India, Himalayas; Burma (Myanmar)
Energetics: Leaves—bitter; flowers—cool, astringent P- V+ (K+ in excess)
Tissues: Plasma, blood, marrow/nerve, reproduc tive
Systems: Circulatory, female reproductive, nervous
Action: Leaves—anti-parasitical, alterative, aromatic, vermifuge, pain reliever. Root—tonic, febrifuge, expectorant, diuretic. Fruit—nervine, cephalic, emmanagogue. Dried fruit—vermifuge
Uses: Hair, eyes, colic, swelling, worms, nausea, ulcers, ear disorders, malaria, hemorrhoids, spleen, uterus, removes obstructions, hemicrania. External: leaves—inflammatory joint swellings in acute rheumatism and of the testes from suppressed gonorrhea or gonorrheal epididymitis and orchitits; sprained limbs, contusions, bites (used as heated leaves or as a poultice). Pillows

stuffed with leaves are slept on to remove catarrh and headache (they are also smoked for relief). Crushed leaves or poultice is applied to temples for headaches. As a plaster on the spleen, it removes swelling; as a juice discharges worms from ulcers. A juice oil is applied to sinuses and neck gland sores (scrofula), or for washing the head for glandular tubercular neck swellings. Oil is also good for syphilis, venereal diseases, and other syphilitic skin disorders. A leaf decoction with *pippalī* is used for catarrhal fever with heaviness of head and dull hearing. A warm bath in a leaf decoction removes pains after child birth. For rheumatism it is taken as a juice, with the juice of *tulsī* and *bhṛiṅgarāj* (eclipta alba), mixed with crushed *ajwan* seeds; or these persons can bathe in a *nirguṇḍī* leaf decoction. A tincture of root-bark is good for irritable bladder and also rheumatism. Powdered root—good for hemorrhoids and as a demulcent for dysentery. Root—dyspepsia, colic, rheumatism, worms, boils, skin disorders. Flowers—diarrhea, cholera, fever, liver disorders, cardiac tonic; seeds—cooling for skin disorders; flowers and stalk powder—for blood discharge from stomach and bowels.
Preparation: Fruit powder—sugar/water or honey paste, decoction; powder, tincture, decoction, poultice

Sanskrit: **Paṣhana Bheda**
पषन भेद

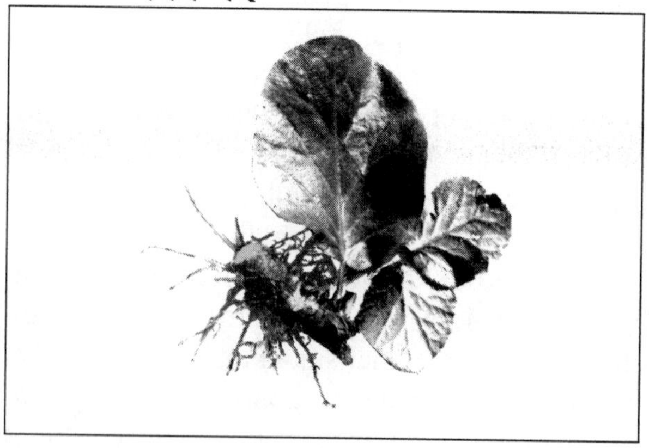

Hindi: Pakhanbed, Dakachru
English: None
Latin: Saxifraga ligulata Wall.
Part Used: Rhizome
Habitat: Found in temperate the areas of the Himalayas, from Bhutan to Kashmir and the Khassia Mountains.
Energetics: Astringent,sweet-cold-sweet PK- V+
Tissues: Plasma, fat, female reproductive
Systems: Female reproductive, urinary
Action: Astringent, demulcent, diuretic, lithotriptic
Uses: Cough, diarrhea, safer (less irritating) diuretic, fevers, vaginal diseases, Vāyu tumors, pulmonary, teething irritation, scurvy, tumors, uric acid, urinary stones/gravel dissolved (especially phosphate; also oxalate); enlarged prostate. External—paste for boils.
Precautions: Amenorrhea
Preparation: Decoction, powder, paste

Sanskrit: **Pippalī**
पिप्पली

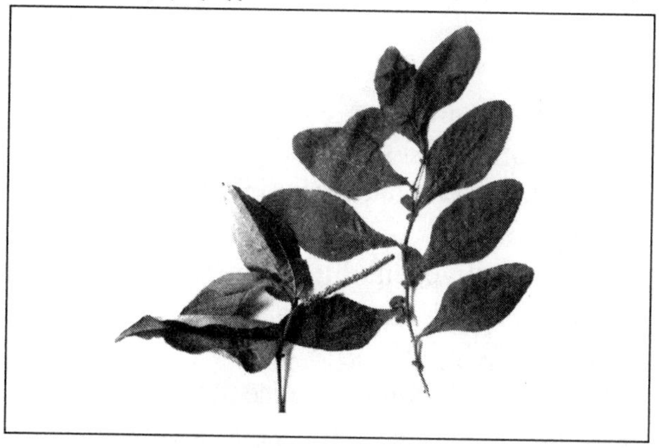

Hindi: Pippalī, Pipal
English: Long Pepper, Dried Catkins
Latin: Piper longum Linn.
Part Used: Fruit
Habitat: Indigenous to North-Eastern and Southern India; Sri Lanka, cultivated in Eastern Bengal
Energetics: Pungent-hot-sweet VK- P+
Tissues: All but bone
Systems: Digestive, reproductive, respiratory
Action: Analgesic, anthelmintic, aphrodisiac, carminative, expectorant

Uses: Abdominal tumors and distention, to improve the digestive fire, Kapha disorders, asthma, bronchitis, colds, coughs, epilepsy, flatulence, gout, laryngitis, paralysis, rheumatic pain, sciatica, worms, immune system, for *āma*.
Spiritual Uses: *Sattwic*
Precautions: Causes high Pitta
Preparation: Infusion, powder, oil

Sanskrit: **Pravāl**
प्रवाल

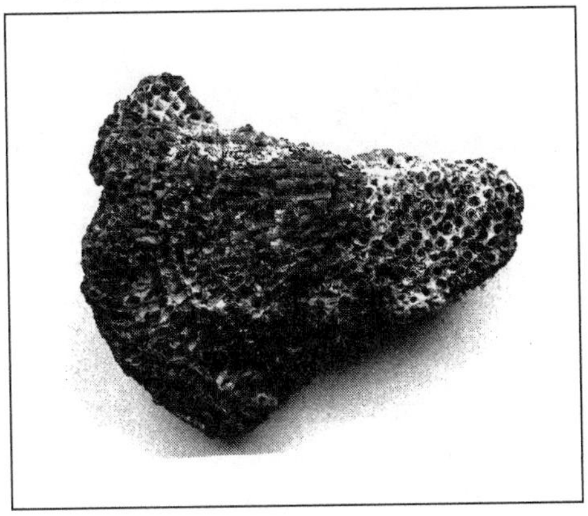

Hindi: Parvara
English: Red Coral
Latin: Corallium rubrum
Part Used: Shell
Habitat: Oceans, seas, and gulfs
Energetics: Its red color is due to large amounts of iron content. Best for Pitta; VPK=
Tissues: Plasma, blood, fat, muscle, reproductive
Systems: Digestive, nervous, excretory, respiratory, circulatory, reproductive
Action: Antacid, astringent, nervine tonic, laxative, diuretic, emetic, antibilious
Uses: It is mainly used for coughs, wasting, asthma, low fever, urinary diseases, carbuncles, scrofula, spermatorrhoea, gonorrhea and other genital inflammation with mucus discharge. Other main uses include nerve headaches, giddiness, and vertigo. Also, it is used for chronic bronchitis, pulmonary tuberculosis, vomiting, dyspepsia, bilious headache, weakness, and debility. It is also used in tooth powders as an astringent. *Pravāl pişhti*—for ulcers.
Preparation: Ash powder

Sanskrit: **Punarnavā**, Raktpunarnava (red) [see also Śhweta punarnarvā (white)]
पुनर्नवा

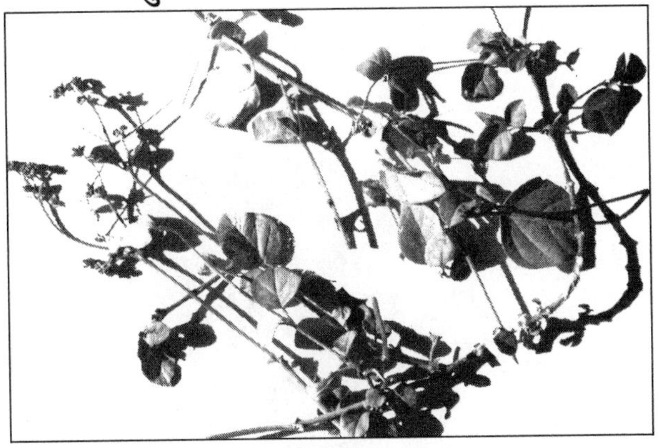

Hindi: Beshakapore, Lal Punarnava
English: Red Hogweed, Spreading Hogweed
Latin: Boerhavia diffusa Linn.
Part Used: Herb, root
Habitat: Throughout India, especially during the rainy season
Energetics: Red—bitter-cool-pungent
Tissues: Plasma, blood, muscle, fat, marrow/nerves, reproductive.
Systems: Digestive, female reproductive, circulatory, respiratory, nervous.
Action: Bitter, stomachic, laxative, diuretic, expectorant, rejuvenative, diaphoretic, emetic Root—purgative, anthelmintic, febrifuge; White—laxative, diaphoretic; Red—vermifuge.
Uses: White—edema, anemia, heart disease, cough, intestinal colic, kidney disorders; same uses as red. Red—nervous system, heart disease, hemorrhoids, skin diseases, kidney stones, edema, rat and snake bites; chronic alcoholism, wasting diseases, insomnia, rheumatism, eye diseases, asthma (moderate doses), induces vomiting in large doses, jaundice, ascites due to early liver and peritoneal concerns; urethritis. Leaf juice—jaundice; Root—decoction or infusion as a laxative, gonorrhea, internal inflammations; Externally—edema, rat and snake bites. Leaf juice with honey, dropped into the eyes for

chronic ophthalmia.
Preparation: Juice, decoction, infusion, powder, paste, oil, sugar water, or honey paste

Sanskrit: **Rasonam** (lacking one taste)/**Laśhuna**
रसोनम, लशुन

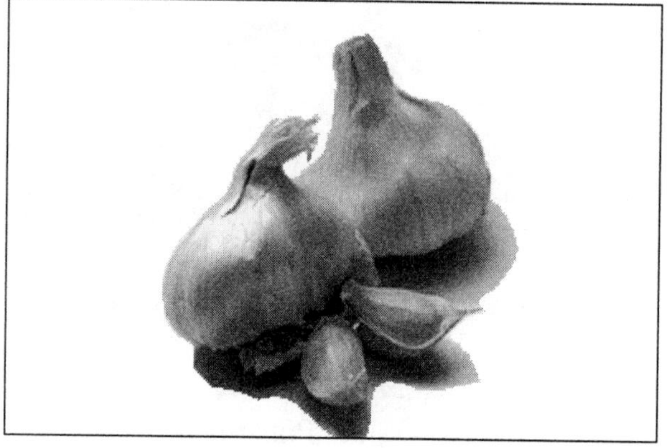

Hindi: Laśhan
English: Garlic
Latin: Allium sativum Linn.
Part Used: Bulb and oil
Habitat: Cultivated all over India, the U.S. and other countries
Energetics: All except sour; pungent-hot-pungent VK- P+
Tissues: All
Systems: Circulatory, digestive, nervous, reproductive, respiratory
Action: Alterative, anthelmintic, antiparasitic, antispasmodic, aphrodisiac, carminative, disinfectant, expectorant, rejuvenative, stimulant
Uses: Arteriosclerosis, asthma, blood and lymph cleanser (anti-*āma*); nerve and bone tissue *rasāyana* (rejuvenative); cholesterol, colds, colic, convulsions, cough, detoxifier, ear problems (external use), edema, flu, gas, heart disease, hemorrhoids, hypertension, hysteria, impotence, indigestion, lung/bronchial antiseptic and antispasmodic, memory, paralysis, rheumatism, skin diseases, T.B., tremor, tumors, Vāyu fevers, Vāyu/Kapha *rasāyana*, worms (round). Used effectively on parasites in dogs.
Spiritual Uses: It is *tamasic*, and only suggested as medicine; not as a food for the healthy. *Harītakī* is its spiritual substitute
Precautions: Hyperacidity, toxic blood heat, excess Pitta, cause mental dullness, not for spiritual devotees—except as medicine.
Preparation: Juice, infusion (don't boil), powder, medicated oil.

Sanskrit: **Rechanaka**, **Raktang**
रेचनक, रक्तन्गा

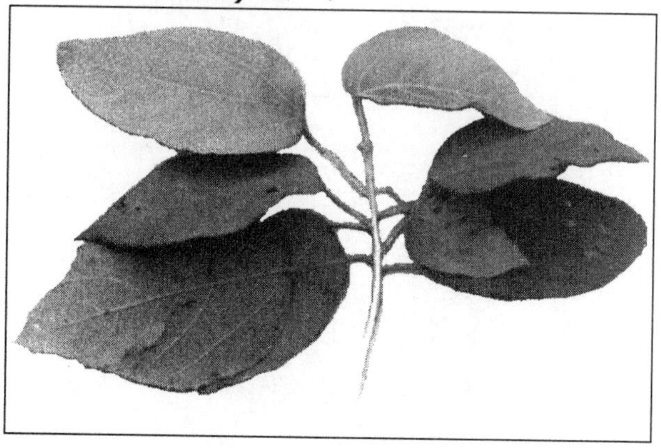

Hindi: Kamala
English: Kamala
Latin: Mallotus philippinensis Muell, Arg. (Croton philippinesis, C. punctatus, C. coccineum (Glandulae rottlerae)
Part Used: Glands and hairs from the capsules or fruits
Habitat: This small evergreen shrub of the Spurge family is found all over India, Sri Lanka, East Indies, Malay Archipelago, Australia, and more.
Energetics: VPK=, P-
Tissues: All, blood
Systems: Digestive, excretory
Action: Cathartic, anthelmintic, aphrodisiac, lithotriptic
Uses: Tapeworms, aperient, purgative (may cause nausea or gripping before purging, but no after-effects; good for children, adults, and pets.
Preparation: Ripe fruits are placed in a cloth and beaten until the glandular pubescence is removed; or fruits are rubbed between one's palms or feet

Sanskrit: **Sālam-miśhrī**
सालम मिश्री

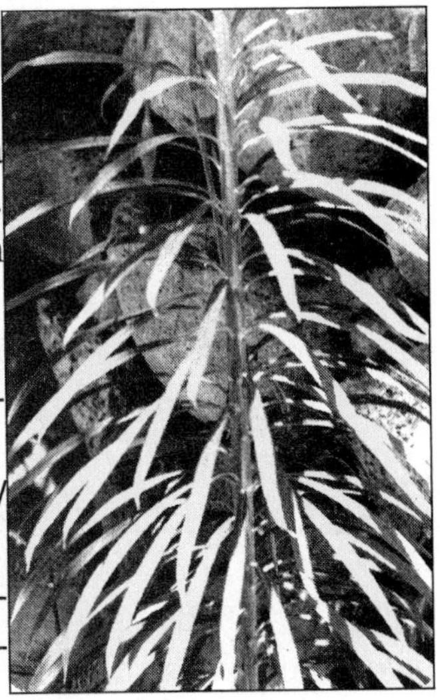

Hindi: Salabmishri
English: Salep Orchid
Latin: Orchis mascula Linn. (O. latifolia, O. Laxiflora, Allium Macleani)
Part Used: Root
Habitat: Iran, Afghanistan
Energetics: Sweet/ sweet/ sweet P-
Tissues: Blood, marrow/nerve, reproductive
Systems: Nervous, reproductive, excretory
Action: Restorative/invigorative tonic
Uses: Wasting diseases, diabetes, chronic diarrhea, dysentery, nervous or sexual debility, hemiplegia, paralysis, general weakness, impotence.
Preparation: One teaspoon of powdered root to one cup of boiled milk
Precaution: Avoid chilies, acids, very spicy foods, intoxicants, staying awake through the night, and sexual acts, when taking this herb

Sanskrit: **Sārivā**
सारिवा

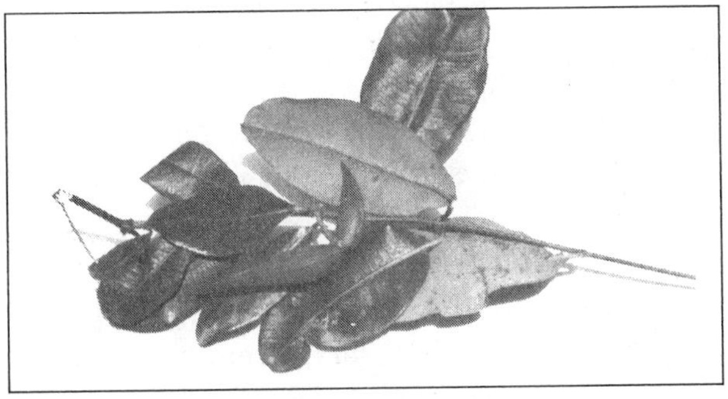

Hindi: Kalisar, Dudhilata, Sugandhi
English: Black Creeper, Sarsaparilla
Latin: Ichnocarpus fruitescens (Apocymene frutescens, Echites frutscens)
Part Used: Root, milk, stalk, leaves
Habitat: A climbing plant throughout India; in the Himalayas under 5,000 feet.
Energetics: Astringent-cool-/astringent P- VK+
Tissues: Plasma, blood, marrow/nerves
Systems: Circulatory, nervous
Action: The root is an alterative tonic, diuretic, diaphoretic
Uses: Stalks and leaves—decoction for skin eruptions, hearing disorders, fevers. Root decoction—skin diseases, syphilis, elephantiasis, loss of sensation, hemiplegia, loss of appetite, blood purifier, kidney and urinary disorders. It is best taken with other herbs.
Preparation: Decoction, powder, pills

Sanskrit: **Sarpa-gandha** (serpentine species)
सर्प-गन्ध

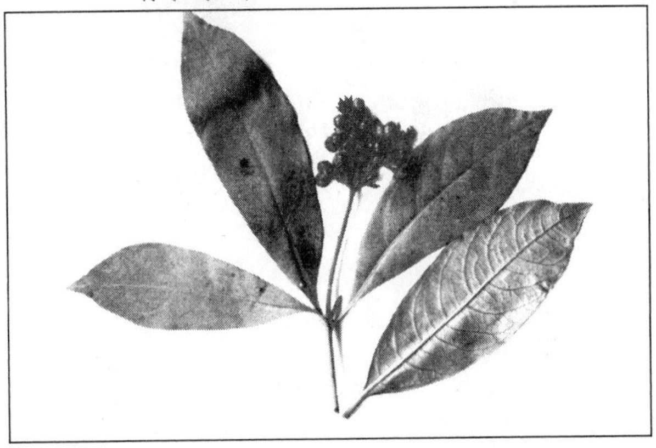

Hindi: Nakuli, Chota-chand
English: None
Latin: Rauwolfia serpentina Benth.
Part Used: Root
Habitat: Climbing shrub in tropical Himalayas; moderate altitudes in Sikkim, North Bihar, Patna, Bhagalpur, Assam, Pegu, Tenasserim, Deccan Peninsula, Sri Lanka, Java, Malay
Energetics: Root—bitter
Tissues: Plasma, blood, marrow/nerves
Systems: Excretory, nervous, circulatory, respiratory
Action: Bitter tonic, sedative, febrifuge
Uses: It contains Reserpine alkaloid which is used for hypertension. This is the main herb for high blood pressure, insanity with violent mania-

cal symptoms (doses; 20-30 grains of root powder), insomnia, insect stings, dysentery, painful bowel disorders, fevers, insanity, sedative, hypochondria, irritative conditions of the CNS (central nervous system); leaf juice—in eyes heals cornea opacities.
Preparation: Decoction, powder, pills
Precautions: Lethal in large doses; not yet allowed in the U.S.
Prolonged use over 10 years can cause sterility

Sanskrit: **Śhaṅkh Puṣhpī**
शंख पुष्पी

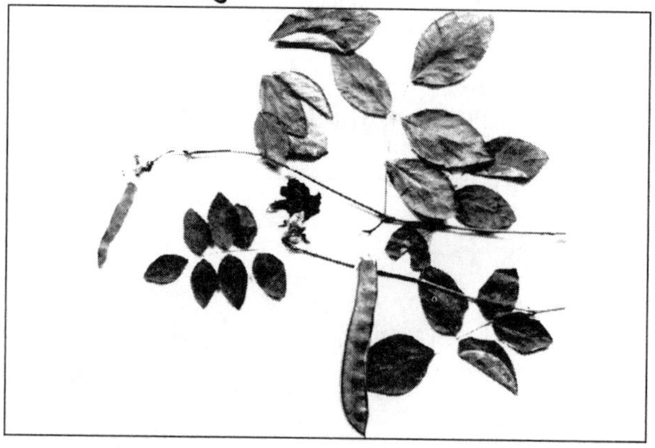

Hindi: Shankhini
English: None
Latin: Canscora decussata Roem. etc. Sch.
Part Used: Entire plant and juice
Habitat: Found throughout India and Burma (Myanmar)
Energetics: Bitter-warm-pungent VPK=
Tissues: Nerves
Systems: Mind, nervous
Action: Alterative, nervine
Uses: Juice for epilepsy, insanity, nervousness, memory. One of the main Āyurvedic nervines with *brāhmī, jaṭāmāṇshī,* and *vachā.*
Preparation: Juice, infusion, decoction, powder, paste

Sanskrit: **Śhatāvarī, Śhatamūlī**
शतावरी, शतमूली

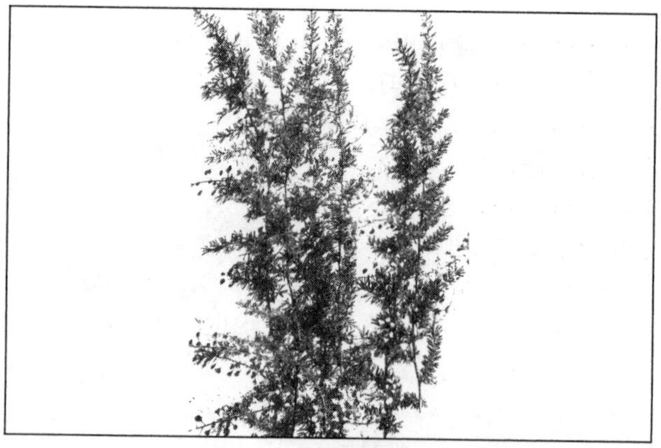

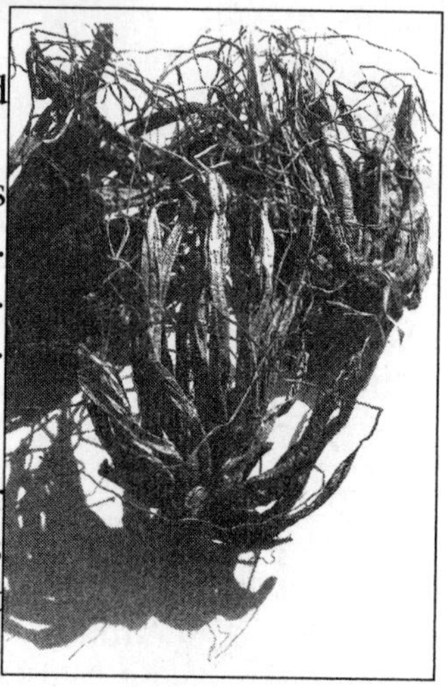

Hindi: Śhatāvarī
English: Hundred Husbands
Latin: Asparagus racemosus Willd. (A. sarmentosus, Willd; A. gonoclados, Baker; A. adscendens, Roxb.)
Part Used: Root
Habitat: This climber is found in the jungles around 8,000 feet throughout India, especially Northern India
Energetics: Sweet, bitter-cool-sweet PV- (K, *āma* + in excess)
Tissues: All Systems: Circulatory, digestive, reproductive, respiratory
Action: Mucilaginous, antidiarrhetic, refrigerant, diuretic, antidysenteric, nutritive, tonic, demulcent, galactagogue, aphrodisiac, antispasmodic, stomachic
Uses: Cancer, convalescence, cough, dehydration, diarrhea, dysentery, female organ debility (main female rejuvenative herb), fevers (chronic), hematemesis, herpes, hyperacidity, impotence, infertility, leukorrhea, menopause, lung abscess, sexual debility, ulcers, rheumatism, soothes dry, inflamed membranes of kidneys, lungs, sexual organs, and stomach. External application—emollient for stiff joints and neck, and muscle spasms. Increases breast milk and semen, nurtures mucus membranes, blood cleanser, supplies female hormones, nourishes

the ovum. Immune system boost—good for AIDS, Epstein Barr, etc., cancer—strengthens one from and for chemotherapy.
Spiritual Uses: *Sattwic*, increases love and devotion, increases *ojas*
Precautions: Do not use if congested or with *āma*
Preparation: Decoction, powder, *ghee*, oil; for serious diseases like cancer, use one or more ounces daily.

Sanskrit: **Śhilājit** (meaning: sweat of the rock)
शिलाजित

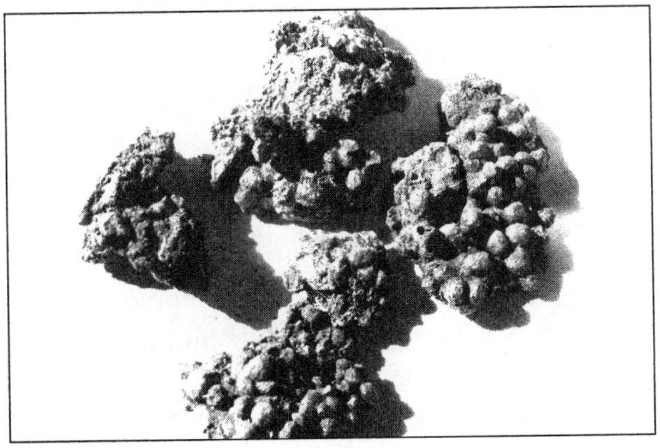

Hindi: Śhilājita
English: Mineral Pitch; Vegetable Asphalt
Latin: Asphaltum
Part Used: The oozing from the rocks
Habitat: Himalayas, near the source of the holy *Ganges* river
Energetics: Pungent, bitter, warm-pungent VPK=, P+ in excess
Tissues: All
Systems: All, especially the urinary and nervous
Action: Alterative, diuretic, lithotriptic, antiseptic, rejuvenative
Uses: Especially useful as a Vāyu tonic and rejuvenative, aphrodisiac, and for the kidneys and diabetes; obesity, jaundice, kidney, and gall stones, dysuria, cystitis, edema, hemorrhoids, sexual debility, menstrual disorders, asthma, epilepsy, insanity, skin diseases, parasites, heals broken bones, mental work. Of the varieties of *śhilājit*, the black is used for healing. Although it is expensive in comparison to herbs, it can heal most diseases
Production: In the Himalayan region known as *Gangotri* (the northern region of the *Ganges* river), *śhilājit* drips from the rocks. In other areas, foot-long scorpions sting the rocks. The poison from their stingers causes the *śhilājit* to ooze from the stones. In still other places, it appears in coagulated form. Monkeys use this natural remedy for various health ailments. They stay healthy and live a long time
Precautions: Do not use with high uric acid count, or with febrile diseases
Preparation: Powder, with milk. 1 oz or more a day for severe diseases; 1/4-1 tsp.- 3 times daily, otherwise

Sanskrit: **Śhweta Musali**
श्वेत मुसलि

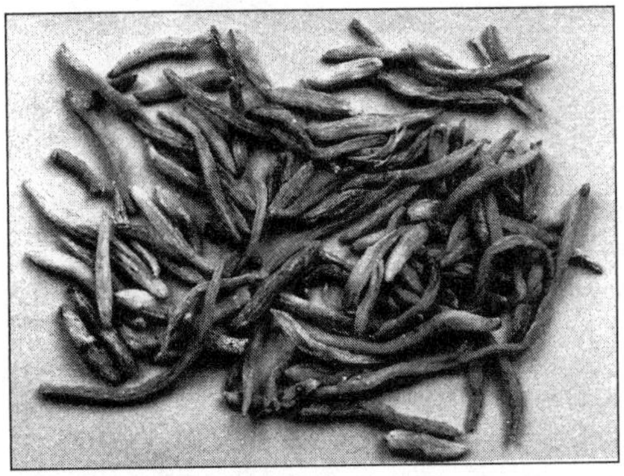

Hindi: Safeta Musali
English: White Musali
Latin: Asparagus adscendens Roxb.
Part Used: Tuberous root or rhizome
Habitat: Western Himalayas, Punjab, Gujarat, Bombay, Oudh, Central India
Energetics: Sweet, bitter-cold-sweet VP- K+
Tissues: Reproductive
Systems: Reproductive, respiratory
Action: Demulcent, galactagogue, nutritive tonic
Uses: Debility (general and sexual), diarrhea, leukorrhea, spermatorrhea, wasting diseases. It helps during pregnancy and postpartum, nourishing fetus and increasing breast milk flow. A

relative of *shatāvarī*.
Precautions: *Āma*, congestion
Preparation: Milk decoction, powder, confection

Sanskrit: **Snuhī, Thohar**

स्नुही, वज्र

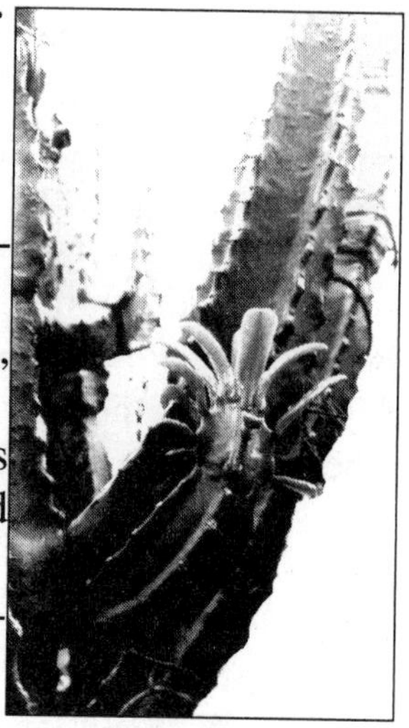

Hindi: Thohar
English: Milk Hedge
Latin: Euphorbia neriifolia Linn. (E. lingularia)
Part Used: Stem juice, root
Habitat: Leafless shrubs are found in Northern and Central India
Energetics: Very hot VK- P+
Tissues: Marrow/nerves, plasma, fat,
Systems: Nervous, excretory
Action: Juice—purgative, expectorant; locally—rubefacient Root—antispasmodic
Uses: Milky juice—cathartic to relieve earache, liver and spleen disorders, syphilis, edema, skin diseases, asthma, cough, remove warts (externally used), with soot of *ghee* lamp as an eye salve for ophthalmia; externally with *ghee* applied to ulcers and scabies; glandular swellings—prevents pus formation and oozing; with turmeric—applied to hemorrhoids. Mainly used externally.
Preparation: Juice, powder, pill, syrup, paste, tincture, decoction, salve
Precaution: It is very irritant and strong alkalis use under the supervision of an Āyurvedic specialist

Sanskrit: **Tagara**

तगर

Hindi: Tagar, Bala-tagra, Sugandh-bala
English: Indian Valerian

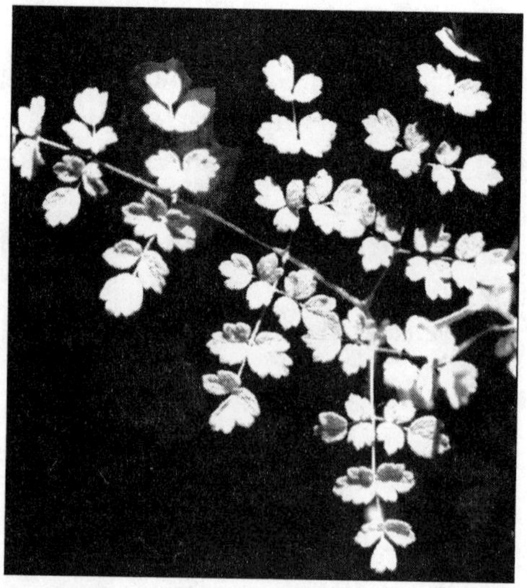

Latin: Valeriana wallichii DC. (V. leschenauitic, V. brunoniana)
Part Used: Rhizome (root)
Habitat: Himalayan temperate regions, Kashmir, Bhutan; Afghanistan
Energetics: Bitter, pungent, sweet, astringent-heating-pungent VK- P+
Tissues: Plasma, muscle, marrow/nerve
Systems: Nervous, digestive, respiratory
Action: Stimulant, antispasmodic, stomachic, sedative, analeptic, carminative, nervine
Uses: Diminishes irritability of the brain and spinal marrow; nervous cough, dysmenorrhea, palpitations, migraine, chronic skin disorders, gas, colic, vertigo, nervous debility, failing reflexes, spasms, menopausal spasms, menstrual cramps, G.I. fermentation, insomnia, delirium, neuralgia, convulsions, nervous exhaustion, mental stress, and overwork; hysteria, epilepsy. One of the best herbs for Vāyu nervous disorders; cleanses undigested toxins (*āma*) from the colon, blood, joints, and nerves; clears nerve channels from excess Vāyu; fainting; mixed with calamus (*vachā*) it is less dulling (4:1). Its relative, *jaṭāmāṇshī,* is tridoṣhic, also a sedative, but not *tamasic* (spiritually dulling).
Spiritual Uses: It is *tamasic*, not recommended for meditation
Preparation: Infusion, decoction, powder, pills
Precaution: Excessive use may dull the mind. Excessive doses may cause central paralysis and other severe conditions. Use only under the su-

pervision of a qualified practitioner

Sanskrit: **Tejbal, Tumbru**
तेजबल, तुम्बरु

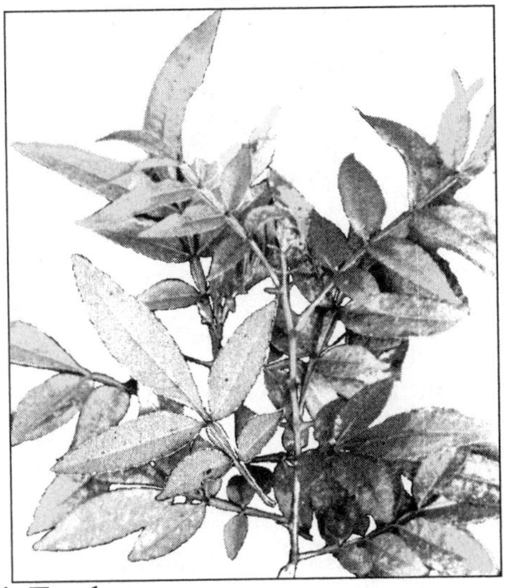

Hindi: Tumbru
English: Toothache Tree
Latin: Zanthoxylum alatum Roxb.
Part Used: Bark, carpels (ovule bearing leaf of pistil on a flower), carpels of fruits, seeds
Habitat: Shrub common in the temperate Himalayas, Bhutan, Darjeeling
Energetics: Sweet, bitter-cold-sweet P- VK+
Tissues: Plasma, blood, bone
Systems: Excretory, circulatory, digestive, respiratory
Action: Bark and seeds—aromatic tonic; branches, fruit and thorns—carminative, stomachic
Uses: Bark and seeds—fever, indigestion, cholera; fruit, branches, and thorns are used to heal toothache and other diseases of the teeth. Good for asthma, bronchitis, Kapha disorders.
Preparation: Bark—infusion, decoction

Sanskrit: **Tila**
तिल
Hindi: Til

English: Sesame
Latin: Sesamum indicum DC. (S. orientale, S. trifoliatum, S luteum)
Part Used: Seed, oil, leaf. There are three varieties; black, white, red (or brown). White has most oil, black is best for healing
Habitat: Small bush throughout India
Energetics: Sweet-heating-sweet V- PK+
Tissues: All, especially bone
Systems: Excretory, reproductive, urinary, respiratory
Action: Seeds—laxative, emollient, demulcent, diuretic, promote *ojas*, nourishing, galactogogue, emmenagogue, nutritive tonic, rejuvenative. Leaves—demulcent
Uses: Seeds—excellent rejuvenative tonic for Vāyu *doṣhas*, bones and teeth; hemorrhoids, dysentery, constipation (decoction or sweets); decoction with linseed for cough, aphrodisiac; as a paste, with butter for bleeding hemorrhoids; powder for amenorrhea, dysmenorrhea (and a warm hip bath with a handful of seeds placed in the water); poultice applied externally to ulcers, burns, and scalds. Applying the oil to the body and head is useful for Vāyu *doṣhas*, calming, giving nutrition, anti-oxidant properties, dry skin, ulcers, oozing wounds, with equal parts of lime juice for burns and scalds, on eyelids for eye problems; cooking/frying. Ingesting oil—gonorrhea. Leaves—mucilage for dysentery, cholera infantum, etc. Decoction from leaves and root—hair wash, blackens hair, promotes hair growth. Sesame stalks are good food for cows.
Spiritual Uses: *Sattwic* (holy)—good for *yogis* (up to one ounce daily)

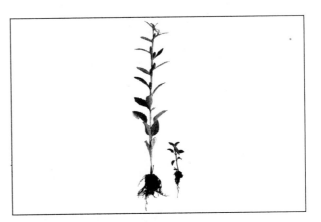

Preparation: Decoction, sweets, paste, poultice, powder, medicated oil
Precaution: Large doses may cause abortion; obesity, high Pitta

Sanskrit: **Trāymān**
त्रायमान

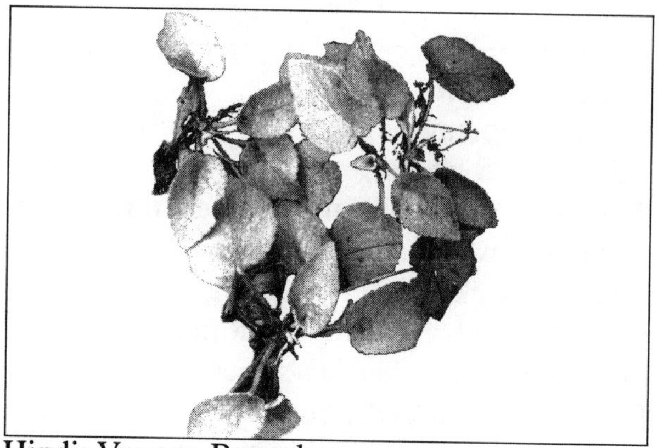

Hindi: Vanpsa, Banaphsa
English: Wild Violet
Latin: Viola odorata Linn.
Part Used: Flowers, root
Habitat: An herb found in the Himalayas over 5,000 feet
Energetics: Flowers astringent; bitter-cold-bitter VPK=
Tissues: Plasma, blood, reproductive
Systems: Respiratory, excretory, female reproductive, circulatory
Action: Emetic, flowers—demulcent, diaphoretic, diuretic, aperient
Uses: Decoction for cough, sneezing, flu, and other respiratory problems. Bile, lung disorders, rectum and uterus prolapse, stops oozing of pus, kidney and liver diseases; diaphoretic for pulmonary disorders, nauseating emetic, large doses—emetic, mixed with almond oil and senna syrup—excellent demulcent and aperient for children, petal syrup—infant coughs and chest tightness; flower infusion—fevers; root is emetic in larger doses.
Preparation: Decoction, infusion, powder, pill, syrup

Sanskrit: **Tulsī, Tulasī, Kṛiṣhṇamul**
तुलसी, तुलसी, कृष्समुल

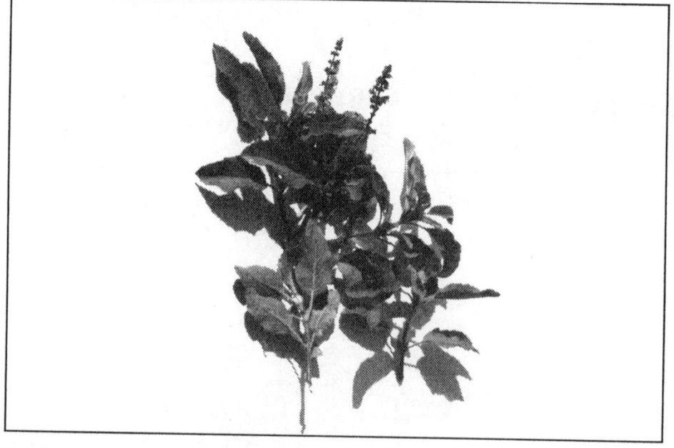

Hindi: Kala Tulasī
English: Basil, Holy Basil
Latin: Ocimum Spp. or O. Sanctum or O. basilicum
Part Used: Herb
Habitat: Small herb found throughout India and cultivated near Hindu houses and temples
Energetics: Pungent-hot-pungent VK- (P+ in excess)
Tissues: Plasma, blood, marrow/nerves, reproductive
Systems: Digestive, nervous, respiratory
Action: Antibacterial, antiseptic, antispasmodic, diaphoretic, febrifuge, nervine
Uses: Coughs, colds, fevers, headaches, lung problems, abdominal distention, absorption, arthritis, colon (air excess), memory, nasal congestion, nerve tissue strengthening, purifies the air (when grown in the house—a natural negative ion machine); sinus congestion, clears the lungs, heart tonic; it frees ozone from sun's rays and oxygenates the body, cleanses and clears the brain and nerves; relieves depression and the effects of poisons; difficult urination, prevents the accumulation of fat in the body (especially for women after menopause), obstinate skin diseases, arthritis, rheumatism, first stages of many cancers, builds the immune system. *Tulsī* contains trace mineral copper (organic form), needed to absorb iron.
Spiritual Uses: *Sattwic*, opens heart and mind, gives love, devotion, faith, compassion, and clarity; sacred to *Viṣhṇu* and *Kṛiṣhṇa*; cleanses the

aura and gives Divine protection. It increases *prāṇa* (life breath). One of the two most sacred plants in India. It develops pure awareness
Precautions: Excess Pitta
Preparation: Juice, infusion, powder, *ghee*

Sanskrit: **Tvak**
त्वक

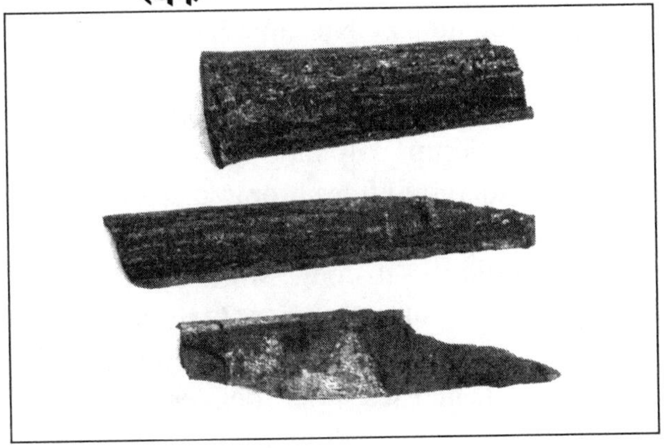

Hindi: Dalchini, Daruchini
English: Cinnamon
Latin: Cinnamomum cassia Blume. (C. zeylanicum; C. saigonicum; C. aromaticum; C. laurus.)
Part Used: Bark
Habitat: Indigenous to Sri Lanka and Southern India
Energetics: Pungent, sweet, astringent-heating-sweet VK- P+
Tissues: Plasma, blood, muscles, marrow/nerves
Systems: Circulatory, digestive, respiratory, urinary
Action: Alterative, analgesic, antibacterial, antifungal, antiseptic, antirheumatic, antispasmodic, aromatic, astringent, carminative, demulcent, diaphoretic, digestive, diuretic, expectorant, germicide, hemostatic, stimulant, stomachic
Uses: Absorption, *agni* (digestive fire) promoting, breathing difficulties, bronchitis, colds, congestion, circulation, generates energy and blood, strengthens one's constitution, diarrhea, dysentery, edema, flu, gas, metabolic (spleen and pancreas) and heart strengthening, hiccup, indigestion, warms and strengthens the kidneys, liver problems, menorrhagia, melancholy, muscle tension, for debilitating pain of the waist, knees, backaches and headaches; palpitations, toothache, uterine muscle fiber stimulant, nausea, vomiting. Assists uterine contractions during labor, menstrual pain from low metabolic function. External—headaches, pain.
Spiritual Uses: *Sattwic*
Precautions: Bleeding disorders, excess Pitta
Preparation: Infusion, decoction, powder, oil

Sanskrit: **Vachā** (meaning: speaking)
वचा

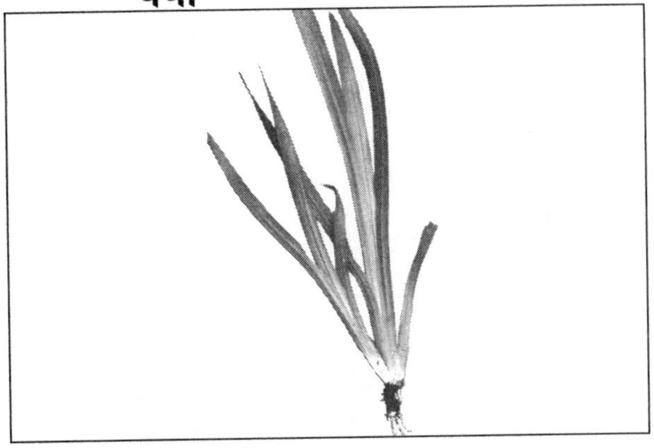

Hindi: Bach
English: Calamus
Latin: Acornus calamus Linn.
Part Used: Rhizome
Habitat: A semi-aquatic perennial cultivated in damp marshy places, or by the edge of lakes and streams in India and Burma (Myanmar)
Energetics: Pungent, bitter, astringent-hot-pungent VK- P+
Tissues: Plasma, muscle, fat, marrow/nerve, reproductive
Systems: Circulatory, digestive, nervous, reproductive, respiratory
Action: Antispasmodic, decongestant, emetic, expectorant, nervine, rejuvenative, stimulant
Uses: Arthritis, asthma, brain rejuvenation, cerebral circulation promoter, colds, coma (as snuff), cough, deafness, detoxifies subtle channels, emetic, epilepsy, hysteria, insanity, memory, mental sharpness, nasal congestion, and polyps (as snuff); nervous system rejuvenation, neural-

gia, shock (as snuff), sinus headaches/sinusitis, transmutes sexual energy to spiritual energy; gastritis, colic pain, laryngitis, Vāyu and Kapha rejuvenator. One of the best mind herbs. It removes the toxic effects of marijuana from the liver and brain. External—paste applied to head for headaches and arthritic joint pain. Powder may be sprinkled in home for removal of insects, fleas; keeps moths from woolens.
Spiritual Uses: *Sattwic*
Precautions: Not to be used with bleeding disorders (e.g., nosebleeds, hemorrhoids) and other Pitta conditions. Excess use may cause nausea, vomiting, rashes, and other Pitta conditions.
Preparation: Decoction, milk decoction, powder, paste

Sanskrit: **Vamśha (Lochana)**
वंश लोचन

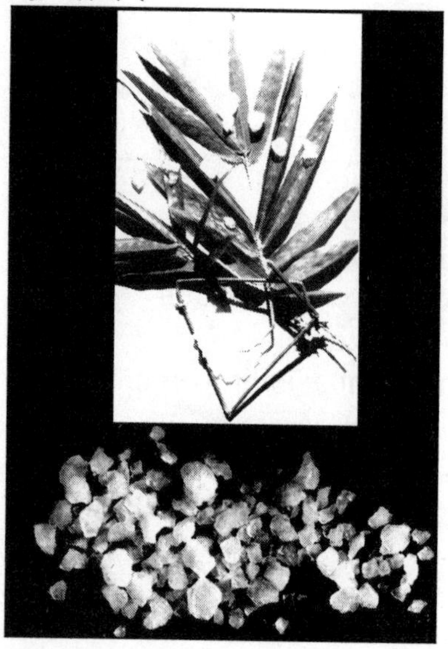

Hindi: Vaṃśh Lochan, Bans
English: Bamboo Manna
Latin: Bumbusa arundinacia Retz. (B. apous, B. orientalls, B. spinosa)
Part Used: [Two varieties (blue, white)] Inner stalks or stems of female plant (silicous deposit)/milky bark; leaves, young shoots, seeds, roots
Habitat: Himalayas; 4,000 feet, and throughout India
Energetics: Sweet, astringent-cold-sweet PV- K+
Tissues: Plasma, blood, marrow/nerve
Systems: Circulatory, nervous, respiratory
Action: Demulcent, expectorant, tonic, rejuvenative, antispasmodic, hemostatic; leaves—emmenagogue, anthelmintic; stimulant, febrifuge, tonic, aphrodisiac
Uses: Excellent for colds, coughs, fevers, and asthma; bleeding, emaciation, debility, dehydration, vomiting, consumption, excellent Pitta reducing herb, lungs. Nurtures heart, liver, and soothes the nervous system; relieves thirst, anxiety, improves the blood, skin disorders, threadworms in children, palpitation, coma, rejuvenative, strengthening after chronic diseases, sedative, tissue deficiency. Leaves—eaten by pets. External poultice—dislodge worms from ulcers. Young shoots—ulcer worms (external—juice poured on bandage). Leaf bud—decoction for discharge of menses after delivery or when scanty.
Preparation: Decoction, milk decoction, powder
Precaution: Increases congestion if not balanced with pungent herbs like ginger

Sanskrit: **Vārāhīkand**
वराहीकन्द

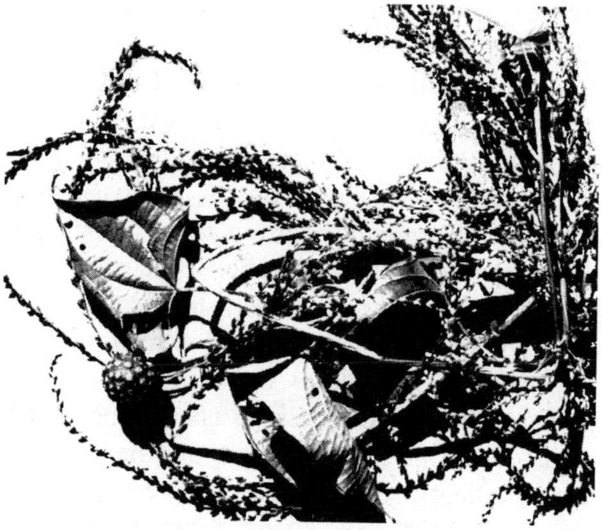

Hindi: Gendhi; Zamin-kand

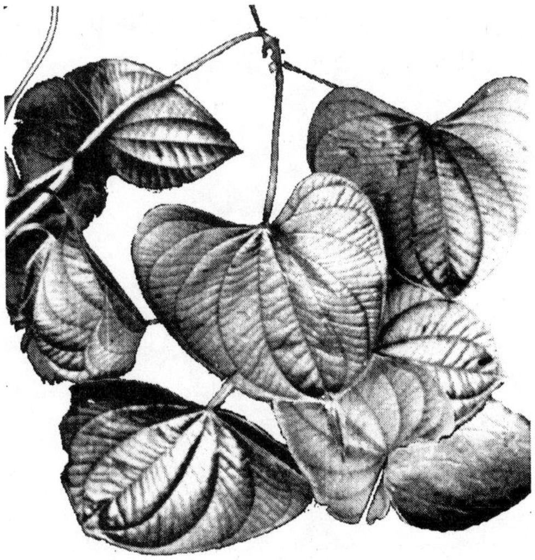

English: Yam
Latin: Dioscorea bulbifera Linn., var.: sativa
Part Used: Tubers
Habitat: Grows in UP, Bihar and Sub Himalayan region of India
Energetics: Sweet, bitter-cold-sweet VP- (K+ in excess)
Systems: Digestive, reproductive, nervous, urinary
Action: Nutritive tonic, aphrodisiac, rejuvenative, diuretic, antispasmodic, analgesic
Uses: Syphilis, hemorrhoids, dysentery, diarrhea, impotency, senility, hormonal deficiency, infertility, colic, nervous excitability, hysteria, abdominal pain and cramps; increases semen, milk (progesterone), and other hormonal secretions (pituitary, thyroid, estrogen); promotes body weight, male/female reproductive tonic, and soothes digestive organs.
Precautions: Glucoside in the plant is poisonous; creates excess mucus and congestion. Only use with the advice of an Āyurvedic specialist
Preparation: Decoction, milk decoction, powder, bolus, candy

Sanskrit: **Vāsāka, Vāsā**
वासाक, वासा
Hindi: Adosa
English: Malabar Nut

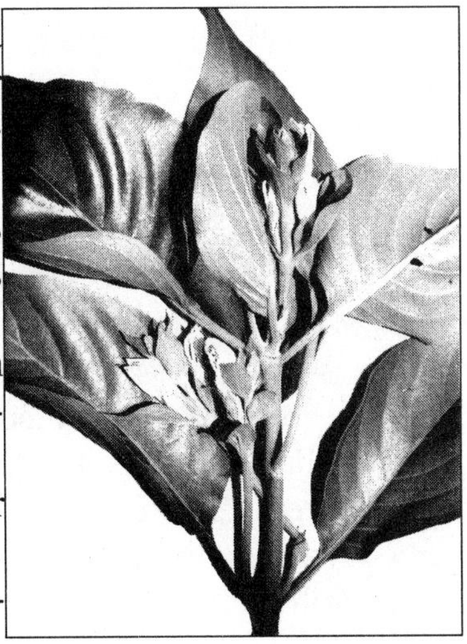

Latin: Adhatoda vasika Nees. (or Adenanthera vasika)
Part Used: Leaves, roots, flowers, bark
Habitat: A bush growing throughout India, especially the lower Himalayan ranges
Energetics: Bitter-hot PK- V+
Tissues: Plasma, blood
Systems: Respiratory, circulatory, nervous, elimination
Action: Expectorant, diuretic, antispasmodic, alterative
Uses: Asthma (bronchodilator), bronchitis, cough, voice, thirst, vomiting, dysentery, diarrhea, wasting, TB, rheumatic pain, swelling, bleeding, urinary disorders including diabetes; neuralgia, skin disorders, fever with cough, epilepsy, hysteria, insanity; repellent for fleas, mosquitos, centipedes, flies and other insects; Kapha disorders, flu.
Preparation: Infusion, extract, decoction, poultice, powder, cigarette

Sanskrit: **Vatsnābh**
वत्सनाभ

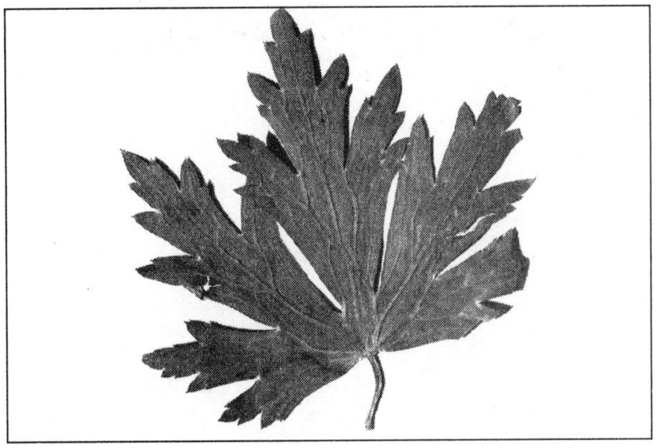

Hindi: Mīdhavis

English: Aconite, Monk's Hood
Latin: Aconitum felconeri Stapf.
Part Used: Leaves, seeds, roots
Habitat: Throughout India
Energetics: VP+ K-
Tissues: All, mainly blood/nerves
Systems: All systems, especially the nervous system
Action: Small doses—Anodyne, antidiabetic, antiperiodic, antiphlogistic, antipyretic, diaphoretic, diuretic. Large doses—poison, sedative, narcotic; metabolized quickly. It is related to and acting with *Vyān* Vāyu
Uses: Enhances the properties of herbs, making them work faster (i.e., for emergencies and immediate relief). Leaves—indigestion, sedative; Externally—neuralgia (especially facial), tetanus (acute and chronic), rheumatism (articular and muscular), gout, erysipelas, heart disorders. Internally—fevers, pain, increase urine flow. Root (external)—*lepa* for neuralgia, muscular rheumatism, itching with erythema, nasal catarrh, tonsillitis, sore throat, coryza, acute gout, leprosy, paralysis (alterative and nervine tonic), spermatorrhea, incontinence, and diabetes (decreases urine and sugar quantity). Root (internal)—fever, rheumatism, cough, asthma, snake bites, inflammations of mucus membranes of the throat, nose, stomach, and intestines.
Preparation: Tincture, extract from fresh leaves and flower tops; external liniment, poultice, homeopathic formula
Precaution: Poisonous without proper purification. The root is not used internally with heart disease. May cause severe headaches. Use only with the advice of a qualified practitioner.

Sanskrit: **Viḍaṅga**
विडङ्ग
Hindi: Viraṅga
English: None
Latin: Embelia ribes Burm. (E. Indica, E. Glandulifera, E. Robusta, Roxb.)

Habitat: Climbers in hilly parts of India ; Central and Lower Himalayas, to Sri Lanka and Singa pore
Part Used: Berries (fruit), leaves, root-bark
Energetics: Pungent, astringent-warm-pungent PK- (V+ mildly)
Tissues: Plasma, blood
Systems: Digestive, excretory
Action: Alterative, anthelmintic, carminative, stimulant
Uses: Main herb for worms (intestinal—especially tape, ring) and fungus [*Kuṭaj* is best for amoebacidal parasites]; good for all abdominal disorders, constipation, gas, indigestion, hemorrhoids. Root-bark powder—toothache. External paste—lung disease (pneumonia). Powdered berry paste— headache or as oil in nose for headache, obesity.
Precautions: Can cause sexual debility
Preparation: Decoction, powder, paste, confections, cigarettes

Sanskrit: **Vidārī-kanda**
विदारी कन्द
Hindi: Bilai-kand
English: None
Latin: Ipomoea digitata Linn. (I. paniculata)
Part Used: Tuberous root
Habitat: The hotter regions of India
Energetics: Bitter, sweet-cool-sweet VP- K+

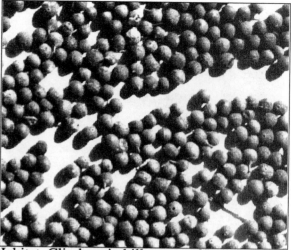

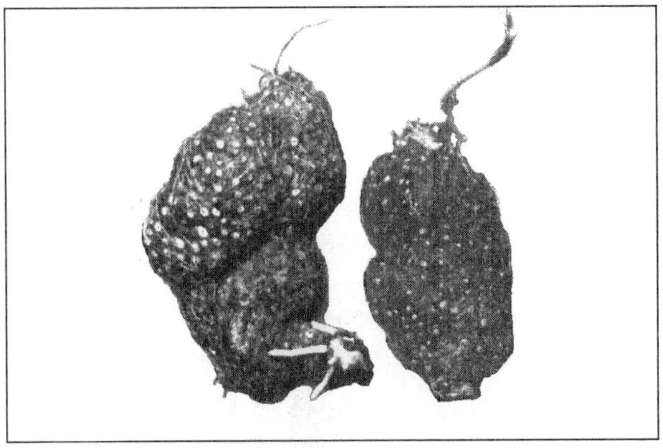

Tissues: Fat, muscle, reproductive
Systems: Digestive, reproductive
Action: Tonic, alterative, aphrodisiac, demulcent, mucilaginous, diuretic, galactogogue, nutritive tonic, cholagogue, emmenagogue, rejuvenative
Uses: Relative of the sweet potato, increases secretion of milk, emaciation, debility, poor digestion, increases weight, enlarged liver and spleen; moderates menstrual discharge, good for weak children.
Preparation: Powder, confection, decoction, milk decoction

Herb: **Yaṣhṭīmadhu**
यष्टीमधु

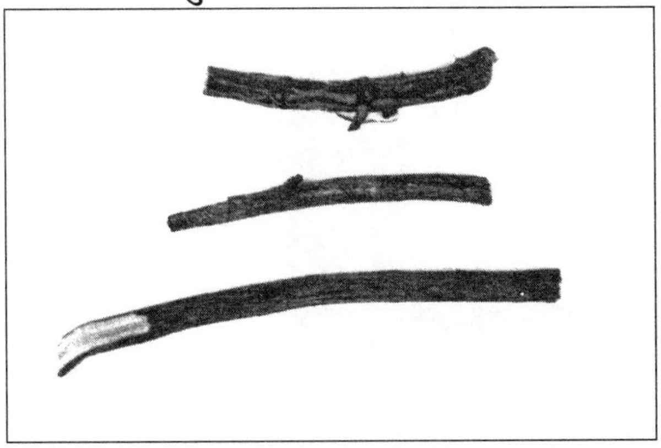

Hindi: Mithi-lakdi, Mulathi
English: Licorice
Latin: Glycyzrrhiza glabra Linn.
Part Used: Root
Habitat: Found in many countries
Energetics: Sweet, bitter-cold-sweet VP- K+ (only if used long term)
Tissues: All
Systems: Digestive, excretory, nervous, reproductive, respiratory
Action: Demulcent, emetic, expectorant, laxative, rejuvenative, sedative, tonic
Uses: Excellent for voice, heart tonic (with warm milk), Vāyu *doṣha*, bronchitis, colds, cough, debility (general), emetic (large doses), hyperacidity, inflammation, laryngitis, laxative, mental calming, mucus liquefying and expectorating, mucus membrane toner and soother, muscle spasms, sore throat, ulcers, urination pain. Cleanses lungs and stomach of Kapha. For colds and flu, mix with ginger (1:1). Blood purification, abdominal pain, nourishes the brain—increasing cranial and cerebrospinal fluid. Improves complexion, hair, and vision.
Spiritual Uses: *Sattwic*; gives contentment and harmony
Precautions: Excess Kapha, edema, stops calcium and potassium absorption, not for osteoporosis, hypertension (increases water around heart). Precautions are removed when taken in boiled milk. Do not use when pregnant.
Preparation: Decoction, milk decoction, powder, *ghee*

Conclusion

Herbs were chosen for this materia medica, based on those most commonly used, and those covering most disorders. Thousands of herbs could be added to the list, but it was felt that a simple, manageable list of herbs was more practical. Other outstanding herbs worthy of mentioning are *Kuṭaj,* the best antiparasitical herb, and *Garcinia* (Tamarind) an excellent weight loss herb for Kapha *doṣhas* (but can cause diarrhea in Pitta people if not blended with additional cool herbs). It is not recommended for Vāyu *doṣhas. Tamarind* is an inexpensive food supplement found in Indian groceries. It is also available in extract form in many new weight loss formulas, though it is more costly. The dose of *Tamarind* (*Garcinia*) extract is to be within the range of 100-500 mg. (9-45 grams) per use.

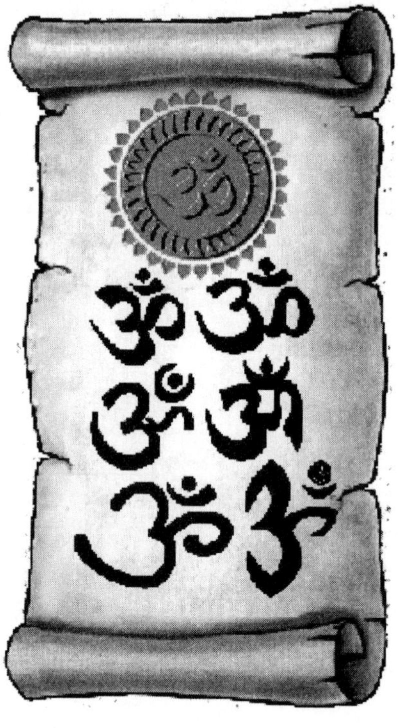

Limited power comes from knowledge and action.
Unlimited everlasting power exists in being.

Swami Narayan Tirtha

Chapter 5
Herb Glossary

The following is a list defining the effects of foods, drinks, and herbs. You may reference them as you read through the herbal materia medica. 'S' stands for *Sanskrit*, and 'H' stands for *Hindi*.

Abortifacient: Induces abortion
Herbs: *chitrak*, aloe, sandalwood

Alterative: [S- *Parivartakas* or *Rakta Shodhana Karma*; H- *Badal-de-ne-wali*] PK- V+; cool, bitter, astringent
Uses: Cleanses and purifies the blood; heals sores, boils, tumors, cancers; reduces fevers and Pitta; detoxifies the liver, kills parasites and worms; helps in the treatment of infectious, contagious diseases and epidemics, flu, acne, herpes, venereal disease, lymphatics. Externally, used on wounds, sores ulcers, etc.
Cool Herbs: Aloe, *neem*, *mañjiṣhṭhā*, sandalwood, red clover, and burdock
Warm Herbs: Bayberry, black pepper, cinnamon, myrrh, and safflower

Amoebicidal: For amoebic dysentery (e.g., *kuṭaj*)

Analgesic: [S- *Vedana shamana*; H- *Pidha harne wali*]
Uses: Reduces or eliminates pain (e.g., digestive, circulatory, respiratory, nervous system, nerve, muscle, tooth pain, nervous digestion, headaches).
Herbs: Camphor, chamomile, cinnamon, cloves, and echinacea

Anesthetics: For surgical anesthesia
Herbs: *Aśhok,* calamus, *guḍmar, jaṭamaṇśhī,* kaṭukā

Anthelmintic: [S- *Krumighana karma* or *Krimighna*; H- *Kire marne wali*]
Uses: Destroys and dispels worms, (round, tape, broad, and thread worms), parasites, fungus, yeast (e.g., candida). See vermicide, vermifuge.
Vāyu—in feces, *Pitta* in blood, *Kapha* in mucus.
Cool Herbs: Pau d'arco, goldenseal, wormseed, wormwood
Warm Herbs: Ajwan, cayenne, peppers, and pumpkin seeds

Antibiotic: PK- V+
Uses: Bitter, antibacterial, and antiviral infections.
Herbs: Turmeric and echinacea

Antidiabetic:
Herbs: *Āmalakī*, blackberry, fenugreek, *guḍūchī, guḍmar*, mica *bhasma*, senna, *shilājit*

Antidiarrhea: An alterative,
Cool Herbs: Blackberry, comfrey, gentian, red raspberry, and yellow dock
Warm Herbs: Black pepper, ginger, *harītakī*, and buttermilk/*lassi*

Antiemetic: [S- *Chherdinashana*]
Uses: Stops vomiting.
Herbs: Cloves, coriander, ginger, *neem*, raspberry, and *vaṃśha lochana*

Antiperiodic: [S- *Visham Jvara har*; H- *Malarial*

Jvara's]
Uses: Prevents the periodic return of attacks of diseases or fevers (e.g., malaria, neuralgia).
Herbs: Barberry, *chirāyatā, guḍūchī, kuṭaj*, and *vacha*

Antipyretic: [S- *Jwarahara*; H- *Bukhar Ko Dur Karne Wa roknewali*]
Uses: Dispels heat or fever (see bitter, febrifuge) by reducing production of heat at its centers; destroying fever toxins; sweating to increase the loss of heat; drawing out the heat (e.g., cold baths).
Herbs: *Āmalakī,* black pepper, *bṛihatī, daśhmūl, mañjiṣhṭhā, nirguṇḍī*, safflower, sandalwood

Anodyne: [S- *Sula-orasa-mana;* H- *Sakornwali*]
Uses: Provides relief from ill-defined pains and general discomfort. Its effects works mostly on the sensory nerves.
Herbs: *Aśhok,* barberry, cedar, ginger, *kuśhṭhā,* licorice, *vatsnab*

Antiphlogistics
Uses: An external application to reduce internal and external inflammations.
Herbs: Aloe, barberry, white sandalwood, *vatsnab*

Antirheumatic: VK- P+
Uses: Relieves or heals rheumatism
Herbs: Warm diuretics: Juniper berries, *guggul, ajwan*, cinnamon, and parsley

Antiseptic: [S- *Śhodhanīya*; H- *Śharir Saph Karne Wali*]
Uses: Removes infection or decay, which micro-organisms live (but does not destroy the organisms themselves)—see bitters.
Herbs: Aloe, *Chitrak, gokṣhura, guḍmar*, sandalwood, *śhatāvarī*, *śhilājit*, turmeric

Antispasmodic: [S- *Vikashī*; H- *Badan Ki Ainthan Wa Maror Ko Dur Wa Kam Karnewali*]
Uses: Relieves or prevents spasms of the voluntary and involuntary muscles (also see nervines) by strengthening nerves and the nervous system; cramps, tremors, convulsions, *prāṇa*, bronchodilators, menstrual cramps, nerve pain, headaches, open mind and senses, high Vāyu, hypersensitivity, nervousness, lumbago, sciatica, paralysis, degenerative nerve disorders, Vāyu emotions cause weak kidneys, insomnia, mental instability, numbness, and ungroundedness.
Herbs: *Vāyu* and *Kapha—Āśhwagandhā,* basil (*tulsī*), calamus, *guggul*, licorice, myrrh, sage, and *vāsāk*

Pitta—*betony, brāhmī* (gotu kola), *bhṛiṅgarāj, jaṭāmāṇśhī, peppermint,* sandalwood, and spearmint.

Antisyphilic: For relief of syphilis (usually alteratives).
Herbs: Black pepper, cedar, *guḍūchī, guggul*

Aperient: [S- *Bhedanīya*; H- *Dast Khol Kar lane wali*]
Uses: Mild purgatives or laxatives—see purgative.
Herbs: Rhubarb

Aphrodisiac: [S- *Vajīkarana*; H- *Namardi-ki-dawa*] gives great power or vitality by reinvigorating the body and sexual organs, if directed spiritually (upward), body, mind, and spiritual growth is gained; revitalizes all seven *dhātus*.

Two types exist: a) tonics, b) stimulants. *Tonics*: Develop tissue substance; *Stimulants*: increase the functioning of the reproductive organs. [Emmenagogues—more specific for women]
Herbs: Angelica, *aśhwagandhā*, asparagus, fenugreek, *fo-ti*, ginseng, *gokṣhura*, hibiscus, *kapikachū* seeds, pippalī, rose, saffron, and *śhatāvarī*

Some enhance spermatogenesis (*śhukrala*) or

Nutritive tonics—increase semen and breast milk: *aśhwagandhā, balā, fo-ti, ghee*, licorice, marshmallow, sesame seeds, *śhatāvarī*, and raw sugar

Sattwic aphrodisiacs—(enhance *ojas*): *aśhwagandhā, ghee*, lotus seeds, and *śhatāvarī*

Appetizer: For stimulating the appetite.
Herbs: Cardamom, coriander

Aromatic: [S- *Sugandhi-tadravya*; H- *Kush-buen*]
Uses: Provides fragrant, spicy tastes, and/or odors that stimulate the GI mucus membrane.
Herbs: Cardamom, cinnamon, cloves, fennel, *musta, nāgkeśhar,* peppermint, and turmeric

Astringent: [S- *Sankeshanīya* or *Stambhana karma*; H- *Bandhej-karnewali*] PK- V+ cool
Uses: Dries secretions (i.e., bleeding), excessive wastes, heals tissues externally, diarrhea, sweat, seminal emissions, urine, (see hemostatic, vulnerary), antidiarrhea herbs).
Herbs: *Āmalakī, arjuna, aśhok,* cinnamon, jasmine, sandalwood, and yarrow

Bitters: PK- V++
Uses: Reduces toxins, toxins in blood and weight; destroys infection and *āma*; high fever, heat, Pitta conditions, fever in blood, internal fever, heated liver, much thirst, sweating, inflammation, infection, bile regulator (hepatitis, jaundice), fat and sugar metabolism regulator (spleen-diabetes), antitumor (malignant and benign); use only until pathogens are destroyed.
Herbs: aloe, barberry, *chirāyatā*, gentian, golden seal, *kaṭukā*, and neem. Three types of bitters:
Bitter aromatics have properties of both bitters (simple) and aromatics

Bitter simple herbs stimulate only the GI tract

Bitter styptic herbs add styptic and astringent properties to those of bitterness

Calmative: For soothing, sedating—see nervines.

Cardiac Stimulant: For promoting circulation when there is a weak heart.

Carminative: [S- *Vata-anuloman* or *Dīpanīya*; H- *Bao Haran*]
Uses: Dispels intestinal gas and distention; increases absorption of nutrients, dispels water, mucus, and *āma* in the GI tract; promotes normal peristalsis; increases *agni*; cleanses *srotas*; relieves spasms and pain; promotes *prāṇa* flow; improves weak digestion from anxiety, nervousness, or depression. May aggravate Vāyu in long-term use.
Herbs: *Cool Herbs*: Chamomile, chrysanthemum, coriander, fennel, lime, musta, peppermint, and spearmint

Warm Herbs: *Ajwan*, basil, calamus, cardamom, cinnamon, ginger, and turmeric

Formulations: *Hiṅgwastāk Chūrṇa, Lavaṅ Bhaskar Chūrṇa, Tṛikatu, Triphalā*

Cathartic: [S- *Bhedana*; H- *Kara Julab*]—see purgatives

Laxatives—(figs, prunes, olive oil)

Simple purgatives—(that stimulate the glands—senna, castor oil, aloe vera)

Drastics—irritate the intestinal mucus membrane

Hydrogogues—cause fluid motions—epsom salts

Cholagogue—purgatives that stimulate the liver—rhubarb, aloe vera

Cholagogue: [S- *Mridubhedana*; H- *Halka Julab*]
Uses: For stimulating liver action, emptying the gall bladder, and promoting or increasing bile secretion or excretion; resulting in free purgation.
Herbs: *Arka, bhṛiṅgarāj, guḍūchī,* licorice, safflower, senna, and sesame

Cordial: For stimulating or exhilarating the heart—aromatic confections.

Decongestant: For relieving congestion—see expectorant.

Demulcent: [S- *Mridukara* or *Kasa-Svasahara*; H- *Tarkarnewali*]
Uses: For softening, soothing, and protecting mucus membranes and skin (i.e., protects stomach and urinary bladder lining).
Herbs: barley, licorice; linseed, olive, and al-

mond oils—see expectorant—moistening.
Dentifrice: For cleaning teeth and gums

Deobstruent: For removing obstructions to the functioning of the body.

Diaphoretic: [S- *Svedana Karma* or *Svedanīya*; H- *Pasina Lanewali*]
Uses: For promoting perspiration, circulation; dispels fever and chills; for eliminating surface toxins; relieving muscle tension, aching joints, and inflammatory skin conditions; bringing water down through urine; cooling and drying in nature; relieving diarrhea, dysentery (dispels damp heat), kidneys, liver, urinary, and gall bladder disorders; dispelling stones of kidney and both bladders (lithotriptic); genitourinary disease (i.e., herpes), edema; painful, difficult ,or burning urination or infections; first step in healing the disease.
Herbs: Two kinds exist: warming and cooling:

Warming: Raise body temperature, dispel chills and colds; stimulants, expectorants, antiasthmatic, and antirheumatic. Warm herbs: *Ajwan*, basil, cardamom, cinnamon, eucalyptus, ginger, juniper berries, and parsley. P+++

Cooling: Bitter-pungent, high fever, sore throat, toxins in blood, alterative, diuretic, cleanses lymph and plasma, subtle channels and capillaries, lungs, respiratory, open mind, *prāṇa,* sinuses, stimulate nervous system, liver, moistens, soothes, and protects kidneys; fevers, infections, liver, gall bladder, steam bath, sauna (keep head out of box), hot bath, etc. Cool herbs: Asparagus, barley, burdock, chamomile, chrysanthemum, coriander, dandelion, fennel, *gokṣhura*, marshmallow, *punarnavā*, spearmint

Digestives: [S- *Dipana-Pachana Karma*]
Uses: For assisting the stomach and intestines in normal digestion.
Herbs: Coriander, cumin, rock salt, turmeric

Disinfectant: [S- *Aguntaka-roganashaka*; H- *Urkar Lagnewali*]
Uses: For destroying disease germs and noxious properties of fermentation; disinfectants, bactericides, or germicides destroy pathogenic microbes (that cause communicable diseases); some antiseptics are disinfectants; all disinfectants are antiseptics.
Herbs: *Apāmārga, arka, guḍūchī, kaṭukā,* sandalwood

Diuretic: [S- *Mutrala Karma* or *Mutra-virehana*; H- *Peshabjari Karnewali*] PK- V+
Uses: For increasing urination; promoting kidney and urinary bladder activity; reducing and removing toxins; reducing water in all tissues (*dhātus*). Three forms of diuretics:

stimulating: stimulates kidneys during their elimination (e.g., pepper, juniper)

hydragogue: raises blood pressure in the glomeruli (e.g., digitalis, caffeine)

refrigerant: washes out the kidneys (e.g., drinking lots of water)
Herbs: *Apāmārga, aṣhwagandhā,* barberry, cardamom, cinnamon, ginger, gotu kola, *gokṣhura, guḍūchī,* licorice, *musta, punarnavā,* sandalwood, *śhatāvarī, shilājit, vacha*

Emetic: [S- *Vamakarīya*; H- *Qai Lanewali*]
Uses: Including or causing vomiting by local action on the nerves of the stomach and mucus membrane.

Three types of emetics:

central: Acts through the vomiting center of the brain (e.g., chamomile)

local: Locally irritates the nerves of the gastric mucus membrane (e.g., mustard, salt water)

general: Acts through the blood on the vomiting center (these are partly local emetics)
Herbs: *Apāmārga, arka, chakramarda, chitrak,* licorice, *pippalī*, rock salt, *vacha*

Emmenagogue: [S- *Rajastha-panīya* or *Raktabhisarana*] Pungent and bitter
Uses: For promoting and regulating menstruation (including PMS, uterine tumors, or infections). Clears blood congestion, blood clot; builds the blood; moistens female reproductive organs; counteracts aging and poor nutrition;

Herbs: Aloe, angelica, hibiscus, jasmine, licorice, myrrh, peony, *rose,* saffron, *śhatāvarī*
Cool Herbs: Menstrual or uterine infections, bleeding; anger, and irritability: Blessed thistle, chamomile, chrysanthemum, hibiscus, *mañjiṣhṭhā*, red raspberry, and rose
Heating Herbs: Delayed menses (from overexposure to cold), overexertion, nervous anxiety: Angelica, cinnamon, ginger, myrrh, safflower; used for antispasmodics, uterine cramps; diuretic for PMS, water retention; hemostatics tonic, rejuvenative.

Emollient: [S- *Snehopaga*; H- *Jalan Aur Sozish Ko Dur Karnewali*] Oils or fats—see demulcent
Uses: Externally—protect, soften, and relax the skin (e.g., oils, honey, bread or bran poultice, carrots, turnips, ointments, hot fomentations).

Epispastic: [S- *Doṣha-ghnalepa*; H- *Uparnewali*] Substances locally applied to the skin—see rubefacient
Uses: Produces blisters and redness on the surface (e.g., mustard).

Errhine: [S- *Śhiro-virechana*; H- *Chink Lanewali Ya Nazla Bahadenewali*] herbs applied to the mucus membranes of the nose
Uses: Increases nasal secretion with or without causing sneezing.
Herbs: *Āmalakī, apāmārga, arka,* black pepper, ginger, *guḍmar,* jasmine, *pippalī, vacha, viḍaṅga*

Exhilarant: Herbs that enliven and cheer the mind.

Expectorant: [S- *Kasa-Svasahara*; H- *Khansi Aur dame Ko Dur Darnewali*]
Uses: Promotes phlegm and mucus discharge; clears lungs, nasal passages, and stomach; respiratory (colds, flu, asthma, bronchitis, pneumonia), digestive problems (from mucus in GI tract) causing poor absorption of nutrients; removes phlegm and mucus that can accumulate and cause growths or tumors (usually benign) or nervous or circulatory ones.
Herbs: Two types: Drying (e.g., ginger) [hot/stimulant/diaphoretic/carminative] and moistening (e.g., licorice) which liquefy—cold and sweet herbs. These are also demulcent and emollients—see demulcent—dispel heat and dryness; liquefy Kapha and *āma* for Vāyu and Vāyu/Pitta respiratory illness; lung tonics, nerves, and heart

Dry herbs: Calamus, cardamom, cinnamon, cloves, elecampane, dry ginger, *pippalī*, and sage

M*oist herbs*: Bamboo, comfrey root, licorice, marshmallow, milk, raw sugar, slippery elm, cough relieving: bayberry, ephedra, eucalyptus, thyme, wild cherry. There are seven ways that they work:
1) Relieving bronchial tube spasms (lobelia, tobacco)
2) Through dislodging, by vomiting (see emetics—large doses)
3) Increasing the flow from the inflamed membrane (see emetics—small doses)
4) Promoting expectoration (onion, *asafoetida*/see expectorant)
5) By soothing the irritation in the respiratory center and promoting expectoration
6) Causing expectoration through stimulating the nerves of the mouth
7) By stimulating the respiratory center and strengthening the expulsive mechanistic muscles

Febrifuge: [S- *Jvarahar*; H- *Bukhar Ko Dur Karne-wa- roknewali*] reduces fever; (see antipyretic, antiperiodic, antiseptic)

Galactogogue: (S- *Stanya-janana*; H- *Dudh Barhanewali*] increases breast milk secretion (internally or externally applied)
Herbs: Cumin, fennel, *musta, pippalī, śhatāvarī,* white musali

Germicide: Destroys germs and worms [see disinfectant]

Germifuge: An agent that expels germs [see germicide]

Hemostatic: [S- *Shonitasthapana*; H- *Khun Band Karnewali*] astringent, alterative PK- V+
Uses: Stops bleeding, purifies blood (styptics).
Herbs: *Cool herbs*: *Dūrba*, goldenseal, *mañjiṣhṭhā,* red raspberry, turmeric
Warm herbs: Cinnamon, ginger; used with nutritives and tonics

Irritant: Causes irritation or inflammation
Herbs: *Arka,* cinnamon, cardamom, ginger, myrrh

Laxative: (S- *Svalpabhedana* or *Virechanīya*; H- *Dast Khol Karlanewali*] mild purgative that relaxes the bowels
Herbs: castor oil, flax seed, psyllium, rhubarb, senna; and *triphalā* (in large doses).

Lithotriptic: Dissolves and prevents kidney, urinary and gall bladder stones (see diuretic;), nervine: nutritive, builds tissues
Herbs: *Arjuna, āmalakī, arka, gokṣhura, paṣhana bheda, punarnavā*

Myotic: [S- *Netra-kaṣhitraroga*; H- *Ankhon Ki Putli Ko Sakornewali*] agents that cause the contraction of the pupil and diminution of ocular tension

Nervine: [H- *Rag-aur-reshon Men Bal Karnewali*] herbs that calm excited nerves and heal nervous diseases and the nervous system
Herbs: Aśhwagandhā, balā, guḍmar, śhaṅkh puṣhpī

Parasiticide: [S- *Krimighna*; H- *Bahar Ke Kire marnewali*] destroys parasites (see germicide, antiparasitic)

Parturifacient: Herbs inducing child-birth
Herbs: Barley, *pippalī, punarnavā* root (wrapped around belly)

Purgative: [S- *Virechanīya*; H- *Kara Julab*] produce, hasten or increase intestinal evacuation from the bowels
Herbs: Aloe, *apāpāmarga, balā, bhṛiṅgarāj, bilwa, chitrak,* epsom salts, *īśhabgol, kaṇṭakārī, kaṭukā*, licorice, *punarnavā,* rhubarb, safflower, senna

Refrigerant: [S- *Dahanaṣhaka*; H- *Pias Bujhanewali*]
Uses: Cools and reduces fevers; quenches thirst and suppresses unnatural body heat.
Herbs: Aloe, *chitrak,* coriander, ginger, hibiscus, orange, lemon, licorice, *musta, pippalī,* sandalwood, *śhatāvarī,* cane sugar, *vacha, viḍaṅga*

Resolvent: Causes the absorption of inflammations and other swellings by stimulating the lymphatics

Restorative: Herbs, cordials or foods that restore nutritive deficiencies

Rubefacient: [S- *Barīyalepana*; H- *Lal Chakatte Kar Denewali*]
Uses: An external remedy that irritates the nerve ends in the skin, causing distention of the capillaries, inflammation and reddening of the skin; increasing blood flow to that area.
Herbs: *Bākuchī* seeds, black pepper, cayenne, *chitrak,* ginger, licorice, *mañjiṣhṭhā,* mustard, *pippalī*

Sialagogue: [S- *Lalavardhaka*; H-*Ral-barhanewali Wa Thuk Barhanewali*]
Uses: Increases or produces saliva, either by local mouth irritation; causing reflex activity of the glands; (e.g., mustard, tobacco), or by exciting the glands during their elimination.
Herbs: *Arka*, black pepper, *chitrak, chirāyatā,* ginger, licorice, *pippalī*

Stimulant: [S- *Agni-sthapanīya* or *Dipana ;* H- *Uksanewali*] VK- P+. Antibacterial, anti-parasitical (also see carminative)
Uses & Herbs: Increases *agni*, destroys *āma*, increases auto-immune system, drying (e.g., pepper, cloves, cinnamon, dry ginger, *and ajwan*). Numerous forms of stimulants exist:

arterial: Cayenne
cardiac: Camphor, cane sugar, ephedra, glucose
cerebro-spinal: *Jaṭāmāṇśhī, kuśhtā*
circulatory: Adrenaline
eyes: Barberry extract, yellow thistle juice
general: a) Diffusible (e.g., antispasmodics),
b) Permanent (i.e., tonics, astringents)
local: Laxatives, emetics, purgatives, diuretics, diaphoretics, rubefacients, expectorants, sialagogues, epispastics
nervine (i.e., exciting the nervous system): Musk, *asafoetida*, caffeine
respiratory: *Bhūmīāmalakī*, cardamom, *jaṭamāṇśhī, mañjiṣhṭhā, nirguṇḍī, tulsī*
rheumatism etc: See rubefacient
skin: Cedar, *chakra marda*, sandalwood
spinal: Barley, dates, figs, pomegranate, rice, cane sugar
ulcers/abscesses: Gotu kola, *nirguṇḍī*
uterine: Cinnamon, *guggul,* myrrh, *vaṃśha lochana*
vascular: Cayenne, cinnamon, ginger, *kaṇṭakārī,* nutmeg, *pippalī, vacha*
stomachic: See aromatics and see below

Stomachic: [S- *Kshudha-vardhanīya*; H- *Bhuk Barhanewali*] digestive stimulant (see stimulant, bitters, carminative)
Uses: Increases or excites gastric juice secretion; improves stomach tone, promotes appetite, and digestion.
Herbs: *Āmalakī, balā, bhṛiṅgarāj, bilwa,* black pepper, cardamom, cedar, *chirāyatā, chitrak,* cumin, ginger, *harītakī, kaṭukā,* licorice, *musta, pippalī,* turmeric, *vacha, viḍaṅga*

Styptic: [S- *Raktha-sthambana*; H- *Khun Band Karanewali*] (See hemostatic)
Uses: Causes vascular contraction of the blood vessels or coagulation of the albuminous tissues of the blood; checks hemorrhage
Herbs: Adrenaline, alum

Tonic (aromatic & bitter): [H- *Taqat Denewali*] coldest: PK- V++ (in most cases)
Uses: Pitta conditions (i.e., fever, heat); blood detox, weight loss, fever in blood; destroys *āma*, liver, and bile regulation (i.e., hepatitis, jaundice); fat and sugar reduction (i.e., spleen-diabetes); anti-tumor (benign and malignant), removes congestion.
Herbs: Aloe, *balā*, barberry, *chirāyatā*, *guḍūchī, kaṭukā, gentian, goldenseal, kaṭukā, musta,* neem, *vacha.* Various forms of tonics exist:
stomachic [H- *Khub Bhuk Laganewali*]
cardiac [H- *Dilko Taqat Denewali*
blood [H- *Khun Barhanewali*]

Tonic (astringent): tissue builders; see nutritives
Herbs: *Harītakī*

Tonic (nutritive): [S- *Bruhangana karma*; H- *Dhatu barane wale*] VP- K+
Uses: Permanently increases the tone of a part of the body, or the entire system by nourishing and increasing weight. They are sweet, heavy, oily, or mucilaginous; increasing vital fluids, muscles, and fat; builds the blood and lymph; increases milk and semen; restoratives for weakness, emaciation, debility, and convalescence; soothing, harmonizing, dispels rigidity, and calms nerves. They are taken with stimulant or carminative herbs (e.g., ginger or cardamom) to assist in absorption; having expectorant, demulcent, and emollient properties; nurtures the lungs and stomach.
Herbs: *Āmalakī, arka, aśhwagandhā, balā, bhṛiṅgarāj, bibhītakī,* cane sugar, coconut, coriander, dates, *ghee*, *gokṣhura, guḍūchī, guggul, harītakī,* honey, *jaṭāmāṇśhī,* licorice, *mañjiṣhṭhā*, milk, raisins, sesame seeds, *śhatāvarī*, turmeric, *vaṃśha lochana, viḍaṅga, vidārī kand*

Rejuvenative Tonics: [S- *Rasāyana karma*]:
Uses: Regenerates cells and tissues (body and brain); promotes longevity—spiritual and physical. For young and old people.
Herbs:
Vāyu—Aśhwagandhā, guggul, harītakī, calamus, and *śhatāvarī.*
Pitta—Aloe, *āmalakī*, gotu kola, *śhatāvarī*, saffron, and *gokṣhura.*

Kapha—Bibhītakī, guggul, pippalī, śhilājit, triphalā, and elecampane.

Vermicide: [H- *Kiremarnewali*] that which kills intestinal worms (see anthelmintic)

Vermifuge: [*Kiremarnewali*] Expels intestinal worms (but may not kill the worms). See anthelmintic

Vulneraries: Astringent, demulcent, emollient PK- V+

Uses: Heals tissue via external use; cool as a plaster or poultice for cuts, wounds, burns, hemorrhage.

Herbs: Aloe, comfrey, honey, licorice, marshmallow, turmeric, and slippery elm.

The doctor of the future will give no medicine but will interest their patients in the care of the the human frame, in diet, and in the cause and prevention of disease.
Thomas Edison

Chapter 6
Nutrition

We have briefly touched upon the topic of tastes, as they are related to the seasons. This may be quite an unusual way to look at the seasons, but nonetheless, a useful one when considering health. To better understand the idea of taste from the Āyurvedic viewpoint, we need to examine it in depth. Its insights offer an explanation of the role of tastes in healing. Unique to Āyurveda is a scientific breakdown of tastes, discussed according to energies—or energetics. Āyurveda classifies herbs, foods, and drinks into five aspects. Each has its own therapeutic effects;

1. Taste
2. Element (property)
3. Heating or cooling effect
4. Post-digestion effect (final taste after digestion)
5. Special properties

Taste: It is considered therapeutic for several reasons. The *Sanskrit* word for taste is *"Rasa"*. It means delight or essence, both of which promote healing. A channel extends from the mouth into the head and brings the essence (one meaning of taste) to the brain. This essence stimulates *prāṇa*, which in turn stimulates the *agni* or digestive fires. If the taste of the food is not pleasing, the gastric fires may not digest the food and thus do not provide proper nutrition. That is why Āyurvedic cooking is a science unto itself, blending the right amount of herbs for the right taste. In our society, we have adulterated our sense of taste with unwholesome (artificial) foods (one of the two fundamental causes of disease we discussed in volume one).

Element: Six tastes originate from the five elements, transmitting their properties: sweet, salty, sour, pungent, bitter, astringent. All tastes essentially originate in the water element, having their origin here. No food consists only of one taste; all five elements are contained in all substances. So when it is said that a food has a certain taste (e.g., sweet), that taste predominates. Similarly, no illness is caused by purely one *doṣha*. However, when a *doṣha* predominates, it is said that an illness is caused by that specific *doṣha*.

Taste	Element	Food
sweet	earth, water	sugar, starch
sour	earth, fire	fermented, acidic
salty	water, fire	salt, alkali
pungent	fire, air	spicy, acrid, aromatic
bitter	ether	bitter herbs
astringent	earth, air	constricting quality with tannin

All persons need some for each of the six tastes in their diet. However, depending on one's constitution and the season, one will adjust their tastes to balance their *doṣha*. The key is to have a moderate amount of each taste.

The benefits listed below result from ingesting foods that develop these healing measures. However, they relate primarily to the *doṣha*(s) listed. If used by a *doṣha* not listed, they will create excess.

Taste (*Rasa*)	Physical Effect	Mental Effect
sweet VP-	builds and strengthens tissues, life sap, complexion, bones	content, pleasure
sour VK-	digestive aid, dispels gas, nourishes, relieves thirst, satiates, helps circulation and elimination of urine and feces; strengthens heart, aids all tissues but reproductive, maintains acidity	wakens mind and senses
salty V-	softening, lubricates tissues, laxative, sedative, digestive aid, promotes sweating, purgative, emetic, softens hard tumors, decongests hard phlegm, maintains mineral balance, holds water, improves taste	calms nerves, stops anxiety
pungent VK-	heals throat diseases and VK allergic rashes, skin diseases, counters water, grease, and fat; digestive aid, dispels gas, removes edema, improves taste, promotes sweat, improves metabolism and organic functions; breaks up stagnant blood or clots and other hard masses; clears channels, relieves nerve pain and muscle tension	opens mind and senses
bitter PK-	heals anorexia, thirst, skin diseases, fever, nausea, burning, parasites, and bacteria; blood purifier, cleanses, detoxifies, reduces fat, tissue, and water excesses; antibiotic, antiseptic, digestive aid, cleanses breast milk, digests sugar and fat	clears senses and emotions
astringent PK-	stops bleeding and cleanses blood, sweat, diarrhea; heals skin and mucus membranes, prolapse and ulcers; expectorant, diuretic, tightens tissues, dries moisture and fat	cools fiery minds and removes lethargy

(V = Vāyu*, P = Pitta, K = Kapha, '-' means reduces)*

Negative Effects Due to Excess

The diseases listed below resulted from ingesting foods that create excesses in the *doṣha*. In excess, eventually any *doṣha* will develop these ailments.

Taste (*Rasa*)	Physical Effect	Mental Effect
sweet K+	excess fat diseases; obesity, diabetes indigestion, malignant tumors, neck gland enlargement	Kapha-leth-argy, Vāyu-anxiety
sour P+	flabbiness, loss of strength, fever, thirst, blindness, itching, pallor, Pitta anemia, herpes, small pox	giddiness, anger, impat-ience
salty PK+	hypertension, baldness, gray hair, skin diseases, wrinkles, thirst, herpes, loss of strength, abscesses	anger, impat-ience, lethargy
pungent P+	thirst, depletion of reproductive fluid and strength; fainting, tremors, waist/ back pain	anger, impat-ience
bitter V+	tissue depletion, Vāyu diseases	anxiety, fear, insomnia
astringent VK+	undigested foods, heart pain, thirst, emaciation, loss of virility, constipation, channel blocks	anxiety, worry, fear, insomnia

It is interesting that Āyurveda is not concerned with naming diseases. Illness is determined according to the excesses and deficiencies of the elements or *doṣhas* (air, fire, and water). When *doṣhas* are balanced, illness does not exist. From this point of view, one can see how, by understanding which tastes mitigate or aggravate which *doṣhas*, nutrition becomes an elemental and effective measure in maintaining the balance of health. The charts shown above also reveal how various diseases are seen to be directly related to tastes and *doṣhas*. Thus, by following an appropriate food plan for one's constitution, a person may maintain health and prevent future illness.

Energy (Vīrya): This energy activates tastes. Foods and drinks possess either cold or hot energy (in the body). Each taste has an associated energy.

Taste	Energy	Food
sweet	cold	sugar
sour	acidic	yogurt*, pickle,
salty	hot	table salt, seaweed,
pungent	hot	pepper, chili, wine, pickles
bitter	cold	alum, golden seal, gentian
astringent	constricting	talum, oak bark

** Yogurt is sour, sweet, and heavy. Pure forms of the tastes will aggravate one's doṣha more easily than complex versions and thus should be used with care.*

Aggravating	Pacifying
sugar	complex carbohydrates
salt	sea weed
hot peppers (cayenne)	mild spices (e.g., cardamom)
alcohol	yogurt, sour fruit
pure bitters (e.g., golden seal)	mild bitters (e.g., aloe)
pure astringents (strong tannins)	mild astringents (raspberry)

Post-Digestive (Vipāka):
Tastes may change at the end of the digestive process. This is due to the digestive *agni* (fire) juices in the alimentary tract (metabolism). For example, foods or liquids, initially sweet, develop an aftertaste. This taste may be any of the six tastes. These aftertastes also affect a person's constitution.

6 Tastes	Post Digestive Taste
sweet, salty	becomes sweet
sour	remains sour
pungent, bitter, astringent	becomes pungent

[Throughout this text, the following abbreviations are used: 'V' 'P' 'K' stand for Vāyu, Pitta, Kapha; respectively. '-' stands for reducing a *doṣha,* and '+' means increasing a *doṣha*]

Sweet VP- K+ (moist) promotes secretion of Kapha, semen, easy and comfortable gas release, and helps the discharge of urine and feces. Produces saliva.
Sour P+ increases the tissues (except the reproductive *dhātu*, which is reduced). It produces bile, acid.
Salty P+ produces saliva
Pungent P+ (in time) causes gas, constipation, painful urine, reduces semen with difficult discharge.
Bitter PK- V+ produces dryness and gas in the colon
Astringent PK- V+ constricts, bothers Vāyu.

Emotions and Taste
Each of the six tastes produces or enhances a certain emotion when eaten. Thus, emotional disorders may be balanced by eating and avoiding foods, according to the tastes.

Taste	Emotion	Deranges
sweet	desire	Kapha
sour	envy	Pitta
salty	greed	Kapha
pungent	anger	Pitta
bitter	grief	Vāyu
astringent	fear	Vāyu

Doṣhas, Nutrition, and the 6 Tastes
Vāyu is balanced by supplementing with moist tastes, sweet, sour, and salty (balancing dryness), and some warm tastes as well. Pitta is balanced by using sweet (moist), bitter, and astringent (cooling) tastes. This helps counter heat-related illness (e.g., infection, rash, anger, impatience). Kapha diseases are removed by using sour and pungent tastes (i.e., they heat and burn up water). Bitter tastes also reduce Kapha by causing a drying action.

Sweet: Generally, food is sweet in taste, neutral in energy, and sweet in its post-digestive effect. It decreases Vāyu and Pitta, and increases Kapha. It nourishes and maintains humors, *dhātus*, and *malas* (wastes).

Sour: Examples of sour tastes include sour fruit, tomatoes, and pickled vegetables. All tissues are nourished by sour tastes, except reproductive tissue (of the sour tastes, only yogurt nourishes all tissues).

Salty: Sea food or condiment. In moderation, salt strengthens all tissues. When used in excess, it depletes tissues.

Pungent: Spices and spicy vegetables do not offer much nutrition, but they stimulate digestion.

Bitter: Vegetables offer little nutrition. They are useful in clearing and cleansing digestive organs, and in aiding digestion, especially if taken before meals (for Pitta and Kapha *doṣhas*).

Astringent: This is mainly a secondary taste. Astringent foods, like green vegetables or unripe apples, provide minerals but do not build tissues.

Energy: Most foods are neutral in heating and

cooling effects. To apply hot or cold therapeutics, appropriate spices and foods are eaten cooked or raw.

Heavy/Light: Most foods tend to be heavy, though many light foods also exist. Spices can make foods lighter. Oils can make them heavier. Foods are also dry or moist. Dryness can be increased by eating dry foods or toast, or made moister by frying foods or adding liquids.

Special Properties: (Prabhāva)

Herbs also have some subtler, more specific qualities, beyond their traditional rules and definitions. For example, basil, although a heating herb, reduces fever. Herbs with similar energies will have different special properties.

Certain external actions affect the herb's *prabhāva*: *mantras*, gems, *yantras*, or just the intention or love imparted by the practitioner alters the herbs beyond the general classifications. For example, *āmalakī (embellica officinalis)* and *barhal* (a variety of *ficus bengalensis, linn.*) both have same taste, property, energy, and final taste after digestion. Yet *āmla* alleviates the *doṣhas* and *barhal* aggravates the *doṣhas*. Also *til* (sesame seeds) and *madan (randia dumetorum, lamk.)* have predominant sweet, astringent, and bitter tastes. Both are oily and sticky. Yet, *madan* is an emetic, sesame is not. Similarly, wearing specific stones like topaz, ruby, sapphire etc., can heal different diseases.

Dual Doṣhas

It is simple mathematics. When *doṣhas* are not in a balanced state, either you must increase the depleted *doṣha* or decrease the aggravated *doṣha*. When a person has a dual *doṣha* (e.g., Vāyu/Pitta) they are advised to ingest foods and herbs that increase the third or deficient element (e.g., Kapha). Simultaneously, one reduces their intake of foods and herbs that increase the two excessive *doṣhas* (e.g., Vāyu and Pitta).

Foods affect the surface nutrition, while herbs aid the subtle nutrition. There also may be instances when one *doṣha* is greatly in excess, and a second mildly aggravated. Thus, proper consideration of degree of derangement is necessary as well.

Tastes and Organs

Each of the six tastes also produces effects on each of the internal organs as well. Again, through ingesting the proper tastes, the health of the organs may be maintained.

Physiology of the 6 Tastes

Āyurveda says that each taste, when found in excess, will adversely affect certain organs in the body. This is used as a cross-reference to the five-element view of health and balance, stated earlier.

Taste	Organ
sweet	spleen, pancreas
salty	kidney
sour	liver
pungent	lungs
bitter	heart
astringent	colon

Thus, Āyurveda offers a unique view of the energetics of taste: six tastes (the initial taste, its hot or cold energy, and its aftertaste), how tastes are related to the *doṣhas*, organs, diseases, and emotions, and their special properties. It is a complete science of the mechanics and energies. Further, it reveals a causal relationship between food and health; how one feels is greatly decided by what one eats.

As discussed earlier, Āyurveda aims to remove the cause of an illness. Rather than 'curing' a specific disease, this science addresses the balance of the whole individual. Along with external causes it always considers the two levels of health: body and mind. In the last chapter, we discussed how the tastes and energies of foods play a direct role in creating health or illness, from the Āyurvedic point of view.

Life habits (external) measures are also considered another essential Āyurvedic healing measure, when lifestyle changes are gradually adapted. In the original Āyurvedic texts, people are cautioned not to start or stop habits too suddenly. In the chapter on the seasons, there was a subtle 7-day transition period between seasons to be noted and worked with to avoid disease during the shift. We find similar wisdom in the spiritual texts about the transition points at sunrise, noon, sunset, and midnight. It is suggested that these are points of weakness; the person is better advised to spend these transitional times in *sādhanā* (meditation).

Even for a healing science that suggests vegetarianism to those who are healthy, Āyurveda does not advise giving up meat cold-turkey (no pun intended). Even if a food is bad for one's constitution (e.g., one's favorite vegetables or desserts), or good for their *doṣha*, gradual stopping and starting of any habits is advised. Gentleness is the key. Similarly, if one undertakes too radically a detoxification program, one may experience bodily discomforts from conditions such as diarrhea or excess toxins. Āyurveda has the unique position of offering a healing process that does not have to make one feel bad before feeling better. Healing is approached in that sense. It will make life better, simpler and more natural, enhancing spiritual growth as well. It may take some months before the effects of healing are manifested. Making one or two changes for health, and consistently following them, is better than experimenting here and there without a foundation for growth and healing. The Āyurvedic motto is, 'no pain—no pain'.

Also, people often look for quick, healing, magic-medicine that allows them to return to their self-harming (bad habits) ways again. In fact, illness is a sign that life is not being lived in balance. Herbs are a food supplement and not magic pills that instantly remove discomfort. Some people may be impatient with this 'gradual' lifestyle development, but it is an enhancement of lifestyle and not a quick cure that Āyurveda achieves.

Chronic indigestion also requires slow change. One week of *kicharī* (rice and beans) may be needed for those with severe conditions. Again, some people may be disinclined about making changes, but the alternatives are not pleasant. Eventually one finds a food plan that is comfortable.

As discussed earlier, food essence rises through the channel to the brain, so it is crucial that wholesome foods are taken for their *sattwic* essence. Organic is also very good. *Sattwic* essence brings the energy of *sattwa* directly into the mind. This is discussed, in detail, in another chapter as the final step before experiencing *samādhi* (*Saibikalpa*).

Dietary Questions

Eat to 1/3 capacity of stomach,
drink 1/3 and leave 1/3 for God.
Aṣhṭāñga Hṛidayam

The Āyurvedic determination of eating habits follows.

Overview

Preparation Eating warm (cooked) foods enlivens the enzymes for easily and quickly digesting food, promoting *Apāna* Vāyu, and removing Kapha. However, when food is overcooked, its life force becomes depleted. Further, cooking with too much heavy oil can weaken the digestive fire. Food is best eaten when cooked or steamed rather than uncooked; it is more nutritive and building. Also, persons on spiritual paths, (i.e., practicing *sādhanā* (meditation) and following a *guru* or spiritual guide), generally need not follow such drastic raw-food measures. Eating raw food causes roughness among persons on the spiritual path. It is true that raw foods have enzymes to remove toxins, but they do not adequately build the tissues. Fruit is better fresh and uncooked. Microwaves damage the life-force. Restaurant food is generally over- or under-spiced, and not as good as a home-cooked meal. Cooking over a wood fire is best. Cooking on a gas stove is better than cooking on an electric stove.

Quality *Sattwic*: organic, fresh, homegrown, fresh-picked, and raw dairy foods are advised. It is not advisable to eat foods that are rotten, under- or over-cooked, burnt, unripe, over-ripe, stale, or junk food. Other harmful foods include those that are canned, artificial, rancid, and prepared with additives, preservatives, or artificial colors. Finally, frozen foods that contain steroids and chemicals (milk and animal products usually have steroids, chemicals and preservatives in them) should not be eaten.

Quantity A proper quantity of food is easily digested, promotes longevity without afflicting the *doṣhas*, and helps *Apāna* Vāyu. Food, when eaten, should fill one-third of the stomach size or capacity. Liquid, when taken after meals, also should fill one-third the stomach size. The time to drink liquids at mealtime varies with the individual. Heavy or obese persons should drink before meals. Underweight or thin persons should drink liquids after meals, and persons of normal weight should drink with their meals. The remaining one-third of space in the stomach helps digestion. The key is moderation and regularity. Vāyu *doṣhas* need to eat every 3 - 4 hours. Pitta persons generally have good digestive fire. Kapha constitutions need to eat less. Ultimately, the stronger the digestive fire, the more one can eat. (Less food is better with a fever.)

When Hungry Eat only after the previous meal has been digested. Otherwise, the digestive product of the previous meal becomes mixed with the new food, instantly aggravating all the *doṣhas*. The digestive fire/enzymes have to act upon the food for a certain period of time in order to digest the food. Then, the body needs time to restore the digestive fire/enzymes for the future. If a person takes food before digesting the previous meal completely, the food will not digest properly. The undigested food is pushed along the GI tract by normal peristalsis, imbalancing and aggravating the *doṣhas*.

Combinations Combining vegetables with fruit or milk can cause digestive problems. One needs to be careful while eating or choosing food. Different combinations may be harmful. Its not advised to combine sour tastes with milk, eat cold items after *ghee*, eat equal amounts of *ghee* and honey, or eat fish products along with dairy (these unhealthy combinations create subtle toxins). Other aggravating foods are too hot and too cold, or too light and too heavy. Stew and curry are more digestible than individual vegetables cooked and eaten separately.

Vāyu— the fewer combinations the better (they like combining foods, though it is not good for them).
Pitta— does best with combinations
Kapha— is between Vāyu and Pitta.

Spices Delicious tastes improve digestion, strength, senses, complexion, and a healthy weight. They are easily digested and help *Apāna* Vāyu. The use of spices stimulates the secretions of digestive enzymes. Over-salted, under-salted, or sour seasoning is to be avoided. Foods that are too tasty increase *rajas* (aggravating the blood). Foods that are too bland cause *tamas* (suppressing *agni*).

Vāyu—does well with rich and moderately strong spices.
Pitta—needs only mild spices.
Kapha—does best with light, strongly spiced foods.

Frame of Mind A relaxed, calm mind promotes easy assimilation of food. This makes the mind more *sattwic*. A nervous, anxious, angry, noisy, and rushed mind makes the food harder to digest. Smoky environments are also harmful when eating.

Silence is good, but there is no need to be too serious. A prayer of gratitude to the Creator and Supplier before a meal, or offering the food to benefit humanity and the creation of beings is advised. Chew food properly to digest and absorb nutrients.

Time daylight hours are the best hours to eat.

Vāyu—dawn and dusk (smaller, more frequent meals—eat every 3 to 4 hours)

Pitta—at noon, largest meal (three meals daily)

Kapha—daylight hours, breakfast is skipped make lunch the large meal

After meals, it is good to take a short, easy walk. Some say napping while lying on your left side helps digest foods This causes breathing through the right nostril or "solar" breathing, which increases the digestive heat or fire in the system. Other authorities say napping after meals is unwholesome. Activities such as exercise, swimming, or sex are not recommended just before or after meals. Smoking disperses and dulls the *agni* (digestive) fire.

Season and Geography Eat foods and herbs according to season (i.e., do not eat cold and dry items in the winter, or hot and pungent items in the summer). Eat foods and herbs according to geography (do not eat hot and dry items in a hot dry desert, or cold and oily items in cold and damp climates).

Miscellaneous Do not ingest equal amounts of *ghee* and honey simultaneously (it becomes a subtle toxin).

Do not break with eating habits (e.g., someone who generally eats cold and sweet things should not suddenly start eating hot and pungent items).

Herbs, diet, and lifestyle are recommended to balance the *doṣha*, but also should be in harmony with one's own habits. Intake of substances that aggravate the *doṣha* and state of one's strength is ill advised.

Eat after clearing the bowel and urinary bladder, and only when hungry.

Drinking (except *lassi* buttermilk [yogurt and water], and medicated herbal wine to stimulate digestion) is not recommended during the meal, but is all right afterwards. Drinking alcohol after meals causes hyperacidity unless it is medicated herbal wines for Vāyu and Kapha. Astringent or herbal teas are all right after meals, but coffee promotes indigestion, hyperacidity or ulcers.

Desserts (especially cold) are heavy and sweet, and suppress digestive fire, causing fermentation and indigestion. They are better before meals, as sweets are the first taste to be digested. Having raw foods and salads at the end of the meal is better for digestion. Other authorities say a little sweet after meals promotes digestion.

Age/Gender these characteristics may bring excess to one's *doṣha*. Therefore, reduction of *doṣhas* may need to be considered at different ages, and for different genders.

Kapha reduction is predominantly used from birth to age 15, and for women.

Pitta reduction primarily from age 15 to 55 years old, and for men.

Vāyu reduction from age 55 and over

Āma: For 1 or 2 weeks, spices and a light and cleansing diet are followed. Spices are given to digest the undigested food or *āma* and cleanse the entire body. Sugars, oils, meat and dairy are avoided. Then, one returns to their *doṣha* diet, staying on the light side until *āma* is completely gone.

Different books offer varying *doṣha* food lists. Ultimately, persons will have to decide whether any specific food is good or aggravating their *doṣha*.

Vegetarianism: Proteins, Vitamins, Minerals

Each year more and more people decide to become vegetarians. Yet the major question asked at our center is how one gets enough protein, vitamins, and minerals in their diet.

It is true that active people who follow a vegetarian diet need sufficient amounts of these nutrients. Proteins are best derived from milk, yogurt, and high-protein content beans like garbanzos (*channa dal*) and *tur dal* (both found in Indian groceries). They can be mixed with *mūngdal*, which also has high protein content, but not as much as the other two beans. Boiled milk can be taken once or twice a day. Yogurt/water (*lassi*) can be taken once or twice a day between 10 a.m. and sunset. Beans can be mixed together and eaten for lunch and dinner.

For an ample supply of vitamins and minerals, a mixture of green leafy vegetables, root vegetables and colored vegetables (e.g., eggplant, yellow squash) need to be eaten daily. The amount of vegetables must be increased as well.

When all the beans and vegetables (each beneficial for various *doṣhas*) are eaten together in one meal, their properties balance, without aggravate any one *doṣha*. However, when a *doṣha* is severely unbalanced, certain foods may be required in smaller quantities—or not at all—until balance is restored.

Foods *When no Sanskrit name exists and a Hindi name is available, it will be marked with an 'H'. V, P, and K stand for Vāyu, Pitta, and Kapha respectivley. Various books offer differing energetics for certain foods. It is up to the individual to determine how each food affects them.*

Fruit

Taste: Sweet and sour (sometimes astringent)
Energy: Cold
Post-Digestive: Sweet
VP- K+ (mildly): Balances the three humors
The most *sattwic* food
Actions: Relieves thirst, refrigerant, alterative, laxative, mildly cleanses and nurtures, *āma* only in excess
Elements: Water, ether (more than any other food group)
Tissues: Builds plasma (*rasa*), cleanses blood, reduces other tissues in excess, lightness and purity in body
Precautions: Its ether and cooling effects can cause spacey, ungrounded symptoms. It can overly diffuse our aura, becoming too sensitive and physically vulnerable (as when living in cities or having stressful lifestyles). Excess can aggravate Vāyu air and Kapha mucus, edema, fatigue
Guṇas: Fruit is the most *sattwic* of all foods, promoting lightness, clarity, harmony, content, intelligence, *sādhanā* (though it does not stimulate us to do mental work)
Preparation: Dry: K- V+
Fruit Juices: P- (sweet) KV+
Cooked: VK- P+
Sour Fruit with Salt: V- PK+
Sour Fruit with Sugar: P ok
Sweet fruits: VP- K+
Sour fruits: VK- P+
Bitter fruits: PK- V+
Combinations: It is best not to combine certain foods. Sour fruits (lemons, grapefruit), pineapples, papaya, cranberries, may be taken with meals. Grains can be eaten with fruit, especially rice. Bananas are ok with milk
Time: Sweet- afternoon
Kapha—fruit is not eaten in the morning, a Kapha increasing time
Season: Fruit eaten in season and ripened naturally is best. It is too cold for a sole diet, especially in winter
Antidote: Warm sweet spices, ginger, cardamom, cloves, cinnamon, nutmeg, cooking fruit also helps

Fruit List

(The taste/energy/post-digestive effects will be listed in this fashion.). Where available, Sanskrit names will be provided for each food.

Apples

Energetics: Sweet, astringent, sometimes sour/ cold/sweet. PK- V+ (in excess, cooked with cinnamon is neutral =)
Action: Astringent, alterative, refrigerant
Indications: Diarrhea, intestinal bleeding or ulcers (pectin binds the stool and promotes healing of damaged membranes), bleeding gums, gall bladder, inflammations, blood cholesterol, de-

toxifies, chronic enteritis, Pitta and Kapha arthritis, herpes, viruses, acid stomach, fiber, chelates metals, protects from x-ray radiation, blood pressure; baked apples or sour apples are better for Vāyu. Apple juice is good for gastritis, colitis, and burning infections. Apple skin is high in calcium.

Apricots

Energetics: Sweet, sour/hot/sweet VK- P+ mildly and in excess

Action: Relieves thirst, anti-cough

Indications: Fever, constipation, cancer, skin, muscle and nerve disorders, fiber.

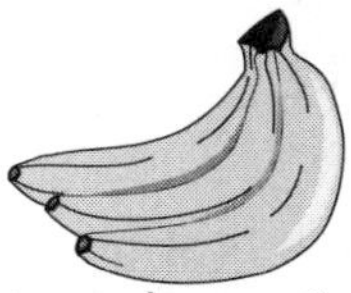

Bananas

Energetics: Sweet, astringent/hot/sour V- K+ P+ in excess or ulcers. (Unripe: astringent PK-, V+)

Action: Astringent, refrigerant, laxative, nutritive, tonic, heavy, strengthening, aphrodisiac

Indications: Unripe—diarrhea, dysentery, cough, lung bleeding, infants and young children, nerves, alcoholism, Vāyu hypertension, heart disorders, protects against strokes, diarrhea, hemorrhoids, high in potassium, vitamin C, and carbohydrates. When taken with *ghee* and cardamom, bananas alleviate hypoglycemia, constipation, and muscle cramps; also build muscle and fat; and nerve and reproductive tissues.

Precautions: Not used for Pitta with ulcers, hard to digest, do not drink liquids for one hour after eating a banana. They are not be be eaten with milk or yogurt, or eaten when suffering from fever, edema, vomiting, or cough with mucus.

Cherries

Energetics: Sweet, sour,astringent/hot/ sweet V- K+ in excess P+ sour ones VK- P+

Action: Alterative (blood cleansing)

Indications: Mental fatigue, insomnia, stress, heart tonic, blood and plasma building, gout, lumbago, motion sickness, poor vision, rheumatism, paralysis, arthritis, stunted growth, obesity, (Black cherries (*Bipem kanta*) better for plasma, tooth decay or loose teeth, diarrhea, glands, detoxifies, gall bladder and liver disorders), juice is stronger. For PMS and menstrual flow, eat 10 cherries on an empty stomach for seven days before menstruation begins.

Cranberries

Energetics: Astringent, sour/hot/pungent. K- VK+

Action: Diuretic, alterative, hemostatic

Indications: Excellent for kidney, urethra, and bladder disorders, asthma, intestinal antiseptic, high in vitamin C. Pitta conditions, burning urine, urinary tract stones and infections, skin rashes, toxic blood, edema, weight reduction (avoid store-bought juices with sugar).

Dates (*Kharjūra*)

Energetics: Sweet/cold/sweet VP- K+ in excess. V+ if dry

Action: Nutritive, tonic, aphrodisiac, one of the best fruit strengtheners, demulcent, laxative, refrigerant, febrifuge

Indications: Tonic with almonds, restorative with milk or kefir, for weak children, lung disease, convalescence, febrile disease, asthma, increase semen, strengthens reproductive systems (may be added to herbal formulas as tonic). Good for wasting diseases and injuries. Date sugar is a good source of iron.

Plantain, Dates, Coconut: Sweet-cold-sweet. VP- K+. relieves burning, lungs, TB, bleeding; increases reproductive fluid, hard to digest.

Figs (*Anjīra*)

Energetics: Sweet, astringent/cold/sweet VP- K+ Dry V+

Action: Nutritive, demulcent, laxative, antibacterial

Indications: Urinary tract and gall bladder stones, liver, kidneys, chronic cough, increase weight, destroys roundworms, hemorrhoids, cancer, digestive disorders, high in fiber. Figs are a good source of iron and an excellent blood builder. Taken in the morning with a pinch of *pippalī,* help asthma. Chewing figs strengthens teeth, tongue, and gums. Research indicates figs shrink cancerous tumors. More calcium than milk, more potassium than bananas.

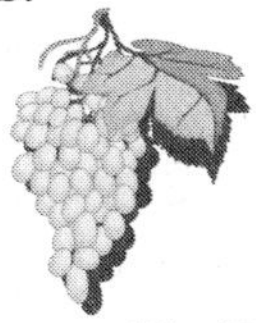

Grapes (***Drakṣha, Mṛidvīkā***)
Energetics: Green: sourt/hot/pungent V- PK+
Purple, red or black: Sweet/cold/sweet V- PK+
Action: Refrigerant, thirst relieving, nutritive, demulcent, diuretic, hemostatic, laxative, aphrodisiac
Indications: They are said to be the best of the fruits; and provide immediate relief from thirst, burning, fever, difficult or painful breathing, bleeding, consumption, wasting, Vāyu and Pitta feces retention, hoarseness, alcoholism, dry mouth, and cough. They help the eyes, blood (rich in iron), and elimination of urine and feces; lungs, TB. They help anemia, heart disease, and palpitations, difficult or burning urine, thrush in children, colds, jaundice, chronic bronchitis, Bright's disease, gout, edema, cancer, detoxification, biliousness, acidity, liver stimulant, energy, skin disorders, constipation, prevents gum disease and tooth decay; and cleanse all tissues and glands. Black grapes build blood. The juice is used for fevers. Raisins taken with herbs are a blood tonic; for debility, sweeten and harmonize stomach; less likely to aggravate Kapha; contains many vitamins and minerals. Eating a handful of raisins daily helps with enlarged liver and spleen. Drinking soaked raisin water and the raisins each morning improves digestion. Research indicates grapes and raisins may prevent cancer.

Grapefruit
Energetics: Sour/hot/sour V- P+ K liquefy/ discharge or +
Action: Stimulant, expectorant, astringent
Indications: Discharges phlegm when taken in the morning, digests sugars and fats, weight reduction, stimulates liver and pancreas, cardiovascular healing, protects the arteries, cancer preventive, cholesterol, high in vitamin C and potassium. Seeds heal candida and are an antibiotic.

Guava (***Perala; Amruta-phalam; Anjīra***)
Energetics: Sweet/cold or hot/
Indications: Excessive digestion and metabolism, anorexia, gout. As a jelly it is a heart tonic and anticonstipative. Soaked in water—relieves thirst due to diabetes. Unripe—diarrhea.
Precaution: When the fruit is raw, the rind and the pulp should be eaten together to prevent constipation. Guava is heavy and hard to digest.

Lemon (***Limpaka***)
Energetics: Sour, astringent/hot/sour V- P+ excess K- fat K+ plasma
Action: Laxative, refrigerant, relieves thirst, expectorant, astringent, digestive stimulant (juice) stomachic, peel-digestive stimulant
Indications: Summer heat, sunstroke (especially with salt), fevers, hot-dry skin; thirst, stops bleeding of lungs, kidney, uterus, and GI tract; inflammation, colds, flu, sore throat, bronchitis, asthma, digestive disorders, diabetes, scurvy, fevers, rheumatism, arthritis, gout, neuralgia; juice —heartburn, sore throat gargle, swollen or bleeding gums; cleanses the blood stream; with honey —rids phlegm discharge and fat reduction; stimulates bile flow; dissolves gall stones; peel—regulates liver, spleen, and pancreas; digests sugars and sweets. It will detoxify balanced Pitta *doṣhas*. Lemon juice and honey relieve nausea, vomiting, indigestion, and mucus. Juice with baking soda and water relieves gas and indigestion. Juice with cilantro juice in water relieves kidney stones and urinary gravel.
External use—insect bites, nerve pain, disinfectant.
Precautions: Do not take with milk, mangos, tomatoes, or when suffering from a peptic ulcer

Lime (***Karkatika***)
Energetics: Sour, slightly bitter/cold/sweet V- P+ in excess—K+, fat, plasma
Action: Juice—digestive stimulant. Peel—stimulant, stomachic, expectorant
Indications: Counters the effects of alcohol, palpitations, malaria fevers, throat gargle, a glass of hot water and 1 teaspoon each of lime and honey,

in the morning, relieves obesity and cholesterol. Peel—increases energy to liver; with salt—sunstroke or summer heat.

Mango (*Āmra*)
Energetics: Yellow-ripe Mangos: Sweet/hot/sweet VP- K+. Green-unripe mangos: sour, astringent/cold/pungent VK- P+ (except when prepared as chutney)
Action: Demulcent, diuretic, astringent, refrigerant, skin-astringent
Indications: Nervous or weak digestion, constipation, vitality, strength, semen, skin, atonic indigestion. Bark infusions, or skin—diarrhea, dysentery, hemorrhoids, high in vitamin C. It is good for pregnancy and improves lactation. Drinking warm milk with *ghee* one hour after eating a ripe mango improves energy and vitality. Unripe or sour aids digestion. Pulp—diabetes, blood pressure. Pickled—for colds; seed powder—vaginal discharge; high in vitamin C. As chutney, they are eaten with meals, improving digestion and enhancing the food's flavor.

Melons
Energetics: Sweet/cold/sweet P- K+ V+ (in excess)
Action: Refrigerant, febrifuge, diuretic, aphrodisiac
Indications: Watermelon (*Chayapula*)—summer heat, sunstroke, fevers, thirst, vexation, irritability, burning urine (taken with a pinch of coriander), or burning sensations; blood purifier, cleans tissues; bleeding gums, canker sores in the mouth; high in vitamin A and C, (with seeds V=); antiseptic for typhoid fever. With cumin and cane sugar the juice helps urinary conditions, intestinal catarrh, and congested liver; Cantaloupe—milder, is better for Vāyu. For acne and rashes, and to promote soft skin—rub melon rind on skin before bed. Watermelon binds the stool and flushes the kidneys, but only eat them 3 hours after meals.
Contraindications: Eat alone. Watermelon—do not eat at night or when cloudy (this causes edema or abdominal pain). Eating them in excess causes respiratory problems. Not eaten with glaucoma

Oranges (*Swadu-naringa*)
Energetics: Sweet or sour/hot/sweet or pungent V- K+ P+ excess or sour variety. Sweet is the best variety
Action: Stimulant, expectorant, appetizer, refrigerant, relieves thirst; peel—stimulant, carminative
Indications: Counters cough, diabetes, bronchitis, liver, heart disorders, vomiting, harmonizes stomach; high in vitamin C and A. A glass of fresh orange juice with a pinch of rock salt restores energy after exercising (Pitta *doṣhas* add 10 lemon drops). A blood purifier, with meals for bile and scurvy; For babies—equal parts with water every 3 hours with mother's milk for stomach disorders. For children with anemia or nervous debility, mix grape and orange juice.
Precautions: Avoid with joint pain or bladder disorders

Papaya (*Papita* - H)
Energetics: Sweet, sour/hot/sweet V- PK+ P+ in excess
Action: Digestive aid, toning, demulcent, stimulant, laxative
Indications: Convalescence, digestive disorders, pancreas, regulates sugar metabolism, cough, worms, asthma, back pain, colon disorders, liver and spleen disorders; chronic illness, seeds—emmenagogue, for abortion; unripe juice—anti-parasitical, blood thinner, prevents heart attack. Externally—the inner skin of the fruit is rubbed on one's skin for eczema and dermatitis.

Peaches (*Aru* - H)
Energetics: Sweet, astringent, or sour/hot/sweet or pungent V- PK+ (V+ sometimes. One peach daily K-)
Action: Demulcent, laxative, refrigerant
Indications: Fever, cough, seeds—anti-cough/laxative, menstruation, colon worms, heal damaged tissues; leaves—allay nausea, vomiting;

high in vitamin A, potassium, fiber; cancer, heart disease, Nectarines are safer for Pitta.
Contraindications: Skin aggravates in excess or acute Pitta conditions (i.e., rash)

Pears (*Arūk*)
Energetics: Sweet or astringent/cold/sweet or pungent PK- V+_(unless baked) K+ (sweet)
Action: Nutritive, demulcent, laxative, tonic, febrifuge, anti-cough
Indications: Lung tonic, diabetes, diarrhea, convalescence from lung disease (with cardamom, cloves, ginger, cinnamon); fevers, poor appetite, biliousness, hyperacidity, chronic gall bladder disorders, excessive thirst, gout, stomach disorders, laxative (eaten on an empty stomach), enlarged liver, gonorrhea, hemorrhoids.
Precautions: Do not eat with arthritis, diabetes, dry cough or sciatica.

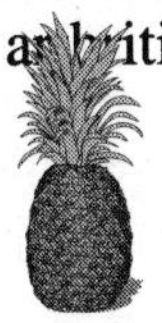

Pineapple (*Ananas*-H)
Energetics: Sweet or sour/cold or hot/sweet or pungent V- KP+ (sour or unripe) sweet in moderation
Action: Diuretic, refrigerant, laxative, digestive stimulant, anti-scurvy, diaphoretic
Indications: Cleanses the liver, biliousness, acidity, jaundice, counters the effects of alcohol. Juice relieves constipation and gastric irritability in fevers. To reduce cigarette smoking and nicotine toxicity, chew small pieces of the fruit with half a teaspoon of raw honey. It digests albuminous (protein) substances. Contains high amounts of easily assimilated manganese (which may prevent osteoporosis).
Precautions: Juice will aggravate Pitta. Not given to children under 7 years old. Not eaten on an empty stomach in the morning. Not taken within two hours of ingesting dairy products. Unripe pineapples may cause abortion

Plums
Energetics: Sweet, sour, astringent/hot/sweet VP- K+ P+ sour European—sweet, Japan-sweet/sour Chinese black plum (*Umeboshi*)—sour (anti-parasitical, anti-cough, digestion)
Action: Refrigerant, relieves thirst, alterative, laxative
Indications: Fever, dry cough.

Pomegranate (*Dāḍima*)
Energetics: Sweet, astringent, sour/hot, cold /sweet, pungent PK- V+ (sweet); (P+ sour)
Action: Astringent, alterative, hemostatic, rind-anti-parasitical
Indications: The sour, astringent, sweet variety is the best. Builds red blood cells (juice), cleanses bile, blood, bilious indigestion, gall stones, hyperacidity, fever, intermittent or malarial fever; diarrhea, dysentery, excessive perspiration, gargle for sore throats; leukorrhea, tapeworm. They are good for the heart, mind, anemia, and as a digestive aid. Pomegranate binds the bowels, cardiac tonic, hoarseness.

Raspberries/Blackberries/Blueberries
Energetics: Sweet, sour, astringent (unripe)/cold/pungent PK- V+
Action: Refrigerant, relieves thirst, astringent; unripe—astringent, leaf—astringent, hemostatic, Blueberries—alterative refrigerant, astringent (unrelated botanical family)
Indications: Unripe—excess urination, nocturnal emission, improves sexual vitality, liver tonic, diarrhea, Blackberries (*Jambul* or *Rajaphala*)— build blood, are good for dysentery and diarrhea; goiter, cholera, hemorrhoids, and insect bites/stings. The bark is used externally on inflammations. The seed powder is useful in diabetes, reducing sugar in the urine and excessive thirst. Raspberry leaf—miscarriage, morning sickness (nausea). For bleeding gums or excess menstruation, 10 to 20 raspberries are eaten on an empty stomach 2 to 3 times daily. Fruit is useful for obesity, gout, arthritis, diabetes, constipation, hypertension, kidney stones, and relieving the delivery pains of childbirth. Blueberries—regulate sugar metabolism and reduce fevers, diarrhea and dysentery; help bladder/urinary tract disorders, contain tannic acid

(destroys viruses).
Precautions: Eating more than two handfuls of raspberries at a time may cause vomiting. Taken with dairy products, they can cause hemorrhoids, skin diseases, and ulcers

Strawberries
Energetics: Sweet, sour, astringent (cold or hot/sweet or pungent VP- K (+in excess)
Action: Refrigerant, relieve thirst, alterative, leaf-mild astringent, antacid as tea
Indications: Similar to raspberries; protects against viruses, cancer, DNA damage, herpes simplex, and skin disorders; high in vitamin C, fiber, potassium, antioxidant. Ten berries daily may help anemia and pulmonary TB. Useful for obesity, gout, arthritis, diabetes, constipation, hypertension, and kidney stones.
Contraindications: Their skin may aggravate Pitta. Eating too many can cause coughing and vomiting. They are eaten alone

Tangerine/Mandarin Orange
Energetics: Sweet, sour/cold/sweet (more sour than oranges) VP- K+ P+ excess
Action: Refrigerant, relieve thirst, expectorant, stimulant
Indications: Peels—warm, aids appetite, settles stomach, vomiting, cough, discharge phlegm—especially mandarin peel
Contraindications: Aggravates acute Pitta conditions

Vegetables
Energetics: Pleasant/even/sweet
Actions: Generally *sattwic* (but less so than fruit)
Indications:
Root— heavier, nutritive, V- K+P= carrots, potatoes, sweet potatoes, artichokes, cauliflower (V+).
Leafy Greens—(including cabbage family) lighter PK- V+ blood-cleansing, vitamins, minerals, not nutritive.
Pungents—onions, chilies VK- P+ *rajasic*.
Nightshades—tomatoes, potatoes, VP- may cause allergies, though if cooked they cause fewer problems.
Diuretics—K- Carrots, celery, lettuce, mustard greens, watercress, broccoli, potatoes.
Preparation:
Vāyu—cooked or steamed, oils and spices, salt and pickled (*rajasic*)
Pitta—raw or lightly steamed, vegetable juices,
Kapha—cooked or steamed. Fresh, organic, home or locally grown is *sattwic*
Canned food is *tamasic*, aggravating all humors.
Combining: Combines well with other foods for one's constitution. Does not combine well with fruit or sugars
Season: It is best to eat vegetables according to season (taking into account one's constitutional requirements)
Spring, Summer—greens, leafy, raw
Fall, Winter—roots, cooked
Antidote—cold and raw—ginger, oil, vinegar (*rajasic*), garlic and onions (*rajasic/tamasic*)
Dry and light—(i.e., cabbage family) oil, butter, sour cream, cheese, whole grains, pasta

Alfalfa Sprouts (*Lasunghas* - H)
Energetics: Astringent, sweet/cold/pungent PK- V+ decrease *agni*
Actions: Alterative, astringent, diuretic
Indications: Cleanse blood and lymph, reduce fat and tumors, acne, boils, skin cancer, arthritis, gout, obesity, edema, vitamins, and minerals.

Artichoke (Globe) (*Kunjor, Hatichuk* - H)
Energetics: Sweet, astringent/hot/sweet PK- V+ (butter or lemon is better for Vāyu)
Actions: Alteratives, hemostatics, diuretics
Indications: Cleanses liver, excess menstruation; high in calcium, phosphorus, iron, vitamin C, and niacin.

—Jerusalem Artichoke (*Hastipijū*)
Energetics: Astringent, bitter/cold/pungent PK- V+
Actions: Tonic, rejuvenative
Indications: Rebuilds reproductive tissue, impotence, infertility, sexual debility, vigor, vitality, *ojas*, emaciation, convalescence.

Asparagus (*Marchuba* - H)
Energetics: Sweet, bitter, astringent/cold/sweet VPK=
Actions: Diuretic, alterative, mild laxative, demulcent, tonic, aphrodisiac, sedative
Indications: High Pitta, bleeding disorders or infections of urinary or reproductive systems (including venereal disease like herpes and for urinary stones), fever, edema (and cardiac edema), gout, arthritis. Drinking boiled asparagus water helps rheumatism.

Avocado
Energetics: Astringent/cold/sweet VP- K+ best taken with spices
Actions: Tonic, nutritive, demulcent, emollient
Indications: Nourishes liver, lungs, skin, builds muscle and blood, emaciation, convalescence, hypoglycemia reduces the risk of heart attacks; high in protein, contains vitamins A, D, E; high in minerals, especially copper and iron; rich in phosphorus, magnesium, calcium, sodium, and manganese; more potassium than bananas.

Beans/Greens
Energetics: Sweet, astringent/hot/sweet PK- V+ excess
Actions: Alterative, diuretic, astringent
Indications: Cleanses blood and liver, gout, normalize liver and pancreas; rheumatism, contain vitamins A, B-complex, C, chlorophyll, carbohydrates, calcium, phosphorous, copper, cobalt, trace source of inositol.

Bean (Mung) Sprouts
Energetics: Astringent, sweet/cold/sweet PK- V+ excess
Actions: Alterative, antacid, febrifuge
Indications: Counter toxins, cleanses liver and bile; alcoholism, hyperacidity.

Beets (*Chukander* - H)
Energetics: Sweet/hot/sweet V- PK+ excess
Actions: Alterative, demulcent, laxative, tonic
Indications: Build blood, promote menstruation; juice more medicinal (and aggravate PK), beet greens have same effects as spinach; lymph functioning, gall bladder, and liver; digestive disorders, anemia (build red blood cells).

Bell Pepper (*Deshomaricha* - H)
Energetics: Sweet, astringent/cold/sweet PK- V+
Actions: Alterative, refrigerant

Bitter Melon (*Karela*)
Energetics: Bitter/cold/pungent PK- V+
Actions: Antipyretic, alterative, antacid, antiparasitical
Indications: Excellent for diabetes; kidney stones, intestinal worms, parasites, cleanses liver, bile, blood, reduces weight, tumors, fever, diarrhea, anemia, summer use, high in vitamin C.

Cabbage Family
Energetics: Astringent, sweet/cold/pungent PK- V+ *rajasic*
Actions: Alterative, may prevent colon cancer

Broccoli—astringent/cold/pungent PK- V+—alterative, blood cleanser, lowers the risk of cancer of the esophagus, larynx, lung, prostate, mouth, colon, pharynx, cervix, and stomach, tumor.

Brussels Sprouts (*Kobi* - H)—astringent/hot/pungent PK- V+—inhibits cancer of the G.I. tract, liver, stomach, and colon; liver tumors, promotes pancreatic insulin; rich in vitamins A, C, riboflavin, iron, potassium, fiber; depresses thyroid function.

Cabbage (*Kobi* - H) and Chinese Cabbage—astringent/cold/pungent PK- V+—gas forming, Chinese variety is easier to digest. Heals ulcers, eczema, infections, heartburn, antibacterial, antiviral, prevents cancer, scurvy, eye diseases, gout, rheumatism, pyorrhea, asthma, TB, gangrene; blood purifier, rashes, high in calcium, vitamin C and A, sulfur. White cabbage juice removes warts.

Cauliflower ***(Phulkobī* - H)**—astringent/cold/ pungent PK- V+—more sweet and *sattwic* than the others, demulcent, nutritive, combines well with dairy; reduces the risk of cancer (especially rectum, colon and stomach). It is better for diabetics than cabbage.

Kale—blood cleanser, one of the best cancer fighting vegetables (lung, stomach, esophageal, colon, mouth, throat, G.I., breast, bowel, bladder, prostate); rich in vitamin A, C, riboflavin, niacin, calcium, magnesium, iron, sulfur, sodium, potassium, phosphorus, and chlorophyll; calcium is easily assimilated.

Carrots (*Śhikha-mulam*)
Energetics: Sweet, astringent/hot/sweet or pungent VK- P+ excess; juice V+ due to its cold nature, sweet nature makes it hard to digest
Actions: Digestive, laxative, diuretic, appetite stimulant, alterative, antiseptic; seeds—stimulant, antispasmodic, emmenagogue
Indications: Increase blood flow, build blood, brighten eyes, rickets, colitis, gout, constipation, worms (eaten raw), arthritis, skin disorders, edema, jaundice, chronic hepatitis, antioxidant, heal skin and tissues; heart disease, reduce the risk of lung cancer; diarrhea, healthy teeth, colon disorders, dehydration, complexion. One cup of juice with 2 teaspoons of cilantro juice, taken twice daily on an empty stomach, relieves hemorrhoids. For chronic indigestion, a glass of juice is taken with a pinch of ginger powder. One half cup of juice mixed with one half cup aloe vera juice, and taken twice daily, helps reduce cancer. Externally—poultice for malodorous, ulcerative sores.

Celery (*Ajmoda*)
Energetics: Astringent, sweet, salty/cold/pungent PK- V+ (needed minerals for all three humors)
Actions: Astringent, diuretic, nervine; seeds and roots—diuretic, seeds are hot, stimulant, carminative, emmenagogue, antispasmodic, (similar to *ajwan*—wild celery seeds)
Indications: Cleanses mind, emotions, perception, increases ether to promote meditation (Closely related to gotu kola/*brāhmī* in this effect); dizziness, headache, eliminates carbon dioxide, Pitta and Kapha arthritis; adrenal disorders, weight loss, blood cleanser, urogenital infections, promotes digestion, kidney and liver disorders; regulates the nervous system, water retention, diabetes, cancer; lowers blood pressure; seeds and roots—dissolve stones, arthritis, gout.

Chilies—Hot Peppers (*Jhal* - H)
Energetics: Pungent/hot/pungent VK- P++ *Agni*++ (*rajasic*)
Actions: Stimulant, diaphoretic, digestive, decongestant
Indications: Burns *āma*, appetite, indigestion, parasites, lungs (asthma, bronchitis, emphysema, tracheal and bronchial cell swelling), blood clots, pain.

Cilantro (Coriander leaf) **(*Dhyanyaka, Kustumbari*)**
Energetics: Sweet, astringent/cold/sweet VPK= (balanced) V+ excess
Actions: Stimulant, diuretic, diaphoretic, febrifuge
Indications: Skin allergies, hay fever, builds the digestive fire, sore throat, hyperacidity, nausea, fever, colds, thirst, cleanses blood, bile and urinary tract infections; juice—burning urine; antidote to hot and sour foods (i.e., salsa, chilies, curries, yogurt). Externally—pulp placed on eyelids relieves conjunctivitis; juice—skin diseases

Corn (sweet) (*Yavanala*)
Energetics: Sweet, astringent/hot/sweet or pungent K- VP+
excess
Actions: Balanced, corn silk- diuretic
Indications: Strengthening, corn silk—jaundice, hepatitis, gall and kidney stones; urinary tract infections, edema, brain and nervous system tonic; helps gain weight; bone and muscle

builder; vitamins A, B, C, potassium, phosphorus, iron, zinc, potassium, magnesium, fiber.
Precautions: Avoid with digestive disorders or obesity

Cucumber (*Sakusa*)
Energetics: Sweet, astringent/cold/sweet VP- K+
Actions: Refrigerant, diuretic; seeds—better diuretics, febrifuges
Indications: Eaten as a raw dessert mixed with lemon juice, pepper, and salt, enables the body to absorb the maximum amount of the cucumber's juice and vitamins. Summer food, thirst relieving, urinary tract infections—difficult or scanty urine, spleen and stomach disorders, acne, blood purifier; seeds—dispels phlegm and heat from the lungs. Antidote to heavy, sticky yogurt properties. Seeds are cooling, diuretic, and highly nourishing.

Eggplant (*Vartāka*)*—listed as a fruit in Charak*
Energetics: Pungent, astringent, bitter/hot/pungent VK- P+ [Only the tender variety] (V antidote with spices)
Actions: Nutritive, demulcent, anticarcinogenic, anticonvulsant
Indications: Long size increase Vāyu and Kapha. Food value, convalescence from febrile diseases; heart tonic, appetite stimulant, mild laxative and diuretic; dull vision, diabetes, cholesterol, arteriosclerosis, immune boosting, convulsions, epilepsy.
Contraindications: Nightshade may aggravate allergies, Pitta, and arthritis

Garlic
See Chapter 4—Herbal materia medica.

Lettuce (*Kahu, Salad* - H)
Energetics: Pleasant, astringent/cold/sweet or pungent PK- V+
Actions: Alterative, astringent, diuretic
Indications: Calms and cleanses mind, emotions, blood, lymph, burning.

Mushrooms
Energetics: Sweet, astringent/hot/pungent PK- V+ *āma*+ (*tamasic*)
Actions: Diuretic, astringent, hemostatic, Some Chinese and Japanese varieties; and wild mushrooms are less *tamasic* and more toning
Indications: Edema, overweight, anti-tumor, anti-carcinogenic, reduce cholesterol, longevity.

Contraindications: Do not eat with boils, carbuncles, pus infections

Mustard Greens
Energetics: Pungent, bitter/hot/pungent VK- P+ moderately
Actions: Stimulant, expectorant
Indications: Seeds discharge phlegm better than greens; high amounts of calcium, iron, vitamin A, and niacin.

Okra (*Tindiṣha*)
Energetics: Sweet, astringent/cold/sweet PK- V+
Actions: Demulcent, emollient, diuretic, alterative, aphrodisiac, tonic, (mallow plant family)
Indications: Difficult, painful, or burning urine; diarrhea, dysentery, spermatorrhea, leukorrhea, strengthening, gonorrhea, intestinal disorders, inflamed or spastic colon, diverticulitis, stomach ulcers, fever.

Onions (*Durgandha, Palandu*)
Energetics: Cooked—sweet/hot/sweet VK- P+ Raw—pungent/hot/pungent K- VP+ *Rajasic* except when thoroughly cooked
Actions: Stimulant, diaphoretic, aphrodisiac, expectorant
Indications: Colds, flu, general debility, sexual debility; with oil or *ghee* strengthening properties of meat, aid for physical exertion. Inhale raw onions (until tearing begins) for fainting and convulsions.

Parsley
Energetics: Pungent, astringent/hot/pungent VPK= P+ excess

Actions: Stimulant, diuretic, alterative, emmenagogoue
Indications: Edema, oozing skin rashes, difficult or delayed menstruation; gall stones, vitamins, hypochondriac pain, kidney stones, minerals, blood and lymph cleanser; urinary tract disorders, kidney, bladder or prostate disorders; adrenal and thyroid gland conditions; corrects vitamin deficiency, high in vitamins A, B1, B-complex, C, potassium, manganese, phosphorus, calcium, and iron.

Peas (Green or Snow) (*Sahīla, Vartula*)
Energetics: Astringent/cold/pungent PK - V+ (green better for Vāyu)
Actions: Alterative, astringent
Indications: Blood cleanser, prevents appendicitis and ulcers, anti-fertility, lowers cholesterol, controls blood sugar, lowers blood pressure, low-calorie protein, anti-carcinogen, high fiber.

Potatoes (*Alu* - H)
Energetics: Pleasant, astringent/cold/sweet PK- V+ (curried is best) [may aggravate VP as a nightshade] V: Use *ghee* or butter
Actions: Nutritive, tonic, diuretic, sedative (grounds), produces breast milk
Indications: Strengthening, diarrhea, absorption, cancer, blood pressure, balances alkalinity and acidity.
Precautions: Avoid with diabetes

Radish (*Mūlaka*)
Energetics: Pungent, astringent/hot/pungent K- P+; V- (long white variety).
Actions: Appetite stimulant, expectorant, anti-cough, diuretic, antiparasitical
Indications: Digests heavy food, colds, flu, respiratory infections, cleanses gall bladder and liver; headaches, laryngitis, sinusitis, gall stones, intestinal worms, contains vitamin A, B-complex, and C.

Sea Vegetables
<u>Seaweed</u>
Energetics: Salty, astringent/cold/sweet VPK= VP- K+ excess
Actions: Alterative
Indications: Minerals, plasma, edema, congestion, thyroid, cysts, benign tumors.
<u>Dulse</u>; Rich in protein, fluoride, iron
<u>Irish Moss/Kelp</u>; High in calcium, potassium, magnesium, iron; excellent for thyroid disorders
<u>Kuzu</u>; Gives quick energy
<u>Nori</u>; Good for prostate and thyroid disorders, high in protein, B1, B2, B6, B12, vitamins C, E

Spinach (*Palak* - H) and Chard
Energetics: Pungent, bitter, sweet, astringent/cold/pungent or sweet K- PV+
Actions: Alterative, refrigerant, demulcent, laxative
Indications: Soothes mucus membranes, fever, cough, dry cough, burning lung sensation, blood cleanser, rich in minerals, intestinal tract disorders, hemorrhoids, anemia, vitamin deficiencies.
Precautions: Do not eat with liver diseases, gall or kidney stones or arthritis. It is difficult to digest

Squash
—Acorn, Summer (Heavy)
Energetics: Sweet, astringent/cold/pungent VPK=
Actions: Demulcent, expectorant, nutritive
—Winter
Energetics: Sweet, astringent/hot/pungent VP- K+
Actions: Demulcent, expectorant
Indications: More nutritive than summer variety, dry cough, laryngitis, high in vitamin A.
—Zucchini and Yellow
Energetics: Sweet, astringent/cold/pungent VP- K; V+ excess *Actions*: Alterative, diuretic, refrigerant, expectorant
Indications: Summer anti-heat food.

Sweet Potatoes and Yams (*Piṇḍālu*)
Energetics: Sweet/cold/sweet VP- K+ P+ excess
Actions: Nutritive
Indications: Convalescence, debility, reduces cancer risk (especially lungs), high amounts of vitamin A/beta carotene, antioxidant properties,

high in vitamin C, low in calories.
Contraindications: Hard to digest, eat without other vegetables. Yams are easier to digest

Tomatoes (*Bilatī, Baigun* - H)
Energetics: Yellow—sweet, sour/heating/pungent VPK+ Red—sour, astringent/hot/pungent the stomach and heat the intestines/sour VPK+ (when raw), VK-P+ when steamed); Tridoṣhic when occasionally eaten along with cumin, turmeric, and mustard
Actions: Refrigerant, relieves thirst
Indications: Circulation, blood, heart, cholesterol, hypertension, lowers cancer risk; appendicitis, digestive disorders.
Contraindications: Aggravates toxic blood conditions, acidity, sciatica, kidney and gall stones, and arthritis. Raw seeds can cause abdominal problems. Nightshade

Turnips (*Raktasarṣhapa*) and Rutabaga
Energetics: Pungent, astringent/hot/pungent K-VP+ *rajasic*
Actions: Alterative
Indications: Blood and lymph cleanser, stops bleeding, Pitta or Kapha arthritis; uric acid, kidney stones, overweight, gout; rich in all vitamins (high in vitamin C) and sulfur.

Watercress (*Chandrasura, Ahalīva)*
Indications: Anemia, calcium deficiencies, blood purifier, catarrh, liver and pancreas disorders, stimulates the appetite, thyroid disorders, arthritis, emotional disorders, TB, high in potassium, sulfur, vitamin A, calcium, and iron; contains copper, magnesium, sodium, potassium, and iodine.

Grains

Sweet/neutral/sweet *Sattwic*, VPK= aggravates in excess. Whole grain is the best staple for all climates and constitutions.
Actions: Gives bulk to stool, easy to digest
Elements: Earth
Tissues: Builds all
Indications:
Diuretics; nutritive, K+, discharge phlegm, barley, pearled barley, corn, rye, buckwheat.
Nutritives; V-, convalescence, wheat, oats, *basmati* and brown rice, (some say barley V-; others say barley V+)
Preparation: Steamed whole grains are balanced and easiest to digest
Breads: Hard to digest, yeast V+, toasted is easier to digest and makes them better for V and K
Pastries: More difficult to digest than bread, especially if made with refined sugars and flour.
Unleavened breads: *Chapatis*, tortillas, matzoh, etc., are better than yeast breads
Pastas/noodles: Good (especially whole wheat)
Cut/ground: Good—lose their properties quicker
Oil Fried: (deep fried) harder to digest, PK *āma*+
Dried: (granola, etc.) V+ K-, corn chips (fried in oil) PK+ & dryness V+, crackers better all around
Antidoting: Some spices may be helpful, use as necessary
Combinations: Do not eat bread with other foods; with steamed vegetables, oil or *ghee*, VPK=; all other grain combinations are ok, but make sure the other foods are combinable (i.e., grain and vegetables are ok, and grain and fruits are ok, but fruit and vegetables may not combine well.)
Season—good during any season due to holding their potency within the seed. Winter is especially a good time

Grains with pointed ends are best.

Grain List

Barley (*Yāva*)
Energetics: Sweet, astringent/cold/sweet
PK- V+ in excess
Action: Diuretic, demulcent, anti-rheumatic
Indications: Lung disease convalescence, cough, fevers, arthritis, edema, water retention, kidneys, absorption, diarrhea, cleanses urinary tract, increases and bulks stool; reduces body fat and mucus; helps difficult breathing, stiff thighs, throat and skin disorders. It is strengthening, stabilizing, heals infections, and removes toxins.

Prevents cholesterol absorption in the intestines and aids the suppression of cholesterol in the liver. Stimulates the liver and lymphatic system. It contains calcium, iron, protein, and potassium.

Buckwheat (*Kaspat* - H)
Energetics: Astringent/hot/sweet K- VP+
Indications: It is not as nutritious as wheat, but is still considered helpful as a food. It is too heating and drying for Pitta and Vāyu *doṣhas*.

Corn (sweet) (*Yavanala*)
Energetics: Sweet/hot/sweet K- VP+ in excess
Action: Diuretic
Indications: Edema, kidney and gallstones, jaundice (corn silk especially), nutritive, liver, kidneys, spleen absorption, solar energy increases perception (especially with *ghee*).
Contraindications: Corn chips, VP+ (blue corn is colder and better for P); corn bread, tortillas, posole V+

Millet (*Soma; Rajika*)
Energetics: Sweet/hot/sweet K- VP+ mildly
Action: Demulcent, diuretic
Indications: Nutritive, convalescence, debility, wholesome but difficult to digest. Millet is high in iron, lecithin and choline, thus preventing some forms of gallstones. It is full of protein and nutrition. It is good for colitis, ulcers, and urinary disorders. Due to its alkaline nature it is good for the spleen, pancreas, and stomach.

Oats
Energetics: Sweet/cold/sweet VP- K+
Action: Demulcent, emollient, laxative (especially cut or rolled)
Indications: Calms and strengthens mind, nerves (especially oat straw), builds all tissues (including reproductive). It normalizes blood glucose in diabetes, helps slow thyroid conditions, neutralizes excess cholesterol, high amounts of iron, vitamin E, thiamine, riboflavin, niacin, and B-complex. Protein is easily assimilated.
Precautions: A little heavy and hard to digest, especially with sugar and milk. May produce skin eruptions or aggravate toxic blood conditions

Rice (*Vrihi, Dhanya*)
Energetics: Sweet, astringent/cold or neutral/sweet VPK=, K+ in excess (especially *basmati*) starch is easy to digest. Highly *sattwic*
Action: Tonic, nutritive, demulcent, laxative
Indications: Vomiting, anorexia, poor digestion, harmonizes the stomach, builds all tissues through plasma, soothes the nervous system and the brain. Helps rid the body of toxins; high in B-complex.

Rice pointed at both ends is best. It relieves thirst and is good for all three *doṣhas*. White *basmati* rice is best, as it is nutritious and easily digested. Brown rice may have more nutrition, but since it is harder to digest, one may not obtain any nutrition from it without an excellent digestive fire.
Contraindications: Bleached, refined white- K+, *āma* +, brown short grain (warming), maybe P+, V- if it can be digested

Rye
Energetics: Astringent/hot/pungent PK- V+
Action: Diuretic
Indications: One of the best Kapha grains. Few allergenic reactions, very high amounts of lysine, helps the glands, good for weight loss.

Wheat (*Godhūma*)
Energetics: Sweet, astringent/cold/sweet VP- K+
Action: Nutritive, aphrodisiac
Indications: Strengthening, children's growth, builds muscle tissue, energy, earth, heart, palpitations, calms mind, insomnia, ulcers, colitis, hemorrhoids, heals fractures; with milk and sugar for bleeding disorders (*rakta* Pitta). Taken as *chapatis* (unleavened bread pancake); wheat bran is a bulk laxative; used as coffee substitute. It is nourishing and strengthening. External poultice—astringent for burns, sores, skin rashes.

Whole wheat restores health and alleviates

Vāyu. It is the best grain for Vāyu *doṣhas*. Pasta (carbohydrate) eaten without protein produces serotonin in the brain that is linked to calmness and cheerfulness. Pasta also contains iron, phosphorous, and magnesium.
Contraindications: Gluten may cause allergies, aggravate arthritis, gout or other *āma* conditions. White flour is an artificial and overly refined food (*tamasic*), K+ *āma*+, clogging channels and dulling mind.

Legumes

Energetics: Sweet, astringent/neutral/sweet PK- V+ (except mung, soy) All beans are *rajasic*—causing gas and irritating body, mind, senses and emotions—and therefore not recommended for *yoga* since they vitiate *sattwa* by aggravating the mind. Mung beans and tofu are the only two exceptions. The mung bean is the only *sattwic* bean.
Indications: Energy for strenuous work
Element: Earth (protein) mostly, and air; heavy and dry, thus hard to digest
Combination: As a protein they combine well with grains for a staple food, containing all the eight essential amino acids; especially split mung bean with long grain or *Basmati* rice *kicharī* (see rice section on previous page). Combine well with vegetables. Legumes do not combine well with other beans, sugars, fruit or diary
Preparation: Well-cooked and properly spiced. Some need to be soaked in water overnight, especially whole beans. When prepared in lard or heavy oils, are hard to digest, PK+
Season: Hold their properties, so can be eaten year-round (because fruits and vegetables lose their energies quickly, seasonal eating is suggested for them) though better in winter
Antidotes: Parboiling and removing water once or twice removes some irritant properties (e.g., for soy or kidney beans); Sspices—onions, cumin, *asafoetida (hiṅg)*, cayenne, and salt help, but will aggravate Pitta
Nutrition: Proteins, iron, B vitamins, trace minerals; as a crop they nourish the soil instead of robbing it and absorb more than 100 pounds of nitrogen from the atmosphere yearly

Bean List

Aduki
Energetics: Sweet, astringent/cold/pungent PK- V+ slightly *rajasic*
Action: Alterative, diuretic, heart tonic
Indications: Heart, blood, circulation, children, convalescence, edema from malnutrition, painful or burning urine; delayed or difficult menstruation; as paste with sugar for confections.

Black Gram (*Maṣha*)
Energetics: Sweet, astringent/cold/sweet P- V+ K+ mildly
Action: Nutritive, demulcent, aphrodisiac, nervine tonic, lactagogue
Indications: The most strengthening bean, diarrhea, dysentery, indigestion, hemorrhoids, arthritis, paralysis, liver disorders, cystitis, rheumatism. Increases semen and breast milk. Externally—plaster for arthritis/joint pain.

Chick Pea/Garbanzo (*Chanaka*)
Energetics: Sweet/cold/pungent PK- V+
Action: Nutritive, aphrodisiac, diuretic, astringent
Indications: Strengthening, increases reproductive tissue, debility, brain, as humus it is easier to digest. Roasted—relieves gas, urine retention or excess; contains calcium, iron, potassium, vitamin A.

Fava/Broad (*Bakla* - H)
Energetics: Sweet, astringent/cold/sweet PK- V++
Indications: Not used as food because some get toxic reactions. Contains calcium, protein, iron, B vitamins.

Flat Bean/Goya (*Simbi*)
Energetics: PK- V+
Indications: Good for phlegm disorders

Precautions: Not good for the eyes, depleting properties

Kidney/Navy/Pinto (*Makuṣhtaka* - S; *Bakla* - H)

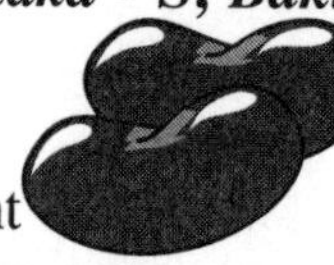

Energetics: PK- V+
Kidney: Astringent/hot/pungent
Navy: Sweet, astringent/hot/pungent
Pinto: Astringent/cold/pungent
Action: Nutritive, digestive, aphrodisiac, cardiac
Indications: Bleeding disorders, bile, fevers, and other Pitta excesses. It is strengthening. Red kidney beans are rich in all nutrients, protein, and fibers.
Contraindications: Hard to digest

Lentils (*Masura*)
Energetics: PK- V+ (in excess)
Red: Astringent/hot/pungent
Sweet: Sweet, astringent/cold/sweet
Indications: Nutritive, strengthening. High in calcium, magnesium, phosphorus, sulfur, vitamin A, proteins. They reduce fat and blood, and absorb water.
Contraindications: Some lentils are hard to digest; though easier if sprouted. (There are differing beliefs on the use of various lentils.) They can cause constipation

Lima (*Cimra* - Bengali)
Energetics: Sweet, astringent/cold/sweet PK- V+
Indications: Easier to digest, especially if fresh. Good for simple diarrhea (but not for Vāyu, Pitta, or mucus diarrhea), constipation. External poultice—cleanses foul ulcers. Rich in potassium, minerals, vitamins, fiber.

Mung (Green Gram) (***Mada, Mudga***)
Energetics: Sweet, astringent/cold/sweet VPK= K+ in excess *Sattwic*
Action: Refrigerant, antipyretic, alterative, hemostatic. Very nutritious and wholesome
Indications: Pitta disorders, summer food, convalescence from febrile or infectious disease (as *kicharī*—see *Basmati* rice), relieves thirst during fevers, febrile disease, liver, drugs, smoking, or alcohol detoxification, cancer, enlarged liver or spleen, bleeding; Tea—high fevers or heat stroke. External paste—burns, sores, swelling, inflamed joints, draws out toxins, swollen breasts, mastitis, breast cancer. It is sometimes called *"mūng-dal"*.

Peanuts (*Buchanaka*)
Energetics: Sweet, astringent/hot/sweet K- VP+
Action: Oily and often classified as a nut
Indications: Strengthening, protein, use raw and cooked (not roasted), add honey or cane sugar
Contraindications: Dry roasted V++, peanut butter hard to digest K+

Soy/Tofu (*Bhatwan* - H)
Energetics: Sweet, astringent/cold/pungent P- VK+ *Rajasic*
Tofu: Sweet, astringent/cold/pungent VP- K-+
Soy cheese: Sour, astringent/hot/pungent V- PK+
Action: Easier to digest as tofu (*sattwic*)
Indications: Tofu after febrile disease, as milk for Kapha or *āma*, lung infections, lymph with fever; taken with *kicharī* VPK=. Tofu is rich in protein, calcium and potassium. It promotes female hormone balance.

Split Peas
Energetics: Sweet, astringent/cool/sweet PK- V+
Action: Binding stool
Indications: Diarrhea.
Contraindications: Hard to digest, better as soup

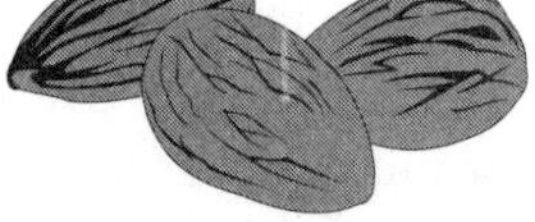

Nuts & Seeds
Energetics: Sweet/warm/sweet V- PK+
Actions: Tonic, nutritive, strengthening, rejuvenative
Indications: The best source of protein and fat from vegetable sources; increase fat, marrow,

nerve tissue, reproductive tissue, *ojas*, build blood and muscles, strengthen memory and creativity; *sattwic*—helps *yoga* and meditation. Seeds—similar yet lighter, less nourishing, easier to digest, V+ excess.
Preparation: Chewed well, not taken in excess drinks—nut milk is best, fermented nut drinks (amasake) easier to digest- use with fresh ginger salt—better for Vāyu; raw sugar—(sucanat, jaggery, dates, raisins) tonic, demulcent for convalescence and debility.

roasting—heavy, oily, hard to digest, roasting takes out oil

light roasting— better for Vāyu.

not roasted—better for PK but check that they are not rancid.

Nut butters are oily and used in small doses.
Season: Properties are stored well. Best taken in fall and winter—oiliness, K+ in spring, P+ in summer
Combination: Do not combine well with beans or starchy vegetables (potatoes); combine well with dairy, most fruit, grain, sugar (though heavier and harder to digest)
Antidote: Mild spices like ginger or cardamom

Almonds (*Badama*)
Energetics: Sweet, slightly bitter/hot/sweet V- PK+
Actions: Nutritive, nervine, aphrodisiac, demulcent, laxative, rejuvenation
Indications: Cough, dry cough, increase marrow, semen, kidney, reproductive organs, brain, convalescence, debility, builds strong bones and *ojas* (life sap); good for the heart, lowers bad (LDL) cholesterol and raises good (HDL) cholesterol; cancer-fighting protease inhibitors. High in potassium, magnesium, phosphorus, protein, fiber, and the trace mineral boron (that may regulate calcium metabolism).

Brazil Nuts
Energetics: Sweet, astringent/hot/sweet; Oily, heavy V- P+ K++
Actions: Tonic strength, nutritive
Indications: Modern research suggests they may improve resistance to cancer and tumors.

Cashews (*Śhoephahara*)
Energetics: Sweet/hot/sweet- see general notes above VPK+
Actions: Expectorant
Indications: Helps deeper tissues. High in potassium, magnesium, vitamin A.

Coconut (*Dīrghavrakṣha*)
Energetics: Sweet/cold/sweet VP- K+
Actions: Refrigerant, diuretic, demulcent, emollient
Indications: High Pitta, lungs, skin, recovery from febrile and infectious disease.

Filberts (*Askhota*)/ Hazelnut (*Findak* - H)
Energetics: Sweet, astringnet/hot/sweet V- PK+
Actions: Lighter, easier for Kapha to digest
Indications: May help restore energy in chronic fatigue syndrome, hypoglycemia, yeast infections. High in potassium, sulfur, calcium.

Flax/Linseed (*Uma*)
Energetics: Warming VK-
Actions: Anti-inflammatory (internal & external)
Indications: Rich in fatty acids, bronchial congestion, constipation.
Contraindications: Taken with lots of liquids and digestive herbs

Lotus Seeds (*Kamala* - white; *Padma*; *Kokonad* - pink; *Induvara* - blue)
Energetics: Sweet, astringent/hot/sweet P- VK+ *āma*
Actions: Nutritive, tonic, calmative, aphrodisiac, rejuvenative
Indications: With sugar and *ghee*—good for Vāyu, increase deeper tissues including *śhukra* (reproductive) and *ojas*, nocturnal emission, leukorrhea, infertility, neurasthenia; combines well with *aśhwagandhā* and *śhatāvarī* .
Contraindications: Very hard to digest

Macadamia
Energetics: Sweet, astringent/hot/sweet V- PK+
Actions: Nutritive

Indications: May reduce weight.
Contraindications: Oily, expensive

Pecan
Energetics: Sweet, astringent/hot/sweet V- PK+
Actions: Nutritive, aphrodisiac, laxative, nervine
Indications: Nourishing the marrow and nerves, reproductive system, laxative for elderly, increases appetite, restores energy. High in potassium, vitamin A.

Pinon
Energetics: Sweet, astringent/hot/sweet *Sattwic* best of all nuts. V- PK+ (but less than other nuts)
Actions: Nutritive, tonic, demulcent, rejuvenative
Indications: Lungs, nerves, reproductive system, debility, wasting, convalescence, good as flour.

Pistachio (*Pista* - H)
Energetics: Sweet/hot/sweet V- PK+
Actions: Tonic, sedative
Indications: Anemia, neurasthenia, builds muscles, energy, may help with alcohol recovery. They are rich in potassium, phosphorus, and magnesium salts; which when combined, help to control hypertension.

Psyllium
Energetics: Astringent/cold/pungent VPK=
Actions: Anti-inflammatory for digestive tract, laxative; may cause gas initially
Indications: Constipation, hardens loose stool
Contraindications: Taken with lots of liquids and digestive herbs.

Pumpkin Seeds (*Punyalatha, Dadhiphala*)
Energetics: Sweet/hot/pungent PK- (light quality) V+ excess
Actions: Antiparasitical
Indications: Parasites including tapeworm and roundworm; gout.
Contraindications: Reduces *śhukra*

Sesame Seeds (*Tila*)
Energetics: Sweet, bitter astringent/hot/pungent V- PK+
Actions: Nutritive, tonic, rejuvenative
Indications: Nourish all tissues, internal organs, and skin; growth of teeth, bones, and hair; debility, convalescence. Black—best for tonic, oil or butter; best used for nourishing effects; white seeds go rancid quickly. Build immunity and life sap (*ojas*); sesame seed milk relieves colitis, gastritis, heartburn, and indigestion.

Sunflower Seeds (*Arkakantha, Suria-mukhi*)
Energetics: Sweet, astringent/cold/sweet VPK=
Indications: Febrile or infectious disease, cleanse lungs and lymph.

Walnuts (*Akṣhota*)
Energetics: Sweet/hot/sweet V- PK+
Actions: Nutritive, aphrodisiac, laxative, nervine; unripe fruit and husk—antiparasitical
Indications: Marrow, calms the nerves, reproductive tissues, laxative for elderly, useful for parasites, ringworm (internal and external use), skin conditions. Leaves are used as a wash for malignant sores, and leukorrhea. High in potassium, magnesium, vitamin A, reduces serum cholesterol.

Dairy

Dairy is most beneficial when raw, from animals that are treated kindly (i.e., free roaming), and who receive no steroid injections or chemicals in their foods.
Energetics: Sweet/cool/sweet VP- K+ *Sattwic*
Tissues: Builds all seven tissues (*sapta dhātus*)—especially increase plasma, fat, reproductive
Indications: Calms the mind, nerves, and emotions. It is good for meditation and *yoga*; emaciation, debility, convalescence, wasting, bleeding, sexual debility.
Contraindications: Heavy, damp, sticky; increases mucus and *āma.* Raw and organic dairy products from healthy, happy cows are best (pasteurized and homogenized dairy products are more *tamasic*)
Preparations: Warm or room temperature, boiled

milk. Refrigerated (i.e., cold) dairy increases *āma*. Milk is better raw and organic, after being boiled for one minute, and then cooled
Combinations: Dairy does not combine well with other foods (or salt). Having milk first thing in the morning is better before other foods are eaten. It is incompatible with meat, fish, yeast bread (which ferment the dairy), sour fruit (which makes the dairy curdle), fruit, nuts, pickles, pickled vegetables, and green leafy vegetables. Yogurt does not combine well with fruit, nuts, meat, or fish. Dairy does combine well with whole grains and raw sugars
Season: Sour dairy (yogurt, kefir, buttermilk, etc.) are not to be taken as much in the summer due to their heating nature (except when taken as *lassi*). Cheese in abundance, and during the winter and spring is not suggested (which are Kapha increasing times). Cheese is also not recommended during the Kapha times of the day. *Antidotes*: Milk—ginger, cardamom, cinnamon; yogurt and cheese—mustard, cayenne, cumin

<u>Dairy Foods</u>

Butter (*Navanita*)
Energetics: Sweet/cold/pungent VP- K+
Indications: Used with Pitta-reduction herbs, nourishing, strengthening, stabilizing, used for debility and convalescence. It improves digestion, complexion, and is an aphrodisiac. For consumption, hemorrhoids, facial paralysis, bronchitis. Suggested for the young and old. It heals Vāyu and Pitta concerns, blood, pulmonary TB, eye problems, and cough.
Contraindications: Heavy, fattening, clogging, increases cholesterol, may be artificially colored, can cause constipation. With salt, it increases heaviness and clogging. Externally—burns

Buttermilk (*Lassi, Takra*)
Energetics: Sweet sour/cold/sweet V-PK+ (Homemade without salt. Store-bought has salt-better to avoid)
Actions: Astringent, digestive stimulant, diuretic
Indications: Appetite, indigestion, malabsorption, debility, emaciation, convalescence, one of the easiest foods to digest. It reduces edema, hemorrhoids, anorexia, phantom tumors, anemia, and nourishes the spleen.

Yogurt is most easily digested when taken with an equal amount of water (and digestive spices), and drunk with meals. For Kapha *doṣhas* —1/4 cup yogurt and 3/4 water.

Cheese (*Panīr* - H)
Energetics: Sweet, sour/hot/sour
Hard: V- PK+ (but still hard to digest for Vāyu)
Soft: VP- K+
Actions: Nutritive, astringent
Indications: Diarrhea, bleeding.
Contraindications: Constipation, congestion, mucus, clogs the channels, salted increases Pitta

Cottage Cheese
Energetics: Sour/hot/pungent VPK=
Indications: Not too difficult to digest.

Cream
Energetics: Sweet/cold/sweet
Actions: Rejuvenative, nutritive, aphrodisiac, calmative, laxative
Indications: Plasma, skin, nourishes all tissues (especially *śhukra dhātu*), lungs, stomach. It reduces bleeding, dry cough, dry throat, fever, thirst. Very similar to milk in its effects.
Contraindications: Heavier and richer, thus, more mucus-forming and harder to digest. Use in small quantities, and avoid combining with other rich foods

Ghee (Clarified Butter) (*Ghrita*)
Energetics: Sweet/cold/sweet VP- K+ mildly
Actions: Tonic, emollient, rejuvenative, antacid, nutritive
Indications: Fattening, increases marrow, semen, and *ojas*. Improves intelligence, vision, voice, liver, kidneys, and brain. The best form of fat for the body. The best oil for Pitta. It balances all *agnis* (digestive fires). Good for memory and digestion. It is used in conditions of insanity and

consumption. *Ghee* promotes longevity and reproductive fluid, good for children and the elderly, supple body, lungs, herpes, injury, Vāyu and Pitta disorders, fevers, TB, and is highly auspicious. Taken with herbs, it transports their nutrients and energies to all seven tissue layers. *Ghee* also reduces the desire for eating animal products. When special herbs like *aśhwagandha* are made into medicated *ghee,* they remove harmful cholesterol from the body. Other herbs are made into medicated *ghees* to enhance their healing effects.

Ice Cream (Kulfi - H)
Energetics: Sweet/cold/sweet P- VK+ *āma*+
Contraindications: Not used with TB, Kapha diseases, *āma,* fever, constipation, alcoholism, cholera. It creates *āma,* weakens the digestive fire, clogs the channels, damages the spleen, pancreas, and deranges the sugar and water metabolism. It causes hypoglycemia, diabetes, tumors. Avoid in the autumn and winter (better in the summer and spring)
<u>Ice Bean</u> is a little better, producing less congestion, but still not very healthful
<u>Frozen Yogurt</u> is also not much better. The less sugar content, the better

Cold dairy and sugar together are not very healthy for the body and mind.

Kefir
Energetics: sour/hot/sour V- PK+
Actions: Lighter than yogurt, heavier than buttermilk
Indications: Improves digestion and absorption, low appetite, relieves anorexia. Fruit-sweetened is not as good.

Milk (*Dugdha, Kṣhīra*)
Energetics: Sweet/cold/sweet VP- K+ Highly *sattwic*. It is invigorating, increasing the *dhātus*.
Actions: May be taken in larger quantities than other dairy. It is a tonic, rejuvenative, nutritive, aphrodisiac, calmative, laxative
Indications: Nourishes plasma, skin, all tissues (especially *śhukra dhātu*). It is a tonic for the lungs and stomach (reduces bleeding from these sites). Milk calms dry cough and dry throat, fever, and thirst. It is a mild laxative with *ghee*. For Pitta conditions. It is excellent for the children and the elderly, debilitation, convalescence, nourishing the brain, nerves, mind, and memory. Boiled milk builds *ojas*, promotes sleep (with warm nervine herbs). Boiled, it reduces Vāyu and Kapha. It produces semen.

Cows: Promotes longevity and rejuvenation. It helps strengthen emaciation after injury, increases intelligence, strength, and breast milk. It is a natural laxative, relieves exhaustion, dizziness, toxins, difficult breathing, cough, severe thirst and hunger; chronic fevers, urinary, and bleeding disorders. It promotes auspiciousness. Cows' milk is said to be the best of the milks.

Goats: Easily digested and heals pulmonary TB, fevers, difficult breathing, bleeding disorders and diarrhea.
Contraindications: It is damp and can weaken *agni*. It generally contains residues of inorganic fertilizers, antibiotics, steroids; and is homogenized and pasteurized; and comes from mistreated cows. Thus, inorganic milk may cause side effects. Dairy allergies may be due to these inorganic substances. However, allergies may also be caused by its heavy nature. Do not take milk at night, unless it being used as a laxative or calmative. Then boil and use the appropriate herbs and oils. May cause colds or rheumatism.
Goats Milk has a warm energy K- VP+.
Antidotes: To remove the heavy nature of milk, digestive herbs such as ginger and cinnamon are suggested. This may alleviate allergies.
AM—aphrodisiac
Noon—KP-; digestive stimulant
PM—for children, calmative, laxative
Surface milk is good for all three *doṣhas*
The foam is good for all three *doṣhas*

Sour Cream
Energetics: Sour/hot/pungent V- PK+
Actions: Stimulant, nutritive
Contraindications: In excess it may cause acidity

Yogurt (*Dadhi*)
Energetics: Sweet, sour/cold/sweet
Sweet yogurt VP- K+. Sour yogurt V- PK *āma* + Very sour yogurt causes bleeding disorders. Sweet and sour yogurt has mixed effects
Actions: Nutritive, digestive stimulant, astringent
Indications: Nourishes all tissues. In small amounts, it aids digestion of all other foods. It replenishes positive flora, decreases vaginal yeast infections and cancer; malignant tumors, boosts the immune system, promotes strength, relieves the flu, colds, anorexia, emaciation, and diarrhea (take with appropriate spices); uric acid, digestive-tract infections, cholesterol, cholera. Yogurt, like milk, is considered sacred (*sattwic*). [See buttermilk].

Yogurt adds weight and fat; and improves digestion when taken during meals. The whey reduces anorexia, weakness, emaciation, malabsorption.

Whey cleanses the *nāḍīs*, increases appetite, and reduces mental fatigue. Yogurt made by hand, mixed with pepper and cane sugar strengthens the body.
Contraindications: Heavy, in excess it causes constipation, clogs *srotas*, aggravates toxic blood (i.e., acne, skin rashes). Do not take after sunset. Yogurt or *lassi* is not to be taken with diseases involving blocked channels (*srotas*)
Antidote: Take with *ghee, āmalakī and water*

Take care of the Earth,
it was not left to us by our parents,
it was loaned to us by our children.
- Kenyan proverb

Animal Products

Meat & Fish

Energetics: Sweet/warm/sweet V- PK+ *tamasic*
Indications: Meat is the most nourishing food, excellent for debility, convalescence, lowering high Vāyu
Contraindications: Most potentially deranging food, breeds toxins or *āma*, feeds infections, fevers, tumors, dulls the mind and senses, reduces love and compassion
Long term effects: Creates bad *karma* (the higher evolved the animal, the worse the *karma*) Red meat of a cow is the most negative *karma*. Poultry yields less bad *karma*, fish even less, shellfish the least, eggs only very slightly. The *Vedic* texts (*śhastras*) state that it is acceptable to take the life of an animal in two instances: if it is your job, i.e., fisherman; and if one is weak and it is needed to preserve or save a human life. Meat is like a drug, inducing energy to get well, but it does not nourish and rebuild the subtler tissues

Non-organic animal products are full of hormones, antibiotics, chemicals. The animals are often diseased and treated badly. Thus, when these products are eaten, the chemicals are ingested and affect one's health
<u>Organs</u> (i.e., liver) are very nourishing to their respective organs, but produce low tissue quality and dull the mind
<u>Bones and bone soup</u> nourish marrow but are heavy, causing toxic blood
Preparation: Cooked properly with digestive spices, raw or not completely cooked *āma*+ and aggravates blood
<u>Salt</u> softens and tenderizes, MSG has many adverse effects
<u>Soups and stews</u> are easier to tolerate
<u>Deep fried</u> are more aggravating
<u>Canned</u> very *tamasic*

Combinations: Do not combine well with other foods, especially milk, bread, or potatoes. Milk is very toxic (mixing milk to nourish a young animal with flesh of one slaughtered)
Season: Avoid in summer due to its warm energy, morning and evening (Kapha times), better for those in high altitudes or northern latitudes
Antidotes: Raw vegetables, leafy greens, vegetable juices, bitter herbs (i.e., aloe gel) may somewhat antidote meat

Beef
Energetics: Sweet/hot/sweet V- PK+
Indications: Nutritious, builds blood and muscles, strength, endurance
Contraindications: Aggravates toxic blood, reduces compassion, dulls the mind *(tamasic)*.

Chicken/Turkey
Energetics: White—Sweet, astringent/hot/sweet PK- V+; Dark—Sweet/hot/sweet V- PK+
Actions: Dry, light
Indications: Easiest meat to digest, improves absorption, anorexia, debility, convalescence (especially as soup). *Tamasic*.

Duck
Energetics: Sweet, pungent/hot/sweet V- PK+
Actions: More nutritive
Contraindications: Harder to digest than turkey or chicken

Lamb/Mutton
Energetics: Sweet/hot/sweet VPK+
Indications: Aphrodisiac.
Contraindications: Irritant, promoting sexual activity, with garlic aggravates the blood. *Tamasic*

Pork
Energetics: Sweet/hot/sweet VPK+
Contraindications: Dullness, heaviness of mind and senses, clogs *srotas* (channels)—bacon, particularly, is difficult to digest and is heavy because of high fat concentration. It increases fat tissue more than any other meat. *Tamasic* ++

Venison
Energetics: Astringent/cold/pungent V- PK+ *Tamasic*
Actions: Nutritive, aphrodisiac
Indications: Kidneys, bones, fertility, growth, or retardation in children.

Fish
Energetics: Sweet, salty/hot/sweet V- PK+
Actions: Tonic, rejuvenative, laxative, lighter than meat, not as dulling or grounding
Indications: Builds plasma; oil nourishes liver, skin, eyes, strengthens heart, reduces cholesterol and arteriosclerosis. Shellfish are generally good for the kidneys, reproductive tissue, and impotence. They reduce Vāyu and increase Pitta and Kapha.
Contraindications: May cause diarrhea or nausea
Preparation: Fresh is important; canned or salted aggravates humors and causes *āma;* steamed or baked is best
Combination: Does not combine well with milk, sugar, meat
Antidote: Mustard, horseradish, ginger, garlic, perilla (shisho), sour sauces P+ aggravate blood, may cause diarrhea

Ocean Fish
Energetics: Salty/hot/sweet V- PK+

Fresh Water Fish
Energetics: Sweet, astringent/hot/sweet VPK= PK+ in excess; less salty, better for Pitta & Kapha
Actions: Trout easiest fish to digest

Animal Oil
Very hard to digest, P,K, *āma* cholesterol, toxic blood

Lard
Energetics: Sweet/hot/sweet K, *āma* ++
Contraindications: Clogs channels, promotes obesity, skin diseases, gallstones

Eggs
Energetics: Sweet/hot/sweet White VPK=; Yolk V- PK+ less *tamasic* than meat and fish because they are not killed. Better yet are the unfertilized eggs. Still, they are considered impure *karma*
Actions: tonic, nutritive, demulcent, aphrodisiac
Indications: Vigor, fertility, convalescence, sexual debility

Oils, Condiments, Spices

Sources: Nuts, seeds, beans, oily vegetables and animal fats like milk, butter, or animal tissue
Energetics: Sweet, bland/warm/sweet V- PK+
Actions: Internal—demulcent, laxative
Indications: Maintain fat, nerve, and marrow tissues, allowing for easy secretion and discharge.
Use: Cooking- adjunct and flavoring
massage—softens skin and muscles, dissolves toxins and congestion, absorbed into skin; thus

lubricating lungs, large intestines, nourish the deeper *dhātus*. Needed by almost everyone, debility, convalescence, *snehana* (oleation therapy-see Chapter 4—*Pañcha karma*)
Contraindications: Not used with *āma*, congestion, toxic blood; massage not done with red or oozing skin diseases; or with severe pain or palpitation—use light oil application to abdomen

Almond (Badam)
Energetics: Sweet, slightly bitter/hot/sweet V-PK+
Action: Demulcent, expectorant, tonic, the same as the nut
Indications: Cough, wasting diseases of the lungs and kidneys; soothes skin and muscles; tension, pain, good massage oil—absorbs well, reduces wrinkles and stretch marks. Builds immunity and life sap (*ojas*).

Avocado
Energetics: Sweet/cold/sweet VP- K+
Action: Same as fruit only more nutritive
Indications: Strengthens muscles and liver, nourishes skin, good massage oil, good for salads.

Canola
Energetics: VK- P+
Indications: Lowers cholesterol, may lower blood pressure.

Castor Oil (Erand)
Energetics: Sweet, bitter/hot/sweet
VP- K+in excess
Action: Purgative, antispasmodic, analgesic
Indications: One teaspoon with a cup of warm milk and 1/2 teaspoon ginger before sleep is a strong remedy for clearing *srotas* and cleansing *āma.* Constipation, used on children, epilepsy, arthritis, nerves, and pain. External—in packs-promotes healing sores, wounds, sprains, and injuries. It detoxifies, reduces abdominal tumors, swellings, and pain, menstrual cramps.

Castor is the best Vāyu-healing oil to ingest and also the best purgative oil, and has been dubbed, the "king of the oils". An Āyurvedic analogy clarifies the role of castor oil. The lion is the king of the jungle. Wherever he goes, all other animals run away. Similarly, when castor oil reaches the internal body, all Vāyu disorders run away; it is one of the major remedies for Vāyu ailments. Taken internally, it heals enlarged prostate, hernia, fevers, pain and swellings of the waist, genitals, abdomen, and back. It is a good purgative (two teaspoons with warm water before bed).

Coconut (Nariyal)
Energetics: Sweet/cold/sweet VP- K+
Action: Tonic, emollient, refrigerant
Indications: Specific for Pitta, nourishes and softens skin, inflammatory skin, psoriasis, eczema, sunburn, burns, chapped lips, dry cough with fevers, burning in lungs, increases *śhukra dhātu*, one of the easiest oils to digest.

Corn
Energetics: Sweet, astringent/hot/pungent K-VP+ mildly
Action: Demulcent, diuretic
Indications: Difficult urination, nourishes skin.

Flaxseed/Linseed
Energetics: Sweet/hot/pungent VK- P+ K+ in excess
Action: Expectorant, lubricating laxative
Indications: Cough, loosens phlegm, draws mucus from system.

Margarine
Energetics: P- V+ K+ mildly
Action: Depends upon vegetable oil used
Indications: Depends upon vegetable oil used.

Mustard (Sarson)
Energetics: Pungent/hot/pungent VK- P+
Action: Stimulant, demulcent
Indications: Excellent for Kapha and Vāyu disorders. For Kapha external/internal, anticough, loosens lung mucus, congestion, cold, joint heaviness, arthritis, abdominal pain.

Olive (Jaitoon)
Energetics: Sweet/cold/sweet VP- K+
Action: Mild laxative
Indications: Liver, softens gallstones, bile, skin, hair, lowers cholesterol, salads, massage (particularly general use or day massage since it is lighter in property). It may help control blood pressure and diabetes. Causes cellulite

Peanut (Mūngphali)
Energetics: Sweet/hot/sweet V- PK+
Action: laxative, demulcent, diuretic
Indications: Cooking oil, not as nutritious as sesame.

Safflower
Energetics: Sweet, astringent/hot/pungent V- P+ K+ mildly
Action: Laxative, emmenagogue, difficult or delayed menstruation
Indications: Lighter—better for Kapha, circulation, heart, blood, immune boosting, contains vitamin E.

Sesame (Til)
Energetics: Sweet, bitter/hot/sweet V- PK+ highly *sattwic*
Action: Tonic, rejuvenative, sedative, laxative, nutritive
Indications: The best oil. When used externally for massage it penetrates into the skin, nourishing and detoxifying the deepest tissue layers. It aggravates Pitta skin and eye conditions as it is hot in potency. It builds thin people and thins heavy persons; is constipating, kills parasites, and when properly processed, it heals all diseases. Frying makes it unhealthy.

Sesame aids all *dhātus*, lungs, kidneys, brain, debility, convalescence, rejuvenation, calms nerves, relieves muscle tension, spasms, and pain, relieves anxiety, tremors, insomnia, convulsions, dry cough, chronic constipation, voice and vision, growth of hair, nails, teeth, bones, children, elderly, most deeply penetrating oil, best for Vāyu, best for *yogic* diet, improves immune system and *ojas*; antioxidant.

Soy
Energetics: Astringent/cold/pungent PK- V+
Action: Demulcent, diuretic
Indications: Skin, high in vitamin E.

Sunflower (Sūryamukhi)
Energetics: Sweet, astringent/cold/sweet VPK=
Action: Nutritive
Indications: Skin, cough, lung heat, high in vitamin E.

Sweeteners

As discussed earlier, we need a certain amount of sweet taste to maintain tissue development. This is because the basic taste of our body is sweet. White sugars are refined, which means they have been stripped of their nutrition. Thus, as they are absorbed into the body, the body expends nutrition and energy to digest the sugars but gains no nutrition from white sugar. Absorption actually may not take place, turning the refined sweet to *āma* in the tissues. Raw sweets, (e.g., cane sugar, maple syrup, etc.) contain nutrition needed for helping the body. Sugars relieve burning, thirst, vomiting, fainting, and bleeding diseases.

Energetics: VP- K+ In excess they derange all humors. Dry sugars (i.e., cookies, dry fruit, dry pastries) derange Vāyu
Action: Tonic, demulcent, diuretic, calmative, refrigerant, laxative, antiseptic, preservative
Indications: Debility, rejuvenation, external—sores, burns, wounds, rashes, inflamed eyes, *nirāma* Pitta and *nirāma* Vāyu; when digestive system is not clogged (if there is significant coating of the tongue, i.e., *sāma,* only fresh raw honey should be used).
Combination: Generally, eaten alone—the first taste digested. Eaten after meals in large quantities, only sugar is digested (no foods), causing gas and *āma* from the undigested food. It does not combine well with salty tastes at all. With milk, *ghee* and ginger or cinnamon—nourishing
Antidote: Spicy sweet spices (i.e., cardamom,

ginger, cloves, fennel) bitters are ok but do not combine well directly (i.e., gentian, barberry, turmeric, *kuṭki,* neem)—it is better to take these herbs in capsules before or after sweets

Brown Sugar
Energetics: It is white sugar with syrup added
Indications: Slightly less deleterious effect.

Cane Sugar
Energetics: Sweet/cold/sweet VP- K+

Laxative, hard to digest, unctuous, builds the body tissues, increases Kapha and urine, an aphrodisiac. Sweet initial and post-digestive taste, cooling in energy. Modern cane sugars are found in the form of Turbinado sugar or Sucanat.

Fruit Sugar
Energetics: Sweet/cold/sweet VP- K+

They still derange sugar metabolism, weaken digestion, and promote *āma* in excess. Date sugar and grape sugar are two of the better fruit sugars. It is also believed that many fruit sugars are made from fruit from 'third world' countries who have bought the American-banned pesticides (like DDT) from the US and spray their fruit with these pesticides. So it is important to know the source of the fruit sugar as well.

Honey (best sweetener)[used raw] **(Madhu)**
Energetics: Sweet/hot/ sweet VK- P+
Action: Demulcent, emollient, expectorant, laxative, nutritive, tonic, rejuvenative; external—demulcent, astringent, antibiotic
Indications: Has some of its flower properties (i.e., sage honey will be somewhat of a nervine, expel phlegm, fat, nourish mind, nerves, senses, immune system, *ojas* (royal jelly and propolis are even better for *ojas*), external—burns, wounds, sores, eyes. It is a vehicle (*anupana*) to bring herbs to the deepest tissue layers, and make tea a tonic, expectorant, or laxative.

Heals the eyes, breaks up hard masses, relieves Kapha, poison, hiccup, and diabetes (in small doses). It further heals skin conditions, parasites, difficult breathing, cough, diarrhea, cleanses and heals wounds, and aggravates Vāyu. It becomes toxic if cooked, if used in hot weather by people with Pitta diseases, if cooked, if used in hot weather by people with Pitta diseases, or with hot foods. Warm raw honey is acceptable (i.e., in warm water); it promotes vomiting, and is good for decoction enemas.
Contraindications: Heating destroys medicinal properties, aggravates Pitta, creates subtle toxins, so it is better not to cook or bake with it. Excess use will derange humors just like white sugar does. It is also a subtle toxin when taken with equal proportions of *ghee* (better to make it 1:2 or 2:1 proportions) which breeds toxins or *āma,* feeds infections, fevers, tumors

Jaggery (Guḍa)
Energetics: Sweet/hot/sweet V- PK+ Indian raw, natural sugar containing vitamins and minerals
Action: Rejuvenative, tonic
Indications: Difficult, painful, or burning urine, anemia, debility, rejuvenation. Turbinado sugar and any whole cane sugar such as the Sucanat brand of cane sugar are similar to *jaggery*, but are cooler for Pitta *doṣhas*. Well washed and stored (old) only slightly increases Kapha, helps elimination of feces and urine.

Lactose
Energetics: Milk sugar
Action: Tonic
Indications: Empowers herbs.

Maltose/Malt Syrup
Energetics: Sweet/cold/sweet
Action: Tonic, demulcent, analgesic
Indications: Chronic colds, lungs, stomach, abdominal and intestinal spasms, colic, children, convalescence.

Maple Sugar
Energetics: Sweet/cold/sweet VP- K+
Action: One of the best natural sugars; nutritive, demulcent
Indications: Cough, fever, burning.

Molasses
Energetics: Sweet/hot/sweet V- PK+
Action: Iron, nutritive, tonic
Indications: Builds blood, muscles, heart, debility, gynecological—pregnancy, postpartum.

Rock Candy (Mishri)
Energetics: Made from sugar—it gives energy
Action: Demulcent
Indications: Cough, burning in the chest, used in *pujas* or rituals to the Deities and then eaten as *prasad* (blessed food). Better than molasses, an aphrodisiac, for emaciation and reducing Vāyu. When taken with ginger in water, it relieves Pitta, a useful summer drink.

White Sugar
Energetics: Sweet/cold/sweet VPK+
It is artificial, overcooked, toxic, *āma+*, *Tamasic*, aggravates blood, feeds infections, leaches vitamins and minerals from the body, deranges water metabolism, upsets sugar and fat metabolism; weakens liver and pancreas; hyperactivity, addictive. In moderation it can build tissues, though better to use whole sugars listed.

Condiments

Carob
Energetics: Sweet, astringent/hot/sweet VPK= *Sattwic*
Action: Nutritive, demulcent
Indications: Weakness, substitute for chocolate.

Chocolate
Energetics: Sweet, sour/hot/sweet VPK+; *rajasic* and *tamasic*
Action: Stimulant, calmative, aphrodisiac
Indications: Depression, hypotension, as herbal tea.
Contraindications: Usually prepared with white sugar so it deranges Kapha

Mayonnaise
Energetics: Sour, sweet/hot/sour V- PK+
Indications: Used on salad as a balance for Vāyu.
Contraindications: Heavy, hard to digest

Salt (*Namak/Lavaṇ*)
Energetics: Salty/hot/sweet V- PK+
Indications: A little softens food and makes more digestible, aids saliva and gastric juices, gargle, soothe and soften mucus membranes and muscles; draws out toxins, relieves muscle tension; large amounts are used in emesis to clear stomach.
Contraindications: Aggravates blood, excess deranges all humors, weakens digestion, nausea, heat, and heaviness; not good with heavy or moist foods (i.e., dairy products)

Sea Salt is better than commercial, refined salt
Black Salt is better than sea salt; P+
Rock Salt is drier, lighter and a better digestive stimulant—better for Vāyu; Tridoṣhic/best
Vegetable Salts are good, they contain many minerals

Vinegar (*Vikankar*)
Energetics: Sour/hot/sour V- PK+ (K mild)
Action: Digestive, circulatory stimulant
Indications: Aids secretion of hydrochloric acid, promotes and eases menstruation (natural forms like apple cider vinegar, are preferred to refined commercial brands. Extract alkaloids from herbs (acetic tinctures, i.e., lobelia), other sour condiments, lemon or lime juice, sour pickles, perform similarly to vinegar.

Liquids

Liquids are very important to our nutrition as we are mainly made up of plasma.

Milk: Is sweet in initial and post-digestive taste; cool in energy. VP- K+. It is invigorating, increasing the *dhātus*.

Cows: Promotes longevity and rejuvenation. It helps strengthen emaciation after injury, increases intelligence, strength and breast milk. It is a natural laxative, relieves exhaustion, dizziness, toxins, difficult breathing, cough, severe thirst and hunger; chronic fevers, urinary and bleeding disorders. It promotes auspiciousness. Cows' milk is said to be the best of the milks.

Goats: Easily digested and heals pulmonary TB, fevers, difficult breathing, bleeding disorders, and diarrhea.

Butter (fresh): Is an aphrodisiac, improves complexion, strength, digestion, absorbs water, heals Vāyu and Pitta concerns, blood, pulmonary TB, hemorrhoids, facial paralysis, eye problems, and cough.

Ghee (clarified butter): Improves intelligence, memory, digestion, longevity, reproductive fluid, eyesight; good for children and the elderly, supple body, pleasant voice, lungs, herpes, injury, Vāyu and Pitta disorders, insanity, fevers, TB, and is highly auspicious.

Yogurt: (made by hand and mixed with pepper and sugar) strengthens the body. [Mixed with water it makes *Lassi,* which promotes digestion when consumed during the meal. One-half water for Vāyu and Pitta; 3/4 water for Kapha.]
Yogurt or *lassi* is not to be taken with diseases involving blocked channels (*srotas*). [See the dairy section for further details—page 146]

Alcohol
Energetics: Pungent, sweet, bitter, sour/hot/sour V- PK+ *rajasic*
Action: Beer—diuretic
Indications: Small amounts of wine aid digestion and circulation (particularly medicated Āyurvedic wines, like *Drakṣha*), relax nerves, promote menstruation; extracting herb properties (especially spicy or bitters).

Beer causes kidney stones. Wine is the best form of light consumption. Hard liquor is very disruptive. Sweet liqueurs are deranging due to the combination of sugar and alcohol.
Contraindications: Excess aggravates all humors, aggravates blood, deranges liver, pancreas, kidneys, addiction, not for *yoga* or meditation; beer—long term—causes edema and overweight

Coffee
Energetics: Pungent, bitter/warm/pungent K- VP+ *Rajasic*
Action: Nervine, cardiac stimulant
Indications: Occasional use for energy, hypotension, depression.
Contraindications: Mild narcotic, addictive

Fruit Juices
Energetics: *Āma+*
Action: Laxative
Indications: Sour or astringent are better (cranberry, lemon, lime, pineapple, pomegranate, Sour V-; astringent PK-).
Contraindications: Weaken digestive fire, not taken with or directly after meals or first thing in the morning

Herbal Teas
Energetics: spicy and astringent
Spicy- ginger, cinnamon, cloves, cardamom, orange peel, mint, chamomile, etc.—stimulate digestion VK-
Astringent—alfalfa, dandelion, chicory, strawberry leaf, hibiscus, etc.—antacid, alterative PK-

Milk & Dairy
Energetics: See Dairy section **(p. 135)**
Milk VP- (with sugar or honey)
Buttermilk V-

Mineral Water
Energetics: Carbonated PK- V+
Action: Oxygenates blood and cells
Indications: Circulation, some mineral supplementing

Soda
Contraindications: Both commercial (Coke, Pepsi etc.) and natural are sweet and usually taken cold. They do not combine well with other foods, weakens *agni*, weaken spleen and pancreas, derange sugar and water metabolism
Indications: Better in hot weather or when very thirsty.

Tea
Energetics: Bitter, sweet, astringent/cool/pun-

gent PK- V+ some feel it is *sattwic*
Contraindications: Refined teas may be artificial and damaging, excess causes insomnia, dry mouth and thirst, overly brewed causes constipation
Indications: Taken with milk and spices like ginger and cinnamon (Indian *Chai*) it is less aggravating to Vāyu. Best taken after meals, as astringent tastes are digested last. Counters hyperacidity, summer drink, counters heat, damp, and sun exposure; migraine headaches, overly brewed causes constipation (so it is good for treating diarrhea).

Vegetable Juice
Energetics: See the vegetable section
Sour (i.e., tomato) P+, blood aggravation
Salty V- (as soup is best)
Green (celery, parsley, comfrey leaf) detox, PK- V+
Carrot- cleansing, strengthening (too sweet, may weaken digestion)
Wheat Grass- highly cleansing, good for *āma*, PK-, cleans blood, counters infection and tumors, V+ unless used with sours—lime, lemon, orange

Water
Energetics: Fresh spring or well is best. Tap water is chlorinated and devitalized; causes disease and *āma* aggravation.

Vāyu—warm or hot, better with milk or spiced due to its lightness

Pitta—taken a little cool or at room temperature

Kapha—warm or hot, not in excess

Cold—astringent—stops bleeding, relieve burning sensation
Warm—stimulant, laxative, promotes sweating, relieves cold sensation
Distilled—devitalized, depletes *prāṇa*, V++, drains toxins from system
Excess—(especially distilled) leaches nutrients and dilutes plasma
Spring—water is preferred over distilled water.

Āyurveda suggests that liquids are best taken in a form other than plain water as water leeches the body of its minerals and nutrients. For example, herbal teas are preferred over plain water.

Vāyu—drink between Pitta and Kapha, sweet, sour, fruit, vegetable juices, and herb teas
Pitta—more, sweet, bitter, astringent fruit or vegetable juices, herb teas
Kapha—drink less, bitter, astringent, diuretic, pungent herbal teas

Meals—1/2 to 1 cup with meals is ok (*lassi* is recommended) to wash and clear taste buds- more than this dilutes digestive juices

Season—General—drink 3 to 5 cups warm (as tea) [summer—more; winter—less]

Water is the great healer described in the *Atharva Veda*. It should be obtained from clean sources: wells, rivers, etc. Āyurveda says that our bodies are mostly made up of plasma. Drinking too much plain water will deplete the minerals and nutrients. Autumn and summer are the two seasons that are best for healthy people to drink plain water (and drink less plain water in the other seasons). Therefore, drinking teas, and fruit and vegetable juice is advised. Some water is acceptable to drink at the beginning, the middle and end of the meal. Drinking water at the end of the meal will have no adverse effects on the person

Precautions: Do not drink water with a low digestive fire, abdominal tumors, or enlarged abdomen; anemia, diarrhea, hemorrhoids, duodenum diseases, pulmonary TB, or edema. Do not drink water at the beginning of the meal (causes stoutness), or at the end of the meal (causes emaciation)

Cold water: Relieves alcoholic intoxication, exhaustion, fainting, vomiting, debility, giddiness, thirst, sun heat causing burning sensations, Pitta excesses, blood problems, and poisoning.

Hot or warm water: Stimulates hunger, helps digestion and the throat, easily digested, cleanses the urinary bladder, relieves hiccup, gas, Vāyu and Kapha imbalances.

Boiled water: Does not overly increase the body's inner moisture content. It is good for Pitta *doṣha*. Do not drink boiled water kept overnight;

it becomes stale and aggravates all three *doṣhas*.

Coconut water: Relieves Vāyu and Pitta *doṣha* concerns.

Benefits of Drinking Water

Boiled Water: Tridoṣhic. It is light, a digestive stimulant; dispels gas, heals pain in the rib area; rhinitis, and hiccup. Boiled and reduced to 3/4—relieves Vāyu; reduced to 1/2—balances Pitta. It is is useful in early and late winter, spring, and rainy season. When water is boiled and reduced to 1/4 it relieves Kapha (but it is also constipative). It is helpful in the summer and fall. When water is cooled after boiling it heals all *doṣhas*, and is wholesome. Boiled water is not to be kept overnight; it becomes stale and impure.

Hot Water: VK- Light. It stimulates digestive power, heals pains in the rib area; rhinitis, gas, hiccup, and cleanses the urinary tract. Taken before bed, it cleanses Kapha sticking to the inner body; eliminates Vāyu, and removes indigestion.

Warm Water: This is not advised for exhaustion, mental fatigue, convulsions, hunger, and bleeding in the upper body areas.

Water Digestion: Unboiled water takes three hours to digest. Water that is boiled and allowed to cool down is digested in 1 1/2 hours. Water that is boiled and drunk when warm is digested in 48 minutes.

Less Water Quantity: For certain diseases, it is advised to drink less water: anorexia, coryza, salivation, edema, consumption, poor digestion, obstinate abdominal diseases, fever, eye diseases, ulcers, and diabetes mellitus.

Spices & Herb Therapy

Spices

Energetics: Pungent/warm/pungent VK- P+
Actions: Light, dry, warm, fragrant, subtle, clear, stimulant, carminative, antispasmodic, diaphoretic, expectorant
Indications: Spices regulate appetite and strengthen the *agni* fire, lungs, head, gastrointestinal, cleanse *srotas*, burn up *āma,* aid mental activity.
Antidote: Counters heaviness, dispels gas, eases digestion
Commercial spices: Most supermarket spices have been irradiated, destroying their *prāṇa* and adding the negative effects of radiation to the spices
Powders: Once powdered, energies begin to diminish after 6 months, although they have been found useful up to two years later
Combinations: Adding them to heated *ghee* or oils empowers spices, as does a bit of honey or raw sugar

Individual Spices

Anise (Sweet Fennel) (*Shatapuṣhpa*)
Energetics: Pungent/hot/pungent VK- P+
Actions: Stimulant, carminative, lactagogue
Indications: Similar to fennel but is more pungent and warm, abdominal pain, gas, indigestion, menstrual cramping, vomiting, dry cough.

Asafoetida (*Hiṅg*)
Energetics: Pungent/hot/pungent VK- P+ *tamasic*
Actions: Stimulant, carminative, antispasmodic, anthelmintic
Indications: Some consider it the best Vāyu spice, best for relieving abdominal distention, pain, cramping and gas, parasites, worms, candida, delayed or difficult menstruation, pain, anxiety, mental disorders—i.e., nervousness, vertigo, anxiety, hysteria, worry, depression, lethargy, cough, asthma, arthritis, headaches, nerve pain, paralysis, circulation; strengthens heart; palpitations, angina, exorcism.
Contraindications: Not for meditation or *yoga*; (*tamasic*), aggravates bile or acid conditions
Antidote: For beans

Basil/Holy Basil (*tulsī*) (see Chapter 4 materia medica)

Bay Leaves
Energetics: Pungent, bitter/hot/pungent VK- P+ mildly

Actions: Stimulant, carminative, analgesic
Indications: Cleansing, headaches, clear *srotas*, cough and congestion, diarrhea, hemorrhoids. Useful as an insect repellent in the kitchen.
Antidote: Dairy, meat, damp sticky food

Black Pepper (*Maricha*)
Energetics: Pungent/hot/pungent VK- P+ *rajasic*
Actions: Stimulant, carminative, decongestant, expectorant
Indications: Burns up *āma* very well, colds, flu, cough, gargle for sore throat, fevers, colon cleanse, digests fat and obesity; metabolism, mucus, expectorant, sinus congestion, cold extremities, raises *agni*, epileptic seizures, with honey, clears Kapha from the system in the morning. External—inflammations, urticaria, erysipelas.

Caraway/Cumin (*Jīraka*)
Energetics: Caraway—Sour, pungent/hot/sweet K- VP+ Cumin—Pungent/hot/pungent VK- P=
Actions: Stimulant, carminative, lactagogue, diuretic (used like fennel and coriander)
Indications: Digests bread, like fennel and dill relatives; colitis, gas, digestion, abdominal pain, distention.
Antidote: Overeating, heavy foods

Cardamom (*Elā*) see Chapter 4 materia medica
Antidote: Ice cream, milk, cold or sweet foods like bananas, coffee

Cayenne (*Marichaphalam*)
Energetics: Pungent/hot/pungent VK- P+ hottest; most *yang*; *rajasic*
Actions: Stimulant, expectorant, diaphoretic, hemostatic, anthelmintic
Indications: A heart strengthener, circulation, gives energy after shock, heart attack or collapse; stops acute bleeding; absorption, chill, abdominal distention, worms, colds, flu, sinus congestion, cleanses colon, helps digest fats, burns *āma*.
Antidote: For raw food

Chamomile (*Babunike-phul* - H)
Energetics: Pungent, bitter/cold/pungent PK- V+ in excess; *sattwic*
Actions: Stimulant, antispasmodic, emmenagogue, emetic, diaphoretic, carminative, analgesic, nervine, calmative
Indications: Pain, headaches; abdominal, children—nerves and digestion; colic, bile, blood, menstrual, ear, neuralgia, and injury pains; external use also; calms nervousness, anxiety, hysteria, insomnia, neurasthenia; poor digestion related to emaciation and nervousness.

Cinnamon (*Thwak*)
Energetics: Pungent, sweet/hot/pungent VK- P-+; *sattwic*
Actions: Stimulant, diaphoretic, diuretic, expectorant, carminative, alterative, astringent, analgesic
Indications: Circulation, cold extremities, heart muscle and palpitations; toothache, facial nerve pain, arthritis in joints, lower backache, menstruation, fertility, post-partum, colds, sinus congestion, bronchitis, dyspepsia, indigestion.
Contraindications: Aggravates bleeding disorders, not used during pregnancy
Antidote: Sugar and fruit (good with apples and pears)

Cloves (*Lavangaha*)
Energetics: Pungent/hot/pungent; *rajasic*
Actions: Stimulant, expectorant, decongestant, anthelmintic, analgesic, aphrodisiac
Indications: Gas, nausea, vomiting, toothache, hiccup, laryngitis, pharyngitis, headache, clears head, sinus and lungs, nerves, toothache, colds, cough, asthma, warms and disinfects the lymphatics, low blood pressure, impotence, indigestion, opens and clears *srotas*.
Precaution: Promotes sexual activity
Antidote: Sugars

Coriander (*Dhyānaka*) (see Chapter 4 materia medica)
Antidote: Hot foods and spices (i.e., as cilantro - coriander leaf)

Cumin (see caraway)

Dill (*Misroya*)
Energetics: Sweet, astringent/hot/sweet VPK= leaves cooler, seeds warmer
Actions: Stimulant, antispasmodic, lactagogue
Indications: Colic, cramps, and diarrhea for children; similar to fennel.

Fennel (*Methica*)
Energetics: Sweet/cold/sweet VPK= perhaps the most *sattwic* spice
Actions: Stimulant, diuretic, carminative, stomachic, antispasmodic, lactagogue
Indications: Abdominal pain (gas or indigestion), menstrual cramps, hernia, diarrhea, colic, vomiting, morning sickness, nausea, anorexia, cough, dry cough, promotes semen, increases vision, raises *agni*, difficult or burning urination, digestion—children and elderly; promotes menstruation, nursing mothers—increases breast milk flow.

Fenugreek (*Medhika*)
Energetics: Pnngent, bitter/hot/pungent VK- P+
Actions: Demulcent, diuretic, tonic, rejuvenative, aphrodisiac, stimulant, antirheumatic
Indications: Longevity, nerves, allergies, arthritis, skin, rejuvenation, diabetes, allergies, bronchitis, flu, chronic cough, dysentery, dyspepsia, convalescence, edema, toothache, sciatica, neurasthenia, counters cold (i.e., extremities, abdominal pain, indigestion, respiratory and reproductive systems, hair growth, promotes breast milk flow, liver hypo-function, seminal debility, debility, outdoor winter work). Do not use when pregnant.

Garlic see Chapter 4 materia medica

Ginger see Chapter 4 materia medica

Horseradish (*Sobhanjana, Sirgu*)
Energetics: Pungent, astringent/hot/pungent VK- P+ like mustard
Actions: Stimulant, expectorant, diuretic, antispasmodic, antilithic (dissolves stones)
Indications: Cleanses lungs, sinuses, colds, flu, sore throat, hoarseness, digestion, circulation, rheumatism. External poultice for facial neuralgia, inflammatory swellings).
Antidotes: Fish and raw vegetables

Marjoram (*Sathra* - H)
Energetics: Pungent, astringent/hot/pungent VK- P+
Actions: Stimulant, diaphoretic, expectorant
Indications: Colds, flu, weak digestion, promotes menstruation.

Mustard (*Rajika*- Brown; *Sarṣhapah* - Black)
Energetics: Bitter (brown) Pungent/hot/pungent VK- P+; best Kapha spice
Actions: Stimulant, analgesic, expectorant
Indications: Laxative, 1 teaspoon ingested as an emetic for drunkenness, poisons. Clears head and sinuses, chronic colds and coughs. Hot mustard bath—as an emmenagogue. Ten-minute external paste—chest troubles, blisters, inflammatory nerve disorders, pain and swelling of the joints, edema, headache, abdominal colic and pain, obstinate vomiting; gout, sciatica, urticaria, arthritis.

Nutmeg (Malathi-phalam; Jati-phalam)
Energetics: Sweet, pungent, astringent/hot/pungent VKP= best sedative of all spices; *tamasic*
Actions: Stimulant, carminative, astringent; use for abdominal pain, dysmenorrhea, insomnia, poor absorption (especially in the small intestine), abdominal distention, incontinence, diarrhea, dysentery, impotence, mental disorders (i.e., nervousness, anxiety, hysteria—prepared in milk decoction)

Oregano
Energetics: Sour, astringent/hot/pungent VK- P+
Actions: Stimulant, diaphoretic, carminative, analgesic, antiseptic
Indications: Colds, cough, nausea, morning sickness, dysmenorrhea, gas, distention, indigestion.

Peppermint (*Paparaminta* - H)
Energetics: Sweet/cold/pungent VPK=
Actions: Stimulant, diaphoretic, carminative, analgesic
Indications: Colds and flu, fevers, and sore throat; clears head, sinuses, allergic headaches, and hay fever; opens mind and senses; promotes emotional harmony.

Poppy Seeds (*Kasa bijam*)
Energetics: Sweet, astringent/hot/ pungent VK- P+
Actions: Stimulant, antispasmodic, astringent
Indications: Diarrhea, malabsorption, cramping pain, cough, aids digestion.

Rosemary
Energetics: Pungent, bitter/hot/pungent VK- P+ mildly
Actions: Stimulant, diaphoretic, excellent emmenagogue
Indications: Eases menstruation, headaches, harmonizes and strengthens heart and emotions.

Saffron see Chapter 4 materia medica

Sage (*Salbia-sefakuss* - H)
Energetics: Pungent, astringent/hot/pungent VK- P+ in excess
Actions: Stimulant, diuretic, nervine, astringent
Indications: Opens the lungs, head, sinuses; sore throat; clears *srotas*, voice, perception, thought; relieves excessive sexual desire, calms heart, digests meat and dairy, reduces excess secretions in body (i.e., stops the flow of milk in nursing women, swollen lymph glands, dries excess mucus in lungs and nose, dries sores, ulcers, and bleeding; and night sweats), is a diuretic for urinary tract problems, calms the brain.

Spearmint (*Pahadi pudina* - H)
Energetics: Sweet/cold/pungent VPK=
Actions: Stimulant, diaphoretic, diuretic, calmative
Indications: Painful, difficult or burning urine (cold), colic, indigestion, and sleep in children, nausea, vomiting, morning sickness.

Thyme (*Ipar* - H)
Energetics: Pungent/hot/pungent VK- P+
Actions: Stimulant, diaphoretic, anticough, anthelmintic, antiseptic
Indications: Severe cough, whooping cough, bad breath, indigestion, gas, menstrual disorders.

Turmeric see Chapter 4 materia medica

Vitamins

Under normal conditions, Āyurveda suggests persons receive their vitamins through herbs and foods because they are easier to digest and absorb in these simple or elemental forms. Each *doṣha* requires a few vitamins that may naturally become depleted more rapidly than the rest. If vitamin pills or liquids are taken, it is suggested coriander or cardamom be taken with them to help digest and absorb the vitamins and minerals. Pitta *doṣhas* have the strongest digestive system, and can better utilize supplements without weakening their digestive fire. Kapha *doṣhas* need the least amount of supplements, and more hot spices to raise their digestive fire. Further, oily vitamins (e.g., E, D, A) are not advised due to their tendency to dampen digestion.

Doṣha	Vitamins	Minerals
Vāyu	A, B3, D, E, C	zinc, calcium
Pitta	A, B, K	calcium, iron
Kapha	B6, D	none needed

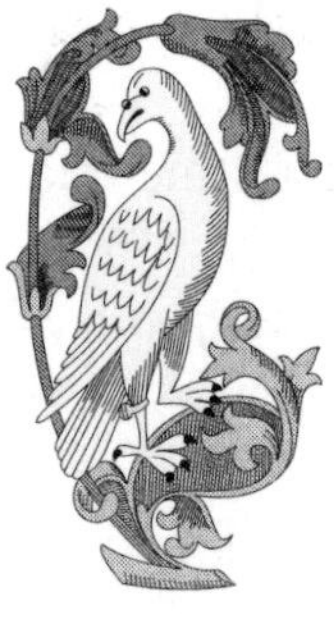

Vitamins	Symptoms of Vitamin Deficiency
A	dry, rough, scaly, itchy skin; wrinkles, pimples, premature aging, dandruff, split nails, night blindness, burning, itching eyes; thickening cornea
B1*	poor memory and digestion, fatigue, edema, ear problems, irritability, heart failure
B2*	itching, burning, bloodshot eyes; light sensitivity, hair loss liver disorders
B3*	poor memory, circulation and metabolism; fatigue, cholesterol
B5*	infections, poor digestion, nerve and heart disorders, hay fever, hair loss
B6*	poor digestion, hormone imbalance, eczema, anemia, water retention, PMS, dandruff
B9*	anemia, G.I. disorders, hair loss
B12	premature aging, fatigue, insomnia, poor memory/concentration; central nervous system disorders
C	bleeding gums, heavy metal poisoning, adrenal weakness, cellulite
D	weak teeth, nails, bones, hair
E	muscle/nerve weakness, weak adrenals, dry skin
F	heart disorders, cholesterol, female disorders, skin disorders, yeast infections, hypertension, cystic fibrosis, liver disorders, malformed tissues, intestinal disorders
K	low energy, premature aging, bleeding

**B1- Thiamine, B2- Riboflavin, B3- Niacin, B5- Pathothenic Acid, B6- Pyroxidine, B9- Folic Acid*

Vitamins	Food Sources
A	dark green or yellow vegetables, corn, soy, lentils, garbanzo beans, whole milk
B1	rice bran, whole grains, molasses, green vegetables, beans, soy flour, nuts
B2	millet, corn, soy, whole wheat, rye, wheat, germ, beans, milk, avocado, nuts, molasses, dark greens
B3	wheat, buckwheat, barley, wild rice, black beans, sesame seeds, nuts, dark greens, milk
B5	whole grains, corn, beans, broccoli, cabbage, cauliflower
B6	brown rice, buckwheat, beans, carrots
B9	whole grains, salad, green vegetables, wheat germ, bran, sprouted grains, soy products, yogurt
B12	asparagus, alfalfa sprouts, cabbage family, potatoes, mustard greens, peas, okra, green peppers, *mūng* beans, tomatoes, berries, citrus fruits, melons, mangoes, papayas, pineapple, dairy, *āmalakī*
C	whole grains, milk
D	sunlight, flax oil, whole grains, dark greens, butter
E	wheat germ, whole grains, dark greens, nuts, seeds, butter, milk, molasses
F	vegetable oils, linseed oil, olive oil, flaxseed oil, soy oil, safflower oil, seeds
K	yogurt, eggs, molasses, milk

Minerals	Symptoms of Mineral Deficiency
Biotin	anemia, depression, poor metabolism, balding, adrenal/testosterone disorders, dermatitis, balding
Choline	fat, low immunity, weak nerves, premature graying
Inositol	eczema, hair loss, cholesterol, constipation
PABA	nervousness, fatigue, indigestion, premature graying, vitiligo
Bioflavonoids	varicose veins, bleeding gums, eczema
Calcium	weak hair, teeth, nails; PMS, insomnia, white nail spots, leg cramps
Chromium	arteriosclerosis, hypoglycemia, memory loss, fatigue, slowed growth, muscle growth
Chloride	pernicious vomiting
Copper	loss of hair color, poor skin tone
Iodine	thyroid disorders, dry skin, cold
Iron	anemia, low vitality, brittle hair, weak nails, frequent infections, itchy skin, short breath
Magnesium	low vitality, tense muscles, psoriasis
Manganese	diabetes, brain weakness, knee problems
Molybdenum	decreased growth, food consumption
Phosphorus	bone loss, muscle weakness, fatigue
Potassium	depression, arrhythmia, indigestion, dry skin
Selenium	premature aging, dandruff, skin elasticity loss
Silica	flabbiness, weak nails
Sodium	anorexia, weak muscles, nausea
Sulfur	eczema, weak nails, scaly skin
Zinc	white nail spots, night blindness, colds/infections, hair loss, loss of taste and smell

Minerals in Foods	
Minerals	**Foods**
Biotin	whole grains, nuts, legumes, cauliflower
Choline	lecithin (in whole grains, nuts, soybeans)
Inositol	molasses, brown rice, barley, oats, legumes, seeds
PABA	brown rice, wheat germ, molasses
Bioflavonoids	the same herbs as vitamin C
Calcium	sea or dark greens, seeds, milk, nuts, dried fruit, yogurt, carob, asparagus, broccoli, tofu, oats
Chromium	whole grains, corn oil, potatoes
Chloride	salt
Copper	kelp, legumes, grains, avocados, raisins, oats, nuts
Iodine	kelp, beans, carrots, tomatoes, pineapple
Iron	leafy greens, parsley, dulse, whole grains, potatoes, fruit, raisins, seeds, nuts, milk
Magnesium	whole grains, yellow corn, soy, nuts, lentils, dried fruits, sea and leafy greens, apples, celery, citrus, dairy, oats, cornmeal, rice, apricots
Manganese	whole grains, green and sea vegetables, nuts, seeds, avocados, blueberries
Molybdenum	legumes, whole grains, leafy greens
Phosphorus	whole grains, beans, nuts, dairy, all vegetables, sesame seeds, sunflower/pumpkin seeds
Potassium	bananas, watercress, all vegetables, dried fruit, oranges, grains, sunflower seeds, dairy, legumes
Selenium	whole grains, beans, tomatoes, broccoli
Silica	horsetail (herb)
Sodium	salt
Sulfur	nuts, cabbage family, apples, cranberries, beans
Zinc	pumpkin/sunflower seeds, grains, soy, vegetables

Menus

Below are sample menus for various health concerns, as well as daily meals for various *doṣhas*.

Vāyu Doṣha

Vāyu (eat every 3-4 hours)

	Spring/ Summer	Fall/Winter
Waking (1/2 hr. before meal)	herb tea (cardamom, (*aśhwagandhā, triphalā*)	hot milk with *ghee*, fresh ginger, turmeric, honey, *chyavan prāśh*
Break-fast	Cream of Rice with *ghee*, cardamom, and honey	Oatmeal or Cream of Wheat with *ghee*, cardamom, and honey
Snack	cane sugar sweet with coriander	almond butter on *chapatis* with cardamom and *ghee*; herb tea
Lunch	white *basmati* rice, split yellow *mūng dal*, *ghee*, sweet potato, *lassi*	same; add whole wheat *chapatis*
Snack	sesame seeds; fennel	baked apple with cinnamon and honey; herb tea
Dinner	artichoke pasta, *ghee*, squash, *lassi*, cardamom	whole wheat pasta, *ghee*, sweet potato, *lassi*, cardamom
Snack	carob brownie	pumpkin pie, herb tea
Bedtime	hot tea, *ghee*, honey, ginger	hot milk, *ghee*, fresh ginger, honey

Vāyu Arthritis

Serves: 4-5 people
Preparation: 30 minutes
*V, P-; K +**

1/2 cup white *basmati rice*
1/2 cup split yellow *mūngdal*
3 medium zucchinis
1 tsp. *balā*
1 tsp. turmeric
5 tsp. *ghee*
1 tsp. cardamom
1 tsp. *tulsī*
1 tsp. *guggul*
2 cups water

Wash the rice and *dal* in water and place in a pot with 2 cups of water; heat until it boils. Reduce the flame to a slow boil and cook for 10 minutes (add more water if needed).

Add a little water in another pot and place a steamer inside. Slice the zucchini, putting the slices in the steamer and boil for 2 to 3 minutes.

When the food is ready, put the *ghee* in a frying pan and turn the heat to high. Put a drop of water in the pan. When it sizzles, lower the flame and add the rest of the spices and stir until the aroma of the herbs is released. Add the rice and *dal* to the mixture in the frying pan and stir.

[For a Pitta- or Kapha-reducing meal, replace zucchini with celery. Add 1/4 tsp. neem to the herbal ingredients]

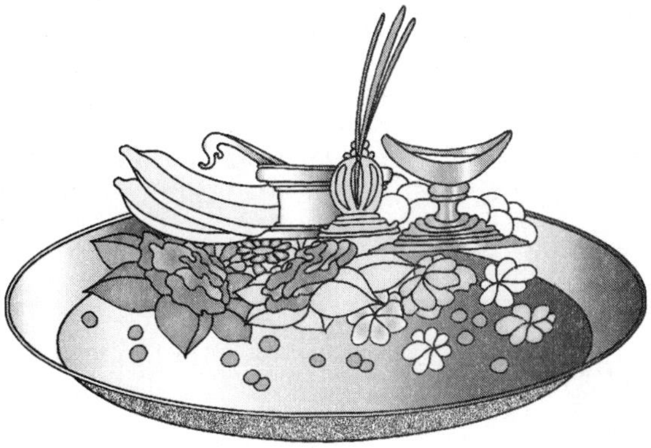

Pitta Doṣha

	Spring/Summer	Winter/Fall
Waking	herb tea (*śhatāvarī,* turmeric, fennel) with *ghee,* cane sugar	hot milk with *ghee*, turmeric, *chyavan prāśh*
Break-fast	puffed rice or wheat with *ghee,* coriander, coconut milk	Cream of Wheat or barley with *ghee,* coriander, soy milk
Snack	sweet or bitter fruit	apple or pear
Lunch	white *basmati* rice, split yellow *mūng dal, ghee,* broccoli, coriander, *lassi,* salad	same; add whole wheat *chapatis*
Snack	sunflower seeds; fennel; lemongrass tea	milk *burfi;* mint tea
Dinner	artichoke pasta, *ghee,* cauliflower, cilantro, *lassi*	barley/garbanzo soup, *ghee,* cabbage, *lassi,* cardamom
Snack	coconut macaroon	pumpkin pie, herb tea

Liver, Spleen, Gall Bladder Disorders

Serves: 4-5 people
Preparation: 30 minutes
V +, P, K -

1/2 cup *basmati* rice	1/2 cup lima beans
2 cups fresh corn	2 cups green beans
2 1/2 cups *mūng* bean sprouts	
1 tsp. turmeric	1 bunch cilantro
1 tsp. *mañjiṣhṭhā*	1 tsp. *gokṣhura*
2 cups water	1 tsp. *bhūmīāmalakī*
5 tsp. *ghee*	1 bunch dandelion root

Wash the rice and lima beans in water and place in a pot with 2 cups of water; heat until it boils. Reduce the flame to a slow boil and cook for 10 minutes (add more water if needed).

Put a little water in another pot and place a steamer inside. Place the corn and green beans in the steamer and boil for 2 to 3 minutes.

When the food is ready, put the *ghee* in a frying pan and turn the heat to high. Put a drop of water in the pan. When it sizzles, lower the flame and add the spices, stiring until the aroma of the herbs is released. Add the rice and *dal* to the mixture in the frying pan and stir for 15 to 30 seconds. Add a *mūng* bean sprout salad to the meal.

[Excellent for recovering from alcohol addictions]

Heart Disorders

Serves: 4-5 people
Preparation: 30 minutes
V +, P, K -

1/2 cup whole wheat	1/2 cup aduki beans*
11/2 eggplants	1 bunch cilantro
1/4 tsp. turmeric	1/4 tsp. *arjuna*
1/4 tsp. *guggul*	5 tsp. *ghee*
3 cups water	
tomato/cucumber/lettuce salad	

Soak aduki beans and wheat overnight. Wash and peel eggplant and cut into slices. Pour salt on both sides of the eggplant and let it sit on a paper towel for about 1/2 hour. This draws out the alkaloid properties (which may cause allergies). Then cut the eggplant into pieces.

Wash the wheat and lima beans in water and place in a pot with 2 cups of water, heat until it boils. Reduce the flame to a slow boil and cook for 10 to 20 minutes (until soft). Add more water to the pot if needed.

Add a little water in another pot and place a steamer inside. Place the eggplant slices in the steamer and boil for 2 to 3 minutes.

When the food is ready, put the *ghee* in a frying pan and turn the heat to high. Put a drop of water in the pan. When it sizzles, reduce the flame to low and add the spices, stiring until the aroma of the herbs is released. Add the wheat or beans to the mixture in the frying pan and stir for 15 to 30 seconds. Add cilantro on top of the meal, and a lettuce, tomato, cucumber salad on the side.

[For Vāyu heart disease, replace aduki beans with mūng beans]

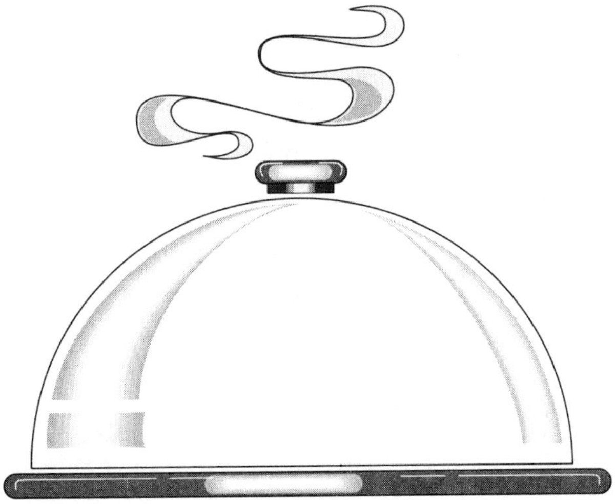

Kapha Doṣha

	Summer/ Spring	Winter/Fall
Break-fast	ginger/licorice tea	*chyavan praṣh*, coffee with goats milk
Snack	cranberries	stewed apricots
Lunch	barley, split yellow *mūngdal, ghee,* celery, coriander, *lassi*	buckwheat *chapatis*, lima beans, brussels sprouts, *ghee,* pepper, mint tea
Snack	raspberries; lemongrass tea	pumpkin seeds, saffron tea with honey
Dinner	artichoke pasta, *ghee,* burdock, cardamom, *lassi*	rye soup, garbanzo beans, beets, cardamom, cinnamon tea
Snack	cranberries	macintosh apple, chamomile tea

Kapha Diabetes

Serves: 4 people

Preparation: 30 minutes

V, K -, P + (moderately)

1/2 cup barley	1/2 cup *mūngdal*
1/2 eggplant	1 bitter gourd (*kerala*)
1 tsp. *guggul*	1 tsp. turmeric
1 tsp. cardamom	1 tsp. mustard seeds
2 cups water	mango *chutney*

3 tsp. *ghee*, mustard or canola oil
1 tsp. *guḍmar* (if there is pancreatic damage)

Wash and peel eggplant and cut into slices. Pour salt on both sides of the eggplant and let it sit on a paper towel for about 1/2 hour. This draws out the alkaloid properties (which may cause allergies). Wash the bitter gourd and cut the gourd and eggplant into pieces.

Wash the barley and *dal* in water. Place the

Food	Antidotes For Indigestion	Food	Antidotes For Indigestion
Alcohol	chew cardamom or cumin seeds	Lassi	black pepper, cumin, salt
Almonds	soak in water overnight and peel the skin. Take with cane sugar.	Legumes	black pepper; cumin; salt
Apples	cinnamon	Marijuana	calamus, milk, ghee
Avocado	turmeric, lemon, black pepper	Meat (red)	cayenne; cloves, chili peppers
Bananas	dry ginger; raw honey and cardamom	Milk	cane sugar
Butter	raw honey; cane sugar	*Mūng* Beans	lemon
Cabbage	cook in sunflower oil, turmeric, and mustard seeds	Nuts	soak overnight
Caffeine	nutmeg and cardamom	Oats	turmeric; mustard seeds; cumin
Cauliflower	ginger	Oil	lemon
Cheese	black pepper; chili pepper; cayenne	Onions	well cooked
Chick peas	*ajwan* seeds	Popcorn	*ghee*
Chocolate	cardamom; cumin	Potatoes	warm water with *ajwan* seeds
Cucumber	*ajwan* seeds; salt	Radish	salt
Eggs	parsley, cilantro, turmeric, onions	Red Pepper	*ghee*
Fish	coconut, lime, and lemon	Rice	salt or black pepper
Garlic	olive oil with lemon juice	Sugar	lemon
Ghee	grated coconut and lemon	Tobacco	*Brāhmī, vachā* root, *ajwan* seeds
Green Beans	*ajwan* seeds; salt	Tomato	lime; *cumin*
Green Salad	olive oil with lemon juice	Vinegar	sweets
Honeydew	grated coconut with coriander; lemon; honey	Wheat	ginger
Ice Cream	cardamom; cloves	Yogurt	cumin; ginger
Kidney Beans	cumin; rock salt		

barley and *mūngdal* in a pot with 2 cups of water and heat until it boils. Reduce the flame to a slow boil and cook for 10 minutes (add more water if needed).

Add a little water in another pot, place a steamer in the pot and put the eggplant and *kerala* in the steamer and boil for 2 to 3 minutes.

When the food is ready, add the *ghee* or oil and three mustard seeds in a frying pan. Turn the heat to high until the seeds pop. Then reduce the flame to low add the rest of the spices, and stir until the aroma of the herbs is released. Add the barley and *dal* into the frying pan and stir for 15 to 30 seconds. Serve sweet mango *chutney* with the meal (about 3 teaspoons per person). This is readily available at Indian grocery stores.

Overweight

Serves: 4-5 people
Preparation: 30 minutes
V, K -, P + (moderately)

1/2 cup barley	1/2 cup garbanzo beans
2 1/2 cups peas	3 carrots
1 tsp. *guggul*	1 tsp. turmeric
1 tsp. cardamom	1 tsp. mustard seeds
1 tsp. *triphalā*	1 tsp. *musta*
3 cups water	3 tsp. mustard or canola oil

Soak the barley and garbanzo beans overnight in water. Wash the peas and carrots. Scrape off the carrot skins and slice into pieces. In separate pots, place the barley and the garbanzo beans. Add 1 1/2 cups of water to each pot and bring to a boil. Lower the flame to a slow boil and cook for 10 minutes or until soft. Then steam the vegetables for 2 to 3 minutes.

Place the oil and three mustard seeds in a frying pan and raise the flame to high. When the mustard seeds pop, reduce the flame to low and add the remaining herbs. Stir until the aromas of the herbs are released, and then add the barley.

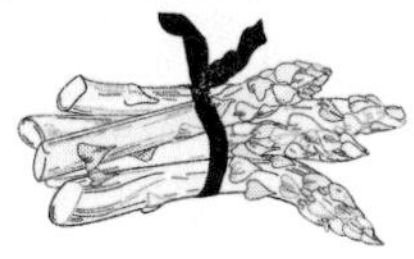

Incompatible Foods

Many diseases are caused by combining foods that aggravate create harmful, subtle chemicals in one's body. Below is a partial list.

1. Honey with *ghee* (in equal amounts)
2. Honey with radish
3. Yogurt with hot foods, milk, bananas, tea (except with balancing herbs)
4. Milk with oil, salt, vinegar, green squash, radish, bananas, lemons, oranges, plums, candy, sesame, yogurt.
5. Vinegar with sesame seeds
6. Honeydew melon with honey, yogurt, or water
7. Cucumber with water
8. Rice with vinegar
9. Meat with dairy, sesame, vinegar, or honey
10. Hot foods and drinks with cold foods and drinks
11. Cold drinks after cucumber or melons

(SEE CHART ON PREVIOUS PAGE)

Suggested Reading

Balch P, Balch J. *Prescription for Cooking & Dietary Wellness*. Greenfield, IN: PAB Books; 1992.

Dash, B., Kashyap L. *Materia Medica of Āyurveda*. New Delhi, India: Insight Publishing; 1987.

Frawley D. *Āyurveda Certification Course*. Santa Fe, NM: American Institute of Vedic Studies; 1992.

Heinerman John. *Encyclopedia of Nuts, Berries and Seeds*. West Nyack, NY: Parker Publishing; 1995.

Lad Usha, Vasant. *Āyurvedic Cooking*. Albuquerque, NM: Āyurvedic Press; 1994.

Nadkarni K.N. *Indian Materia Medica*. Bombay, India: Popular Prakashan; 1993.

Mindell Earl. *The Vitamin Bible*. New York, NY: Time Warner Books; 1991.

Sachs Melanie. *Āyurvedic Beauty Care*. Twin Lakes, WI: Lotus Press; 1994.

Sharma RK, Dash B. *Charak Saṃhita* (vol.1). Varanasi, India: Chowkhamba Sanskrit Series; 1992.

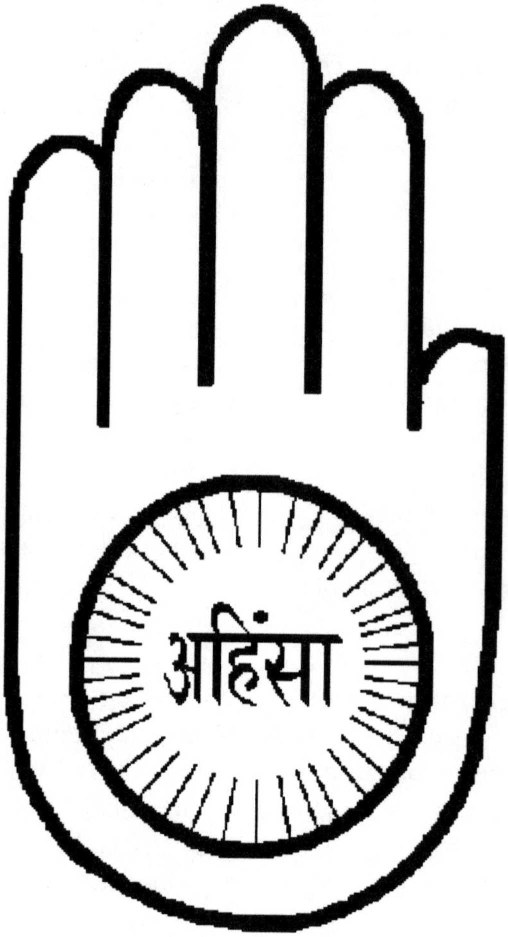
अहिंसा

लङ्घनं बृंहणं काले रूक्षणं स्नेहनं तथा ।
स्वेदनं स्तम्भनं चैव जानीते यः स वै भिषक् ।।४।।

Laṅghanaṃ bṛiṃhaṇaṃ kāle rūkśhaṇaṃ snehanaṃ tathā.
Svedanaṃ stambhanaṃ chaiva jānīte yaḥ sa vai bhiṣhak.

One who knows how to reduce, nourish, dry, oleate, foment,
and use the astringent therapies is the real physician.
Charak Sū:Ch. 22 verse 4

Chapter 7
Pañcha Karma

Āyurveda offers unique therapeutic measures that heal mild and chronic diseases. Even diseases that are believed to be incurable by modern medicine have been healed. Stories abound of people being carried into *pañcha karma* centers, and a few weeks later, walking out on their own two feet, healthy and rejuvenated. Āyurveda is not based on magic; rather, it is based on understanding medical principles and the six stages of illness.

The most deeply seated toxins that cause disease are heavy and sticky, lodging in the deepest tissue layers. *Pañcha Karma* permanently eliminates these toxins from the body, allowing healing and restoration of the tissues, channels, digestion, and mental functions.

Six therapies are divided into two categories: 1) Toning or nourishing (*bṛiṃhaṇa* or *saṃtarpaṇa*), and 2) Reducing or detoxifying (*laṅghana* or *apartarpaṇa*)—those that cause lightness.

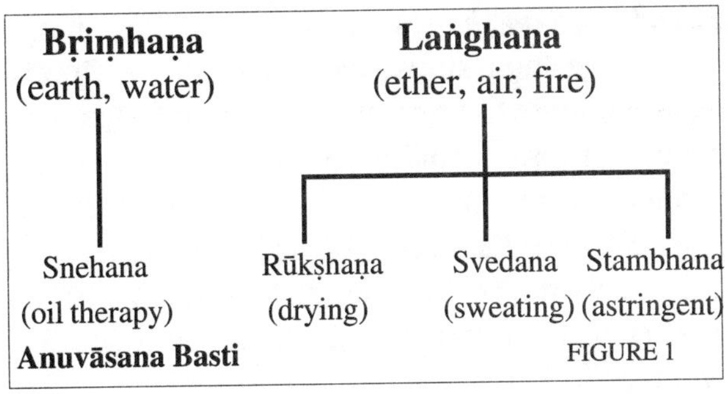

FIGURE 1

Bṛiṃhaṇa tones because it uses therapies that promote earth and water elements, while *laṅghna* lightens by using ether, air, and fire elements to reduce. Illness is relieved as *doṣhas* become balanced through these therapies.

The six major therapeutic categories are either toning or reducing in nature.

1. Reducing (*laṅghana* or lightening) the body, making it light.
2. Nourishing (*bṛiṃhaṇa* or expanding) the body by adding corpulence.
3. Drying (*rūkṣhaṇa*) or producing roughness in the body.
4. Oleation (*snehana*) or applying oil to the body creates softness, fluidity, and moistness.
5. Sudation (*svedhana*) or sweating, removes stiffness, heaviness, and coldness.
6. Astringent (*stambhana*) balances the flow (slow or fast) of bodily fluids (e.g., diarrhea, bleeding, etc.), and prevents mobility.

The therapeutic measures involved for each category primarily include herbs, foods, internal and external application of oils; fasting, and exercise. Below are listed the respective therapeutic measures,

1. Lightening (*laṅghana*)—light, hot, sharp, non slimy, rough, subtle, dry, fluid, hard.

Two forms of lightening exist: strong (*śhodhana*) and mild (*śhamana*). *Śhodhana* expels the *doṣhas* out of the body through decoction enema, emesis, purgation of the body and head, and by bloodletting. *Śhamana* is a palliative approach that, rather than expel the *doṣhas*, merely normalizes them through seven approaches. 1) Digestive, carminative herbs, 2) Hunger-producing herbs, 3) Avoidance of food, 4) Avoidance of drink, 5) Physical exercise, 6) Sunbathing, 7) Exposure to wind.

Palliative therapy is used by people with diabetes, poor digestion, excess watery conditions (e.g., congestion, overweight), toxic buildup (*āma*), and fevers. These measures are also used for stiff thighs, skin diseases, herpes, abscesses, spleen, head, throat and eye problems; and are provided to people during the cold season (*Śhiśhira*—mid Jan. to mid March).

Pitta and Kapha disorders follow *śhodhana* (strong) therapies of purgation and emesis. Symptoms include the presence of toxins, obesity, fever, vomiting or nausea, diarrhea, heart disease, constipation, heaviness, and excess belching.

People with moderate symptoms of weight gain and medium strength are first given digestive herbs like ginger, cardamom, or cinnamon. Persons who need to boost their appetites are also given hunger-producing herbs like *bibhītakī* and *guggul*. Once the person is strengthened and digestion is improved, then both groups of herbs are administered, along with the other purificatory therapies, for a more thorough detoxification.

Those people who are only mildly overweight, and of medium strong, and those who have medium strength and have *doṣha* excesses, are advised to control their thirst and hunger. For people who are weak and ill, and are not yet able to withstand the stronger therapies, mild therapies are initially suggested (i.e., sun and wind bathing and mild exercise).

Excess use of reduction therapies cause joint pain, body aches, cough, dry mouth, thirst, loss of appetite, anorexia, weakened hearing and sight. Further disorders include mental instability, excess fasting, a desire to enter dark places, emaciation, weakened digestion and depleted strength. Other imbalances are giddiness, cough, indigestion, insomnia, depletion of life sap (*ojas*) and semen; hunger, fever, delirium, and belching. Additional disorders include pain in the head, calves, thighs, shoulders, ribs, fatigue, vomiting, constipation, and difficult breathing.

2. Nourishing (*bṛiṃhaṇa*)—heavy, cold, soft, unctuous, thick, bulky, slimy, sluggish, stable, smooth. This is also a *śhamana* (palliative) therapy because it alleviates and/or mitigates both Vāyu and Vāyu/Pitta imbalances. This is mostly applied to the very weak or those with Vāyu excesses. Included here are the very young, very old, emaciated, people suffering from lung injury, those experiencing grief, strain, dryness, excessive emission of semen or excess travel. Nourishing therapies may be given to everyone in the summer, depending upon the condition of their health. Nourishing therapies include bathing, oil massage, oil enema, sleep, nutritive enemas, warm milk with whole sugar, almonds, tahini, organic dairy and *ghee*.

Excessive use of nourishing therapies causes obesity, congestion, difficult breathing, heart problems, diabetes, fever, enlarged abdomen, fistula-in-ano, and *āma*. Other developments include skin disorders, cough, fainting, dysuria, poor digestion, and scrofula (TB of the neck lymph nodes). Further, if toxins are in the body, they should be eliminated before toning.

To counter excessive use of nourishing therapies, antidotes include less sleep and the herbs *guḍūchī*, *guggul*, *śhilājit*, *āmalakī*, *viḍaṅga*, *tṛikatu*, and *chitrak*, with honey.

3. Drying (*rūkṣhaṇa*)—rough light, dry, sharp, hot, stable, non slimy, hard. Herbs and foods having pungent, bitter, and astringent tastes produce dryness. Usually, this therapy is applied when there are Kapha excesses and obstructions in the *srotas* (channels). These therapies are also used with major diseases involving the heart, urinary bladder, spastic thighs, gout, urinary disorders.

Excessive use of drying therapies causes the same symptoms as excessive *laṅghana* therapies.

4. Oleation (*snehana*)—these qualities are liquid, subtle, fluid, unctuous, slimy, heavy, cold, sluggish, and soft. Medicated oils are used. Therapy lasts for 3 to 7 days. This is discussed later in the chapter (*abhyañga* section, p. 207).

5. Fomentation (*svedhana*)- these properties are hot, sharp, fluid, unctuous, rough, subtle, liquid, stable, and heavy. Sweating techniques such as warm water, poultice, and steam; and medicated lotions are used. This is discussed later in the chapter (*abhyañga* section, p. 207).

6. Astringent (*stambhana*)—qualities include cold, sluggish, soft, smooth, rough, subtle, liquid, stable, light VK+. Although this approach seems similar to lightening, astringents are used more for Pitta excesses, while lightening may be required for any *doṣha*.

Indications for using this therapy include excess Pitta, blackish complexion, bradycardia (less than 60 heart beats per minute), alkali, diarrhea, vomiting, poisoning, and perspiration.

Excessive use of astringents develops stiffness, anxiety, stiff jaw, cardiac arrest, constipation, cracked skin, dry mouth, thirst, and decreased appetite. Other conditions include memory loss, increase of upward moving Vāyu, and malaise.

All therapies fall into one of two categories, nourishing (santarpana), and depleting (apartarpaṇa).
Aṣhṭāñga Hṛidayam Sū: Ch 12 verse 1

Generally speaking, Kapha *doṣhas* need reducing or depleting therapy to reduce earth and water excesses (toxic Pittas need a milder form of detoxification). Kaphas also need nourishing therapies for the ether, air, and fire elements of Vāyu and Pitta. In fact, each *doṣha* may need some form of detoxification, depending upon its condition.

It is a unique insight of the Āyurvedic system that healing requires a removal of the toxins through one of the various reduction therapies. Then a nurturing therapy to build healthy new cells and tissues follows. To nourish before detoxifying would be adding to the preexisting toxins. In other words, nourishing therapies would only nourish the toxic condition. Only after toxins are removed can one begin to rebuild their system.

Reduce - then Tone: Most people can use some degree of reducing, whether it is with herbs, fasts, sweating, etc., purifying the body, and preparing it for toning.

When Not to Reduce: Some people, who are already weakened by illness—or the very old or very young—become even weaker through reduction. In these cases, a combination of the two methods is employed so the person's strength is not depleted completely. Reducing and toning are used especially for long term therapies.

Excess application of nourishing or depleting will cause diseases of the opposite nature. Generally, being too thin is better than being too heavy because gaining weight is easier than losing it.

Summary

Therapy

Doṣha	Main Use
Kapha	reduction
Vāyu	toning
Pitta	both

Reduction

Doṣha Reduction	*Doṣha* Therapy
Kapha	strong/fasts, emesis
Pitta/ Blood	moderate/purgation
Vāyu	mild/enema

Kapha is already heavy and needs to become lighter. Vāyu is already light and needs to develop.

Nourishment

Doṣha	Type of Therapy
Kapha	mild/light herbs like elcampane, *pippalī*
Pitta	moderate/cooling herbs like *ŝhatāvarī,* aloe gel
Vāyu	strong/*aŝhwagandhā*, ginseng, rich diet, oils

When Used

Reduce	strong energy, strong pulse, good muscle tone or muscle tension, prominent tongue coating
Nourish	chronic low energy, weak pulse, emaciation, lack of muscle tone, flaccid or weak, obesity

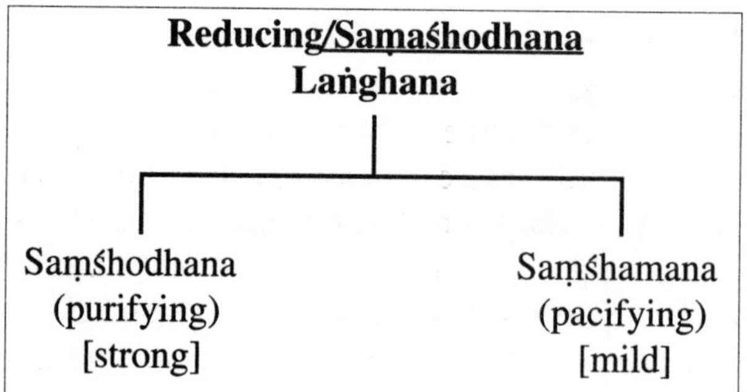

FIGURE 2A

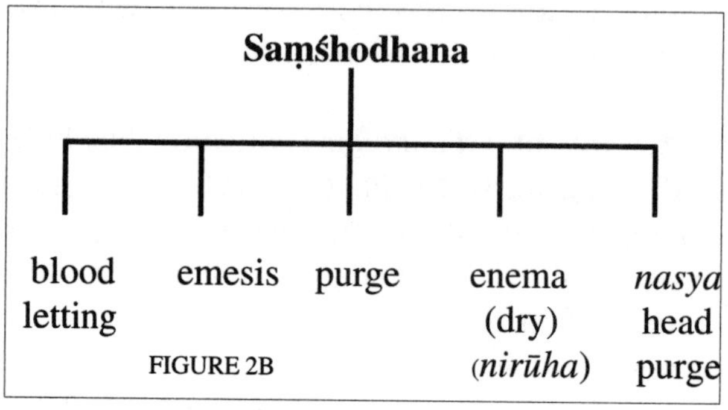

FIGURE 2B

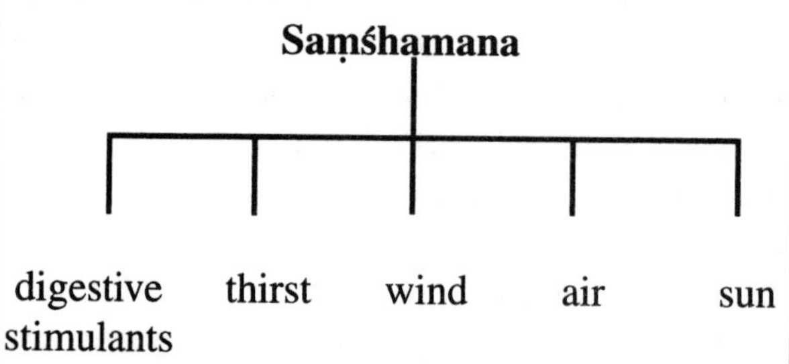

FIGURE 2C

Results of therapeutic reducing include sharp, clear senses, removal of toxins, light body, appreciating the taste of foods, normal hunger and thirst. Other results include normal or healthy feeling in the heart and throat, little or no belching, reduction of disease severity, more enthusiasm, and removal of laziness. Excess reducing produces emaciation, weakness, etc.

Results of therapeutic toning include strength, a nourished mind and body, and healing of diseases related to being underweight and to having a weak immune system. Symptoms of excess toning include profound obesity, diabetes, fever, enlarged abdomen, cough, toxins, skin diseases, fistula.

Note the difference between purification and palliation. If the aggravated humors are in the GI tract, they are ready for purification (*pañcha karma*). If they are still in the *dhātus, malas* or *āma* (tissues, waste or undigested foods) they cannot be directly eliminated and palliation or pacifying methods are first needed.

Toning/*Ŝhamana*, *Bṛiṃhaṇa*, and *Snehana*
For Vāyu and Pitta

Saṃŝhodhana, [bloodletting, emesis (*vamana*), purgation (*virechana*), dry enema (*nirūha basti*), and head purgation (*nasya*)] are all elements of the unique cleansing called *pañcha karma.* This will be discussed later as the main healing approach for chronic disease. It is used for excess Kapha, Pitta, fat, blood, wastes, minor Vāyu disorders, along with the other *doṣhas.* These therapies are useful with diabetes, *āma*, poor digestion, fever, water retention, obesity, and stiff thighs. They are also used for skin disorders, herpes, abscesses, spleen, throat, head, and eye disorders, and used by everyone in the cold seasons. For skin diseases, diabetes, and high Vāyu, reduction is not used between November and February. It is said that by undergoing *saṃŝhod-*

hana treatments, disease will not recur.

Saṃśhamana, [digestive stimulants (including spices, fasting, and exercise), thirst, sun or wind bathing, and fresh air] are gentler therapies to pacify mild disorders. Strong persons may be healed just from exercise, sunbathing, and fresh air. Those with moderate strength begin with digestive stimulants including herbs. These therapies are used for vomiting, diarrhea, heart diseases, cholera, intestinal disorders, fever, constipation, heaviness, belching, nausea, anorexia, Kapha, and Pitta.

Śhodhana reduces excess wastes, while *śhamana* heals excess *doṣhas*. These therapies eliminate the wastes and balance the *doṣhas*.

Summary

Preliminary Therapies (Purva Karma)

Before *pañcha karma* is employed, persons first reduce the excessed *doṣhas* and cleanse *āma* (toxins) from their system. This is achieved by eating lightly spiced meals according to their *doṣha* (see Chapter 6).

Ten therapies are useful in *Purva karma,* also known as palliation or *Śhamana.*

1. Body Oiling	6. Food
2. Sweat Therapy	7. Aromatherapy
3. Herbal Tonics	8. Colors/ Meals/ Environment
4. Oils and *Ghee*	9. Lifestyle
5. Exercise	10. *Sādhanā*

Herbs were discussed in detail in Chapter 4, and foods, nutrition and *ghee* were reviewed in the last chapter. Now, we take a closer look at body oil and sweat therapies. Later chapters will detail the remaining topics. Taking herbs and eating the proper diet according to one's *doṣha* are a long-term form of *pañcha karma*. These 10 applications can be used independently of preliminary palliation to heal and help maintain one's balance of physical and mental health.

Palliation generally lasts for three months, one month, or one week. When an illness is chronic or strong, palliation may be shorter since the humors may be ready to be eliminated. Conversely, healthy persons undergoing *pañcha karma* merely for enhancement or prevention may skip the palliation therapies.

Long term palliation	3 months
Moderate palliation	1 month
Short term palliation	1 week

Snehana & Svedhana (Oleation & Sweating Methods): After palliation therapies remove toxins, two main preliminary therapies are used, oleation and sweating. Both begin to unseat the toxins that have moved and situated themselves in places they do not belong. These relocated toxins are the cause of ill health or imbalance.

Below is an overview of the 10 therapies and what measures are suggested for each *doṣha*. Readers are advised to see their respective chapters for a complete understanding of their procedures.

Śhamana - Palliation

1. Oil Massage [*Snehana*]

Vāyu—lots of sesame oil with *mahānārāyan* and castor oil are best. Massage should be warm, gentle and firm. Oils are only used after most of the *āma* is removed by eating hot spices.

Pitta—touch is soothing, light, gentle, slightly cool with a moderate amount of oil (cool coconut, *ghee*, safflower), *brāhmī* (gotu kola), or *mahānārāyan* oil is also applied.

Kapha—strong, dry, or with light and hot oils (i.e., mustard, canola, olive), deep tissue, perhaps with some slight pain. Also, *daśhmūl* oil is helpful for Kapha *doṣhas*.

2. Sweat Therapy [*Svedhana*]

Vāyu—(mild) brief steam baths or hot tubs (head is kept out of the heat), or ingesting mild diaphoretics like *nirguṇḍī*, cinnamon, and ginger, or tonics like *balā*, comfrey, or *daśhmūl*. They need to drink plenty of liquids to replenish the water (during and after sweating) or they will become too dry. Too much sweating may lead to dizziness, convulsions, fainting, or vertigo.

Pitta—cool or mild sweating using cool and dispersing herbs (i.e., *kuṭki*, yellow dock, burdock) followed by a cool shower. During excess sweating one may feel thirsty, develop burning sensations, feel dizzy, or develop a fever.

Kapha—strong, dry heat, hot diaphoretics and expectorants (i.e., ginger, sage, *pippalī*, cinnamon). One sweats until one begins to feel uncomfortable, but not exhausted.

3. Herbal Tonics

Vāyu—*śhatāvarī*, *aśhwagandhā*, *balā*, *triphalā* with digestive spices like ginger or cinnamon, and herbal wines like *drākṣhā* are useful. Excessive use of these herbs aggravates Vāyu, coats the tongue, distends the abdomen, and may cause constipation.

Pitta—cool, bitter, astringent alteratives, aloe gel, barberry, dandelion, burdock, red clover, pau d'arco, *brāhmī*, *mañjiṣhṭhā*, comfrey, and coriander. These are all blood and bile cleansers, and drain the excess heat from the body.

Kapha—hot, dry, pungents (i.e., ginger, *pippalī*, myrrh, *ṭrikatu*), bitters (i.e., aloe, turmeric, barberry) reduce fat. Herbs are most effective when taken with a little raw honey (which helps loosen phlegm).

4. Oils & *Ghee*

Vāyu—(daily use of sesame or *ghee*—1 to 2 tbs.—taken internally). This moistens the dry Vāyu membranes and tissues, and softens and loosens dry and hardened toxins in the body tissues.

Pitta—*ghee*, internal (1 to 2 tbs. daily) and external (especially in eyes). *Triphalā* or *brāhmī ghee* are the suggested medicated *ghees.*

Kapha—1 to 2 tsp. daily of mustard, canola, and flax seed oils are taken internally. These oils loosen phlegm.

5. Exercise

Vāyu—mild exercise, calming *yoga* postures (sitting or lying down) and gentle breathing exercises also strengthen (see *the haṭha yoga* chapter). Mild sunbathing (avoiding wind and cold) and daily *sādhanā* (meditation) automatically heal the mind and body.

Pitta—moderate amount, in cool air or wind, walks taken during the full moon and other moderate activities like flower gardening. Cooling *Yoga* postures, like shoulder stands or sitting and lying down, and *prāṇāyām* are suggested. People with heart problems are advised not to do shoulder stands. The best *prāṇāyām* for Pitta is *śhītalī* and lunar practices (see Chapter 9). Both are best taught by a qualified *yoga* or *prāṇāyām* instructor, rather than by clients trying on their own. Exercise that creates excess heat and sweating (i.e., aerobics, heavy exertion, exercising under a hot sun) are contraindicated.

Kapha—strong aerobics (e.g., jogging in the wind and sun), long hikes, camping, and strong physical labor. One must first be healthy and strong enough to exercise at this level. If persons sweat or exercise too much they feel tired afterwards.

6. Food

Vāyu—adequate, nutritious, Vāyu reducing- (i.e., dairy, nuts, grains of *basmati* rice, oats, and wheat, root vegetables, sweet fruits, boiled milk with ginger, cardamom, cinnamon, fennel). One should eat nutritiously; overeating should be avoided. Fasts for 1 to 3 days, with ginger and cinnamon tea, are all right for those who are strong enough. (Meat is used when one is recovering from a debilitating illness).

Pitta—moderate and cool Pitta reduction, sweet fruits, raw or lightly steamed vegetables, green vegetable juice, cool grains like rice, oats, and wheat, and yellow split *mūngdal* (or whole mūng beans). Spices include coriander, cumin, fennel—cool spices. Hot spices should be avoided, as are salt and vinegar. Moderate fasts with cool herbs (i.e., dandelion or burdock), green vegetable juices or fruit juices (i.e., pineapple or pomegranate) are also suggested. Weak Pittas may take more dairy (preferably organic—no drugs or steroids fed to the animals, and from contented animals—not factory-herded ones).

Kapha—light, anti-Kapha, steamed diuretic vegetables, diuretic grains, beans, hot spices, reduce water and juice consumption. Fasting on spices and honey from 3 to 7 days is suggested. Overall, sugar, sweet foods, dairy, heavy oils. and meats should be avoided.

7. Aromas

While aromatherapy is not technically a consideration of *saṃśhamana*, it is incorporated here for additional therapeutic value. Aromas work more on the mind than the body, so they help balance psychological causes of illness.

Vāyu—sandalwood, frankincense, cedar, and myrrh, are calming and grounding.

Pitta (cool)—oils, incense, soaps, sachets of sandalwood, rose, geranium, and other flower scents open the heart and reduce fire.

Kapha—oils, incense, soap, sachets etc. of myrrh, frankincense, cedar, eucalyptus, sage.

8. Colors/Environment/Meals

Fresh air, wind, and sun help stimulate digestion in mild cases of illness. While color therapy is not technically a consideration of *saṃśhamana*, it is incorporated here for additional therapeutic value. Colors work more on the mind than the body, so they help balance psychological causes of illness.

Vāyu—balancing therapies include short fasts (1 to 3 days), being warm and comfortable inside and outside the home, moist air (for one living in a dry climate), and mild sunbathing. Wear warm colors of red, orange, and gold. White (a moist color) also balances mild Vāyu excesses. The bed should be soft and comfortable. The environment should be pleasing. One must adopt measures for self-care.

Pitta—mild fasts (about one week), air and wind bathing reduce excess heat. Cool-colored clothing (i.e., white and pale shades of green, pink, and blue) are also balancing.

Kapha—sunbathing, fresh air, long fasts, warm color therapy—red, orange, yellow in clothes, furniture, and decor—in both home and office—balances excess Kapha.

9. Lifestyle

Vāyu—resting the body and mind. Excess traveling, noise, distractions are avoided, sleeping during the day, if tired, and having a secure and stable lifestyle—with happiness, contentment and joy—is suggested. Mild exercise (stop when perspiration begins) is useful.

Pitta—cool, pleasing environments, cool breezes, moonlight, avoiding sun, heat, and fire. Relaxation is advised, doing various or diverse things, allowing time for amusement and play, practicing sweet, affectionate, loving, friendly behavior; being near water and gardens. Conflict, arguments, aggression, ambition, strain, and overwork, and effort are avoided. Moderate exercise is useful (stop when perspiration begins).

Kapha—dry, rough clothes and environment (i.e., austere life—sleeping on the floor, physical labor, staying up late at night, not napping or sleeping late), avoiding cold and damp; and being in hot, dry, sunny, fiery, and warm breezy places. This is a time one when breaks attachments and habits—giving up the past (mentally) and possessions. Strong exercise is useful (exercise a little past the point of fatigue).

10. *Sādhanā*

Vāyu—for calm and peace—allows one to be less talkative, or even silent, emptying the mind of thoughts, worry etc.; surrendering fears, and anxieties is also practiced.

Pitta—one focuses on positive energies of love, peace, forgiveness, visualization, and artistic creativity.

Kapha—practices active meditation, (e.g., study, thinking, inquiring, reading scriptures, chanting aloud, dancing, and singing) stimulates and activates the mind until one feels strained.

Purification Therapy (Śhodhana)

Unique to Āyurveda is a process of completely expelling toxins from the body. First, through palliation and purification, one loosens toxins lodged in the body. This allows the toxins to return through the bloodstream to their origin sites in the gastrointestinal tract. Once there, the toxins can be completely expelled from the body through five methods known as *pañcha karma*. *Pañcha karma* (five actions) actually includes three stages (see table below).

Therapy	Description
1. Preliminary (palliative)	employing oil and sweating methods (*snehana* and *svedhana*). [often used throughout the year as a general maintenance and preventive program]
2. Primary purificatory practices (*pañcha karma*)	uses emesis, purgation, enemas, nasal therapy.
3. Post PK therapies	rejuvenation and tonification.

Oil Therapy (Snehana)

Using oils, both internally and externally, is a very important Āyurvedic therapy

Warm, medicinal oils are applied in large amounts all over the body. Some practitioners use sesame oil for all three constitutions. Others use medicated oils like *mahānārāyan* oil. Still others use medicated oils in specific body sites, such as on the *chakras* and *marma* points, or at specific trouble spots. Essential oils may also be employed according to the *doṣhas*. It is the use of the oil that is important, and not the massage technique or training. (Actually, a professional massage produces the same effects as *snehana* and *svedhana).* Specific Āyurvedic massage-like techniques *(abhyañga)* will be discussed later. Along with the application of oil, intake of oil or *ghee (snehapāna)* is also recommended. Sesame oil or *ghee* is used for Vāyu, sunflower or *ghee* for Pitta, and mustard, canola, or flax seed oils for Kapha.

Oil Uses: Oils help loosen and liquefy toxins and humors in the skin and blood (called the outer disease pathway), dislodging and removing the heavy, sticky toxins from the smallest channels. Thus, toxins begin to drain from the central disease pathway (deeper tissues) and start to flow into the GI tract. Secretions are also activated, enabling easier *doṣha* transport of toxins (*āma*) and wastes (*malas*) as they return to the GI tract for elimination. Oil lubricates and protects tissues from damage, as *āma* returns to the GI tract. Finally, since Vāyu is responsible for movement, oil lubrication restores proper Vāyu functioning, allowing for proper flowing of wastes and toxins to their removal sites.

Special herbs blended with the oils enable the tissues to expel the oil from tissues. Therefore, oil does not accumulate in the body. Herbs like *guḍūchī, kaṭuka, harītakī, yaṣhṭīmadhu* (licorice), and *chitrak* have bitter properties that cause oils to be expelled. Specific oil massage (*abhyañga*) therapies are discussed later in this chapter.

Oils and purificatory therapies are useful for arthritis, insomnia, paralysis, tremors, convulsions, nervous exhaustion, dry cough, constipation, and other Vāyu derangements. Oil is also useful for alcohol addiction, the elderly, children, eye problems, tumors, sinus conditions, worms, ulcers, memory, dryness, poisons, Vāyu, Pitta, and Kapha diseases. Such therapies promote alertness, slimming, toning, and sturdying the body; improving strength, voice, complexion, and they cleanse the female genital passage. Oil builds plasma, reproductive fluid and *ojas* (life-sap). Kapha *doṣhas* use oil for worms and gas.

Sesame is the best oil. Overall, oil reduces Vāyu, is neutral for Kapha, and increases Pitta. Oils are used during the rainy season.

Contraindications: There are some people for whom oleation is not recommended. They include people who have very weak or very strong digestion, who are very obese, who have stiff thighs, or who suffer from diarrhea and toxins (i.e., they must be expelled first). Oleation is also not used to treat throat diseases, enlarged abdomen, fainting, vomiting, anorexia, abnormal child delivery, Kapha excesses, or inebriation. Instead, clients are given nasal, enema, and purgative therapies. *Charak* notes that while oil reduces Vāyu, it does not aggravate Kapha (as long as oils are warmed).

Ghee Uses: *Ghee* is best used for improving intellect, memory, and intelligence; plasma, reproductive fluid, and *ojas* (life-sap). It helps soften the body, and promotes clear voice and complexion.

Vāyu: Medicated *ghee*, or *ghee* and black salt. Its moistness balances Vāyu.

Pitta: Plain *ghee*. Its cool and sweet nature balances Pitta.

Kapha: *Ghee* with barley and *tṛikatu* (empowers the herbs).

Ghee is used in the autumn. For Vāyu/Pitta imbalances in the summer, evening oleation is advised. For aggravated Kapha, and throughout the winter, unction on sunny days is advised. In emergencies, and for those with extreme Vāyu disorders, oleation may be used anytime. Ingesting *ghee* (*snehapāna*) follows the same schedule.
Precautions: Do not use *snehana* for ascites, fever, delirium, drinking or with alcoholism, loss of appetite, vomiting, fatigue, on cloudy days, rainy season, after *basti*, purgative emetics or *nasya*, after premature birth, for too strong or weak digestion, stiff thighs, diarrhea, *āma*, throat diseases, artificial poisoning, enlarged abdomen, fainting. Do not use oil for coma, thirst, anal secretions, pregnancy, and excess salivation. Use drying herbs for 10 days following childbirth.

After taking *ghee*, one drinks hot water. After oil, one drinks boiled rice water. This should cause belching and a desire to eat. If one feels thirsty, they may stimulate the regurgitating reflex. Afterwards, cool baths, head plasters, or towels are used. Those with strong digestion can take more oleation. Those with moderate digestion can use moderate amounts of oil or *ghee*, and those with weaker digestion use less unction. Results of *snehana* include proper flow of Vāyu, improved digestion, proper feces, moistness, and initial fatigue.

As the *snehana* begins to get digested, one may experience thirst, vertigo, lassitude, mental disturbance, and burning sensations. After oleation, one needs to rest, get to sleep early, avoid exposure to wind and hot sun. One should observe celibacy, and eat light, simple foods, according to one's *doṣha*, and not suppress bodily urges. If this is not followed, serious diseases may develop. After *snehana* is digested, one takes a hot shower, then eats a small portion of plain rice or barley (at room temperature).

Snehana therapy lasts an average of 3 to 7 days, or until the symptoms disappear. The elderly, the weak, the very young, and those with thirst should take such therapy with lunch. Persons currently drinking wine are not eligible for *snehana*. Vāyu *doṣha* follows *snehana* for 7 days, Pitta for 5 days and Kapha for 3 days.

Snehana Therapy Schedule

Doṣha	**Days for Therapy**
Vāyu	7
Pitta	5
Kapha	3

Dose: There are 3 doses of drinking *snehana*, according to the strength of the *doṣha* .

Mild Strength: Vāyu—oil stays in the system for 9 hours. This dose is for slight aggravation.

Its application develops the appetite. Use for 3 days.

Medium Strength: Pitta—oil stays in the system for 6 hours. It is for moderate aggravation, and builds and tones the system. Use for 4 to 6 days.

High Strength: Kapha—oil stays in the system for 3 hours. It acts as an emollient for extreme aggravation. Use for 7 days.

Doṣha	**Hours**
Vāyu	9
Pitta	6
Kapha	3

त्र्यहेण श्लेष्मिकः स्नीह्यात् पंचरात्रेण
पैतिकः

वतिकः सप्तरात्रेण सात्म्यतां परम्

Tryaheṇa śhleṣhimikaḥ snīhyāt
pañcharatreṇa paitikaḥ
Vatikaḥ sapta rātreṇa sātmyatāṇa param

[Reference Bhog]

Drinking Snehapāna

Day	Dose	*Doṣha*
Test Dose	1 oz.	Kapha *doṣhas*
1	2 oz.	
2	3 oz.	
3	4 oz.	Pitta *doṣhas*
4	6 oz.	
5	8 oz.	Vāyu *doṣhas*
6	10 oz.	
7	12 oz.	

Various authors offer other suggestions.

Doses: Depending upon the strength of the person and the severity of the disease, mild, moderate or high doses are used. *Snehana* is ingested either first thing in the morning or late in the afternoon (ideally 3:00 to 6:00 a.m. or p.m.) on an empty stomach. Only when the appetite returns does one eat.

Mild: One to 4 days. The diet during snehana involves 3 days of avoiding very fatty foods, eating simply, no food combining and eating warm, regular quantities (according to one's constitution or *doṣha*). Before and after *snehana*, take warm baths and drink warm water; be celibate. Avoid becoming stressed, angry, or grief stricken. Avoid exposure to cold, sun, travel, talking, naps, and pollution. Do not suppress natural urges. Take the dose just after sunrise.

Moderate: Four to 6 days. Avoid sticky, oily, and incompatible foods.

High: Seven days/with hard bowels or until healthy symptoms appear. The high dose always causes intolerance, but persons are made to drink by holding their nose and closing their eyes while drinking.

Some authorities suggest always using 7 days of oleation in order to reach all 7 tissue layers. Others follow the mild, medium, and high doses, depending on which *dhātus* are unbalanced. Signs of effective oleation include soft, shiny skin, softer skin and hair, healthy elimination of stool that looks yellowish, shiny, oily, and softer; urine may look brighter, and urine and stool smell like *ghee*. Eye, ear, and nose secretions shine slightly. Mental clarity, enthusiasm, energy, and strength increase.

If diarrhea results from *snehana*, then persons have only moderate or mild symptoms; for the 3rd and 4th days of *snehana*, lemon juice is added to the *snehana* formula (*ghee* with hot water may be used. Oil with vegetable soup or hot water is an alternative).

Śhodhana (purification): Drink alone, soon after digestion, drink the large or maximum dose.
Śhamana (removal of mild dosha/disease symptoms): Use a medium dose with fasting.
Brimhana (toning): Take the minimum dose (a small quantity) with food.
Precautions: *Snehapāna* is not used for indigestion, abdominal enlargement, acute fever, weakness, anorexia, obesity, fits, intoxication, immediately after *basti* (enema), *vamana* (vomiting), *virechana* (purgation), with thirst, fatigue, after premature delivery, or on rainy days.

Depending on when *snehana* is taken, different parts of the body will be affected.

Meal	Body Part Affected
Before	Lower
During	Middle
After	Upper

Unctuous Substances: Those who cannot comfortably ingest plain oil or *ghee* may begin by eating unctuous items. These substances include porridge (*odana*), gruel (*vilepī*—grain with 4 to 8 times as much water), gruel (*yavāgu*—grain with 6 times as much water), legumes, curry, vegetable soup, *kāmbalika* (curd, rock salt, sesame oil, and *ghee*), sesame oil or sesame butter, sugar, organic milk, *ghee, lassi, pippalī,* and *śhatāvarī.*

Vāyu *doṣhas* do well with a little rock salt.

Pitta *doṣhas* do well with *ghee*.

Kapha doṣhas do well with *ṭrikatu*.

For worms, a large dose of sesame oil is used.

Seasonal Use of Oil and Ghee

Fall	cow *ghee*
Rainy	oil
Summer	Vāyu and Pitta excesses, joint pain—oil used in evenings
Winter	Kapha/Vāyu and Kapha/Pitta excesses or joint pain—oil used in the afternoon
Cold Winter	15 to 30 minutes after sunrise and for joint problems—oil

Herbs for particular diseases may be cooked in the *ghee* or oil to apply *snehana* more effectively. For example, *gokṣhura* may be added to oil for urinary problems.

Three Degrees of Boiling Oil and Ghee

	Boil	Consistency	Use
Errhines	mild	hard/dry	with food/drink
Drinks\ *Basti*	medium	wax- like	errhines/ salves
Anoint	hard	clear/black	*basti*/ear drops

Ghee is ready when froth and cooking sounds disappear, and the *ghee* emits an aroma. Oil is ready when it becomes frothy on the surface, and an aroma develops.

Sample Recipes

1. *Pippalī*, rock salt, yogurt, sesame oil, or *ghee*. This *sneha* produces quick results.
2. Barley with milk, and a small amount of rice and *ghee*.
3. Milk, *ghee*, cane sugar. This is an instant emulsive preparation.
4. Barley fried in sesame oil, 1/2 boiled molasses, rice, green *dal*, milk, *ghee*, *lassi*, *jaggery*, and salt. This preparation causes tissues to exude,

entering minute pores, not drying, and spreading throughout the body warming and transforming) [i.e., for immediate oleation effects].

Precautions: Do not use this formula for skin diseases, edema, diabetes. Instead use,
4a. *Triphalā, pippalī, guggul, śhilājit, gokṣhura, ghee.*

Oil *snehana* is very good for tumors, sinus ulcers, worms, excess Kapha, fat, and Vāyu. It improves digestion, clears the digestive tract, strengthens the tissues, senses, slows the aging process, and improves complexion.

Other *snehana* therapies include oil massage, enema, douche, gargle, nose, ear, and eye drops, (See pages 197 - 201 and 242 - 244)

Inadequate *snehana* administration: Causes dryness, burning, weakness, and slower digestion.

Excess *snehana* administration: Causes yellow complexion, heaviness, stuffiness, undigested food in the stool, dullness, anorexia, nausea, vomiting.

Complications: Indigestion, thirst, fainting, dullness, nausea, tympanitis (inner ear inflammation), fever, stiffness, anorexia, abdominal pain, slowed digestion. If *ghee* causes abdominal pain, hot water should be drunk to produce vomiting. For severe thirst due to excessive digestive fire, cold water should be drunk after *sneha.*

Chronic Symptoms: Dry skin, itching, anemia, edema, GI diseases, sprue (malabsorption of nutrients in the intestines, leading to diarrhea, emaciation, and anemia), hemorrhoids, numbness, difficult speech.

Other forms of oleation include *abhyañga, lepa, gandūṣha* (mouth gargling), head, ear, and eye baths. These will all be discussed later under *Kerala abhyañga* (except for *gandūṣha,* which is discussed in Chapter 19 under mouth conditions and therapies). Application of oil and oil pastes are discussed below.

Sudation or Sweat Therapy (Svedhana)

स्निग्धस्य सूक्ष्मेष्व यनेषु लीनं
स्वेदस्तु दोषं नयति द्रवत्वम् ।

Snigdhasya sūkśhmeṣhva yaneṣhu līnaṃ
svedastu doṣhaṃ nayati dṛivatvam

Sweat applied to uncted persons liquefy impurities hidden in minute channels.
Charak: Sidd. Ch. 1, verse 8

According to *Aṣhṭāñga Hṛidayam*, after oleation, steam or sweating therapies are employed for effective dislodging and liquefying of toxins and improving digestion. *Svedana* causes the body's channels to widen, enabling *āma* to easily flow from the tissues back to the GI tract and improve circulation. Heat allows the skin and blood (outer disease pathway) to be cleansed. This relieves, cleanses, and reduces fat tissue and muscle tension.

Heat also restores balance to Vāyu and Kapha (i.e., removing coldness and stiffness) and reduces the heavy, sticky nature of *āma*. Once toxins are back in the G.I. tract, they are ready to be completely expelled from the body through *pañcha karma* (five purificatory actions).

Internal (e.g., spicy herbs) and external (e.g., jacuzzi, sauna) heat are used to dislodge wastes and toxins. Castor, *arka, red punarnavā,* sesame, and barley all induce sweat.

Four types of *Svedhana* therapies exist,
1. *Tāpa* or fomentation—placing a heated cloth, a metal object or warm hands on the body. This therapy is best for Vāyu and Kapha *doṣhas*.

2. *Upanāha* or applying a hot poultice to the body (before bed) made with the appropriate herbs and foods to reduce the respective aggravated *doṣhas*. After the poultice is applied, an oiled and heated silk or woolen cloth is wrapped around the body,

and the person goes to sleep for the night. It is removed in the morning (in the winter it may be kept on longer). This therapy is best for Vāyu disorders. General ingredients include wheat, barley, unctuous substances, *kuṣhṭa*, *kākolī,* and *kṣhīr-kākolī.*

Vāyu: Poultices include *vachā*, aromatic herbs, yeast, licorice, cedar, castor oil, *ghee*, *lassi*, milk.

Vāyu/Kapha: *Triphalā, tṛikatu.*

Vāyu/Pitta: *Guḍūchī,* licorice.

Upanāha Recipe: General suggestions include Vāyu-reducing herbs, sour juice, milk, and a little rock salt. Boil until it becomes a thick liquid and apply to the whole body (in the direction against the hairs). When it becomes cold, reapply. This process is repeated many times.

Other heating therapies include exercise, staying in warm, draftless rooms, wrapping oneself in heavy clothes, and sunbathing.

3. *Ūṣhmā* or warm steam is used by boiling the appropriate foods and herbs for a *doṣha*, and allowing the steam to surround the body. Steam may be applied with a sweat box (with the head kept free from heat) or apparatus like a pressure cooker. Appropriate herbs are added to the water in the pot. The steam is applied locally to an illness spot, like arthritis. This therapy is used for Vāyu and Kapha imbalances.

Stones, pebbles, mud, leaves, and sand are also heated and applied to specific body parts. They are more useful in Kapha disorders as they are a form of dry heat.

4. *Drava or Dhārā* means pouring warm, medicated liquid over the body. Again, herbs and foods are used to reduce the respective excessed *doṣhas* (or for specific health concerns). This method is useful for *āma*, Kapha, and fat excesses, stiff thighs, and breast milk disorders. The part of the body needing attention is covered with a cloth, and then the medicated water is slowly poured over the cloth. When Vāyu disturbs the entire body, a medicated water bath is used. The water temperature is 85 to 100 degrees. This is also useful for all diseases of the rectum and urinary tract. *Drava* is used for Vāyu/Pitta disorders. Useful herbs include castor, *vāsā, vaṃśha, arka,* turmeric, and licorice.

Two types of *drava* exist,

1. *Pariṣheka*: Medicated liquid is applied to specific body parts (that are covered in cloth).
2. *Avagāhan*: Persons soak in a tub filled with a medicated decoction.

Svedhana is best used for Vāyu disorders (i.e., nervous conditions). It is used only after one has undergone *snehana* (internal and external oil application), is in a warm room protected from breezes and has fully digested their last meal. Sudation is applied in strong, moderate, or mild measure, depending upon the strength of the person undergoing therapy.

Sessions last 5 to 10 minutes for Vāyu and Pitta *doṣhas*, and 10 to 15 minutes for Kapha *doṣhas*. Alternately, a strong intensity is used for strong persons or severe diseases; moderate intensity is used for persons with moderate strength or moderate diseases; and a minimum intensity is used for persons with minimal strength or minor diseases.

Kapha *doṣhas* use a dry sudation (dry heat and warming oils—for example, sitting under a blanket with a space heater). Kapha/Vāyu *doṣhas* use both dry heat and oily liquids (e.g., *ghee*). They can sweat in warm rooms or in the sunlight. *Ghee* is used in situations such as a Vāyu excess in the stomach and a Kapha excess in the colon. If used, sudation should be administered very gently on the testes, heart, and eyes. A cool cloth should be placed over these areas to prevent exposure to heat.

For Vāyu/Kapha excesses, (e.g., Vāyu in the stomach) first clients sweat without oil, then with oil. For Kapha/Vāyu excesses, (i.e., Kapha in the colon) first clients are given oil/steam, then a steam treatment without oil).

Svedhana is suggested for cough, cold, earache, headache, monoplegia, hemiplegia, paraplegia, constipation, absence or retention of urine. It is also indicated for stiffness and tetany arthritis (muscle spasms and tremors caused by poor metabolism of calcium, and associated with poor parathyroid gland functioning). It is also good for enlarged spleen, *fistula-in-ano*, hemorrhoids, renal calculi, and before surgery. *Svedhana* is also advised after an operation that removes a foreign object, or after abnormal, premature or normal delivery.

शीतशूलव्युपरमे स्तम्भगौरवनिग्रहे ।
संजते मार्दवे स्वेदे स्वेदनाद्विरतिर्मता ॥१३॥

Śhītaśūlavyūparame stambhagauravanigrahe.
Saṃjate mārdave svede
svedanādbhiratirmatā.

Svedhana is stopped only when cold, colic pain, stiffness and heaviness subsides in the body, or until softness and sweating are produced.
Charak Sū, Ch. 14, verse 13

Three Types of Sweat

1	External heat (e.g., steam)—use fire
	Internal heat (exercise, warm clothes, etc.) —no fire
2	Whole body (external heat)
	Part of the body (e.g., shoulder—*nāḍī, pariṣheka)*
3	With oil (wet)—for Vāyu—fire/no fire
	Without oil (dry)—for Kapha—fire/no fire

13 Sveda Forms

According to *Charak Saṃhitā,* 13 forms of *sveda* (sweat) are available; some use fire to generate heat, some do not. Oil *abhyañga* is required before initiating any of the methods.

Whole Body *Svedas*

1. *Sankara Sveda*: (use of bolus). *Piṇḍa Sveda* is such a therapy. It is discussed in detail on page 235.

2. *Jentāka Sveda*:, 3. *Prastara Sveda*: Similar to sauna rooms.

4. *Avagāhan Sveda*: Persons lie in a tub filled with a medicated decoction, milk, oil, or *ghee*. It is administered every other day or every two days. This process dilates the veins, arteries, hair follicles, and strengthens the body. It is useful for Vāyu disorders, hemorrhoids, dysuria, and other painful diseases.

A person either sits in a tub filled with a decoction until they begin to sweat, or sits in a tub and has oil, milk, or *ghee* poured over their shoulders until the liquid reaches six inches above their navel.

After the medicated bath, persons are first massaged, then take a warm bath (in plain water), and eat nourishing foods according to their *doṣha*. They rest for the remainder of the day.

The therapy sessions cease after one feels relief from cold, pain, stiffness, heaviness, and develops a good appetite and softness of body parts.

5. *Aṣhmaghana Sveda*, 6. *Karṣhū Sveda*, 7. *Kutī Sveda*, 8. *Bhū Sveda*, 9. *Kūmbhī Sveda, 10. Kūpa Sveda*, 11. *Holāka Sveda*: Other ancient forms that can be replaced by modern steam tents.

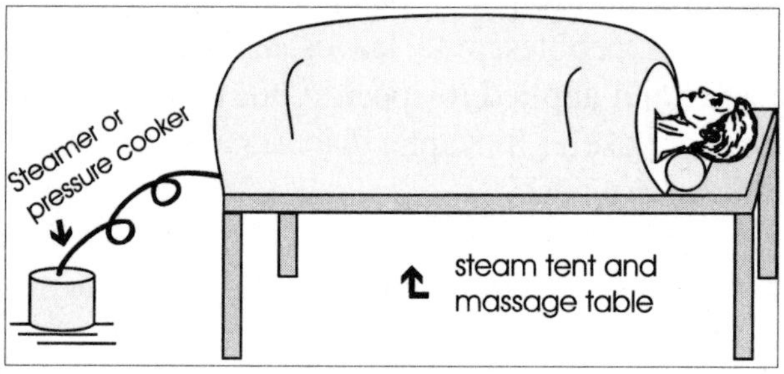

MODERN SWEAT-TENT

Partial Body *Svedas*

12. *Nāḍī Sveda*: Herbal decoctions are heated over a low flame in a pressure cooker, steamer, or covered pot with a hose placed over a hole in the top, and pointed at the sore spot (e.g., bursitis), joint pain, or other local condition.

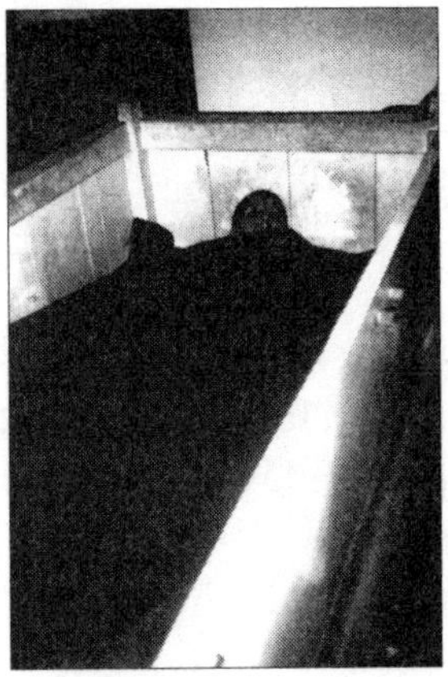

Sweat Box:
Woman with psoriasis undergoing svedana in India

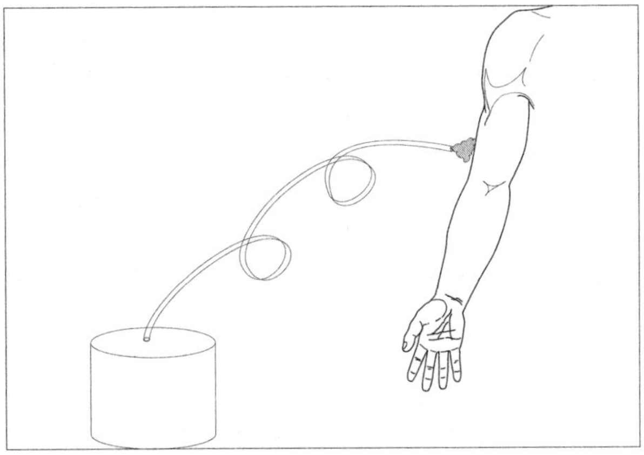

NĀḌĪ SVEDA

The tube has two or three curves to lessen the heat of the vapor. Traditionally, the hose lengths are either 91.44cm/@36" (high dose), or 45.86cm/@18" (low dose). The circumference of the tube is 22.86cm/@9" at the steamer and 11.43cm/@4.5" towards the body joint.

Aromatic, channel-clearing herbs (eucalyptus, cinnamon, camphor, calamus, sage, *daśhmūl* (10 roots) are used with emollient tonics (i.e., *śhatāvarī, balā, aśhwagandhā*, comfrey root, or marshmallow). Emollients are used to soften, protect and heal. Steam burns up localized toxins and restores or stimulates circulation at these sites.

Vāyu/Kapha—*daśhmūl*

Kapha—*varuṇa, guḍūchī, erand, vāsā, vaṃśha,* and *arka*.

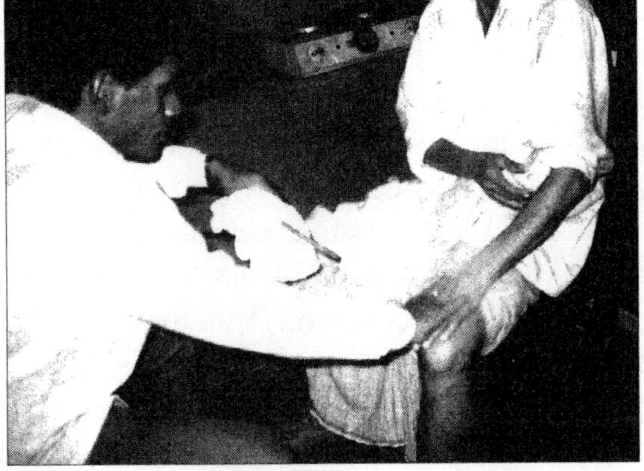

Man with hemiplegia undergoing
Naḍī Sveda in India

13. *Pariṣheka Sveda*: The specific body part that needs therapy is covered with a thin cloth. Then, a decoction made with herbs suitable for the condition is heated and poured into a pitcher that has small holes in its bottom. The pitcher is held over the body part and the decoction sprinkled over the cloth. Suitable ingredients include grape juice, sugar-cane juice, rice water, sugar water, yogurt, honey water, barley, cedar, *ghee*, acidic herbs, milk, and sweet herbs.

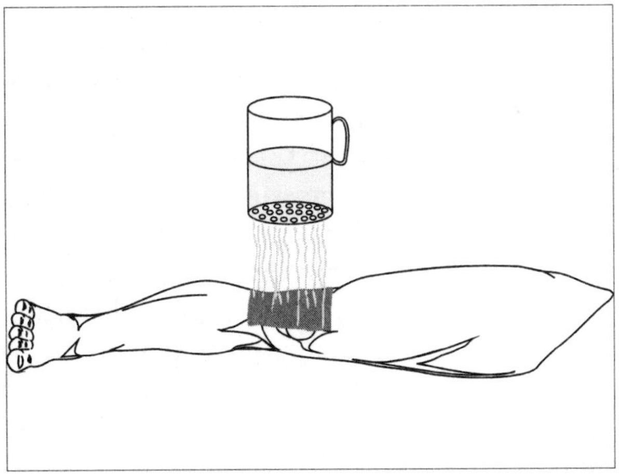

PARIṢHEKA SVEDA PITCHER

<u>*Sveda* Preparations</u>: Vāyu people must drink enough fluids before sweating. Sour juices like lemon or lime with a little rock or sea salt prevent dehydration and excess sweating. Caution is advised not to allow the steam to create excess dryness for Vāyu *doṣhas.* Kapha *prakṛiti* can promote stronger sweating by the use of long pepper, black pepper, and ginger (*tṛikatu*), or

some similar formulas. For Pitta *doṣhas* who have no Pitta diseases, burdock, dandelion, or red clover teas are drunk. This helps cleanse the blood. Hibiscus or other astringents help prevent excess sweating or heat buildup. It is advised not to overheat the Pitta *doṣha* with steam. All are advised to keep the head (and eyes), heart, and groin cool throughout the therapy. Cold, wet towels may be placed on these sites to prevent them from becoming overheated. A pearl necklace may also be placed on these sites to keep them cool.

Signs of Proper *Svedhana*: Sweat, reddish skin, body warmth and lack of chill or stiffness. Persons will feel more enthusiastic and light.

Contraindications: Sudation is not administered to the very obese, dry, weak, those with debilitating chest injuries, those suffering from emaciation, or to those with diseases stemming from alcohol usage or with alcoholism. It is not used for blindness, abdominal disorders (*udara roga*), herpes, skin diseases, TB, gout, or administered to those who have just eaten dairy, fats, and honey; nor is it used after purgation or for prolapse and burns of the rectum. Further symptoms requiring avoidance of sudation include heart disease, high blood pressure, blood disorders (e.g., anemia, leukemia), exhaustion, anger, grief, fear, excess hunger, thirst, sweat; and jaundice, Pitta diabetes, or Pitta diseases (chemical). Sudation is also not administered to pregnant or menstruating women (or those who have recently given birth). It is not given to one who has fainted, undergoing *sthambhana* (astringent) therapy, wasting, bleeding, diarrhea, low *ojas*, starving. In emergencies, people with these diseases are given mild sudation or *nāḍī sveda*.

Uses: *Svedhana* is given to those suffering from difficult breathing, cough, runny nose, hiccup, constipation, or hoarseness. It is used for Vāyu or Kapha diseases, *āma*/toxins, stiffness, heaviness, body aches, pain in the waist, ribs, back, abdomen, or lower jaw. *Svedhana* is used for an enlarged scrotum, toe or finger contraction, tetanus, sprains, or difficult urination. It is used for cancer or benign tumors, obstructions of semen or urine flow, obstinate Pitta urinary disorders, rigid thighs.

Although the main *pañcha karma* practices may take only a few days, these preliminary practices require 3 days to 3 months to work the toxins to the GI tract.

Once persons feel that heaviness, coldness, pain, and stiffness have been removed, they should rest for at least 3/4 of an hour before eating or drinking. No physical exercise should be done that day.

Cautions: Heavy application of oils can depress the digestive fire and cause digestive disorders (i.e., loss of appetite, constipation etc.). Beyond moderate use of oil, digestion-promoting herbs are suggested, like ginger, fennel, cardamom, or pepper. Further, the same effects may be gained by mild, daily oil application, and mild sweating herbs like diaphoretics and expectorants (e.g., ginger, calamus, cinnamon). These methods may be used over a longer time. Even if one follows this life regime of oils and sweating, it is suggested that one occasionally have a major *pañcha karma* therapy to. This can be done seasonally or yearly for to maintain good health.

Results of excess sweat therapy: Pitta and blood excesses, thirst, fainting, weak voice and body, giddiness, joint pain, fever, blue, black, or red skin patches, vomiting. To antidote the excesses, astringent therapy (i.e., light, cool, dry, bitter, astringent) and sweet therapy are used.

If one only follows the preliminary practices, then the toxins return to their site of accumulation, but are not removed. This may cause distress or disease as toxins can be reabsorbed and return to their site of accumulation.

For Vāyu *doṣhas*, failure to follow oil and sweating with an enema may create a variable appetite, gas, distention, constipation, and insomnia. Incomplete Pitta practices may cause irritability, fever, and hyperacidity. For Kapha *doṣha*, it may cause loss of appetite, fatigue, or constipation.

Post Svedhana

After sudation, persons receive a slow and gentle massage followed by a warm water bath (to calm the person and to wash off the toxins that have been expelled through the skin). A wholesome diet is followed thereafter. Exercise and drinking of cold water is are avoided on this day. Fresh air, a warm bath or shower, and a nap after lunch is advised.

Pañcha karma therapies (see below) are begun a set number of days after *svedhana,*

Vamana—second day after svedhana
Virechana—third day after svedhana
Basti, Nasya, Rakta Mokṣha—just after

Pañcha Karma (five actions) returns toxins to their sites of origin to be properly eliminated. This differs from most other healing systems that mainly flush the various organs or body systems regardless if the toxins are present. Once the toxins are removed from the organs and systems, no method exists to remove them from the body gently. Thus, many healers tell clients that they will feel bad for a few days as they detoxify, then they will feel better. With *pañcha karma*, the detoxification process happens without discomfort or withdrawal symptoms, and the body is completely rid of toxins.

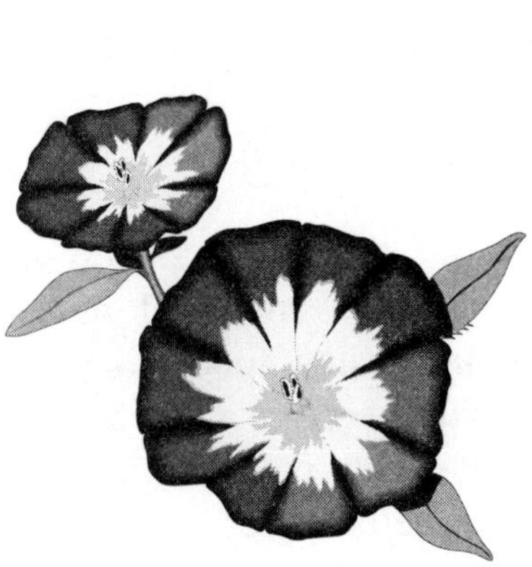

Pañcha Karma

Primary Practices (Pradhana Karma)

Pañcha karma consists of five cleansing aspects: emesis, purgation, medicated enemas, medicated nasal oils, and toxic bloodletting. These therapies are employed for acute diseases as well. For example, emesis (vomiting therapy) may be used during acute asthma attacks, obesity, and acute Kapha disorders. As mentioned before, the person needs to be strong before undertaking *pañcha karma* because these reducing therapies temporarily weaken the system.

Additionally, *pañcha karma* is used to prevent the accumulation of the humors, or as a seasonal health maintenance and a longevity/rejuvenation program. What is unique about this Āyurvedic approach is that it is used not only for healing, but also for prevention and rejuvenation (longevity).

Enemas that include tonics and nutritive herbs are also used in supplementation therapy, as they build tissues rather than reduce humors. Thus, *pañcha karma* offers various therapies that may be used in various ways, depending upon the person, disease, season, culture, etc. The milder therapies may be used seasonally in self-healing, prevention, and rejuvenation.

Therapeutic Vomiting (Vamana)

Of all the five *pañcha karma* therapies, this is the most dangerous; one can strain to vomit and damage the nerve reflexes. With proper guidance one learns the method for oneself or consults a qualified *pañcha karma* specialist. It is done regularly to cleanse the stomach and remove *āma* (toxins) and mucus from the *nāḍīs* (channels) and chest. It is used for relieving recent fever, diarrhea, pulmonary TB, and all lung conditions, skin diseases (e.g., eczema, psoriasis, leukoderma), diabetes mellitus, goiter, tumors, cough, asthma, and difficult breathing. *Vamana* is also useful for nausea, herpes, head and sinus diseases, allergies, chronic colds, rhinitis, rheumatic diseases, arthritis, viral disorders (e.g., herpes zoster), insanity, parasites (filariasis), bleeding of a downward nature, and excess salivation. It helps heal hemorrhoids, anorexia, cervical adenitis, edema, epilepsy, confusion, abscesses, and sore throats.

Vamana helps heal obesity, ear discharge, epiglottis, uvulitis, stiff neck, acute fever, Kapha fever, and nasal discharge. It is also useful for indigestion, gastro-enteritis, *alasaka*, poison, chemical burn, and diseases due to bad breast milk. When vomiting or heart diseases are due to Kapha, then *vamana* is also used (but never when Pitta causes these two diseases—as per the below caution).

छर्दिषु बहुदोषसु वमनं हितमुच्यते

Chardishu bahudoṣhasu vamanaṃ hitamuchyate - *Suṣhrut Saṃhitā.*

Vamana is used with Kapha excesses alone, or when Kapha is predominant while being associated with Vāyu or with Pitta.

Precaution: *Vamana* is not recommended for pregnant women, with other Vāyu excesses, before oleation, when hungry, under constant grief, for children, elderly, emaciated, Vāyu obesity, wounded, heart problems, high blood pressure, and vomiting (Pitta or Vāyu imbalances). It is not practiced with weakness, enlarged spleen or abdomen, blindness, intestinal parasites, upward movement of Vāyu (reverse peristalsis) bleeding, immediately after an enema, loss of speech, urine retention, or abdominal tumors. *Vamana* is not for those having difficulty with emesis, with strong digestive fire, hemorrhoids, giddiness, enlarged prostate, rib and chest pain, catchexia, thrush, fatigue, with excess sex, study or exercise; neurasthenia, constipation, helminthiasis, G.I. disorders, prostatitis, aphonia, cataracts, headaches, earache, eye pain, confusion, neuromuscular disorders, deficient emesis, or belching with edema.

Two types of *vamana* herbs exist:

a) Those that induce vomiting (*vamaka*). They are hot (circulating throughout the body, loosening and liquefying), sharp (separating qualities), and penetrating (throughout the body). Therapies include *kuṭaj,* salt water, licorice, and *vachā*.

b) Herbs that further help or enhance the inducing herbs (*vamanopaga*). Herbs include *pippalī, āmalakī,* rock salt, neem, and *madan phal.*

Time: The best time to practice is during the late spring or early summer (Kapha- provoking time) and close to the full moon when the water element is high, one day after *snehana* and *svedhana*, after a good sleep, after food is digested, or after sunrise—6:00 to 900 or 10:00 a.m. (Kapha time).

After 7 days of oleation and sweating, the skin should look shiny, soft, and slightly oily. Feces also should look shiny and oily, and increased in quantity. The smell of oil should be emanating from the skin and stool. These are indications that persons are ready for *vamana*.

Disease Origin	Ingredients
Kapha	*pippalī,* rock salt, warm water
Pitta	*vāsā,* neem, *pāṭola* cold water
Kapha/Vāyu	*mandan phal*, milk
Indigestion	rock salt

Method: Two to three days after *svedhana* (and after oleation), the evening before *vamana*, one eats Kapha-increasing foods like sugar, dairy, bananas, sesame seeds, and *urad dal*; causing Kapha excesses that make *vamana* more easily applied. Just before sleep persons can take 1/2 to 3/4 gram of *vacha* to stimulate secretions, further increasing stomach volume of Kapha. The heating effect of *vacha* begins to reduce the *āma* and, because heat rises, prepares the body for emesis.

The next morning the stomach remains empty (i.e., don't eat), causing further secretions to develop in surrounding tissues, promoting secretion movement to the stomach. After meditation persons undergo mild *snehana* and *svedhana*, increasing body temperature and insuring expansion of tissues and subtle channels.

Next one eats 1 1/2 cups of a thin, sweet-tasting porridge of rice or wheat cooked with milk, salt, and a little *ghee*. The use of Kapha-increasing foods and liquids coats the inner membranes and induces the need to vomit. After about an hour, one prepares a strong emetic tea like licorice, calamus, chamomile, or *madan phal*. This will promote immediate emesis. When the tea is properly prepared, persons will not feel sick or uncomfortable. The entire process lasts about one hour.

Recipe: The dose is 1 ounce of herbs to 2 cups of water. Alternatively, 2 tbs. of salt added to each cup of warm water may also be used. A third option is to soak *madan phal* powder in honey overnight and make into a paste. The next day 1/2 tsp. is licked with the tongue. These methods are emetic—or vomit-promoting. *Vamana* is not done on a full stomach (after eating). Another recipe using *madan phal* adds 4 parts of the herb with *vachā* (2 parts), rock salt (1 part), and is used with raw honey as its vehicle (*anupāna).*

If no urge to vomit exists, *pippalī*, *āmalakī*, *vachā* and salt are added to the tea. The properties of honey and rock salt liquefy the mucus. In order for *vamana* to proceed easily, persons can drink large quantities of licorice tea prepared the night before as a cold infusion (soaking the herb in room-temperature water). Licorice collects toxins from tissues without it being absorbed into the body itself.

a) Milder liquids include one or two cups of mild carminative tea (mint, fennel, etc.—2 tsp. herbs are infused into 1 cup of water). Children, the elderly, debilitated, impotent, and frightened people drink milk with raw sugar, honey, and rock salt. The amount ingested depends upon the severity of the illness. A moderate dose is 2 3/4 ounces of a decoction, fresh juice extract, or infusion; 1 3/4 ounces for powders or paste.

While facing the east, one should recite a prayer of health. (e.g., "May *Brahma, Dakṣha, Aśhwinīs, Rudra, Indra*, Earth, Moon, Sun, Air, Fire, Sages, medicinal plants, and all the creatures, protect me. May this therapy prove an effective rejuvenative for sages, nectar for the gods, and ambrosia for the best among serpents.") Then the liquid is drunk.

b) After drinking mild liquids the person waits 48 minutes before vomiting. Sitting on a seat parallel to the knees (some suggest squatting), one feels the reflex, then attempts to vomit. If unable to vomit, the person places a spoon or finger in the back of the throat (without harming the throat) to stimulate the emetic reflex. The head and ribs are supported by another person, and the navel and back are massaged in an upward direction. If excess Kapha exists, then Kapha-reducing herbs (e.g., hot or pungent) are also drunk. When excess Pitta exists, sweet and cold herbs are used. For Kapha/Vāyu diseases, salt, oily, and sour herbs are used. If Kapha is deficient, emetic herbs are used.

c) One makes sure the stomach is empty from vomiting. Once the vomit reflex occurs, it is advised to let it proceed all the way. Allowing for a few good reflexes is easier than many weak ones. This ensures the likelihood of not developing side effects. Four, six, and eight regurgitations define minimum, medium, and maximum bouts. Alternately, when the mucus and phlegm are released and bile begins to be expelled, or until there is a bitter, sour, or pungent taste in the mouth, one stops the process. If some of the licorice has entered the small intestine, persons may experience two or three loose stools over the next 12 hours.

The amount expelled during *vamana* is measured by the practitioner to determine proper elimination. For example, if persons drink 2 quarts of licorice decoction and expel 3 quarts, this last quart is the *āma* and excess Kapha. The color, consistency, and odor are also observed to provide more information on the effectiveness of the treatment.

Persons can follow a long-term emesis alternative with the daily use of expectorants like ginger, cardamom, and calamus or *ṭrikatu*. These herbs are taken with a mucus/Kapha-reducing diet and lifestyle.

Additional Decoctions

1. *Triphalā* may be added to the tea for excess salivation, gland disorders, fever, anorexia, and abdominal disorders.
2. Boiled milk is used for internal bleeding in a downward direction or burning sensation in the heart area.
3. Yogurt is used for Kapha-vomiting disorders, bronchial asthma, and salivation.
4. Cold yogurt (about 51/2 ounces) is taken to reduce pain in the chest, throat, or heart.
5. Butter is added for low digestive fire due to Kapha or when the body is dry.
6. Neem, *guḍūchī*, *bhṛiṅgrāj*, *pippalī*, *chitrak*, ginger, sesame seeds, and rice flower are used to reduce Pitta in a Kapha organ.

Results/Post *Emesis*: Outcomes of correctly administered emesis include calmness, ease, clarity, improved digestion, absence of symptoms of the illness, and not too much discomfort. After emesis, persons wash hands, face, and feet; and inhale herbal cigarettes. Sleep or rest is very important. After sleeping, hands, face, and feet are again washed. If hungry, light food is taken in liquid form (solid food is not taken for at least 4 hours when *manda* or rice water is ingested).

1. *Manda*: Is drinking only the lukewarm water in which white *basmati* rice is boiled. Some authorities suggest that a small amount of *ghee* and a pinch of black salt may be added to *manda*.

2. *Peyā*: The next meal is taken two hours later. *Peyā* is a slightly thicker rice liquid made of 8 parts water to 1 part white *basmati* rice. Rice is cooked until it is very soft, thin, light, and porridge-like. (Two or three meals of *peyā* are taken depending upon the degree of purification used.)

Rest is required for the remainder of the day, avoidance of speaking, strong emotions (e.g., worry), drafts, travel, sex, sun, and suppressing natural urges are required.

For mild purification, only 1 meal of *peyā* is required.

For moderate purification, 2 meals of *peyā* are required.

For strong purification, 3 consecutive meals of *peyā* are required. Meals are taken only twice daily, lunch (noon) and dinner.

3. *Vilepī*: After this, *vilepī* or thick rice soup, is served, consisting of 4 parts water to 1 part white *basmati* rice. A little sugar cane powder (e.g., turbinado sugar or Sucanat) and a pinch of black salt can be added for taste. A small slice of fresh ginger can be sautēed with turmeric, cumin, coriander, or fennel in a small amount of *ghee* to build the digestive fire. This is taken in the same manner (once, twice, or thrice).

4. *Odana*: The next meal is soft, plain *basmati* rice (*odana*), and vegetable soups. (Some authorities suggest omitting the vegetables.)

5. *Yuṣha:* Or rice and split yellow *mūng dal* soup meals are next taken with *ghee*, rock salt, and sour tastes added (some practitioners suggest avoiding the sour tastes). This meal begins on the third day after *vamana*.

6. *Kicharī*: Meals include *ojas*-increasing herbs (e.g., *guḍūchī*, *balā*, *aśhwagandhā*, *śhatāvarī*), depending upon one's *doṣha*. *Kicharī* starts thin (3 parts water to 1 part *basmati* rice and 1/4 part *mūng dal*). Next, it is prepared thicker using only 2 parts water to 1 part rice.

After this, regular meals are gradually introduced as the digestive fire grows stronger. Just as a fire is gradually increased from paper and twigs, to sticks, and then to logs until there is a strong flame, so then is food gradually increased after emesis naturally strengthening the digestive fire until it is strongly and healthily. The general rule of thumb is to eat only when hungry.

Alternative post-*pañcha karma* or *samsarajana* diets are listed below.

Meals	Food
1-3	thin gruel (*manda/peyā*)
4-6	moderate gruel (*vilepī*)—little or no *ghee* and salt with the meal. Drink warm water after the meal until the end of the 18 meals.
7-9	porridge and thin soup, *ghee,* and salt (*yuṣha/odana*)
10-12	thicker meal (grain and bean-*kicharī*), *ghee*, salt; drink warm water after meals
13	same, and add a sweet taste to the meal
14	same, and add a sour taste to the meal
15	same, and add a salty taste to the meal
16	same, and add a pungent taste to the meal
17	same, and add a bitter taste to the meal
18	same, and add an astringent taste to the meal
resume normal meals	

Post-Strong Dose Purgation Meal Plan

Day	11:00 a.m. - Noon	4:00 - 6:00 p.m.
1	*vaman*	thin gruel (*madan*)
2	thin gruel/*peyā*	thin gruel/*peyā* or /*vilepī*
3	moderate gruel/*vilepī* or *odana**	moderate gruel/*vilepī or odana**
4	moderate gruel/*odana**	mūng soup/*yuṣha*+
5	*mūng* soup/*yuṣha*+	*mūng* soup/*yuṣha*+
6	thicker *kicharī*	thicker *kicharī*
7	thicker *kicharī*	taste 1—sweet**
8	taste—sweet	taste 2—sour
9	taste 3—salty	taste 4—pungent
10	taste 5—bitter	taste 6—astringent
11	*normal meals from now on*	

*Moderate thickness gruel (*vilepī/odana*) is taken with little or no *ghee*. Drink warm water after all meals from this point until the end of the seven days.

+ *Mūng/yuṣha* soup is taken with a little *ghee* and salt; all remaining meals (of the seven days) will include *ghee* and salt.

** Some say to begin normal meals at this time.

Inadequate *Vamana*: If vomiting does not occur, or if it is only partially eliminated, symptoms develop such as itching, excess expectorating, itching, skin rashes, or fever.

Purgation (Virechana)

This is the simplest method of *pañcha karma* and has most easily observed effects. It is an excellent method to heal various conditions, including abdominal tumors, hemorrhoids, smallpox, patches of skin discoloration on the face, jaundice, chronic fevers, and enlarged abdomen. *Virechana* heals poisoning, vomiting, spleen diseases, abscesses, blindness, cataracts and other eye problems, colon pain, and colitis. It further heals vaginal diseases, diseases of the semen, intestinal parasites, ulcers, gout, bleeding diseases in the upward direction, blood toxins and diseases, suppression of urine, and obstructed feces.

Purgatives eliminate excess Pitta from its site in the liver, gall bladder, and small intestine (it does not deal with the large intestine). The bitter purgatives like rhubarb, senna, or aloe also clean the liver and gall bladder, decongest bile and remove obstructions to its flow. They are preferred for Pitta and liver disorders (e.g., gall stones). Because this cleansing weakens the digestive fire, it is not always recommended for Vāyu *doṣhas*. Kapha *doṣhas,* however, benefit from this therapy, as they have excess bile, congestion, fat, or phlegm. It also helps constipation, old fevers, acute diarrhea, dysentery, food poisoning, kidney stones, boils, carbuncles, excess bile, or toxic blood conditions.

For those who have not had *vamana* (emesis), there are 3 days of *snehapāna*, followed by 3 days of body oleation and sudation before beginning *virechana* (purgation). If *virechana* follows a *vamana* therapy, then after the 7 days of proper diet (*samsarjana*), 2 days of regular meals are eaten. On the 9th day, *snehapāna* (drinking *ghee)* is begun for 3 days. The following 3 days persons receives oil *abhyañga* and sudation for three additional days. On this 15th day (since starting *samsarjana*) *virechana* is begun. If sudation (sweating) is contraindicated, then *virechana* begins after the third day of *snehapāna* (drinking *ghee*).

Precautions: *Virechana* is not recommended for those people with recent fevers, poor digestion, bleeding diseases of a downward nature (e.g., hemorrhoids), ulcers, rectum ulcers, and diarrhea. Nor is it recommended for those who have recently received a decoction enema, have hardened feces, suffer from TB, and are greatly lubricated. It is not used for the very young or very old, the weak, debilitated or emaciated, while pregnant, during or immediately before menstruation, or with prolapse of the stomach or uterus.

Method: The stool is examined to determine the nature of the purgation therapy to be used. Soft stools suggest mild *virechana* (e.g., boiled milk, *ghee*, honey, and cinnamon), while hard stools will require stronger purgative herbs (like *triphalā*, castor oil, rhubarb, or senna). For Pitta disorders, herbs of astringent, and sweet tastes are added. Kapha excesses require pungent herbs. Vāyu disorders require rock salt, *ghee,* and hot herbs. It is important for persons to undergo 3 to 7 days of oleation (internal and external) before purgation if they haven't already gone through the process for *vamana*.

Time: According to *Aṣhṭāñga Hṛidayam*, the time of purgation is after *vamana* (emesis), and after 9:00 a.m. (the end of the Kapha time of day). This is done with rapidly acting purgatives. Others suggest medium to mild doses to be taken just before sleep. Still others suggest eating dinner around 7:30 p.m. and taking *virechana* 9:30 p.m., then retiring to bed. Some pundits say food should be fully digested while others suggest waiting two hours after the meal, until food passes out of the small intestine (fasting is advised for stronger people). The best season for *virechana* is late spring to early summer.

Sample Ingredients: A strong purgative like rhubarb root (it may produce gripping). A mixture of rhubarb (4 parts), fennel, ginger, and licorice (1 part each), taken with 2 to 5 grams honey or warm water before sleep to prevent gripping). Castor oil is a moderately strong purgative (2 tsp. in warm water). *Triphalā* (10 to 30 grams with warm water, or boiled milk with *ghee* and cinnamon) is a mild purgative. The first approach is the strongest and not suggested for those who are somewhat weakened or of Vāyu *doṣha*. [The *Suṣhrut Saṃhitā* devotes an entire chapter of additional purgatives (*Sūtrasthāna* - Ch. 44).]

Doṣha Excesses	Therapeutic Purging	Example Purgatives
Vāyu	hot, salty, oily	*triphalā, jaiphal, īśhabgol,* rock salt, ginger
Pitta	astringent, sweet	castor oil, *niṣhottar* rhubarb, *kaṭukā*
Kapha	pungent	rhubarb, senna, *tṛikatu, triphalā*

Result: The next day (or later that morning), about five stools (movements) are passed, flushing toxins from the small intestine. The number of stools can range from 4 to 15, depending upon the *doṣha*, health condition, etc. If one has fewer than 4 stools, the process is repeated within a few hours. Stools may be loose, but if cramping or griping results, a little medicated *ghee* can be taken, and cardamom or fennel should be added to future purgatives. Traditional stool amounts are 30 (maximum or ideal), 20 (moderate), and 10 (minimum), or until Kapha is expelled in the stool. An example of a quick acting purgative is castor oil with two times as much *triphalā*. Purgation can be done for 2 to 3 days in a row in severe conditions, or 2 to 3 times every other day. If one can schedule this day for a weekend or other calm day, it will be more beneficial, practical, and more relaxing. Mild, short-term purgation may also be used, as needed.

Successful purgation: This results in clear mindedness, keen senses, stable tissues, strong digestion, light, clean, strong, removal of symptoms, and slowed aging.

Abnormal Bouts: These are noted by symptoms of abdominal and heart discomfort, anorexia, expectorating bile and mucus, itching, burning, skin eruptions, rhinitis, gas, and no elimination of stools.

Excess Bouts: Symptoms include watery stool that are white, black, or red in color, rectum prolapses, thirst, giddiness, and sunken eyes.

Follow-up: Purgation is followed by hot spices to increase the digestive fire (e.g., ginger, *tṛikatu*). They are especially useful in the winter or, if the appetite does not return to normal, after the therapy. Meals are given as described for *vamana* (emesis) on page 189. After purgation and before any other purificatory therapies, oleation is again given to strengthen the person.

Lack of results: The person eats that day, and purgation is given again on the next day. For weaker people or those with unlubricated alimentary tracts, oleation and sudation are given for 10 days, and then purgation is re-administered.

Exceptions: Vāyu *doṣhas*, people who exercise vigorously, those with a strong digestive fire and those with dry alimentary tracts find that purgatives are digested before they produce the desired results. For these people, an enema (*basti*) is given first (see below).

Those suffering from trauma, skin problems, edema, herpes, jaundice, anemia, poisonous intake, and diabetes are given mild oleation, as this alone may produce the purging action.

Post-Virechana: Symptoms of successful *virechana* include feeling lightness in body, calmness of mind and in whom gas moves in a downward direction. Rice and a lentil *dal* soup are suggested as restorative meals.

Enema (Basti)

Enema is half of the medicinal therapy,
or even the complete treatment.
Charak- Sid. Ch. 1 verse 39

Basti therapy is primarily used for Vāyu

excesses, either alone, or as the predominant *doṣha* deranged. *Basti* is the *Sanskrit* name for urinary bladder. Originally the bladders of larger animals, like buffaloes and goats, were used as enema bags. The colon is related to all other organs and tissues, so by cleansing and toning the colon, the entire body is healed and rejuvenated. The colon is the main organ that absorbs nutrients. A healthy, functioning colon is imperative for proper assimilation of nutrients.

Basti is unlike Western enemas or colonics. Enemas only cleanse the rectum and sigmoid colon (only the lower eight to ten inches of the colon) causing an evacuating effect. Colonics remove feces blocks but may weaken the mucus membranes and dry the colon. This further imbalances Vāyu's normal elimination process. *Basti*, however, treats the entire length of the colon from the ileocecal valve to the anus. Not only is feces flushed from the system but also *āma* is removed from the tissues. Furthermore, balanced and healthy colon function is restored as tissues and organs are rebuilt.

General Benefits: *Basti* is useful for many disorders including chronic constipation, sciatica, lower back pain, arthritis, gout, and rheumatism. It also heals numerous neurological disorders like Parkinson's, MS, muscular dystrophy, paraplegia, hemiplegia, poliomyelitis, osteoporosis, and muscle and nerve atrophy. Further, *basti* helps with mental conditions such as Alzheimer's, epilepsy, mental retardation, and sensory disorders.

General Precautions: *Basti* is not used for babies, for diarrhea, ulcerative colitis, colon cancer, diverticulitis, rectal bleeding, polyps, fever, and some forms of diabetes.

Three types of *bastis* exist:

1. *Anuvāsana* (unctuous)—this enema remains in the body for some time without causing harm. Mainly herbal medicated oils and *ghee* are used. The amount of oil used in *anuvāsana basti* is 48 or 96 grams (1.7 oz. or 3.4 oz.). It is administered through the rectum. It is given to all those who are suited for *nirūha* (nonunctuous *basti*), especially those having strong digestion, to those not receiving oleation, and those with Vāyu diseases (only). This form of enema is given before *nirūha*.

This enema moistens dry tissues and organs, reduces hyperactive digestion, and Vāyu disorders, including nervous conditions. It is done in the day during the spring and on colder winter days; and in the night during the summer, the rainy season, and on milder winter days.

Anuvāsana Doses

Strength	*Basti* Dose	Rock Salt & Fennel
Maximum	10 oz.	4.5 gms.
Moderate	6.8 oz.	3 gms.
Minimum	3.4 oz.	1.5 gms.

The day after *basti* a warm ginger/coriander decoction is drunk to prevent any adverse effects from oleation.

2. *Nirūha* or *Āsthāpana* (non-unctuous)—This is a highly beneficial herbal decoction enema mixed with milk and a little oil. *Nirūha* is given to those with abdominal pain, distention, tumors, gout, splenic diseases, diarrhea (without other associated diseases), chronic fever, runny nose, obstructed semen, gas, or feces; enlarged scrotum, urinary stones, amenorrhea, or severe Vāyu disorders. It provides health to the healthy and gives strength to the tissues that are weak.

Strength	*Basti* Dose
Maximum	33.9 oz.
Moderate	27.7 oz.
Minimum	20.3 oz.

Symptoms of proper *basti* include feeling lightness in the body. Two, three, or four *nirūha bastis* can be given in a row.

Basti	Purpose	Ingredients
1st	to aggravate *doṣha*	rock salt, *vachā*, *pippalī*, licorice
2nd	pacify *doṣha*	licorice, *bilwa*, *kuṭaj*
3rd	normalize *doṣha*	licorice, *musta*, *prīyaṅgu*, milk

Simple Nirūha Basti
-1-3/4 cup *daśhmūl* herbal decoction
-1-1/2 oz sesame oil
-a little honey
-a pinch of black salt to increase colon secretions

3. Uttarabasti—is an upper-tract enema that uses a combination of decoction and medicated oils. It is delivered through the urethral and vaginal passages for the particular problems associated with these organs (page 197).

Precautions:
Enemas are not given for the following reasons,

Nirūha—This is not used for excess oleation, chest injury, severe emaciation, diarrhea with *āma* (toxins) or of a recent onset; vomiting, just after purificatory therapies, or just after *nasya* (nasal oil therapy). It is also contraindicated for asthma, coughs, salivation, gas, poor digestion, rectal swelling, taken before food is digested, or with an enlarged abdomen due to intestinal obstructions. This enema should not be used when clients suffer from perforated alimentary tracts and water, skin diseases, diabetes mellitus, or when women are in their seventh month of pregnancy. Other conditions when *nirūha* is not advised include after drinking *ghee*, with aggravated *doṣhas*, when fatigued, hungry, thirsty, overworked, angry, anxious, frightened, or drunk. It is also not used when there is difficult breathing, hiccup, *alasaka*, cholera, dysentery, urinary disorders, hemorrhoids, anemia, edema, anal inflammation, confusion, anorexia, coma, obesity dry throat, or lung injury. *Nirūha* is not used on the very young or very old.

Anuvāsana—This is not for persons unsuited for *nirūha*, nor for anemia, jaundice, diabetes, rhinitis, fasting, splenic diseases, diarrhea, constipation, and an enlarged abdomen from Kapha excesses. It is not suggested for those with eye problems, obesity, intestinal parasites, gout, goiter, lymphatic TB (swollen lymph glands), blood or tissue parasites, or for those who have consumed poisons.

Anuvāsana basti can be done the same day as *nirūha*. If symptoms persist, a second application can be given the 2nd, 3rd, or 5th day. The second *anuvāsana* can be stronger if stool is not passed within 48 hours.

Quantity:
Birth until 2 years old, 48 grams (@1.7 oz.) of liquid are used. [For emergency cases only]
2 to 13 years old, each successive year it should be increased by 48 grams (until it reaches 576 grams or about 20 oz.).
13 to 18 years old, each successive year by 96 grams/@ 3.4 oz. (until it reaches 1,152 grams or approximately 41 oz.).
18 + years old, 960 grams (@34 oz.) are used.

The amount of oil used is 1/4 that of a decoction, according to each age group.

Herbs

Vāyu	cedar, licorice, *vachā, bilwa, śhatāvarī, aśhwagandhā*
Pitta	licorice, *bilwa śhatāvarī*
Kapha	cedar, *vachā, bilwa, aśhwagandhā*

Method: After oleation (*snehana*), sudation (*svedhana*), (and if necessary) emesis (*vamana*), and purgation (*virechana*); after elimination, on an empty stomach, after performing prayers; considering one's *doṣha*, the proper herbs, the practitioner, and having other *basti* experts present, *basti* (enema) is given. If a person is strong and is so suited, an oil enema is given first. [According to the *Aṣhṭāñga Hṛidayam*, from September through March, enemas are given during the afternoon. In the remaining months, *bastis* are administered in the evening. Some suggest it be always given in daytime. Regarding time of year, some suggest *basti* during the late summer or early fall]. *Charak* says non-unctuous enemas can be given during the day in the winter and spring, and in the evening during the remainder of the year.

1. An oil massage (*abhyañga*) and bath are given, followed by an easily digestible meal (1/4 less the usual quantity). Afterwards, they drink a liquid then take a walk. Meditation or prayers are performed as well. Next the person evacuates stool and urine and then lies on a comfortable bed, neither too high nor low (*Charak* adds, on white sheets with head facing the East). They lie on their left side, with the left leg extended and the right leg bent (knee close to chest) for easier administration. A lubricated nozzle is inserted into the rectum, approximately six inches, after the air has been expelled from the enema bag. Fluids are slowly released into the colon. Some liquid is left in the bag to prevent air from passing into the rectum. Different herbs are made into a decoction to be used in the *basti* with the oil.

Symptoms	***Basti* Herbs**
legs, thigh, shoulder, neck	*vidārī kand, guḍūchī, harītakī,* ginger
sciatica, urinary problems, hunchback	*guggul, śhatāvarī*
Pitta diseases	*vāsāk, kaṭukā, mañjiṣhṭhā*
Kapha diseases	*triphalā*, neem

If stool, urine, or gas blocks the *basti* flow, a smaller dose is given to ensure the oil enters into the body (and not just the water).

2. After the *basti* is administered and the nozzle is removed, the person lies on their back while the practitioner gently hits the person's buttock several times. The person then slightly raises the heels and buttocks and gently pounds against the bed. Next, the foot of the bed is raised three times, followed by extending both legs. A pillow is then placed under the legs, and the person receives an oil massage, working out any painful or knotted spots. This helps the enema to stay in longer (if the enema is soon expelled, another oil enema is immediately given).

3. *Nirūha* or water-based *basti* is held in the body for about 48 minutes. *Anuvāsana* or oil *basti* must remain in the body for 9 hours. Should the elimination reflex cause early release of the fluids, they are re-applied.

If, after *anusāna,* the person has regained a strong digestive fire, they can eat a light meal in the evening. If the oil does not come out due to the excessive dryness inside the body, and the person feels good, it can remain inside overnight. It is expelled in the morning by drinking warm water. If it does not come out after 24 hours, the person is administered an herbal (fruit) rectal suppository or strong decoction enema. Signs of proper administration of enema include feeling relief from the toxins, and finding the oil being expelled along with the feces, followed by gas.

4. *Basti* is repeated on the 3rd or 5th day, or until the fat is well digested. Those with excessive dryness, or who exercise daily and have good digestion, receive daily oil enemas.

5. When the body becomes well lubricated, a purificatory decoction enema is given to clear the channels (*srotas*) 3 or 5 days after the unctuous enema (*Suṣhrut* suggests the same day). It is given in the afternoon, after the person digests a light meal, and after oleation, sudation, elimination of feces, urine, and meditation. The strength of the decoction depends on the strength of the client.

After receiving an oil enema, a decoction enema is given to restore balance between toning and reducing. This balances all three *doṣhas.* Oil enemas are given after a span of three days so as not to impair the digestion. For extreme Vāyu excesses and dryness, oil enemas may be given daily.

Doṣha	Enemas	Basti Herbs
Vāyu	9-11	*daśhmūl, balā, punarnavā, bilwa, guḍūchī, śhatāvarī*
Pitta	5-7	sandalwood, *mañjiṣhṭhā, musta*
Kapha	1-3	rock salt, *vachā, bilwa, pippalī*

Oil is used for unctuous enemas.
Pitta *doṣhas* may use *ghee.*

Results of Nine Bastis

An ideal therapy consists of a series of nine enemas.

1st permeates the inguinal and pelvic region with demulcent properties
2nd restores Vāyu in the cephalic part of the head
3rd improves body strength and complexion
4th permeates the plasma (*rasa*)
5th permeates the blood (*rakta*)
6th permeates the muscles/flesh (*māṃsa*)
7th permeates the fat (*medas*)
8th permeates the bones (*asthi*)
9th permeates the marrow (*majjā*)

This series is repeated twice; once without oil, once with oil.

Non-unctuous *(nirūh*a) enemas promote longevity, intelligence, voice, complexion, and draw out feces, mucus, bile, and urine. Unctuous (oil) enemas (used after non-oil enemas) help the complexion, strength, Vāyu, mental clarity, energy, and weight. After oil enemas, fasting is advised for the rest of the day. Oil enemas are best for conditions of the head, heart, bladder, and Vāyu excesses. Pain, numbness, and swelling may develop when Vāyu is obstructed by fat or Kapha. For these situations, unctuous enemas are not advised as they will aggravate the fat and Kapha conditions.

The number of enemas suggested are traditional, but in today's fast-paced life, it may not be practical or necessary for persons to take so many enemas. Readers and practitioners are advised to use intuition and evaluate the results even one or two enemas produce before possibly forcing more sessions. Just as the dose of herbs has been found to be much less in the west than in India, so too *vamana, virechana*, and *basti* may need to be applied in moderation.

Post-Enema Precautions: It is always best to stay on a wholesome diet, but if this is not possible, persons should eat properly for at least double the length of the *basti* therapy. For example, if one undergoes a nine-day *basti* program, healthy foods should be eaten for at least 18 days immediately afterwards. Otherwise, persons may feel worse than they did before they began the *basti* therapy.

After *basti* one is also advised to avoid excesses of any kind, such as prolonged sitting, standing, speaking, travel, naps, coition, cold, sun, grief, wrath, and suppression of natural urges.

If too much oil has been administered during *basti* and excess pressure exists, one may experience aversion to food, an oily or greasy complexion, an oily smell in the mouth, coughing, difficult breathing, and dull senses. Also, each person may develop symptoms specific to their *doṣha*.

Vāyu— astringent taste in mouth, yawning, shivering, limb pain, Vāyu discharges, *viṣhamsa* fever (i.e., malaria, viral fever, or fever due to injury).

Pitta—fever, burning, thirst, perspiration, pungent taste; yellowish complexion, urine, and eyes.

Kapha—water brash, sweet taste in mouth, heaviness, vomiting, difficult breathing, mucus, fever, food aversion.

Receiving inadequate or cold enemas (either dry or oily) without proper pre-cleansing can produce scanty stools, cramps, heaviness, distended intestines, or constipation.

Enemas after a heavy meal cause cramps, a heavy stomach, no release of gas, heart problems, bad taste or food aversion. If oleation, sudation, proper diet, and elimination of stool have not been done properly, one may experience heavy limbs, colic, abdominal distention, difficult breathing, or heavy intestines.

Decoction Enema (Nirūha Dravya Kalpanā)

Preparation: (The recipe in *Aṣhṭāñga Hṛidayam* Sū.; Ch 19, verse 381/2-40, is as follows), 960 grams (34 oz.) of the herbs appropriate for ones *doṣha* (constitution) are made into a decoction. [Herbs are boiled with 16 parts water (approximately 4.2 gallons over a low flame) until 1/4 of the water remains (about a one-gallon decoction). Next oil or *ghee* is added to the decoction, in the amount of 1/4 of the decoction for Vāyu, 1/6 quantity for Pitta, and 1/8 quantity for Kapha. 1/8 quantity of medicated paste is sometimes added, making the decoction neither too watery nor too thick. Lastly, 48 grams (@1.8 oz.) of raw sugar cane (*jaggery*) or molasses is added, along with similar doses of honey and salt, depending upon the *doṣha*].

(The author *Vāgbhata*, notes other views: oil and honey are each 144 grams (5.1 oz.), salt for the strong person is 12 grams, (.42 of an ounce) medicinal paste is 96 grams (3.4 oz.). All other liquids are 480 grams (17 oz.). Further, *Charak* offers a breakdown similar to the *Aṣhṭāñga* formula for oil enemas:

1 year old 40 grams (@1.5 oz.).

2 to 12 years old—each year an additional 40 grams is added.

12 to 18 years old—80 grams (@3 oz.) are added each year until it reaches 960 grams (@34 oz).

18 to 70 years old— 960 grams.

70 +— 800 grams (@28 oz.).

The order of mixing ingredients is honey, salt, oil (or *ghee*), paste, and decoction. The ingredients are well mixed and mildly warmed before being administered to the person.

The flow of the enema should be moderate (i.e., not too forceful). After receiving the enema, the person lies on their back with a pillow under their head, concentrating on the enema. When the elimination urge presents itself, they should squat on their heels to expel the enema and wastes. If the enema should stay in for 48 minutes, it becomes critical to expel it. Various substances, including oils, alkalis, hot and sour properties, are immediately given. Alternatively, an herbal (from fruit) suppository is given, along with sudation and—even frightening the person, so as to expel the enema.

Decoctions may be given several times until the person feels relief from the toxins. Once they are feeling better they take a warm bath to remove any lingering complications due to the enemas. Food consists of rice and soothing herbal teas with *ghee*. If the enema increases Vāyu, an oil enema is immediately given.

Charak suggests, that once the enema is expelled, the person should be sprinkled with cool water and given boiled rice. Later in the evening, after the earlier meal is digested, the person eats a small and easily digestible meal. Then an oil enema is given to restore bulk.

Herbs used in decoctions by *Charak* include *guḍūchī*, *gokṣhura*, sandalwood, *triphalā*, *daśhmūl*, *bilwa*, *vachā*, *musta*, *pippalī*, also *jaggery*, honey, *ghee*, oil, and rock salt.

Sample Decoction Basti

Calamus, ginger, fennel, 1-2 tsp. rock salt, and up to 1/2 cup sesame oil, per quart of decoction. Licorice, other demulcents, or oil is used because the enema may be too drying or depleting. Cleansing enemas are followed with an oil enema (1/2 cup sesame oil in 1/2 cup warm water). This balances all three *doṣhas*.

Helps: Chronic constipation, colitis, arthritis, epilepsy, paralysis, anxiety, neurosis, insomnia, sciatica, lower back pain, kidney disorders, neuralgia, and Vāyu disorders.

Note: *Vamana, virechana,* and *basti* are not given to people before age 10 or after age 70.

Urethral Basti (Douche)

For complications of urine, genital tract pain, prolapsed uterus, urine retention or incontinence, menorrhagia, and during the menstrual cycle, douches are advised. During menstruation the uterus is not covered; therefore, it receives unction very easily. This allows for easy release of Vāyu.

After a meal (with *ghee*), passing stool, urine, and after bathing, a person sits comfortably on a straight, soft, knee-high seat. The catheter is introduced gently into the orifice, neither too deep nor too shallow. The nozzle is greased with *ghee* and 20 grams (.7 of an ounce) of a decoction and is inserted into the body. As the decoction is expelled, the process is repeated another two times. If the third decoction is not released, it is all right. Decoction herbs include *pippalī*, black salt, *apāmārga*, mustard, *nirguṇḍī*, and cane sugar. The same procedures, restrictions, complications, and signs of proper application of unctuous enemas apply to douching.

For women, the catheter is 10 finger-widths long. It is inserted into the genital tract up to four finger-widths deep. In the urethra, it is inserted up to about two fingers deep. The catheter is easily inserted while the woman lies on her back, with legs fully flexed. Douche is given 2 to 4 times over the course of 24 hours. After the douche, a somewhat thicker suppository is inserted. This therapy continues for 3 days, with the dose gradually increased. After a 3-day rest, the procedure is repeated.

Nasal Therapy or Snuff (Nasya)

Āyurveda suggests that the nose is the gateway to the head. Thus, nasal herb therapy is used for healing diseases of the throat, neck, head, and senses (e.g., ears, nose, eyes, etc.). *Nasya* is also used for toning and strengthening these areas.

Nasya is useful in relieving stiffness in the head, neck arteries, throat, and jaw obstructions, coryza, uvulitis, tonsillitis, cornea, vision and eyelid disorders, migraines, disorders of the neck, shoulders, ears, nose, mouth, head, cranium, and scapula. It helps facial paralysis, convulsions, goiter, pain, tingling sensation, loose teeth, tumors, hoarse voice, speech disorders, and Vāyu disorders of the mind, head, neck, and throat. *Nasya* is also helpful in head diseases caused by Kapha (e.g., stiffness, numbness, heaviness). Saturating *nasyas* are recommended for Vāyu disorders (e.g., facial paralysis, trembling head). Pacifying *nasyas* are useful for internal bleeding and other Pitta head and neck disorders.

Snuff is suggested three times daily in the rainy, autumn, and spring seasons when there are no clouds in the sky. Snuff is said to improve vision, smell, and hearing; keep hair from graying and falling out; prevent stiff neck, headache, and lockjaw. It is also said that snuff relieves chronic rhinitis, and head tumors. The veins, joints, ligaments, and tendons of the skull gain greater strength. The face becomes cheerful and well developed; the voice becomes more melodious. (See *Charak: Sū.* Chapter 5; verse 56-62 and *Suṣhrut:* Chapter 50 for further information.)

Nasya herbs include *balā, viḍaṅga, bilwa* and *musta*. They are made into an oil decoction with various other ingredients.

Three kinds of *nasyas* exist:

<u>1. *Virechana*</u> (purgatives)—for headaches, eye problems, throat problems, swellings, enlarged glands, parasites, tumors, skin diseases, epilepsy, rhinitis, and loss of head movement. Ingredients include the appropriate oil, herbal powders, pastes, or decoctions; and are mixed with honey and salt.

Virechana is of two types: *avapīda* (fresh herb juices) and *pradhmāpana* (blowing of herb powders through a tube). For formula, see below.

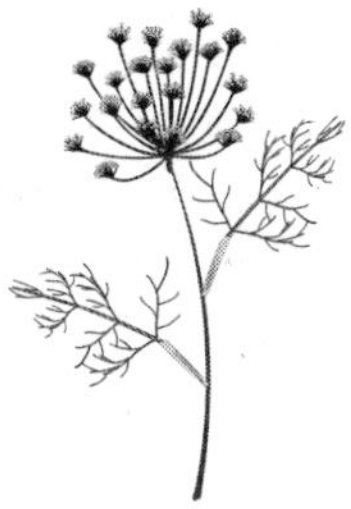

Ingredient	Dose
pungent herb (e.g., *pippalī*)	3 gms.
hiṅgu	31.25 mgs.
rock salt	750 mgs.
milk, water, or decoction	24 gms.
sweet: raw honey, or sugar	12 gms.

2. Briṃhaṇa (nourishers)—for Vāyu headaches, migraines, loss of voice, dry nose and mouth; difficulty speaking, opening eyes, or moving the arms. Medicated oils help with premature graying and hair loss; ringing in ears, neck, shoulder, and arm disorders; dental problems, and headache on either side of the head. It is also highly beneficial for degenerative brain disorders such as Alzheimer's, MS, epilepsy, and mental retardation. Ingredients include medicated *ghee* and extracts from plants.

3. Śhamana (palliatives)—for discolored patches on the face, blue patches on the skin and for hair and eye diseases. Ingredients include medicated *ghee*, milk, or water.

There are two general methods to administer *nasyas*: powder form (blown through a tube); and liquid drops (4, 6, 8 drops—minimum, moderate, maximum). Traditional powder quantities are 6 grams, but even 1/2 gm. may be effective for westerners. The tub length is 6 *aṅguli* long (6 finger widths).

Five forms of *nasya* are used: snuffing, pressing, blowing, smoking, and smearing. Two categories of snuff exist: uncting and evacuating. Also, 2 types of pressing are available: evacuating (*śhiro virechana*) and retaining *(nasya)*. Blowing of powders into the nose cleans the body channels (*srotas*). Smoking has 3 categories: pacifying, evacuating, and saturating. Smearing promotes both evacuating and pacifying results. The two most effective methods are powder (inhaled through a tube) and liquid drops (4, 6, 8 drops—minimum, moderate, maximum).

Nasya

Snuff	Press	Blow	Smoke	Smear
unct	retain	cleanse	saturate	
			pacify	pacify
evacuating	evacuating		evacuating	evacuating

Snuff—uncting *(nasya)* and evacuation (*śhiro virechana*) are the most effective forms of *nasya*. Snuff is subdivided into five categories, as shown in the chart above.

1) Uncting *(Sneha)*: Oil increases deficient oily matter of the brain, reduces feelings of void or emptiness, tones nerves and muscles in the neck, shoulders, and chest. It improves eyesight, balding, premature graying, loose teeth, earaches, cataracts, dry mouth, nose disorders, loss of voice, Vāyu-head disorders, and wrinkles. Vāyu- and Pitta-reducing herbs are used. Four, 6, or 8 drops constitute the minimum, moderate, and maximum doses. Other sources suggest using only 3 drops.

2) Evacuating *(Śhiro-virechana)*: Powders of *pippalī, viḍaṅga, apāmārga*, or any oil mixed with these herbs, is used to reduce Kapha and mucus in the throat, palate, or head. This procedure helps with food aversion, headache, heavy head, cold, coryza, hemicrania (headache on one side of the head), edema, skin disorders, epilepsy, laryngitis, worms, and hysteric convulsions. Four, 6, or 8 drops are the minimum, moderate, and maximum doses.

3) *Pratimarṣha*: This is also an uncting procedure in which oil is dropped into the nose and expelled through the mouth. *Suṣhrut* says, 1 to 3 drops, or whatever amount it takes for the oil to move through the nose and reach the mouth. *Suṣhrut* also suggests that oil be used for Vāyu and Kapha *doṣhas*, and *ghee* be used for Pitta *doṣhas*. However, any medicated Pitta-reducing oil is also

suggested by other writers (e.g., *brāhmī* oil). *Pratimarṣha* is useful for those who are wounded, emaciated, children, and the elderly; and at all times and seasons (including rainy weather). It strengthens the senses, helps prevent premature graying and hair loss, thirst, head and mouth diseases, and all disorders above the shoulders.

4) *Avapīda*: This is an evacuative procedure. Fresh pungent herbal juice is dropped into the nose. Then the nostrils are pressed with both palms. Four, six, or eight drops constitute the minimum, moderate, and maximum doses. This method helps with tridoṣhic fevers, throat disorders, excess sleep, parasites, and mental disorders (including epilepsy and insanity). Some ingredients, for example, are licorice, black pepper, *vachā,* and rock salt, made into a liquid with warm water.

5) *Pradhmāpana*: (or *pradhamana*) This is another evacuative method. Here, evacuating six gms. of herbal powders are blown into the nostrils through a tube six *aṅguli* (six finger widths). It is useful for those with extreme *doṣha* imbalances (e.g., unconsciousness). Ingredients include rock salt and *tṛikatu.*

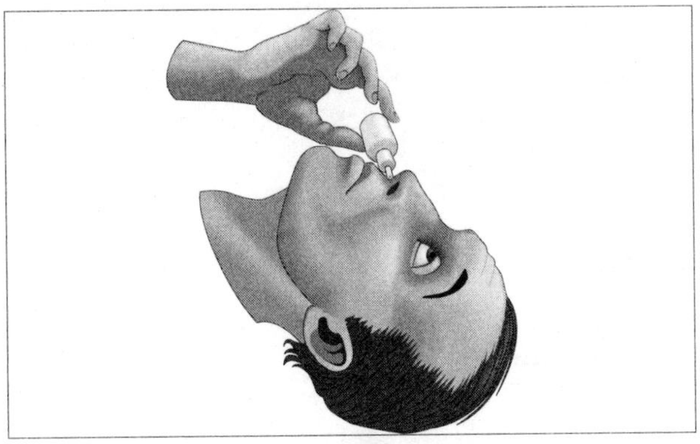

NASYA

Precautions: It is not advised to take *nasya* when thirsty, after a meal or a fast, just before or after bathing, with acute rhinitis, the last few months of pregnancy, during menstruation, just after asthma attacks or with difficult breathing, colds or coughing. *Nasya* is also not used just after oleation, emesis, purgation, *basti*, after sex or drinking too much water or alcohol; on sunless days, with acute coryza, anger, grief, fatigue, when excited or suppressing natural urges. Further, it is not used during bad weather or for children under 7 years old, and the elderly over 80 years of age.

Pratimarṣha is not used after wine, when weak, with head-worms, and when *doṣhas* are greatly excessed and move around.

Time: *Nasyas* are taken before meals. Kapha *doṣha* take these *nasyas* in the morning, Pittas in the afternoon, and Vāyu *doṣhas* in the evening or night. Healthy persons take snuff in the morning in the summer, afternoons in the winter and rainy seasons (when it is not cloudy). Snuff is not taken during the early rainy season, fall, and spring, except during emergencies. Then, it is taken in the morning.

Nasya is taken daily, both morning and evening, for Vāyu head disorders, hiccup, tetanus, convulsions, stiff neck, and for a hoarse voice. For all other diseases it is taken only once daily for 7 days.

Method: *Nasya* is taken after elimination of stool and urine, brushing teeth, smoking herbs and receiving oleation (oil massage) to the neck, cheeks, and forehead. The palms are first rubbed together until warm and then placed over the face (as fomentation). Alternatively, a warm wash cloth may be placed over the sinuses. This process begins to loosen toxins and expand the channels for easier toxin elimination.

Next, the persons lie on their backs on a bed in a room with no drafts. Feet are slightly raised and the head is slightly lowered. The limbs are extended.

Nasya oil is slightly warmed and then inserted into the nostrils, (right nostril first), while the other nostril is kept closed. Oil is sniffed up into the head. To better achieve this effect, nostrils may be closed with the fingers while inhaling through the nose begins. Then fingers are released, causing a sudden rush of air into the nostrils. This process can be done five to ten times.

Afterwards, the soles, neck, palms, ears, and face are fomented again with warm palms, and gently massaged. Turning to the side, persons spit out any oil that may have reached the mouth and throat. This procedure is taken two to three times. Should fainting occur, cold water is sprinkled over the body (but not the head). After a purgative *nasya*, a medicated oil *nasya* is administered (according to one's *doṣha*). Persons lie on their backs for about two minutes, inhale smoke from various herbs, then gargle with tepid water several times to cleanse the throat from the *nasya*.

Doses - Drops per nostril

Nasya	Small	Medium	Large
Snuff	8/8	16/16	32/32
Evacuative	4/4	6/6	8/8
Pratimarṣha	2/2	2/2	2/2

In the above chart, *Suṣhrut* suggests the number of drops applied in each nostril, for small, moderate, and high *nasya* doses.

Results of effective *nasya* include feeling lightness in the head, clear passages, easing of the original symptoms, clear mind and senses. If *nasya* has been done in excess, dry foods are eaten to restore balance. If *nasya* has been insufficient, *ghee* is taken.

For more serious health concerns, the process is followed for 7 days. After a few days rest, the process can again be repeated for 14 days. After a few days rest, *nasya* is again give for 21 days.

Suggested times for therapeutic administration are shown below.

Doṣha	*Nasya Time*
Vāyu	3:00 - 6:00 a.m./p.m.
Pitta	Noon and/or midnight
Kapha	6:00 - 9:00 a.m./p.m

Remedies	Disorders
Sweets (e.g., honey raw sugar, *śhatāvarī*), medicated oils	neck, shoulders, anus, dry mouth, ear ringing, Vāyu and Pitta excesses, premature gray hair, balding, fright, females, children, weak persons, head, nose, eyes, migraines, teeth, hemicrania
Pungent herbs	above shoulder diseases, loss of voice, anorexia, cold, headache, chronic rhinitis, edema, epilepsy, skin disorders
Avapīda (fresh pungent herb juice)	throat, toxic/tridoṣhic fever, excess sleep, remittent fever, mental disorders, parasites
Pradamana (e.g., rock salt, *vachā*, black pepper, ginger,	serious disorders (e.g., unconsciousness)
Cane sugar, *pippalī*, black salt, ginger	eye, ear, nose, head, neck, lower throat, jaw, shoulders and back diseases
Vachā, black pepper, black salt	insanity, epilepsy, severe (tridoṣhic) fevers, tetanus

Results: Generally, all nasyas promote clarity, sharp senses, and improved sleep patterns. The use of purgatives includes relief of eye strain and tension, clean mouth, and clear voice.

Results of Pratimarṣha Nasya

Time of Use	Benefits
Upon waking in the morning	removes waxy mucus in the nose, cheerful mind
after brushing teeth	sweet aroma, taste, firm teeth
before leaving home	safeguards from smoke, dust, pollution
after exercise, coition, travel	removes fatigue
after stool/urine	removes dull/heavy vision
after gargling, eye salve	invigorates the eyes
on an empty stomach	cleans/lightens inner channels
after emesis	cleans mucus in ducts, stimulates appetite

Specific Therapies

The *Śhāṅgadhara Saṃhitā* outlines therapies for specific health concerns and their doses. *Virechana,* or evacuative *nasya,* is divided into two kinds, *avapīda* (fresh pungent herb extract juice) and *pradhmāpana* or *pradhamana* (blowing pungent herbal powders in the nose).

Ingredients: Various cleansing herbs are used as snuffs, decoctions, oils, *ghee*, and smoking to heal the nasal passageways and head. Herbs used are calamus, cloves, gotu kola, bayberry, sage, and basil. *Nasya* works directly on the *prāṇa* and brain, and it is good for all *doṣhas*, though smoking may aggravate Vāyu or Pitta. It is useful in helping the sinuses by using expectorant herbs, including *vāsāk*, ginger, and black pepper.

Sinuses and brain: Gotu kola or calamus oil, or *ghee* are used.

Nasal passages: Cloves, calamus, and bayberry are smoked.

Doṣhas:

Vāyu persons take nutritional *nasyas*.

Pitta/Vāyu persons use herbal sedatives.

Nasal massage is also suggested to release emotions that can be stored in the nose.

Kapha *doṣhas* use calamus or gotu kola to relieve headaches, heavy or lethargic heads, colds, running noses, sticky eyes, hoarseness, sinusitis, tumors, epilepsy, chronic rhinitis, attachment, greed, and lust.

Nutritional *Nasya*: For Vāyu *doṣha*. *Ghee*, oils, or salt are used for migraines, dry voice or nose, nervousness, anxiety, fear, dizziness, emptiness, negativity, stiff neck, dry sinuses, or loss of sense of smell.

Sedative *Nasya*: For Pitta *doṣha*. Use aloe vera juice, warm milk, *aśhwagandhā,* or gotu kola juice/oil; for hair loss, conjunctivitis, or ringing in the ear.

Oil *Nasya*: For all *doṣhas*. Decoctions and oils together are used.

Complications: Symptoms of inadequate *nasya* include deranged senses and dryness. As an antidote to this, *nasya* is repeated using the proper amounts. Excess, deficient, cold, hot, or sudden *nasya* may cause thirst, belching, and aggravation of the condition.

Nasal Massage: Pinky fingers are dipped into the oil needed and gently inserted into the nostrils (one at a time) as deep as comfortably possible. The passage becomes lubricated through a gentle massage. This relaxes the deeper tissues and can be done every day or whenever under stress. First the massage is done clockwise, then counter-clockwise.

Blood-letting
(Rakta Mokśha)

(Therapeutic toxic blood-letting) involves releasing toxic blood from various body sites, although mainly from the back. At first, blood should be dark or purplish. When it turns bright red, therapy is complete. Two to 8 ounces is the general amount of blood released. Sometimes various sensitive sites require only a prick to relieve problems. For example, at the eyebrow a prick relieves headaches, and eye inflammation. This process is no longer used in India as often as it once was. In some countries a professional license is required in order to practice this therapy. Blood-letting is useful when wishing for immediate results with Pitta disorders such as skin, liver, spleen, and conditions like gout, headaches, and hypertension. Late summer through early fall is the best time for this procedure.

<u>Precautions</u>: *Rakta mokśha* is not used on babies, the elderly, during pregnancy or menstruation, or with anemia, edema, leukemia, bleeding, or cirrhosis.

Smoke Inhalation Therapy
Dhūma

Daily use of smoke inhalation is used for cough, asthma, chronic rhinitis, voice disorders, bad smell in the nose or mouth, pallor, hair disorders, mucus, itching, and pain. It is also used for loss of hearing, taste, or sight; stupor, hiccup, heavy head, head or neck pain, hemicrania, earache, eye pain, throat or jaw spasm, weak teeth or toothache, ear, eye, or nose discharges, worms, sneezing, fatigue, dull intellect, Vāyu or Kapha diseases, and excess sleep.

Vāyu *doṣhas* use lubricating smoke (*snigdha*), Vāyu/Kapha *doṣhas* use medium or *madhya* smoke, and Kapha constitutions use *tikṣhna* or strong smoke therapies. Like other therapeutics discussed, the categories of smoke fall into the categories of mild, palliative, purificatory, or purgative.

Strength	Herbs
Mild (lubricate)	*guggul, musta, bilwa,* cardamom, *madanaphal,* saffron, sesame oil, and *ghee*
Medium (palliative)	*utpala*, licorice, *kuṣhtha,* aromatics
Strong (purgative)	frankincense, *vachā, daśhmūl, triphalā*

Others suggest two medicated smokes, and one oil smoke daily. The result is the cleansing of the heart, throat, senses, lightness of the head, and pacifying of the *doṣhas*. For calming the mind, sandalwood, *jaṭāmāṇśhī*, etc. are useful.

<u>Mild</u> (lubricating) herbs are inhaled after sneezing, yawning, defecation, urination, copulation, surgery, laughing, and brushing teeth. It is done once a day. Ingredients include *guggul, musta*, sesame, and *ghee*.

<u>Medium</u> (palliative) herbs are inhaled at the end of the night, after meals, and after *nasya* therapy. Inhalation is done only once a day. Herbs include licorice and (naturally) perfumed scents.

<u>Strong</u> (purgatives) are used upon waking from sleep, after *nasya*, washing eyes, bathing, and vomiting. Smoke is inhaled four times daily. Herbs used include *triphalā*, *vachā* (calamus), and frankincense.

6 Forms of Dhūma

Bṛiṃhaṇa (toning)
Rechana (purgative)
Kāsaghna (cough-reducing)
Vamana (emetic)
Vraṇadhūpan (ulcer fumigation)
Śhamana (palliative)

Time: The procedure is to take 3 puffs 3 times. Some authorities suggest smoking 8 times during the day for Vāyu and Kapha excesses, after bathing, meals, vomiting, sneezing, brushing teeth, after snuff, eye-salve application, and sleep.

Others suggest two medicated smokes and one oil smoke daily. The result is the cleansing of the heart, throat, senses, lightness of the head, and pacifying of the *doṣhas*.

Precautions: Smoke inhalation is not recommended for people who have bleeding disorders, have completed purgation therapy (*virechana*), or enema (*basti*); or who suffer from enlarged abdomen, diabetes, blindness, Vāyu moving upward (e.g., belching), flatulence, or have just eaten fish, wine, yogurt, milk, honey, *ghee,* or oils, or have ingested poison, or have head injuries, anemia, and insomnia. Smoking at improper times results in bleeding disorders, blindness, deafness, thirst, fainting, delusions, and intoxication (they are countered by cold). Exhalation through the nose causes loss of vision; exhale only through the mouth.

Herbal smoke inhalation is not given until 18 years of age (some say after age 12). [Mouth gargle begins at age five].

Excess/Untimely Smoking: Symptoms include deafness, blindness, dumbness, vertigo, internal hemorrhaging. Antidotes include using *ghee* snuff, and eye salve. Cooling herbs are used for blood disorders. Rough herbs are used for Kapha and Pitta disorders (e.g., cardamom, *kūt*, black pepper).

Preparation of Smoke Wick: A reed, 12 finger-widths in length, is soaked in water for 24 hours, then wrapped in 5 layers of cloth and smeared with a thin paste of the appropriate herbs.The herbs are left to dry; then the reed and cloth are removed. *Ghee* or sesame oil is added to the herbs. Then, herbs are inserted into a pipe, and lit. Others suggest that the tube be in 3 pieces, one fitting snugly into the other, and that the inner tube be the thickness of the pinky finger. For coughs, powdered herbs are placed on hot coals, and a tube is used to inhale the smoke.

Pipe lengths vary. For evacuative purposes it is 24 finger-width long (*aṅguli*). For oil, it is 32 *aṅguli*. Regular therapies require 36 *aṅguli*. The pipe is straight, having three filters near the mouth, ending with a nozzle. Tube thickness is as wide as the little finger. Excess smoking may cause dryness and heat in the head and throat, fainting, thirst, bleeding, giddiness, and poor sense functioning.

Specific lengths of smoking tubes are assigned for the three types of herbs, and methods of soaking reeds (wicks).

Method: The person sits erect.

Slight congestion (movement): With the mouth open, as smoke is inhaled through the nose, alternating nostrils (one nostril open, the other closed). Inhalation is through the nose, exhalation is through the mouth. This is repeated three times.

Clogged (non-moving): Inhaled through the mouth (to decongest or create movement). Exhale through the mouth.

Throat congestion: First inhale through the nose, then later through the mouth. Exhale through the mouth.

The therapy used determines the reed length (see table below).

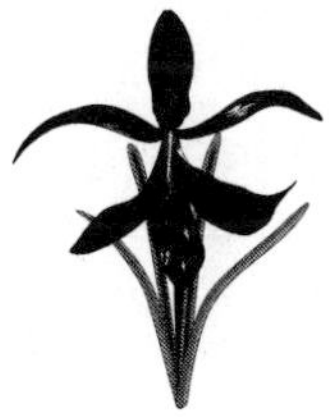

Aṅguli	Therapy	Herbs
40	palliative	cardamom
32	nourishing	*ghee*, oil
24	scraping, cleansing	evacuates
16	cough suppressing	black pepper
12	emetics	*vachā,* neem
*	ulcers	appropriate herbs

** the tube needs to reach the ulcer*

A length of two *aṅguli* (finger widths) must be left free. Paste is applied to the end of the nozzle and smoked.

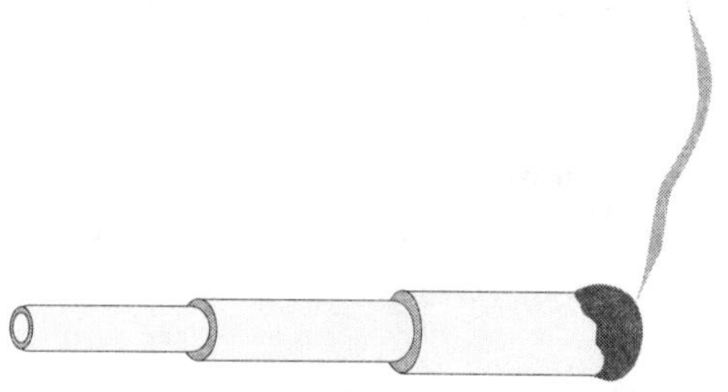

Signs of effective *dhūma* include clarity of the senses, speech and mind; strong teeth, and a pleasant odor in the mouth.

Follow-up Practices to Pañcha Karma (Uttara Karma)

1. *Pañcha karma* is sometimes repeated, for it may take several times to cleanse deeply seated toxins. This is especially true when following short term methods. Also, it may be repeated after 1 to 3 months. *Pañcha karma* is recommended at least once a year.

2. It is important to resume or establish a diet and lifestyle that is harmonious with one's constitution. If a person returns to old, bad habits, they may worsen their condition by suppressing the renewed healing energies. The toxins may then directly enter cleansed tissues and go deeper than before, causing severe diseases. During convalescence, persons avoid loud talking, bumpy rides, long walks, excessive sitting, and eating, if experiencing indigestion.

To avoid aggravating the humors, persons also avoid eating unwholesome food, day naps, and sexual relations. If any of these harmful experiences are followed, follow-up toning and rejuvenation processes are used to counteract the ill effects.

3. Once therapy is successful or complete, the next step is rebuilding the tissues damaged by the disease, giving them a new level of strength and purity. Oil or *ghee* is first taken with gradual re-introduction of the six tastes. First, sour, sweet, and delicious tastes are taken. Then one takes sour and salty tastes. Next bitter and sweet tastes are introduced. These dual tastes are used in these combinations to make food delicious. Lastly, astringent and pungent ones are taken in small quantities as a hygienic measure to clean the mouth and sliminess. Rebuilding the healthy cells and tissues is known as rejuvenation, and is the basis of the Āyurvedic approach to longevity. Deeper tissue rejuvenation is most important because this is the source of the body's energy or life-sap (*ojas*). Herbs that increase *ojas* for each *dhātu* (tissue) layer are included in the chart at the top of the next page. *Brāhmī rasāyana,* a mixture of gotu kola, *ghee*, and other herbs is an important rejuvenative.

Organs and Herbs

Herbs and foods can be used specifically to rebuild tissue layers, and herbs can also have a direct rejuvenative effect on the various body organs and tissue layers. (See lower chart on next page).

Life-Sap (Ojas) Increasing Herbs

To prevent future illness and develop a general sense of well-being or balance, rejuvenation may

Organ-Building Herbs	
Organs	**Herbs**
Lungs	*bibhītakī*
Heart	cinnamon, *drākṣhā*, ginseng, hawthorn berries, lotus seeds, rose, sandalwood, saffron
Stomach	licorice, marshmallow, *ṡhatāvarī, vaṃṡha lochana*
Small Intestine	cardamom, cinnamon, *drākṣhā,* fennel, *galangal*, ginger
Liver	aloe gel (with turmeric), dandelion root, *mañjiṣhṭhā*
Spleen	*astragalus, balā*, ginseng, licorice
Colon	*triphalā*
Kidney	*fo-ti, gokṣhura*, gotu kola, *ṡhilājit*
Brain	calamus, *brāhmī*, *harītakī, jaṭāmāṇṡhī, ṡhaṅk puṣhpī*
Uterus	aloe vera gel, *kapikachhū*, saffron, *ṡhatāvarī*
Testes	*kapikachhū, balā*, black musali

Plasma	**Blood**	**Muscle**	**Fat**	**Bone**	**Marrow**	**Semen**
comfrey root	*āmalakī*	*āmalakī*	*ghee*	comfrey root	*ghee*	*fo-ti*
marshmallow	*chyavan prāṡh*	*aṡhwa-gandhā*	*aṡhwa-gandhā*	*aṡhwa-gandhā*	*aṡhwa-gandhā*	*aṡhwa-gandhā*
irish moss	*ghee*	*balā*	*balā*	*guggul*	*brāhmī*	saw palmetto
slippery elm	saffron milk	ginseng	sesame oil	solomon's seal	*harītakī*	lotus seeds
ṡhatāvarī	*ṡhatāvarī*		*ṡhatāvarī*	*ṡhatāvarī*	sandalwood	*ṡhatāvarī*
	turmeric			myrrh	licorice	*balā*

become a part of a person's lifestyle. One should also follow an appropriate nutritional food plan (see Appendix 3). Āyurveda offers rejuvenative therapies that achieve balance through each of the five senses. Herbs and foods harmonize the sense of taste. The next few chapters describe therapies of touch (*abhyañga*), the senses of smell (aromas), sight (colors), and sound (*mantras* and music).

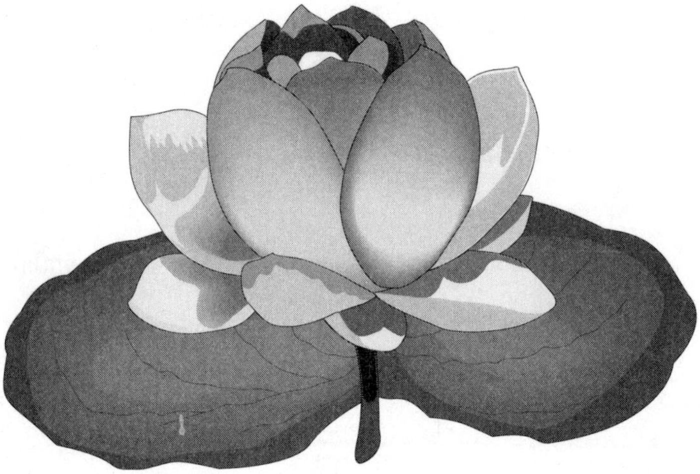

Oil Application (Abhyañga)

Other aspects of *pañcha karma* include *śhiro dhārā* (hot oil poured on the head), meridian cleansing, *abhyañga* (pouring oil on the body), and *marma* balancing (applying oil on sensitive points). Because every practitioner has their own style of this traditional therapy, both traditional and modern approaches will be discussed.

History

More than 2,000 years ago in India, oils were found that not only healed illness, but also prevented future imbalances. These therapies were traditionally given (to oneself or to others) on a daily basis. Oil was poured onto the entire body (also called *abhyañga*), head (*śhiro bhyañga* and *śhiro dhārā*), ears (*karna pūrana*), feet (*pāda bhyañga*), or specific sites that required attention (*marma bhyañga*).

Lymphatic System: One important benefit from *abhyañga* is the stimulation of the lymphatic system. The lymph system is pervasive throughout the body, except in the brain, bone marrow, and deep skeletal muscle (though some scientists believe they may extend there as well). The role of this system is to carry nutrients to and remove toxins from the cells. Some cells in the nodes destroy bacteria, viruses, and other potential harmful particles. Other vessels send fresh fluids from the other side of the node to the heart.

Lymph contains about half the concentration of proteins in the plasma, and returns the serum proteins to the blood. Thus, this is a sort of self-feeding, pre-processing system that means the body prepares its own food and feeds itself. Additionally, it contains many white blood cells that help maintain the body's resistance to immune disorders, forming these infection-fighting cells in the nodes.

This system contains various amino acids. One amino acid called tryptophan is needed for producing energy and balancing the hormonal and nervous systems. Melatonin a brain hormone synthesized from tryptophan within the pineal gland, is believed to be related to the thyroid, adrenals, and gonads. It has been found to help calm excess mental activity. An enzyme, dopamine beta hydroxylase, is believed to be related to schizophrenia and other mental disorders. Histaminase, another enzyme, breaks down histamine. If histamine is in excess, it may cause gastric acidity, lethargy, itching, headaches, pain in muscles and nodes; and allergies. Thus, *abhyañga* may help the body produce its own natural antihistamines. Lymphs also play a role in the various forms of edema.

The lymph system is Kapha in nature. *Śhleṣhaka* Kapha is a mixture of lymph and synovial fluid found in the joints and also runs through the nervous system. Lymph provides the nerves with receiving and transmitting signals. It also helps develop antibodies that are important for the immune system.

By rubbing the joints in a circular motion, circulation is enhanced and fluid is secreted from the lymph nodes. This causes more protein, glucose, minerals oxygen, and antibodies, involved with the lymphatic system, to circulate in the blood.

Benefits of *Abhyañga*:

The *Aṣhṭāñga Hṛidayam*, one of the triad of the classical Āyurvedic texts, suggests *abhyañga* be given on a daily basis to prevent and heal illness. Many benefits arise from daily *abhyañga*. Let us look at each benefit individually.

1. Reverses/prevents aging and increases longevity
2. Removes fatigue and stress from work and life overall
3. Heals andprevents nervous system disorders
4. Promotes good vision
5. Nourishes the body and promotes sturdiess
6. Remedies insomnia
7. Creates an electrochemical balance in the body.
8. Oil rubbed into the skin prevents dehydration and strengthens the nerves.

9. Oil helps the electromagnetic field of the body.
10. Stimulates antibody production, thus strengthening the immune system.

Aging (*Jarā*) is a natural process of the body, and surely death is one of life's certainties. Nevertheless, the diseases caused in the aging process are removed through *abhyañga.* Symptoms of aging include gray hair and wrinkles; loss of sleep, teeth, impairment of sight and hearing; weakened digestion and elimination; and brittle bones (osteoporosis, arthritis, weakened spine, calcification, stiffness, etc.). Other signs of aging include pains, giddiness, Parkinson's disease, heart, artery, and blood pressure problems; decreased mental function (memory, concentration, etc.), and diseases of the various organs. Through daily *abhyañga* life is maintained and people can live a normal life span (longevity or *Āyuṣh*).
Method: Sesame, mustard, or almond oil, applied to the spine, head, and feet, remove effects of old age and increase longevity.

Fatigue (*Śhrama*) results from hard work, stress, poor diet, lack of exercise, not protecting oneself from the environment, etc. These habits weaken the muscles, nerves, and joints. *Abhyañga* provides a passive exercise, cleanses stress from the muscles, removes toxins from the organs, cells, tissues, and blood; and tones the muscles and nerves.
Method: Rubbing, patting, squeezing of muscles. Add sandalwood oil to the oil mixture.

For fatigue caused by straining muscles add a pinch of salt to warm water and soak the limb.

Fatigue due to toxin accumulation is helped by adding a heating oil such as mint, eucalyptus, or mustard.

Nervous disorders (*Vāyu Roga*) occur due to excess air (Vāyu), which is the element that regulates sensory-motor skills. It is also the most important element because it regulates the other two *doṣhas* (Pitta regulates the metabolism and enzyme and digestive functioning. Kapha regulates the body organs). So, balancing Vāyu is necessary; daily *abhyañga* achieves this balance.
Method: *Mahānārāyan* oil removes air imbalances that aggravate the nervous system.

Eye (*Driṣhti*) sight is weakened by poor lighting, poor posture, reading print that is too small, excessive television, gazing at overly bright or flashing lights, (e.g., the sun, neon, and flashing signs), receiving excess sun, heat, or cold to the head; excess eating and drinking of pungent and oily foods. Additionally, old age causes impairments such as cataracts, near- and farsightedness, night blindness, optic nerve problems, etc. Poor or improper diet creates an inflamed or detached retina, atrophy of the optic nerve, etc. Āyurveda also believes that constipation causes various eye problems. Again, *abhyañga* heals these impairments and corrects the visual problems associated with the aging process.
Method: Attending the spine, neck, head, and feet. Before bed

a) massage the navel clockwise using sesame or coconut oil.
b) foot massage, including pressing between the big and index toes.

Other helpful measures for the eyes include staring at a candle flame (at eye level), massaging the temples, using a *neti* pot, massaging the nostrils with *ghee*, ingesting *triphalā* each morning, washing the eyes with *ghee.*

Nourishing (*Puṣhti*) the tissues (*dhātus, i.e.,* plasma, blood, muscle, fat, bones, nerves/marrow, reproductive fluid), are affected by poor eating habits, digestion, and metabolic functioning. The result is that foods are not digested and properly eliminated. Undigested foods become toxic waste in the body (*āma*) and hamper the natural absorption of nutrients. Through *abhyañga* wastes are loosened, flow to their sites of elimination, and are expelled as urine, feces, and sweat.
Method: Rubbing, pressing, kneading.

Sturdiness (*Dārdhya*) of the body is diminished by stress, trauma, shocks, and accidents. The inability to overcome these blows to the system results in many diseases and impairments. *Abhyañga* relieves these problems, allowing persons to recover and heal, and prevents further weakening of their system. For those who are physically incapacitated *abhyañga* provides a passive form of exercise.
Method: Rubbing, pressing, kneading.

Sleep (*Swapna*) or rest is needed to recover from the mental, physical, and emotional activities of the day. Persons deprived of sleeping and dreaming develop physical and mental diseases. Some people sleep too much, some sleep too little. Sleeping pills, caffeine, etc. are artificial attempts to balance one's unhealthy sleeping habits. Bad foods, overeating, drugs, overwork, worry, anger, lethargy, fear, etc. create these situations of insomnia and oversleeping. *Abhyañga* removes toxins, calms the nerves, brings the body and mind back into balance with nature, and helps the person naturally adjust to daily rhythms.
Method: Rubbing of oils to the feet and tense areas before bed.

Abhyañga and the Doṣhas:

Besides removing general aging problems, *abhyañga* provides specific benefits for people of different constitutions.

Vāyu *doṣhas* tend towards excess dryness, both on the skin (including wrinkles) and internally. They may develop nerve and bone disorders, constipation, anxiety, and weak immune disorders. Oil application restores moisture to the skin, soothes the nerves, strengthens the bones, and nourishes the tissues. Some authorities suggest *abhyañga* against the direction of the hair to open the pores, then reversing the direction. Others suggest *abhyañga* only in the direction the hair grows. Sesame oil is blended with general Vāyu-reducing herbs and essential oils or herbs and oils for a specific health condition.

Pitta constitutions generally have heat excesses such as skin rashes, ulcers, infections, eye, heart, and blood disorders; impatience, and hot temper. Applying oils that are sweet and cooling brings balance, and also heals and prevents further occurrence of these situations. Sesame oil is blended with general Pitta-reducing herbs and essential oils or herbs and oils for healing a specific condition.

Kapha people retain an excess of water, and tend to suffer from symptoms such as weight retention, edema, mucus, lung and sinus congestion; and sluggish minds. Warm oils help remove the excessive amounts of water and restore balance. *Aṣhṭāñga Hṛidayam* also mentions the applying of fragrant powders to reduce Kapha, liquefy fat, promote compactness strength of the body parts; and create good skin tone. Sesame, mustard, or canola oil is blended with general Kapha-reducing herbs and essential oils, or herbs and oils for specific health conditions.

Pressure during *abhyañga* varies according to one's *doṣha*. Vāyu people need a light, gentle touch. Pitta *doṣhas* prefer a moderate touch. Kapha constitutions enjoy deep muscle *abhyañga*. Further, a slow, pressure is applied around the waist with slightly more pressure exerted around the face and neck. The head and feet receive even more pressure, and more time is spent on these two areas. Soft, less fleshy, and less muscular areas are also gently pressed (e.g., navel region, temples, heart, and ribs).

Abhyañga Time:

Daily *abhyañga* is done 1 to 2 hours after eating, preferably *yoga* or exercise (until persons break a sweat) is practiced after *abhyañga*. It is best to wait at least 1 hour after *abhyañga* before taking a bath to let the oil nourish and detoxify all the tissue layers. The oil also keeps the body and skin flexible. Oil is applied at room temperature in the summer and warmed in the winter. Herbal decoctions and essential oils, according to one's *doṣha*, may be added to the oils.

Sesame oil (i.e., unscented), when used by itself, is best applied on Mondays, Wednesdays, and Saturdays, for auspiciousness, wealth, and longevity. *Abhyañga* with unscented oil or without herbal oil is not recommended on the lunar days, 3, 6, 8, 10, 11, 13, 14 (i.e., counting from the first day of the new moon to the full moon. It is also not recommended on the same days from the full moon to the new moon). Infants and elderly may receive care on all days.

All days are favorable for abhyañga when the base oil is mixed with essential flower oils, herbal plants, or using mustard oil (for Kapha doṣha).

Abhyañga is not be given immediately after enemas, emesis, or purgation therapy; during the first stages of a fever, or with indigestion. It should also not be given to persons with excess Kapha (*āma* or toxic) disorders, such as obesity, unless the oils or powders are specific to reduce *āma* and Kapha.

One unique advantage of medicated oil *abhyañga* is that their healing properties are absorbed into the system within two minutes. It nurtures all seven tissue elements in less than 14 minutes. Ingesting herbs takes a longer time because they pass through the digestive system.

Specific *Abhyañga* Therapies:

Besides the general benefits of healing difficult diseases and promoting longevity, each special *abhyañga* method offers unique therapeutic properties. Some of the approaches offer both traditional and modern uses. Traditional methods are used along with *pañcha karma* practices. Modern approaches are generally from India's *Kerala* state. These modalities can be used for healing by themselves; there is no need for emesis, purgation, and enemas.

Pressure: Two views on *abhyañga* pressure exist: According to *doṣha* and according to *guṇa* (quality). As mentioned above, a person can receive *abhyañga* with light, moderate, or deep touch, depending on whether they are Vāyu, Pitta, or Kapha *doṣhas*, respectively. A second option is to apply pressure according to how much purity (*sattwa*), heat/energy (*rajas*), and grounding (*tamas*) one needs. For example, if a person is experiencing mild imbalances (e.g., the start of a cold), then a gentle, *sattwic* touch is used. If a moderate imbalance exists (e.g., a full-blown cold) then more heat and energy (*rajas*) is used. Lastly, if the imbalance is great (e.g., chronic bronchitis), then an even deeper pressure (*tamasic*) must be exerted.

Another dimension is also considered. If a person is experiencing a Vāyu (air) excess (e.g., constipation), then moderate, warming (*rajas*); and deep, grounding (*tamas*) pressures may be used. Likewise, if one's imbalance is too grounded (i.e., excess Kapha/overweight) then moderate and light touches energize and enlighten the overly grounded imbalance. Lastly, if there is too much of the *rajasic* (heat) imbalance (e.g., skin rash), then cool (mild/ *sattwic*) and moist (deep/*tamasic*) pressure is exerted. The practitioner chooses the most comfortable and balancing methods for each client.

Yet another view suggests that for serious disorders like high blood pressure, light *abhyañga* (done only with the fingers from the middle of the chest out to the sides), or no *abhyañga* at all is to be done over the chest. Persons with low blood pressure receive only foot *abhyañga*. *Abhyañga* is not advised for fevers or skin diseases. *Abhyañga* is avoided over troubled areas such as stomach diseases or bone injuries.

Āyurveda suggests that *abhyañga* be given and received by members of the same gender. This allows for a better exchange of energy. Of course, family members will enjoy giving and receiving *abhyañga* to each other. This develops a greater bonding experience.

One or Two-Person Abhyañga

One very popular Āyurvedic *abhyañga* is done with two practitioners. As one person works one arm (leg, head, or torso side), the second person works with the corresponding body part, with identical movements and pressure. Apart from receiving a harmonious or balancing session, the feeling is most pleasurable and pampering. Traditional *abhyañga* involves six people, four to give the *abhyañga*, one to keep the oil warm (and supply the practitioner with fresh warm oil) and one to supervise. The person receives *abhyañga* in seven positions for approximately 15 minutes per position.

Abhyañga Sequence
1. Sitting
2. Lie on Back
3. Lie on Left Side
4. Lie on Right Side
5. Lie on Right
6. Sitting Again
7. Lie on Back Again

As with all Āyurvedic *abhyañga*, the main emphasis is on feeding the skin rather than on massage techniques. Oil penetrates the skin, all the tissues are fed, and the toxins contained within the tissues are released. Oil takes five minutes to permeate the skin completely. Then it spreads through the seven *dhātus* (tissues). Oil moves through each *dhātu* in less than two minutes (100 seconds).

The method suggested below describes a general overview. For every practitioner differences in style will exist. As *abhyañga* is practiced on family members and clients, persons will slowly develop their own style.

Two-person *abhyañga* uses approximately 1 1/4 cups of oil (appropriate to one's constitution). One method of *abhyañga* suggests a time schedule lasting approximately five minutes per set of body parts (i.e., both arms, shoulders, neck, torso, back, legs, and feet). This lasts about a 45 minutes.

Various techniques, such as rubbing, sliding, kneading, etc., may be employed. Joints are massaged in a circular motion. Generally, the hands follow the contour of the body. One view suggests massaging only in the direction of the hair. Another belief considers massaging in the direction that the blood flows. The key factor is that one practitioner determines the style, speed, and pressure, while the second practitioner mirrors these movements and amount of pressure.

When oil is applied and rubbed in, toxins are dislodged from the tissues and returned to the blood system. Certain *abhyañga* strokes match the movement of the five Vāyus.

1. Strokes that begin at the head and move to the navel remove excess *Prāṇa* Vāyu and improve the senses.

2. Strokes that start at the navel and end at the head remove excess *Udāna* Vāyu, carbon dioxide, mucus, and saliva.

3. Clockwise strokes around the navel balance *Samāna* Vāyu, improving digestion, metabolism, the small intestine, and liver.

4. Strokes that move from the heart to the periphery and back balance *Vyāna* Vāyu, improving blood circulation and the lymphatic system.

5. Moving the hands from the navel to the anus and urethra balances *Apāna* Vāyu, improving discharge of urine, feces, and menstrual fluid; and improving parturition in women.

Alternative Abhyañga Sequence
1. Strokes begin from navel, moving to head
2. Strokes return from head to navel
3. Strokes move from navel to feet
4. Strokes return from feet to navel
(the process is repeated three times: on the front, back, and sides of the body)

Steam therapy is employed immediately after *abhyañga* to sweat the toxins out through the skin. The remaining toxins flow back to their sites of origin in the GI tract (stomach, small intestine, colon). From these sites the toxins are removed from the body through the various *pañcha karma* therapies discussed earlier in this chapter.

One needs to be very careful and gentle when working the temples, heart, and spine. It is also important not to get oil in the client's eyes.

For healthy persons *abhyañga* begins at the feet and ends at the head. Some suggest that, for high blood pressure, *abhyañga* be done on the head for 20 minutes. Points 11 and 12 in the Head *Abhyañga* diagram [part 2 on page 214] reduce high blood pressure, along with gently rubbing up and down the sides of the neck. It is useful to place a cool towel on the head and heart during *abhyañga*. If any person's pulse is 100 beats or more per minute, no *abhyañga* is given at all.

A third school of thought suggests moving from the soles of the feet and working toward the heart to move impure blood to the heart for better functioning.

3rd Alternative Abhyañga Sequence	
feet	prone
legs	prone
arms	prone
chest	prone
abdomen	prone
back	prone
hips	prone
head	sitting
neck	sitting
face	sitting

Āyurvedic Abhyañga Techniques

Following one's intuition during *abhyañga* is important; notice whether the client is comfortable. The person giving the *abhyañga* also needs to be comfortable, neither bending too low nor raising their arms too high. If *abhyañga* is done on the floor, then one should feel comfortable squatting or sitting in *siddhāsana/siddha yoni āsana* position. After the *abhyañga*, both people should feel recharged.

Oil should not be cold when applied to the person's skin, or it will shock them, preventing relaxation. Also, the practitioner's hands should not be cold. Rubbing the hands together will bring warmth and healing energy. Working the muscles relaxes and tones them, while working the bones strengthens the skeletal system.

Techniques: Tapping, kneading, rubbing, squeezing.

Tapping is first introduced to inform the body it is about to receive *abhyañga*. It increases circulation and strengthens muscles. Tapping is done with open palms and relaxed fingers.

Kneading is done as if kneading dough. It increases the energy flow, relaxes, removes stress, and rejuvenates the body.

Rubbing is best done with oils according to one's *doṣha* (only Kaphas can have a dry *abhyañga*); otherwise, dry rubbing creates friction and aggravates Vāyu. Gentle rubbing is more relaxing, whereas vigorous rubbing creates passive exercise. Oil rubbed under the joints works the lymph system. Circular motion on specific points (*marmas*—discussed later) releases growth hormones. Comfortable pressure is always be applied during *abhyañga*. Creating a rhythm is another important part of the rubbing technique.

Squeezing is the fourth phase in this *abhyañga* process. Both hands are used to squeeze all the areas that were rubbed using comfortable pressure. Cross movements are also employed. Hands slide in the opposite directions). Pressing special points (*marmas)* is also advised. Applying oil to the fingernails is the final stage in this process. Fingers are squeezed one at a time; this ensures that the oil seeps into the cracks between the nail and the cuticle.

Some authorities suggest that healthy persons can receive the circular portion of the *abhyañga* both clockwise and counterclockwise, while persons with an illness can receive only clockwise *abhyañga.*

Post *Abhyañga*: When the session is complete it is advised that both practitioner and client lie in the corpse *āsana* pose (Chapter 9) and rest for some time. *Sādhanā* (meditation) is recommended. *Aum*, the *Gāyatrī mantra,* personal *mantra*, or prayer may be used.

Abhyañga Length: Depends upon the health and age of the person.

Age	*Abhyañga* Time
6 days - 6 months	15 minutes
Infants (until 3 yrs.)	15 - 20 minutes
3 - 18 years	30 - 45 minutes
18 - 40 years	40 - 45 minutes
40 + years	according to health
People with diseases	15 - 20 minutes

Lymph: Working the areas where lymph glands exist will cleanse and stimulate this system. Circular motion all around joints stimulates the lymph.

Pregnant Women: *Abhyañga* is applied very carefully and gently. Traditionally, *abhyañga* was received on a daily basis during pregnancy. It was found that proper *abhyañga* would result in a painless delivery.

Post Partum: Traditional Āyurvedic care suggested that the woman who had just given birth would receive *abhyañga* for the next 40 days, while she rested. This *abhyañga* would help return the body to its normal size. Although this is not usually possible in today's world, it is advised the new mother should receive *abhyañga* as frequently as possible.

New Born: Six days after birth, the baby would receive traditional Āyurvedic *abhyañga* when they were bathed. A dough ball of whole wheat flour was made (tennis ball size), mixed with sesame oil (mustard in the winter), and gently rubbed across the baby's body. This cleansed and strengthened the child.

Described below is a head *abhyañga* discussed in Ancient Indian Massage, by Hariṣh Johari.

The hand contains all healing qualities;
gentle touch brings wholeness.
Ṛig Veda

Head Abhyañga

pour oil at point 1 (optionally point 2 also)
spread with fingers only (not palms)

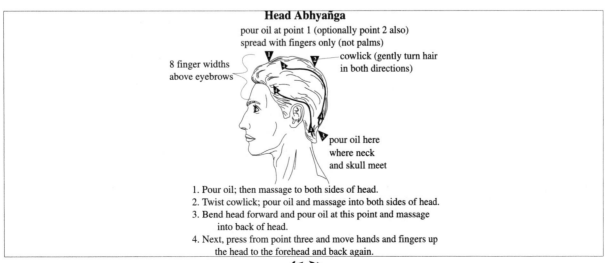

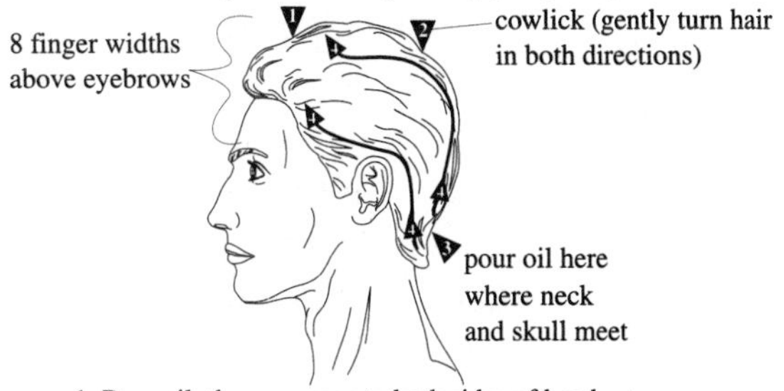

1. Pour oil; then massage to both sides of head.
2. Twist cowlick; pour oil and massage into both sides of head.
3. Bend head forward and pour oil at this point and massage into back of head.
4. Next, press from point three and move hands and fingers up the head to the forehead and back again.

Head Abhyañga - [part 2]

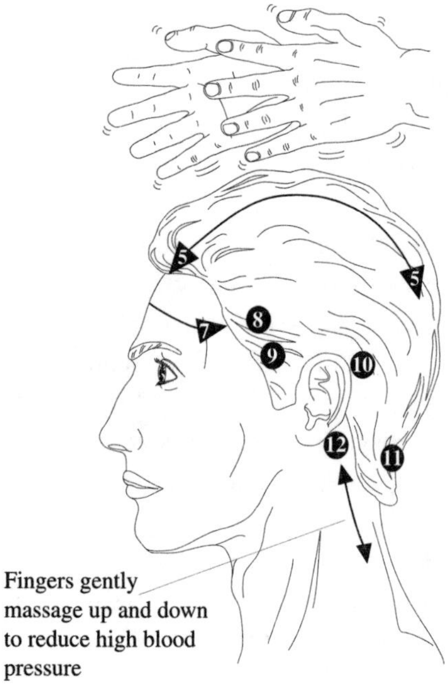

Fingers gently massage up and down to reduce high blood pressure

5. Gently pound the top-middle of head from back to front, and back again. This stimulates the circulatory and nervous system's capillaries.
6. Twist and gently pull the hair in all three spots (see diagram 1) to increase the flow of the cerebral spinal fluid.
7. Press and rub forehead from the middle to the sides to improve alertness, memory and balance of the pituitary and pineal glands.
8. Rub *Utkṣhepa marma* counterclockwise to balance the eyes, lungs, and heart.
9. Gently rub the temples (*Sthapani marma*) counterclockwise to improve the colon, intestines and balance Vāyu.
10. Rub behind the ear (clockwise) to balance the intestines, colon and brain.
11. Gently press at the junction of the neck and head to balance the nervous system, promote stability and lower high blood pressure.
12. Rub the *Vidhura marma* behind the earlobe (clockwise) to lower hight blood pressure.
13. Rub finger tips along the top middle of the head (back and forth, pressing the skull (#5 line).
14. Twist and pull the hair in the three places, starting at the base of the scull and ending with the point eight *aṅgula* above the forehead (see diagram 1).

Head Abhyañga - [part 3]

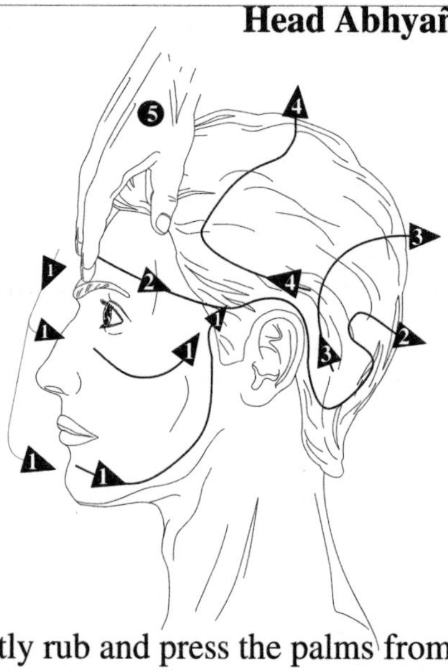

1. Gently rub and press the palms from the middle of the forehead, moving over the eyebrows, eyelids, nose and chin. Then move towards the jaws and up, in front of the ears.
2. Press along the sides of the head, behind the ears, to the lower back of the head. Then twist and gently pull the hair (see arrow #2).
3. 4. Follow the arrows in the picture, twisting and pulling the hair where shown.
5. Gently clap over the top of the head.

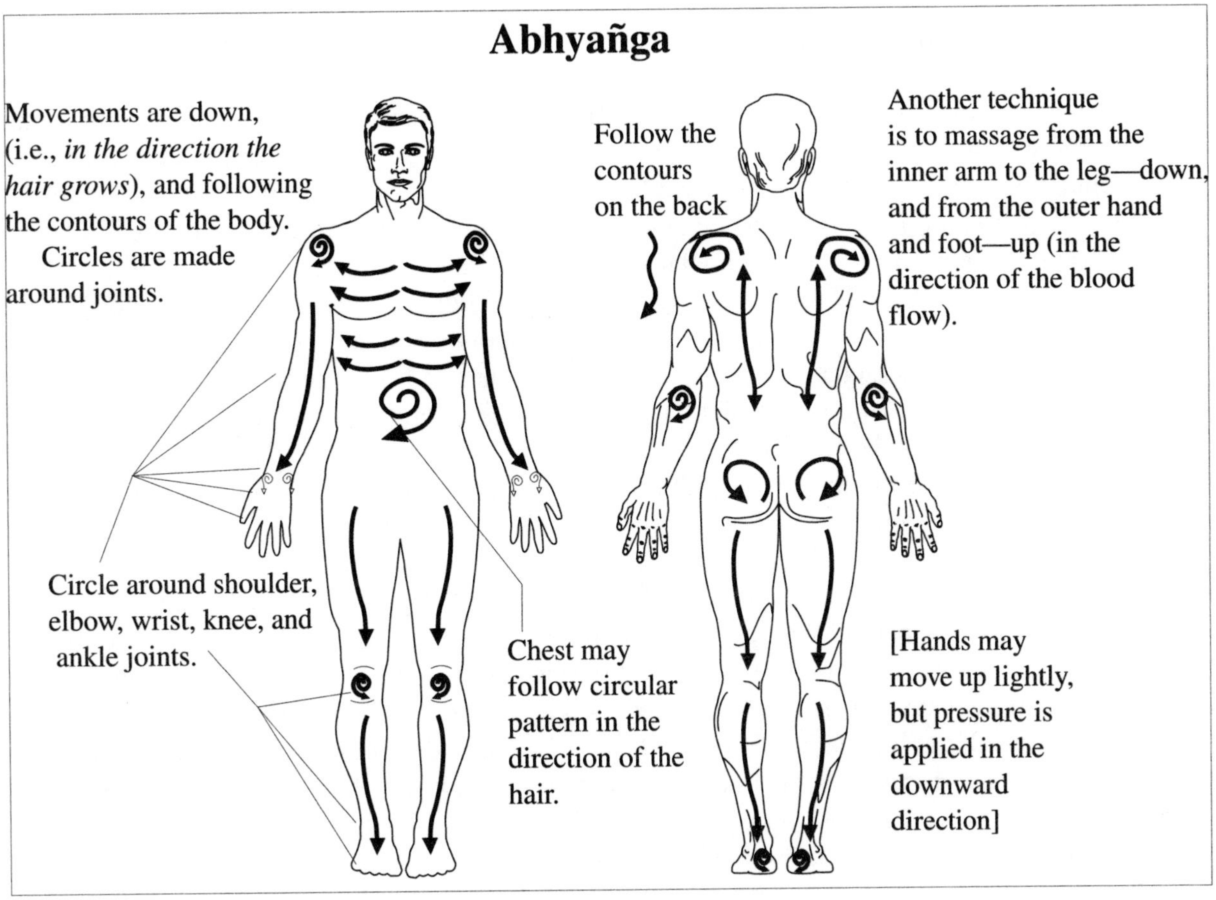
Abhyañga
Movements are down, (i.e., *in the direction the hair grows*), and following the contours of the body.
Circles are made around joints.
Follow the contours on the back
Another technique is to massage from the inner arm to the leg—down, and from the outer hand and foot—up (in the direction of the blood flow).
Circle around shoulder, elbow, wrist, knee, and ankle joints.
Chest may follow circular pattern in the direction of the hair.
[Hands may move up lightly, but pressure is applied in the downward direction]

Marma Abhyañga

Another form of *abhyañga* is the use of the major and minor *marma* points. *Marma* is discussed in one of the four main *Vedas,* and also detailed in the classical Āyurvedic text, *Suṣhrut Saṃhitā*. The *marma* points are similar to Chinese acupuncture, only no invasive use of needles is involved.

Marma points are positions on the body where flesh, veins, arteries, tendons, bones, and joints meet. They may be seen as the junctions where Vāyu, Pitta, and Kapha meet; where *sattwa, rajas,* and *tamas* meet; or where eternity and relativity meet. Some say they are also the points where the three aspects of Self-realization meet, i.e., inner Self, outer world, and between the two (knower, known, and process of knowing). They may also be the junctions between the physical, astral, and causal bodies. In short, they are points that have great importance to a person's body, mind, and spirit.

Although the *marmas* are the junctions of all five principles (i.e., flesh, veins, arteries, tendons, bones, and joints), at each point a predominance of one principle exists. It is at these points where *abhyañga* can most effectively restructure or rebalance the system to function most healthily. Further, *abhyañga* helps develop the preventive health and longevity of the body and mind by ensuring the proper balance and flow of hormones, fluids, immune factors, etc.

One hundred seven *marma* points exist on the body. This makes it much easier to remember and work with, compared with the thousands of points in Chinese acupuncture. Āyurveda details major (*mahā*) and minor *marma* points. The major points correspond to the major *chakras* (secret energy points) on the body, while the minor points are found around the torso and limbs. Thus, healing through *marma abhyañga* affects the *chakras,* physical health, and the *doṣhas*.

The purpose of a *marma abhyañga* is to stimulate the various bodily organs and systems. Like acupuncture, these points are measured by finger units (*aṅguli* or *aṅgula*) to detect their correct locations. Many *marma* points are larger than acupuncture points. Thus, they can be found more easily.

One school of thought suggests that *marmas* are not so much points as they are circular bands around certain parts of the body. For example, a *marma* exists just above the knee (the width of the client's four fingers above the middle of the knee), known as *Ani Marma*. This *marma* relates to the small intestine. It is also situated on the back of the leg, directly behind this spot. If one were to move the hands from the front *Ani Marma*, in a straight line to the back (i.e., by working the sides of the leg that are in line with *Ani Marma*) this *marma* would also be stimulated. So when one works a *marma* point, they can affect the front, sides, and back of a *marma* (i.e., encircling the area around the arm or leg).

In ancient India, it was cautioned that these *marma* points were to be guarded from harm. If these points were pierced by arrows or hit forcefully, it could result in disease, trauma or even death. Obviously, places like the heart, forehead, and throat are vulnerable areas, whereas sites on the arms and legs are less vulnerable to severe injury. When imbalances exist in the body, these same spots become sore. Through *marma abhyañga* health is restored.

Marma points are grouped according to the region of the body (arms [22 points] and legs [22 points] 11 per limb), abdomen [3 points], chest [9 points], back [14 points], and head and neck [37 points]). They are also grouped according to muscles [10 points], tendons/ligaments [23 points], arteries [9 points], veins [37], joints [20 points], and bones [8]. (Some group these points slightly differently.)

Traditionally, *marma* points are grouped into three categories: those on the legs and feet (*Śhankha Marma*), those on the trunk (*Madhāyamañga Marma*), and those on the neck and head (*Jatrūrdhva Marma*).

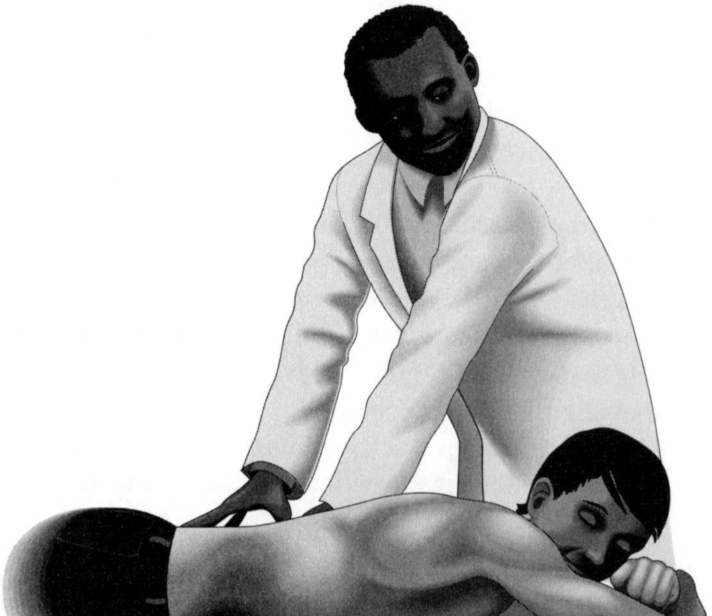

Marma Points

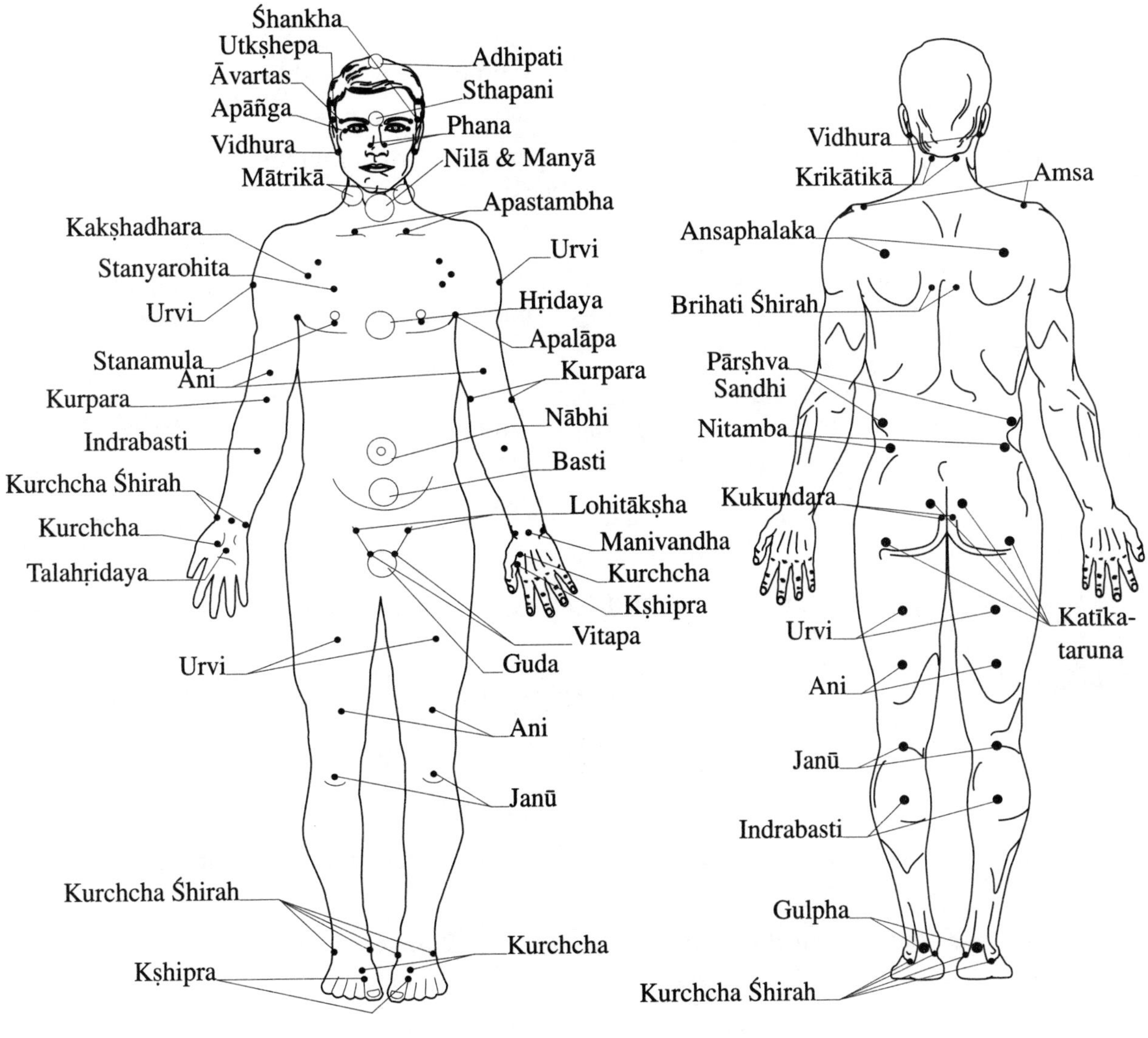

Marma	Arm & Leg *Marma* Location, Number, Size	Governs
Tala Hṛidaya	center of palms and soles (4 points/i.e., 1 per limb) 1/2 finger width	lungs
Kṣhipra	between big toes/fingers & first toes/fingers (4 points) 1/2 finger width	heart, lungs
Kurchcha	2 finger widths (aṅguli) of client, above *Kṣhipra*—of feet and thumb roots (4 points/i.e., 1 per limb) 4 finger widths	*Alochaka* Pitta
Kurchcha Śhirah	just below the ankles (8 points/2 per limb) 1 finger width and sides of wrists	muscle spasms
Indrabasti	center of the calf muscle (in line with the heel—12 fingers above it) 1/2 or 2 finger widths (varying views)	digestion, intestines
Ani	four fingers above *Janū* (just above kneecaps) front and back. 1/2 finger width	muscle tension
Urvi	thigh center (front and back) 1/2 finger width	*Udakavaha Srota*
Lohitākṣha	joint of groin and thigh (2 points) 1/2 finger width	leg blood supply
Manibandha	center wrist joint (2 points) 2 finger widths	relieves stiffness
Kurpara	on elbow joint (2 points) 3 finger widths	heart, spleen liver
Kakṣhadhara	between chest and shoulder (2 points) 1 finger width	muscle tension
Gulpha	foot/calf junction (Achilles tendon area) 2 finger widths	relieves stiffness
Janū	calf/thigh junction (center of kneecap and directly behind it on the back of knee)(2 points) 3 finger widths	heart, spleen liver
Vitapa	between groin and scrotum (measure from *Lohitakṣha*, down & angled towards scrotum, length—index finger tip to its midjoint—2 *aṅguli)* (2 points) 1 finger width	belly muscle tension, impotence, semen

Marma	Trunk Points Thorax/Back Location, Size	Governs
Guda	perineum, 4 finger widths (*aṅguli*)	reproduction, colon, urine, gas, stool, 1st *chakra* stimulation
Basti	between pelvis/navel, 4 finger widths	urinary, Kapha
Nābhi	navel, 4 finger widths	seat of all veins transfer points, small intestines
Hṛidaya	between nipples, 4 fingers widths	main Pitta marma, *Sadhaka* Pitta, *Vyāna* Vāyu
Stana-mula	just below nipples, 2 points, 2 finger widths	Kapha, Pitta, blood circulation
Stanar-ohita	above breast nipple (from *Stanamula*, from the index finger tip to mid joint), 2 points, 1/2 finger width	Kapha, Pitta, arm muscles
Apa-stambha	either side of trachea base— mid collarbone area, 2 points, 1/2 finger width	blood, sympathetic/ parasympathetic nerve, lungs
Apalāpa	the armpit, 2 points, 1/2 finger width	blood, sympathetic/ parasympathetic nerve
Katīka-taruna	sacrum top by spine/lower buttocks, 4 points, 1/2 finger width	fat, constipation, Vāyu
Kukun-dara	just above buttocks, both sides of spine, 2 points, 1/2 finger width	reproduction, elimination, leg mobility, controls 2nd *chakra*
Nitamba	5 fingers above & lateral Kukundara, over hip bone (on back), 2 points, 1/2 *aṅguli*	Vāyu & Pitta digestion, vitality, RBC
Pārśhva Sandhi	from *Nitamba*, measure from the index finger tip to the mid joint, and lateral (about 1" up and 1" to the side), 2 points, 1/2 *aṅguli*	Pitta, digestion, elimination
Brihati Śhirah	between shoulder blades, on both sides of spine (directly behind Stanamula), 2 points, 1/2 finger width	a major Pitta accumulation site. Controls 3rd *chakra*
Ansa-phalaka	above *Brihati* (arm root - mid shoulder blade), 2 points, 1/2 finger width	Vāyu touch/sensation, atrophy, 4th *chakra*
Ansa	5 finger widths above Ansaphalaka	between shoulder bones—between shoulder & neck, 2 points, 1/2 finger width
The first eight are located on the thorax & trunk. The last seven are located on the back.		

Marma	Head & Neck Marmas	Governs
Dhamani (Nilā & Manyā)	both sides of the trachea (posterior/anterior sides of larynx, respectively, 2 points, 4 finger widths	speech, taste, perception, blood, transfer *marma*
Mātrikā	4 points on each side of the throat, 4 finger widths	blood circulation
Krikātikā	head/neck junction (back of head), 2 points, 1/2 finger width	tremors, disability, stiffness
Vidhura	just below the back of both ears, 1/2 finger width	hearing, head support
Phana	both sides of the nostrils, 1/2 finger width	smell, sinus, ears, stress
Apāñga	outer corners of both eyes-ends, 1/2 finger width	vision, stress
Āvartas	above both outer eyebrows, 1/2 finger width	depression, vision, posture
Śhankha	temples—front bone (above eyebrows), 1/2 finger width	colon
Utkṣhepa	1 finger width above *Śhanka*, 2 points, 1/2 finger width	colon
Sthapani	center of eyebrows, 1/2 finger width	main Vāyu *marma*, mind, nerves, hypothalamus
Śhringataka	[4 points] cleft, under nose, outside eye bones, nose tip	eyes, ears, nose, tongue, nerves
Simanta	sideways and upwards on the skull, 4 finger widths	sanity, grounding, intelligence, blood
Adhipati	crown *chakra* (baby's soft spot), 1/2 finger width	mind, nerves, epilepsy

Marmas and Chakras

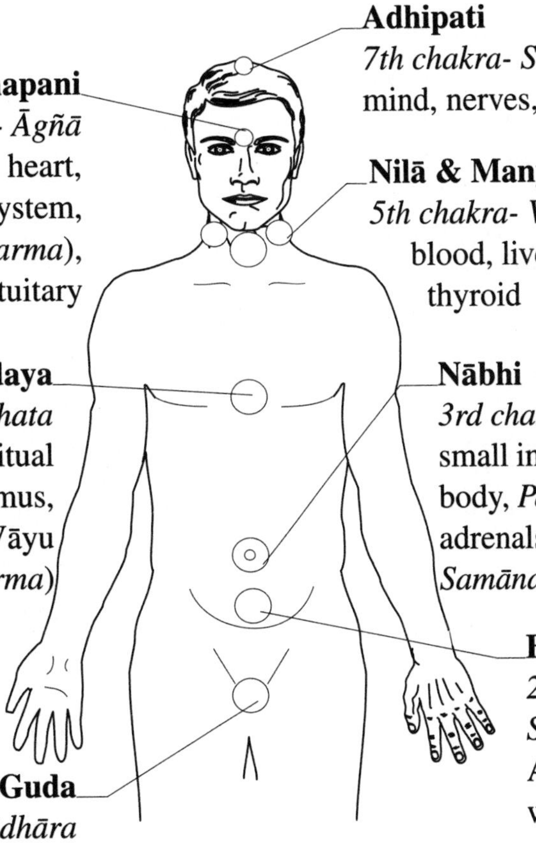
Adhipati
7th chakra- Sahasrāra
mind, nerves, ether, pineal
Sthapani
6th chakra- Āgñā
mind, nerves, colon, heart, lungs- respiratory system, bones (main Vāyu *marma*), pituitary
Nilā & Manyā
5th chakra- Viṣhuddha
blood, liver, spleen thyroid
Hṛidaya
4th chakra- Anāhata
circulation, blood, spiritual goals, discrimination, thymus, Sadhaka Pitta, Vyāna Vāyu (main Pitta *marma*)
Nābhi
3rd chakra- Manipūra
small intestine, subtle body, *Pachaka* Pitta, adrenals, pancreas *Samāna* Vāyu
Basti
2nd chakra- Swādhiṣhṭhān
All Kapha functions, water metabolism, urinary system, pituitary, gonads (testes & ovaries), (main Kapha *marma*)
Guda
1st chakra- Mūlādhāra
reproductive, urinary, menstrual systems, obesity, prostate, excretory, Apāna Vāyu

Marma Points and the Srotas (Bodily Systems)		
The various bodily systems (srotas) are also balanced with marma work.		
Srota	***Marma***	**Governs**
Prāṇavaha	*Sthapani*	respiration, heart, lungs/asthma
Annavaha	*Indra Basti*	digestion/ indigestion, gas, nausea, diarrhea, stomach, intestines
Udakavaha	*Basti/Urvi*	water metabolism, pancreas, diabetes
Rasavaha	*Nilā/Manyā*	lymphatic/lymph glands, Kapha disorders
Raktavaha	*Hṛidaya/Nilā/Manyā/Brihati Śhira/Mātrikā*	blood, hemoglobin/liver, spleen, skin rashes, bleeding disorders
Māṃsavaha	*Tala Hṛidaya/Guda/ Stanarohita/Indrabasti*	water metabolism/pancreas, diabetes
Medavaha	*Guda*	fat (adipose)/ kidneys, visceral membrane
Asthivaha	*Sthapani/Adhipati/ Śhankha/Utkṣhepa*	skeletal/bones, colon, hair, nails
Majjāvaha	Simanta/Śhringataka/ *Sthapani/Adhipati*	nervous system—marrow/ bones, joints, memory, insomnia, anxiety, worry
Śhukravaha	*Guda/Kukundara/Vitapa*	male reproductive/genitals, impotence, prostate, TB
Mūtravaha	*Katīkataruna/ Kukundar/Basti*	colon, urinary bladder
Purīshavaha	*Krikātikā/Guda/ Sandhi/Urvi/ Adpathi/Śhanka/Basti/Kartīka-taruna*	rectum, anus, diarrhea, constipation, colitis, blood in stool, hemorrhoids
Swedavaha	*Stanamula/Stanarohita/ Kakṣhadhara/Basti*	adipose tissue, skin pores, sweating
Artavavaha	*Katīkataruna/Kukundar/Basti*	Females—uterus, fallopian tubes/PMS, menstruation problems, menopause, fertility/*Apāna* Vāyu
Stanyavaha	Stanamula/Stanarohitam */Kaṣhadhara/Basti*	Females—breasts, nipples/lactation, breast tumors and abscesses

Three of the seven *marmas* relate specifically to the three *doṣhas*, and are the primary *marmas* worked with.

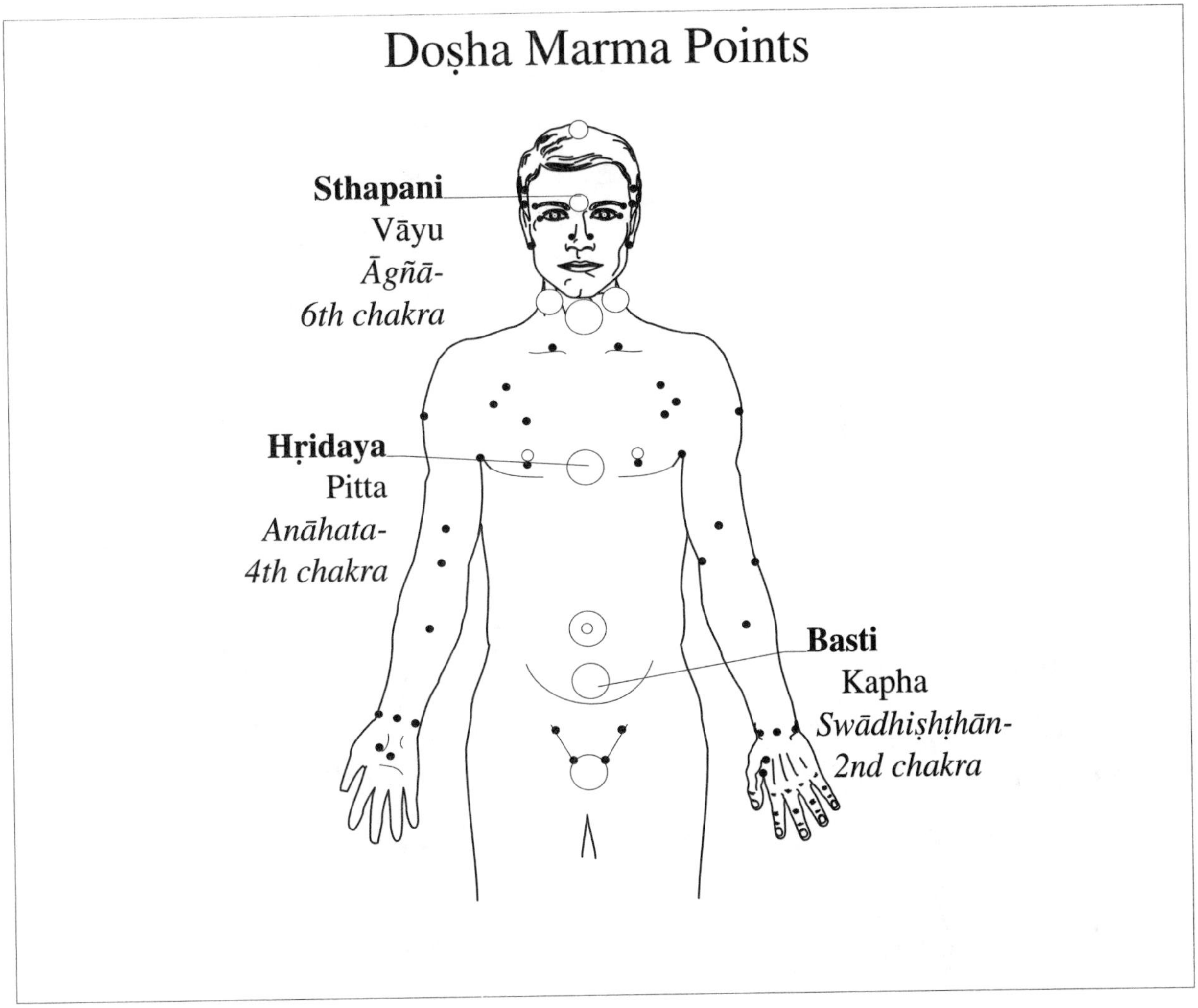

We have detailed the three *doṣhas*, Vāyu (air), Pitta (fire), and Kapha (water). A *doṣha* excess means an increase of that element in the body and/or mind. These excesses or imbalances are mild or severe diseases (depending upon the degree of the excess). For example, excess Vāyu can develop into constipation, dry skin, anxiety, etc. Further, most illnesses can be caused by any *doṣha* excess (e.g., asthma can be caused by any of the *doṣhas*. Each *doṣha* has its own unique set of symptoms. This enables one to detect the *doṣha* causing the disease). This *yogic* or spiritual tool is unique to Āyurveda. Thus, one can fine tune or note distinctions instead of merely working with generalizations. This insight into individualized symptoms is an invaluable tool in determining the root cause of an illness.

Each *doṣha* has five aspects—or sub-*doṣhas*—that further describe the different activities that each *doṣha* performs. The sub-*doṣhas* govern various body functions. For example, we know that one function of Vāyu is related to stool elimination. One sub-*doṣha* exists to specifically govern the downward movement of the air, called *Apāna* Vāyu. This added insight allowed the ancients to know which *marma* points were related to downward moving air, and to properly stimulate or reset this downward flow. Through *abhyañga* and stimulating *marma* points the downward flow air flow can be restored or balanced.

Vāyu Major Marma Points

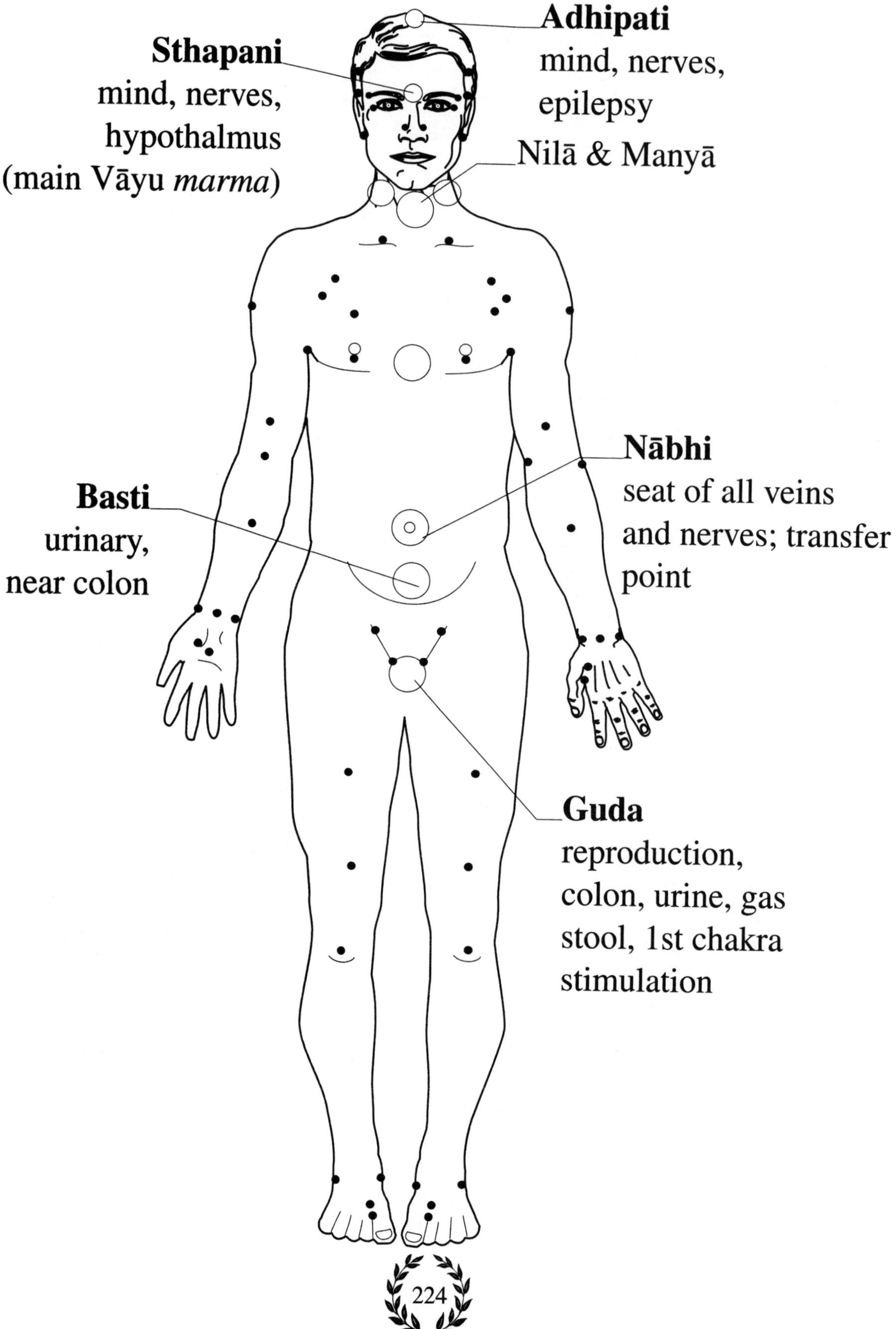
Adhipati
mind, nerves,
epilepsy
Sthapani
mind, nerves,
hypothalmus
(main Vāyu *marma*)
Nilā & Manyā
Nābhi
seat of all veins
and nerves; transfer
point
Basti
urinary,
near colon
Guda
reproduction,
colon, urine, gas
stool, 1st chakra
stimulation

Secondary *marma* points exist for Vāyu; these points are used with the main *marmas* as assisting points. One traditional Vāyu method involves the use of one hand on the main Vāyu *marma* point (*Sthapani*), while the other hand is used on the minor Vāyu *marma* points. This approach is similar to polarity therapy, which was derived from Āyurvedic *marma abhyañga*. Persons will also notice that a 'mirroring' effect occurs; some of the same points are sited on both the arms and legs.

Secondary Vāyu Marmas

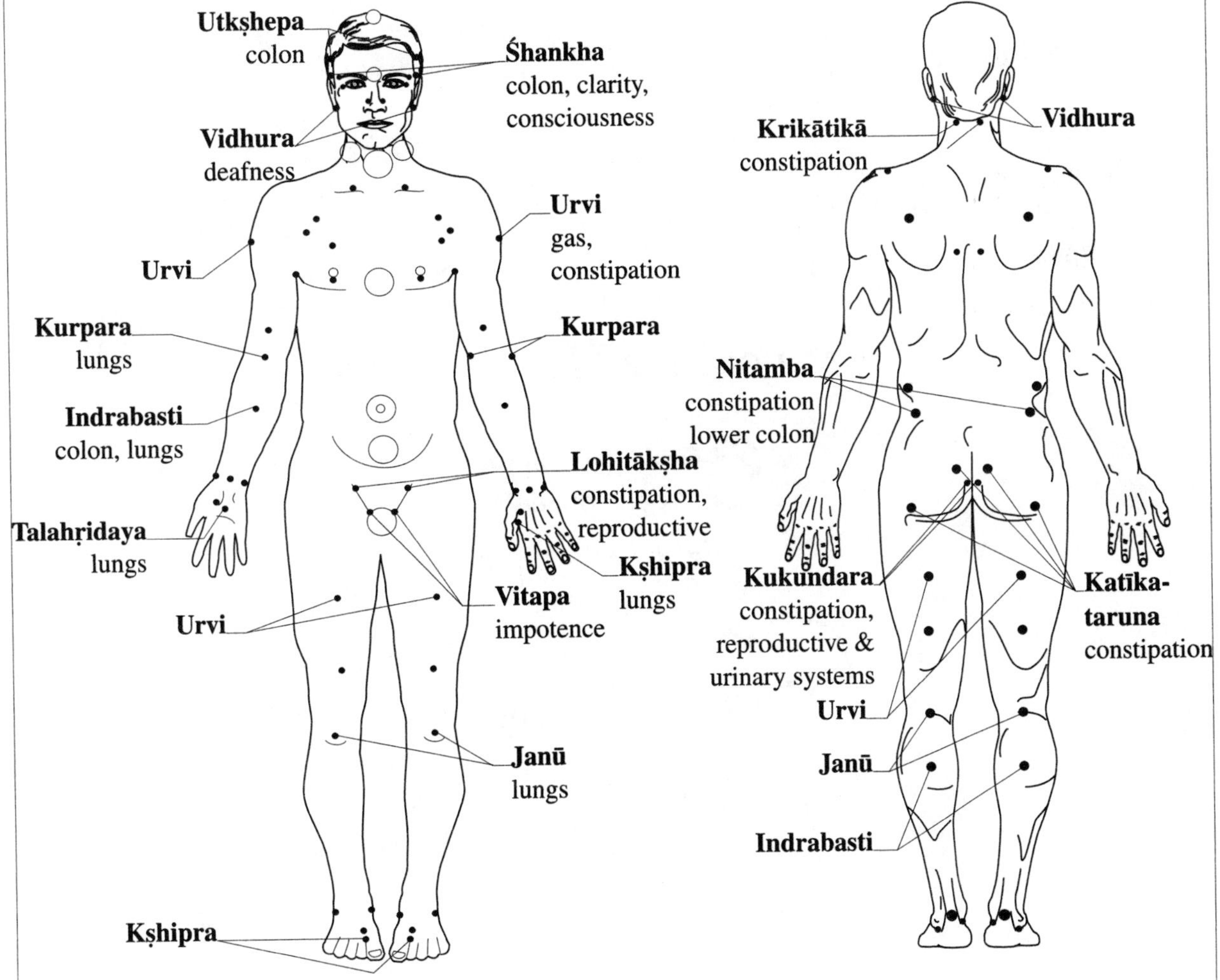

Marma Points and the 5 Vāyus

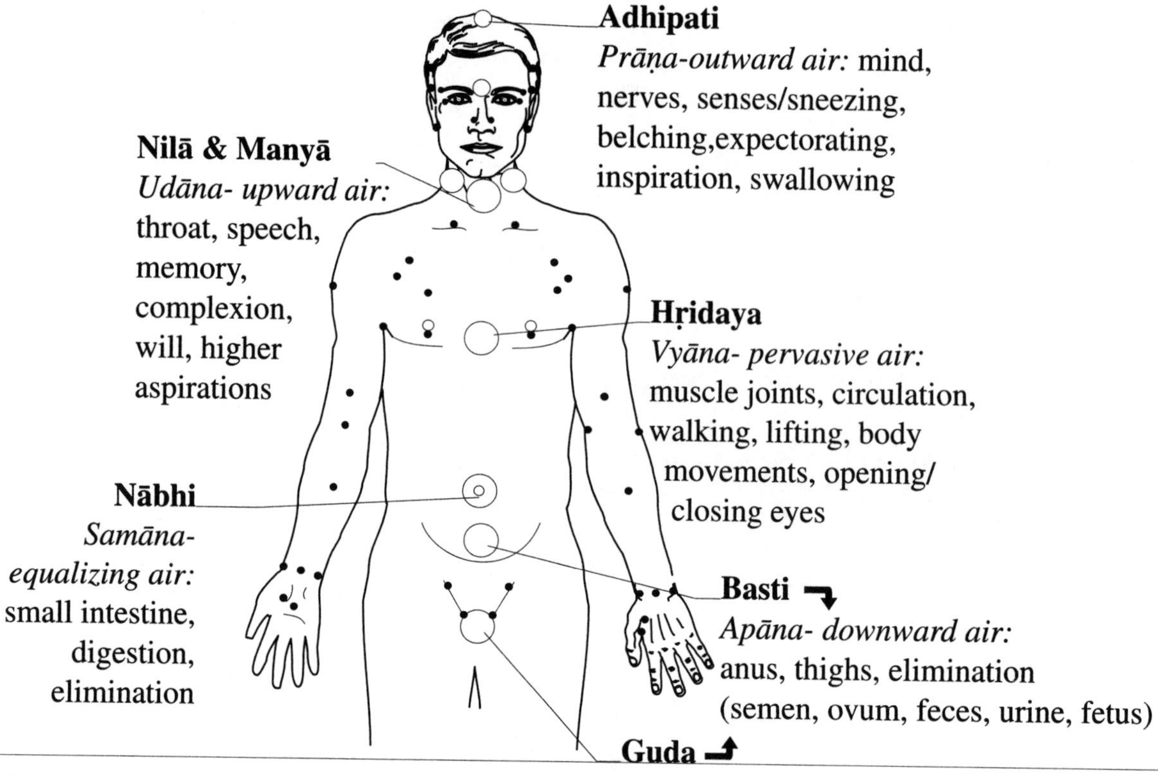
Adhipati
Prāṇa-outward air: mind, nerves, senses/sneezing, belching,expectorating, inspiration, swallowing
Nilā & Manyā
Udāna- upward air: throat, speech, memory, complexion, will, higher aspirations
Hṛidaya
Vyāna- pervasive air: muscle joints, circulation, walking, lifting, body movements, opening/ closing eyes
Nābhi
Samāna- equalizing air: small intestine, digestion, elimination
Basti
Apāna- downward air: anus, thighs, elimination (semen, ovum, feces, urine, fetus)
Guda

Major Pitta Marma Points

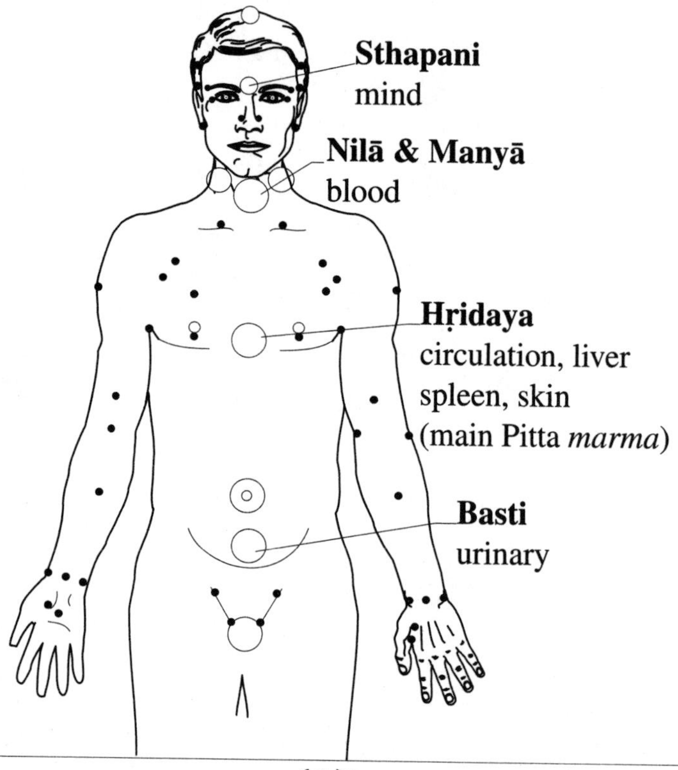
Sthapani
mind
Nilā & Manyā
blood
Hṛidaya
circulation, liver spleen, skin (main Pitta *marma*)
Basti
urinary

Minor Pitta Marma Points

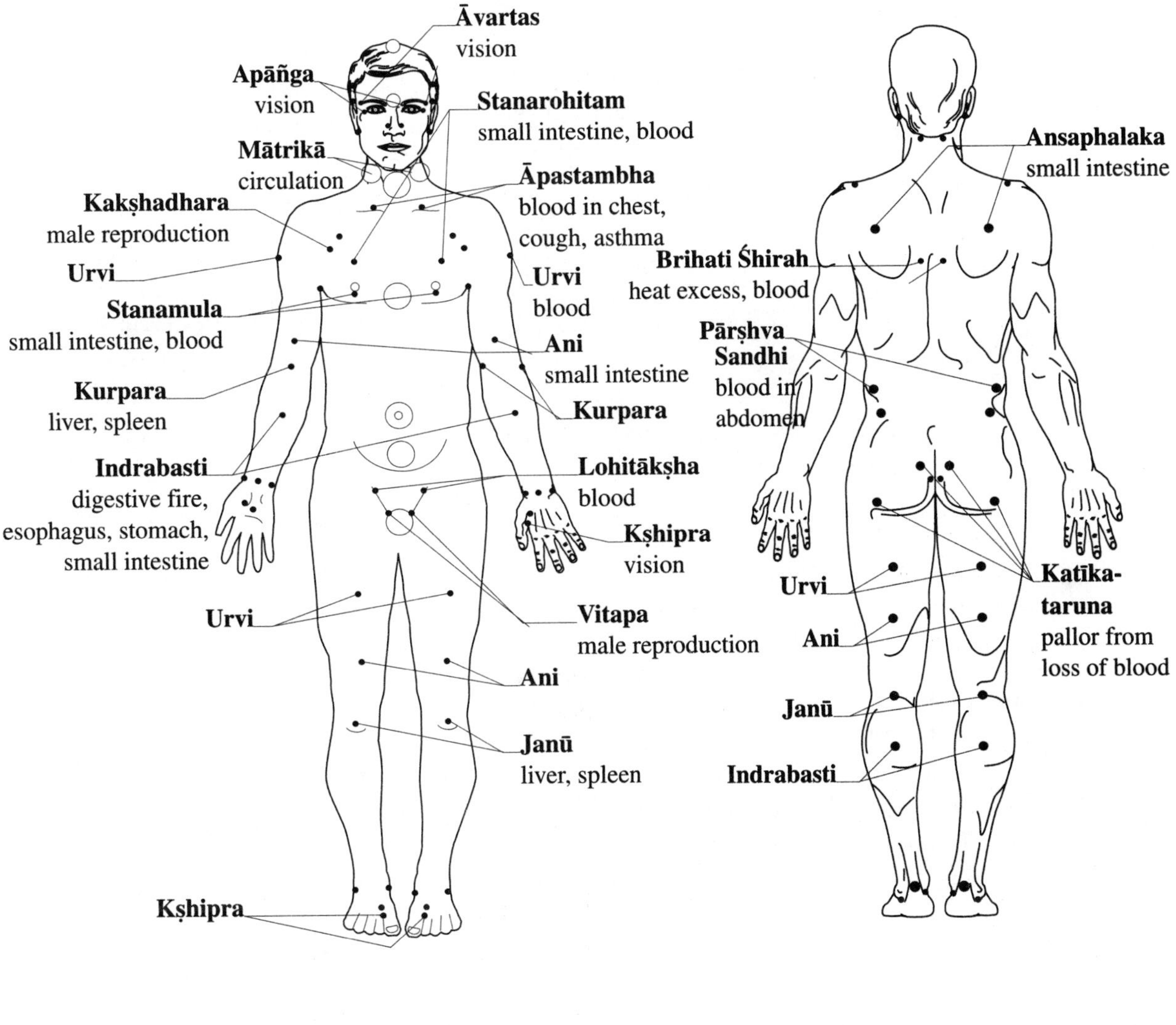
Āvartas
vision
Apāñga
vision
Stanarohitam
small intestine, blood
Mātrikā
circulation
Āpastambha
blood in chest,
cough, asthma
Kakṣhadhara
male reproduction
Urvi
Urvi
blood
Stanamula
small intestine, blood
Ani
small intestine
Kurpara
liver, spleen
Kurpara
Indrabasti
digestive fire,
esophagus, stomach,
small intestine
Lohitākṣha
blood
Kṣhipra
vision
Urvi
Vitapa
male reproduction
Ani
Janū
liver, spleen
Kṣhipra
Ansaphalaka
small intestine
Brihati Śhirah
heat excess, blood
Pārṣhva
Sandhi
blood in
abdomen
Urvi
Ani
Janū
Indrabasti
Katīka-
taruna
pallor from
loss of blood

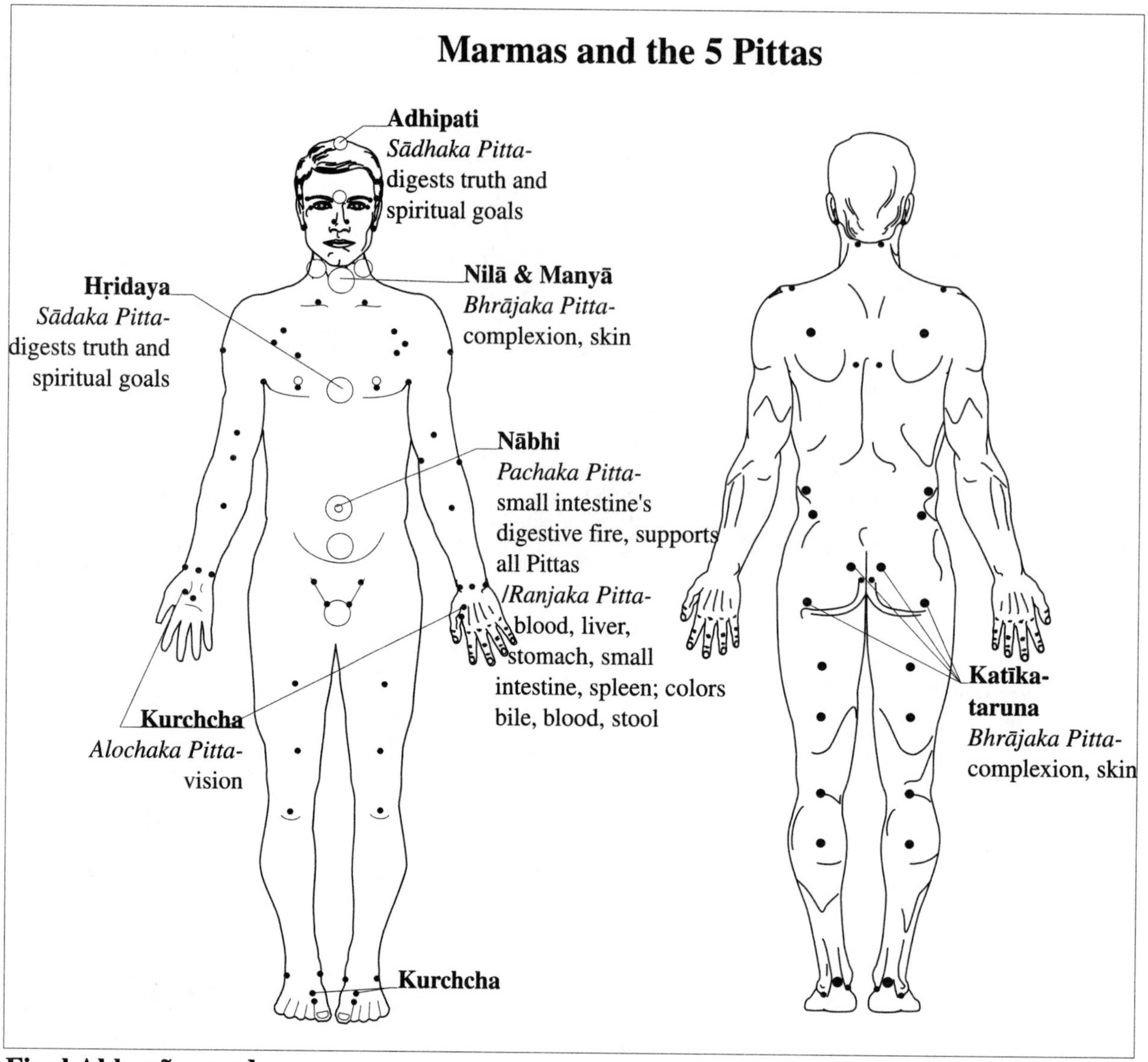

Final Abhyañga and Energy Transfer Marmas

After *abhyañga* the practitioner checks the major *doṣha marma* points (*Sthapani*—third eye, *Hṛidaya*—heart, *Basti*—below the navel) feeling for energy and heat comparisons. If one *mahā marma* still feels out of balance, additional time is spent balancing the transfer *marmas*, the throat (*Nilā* and *Manyā*), and navel (*Nābhi*) *chakras*.

The process begins with one hand on, or over the crown *chakra* (*adhipati*) and the other hand on, or over the main *doṣha marma* of the client.

Next, one palm lightly rests on, or is held slightly above one of the *mahā marmas*. The other palm is placed on, or over the throat transfer point, then after a while, moves to the navel transfer point. For example, if there seems to be too much air in the region between the eyebrows (*Sthapani Marma*), the practitioner keeps one palm on, or over this *marma*. The other palm is on, or over the throat. This position is held for some time, then the hand over the throat moves on, or over the navel. When the hand is by the throat, excess air transfers out of the head and sends in extra warmth or fire from being near the heart *marma* (Pitta *mahā marma*). Similarly, when the hand is by the navel, it sends moisture from the nearby *Basti marma* (a Kapha *mahā marma*) in the direction of the head.

Kapha Major and Minor Marma Points

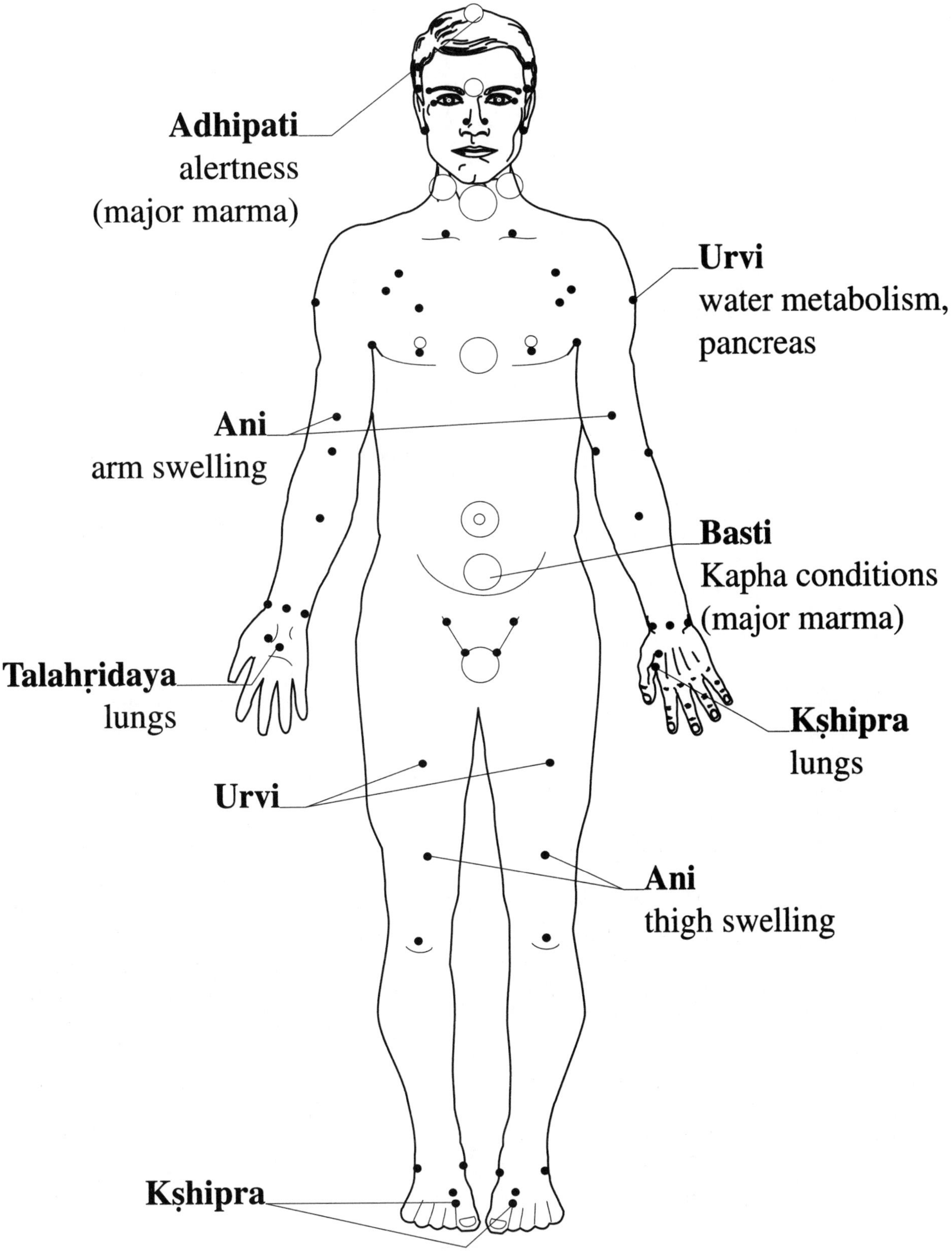

Marma	Definition	*Marma*	Definition
Talahṛidaya	Center of palms and soles	*Brihati Śhirah*	large region of the back
Indrabasti	*Indra's* bladder: mid-forearms and calves	*Ansaphalaka*	Shoulder blade
Ani	Lower region of upper arms and legs	*Ansa*	Shoulder
Lohitakṣha	Red eyed: lower frontal area of arm and leg joints	*Krikātikā*	Neck joint
Stanarohita	Upper region of the breast	*Vidhura*	Distress from sensitivity
Apastambha	Upper sides of the chest (carries the life force)	*Phana*	Serpent's Hood: nostril sides
Apalāpa	Unguarded: the armpits	*Apāñga*	outer eye corners
Katīkataruna	Rising from the sacrum: center of the buttocks	*Avarta*	Calamity from sensitivity
Kunkundara	Loin marking both sides of spine base where buttocks meet	*Utkṣhepa*	Thrown upwards: above temples
Nitamba	Upper buttocks region	*Sthapani*	Giving support
Pārśhwasandhi	Sides of the waist	Adhipati	Overlord: crown of the head

The sizes of the *marmas* are measured by finger breadth, called *aṅguli or aṅgula* (e.g., 1 *aṅguli* is the width of one's own finger). All *marma* measurements are made with the client's own fingers, not the fingers of the practitioner. Most of the *marmas* have the same meaning as their position, making it easy to remember their location. The charts below group the *marmas* according to size.

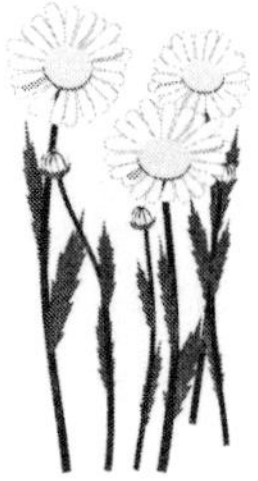

1 aṅgula

Marma	Definition
Vitapa	perineum
Kakṣhadhara	upholding flanks top of shoulder joints
Urvi	wide mid-region of thighs and forearms
Kurchchaśhira	head of *Kurchcha* base of thumb/big toe

2 aṅgula

Marma	Definition
Manibandha	bracelet
Gulpha	ankle joint
Stanamula	breast root
Śhankha	conch: temples

3 aṅgula

Marma	Definition
Janū	knee joint
Kurpara	elbow joint

4 aṅgula
(Some say the size of one's own palm)

Marma	Definition
Guda	anus
Basti	bladder
Hṛidaya	heart
Nābhi	navel
Nilā	dark blue: color of veins at this location
Simanta	summit: skull & surrounding joints
Mātrikā	blood vessel's mother: arteries flow to head from here
Kurchcha	knot: muscles or tendons at base of thumbs/big toes
Śhringataka	crossroads of four streets: soft palate of mouth
Manyā	honor

Reference: *Aṣhṭāñga Hṛidayam* Ch. 4; v.60-63.5
Different authorities use slightly different measurements

Abhyañga Oils

Āyurveda offers numerous oils for various *pañcha karma, abhyañga,* and *nasya* treatments. Presently many of the oils are not readily found in the US. *Brāhmī, chandan*, neem, and *mahānārāyan* oils seem to be among the main oils used. Below is a sample of some Āyurvedic oils and which diseases they help. Oils often can be applied externally, taken internally, and as nasal drops.

Oil	Use
Brāhmī	Head & eyes
Chandan	Fever, alcoholism, confusion, burning, rheumatism, jaundice, mental diseases
Dūrba or Neem	Dandruff
Gandha	Sprains, fractures
Kshīraba	Hemiplegia, nervous disorders, acute gout, rheumatic pain, paralysis
Mahānārāyan	Hemicrania, glands, facial paralysis, conception, arthrits, pain
Mahāmaṣha	Hemiplegia, facial or arm paralysis, lockjaw
Kumkum	Acne, pimples
Nararsas	Nasal polyps

Doṣha Marma Oils

Essential oils appropriate to one's *doṣha* are placed on the *marma* points that relate to their *doṣha*. On the next page is a partial list of these oils. For further explanations about oils, see Chapter 8 on aromatherapy.

Doṣha Marma Oils		
Vāyu	**Pitta**	**Kapha**
Sandalwood	Sandalwood	Sandalwood
Rose	Rose	
Jasmine	Jasmine	
Lily	Lily	
Vanilla	Vanilla	
Lavender	Lavender	
Patchouli		Patchouli
Basil		Basil
Frankincense		Frankincense
Myrrh		Myrrh
Sage		Sage
Cedar		Cedar
Musk		Musk
Lotus		Lotus
Eucalyptus		Eucalyptus
Cinnamon		Cinnamon
	Geranium	
	Lemongrass	
	Gardenia	

Keralīya Āyurvedic Abhyañga

Contemporary Methods

Kerala is a state in southern India where *pañcha karma abhyañga* has been preserved. However, unlike *pañcha karma*, it is used more for rejuvenation purposes than for cleansing. Various contemporary forms of *abhyañga* are used in *Kerala*, and are very effective. Some modern authorities note that some of these practices are especially useful in healing serious mental disorders. However, other modern authorities believe they aggravate the condition. Practitioners have noted that procedures such as *śhiro dhārā* have evoked troubling past emotions in some persons. Therefore, persons who have very deep emotional problems may be advised by some practitioners to heal through herbs, aromas, and professional counseling first.

Several important differences exist between *Kerala* and ancient *pañcha karma* therapies.

Ancient Rules	*Kerala* Rules
pañcha karma must be done only during certain seasons	*pañcha karma* can be done in all seasons
oil and sweat are preliminary therapies	oil and sweat are the principle therapies
treat the constitution	treat the illness
purification/reducing oriented	palliation/toning oriented
only five therapies	more than five therapies
not done when too hot or cold; or when cloudy (or rainy)	especially effective when rainy

Even though there are numerous treatments in *Keralīya Pañcha Karma* they all fit into five major categories.

5 Keralīya Pañcha Karma Categories

Therapy	Benefits
1. *Dhārā Karma* (*Śhiro Dhārā*) *Avagāhan Parişheka*	diseases of the mind, *Prāṇa* Vāyu, CNS, ears, eyes, nose, and throat; facial palsy, insomnia, nervous disorders, memory, psychosis, fainting, confusion, excess perspiration, alcoholism, coma, etc.
2. *Kāya Seka* (*Pizhichil*)	promotes tissue strength, biological fire, luster, complexion, *ojas*, clear senses, Vāyu disorders, muscle spasms, degenerative muscle disorders
3. *Piṇḍa Sweda*	heals neuromuscular (facial paralysis, MS, muscular atrophy, and some systemic diseases/ most useful of the therapies
4. *Anna Lepa*	used when *Piṇḍa Sweda* does not work (medicated grains)
5. *Śhiro Lepa*	mental and brain disorders

Both *dhārā* and *lepa* are palliative measures that eliminate excessed *doşhas*. They remove stagnant, sticky toxins from the body's channels (*srotas*) without applying traditional reducing methods (*śhodhana*). Both can be given at all times in all seasons.

1. Dhārā Karma

Three forms of this therapy exist.

1. head baths (*śhiro dhārā*)
2. whole body baths (*sarvānga dhārā*)
3. local bath (*ekānga dhārā*)

Dhārā karma makes use of medicated oils,

milk, *ghee*, etc. (see page 246). *Sarvānga Dhārā* (*Avagāhan*—medicated baths) and *Ekānga Dhārā* (*Pariṣheka—liquid sprinkling*) were previously discussed under sudation therapy on pages 182 to 183.

Dhārā karma makes use of medicated oils, milk, *ghee*, etc. (see page 246). *Sarvānga Dhārā* (*Avagāhan*—medicated baths) and *Ekānga Dhārā* (*Pariṣheka—liquid sprinkling*) were previously discussed under sudation therapy on pages 182 to 183.

Medicated oils include *bhṛingarāj, balā, musta,* sandalwood, licorice, medicated milk, and medicated decoctions. Examples of ingredients for each *doṣha* include the following:

Vāyu—*balā, daśhmūl, bhṛingarāj,* sesame oil.

Pitta—sandalwood, coconut water, *bhṛingarāj, musta.*

Kapha—licorice, *balā, bhṛingarāj.*

2. Kāya Seka (Pizhichil)

This form of *abhyañga* is said to be most beneficial for rejuvenating the nervous system. In this method, the medicated oil used during *dhārā karma* is poured over the person's body from a height of 15 *anguli* (head) and 13 *anguli* (body), while simultaneously being rubbed into the body. These heights may cause the oil to splash on practitioners, so old clothing is worn. *Pizhichil* is also known as *Taila Seka* or *Sarvānga Senchana*. This method strengthens the tissues and promotes the biological fire.

Oil and *ghee* can be reused for another 3 days, but must be replaced on the 4th day. When milk and vinegar are used they are replaced daily.

Healthy persons can receive *kāya seka* twice daily, using a mixture of sesame oil and *ghee*. For weaker persons a 2- to 6-day interval between sessions is advised. The body's luster and beauty are enhanced, *ojas* becomes stabilized, and sense organs are cleared. The process also promotes longevity, regeneration, and rejuvenation of the body. It is especially good for Vāyu disorders. The same massage table, eye protection, and other oil requirements used in *pinḍasveda* and *śhiro dhārā* are applied here (see page 240).

For healthy persons, warm sesame oil and/or *ghee* are used along with rejuvenating herbs (e.g., *śhatāvarī, aśhwagandhā, guḍūchī*). Medicated milk or sour vinegar can be used in place of medicated oil. For Pitta disorders, oil or *ghee* can be unheated. Kapha and Vāyu disorders require warm oil. However, unheated oil is used on the head in all cases.

Four practitioners attend the seated person. Two practitioners massage from the shoulders to the navel, and the other two practitioners massage from the navel to the feet. In this approach, cloths are soaked in *ghee* or oil and squeezed on the body (or oil is poured on the body from vessels) with the right hand. The left hand rubs the oil into the body. Again, insuring uniform pressure and movement, at a moderate speed, among all the *abhyañga* practitioners is important. Hand strokes start from the upper portion of the body and move downward.

A cloth is tied around the eyebrows to prevent liquids from dripping into the eyes. Again, oil applied to the body is lukewarm, while the oil applied to the head is at room temperature. A fifth practitioner keeps the cloths in warm oil and replaces them as they cool off. When lying down, the head faces the east in the morning and the west in the evening. The person receives massage for 1 hour in the same seven positions as in *pinḍasveda* (page 236).

If the treatment lasts for 14 or 21 days, the hour-long session is gradually increased by 5 minutes from the 2nd day on, until it reaches 11/2 hours. When it reaches 11/2 hours (i.e., the 7th day), the time of each session is shortened by 5 minutes. For the 21-day series, upon reaching the 7th day(11/2 hours), the sessions remain at the 11/2 hour time through the 14th day. From the 15th day on, each session is reduced another 5 minutes. It is stated that the oil fully penetrates one tissue layer (*dhātu*) a day. Thus, on the 1st day the oil is absorbed only into the skin. Since there are seven *dhātus*, it takes seven days for oil to completely penetrate all the tissue layers.

Some authorities suggest that Vāyu disorders

require a 2-hour session and Vāyu/Kapha disorders only require 1 hour. In these cases, the oil is applied first and absorbed for a 100 to 300 count before massage begins. These times should correspond with the forehead, chest, and armpits beginning to perspire. The *abhyañga* is then over.

At the end of the session the client sits again while their shoulders and back are massaged vigorously. While this is happening, the oils are wiped off with a towel.

If persons feel tired after receiving the *abhyañga*, they may be lightly fanned, sprinkled with cold water; then rest. Afterwards, the body is massaged, and the excess oil is rubbed off with a towel. Fresh oil is then applied to the body and head, and chick-pea flour (*besan*) is sprinkled over the oil to remove the excess. The head and body are then cleansed again of excess oil by wiping off the flour. Persons then bathe in lukewarm water (room temperature water for the head) to wash off the flour. After bathing, they put on clean clothes and drink a cup of ginger/coriander tea. If hungry, they may eat a light, boiled meal with carminative herbs (e.g., turmeric, cardamom) for Vāyu and Kapha *doṣhas*, or coriander and fennel for Pitta *doṣhas*.

Following *kāya seka*, persons remain on this diet for as many days as they have received treatment. The number of *abhyañgas* depends upon the strength of the person and the strength of the disease they have. They may receive *abhyañga* daily, or on every second, 3rd, 4th, or 5th day; *abhyañga* requires 14 days for one course of treatment.

3. Piṇḍa Sveda (Navarakizhi)

This is considered the most important of all the *Keralīyan* methods. It is also used in traditional *pañcha karma*. *Piṇḍa sveda* is a rejuvenation technique that causes the entire body to perspire by using medicinal puddings followed by *abhyañga*.

Piṇḍa sveda makes the body supple, and removes stiffness, and swelling in the joints. It heals Vāyu diseases, clears obstructions, improves blood circulation, removes wastes from the body, improves complexion, increases Pitta, strengthens digestion, and restores vigor. It also prevents excessive sleep while promoting sound sleep. This therapy is very effective in healing disorders of the nervous system and brain (e.g., paralysis, MS, chronic rheumatism, osteoarthritis, gout, muscle emaciation, and toxic blood). It makes the entire body strong, sturdy, and well developed. The senses are sharpened and the aging process is slowed. Insomnia, high blood pressure, diabetes, skin disorders, balding, premature graying, and wrinkles are prevented. It is helpful for all neuromuscular diseases and some systemic (whole body) diseases.

In this procedure a warm bolus of medicated grain is applied to the body. *Snehana* or body oil application is a prerequisite for *piṇḍa sveda*. A cloth is tied around the eyebrows to prevent oil from dripping into the eyes.

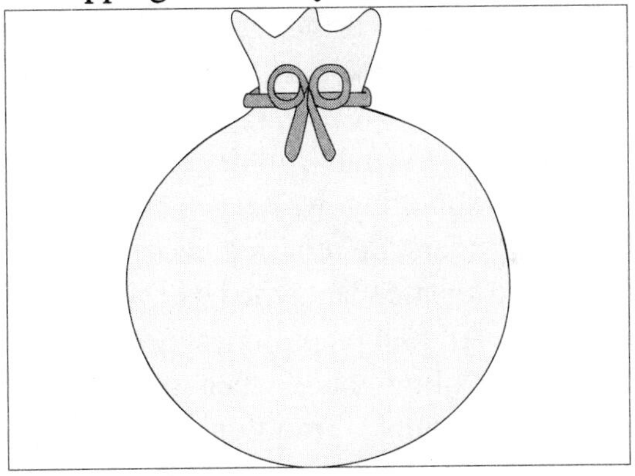

PIṆḌA SVEDA BOLUS

Preparation of Decoction and Pudding: About 17.5 ounces of *balā* root (crushed chips) are poured into two gallons of water and boiled until only 1/4 of the water remains. This decoction is then strained, leaving a 1/2 gallon quantity. One quart of this decoction is mixed with one quart of cow's milk. The other quart is retained for later use. Next, about 17.5 ounces of dehusked and crushed rice is added and cooked until the decoction becomes a semi-solid pudding (*pāyasam*).

Eight pieces of soft and strong cloth, about 15 square inches in size, are used to hold the pudding. The pudding is divided equally into 8 portions and placed in the cloths. The edges of the cloths are wrapped together and tied with string.

For Vāyu diseases, some authorities suggest using black gram, *ghee*, oil, porridge, or puddings. *Piṇḍa* Kapha disorders can be done with barley or sand.

Pre-*Piṇḍa sveda*: Traditionally, persons giving *abhyañga* offer some prayers and meditate before beginning the therapy. Then, oil is applied over the head and body of the client. Head oil is not very greasy; body oil is greasy (medicated oils differ according to illness). Oil application helps maintain the uniformity of the heat of the pudding ball (bolus) and protects the skin from sudden evaporation and perspiration. Experiencing sudden cold or draft after the treatment may cause various forms of respiratory diseases.

A piece of cloth is tied around the eyebrows to prevent oil from dripping into the eyes and irritating them. A special *abhyañga* table is used, just like the *śhiro dhārā* table (see p. 239). Practitioners use a table with or without legs; standing or squatting while giving *abhyañga*. Four practitioners are required, along with a supervisor and an attendant who heats and replaces the boluses. All four practitioners need to use the same degree of pressure when rubbing. The atmosphere is quiet. Traditionally men do *abhyañga* on men and women on women. All clothing is removed except undershorts. The room is well ventilated, with soothing lighting. Drafts, dust, and direct sunlight are to be avoided.

Four bundles are removed from the simmering liquid and left to cool for five minutes. The bolus is held by the tuft in the right hand and placed on the back of the left hand to check the temperature.

Method: The session always begins at the neck, and the movement is always in the downward direction. Two practitioners are on each side of the person. Two persons work in simultaneous motion, at the same temperature and pressure, from the neck to the hip. The other 2 persons work in unison from the hip to the soles of the feet. While the first 4 bundles are used, the remaining 4 are kept heated in the decoction. As the bundles cool, the attendant replaces them with the warm ones and re-heats the cool boluses. The attendant ensures that no interruption during *abhyañga* occurs. The attendant constantly replaces the practitioners' cooled boluses with warm bundles.

Persons receive *Piṇḍa sveda* in seven alternating positions. *Abhyañga* continues for 15 minutes in each position.

1. sitting	5. lying on their back
2. prone (lying on one's back)	6. lying on their left side
3. lying on their right side	7. sitting
4. lying on their left side	

When the liquid in the bowl is used up, the boluses are opened and the pudding is applied over the body and rubbed for 5 minutes. It is then gently scraped off with a blunt edge and the head is gently wiped dry with a towel.

The head and body are then anointed with the appropriate medicated oils (according to the nature of the illness or *doṣha*).

Post-*Abhyañga*: Next, the client takes a lukewarm bath with the appropriate herbal decoction added to the water. The head is not washed or submerged in the bath water; water at room temperature is used to wash the head. Chick-pea flour is rubbed on the body and head to remove the excess oil.

After the bath, persons are wrapped in cotton or wool and rest for about an hour (but do not sleep), avoiding drafts, sun, noise, dust, cold, and smoke. At this time persons are advised to meditate or mentally recite holy scriptures of their respective faiths. After an hour, persons may eat a light meal.

Depending upon the strength and nature of the disorder persons are experiencing,

Pinḍasveda may be applied daily,
or on alternating days for
7, 9, 11, or 14 days.

Pinḍa sveda is good for persons of all ages, but caution is advised for those with heart diseases. However, if boluses are applied with uniform temperature, no adverse effects will develop.

Lepas
Medicinal Plasters

These methods are considered the most important method to reduce inflammatory swellings. All plasters are applied against the direction of the hair (i.e., in an upward direction). Plasters are removed as soon as they dry (except when drawing pus to a head). For a further introduction to plasters, see the earlier discussion under sudation on page 180.

Lepas can include a number of ingredients: *kuṣhṭha, vachā*, barley, oil, *āmalakī*, and mixed with water. The consistency of *lepas* is semisolid, and is neither too thin nor too thick.

If oil or *ghee* is included in the *lepa*, 1/4 the amount of the herbs is added for Vāyu *doṣha*, 1/6 the amount of herbs is used for Pitta *lepas*, and 1/8 the amount of herbs is mixed for Kapha *doṣha*.

Three forms of this procedure exist.

1. Pralepa: These pastes are thin and cold, and have either absorbing or nonabsorbing properties. They restore deranged blood and Pitta.

2. Pradhena: These pastes are applied either thick or thin, cold or warm. They have nonabsorbing properties. They reduce Vāyu and Kapha excesses; purify and heal ulcers; and reduce swelling and pain (in either ulcerated or nonulcer conditions).

3. Alepa/Ātepanam: These pastes are applied over ulcers. They are either arrestive or astringent. Results include stopping local bleeding, softening ulcers, withdrawing local bad flesh, stopping pus from forming in ulcers, correcting *doṣhas*, relieving Pitta-burning sensations, Vāyu aches and pains, severe itching caused by Kapha, and cleansing the skin, blood and flesh.

The *Śhārṅgadhar Saṃhitā* discusses these types of *lepas* and their respective paste thickness.

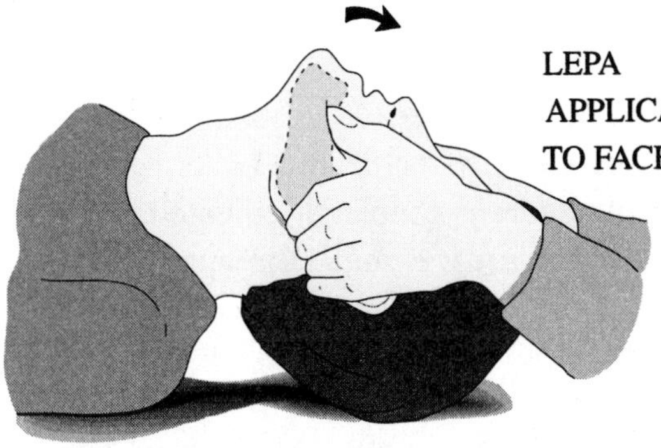

Lepa	Thickness
1. *Doṣha*-reducing (*doṣhaghna*)	1/4 *aṅguli*
2. Poison removal (*viṣhaghna*)	1/3 *aṅguli*
3. Cosmetic (*vaṛinya mukhalepa*)	1/2 *aṅguli*

aṅguli is a finger width

An example of a *lepa* for all forms of edema includes ingredients like *punarnavā*, cedar, and ginger.

A *daśhmūl* and milk plaster is useful for acute pain. *Ghee* is added in plasters for Vāyu rheumatism. Unlike *abhyañga* oil, plaster is not reused.

Anna Lepa

When *Pinḍa Sveda* is contraindicated or ineffective, *Anna Lepa* is used. This *Keralīyan* therapy is not merely contemporary treatment. Its use is discussed in the ancient Āyurvedic texts, *Charak Saṃhitā* and *Aṣhṭāñga Hṛidayam.* Preparation of ingredients, methods, and proportions for *Anna Lepa* are the same as for *Piṇḍa Sveda*; only medicated grains are used without the oil application.

Śhiro Lepa

The use of herbal pastes to treat brain disorders, and head and neck diseases is also discussed in the traditional Āyurveda texts, *Charak Saṃhitā, Aṣhṭāñga Hṛidayam* and *Suṣhruta Saṃhitā*. Herbs include sandalwood, *kuṣhṭā, balā, musta*, licorice, *triphalā, daśhmūl*, and are chosen according to the health concern.

The procedure is simple. Medicated oil (e.g., *brāhmī, bhṛiṅgarāj, āmalakī*) is applied to the hair and scalp before the herbal paste is applied to the hair (not on the forehead). It is removed from the hair after 11/2 hours. Steam therapy is then applied to the body. After *śhiro lepa* a lukewarm medicated bath is given (as described under *Piṇḍa sveda*).

Śhiro Lepa:
1. Oil is kept in hair for 11/2 hours
2. Steam therapy
3. Lukewarm medicated bath

Śhiro Lepa is given either:
1. Once
2. Alternating days or daily for 1 week

Other forms of *abhyañga* exist in *Kerala* and throughout India; there are too many to mention here. Āyurveda, like most professions in India, is a family tradition passed on from parent to child. Thus, many methods are unique to each family.

Śhiro Dhārā
(Hot Oil Flow On The Head Abhyañga)

Unique to Āyurveda is the hot oil flow on the head. Warm oil poured on the forehead is one of the most divine, relaxing therapies one can experience. '*Śhiro*' means head, and '*dhārā*' means flow. When people get up from this therapy, a healthy glow radiates from their skin. People look 20 years younger. Eyes gleam with tranquillity while lips wear a smile of serenity.

Śhiro dhārā helps with diseases of the head, *Prāṇa* Vāyu, neck, eyes, ears, nose, throat, and nervous system. It also relieves insomnia, asthma, cholesterol, enlarged prostate, ulcers, rheumatism, etc., and is used to heal difficult diseases like diabetes, schizophrenia, and epilepsy. Various methods of *śhiro dhārā* exist. The traditional approach includes giving the client a short haircut and combing the hair. A modified version is described here, taking into consideration modern day practicalities of time and finances.

General Method: The client lies on an *abhyañga* table or a specially built oil table which drains the excess oil. The oil is held in a quart-sized bowl. A small hole, a little less than 1/2 inch, is in the bottom-middle of the bowl. A spigot might be attached to the bottom of the bowl to more accurately control the oil flow.

The bowl material retains heat, so the oil does not cool before it is poured on the client's head. If the bowl hangs over the client's head, the therapist doesn't have to hold the bowl for the entire session (45 minutes, to 1 1/2 hours). Three holes must be in the top of the bowl so that a chain or string can be used to suspend the bowl from the ceiling or mobile stand. The distance from the hole or spigot to the forehead is 2 to 3 inches.

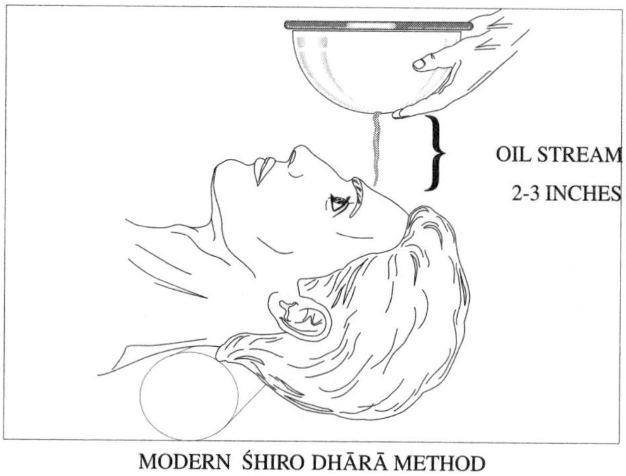

MODERN ŚHIRO DHĀRĀ METHOD

A traditional bowl was set up a little differently. Inside the bowl, half a coconut shell was placed open-side down. It too had a hole at its base. A string, about 6 finger-widths long was placed through the hole and tied to a stick (2 to 3 inches wide). The other end of the string was threaded through the hole in the bottom of the bowl, and hung 2 to 3 inches above the person's forehead (see diagram to right).

Below the table was another wide-mouthed bowl or pan to catch the oil that falls from the head after being poured. Having a heater under this pan to keep the oil warm may be useful if it will be reused during the session.

The bowl is filled with enough warm oil to continue the flow for an entire session. If this is not possible, then one stops every so often to replace the drained oil (oil is reheated if necessary before re-applying).

Ideally, the client with a severe illness will be vacationing at the Āyurvedic resort and receive daily sessions for 7 to 14 days. Weekly sessions are useful and sometimes more practical.

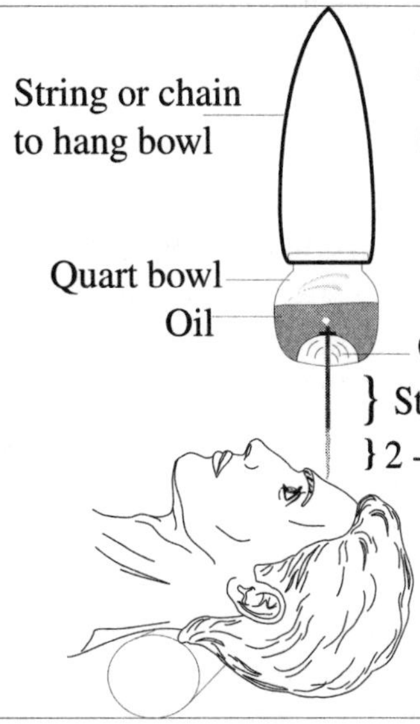

TRADITIONAL ŚHIRO DHĀRĀ BOWL

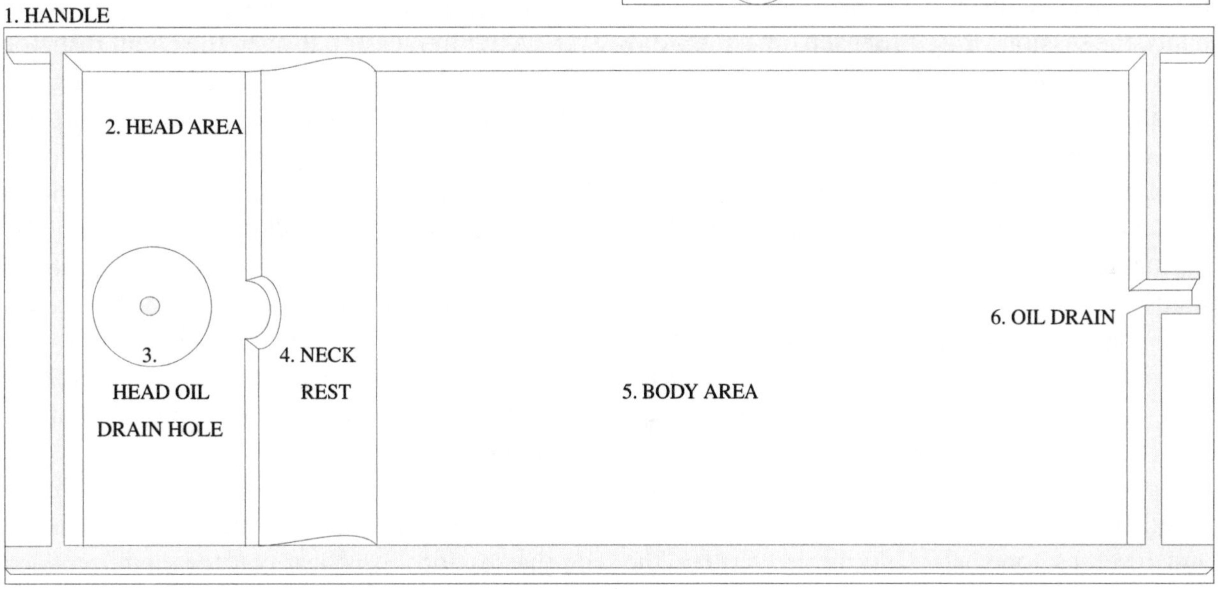

TRADITIONAL ABHYAÑGA TABLE

<u>Fourteen-day treatment</u>: The first session lasts for 1 hour. From the 2nd day to the 7th day of the treatment, 5 minutes are added to each session, with a maximum time of 1 1/2 hours. From the 8th day through the 14th day, the time is reduced by 5 minutes. In this way the 14th session lasts for 1 hour again.

<u>Twenty-one-day treatment</u>: The 7th through 14th day times are kept at 1 1/2 hours. Then, from the 15th day on, the session is reduced by 5 additional minutes. *Śhiro dhārā* is usually never given more than 21 days. It is believed that the medicated oil flow completely affects the entire body in 21 days.

Early morning is the best time for *śhiro dhārā;* spring and fall are the best seasons for *śhiro dhārā* .

Śhiro Dhārā:
A 14 - or 21-day series is ideal
Weekly or monthly sessions are more practical
Best Time: Early morning
Best Seasons: Spring and fall

Procedure

Śhiro dhārā is ideally practiced on auspicious mornings (according to the Indian astrological almanac—*pañchang*). It is best not to have eaten for at least an hour before the therapy. The room should be clean, quiet, have fresh air, and no drafts. Any windows should have curtains to prevent sun glare and to ensure privacy. Soft-colored lights, incense, or aromas suitable for the client help create a healthy and calming environment, even before the session begins. Soft spiritual music, like classical Indian *ragas;* can enhance the session. *Ragas* for each time of the day exist to further harmonize the relaxation and healing process.

Before therapy, the practitioners meditate, preparing themselves to be effective healers. Clients and practitioners practice *mantra* meditation during the session to keep their minds spiritually focused.

Whether clients stay at an Āyurvedic resort for several days or weeks, or make daily visits for *śhiro dhārā,* they are advised to follow their Āyurvedic lifestyle. Appropriate foods, baths, exercise, spiritual studies, *yoga*, etc. are recommended. This further balances one's constitution and develops good habits. Thus, persons feel the maximum healing effects and find it easier to follow their program once they return home.

Clients receiving weekly sessions, will find relief from the stress and strain of their daily work schedules. This is truly a constructive form of pampering.

In a traditional session the client sits on the massage table facing east. Room-temperature oil is poured through the hair three times. Then, the body is massaged below the neck (i.e., from the shoulders down) with slightly warm oil. A cloth is placed or tied over the eyes to prevent oil from leaking into them during *śhiro dhārā*.

Practitioner and client can meditate before and during śhiro dhārā to bring the highest spiritual energy into the healing session

The client is supine on a massage table with a pillow under their neck for comfort. Oil is released from the bowl onto the forehead. Traditionally, oil is circled on the third eye (just above and between the eyebrows). Modern experience finds that many people find this directed application too powerful. Thus, oil must be moved around the entire forehead and temples.

When the oil in the bowl (or funnel) runs out, it is once again placed in the bowl and reused. If the oil is cool, it can be reheated during the session or just after the bowl is empty.

After the session is over, the client rests for a few minutes on the table. The oil in the hair is pressed into the scalp as its warmth further soothes the client. Then a towel is placed over the head and the practitioner helps the client sit up, making sure the head is covered with the towel to prevent the oil from dripping. The client is given a few minutes to adjust to the seated position. Then, they are helped to stand up. Sometimes they are so relaxed that they feel disoriented upon standing, so helping up them is important.

If the weather is cool—to avoid catching a cold—a warm hat and scarf are worn when leaving the session. It is best that for the remainder of the day the client rest, taking light meals, and retire to bed early.

Head-Soaking Oils
Śhiro Basti

Śhiro basti, like *śhiro dhārā*, is another head oil application. However, in this method the oil soaks on the top of the head for some time. *Śhiro basti* is useful in healing facial paralysis, insomnia, dry mouth or nose; cataracts, headaches, and other head diseases. It prevents and stops hair loss, balding, and premature graying. This therapy also strengthens hair roots and makes the hair soft and glossy, heals eye problems, improves complexion and sinus disorders. *Śhiro basti* balances the air and fluid (Vāyu and Kapha) in the space between the brain and skull.

The head oil (*dhārā drava*) is prepared in different ways for different situations. Basic oils listed below are useful for *śhiro dhārā* as well.

Dry hair: Coconut and sesame oils.
Memory: *brāhmī, āmalakī, bhṛiṅgarāj* oils.
Young Women: Black sesame, *bhṛiṅgarāj, āmalakī* oils.
Women 40 to 50: Black sesame, wheat germ, almond oils.
Women 50+: Black sesame, coconut, wheat germ, sandalwood oils.
Newlyweds: Coconut, jasmine, almond, wheat-germ oils.
Ear Pain: Mustard oil
Vāyu: Sesame, coconut, canola, *brāhmī* oils
Pitta: Sunflower, coconut, *brāhmī* oils
Kapha: Canola, mustard oils
All: Sesame, *brāhmī, bhṛiṅgarāj, āmalakī* oils

Many complicated formulations, such as *takra dhārā, kṣhīr dhārā*, can be prepared. Since these products are scarce outside of India (and also for the sake of simplicity), plain oil or any of the above-mentioned medicated oils can be used.

Precaution: In some cases Vāyu becomes aggravated during extended treatments. To counter this, clients receive a warm oil *abhyañga* followed by a warm medicated bath.

Definition: *Basti* is defined as a bladder or container that holds medicated herbs and oil. *Śhiro basti* is somewhat similar to *śhiro dhārā* in that the oil is placed on the head. The differences are that in *śhiro basti*, the oil is kept soaking on the head.

The bladder can be made of a flexible plastic, approximately 3 feet high. The circumference is wide enough to fit around the head. Whole-grain flour is mixed with warm water (2:1) and kneaded into dough. It is used between the head and bladder to prevent the oil from leaking. The dough is placed in a circle parallel to ear level. A belt or rope is used to secure the bladder to the head.

Method: After a person completes the appropriate *pañcha karma* therapies, oleation and fomentation are given. Next, the person sits on a stool or chair (knee-height). The paste is applied to the head under the cap to prevent the oil from leaking. The flour, cap, and belt are placed on the head. The medicated oil is heated to a lukewarm temperature and is then placed in the bladder on the head. Oil should be about six inches above the scalp (one finger width).

It remains on the head for about 2 hours, 45 minutes; 2 hours, 15 minutes; 1 hour, 40 minutes; or until the mouth and nose begin to expel secretions and clients feel relief from their symptoms. The length of time the oil remains on the head varies according to the *doṣha* causing the disorder (Vāyu, Pitta, Kapha respectively).

For healthy persons who are merely receiving preventive measures, oil remains on the head only for approximately 17 minutes. The therapy lasts no more than 7 days.

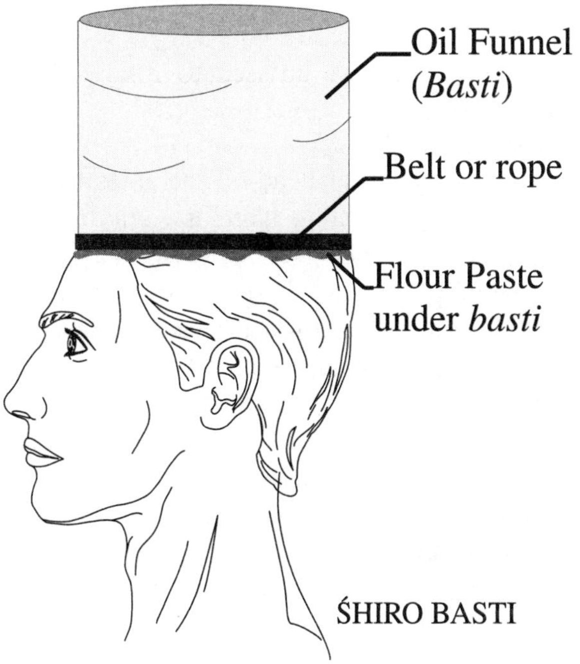

ŚHIRO BASTI

Śhiro Basti Duration

Disease	Time
Vāyu	about 2.45 hours
Pitta/Blood	about 2.3 hours
Kapha	just over 1.3 hours
Healthy	17 minutes

The oil is taken out of the cap, the belt is removed; then the cap and paste are taken off. The head, neck, shoulders, and back then are rubbed gently. Afterwards, persons take a lukewarm bath. A wholesome diet according to one's constitution is then taken. *Śhiro basti* is repeated daily for three, five, or seven days.

Post Śhiro Basti:
1. Gently rub head, neck shoulders, back
2. Lukewarm Bath

Śhiro Basti:
Taken daily for 3, 5, or 7 days

Head Oil
Mūrdha Taila

The Benefits of head-oil therapies include preventing and healing hair loss, graying, and hair matting, cracking of the scalp, Vāyu head disorders; producing sharpness of the senses, improving the strength of the voice, lower jaw, and the head. Two other methods of applying oil to the head are worth mentioning:

1. Pouring oil in a continuous stream (*pariṣheka*) removes scalp ulceration and boils, burning sensations, and wounds.

2. Wrapping a cloth over the head and soaking in oil (*picu*) prevents hair loss, cracking of the scalp, and burning sensations.

Ear-Oil
(Karna Pūrana)

This procedure involves placing oil into the ears. Some authorities suggest 1 to 2 drops. Others suggest filling the entire ear cavity with oil. Ear oil heals disorders of the sense organs such as earaches or pain, deafness, ringing in the ear, all ear diseases and headaches; lockjaw, giddiness, twisted (wry neck), and diseases of the gums and teeth. Certain nerves connect the eyes and ears with the feet. Thus, this treatment also relieves burning sensations in the feet. *Karna pūrana* is done during the day, before meals.

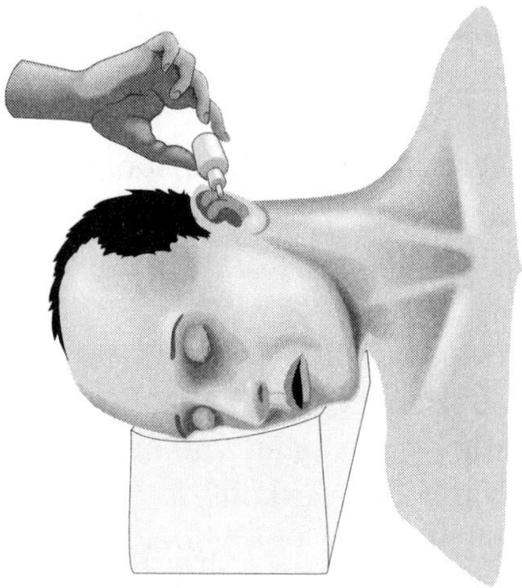

EAR BASTI (KARNA PŪRANA)

Karna Pūrana
is done before meals

Method: Lukewarm sesame oil or medicated oil is poured in the ear canals, filling them up. Oil remains in the ears for 10 to 20 minutes. For preventive care, oil remains in the ear for about 17 minutes. For ear pain, the root of ears can be massaged until the pain subsides.

Ear (and eye) therapies always begin with the right side. A tissue is kept nearby to wipe up any dripping oil. Clients first lie on their left side while the oil is poured into their right ear.

After the process is complete, a small bowl or cup is placed behind the ear to catch the oil as it comes out. The client slowly turns their head to the right and the oil pours out of the ear and into the cup. They may then roll onto their back in order for the remaining oil to be released. A tissue is placed on the ear to prevent any excess oil from dripping. The process is then performed on the left ear.

Eye Therapy
(Āṣhcotana - Anjana Vidhi)
(Also discussed in Chapter 19)

Āyurveda employs eye drops and eye salves for prevention and healing diseases of the eyes, like bleeding, itching, tearing, burning sensation and redness.

Eye drops: (*Āṣhcotana*) are warm for Vāyu diseases, lukewarm for Kapha disorders, and cold for Pitta ailments. The person lies on a bed in a draftless room. Their eyes are opened with the practitioner's left hand, while the liquid is dropped in the eye with the right hand. Ten to 12 drops are placed in the eye from a distance of 2 finger widths from the inner angle of the eye.

A soft, clean cloth is placed over the eyes for a few minutes (a warm cloth is used for Vāyu and Kapha disorders).

Eye salve: (*Anjana*) is used after a person has undergone *pañcha karma*, and the illness is localized only in the eyes, when diseases are matured, such as in edema, severe itching, sliminess, and thick excretions.

Three types of *anjana* exist:

1. Scraping (*lekhana*) using astringent, sour, salty, and pungent tastes
2. Healing (*ropana*) with bitter tastes
3. Vision clearing (*prasādana*) using sweet tastes

Time: The recommended time for salves is morning or evening. Application is not recommended before evening sleep, at noon, and when the sun irritates the eyes—because it increases the illness and spreads it elsewhere. For Kapha diseases that require scraping eye salve, daytime application is acceptable if it is not too hot a day. During very cold weather, night application will further aggravate the illness.

Precautions: *Anjana* is not used on those suffering from fear, after emesis and purgation, when hungry, when having the urge to urinate or defecate; when angry, when feverish, or when the eyes are tired. It is also not used with a headache, when experiencing grief and insomnia; when cloudy, after smoking, when drinking alcohol, or just after washing hair. *Anjana* is not suggested with indigestion, when tired due to excess exposure to fire or sun, just after day naps, or when thirsty. This therapy may bring up strong emotional issues.

Post-Application: Eyeballs are gently and briefly rubbed and slowly rotated up. The eyelids are also gently massaged. This is to spread the salve throughout the eye. It is not recommended to open, close, squeeze, or wash eyelids. When the salve no longer has an effect, the eyes are washed (water temperature is according to the disease, *doṣha* and season). This removes the disease cleansed from the salve. The left eyelid is lifted and held with a piece of clean cloth in the fingers of the practitioner's right hand, and vice versa. If there is itching or a lack of results from the salve, a stronger salve or strong smoke inhalation is used. Persons are strongly advised to rest in a darkened room for at least one hour before exposure to light and activity.

Eye-Bath (Netra Basti)
(Also discussed in Chapter 19)

This therapy involves washing the eyes with medicated oils or *ghee*. Benefits include relieving tension in the eye sockets that may lead to loss of vision, pain, fatigue, glaucoma, cross-eye, conjunctivitis, night blindness, cornea inflammation, sunken eyes, and other eye disorders. Further, it nourishes the nervous system, brain, memory, and develops one's linguistic abilities. It makes the eyes lustrous, removes wrinkles, improves complexion, reduces physical tension.

Method: Dough is prepared using flour and water (2:1). The dough is made into two rings to fit around the eyes, 11/2 inches in height. One half cup of lukewarm *ghee* is kept warm nearby. Oleation and fomentation of the face are done in advance. The lights are dimmed so as not to disturb the session. Next, the temperature of the *ghee* is tested (several drops may be placed on the wrist, or a finger is swirled in the *ghee*). *Ghee* should be lukewarm. The dough dam is placed around the eyes, the base pressed onto the face to prevent oil from leaking. *A little ghee* is then poured into the dough-dam (around the eyes) while eyes are closed. If the temperature is comfortable, the remaining oil is poured into the dam until it covers the eyelashes. Eyes are then opened when comfortable (initially it may take some time adjusting to the liquid). The eyes may be slowly rotated clockwise, counterclockwise or moved in the 8 compass directions.

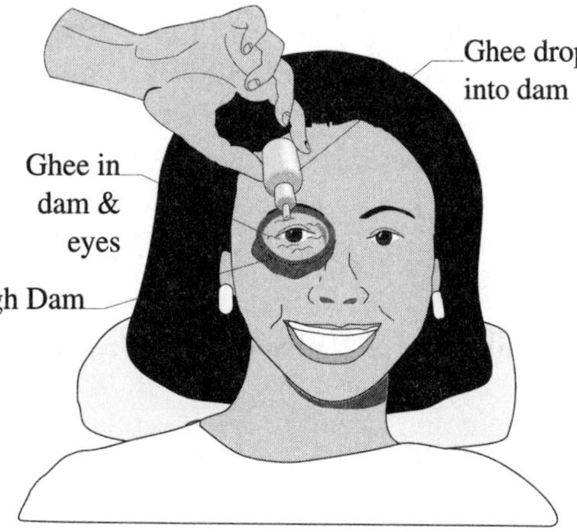

EYE BATH (NETRA BASTI)

Some authorities suggest that the *ghee* be kept in the eye for 20 minutes. Others say that for Vāyu disorders it is kept in for 6 minutes. For Pitta disorders and healthy persons oil remains in the eye for 31/2 minutes and only for 2 minutes, 45 seconds for Kapha diseases. Afterwards, persons need to rest for 1 to 2 hours in a dark room. When going outside, if it is bright sunglasses should be worn.

Eye Condition	Length of Eye Bath
eyelid disorders	30 seconds
eye joint circles	95 seconds
white circles	3 1/2 minutes
black circles	4 minutes
refractive disorders	4 1/2 minutes
glaucoma	5 minutes, 5 seconds
Vāyu disorders	done daily
Pitta disorders	alternate days
Kapha /healthy eyes	done every two days

If *netra basti* is overdone, one experiences itching and Kapha disorders. This therapy can cause strong emotional releases. It is not advised for those with emotional disorders.

Lower Back Bath (Katti Basti)

The main benefits of this therapy are for muscle spasms and lower spine rigidity, and strengthening the bone tissue of the lower back. The same method of preparing dough as in the eye bath is used here. Placement of the dough dam is however around the spine of the lower back.

Chest/Heart Bath (Uro Basti)

This therapy strengthens the heart and reduces sternum pain. Again, the dough dam is prepared in the same manner as the eye bath. The dam is placed over the heart (left breast)

Body Powder-Rub (Udgharṣhana)

Herbal powders may be applied to the body to promote healing. They heal itching, Vāyu disorders, hives, and develop a stable, light body. Rubbing the skin after water is sprinkled on the body removes dirt, opens the sweat glands, and activates the enzymes in the skin. Afterwards, water is again sprinkled on the body and the skin rubbed to remove the powder.

Āyurvedic Foot Massage Pādābhyañga

Abhyañga applied to the feet is a simple, enjoyable and healthy thing to do. It prevents dryness, cracks, and roughness of the skin; numbness, fatigue, sciatica, cramps; and contraction of ligaments, vessels, and muscles of the feet and legs. It removes Vāyu from the body, promotes sturdy limbs and feet, strength for walking, and sound sleep. Further, nerves from all the organs in the head and body terminate in the feet (also in the hands, ears, and head). Thus, by rubbing the feet, persons tone the whole body. A close relationship exists between the feet, eyes, and ears. Foot *abhyañga* helps heal and prevent disorders of hearing and sight. Four important nerves in the soles are connected to the head. Constant friction and pressure on the nerves in the soles reduce eye sight. *Abhyañga* on a daily basis, or at least several times a week, restores health to these nerves. It is best done before bedtime, rubbing the soles and tops of the feet with some warm sesame oil. This also fosters sound sleep.

General Suggestions

After all *abhyañgas,* clients are advised to rest for 1 to 2 hours before returning home. It is best if another person drives them home to avoid the stress of driving. If this is not possible, then when reaching home, they rest. Light meals and rest are advised for the remainder of the day. An early bedtime that evening is strongly suggested. Some people find *abhyañga* so relaxing that they sleep through the next day, releasing deep-seated stresses.

As discussed earlier in this section, persons with emotional problems may find the *abhyañgas* too powerful. Therefore, it is advised to achieve mental balance slowly through herbs, foods, aromas, colors, and, if needed, professional counseling.

Doṣha Beauty Care Facial Abhyañga

Depending upon one's *doṣha* different facial oils are used.

Doṣha	Oils
Vāyu	*ghee*, sesame, avocado
Pitta	coconut, safflower, sunflower
Kapha	canola, almond, olive
Tridoṣhic	sesame, jojoba, almond

For various skin disorders, essential oils may be used, see the "*Doṣha Marma* Oil" chart (page 232) in this chapter, and Chapter 8 on Aromatherapy.

Face Care

Conditions	Essential Oil Mixtures
Wrinkles	fennel, lavender, rose, frankincense, cypress
Acne	bergamot, juniper, cypress, tea tree, lavender

Miscellaneous Skin Care

Conditions	Therapy
Eye care	*triphalā, kajal*
Stretch marks	almond oil

Cosmetic Plasters
(Varṇya Lepa)

To improve complexion and color, medicated herbal pastes are applied to the skin. The applied paste is 1/2 *aṅguli* (1/2 one's finger width).

Complexion, pigmented patches on face: Red sandalwood, *mañjiṣhṭhā. kuṣhṭha.*

Acne: Coriander, *vachā,* black pepper

Dandruff: *Kuṣhṭha,* licorice, rock salt, mixed into a paste with honey.

Facial Hair: Excess Pitta unbalances the hormones. A mixture of *aśhok,* fennel, *śhatāvarī,* cardamom, *triphalā*, rock candy are taken internally, and sandalwood and *multani methi* clay are mixed with water to form a *lepa* for the face. The *lepa* is left on from 4 hours to overnight (2 times weekly). Hot spices and steroids aggravate this condition.

Properties of Paste Liquids

Ghee: PV- K (neutral). Unctuous/Cool
Uses: It promotes taste, semen, and *ojas*, alleviates burning, develops a soft body, voice, and complexion; and strengthens the metabolism and digestion. *Ghee* improves the voice and complexion, and has a special property of transporting herbal properties to all the *dhātus* (tissues).

Oil:
Uses: Oils promote strength, health, and a stable body. They improve the skin and cleanse the urogenital tract (especially for females).

Sesame Oil V- KP+ in excess

It gives strength, intelligence, digestive power, helps the skin, and has antioxidant properties. When taken with the appropriate herbs, it heals all disorders.

Castor Oil: Sweet, astringent-hot P+

Castor is a digestive stimulant and a purgative. It helps with obstructed abdominal diseases, gas, tumors, stiff lumbar region, colic pain, ulcers, edema, *āma*, abscesses, clears vagina and semen.

Coconut Oil: Sweet-cold-sweet VP- K+

This oil is best for Pitta *doṣhas*, nourishing and softening the skin. It is useful for inflammatory skin conditions, psoriasis, eczema, sunburn, burns, rosacea. [Sample skin oil: coconut oil 100 ml.; almond oil 50 ml.; sandalwood oil 5 ml.]

Milk (Dugdha): VP- K+ Sweet/Cold; unctuous
Uses: (Cow's) Milk is best when it is organic and raw (if possible). It gives rejuvenation, strength, intelligence, and *ojas*. Milk heals semen and blood diseases, difficult or painful breathing; consumption, hemorrhoids, complexion, and giddiness. It is considered holy (*sattwic*).

Goat Milk: Light

This form of milk is better for Kapha *doṣhas*. It is a digestive stimulant, heals hemorrhoids, diarrhea, menorrhagia, toxic blood, giddiness, and fever. Some say it heals all diseases.

Yogurt/Curd (Dadhi): V- PK, Blood+ Astringent/Hot/Pungent unctuous. Again, organic yogurt is advised.
Uses: This is a digestive stimulant and gives strength. It heals dysuria, coryza, and coldness in the body; diarrhea, anorexia, and emaciation.

Sweet yogurt reduces Vāyu and Pitta. Sour yogurt increases Pitta, Kapha, and blood toxins. Very sour yogurt causes bleeding disorders. Sweet and sour yogurt has mixed effects.

Water: P- Cold
Uses: It is a cardiac tonic, heals poisoning, giddiness, burning, indigestion, exhaustion, vomiting (cold), intoxication, fainting, and alcoholism.

Liquid, Paste and Oil Preparation

The general formula for mixing these three ingredients is,

1 part paste (herb powder)
4 part oil
16 parts liquid (e.g., milk, decoction, herb juice, water)

For decoctions, paste is 1/6 its quantity.

For plant juice, paste is 1/8 its quantity.

When a recipe calls for 4 or fewer liquids, the amount of each is 4 times that of the oil.

When there are more than 4 liquids in a recipe, then each is in equal proportion to the oil.

Preparation: The herbal paste and liquid are mixed together; then oil is added and the entire mixture is boiled. As it is cooked, the mixture is constantly stirred to prevent paste from sticking to the bottom of the pot.

Āyurvedic Beauty Suggested Reading

Kuṣhi A, Tawari M. *Diet for Natural Beauty*. New York, NY: Japan Publications; 1991.

Murthy KRS. (transl.) *Śhārṅgadhar Saṃhita*. Varanasi, India: Chaukhambha Orientalia; 1984 [Section 3; Ch. 11].

Sachs M. *Āyurvedic Beauty Care*. Twin Lakes, WI: Lotus Press; 1994.

Pañcha Karma Suggested Reading

Bhishagratna KL. (transl.) *Suṣhrut Saṃhita*. Varanasi, India: Chowkhamba Sanskrit Series; 1991.

Dash B. *Abhyañga Therapy in Āyurveda.* New Delhi, India: Concept Publishing ;1992.

Devaraj TL. *The Pañchakarma Treatment of Āyurveda*. Bangalore, India: Dhanwantari Oriental Publications; 1986.

Institute for Wholistic Education. *Marma Point Therapy* [video]. Twin Lakes, WI: 1989.

Govindan SV. *Massage for Health and Healing*. New Delhi, India: Abhinav Publications; 1996

Gray H. *Gray's Anatomy*. Philadelphia, PA: Running Press; 1974.

Guyton A. *Textbook of Medical Physiology*. Philadelphia, PA: Saunders Co.; 1981.

Johari H. *Ancient Indian Abhyañga*. New Delhi, India: Munshiram Manoharlal Publishers: 1988.

Joshi SV. *Āyurveda & Pañcha Karma*. Twin Lakes, WI: Lotus Press; 1997.

Merck Manual. Rahway, NJ: Merck Research Laboratories; 1992.

Murthy KRS (transl.) *Aṣhṭāñga Hṛidayam*. Varanasi, India: Kṛiṣhṇadas Acadamey; 1991.

Murthy KRS. (transl.) *Śhārṅgadhar Saṃhita*. Varanasi, India: Chaukhambha Orientalia; 1984.

Ranade S. *Natural Healing Through Āyurveda*. Salt Lake City, Utah: Passage Press; 1993.

Sharma RK, Dash B. *Charak Saṃhita*. (editors) Varanasi, India: Chowkhamba Sanskrit Series; 1992.

Singh RH. *Pañcha Karma Therapy*. Varanasi, India: Chowkhamba Sanskrit Series; 1992.

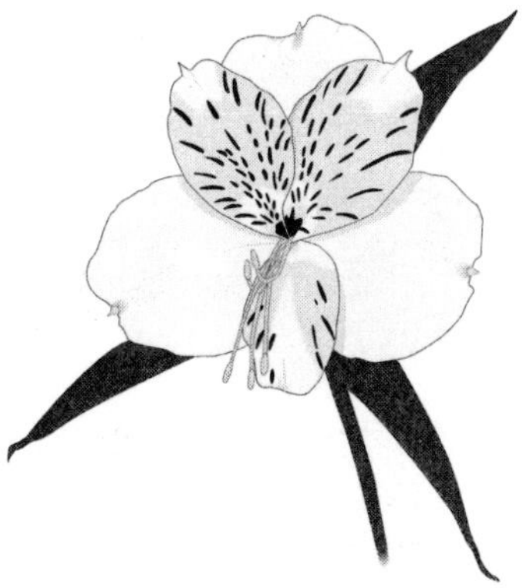

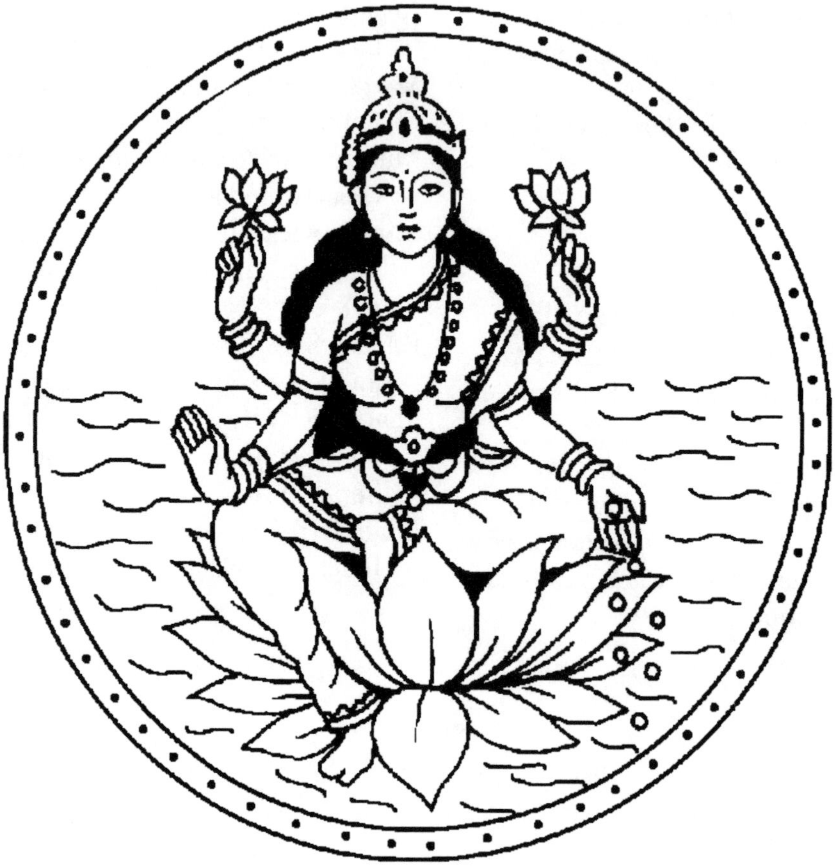

As bubbles and foam are non-existent without water
This world is non-existent without eternal Divinity (Brahman).
Vedic saying

Chapter 8
Aroma Therapy

As mentioned earlier, Āyurveda's main therapy is herbal, with a secondary emphasis on food or nutrition. These therapies work predominantly on the gross, or outer physical, level. Aroma therapy, gem therapy, color, and *mantra* (or sound therapies) work on a more subtle level, healing through the mind, the senses, and the absorption of subtle impressions.

Aromas

Pure fragrances are used for healing. Aromas are commonly used in the forms of incense, flower essences, and essential oils. Other methods of aromatherapy include pure scented candles, soaps, and sachets. Aromas are most effective when pure (i.e., not diluted with chemical substances). They are used externally, and unless mixed with a diluting or base oil, some oils burn the skin. If taken internally, the mucus membranes would be harmed. They should not be placed too close to the eyes or any bodily orifice. A suggested base oil for each *doṣha* is provided in the table below.

Doṣha	**Base Oil**
Vāyu	sesame
Pitta	coconut or sunflower
Kapha	canola or mustard

A generally accepted ratio of essential oil to base oil is the following:

25 ml. (12-13) drops: 1 fluid ounce base oil

It is especially useful to place drops of oil on various body sites: the crown, third eye, temples (for headaches), at the root of the nose (for sinus problems), or at the heart. Oils are more practical to use while in the company of others who may not like to breathe any kind of smoke (e.g., at the office).

Āyurvedic Marma Points

These are specific sites on the body that balance the *doṣhas* and their associated health situations when oils are applied to them. *Marmas* were discussed in detail in the last chapter. To summarize, the main *marma* points for each *doṣha* are given in the table below.

Doṣha	**Main *Marma***
Vāyu	third eye (between eyebrows)
Pitta	heart *chakra* (chest center)
Kapha	between the navel and pubic bone

Steam/Sweat Therapy

Aromatic oils are used in these therapies as well, being directed at specific sites (e.g., arthritis in the hands).

Aromas balance the three humors and *prāṇa*, *ojas*, and *tejas*. Below is a list of commonly used essential oils:

Primary Oils

Aromatic oils have the same properties as the herb and plant.

Basil: **(*Tulsī*)** VK- P+
Uses: Cleanses mind, phlegm, colon, purifies air, reduces fever and viruses, removes *Apāna* Vāyu (downward air), increases devotion and intuition

Camphor: **(*Karpūr*)** VK- P+
Uses: Opens the mind, senses, lungs, increases perception and meditation, alleviates headaches and arthritis, can be used for *pūja* (devotional ritual), calms hysteria, neuralgia, and other nervous ailments; insect repellent. External—sprains, inflammations, rheumatism. Precaution—large doses are toxic

Cedar: (***Devadaru***) (Juniper - *Hapuṣha*) VK- P+
Uses: Diabetes, arthritis, edema, air cleanser

Eucalyptus: VK- P+
Uses: Opens the mind, senses, lungs, removes phlegm and alleviates depression, cleanses negative psychic thoughts. Insect/roach repellent

Frankincense: **(*Kapitthaparni*)** VK- P+
Uses: Heart, head, blood, and nerve cleanser; pain reliever, strengthens joints, calms mind, increases faith, virtue, detachment, and devotion, removes negative psychic thoughts and fears

Gardenia: P- (VK+ in excess)
Uses: Cleanses the blood, kidneys, heart, fevers, and infections (including uterine)

Ginger: **(*Sunta*)** VK- P+
Uses: Colds, flus, headache, lung congestion, joint and muscle pain, improves pulse and appetite, enhances joy and creativity

Iris: P- VK+
Uses: Cleanses the blood, lymphatic, liver, heals infections, helps remove jealousy, envy, anger, and hate

Jasmine: **(*Mallika*)** P- K+ (V+ in excess)
Uses: Heals breast and uterine infections, also heals cancer (especially lymph), strengthens a woman's reproductive system and makes her more attractive; removes depression (P+ men)

Lavender: **(*Dharu* - H)** VPK=
Uses: Calms emotions and nerves (good for hyperactive children), PMS, bug repellent

Lily: **(*Kumuda*)** VP- (K+ in excess)
Uses: Calms heart, nerves, and emotions (irritability, anxiety, insomnia), dry cough, tonic for stomach and lungs, increases faith, devotion, and virtue

Lotus: **(*Padma, Śhatapatra*)** VPK=
Uses: Calms mind and heart, effects deep sleep, increases love, faith, devotion, compassion, builds *ojas* (i.e., strengthens the reproductive system and nerves), is antiallergenic, calms nerves, relieves spasms. It is the symbol of Self-Realization

Mint: (Peppermint: ***Paparminta* - H;** Spearmint: ***Pahadi pudina* - H**) VPK=
Uses: Clears mind, head, and sinuses

Musk: (***Kasturi***) VK- P+
Uses: Revives those who are comatose or near collapse, strengthens heart and reproductive system, awakens senses, is the most *rajasic* oil

Myrrh: **(*Bola*)** VK- P+
Uses: Blood cleanser, relieves infections, decreases tumors, strengthens bones, heart, uterus, and nerves; reduces excess fat, helps tissue healing

Patchouli: **(*Pacholi* - H)** VK- P+
Actions: Stimulant, diaphoretic, expectorant, diuretic, carminative
Uses: Cleanses digestive system, stimulates senses, gives joy (removes depression), is especially good for Kapha. Externally—insecticide (moths, ants, gnats, flies, mosquitoes)

Rose: **(*Rudhrapuṣhpa, Japa*)** (flower of the heart) P- VK+
Uses: Eye tonic (as rose water), increases love, compassion, devotion, acts as female reproductive tonic, urogenital tract, fevers, cough

Rosemary: PK- V+
Uses: Blood, heart, circulatory system, tonic, helps headaches and emotional tension, promotes menstruation

Sandalwood: **(*Chandan*)** (best aroma for the mind) VP- K+ in excess *Sattwic*
Uses: Heart and lung tonic, cleanses kidneys, reduces fever, irritability, and anxiety; promotes meditation

Āyurvedic Aromatherapy

As mentioned above, essential oils must be mixed in base oils before application to the skin.

Aches & Pains
Oils: Myrrh, cinnamon, *mahānārāyan*
Base: Rubbing alcohol, beeswax (*mahānārāyan* oil is mixed with sesame oil)
Use: Headaches, neuralgia, arthritis

Antibacterial
Oils: Sandalwood, myrrh, jasmine, gardenia, iris
Uses: Cools blood, fevers, infections; builds the immune system, removes thirst and delirium

Congestion
Oils: Eucalyptus, sage, basil, mint
Base: Alcohol
Use: Near nose, or inhaling as steam

Digestive Aids
Oils: Cardamom, cloves, fennel, ginger
Use: Promotes *agni*/digestion

Digestive Stimulants
Oils: Cardamom, clove, fennel, ginger
Use: Promotes *agni*/digestion

Gynecological Disorders
Oils: Rose, rosemary
Use: Regulates menstruation (apply to problem site, or soak in an aroma-bath)

Immune Functions
Oils: Myrrh, frankincense, rose, lotus
Use: Strengthens immune system, build *ojas*, (external infections)

Infections
Oils: Eucalyptus, cedar
Use: Parasites, repel insects/insect bites, cleanses the skin, air, and aura

Rejuvenatives (Rasāyanas)
Oils & Use:
frankincense—blood and brain
guggul—brain and bones
myrrh—blood, heart, uterus
rose—heart and uterus
lily—heart and brain
sandalwood—nerves and brain
lotus—heart and reproductive system
gardenia and sandalwood—kidneys
basil—nerves and lungs
gardenia and iris—liver

Soothing
Oils: Sandalwood, rose, lotus, lily, lavender, frankincense
Use: Calming, prevent negative dreams, worry and agitation, insomnia

Insecticide
Oils: Eucalyptus, patchouli, lavender

Aroma Therapy & The Three Doṣhas

Aromas can be derived from essential oils, incense, soaps, or sachets. Some examples follow.

DoṣhaOils
Vāyu: Mix musk, frankincense, basil, camphor, or cinnamon with sandalwood or rose

Pitta: Sandalwood, rose, lotus, iris, gardenia, lily, lavender, honeysuckle
Kapha: Cinnamon, musk, sage, cedar, frankincense, myrrh

Aromatherapy & Specific Uses

(All oils are diluted as recommended in the previous section)

Acne: Camphor, eucalyptus, lavender; applied at night (12 drops cypress to 12 drops lemon in 2 fl oz. (50 ml.) coconut oil or *brāhmī* oil)
Air Purification: Camphor, frankincense, basil, sandalwood, lavender
Athletes foot: Lavender—2 drops massaged into feet; tea tree oil also works but has less pleasant odor. For verruca (wart-like), lavender, eucalyptus, rosemary, or camphor is applied several times daily
Burns: Lavender
Depression: Ylang-ylang, clary sage, jasmine, patchouli
Earache: Lavender, 1 drop placed on a cotton ball and applied to the outer ear
Fainting: Peppermint, rosemary, wafted under patients nose
Feet: Baths: Use 5 drops peppermint oil to one lukewarm bowl of water; or massage feet with sesame oil
Gums: Sesame oil
Headache: Lavender on muscles at back of neck, on temples, forehead etc.; sick headaches—use of peppermint oil, sniffed frequently, may help; also sandalwood, calamus, *guggul*, lily, frankincense; sometimes just taking a nap or going to sleep early helps—a drop of oil may be put on the pillow
Hemorrhoids: Cypress oil: 5 drops in a bowl of warm water or bath, mix well as 'sitz' bath
Hypertension: Lavender, myrrh, frankincense, saffron, rose, sandalwood, lotus, lily
Mouth ulcers: Myrrh, drop of oil on the sore
Nausea: Lavender, rose, geranium: a few drops in a bowl of hot water—inhale
Post Partum:Perineum Healing: (Especially if episiotomy was torn): Sitz bath: 2 drops cypress to 3 drops lavender in large bowl of warm water or shallow bath water. Cypress, with its constricting properties, is an astringent that closes the raw blood vessels. Lavender heals and gently encourages new skin growth, while protecting raw areas.
Sore Nipples: Diluted rose oil, but wash off completely before each feeding so no harm will come to the baby during breast-feeding; 1 drop rose oil to 3/4 fluid ounce sweet almond oil (20 ml.).
Post-Natal Depression: It is believed to be a hormonal adjustment; jasmine bath; jasmine drop on the pillow edge; Ylang-ylang, patchouli, or clary sage are secondary substitutes.
Lactation: Two drops fennel oil in honey water every 2 hours increases milk flow. (Herbs are also ingested in this case, including *śhatāvarī, balā,* and fennel.)
Mastitis: (Breast inflammation) compress: 1 drop geranium, 1 drop lavender, 2 drops rose in 1 1/2 pints (850 ml.) cold water.
Fatigue: Morning: Rosemary baths; naps, oil massage with rejuvenatives mentioned above.
Sore throat/Laryngitis: Three to four drops of lavender for steam inhalation
Sunburn: Lavender or peppermint oil bath, or mist
Toothache: Clove, peppermint, prickly ash
Weight loss: Juniper oil in bath once a week, if depression is the cause of overeating, see above

Pregnancy:
Stretch Marks: Twice daily breast and belly massage; 20 drops lavender to 2 fl. oz. wheat germ oil; plain almond oil may also be used.
Labor Pain: By hand—hot compress massage to lower abdomen as needed; 14 drops clary sage; 5 drops rose; and 6 drops ylang ylang in 2 fl oz. sunflower oil
Heartburn: Sandalwood applied to belly or ingesting one drop with a spoon of sunflower oil
Constipation: Twenty drops marjoram; 5 drops rose; 2 fl oz. sesame oil

Conversions:
1 ml. = 20 drops/5 ml. = 1 teaspoon

Aromas and Chakras

Refer to Chapter 7 for doṣha-specific aromas and for chakra locations

Chakra	Oil
7 - crown	Sandalwood, frankincense, myrrh
6 - third eye	Sandalwood, basil, lavender, jasmine, eucalyptus
5 - throat	Sandalwood, tea tree
4 - heart	Rose, lavender, sandalwood
3 - solar plexus	Sandalwood, lavender, fennel
2 - groin	Cedar, sage, ylang ylang, patchouli

Suggested Reading on Aromatherapy

Davis P. *Aromatherapy A-Z.* Essex, England: C.W. Daniel Ltd.; 1988.

Frawley D. *Āyurveda Certification Course.* Santa Fe, NM: American Institute of Vedic Studies; 1995.

Miller L, Miller B. *Āyurveda and Aromatherapy.* Twin Lakes, WI: Lotus Press; 1995.

Nadkarni AK. *Indian Materia Medica.* Bombay, India: Popular Prakashan; 1993.

Tisserand M. *Aromatherapy for Women.* Rochester, VT: Healing Arts Press; 1988.

Tisserand R. *Aromatherapy to Heal and Tend the Body.* Santa Fe, NM: Lotus Press; 1988.

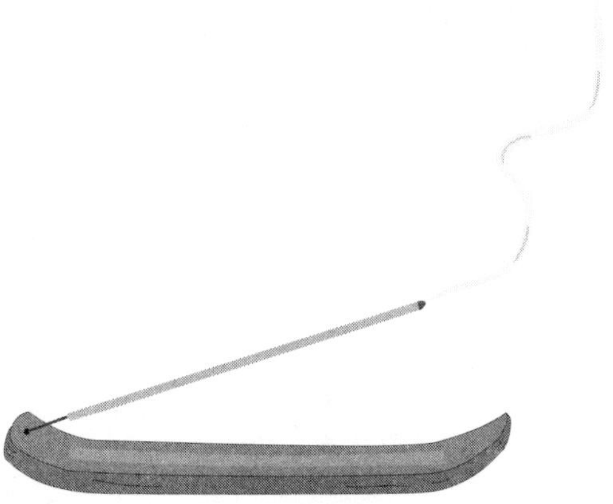

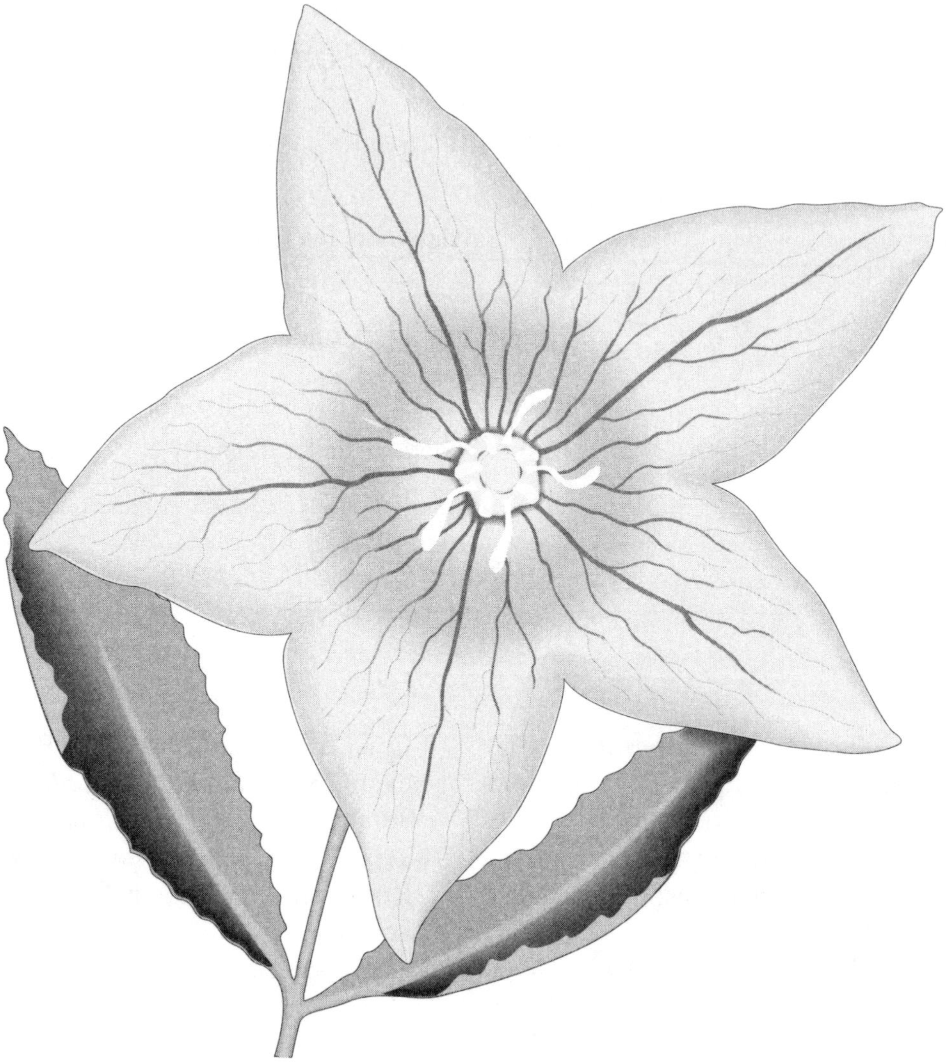

Chapter 9

Haṭha Yoga, Prāṇāyama, Nāda, Mudrā, Bandha

Chapter Overview

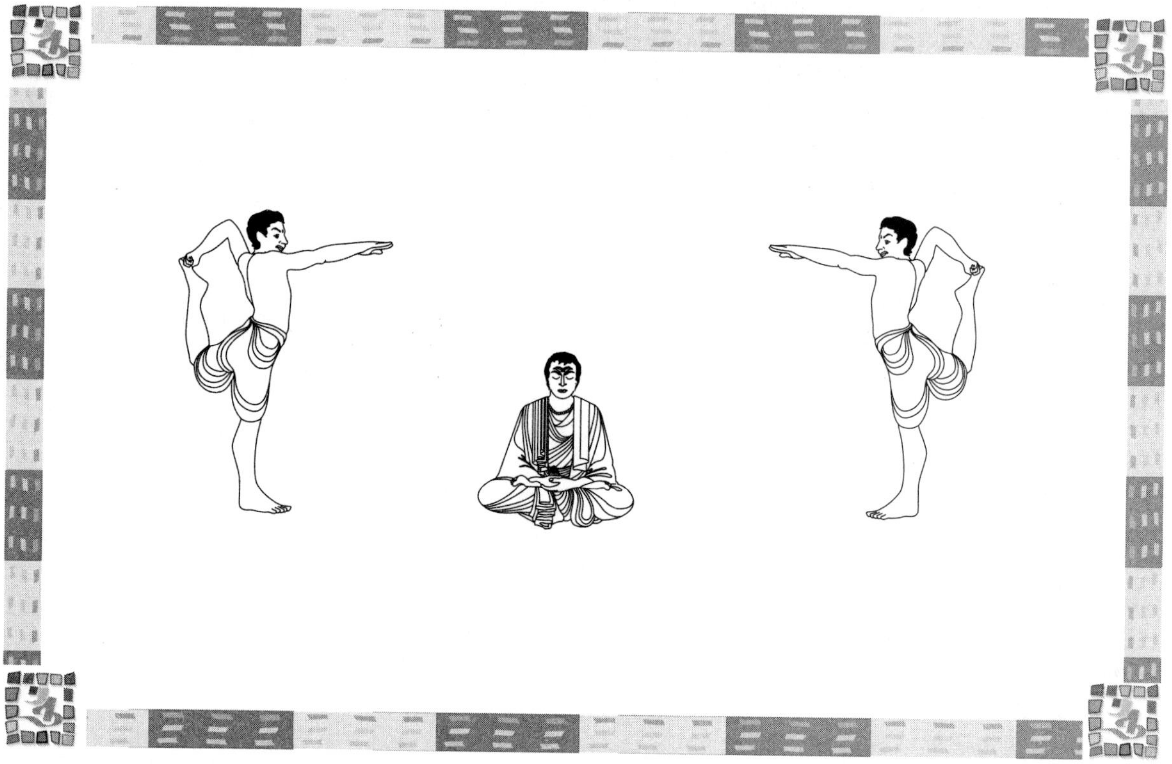

Be the change you want to see.
Gandhi

Chapter 9
Haṭha Yoga, Prāṇāyāma, Nāda, Mudrā, Bandha

From the ancient *Vedic* literature, four texts on *yoga āsanas* (postures) are the most respected: *Haṭha Yoga Pradīpikā, Gorakṣha Saṃhitā, Gherand Saṃhitā*, and *Hataratnavali*. These scriptures were written between the 6th century, when *haṭha yoga* and *prāṇāyāma* began to emerge in India, and the 15th century A.D. This chapter correlates the information in these books with Āyurvedic physical and spiritual benefits.

Many approaches to *yoga āsanas* exist. Three well known methods are *haṭha, kuṇḍalinī*, and *aṣhṭāṅga*. This chapter discusses and integrates these three *yoga* methods.

Interestingly, *haṭha yoga* was also found in pre-Colombian culture—not just confined to India. In St. Augustine, Columbia, ancient stone statues of people in *yoga* postures still exist today.

General Information

The underlying ideas to practicing yoga are the following:

Be gentle, do not force any posture
Forcing is against nature.

Feel complete at whatever stage
of the position one can attain.

Completeness or union is the goal,
not physical perfection of any posture

Yoga āsanas have three purposes. First they can be used as a means to prepare the student (along with *prāṇāyāma* breathing) for advanced spiritual practices like *mantra sādhanā* (meditation). This is especially true for *haṭha yoga.*

Second, when practicing non-forceful meditation, *āsanas* may occur automatically, cleansing and integrating the mind, body, and spirit. Finally, Āyurvedic practitioners may recommend these postures for healing specific diseases.

Haṭha yoga has healed diseases—some thought to be incurable—from ancient eras in India through modern times. Its healing methods are explained in its definition. Spiritually, *yoga* means the union of the red spirit force at the base of the spine with the white spirit force at the crown of the head; the union of the sun-spirit at the navel with the moon-spirit at the head; and the union of the small self with the Divine eternal Self.

Physically, *yoga* means the union of *prāṇ* (inward moving air) with *apān* (downward/outward moving air); the union in which all the energy currents in the body flow up the *suṣhumnā* or main inner tube of the spine. On either side of the *suṣhumṇā* are two secondary tubes. *'Ha'* is the solar or right tube *(piṅgalā)*—Pitta predominant. '*Ṭha*' is the lunar or left channel or *nāḍi,* called *iḍā*—Vāyu/Kapha predominant. Thus, *haṭha yoga* means the union of all physical energy currents into these two channels, which subsequently flow into the *suṣhumṇā.*

Each school of *yoga* emphasizes different things. *Patañjali* suggests that ethics (*yama* and *niyama*) is the way to cleanse the mind, body, and spirit; he emphasizes a more psychological approach to healing and Self-Realization. The book *Haṭha Yoga Pradīpikā* suggests the body's organs and systems are to be cleansed first through *āsanas* and *prāṇāyām*. Āyurvedic practitioners allow each client to choose that healing path for which he or she is best suited.

Yoga āsanas and *prāṇāyām* have, along with meditation, become popular in the 1960's in the west. However, along with their introduction they have also become westernized. Postures began to be taught as ends in themselves, merely to heal an illness, to reduce stress, or to look better; the idea that these postures are a foundation for Self-Realization was generally ignored. The *Haṭha Yoga Pradīpikā* spends the first chapter reminding the student that *Haṭha Yoga* is specifically used as the first step in Self-Realization; this goal must not be forgotten.

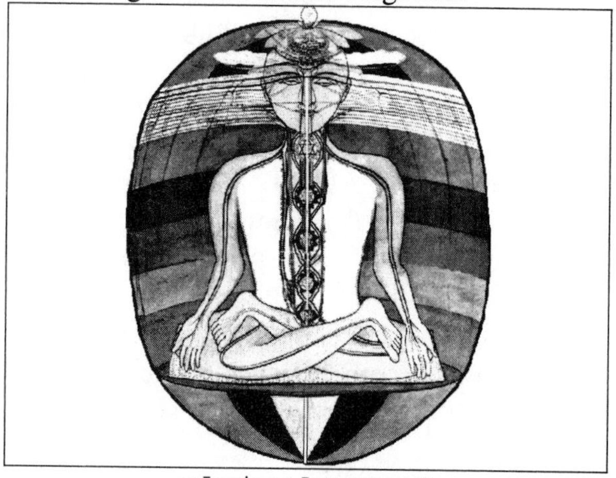

IḌĀ/PIṄGALĀ/SUṢHUMṆĀ

Precautions For Beginners

1. A soft, comfortable mat, blanket, or rug is used when practicing *āsanas*.
2. Persons whose backs, spines, or necks are bad or stiff should practice very gently.
3. Pregnant woman are advised to cease all strenuous and inverted poses, and not to lie on their bellies.
4. Inverted postures (e.g., shoulder stands, head stands) are life threatening to persons with heart problems, and should not be practiced by anyone with pressure problems (e.g., ear, nose, head, heart).
5. The yoga room is to be pleasant, clean, ventilated, and free of drafts.
6. It is always best to learn positions from a qualified *yoga* teacher.
7. *Yoga* is first learned in the spring or fall; starting a course of yoga during winter or summer may cause health imbalances.
8. The practice of moderation and healthfulness in diet prevents health imbalances. Foods that are difficult to digest, stale, very hot, or cold are not recommended.
9. *Yoga* is not to be practiced on a completely empty stomach, nor on a full stomach. Beginners are advised to take a little boiled milk and *ghee* before practicing *prāṇāyām.*

Part 1
Postures (Āsanas)

Eighty-four million seated āsanas exist, as described by Lord Śhiva. Of them 84 are best, and of these, 32 are useful for mankind.

Gherand Saṃhitā: Ch. 2; verse 1

Haṭha Yoga Pradīpikā: Ch. 1; verse 33

Of these 32, four were chosen as the best; siddhāsana (perfect), *padmāsana* (lotus), *simhāsana* (lion), *bhadrādsana* (gracious pose).

Haṭha Yoga Pradīpikā: Ch. 1; verse 34

[The *Śhiva Saṃhitā* lists *siddhāsana, padmāsana, paschimottanāsana* (back stretch), and *swastikāsana* (auspicious) poses. *Gorakṣha Satarka* says only two poses are best; *siddhāsana* and *padmāsana.*]

Siddhāsana is the most important of the āsanas. It should always be practiced as it purifies the 72,000 nāḍīs.

Haṭha Yoga Pradīpikā: Ch. 1; verse 38-9

When perfection is attainable through siddhāsana, what is the use of practicing many other āsanas?

Haṭha Yoga Pradīpikā: Ch. 1; verse 41

This last question relates to *āsanas* as a preparation for deeper meditative practice. From the point of view of Āyurvedic health, the various postures help heal specific health concerns. To that end this chapter describes some of the most effective *āsanas* for healing various diseases.

1. Siddhāsana (Perfection Pose)

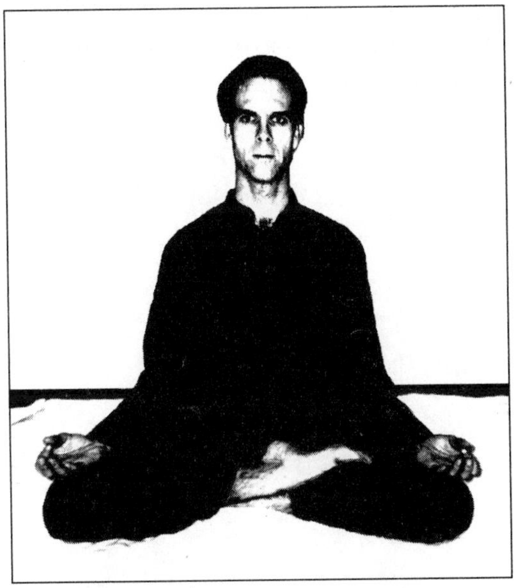

SIDDHĀSANA (MALE—PALMS UP)

This is the most important of the postures. Men practice this posture while women follow its counterpart, *Siddha Yoni Āsana* (see below).

Method:

A) Sit comfortably
B) Place the left heel at the perineum (or anal aperture).
C) Place the right heel directly over the left heel, pressing against the root of the generative organ. (Traditionally the upper heel would press at the root of the generative organ, at the pubis root).
D) Push the toes and the edge of the right foot between the left thigh and calf muscles.
E) Sit comfortably, steady, with spine erect.
F) Lower the chin towards the collarbone, relaxing the head (today some practice with the head upright and eyes closed).
G) Gaze into the *ājñā chakra* (third eye). [When the eyes become tired, close them and gaze at the space in front of the eyes.]
H) Place the hands in the '*Jñyān mudrā*'. (The tips of the thumb and index fingers touch, forming a circle with the fingers. The three remaining fingers remain outstretched or uncurled—palms face upward.) This hand position is said to prevent the energy from flowing out of the body via the fingers. Alternatively, one practices the '*Chin Mudrā*'. (Place the tips of the index finger at the root of the thumbs, and place the palms on the knees.)

1A. Siddha Yoni Āsana

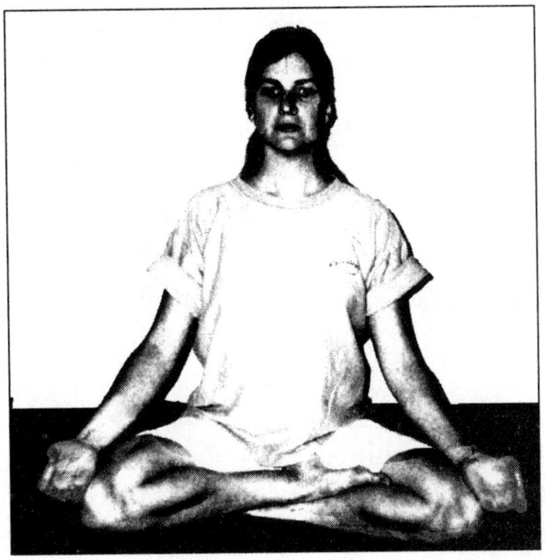

SIDDHA YONI ĀSANA

This method is practiced by women; the pose is almost identical to *siddhāsana*.

Method:

A) The heels press against the lower and upper areas of the reproductive organ.
B) The toes of both feet are inserted between the thighs and calf muscles.
C-H) See *siddhāsana*.

Spiritual Benefits of Both Poses:

1. Stimulates the *ājñā chakra* (develops pure consciousness).
2. Controls nervous and *prāṇic* energies from the

mūlādhāra and *swādishṭān chakras*.
3. Balances one's energy level by equalizing mental and *prāṇic* forces.
4. Pressing the heels at the perineum prevents the *kuṇḍalinī śhakti* (life-force) from escaping out of the *mūlādhāra chakra*.
5. Pressing the heels at the perineum stimulates the *mūlādhāra* where the three major *nāḍīs (iḍā, piṅgala, sushumṇā)* originate.
6. These postures purify the *sushumṇā*.
7. Electrical impulses flow up to the brain, purifying *nāḍīs,* and removing all internal blocks.
8. The three *bandhas* (contractions) automatically occur (Mūla Bandha—contraction of the perineum; Uḍḍīyāna Bandha—contraction of the lower abdomen; Jālandhara Bandha—contraction of the neck [chin lock]). These *bandhas* accumulate greater *prāṇic* energy supply in the body. They are discussed in detail later in this chapter.
9. The poses lead to Self-Realization.

Organs Helped: Stomach, gall bladder, liver, spleen, kidneys (i.e., blood purifying organs).

Physical/Mental Benefits: Heals nervous depression, balances blood pressure, cardiac function, and, in men, male hormones (testosterone). These postures maintain inner body temperature and redirect *prāṇic* energy upwards, activating the *sushumṇā* by balancing the *iḍā* and *piṅgalā*.

Bandha Benefits:
Mūla: Removes senility, creates equilibrium of *prāṇ* and *apān* (life fluid and lower fluid).
Uḍḍīyāna: Purifies the breath and its channels. (This can be practiced alone by fully emptying the stomach and contracting the navel towards the spine.)
Jālandhara: The flow of nectar from the *sahasrāra* (top or crown *chakra*) is consumed by the sun (fire) at the navel *chakra*. *Jālandhara* checks the flow so the fire cannot consume the nectar. This results in mesmerized *sādhanā*.

Doshas: All; especially P- (reducing)

Alternatives: With slight variation of the feet and legs, *Siddhāsana* is also called *Vajrāsana, Muktāsana*, and *Guptāsana*. They are presented here for consideration.

Vajrāsana (thunderbolt)—kneel and place the buttocks between the heels, with the right big toe overlapping the left one.

Muktāsana (liberation)—place the left heel under the anus and the right heel on top of the left.

Guptāsana (secret)—place the feet between the thigh and calf muscles so that the heels press against the anus.

2. Padmāsana (Lotus Pose)

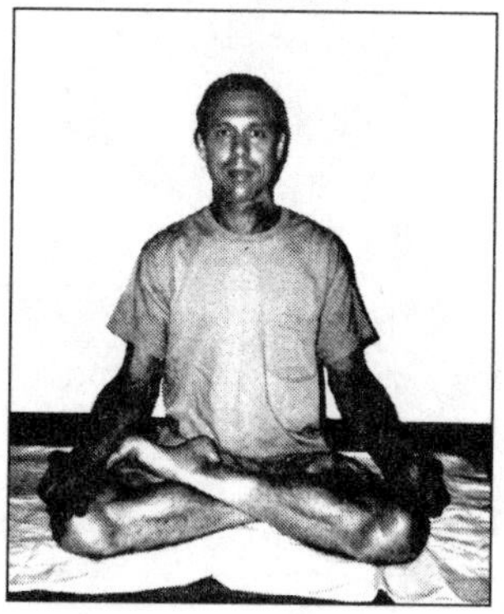

PADMĀSANA (LOTUS POSE)

This is a more difficult posture. Fortunately it is not considered as important as *Siddhāsana.*

Method:
A) Place the right foot on the left thigh and the left foot on the right thigh (soles facing up).
B) If possible, cross hands behind the back and firmly hold the toes.
C) Press the chin against the chest and keep the back straight.
D) If toes cannot be held from behind the back, place hands in *jñyān, chin, bhairava*, or *yoni mudrā*. *Bhairavi* (females)—place fingers of left hand on the top of fingers of the right hand, with both palms facing up, and hands placed in the lap. *Bhairava* (males)—finger placement is the exact opposite of *bhairavi*. *Yoni mudrā*—the last three fingers are interlaced, while the index and thumb

fingers join at the tips. Thumbs point upward, while the index fingers point forward (forming a triangular space between the index and thumb fingers). See photo below

E) Eyes focus on the tip of the nose (*nasakagra drishti*). Alternatively, one can lean forward, eventually resting the forehead on the ground.

F) The tongue is pressed against the root of the upper teeth.

G) Slowly raise *prāṇa* upward.

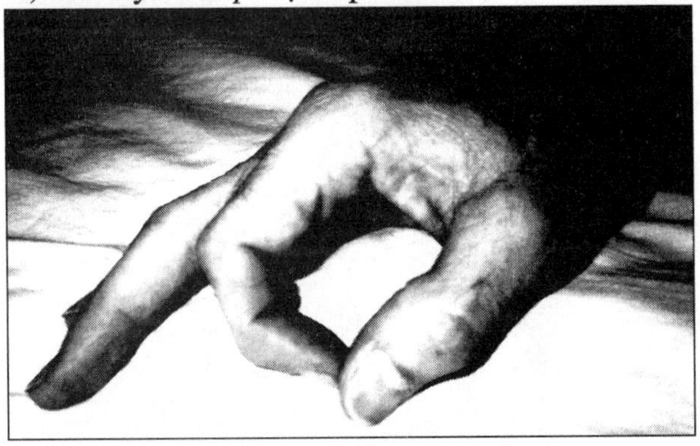

JÑYAN MUDRĀ

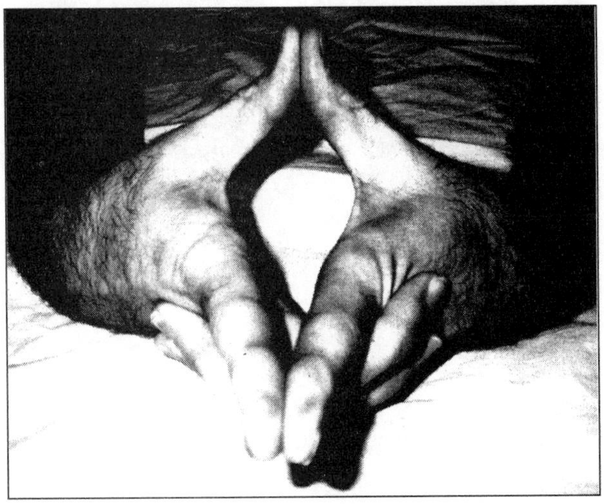

YONI MUDRĀ

Benefits: *Padmāsan* is the destroyer of all diseases, balancing *prāṇa* and mental forces. It also tones sacral and coccygeal nerves through increased blood flow. Blood flows to the abdominal region, helping with mental, emotional, and nervous disorders. Leaning forward helps constipation, depression, wrinkles, headaches, and menstrual disorders.

Organs Helped: This pose stimulates acupuncture meridians of the stomach, gall bladder, spleen, kidneys, and liver; changes the metabolic structure and brain patterns, creating balance in the entire system.

Precautions: Do not practice with sciatica or sacral infection.

Doṣhas: All

The yogi who, seated in padmāsana,
inhales through the entrance of the nāḍīs
and fills them with prāṇa, gains liberation;
there is no doubt.
Haṭha Yoga Pradīpikā

Alternative: Raised Lotus

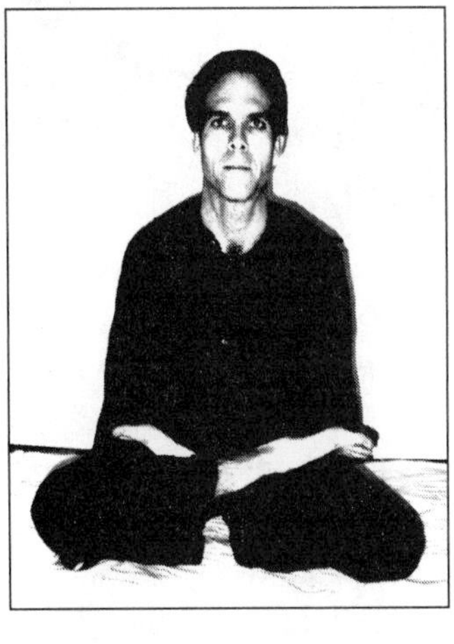

RAISED LOTUS

Method:

A) Sitting in full lotus, palms are placed on the floor beside the thighs.

B) Inhale and raise the body off the floor; breathe naturally.

C) Exhale and return to the floor.

Benefits: This posture strengthens the reproductive system.

Organs Helped: Reproductive organs

So we see several reasons why *Siddhāsana* is

the posture preferred over *Padmāsana*. The former requires less work and mental concentration (i.e., the *bandhas* occur automatically due to the heel pressure, lower abdomen pressure, and the neck-lock; and prevents *kuṇḍalinī* energy from escaping while automatically increasing *prāṇa*). Thus, one can more easily engage in *mantra* meditation while sitting in *Siddhāsana*; *Padmāsana* requires more thought and practice.

3. Simhāsana (Lion's Pose)

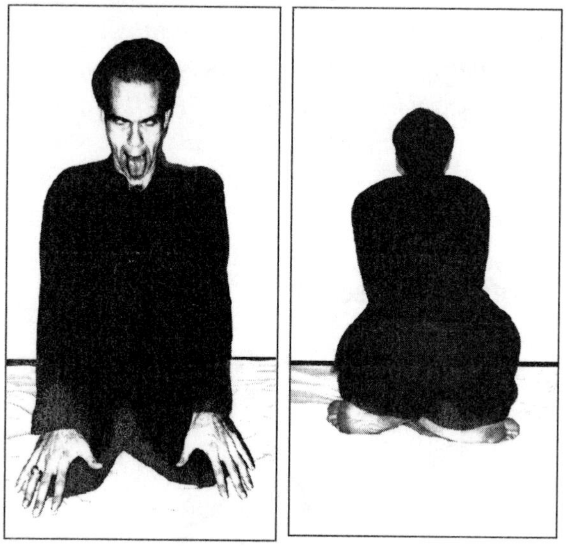

SIMHĀSANA (LION'S POSE)

Method: (Feet and ankles must be very flexible to perform this pose)
A) Sit on crossed ankles
B) Press the left heel on the right side of the perineum—males; right side of the reproductive organ—females.
C) Press the right heel on the opposite side of the perineum or organ.
D) Place palms on knees and spread fingers apart.
E) Lean the head forward with chin almost touching the collar bone.
F) Focus the eyes on the tip of the nose.
G) Open the mouth (i.e., as if yawning), extending the tongue as far out as possible .

The position of the feet induces a natural practice of *mūla bandha* due to the pressure on the perineum or generative organ. The bent head stimulates the neck lock (*jālandhara*). *Uḍḍīyāna bandha* is induced from bending forward. This pose is best performed outside, facing the sunrise.

Benefits: This pose is beneficial for singers and speakers; sore throats, Kapha sinus headaches.

Organs Helped: Ears, nose, throat, and mouth disorders.

Doṣhas: All; especially Kapha

Variation: Seated Simhāsana

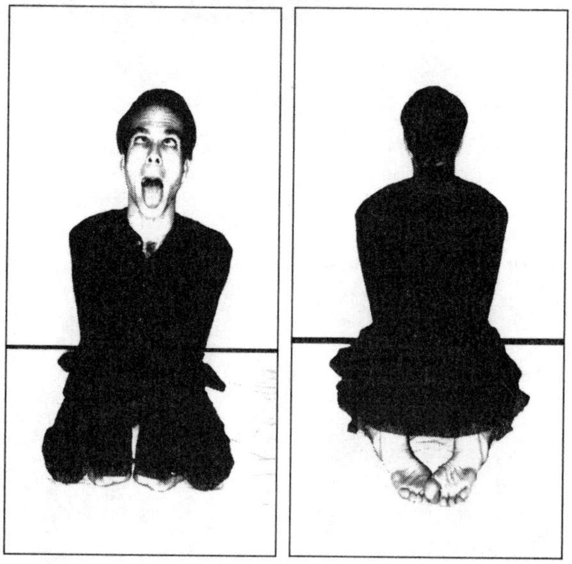

SEATED SIMHĀSANA

Method:
A) Separate knees and lean on them.
B) Place the right foot under the right buttock and the left foot under the left buttock.
C) Seat the buttocks between the heels.
D) Hands can rest on the knees or on the ground between the heels; palms facing down and fingers pointing in towards the body. Put pressure on the balls of the palms.
E) Raise the chin two or three inches and gaze at the third eye (*ājñā chakra*)—this is known as *Śhāṃbhavī Mudrā*.
F) Extend the tongue out as far as comfortable.
G) Inhale deeply through the nose. Exhale, mak-

ing a roaring sound like a lion ("aaahhhh").
H) Move the tongue from side to side to stimulate the throat further.

4. Bhadrāsana (Gracious Pose)

This posture, though an important pose, will not be discussed; it is a more difficult, advanced posture.

5. Swastikāsana (Auspicious Pose)

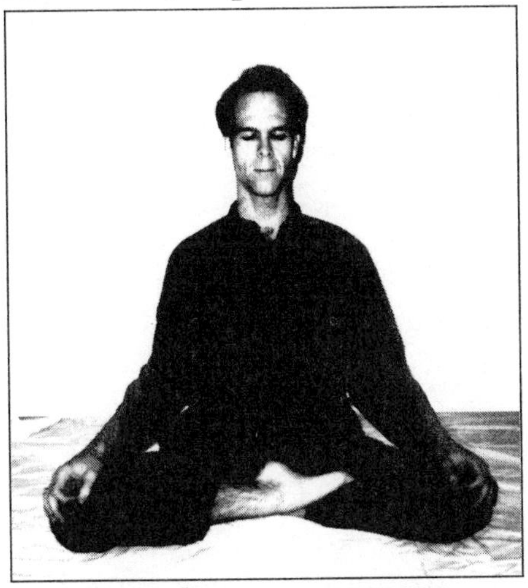

SWASTIKĀSANA (PERFECT POSE)

Method:
A) Sit cross-legged and bring feet up between the thigh and calf muscles. (Beginners—place pillows under the feet to keep the feet propped to stay inside the thigh and calf muscles.)
B) Place hands in *jñyān* or *chin mudrā*.
C) Sit up straight and comfortable.

Benefits: *Nāḍīs* (actual acupuncture meridians) inside the back of the legs are stimulated. The sciatic nerve is gently massaged; lumbar region and abdominal muscles are toned, and the inner body temperature is balanced. In *Vedic* culture the *swastika* is the symbol of fertility, creativity, and auspiciousness; therefore, practicing this posture develops these attributes. It dispels miseries and stabilizes the mind and body. Breath is quickly controlled by this posture.
Doṣhas: All; especially Vāyu and Pitta

6. Paschimottanāsana [Ugrāsana] (Back Stretching Pose)

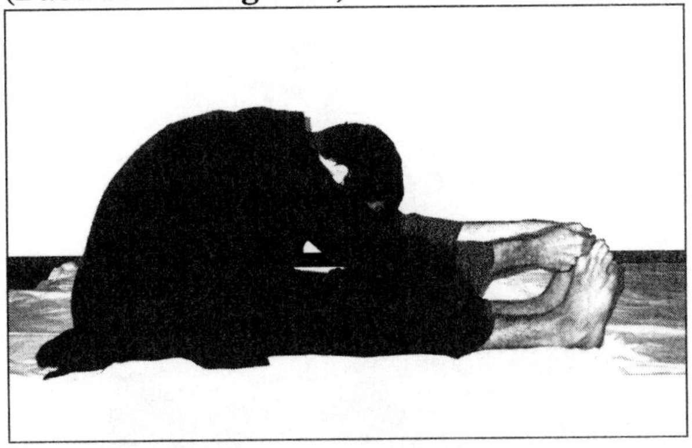

PASCHIMOTTANĀSANA (BACK STRETCHING POSE)

Method:
A) Stretch both legs straight out in front of the body.
B) Inhale and raise hands over head, keeping the back straight.
C) Exhale and bend forward from the hips, stretching the hands out towards the toes (if toes can be comfortably touched or held, do so. Otherwise, feel a sense of completeness regardless of how far you can stretch—e.g., holding knees, calf muscles, etc.). The spinal cord should feel stretched. The back should be straight—not curved or hunched. One may use a towel or rope around the toes to begin to sit properly.
D) Place the forehead on the knees if comfortably reached. Keep the knees on the floor.
E) Breathe normally, concentrating on the navel or on a *mantra*.
F) Inhale and gently raise the arms up over the head while sitting upright.
G) Exhale and bring the hands to the knees.

Benefits: Increases digestive power, physical lassitude vanishes; the breath is soon controlled and miseries are dispelled, diabetes. *Prāṇa* enters the *suṣhumṇā* (the western or inner path).

Precautions: Practice other postures first to loosen the back's muscles and nerves; and the hamstrings and spine.

Doṣhas: All; also for Kapha sinus headaches.

Alternative 1:
Mahā Mudrā (Great Sealing Pose)

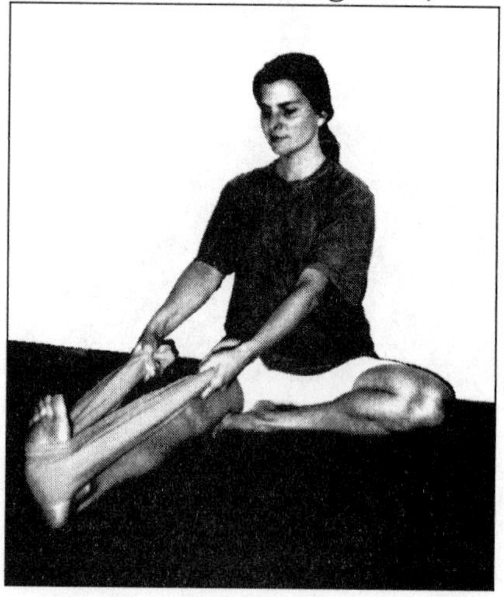

MAHĀ MUDRĀ (GREAT SEALING POSE)

Method:
A) The left heel is pressed against the anus; the sole is pressed against the right inner thigh (or vice versa).
B) Inhale, raising the hands over the head. The spine is erect.
C) Exhale and lean forward, hands grasping the knees, calves, or feet of the outstretched leg. Beginners may use a towel or belt for help.
D) The forehead should be close to the outstretched knee; touching it if possible.
E) Inhale, raising the hands over the head and sitting up straight.
F) Exhale, lowering the hands to the knees.

Benefits: *Bindū* (semen or ovum) is kept from moving downward; physical lassitude is removed, physical ailments are healed; digestion is increased. The body becomes charming, symptoms of aging are dispelled, senses become controlled. Wasting diseases, skin diseases, hemorrhoids, indigestion, tumors, and abscesses are healed.

[see page 294 for more complete version]

Alternative 2:
Mahā Bandha (Great Lock Pose)

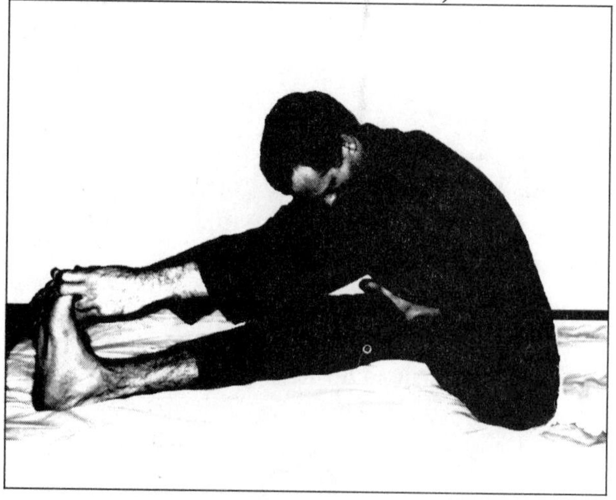

MAHĀ BANDHA (GREAT LOCK POSE)

Method:
A) Left heel is pressed against anus (as in *Mahāmudrā*); right foot is placed on the left thigh.
B) The stomach is filled with air, while in *Jālandhara* pose, and the breath is held.
C) Air is slowly exhaled when air can no longer be comfortably retained.

Benefits: The life breath enters the *suṣhumṇā*. The body becomes robust. Bones and ribs are strengthened.

Doṣhas: VP-; Best for Vāyu

[see page 295 for more completeversion]

Alternative 3: Mahā Bedha

Method:
A) While in the *Mahābandha* pose, hold the breath and practice *uḍḍīyāna bandha* (contraction of abdominal muscles).
B) The hands gently strike into the lower armpit area.

[see page 296 for more complete version]

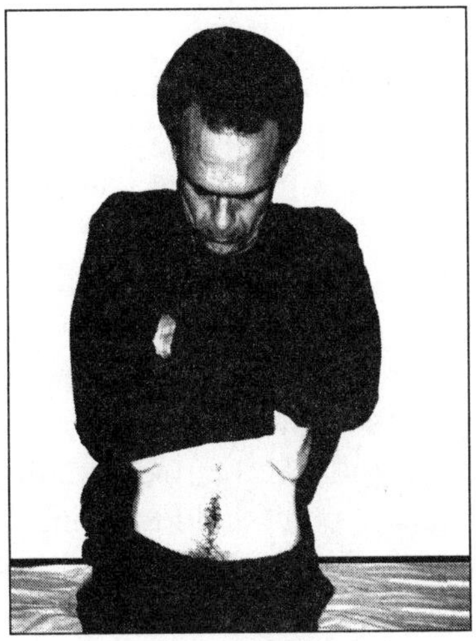

MAHĀ BEDHA

Benefits: The life breath enters the *suṣhumṇā*, leaving the *iḍā* and *piṅgalā nāḍīs*. The three knots are penetrated and *kuṇdalinī śhakti* proceeds to the *sahasrāra* (crown *chakra*) uninterrupted. Breath is controlled and old age weaknesses are removed.

7. Vīrāsana (Hero's Pose)

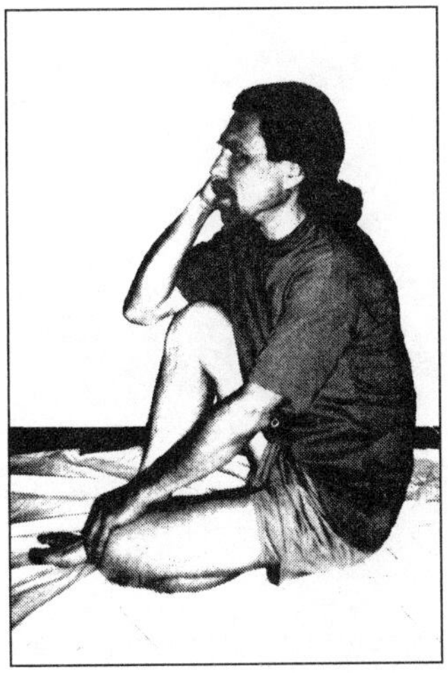

VĪRĀSANA (HERO'S POSE)

Method:
A) Sit on the left heel. Bend the right knee, placing the right foot by the left knee.
B) Place the right elbow on the right knee and the palm against the right cheek.
C) Place the left palm on the left knee.
D) Close eyes and concentrate on the breath.

Benefits: This posture develops the heroic power of *Hanuman* (monkey god; *Mahavīr*). It increases will power and strengthens the body. The pose is also excellent for immune disorders like AIDS, MS, Epstein Barr, etc.

Organs Helped: The pose stabilizes the energy flow to the reproductive organs and controls sexual energy; it also stimulates the reproductive organs and their associated brain centers (this is achieved by activating the *nāḍīs* found in the legs and connected to the reproductive glands).

Doṣhas: VP-

8. Visāsana (Alternative to *Vīrāsana*)

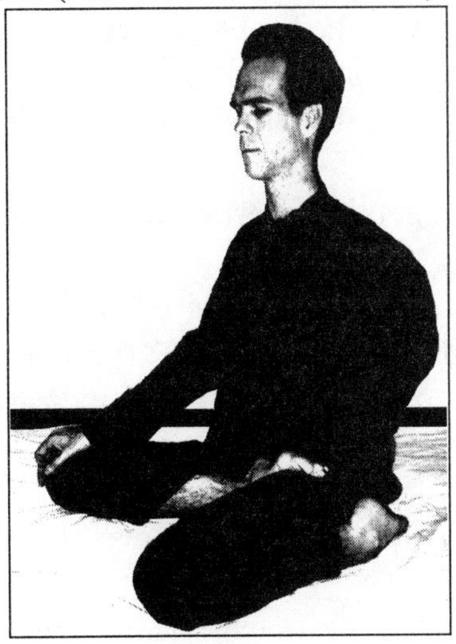

VISĀSANA

Method:
A) Sit on the left heel, while the right foot rests on top of the left thigh. Knees are spread wide apart. Optional—place the big toe under the buttock.
B) Optional—keep hands in the *jñyān* or *chin mudrā.*

Benefits: This pose heals rheumatism, hemorrhoids, and other diseases of the anus.

9. Bhujaṅgāsana (Serpent Pose)

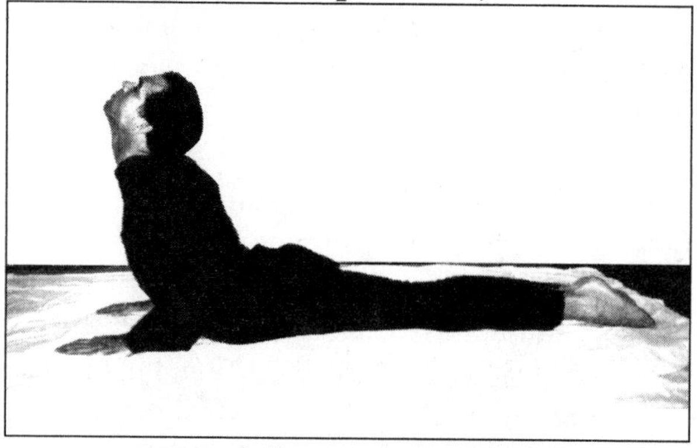

BHUJAṄGĀSANA (SERPENT POSE)

Method:
A) Lie on the stomach with hands parallel to the shoulders and palms placed on the floor.
B) Inhale, gently raising the head and upper torso up (lifting with the back muscles, not the hands). The lower torso and legs remain on the ground (navel to toes). The head is upright and the back is curved.
C) Exhale, gently lowering the body to the floor.

Benefits: *Kuṇḍalinī* is raised, digestion is increased, diseases are healed. Asthma, gastrointestinal disorders, hypertension, menstrual disorders, and insomnia are relieved.

Doṣhas: VPK=

10. Śhalabhāsana (Locust Pose)

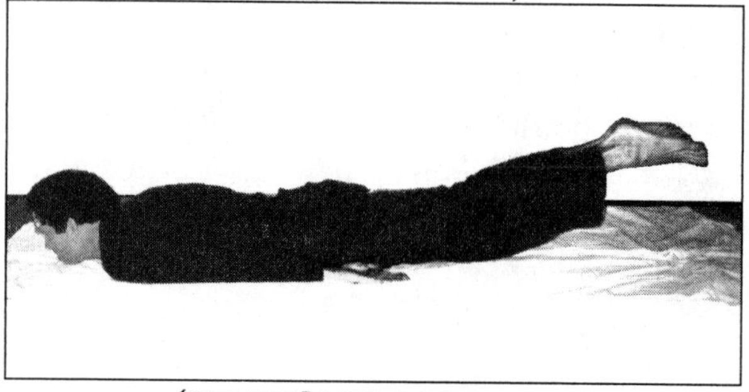

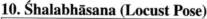

ŚHALABHĀSANA (LOCUST POSE)

Method:
A) Both arms are placed on the ground (palms facing up) while the head is placed on them. (Some practitioners place the hands beside the shoulders under the chest (palms down).
B) Inhale, raising legs off the ground. Contract the buttocks muscles and stretch the thigh muscles. The back and stomach muscles are doing the lifting, not the hands and head.
C) Breathe naturally; if the body begins to tremble, the posture is being held too long.
D) Exhale, gently lowering the legs to the ground.

Benefits: This pose improves digestion and heals physical weaknesses. The sun-fire at the navel that draws the nectar flow from the crown is blocked. This removes the effects of old age; thus retaining a youthful appearance. The posture is good for malabsorption, the gastrointestinal system, and sore throats.

Doṣhas: VK-

11. Vajrolī Mudrā (Thunderbolt Pose)

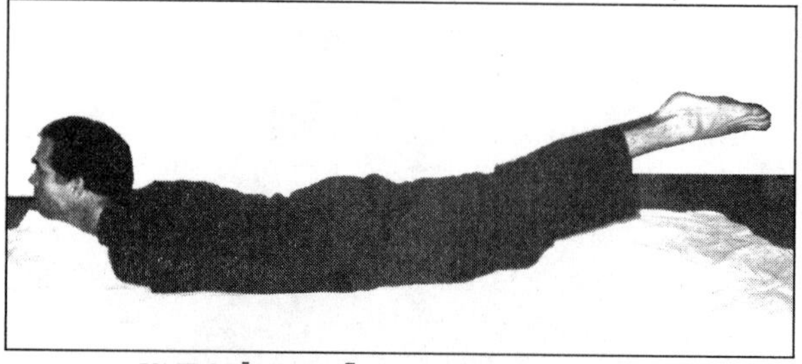

VAJROLĪ MUDRĀ (THUNDERBOLT POSE)

Method:
A) Begin in *Śhalabhāsana,* then place the palms on the ground beside the shoulders or under the thighs.
B) Lift the head and upper torso into the air by pressing the hands to the ground. Feel a gentle pressure in the small of the back, urinary tract, and reproductive organs.
C) The legs are also lifted as in *Śhalabhāsana.*

Benefits: Semen/ovum (*bindū*) is prevented from being discharged; the power to retain this fluid is developed, enhancing long life. The *Gherand Saṃhitā* says this pose is one of the best because it develops liberation.

Organs Helped: Urinary tract, reproductive organs.

Doṣhas: All

12. Dhanurāsana (Bow Pose)

This is similar to *Vajrolī* , but the hands are kept off the ground.

Method:

Beginner: Half Bow

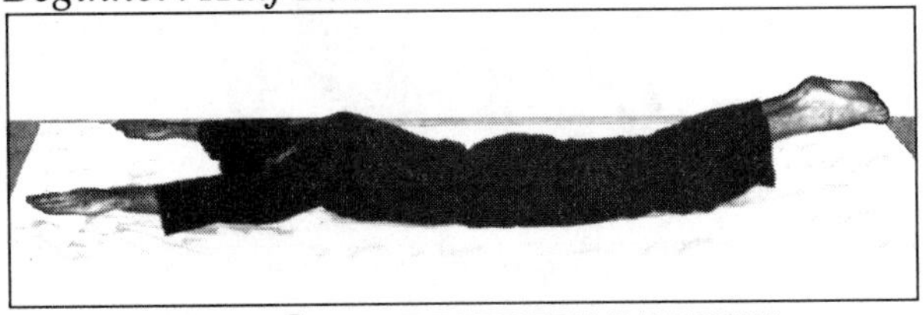

DHANURĀSANA (BEGINNER'S HALF BOW)

A) Lie on the stomach, forehead resting on the ground and arms straight overhead.
B) Inhale, raising the arms and legs straight up, using the lower back and buttocks muscles. Breathe normally.
C) Exhale, slowly lowering limbs to the ground. Note that a slow release tones muscle groups that would not normally be toned if one were just to drop the limbs.

Intermediate: Bow

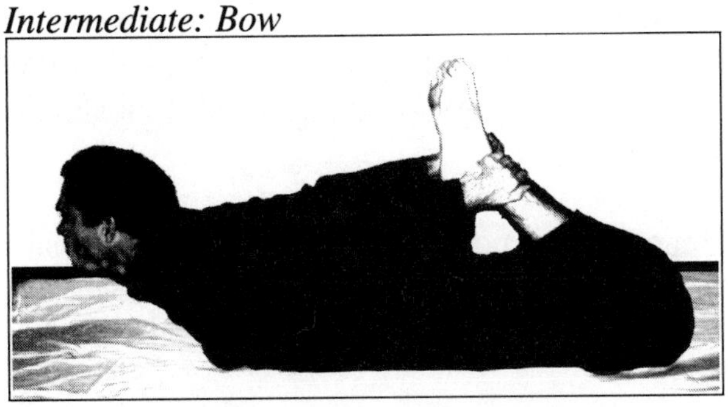

DHANURĀSANA (INTERMEDIATE BOW)

A) Lie flat on the stomach, forehead on the ground, and arms by your sides.
B) Inhale, bending knees; then grasp both ankles.
C) Separate the knees and exhale.
D) If the body begins rocking, it is alright.
E) Exhale, slowly while lowering the body and limbs to the ground.

Advanced: Bow—same as above only

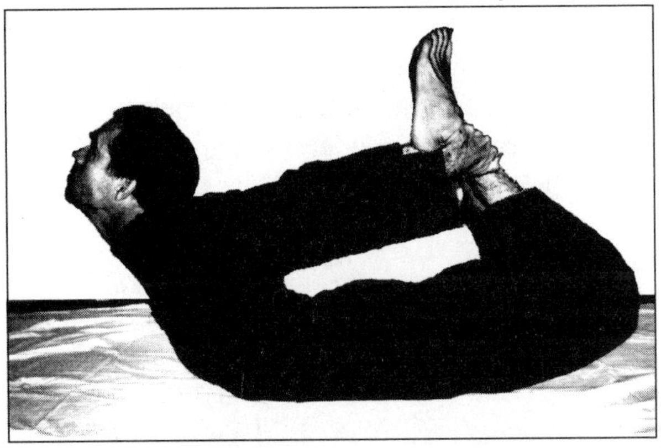

DHANURĀSANA (ADVANCED BOW)

D) Inhale, slightly raising the knees, head, and chest simultaneously, while pulling the feet away and up from the hands (the whole body should be moving together at one time). Breathe naturally. Concentrate on the back of the neck (*viṣhuddha chakra*), on the abdominal area (*manipūra chakra*), or on the midpoint where the back is bent.

Benefits: This pose alleviates diabetes and chest ailments; it produces cortisone in the adrenal glands (for inflammatory, allergic, or excess tissue or tumor growth); adjusts the vertebrae, and straightens hunched back and drooping shoulders. The posture regulates the menstrual cycle and corrects infertility (if not due to deformed reproductive organs—i.e., if not hormonally caused); helps Kapha—asthma, Pitta—hemorrhoids, colitis, hypertension (half bow), rheumatism; Vāyu—arthritis. This is one of the best postures for all digestive disorders. All the *nāḍīs* run through the navel. The navel becomes uncentered if a person lifts heavy items with only one arm. This creates a disturbance in the flow of the *nāḍīs,* and causes digestive troubles. Three minutes of practicing the bow pose (along with two other poses discussed on page 310) realigns the navel within three days. Signs of proper digestion will be noticed immediately thereafter. [See page 309: how to test for navel displacement].

Organs Helped: This pose stimulates the solar plexus, digestive, eliminatory, and reproductive organs; massages the heart, liver, and pancreas; stimulates the kidneys and tones the alimentary canal. It regulates the endocrine glands (especially the thyroid and adrenals).

Doṣhas: All

13. Matsyendrāsana (Spinal Twist Pose)

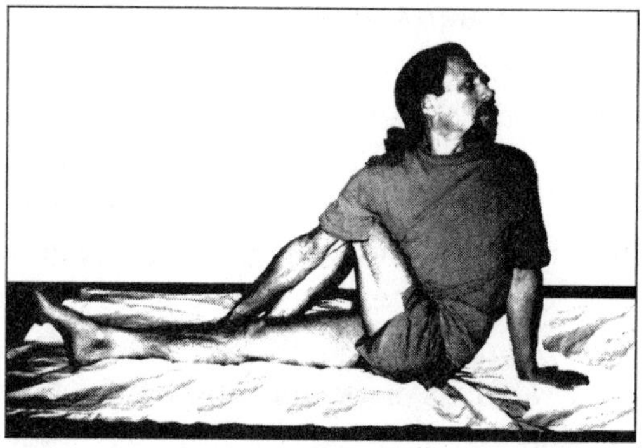

MATSYENDRĀSANA (SPINAL TWIST POSE)

Method: *Beginner*
A) Fully extend the right foot. Cross the left foot over the right knee, placing it on the ground next to the knee.
B) The right arm rests against the outer left leg. The hand is placed on the right knee or on the floor by the left side of the body.
C) The left arm is wrapped around the back, or the palm is placed on the floor behind the left buttock.
D) Inhale, gently and slowly rotating the spine and head as far to the left as comfortable. The position is held with the hands or with the stomach and back muscles. Breathe naturally.
E) Exhale, gently and slowly releasing the pose, and return to the starting position.
F) Repeat in the reverse position.

Precautions: It is very important not to strain the spine or neck in this pose; especially for those with bad backs or necks. Remember, once hurt from a *yoga* pose, healing takes a very long time.

Alternate: Pāṣhāsana (Chord Pose)

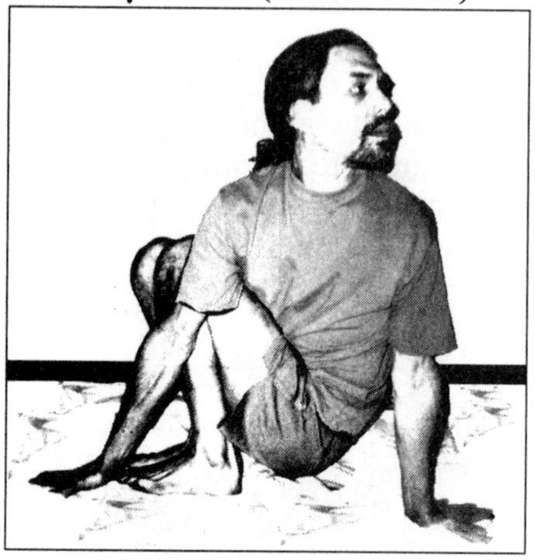

PĀṢHĀSANA (CHORD POSE)

Method: *Beginner*
A) Squat on the floor (keeping the soles and heels flatly on the ground). Knees and feet are close together. Achieve a balanced squat.
B) Twist the trunk until the right arm reaches around the outside of the left knee. The right shoulder touches the left outer knee or thigh.
C) With hands or fingers on the floor, exhale; gently continue the twist as far as the arms will reach. Hold this position while breathing naturally.
D) Release the posture, exhaling and slowly untwisting to the starting position.
E) Repeat the pose, twisting in the opposite direction.

Benefits: This poses strengthens the ankles, making them more elastic; it helps to release gas, to tone, and to help people who stand on their feet all day.

Both poses improve spine agility, strengthen

the shoulders, reduce abdominal fat, massage abdominal organs, expand the chest; help diabetes, and improve digestion.

Organs Helped: Liver, spleen, pancreas sluggishness.

Doṣhas: All

Intermediate: Ardha Matsyendrāsana

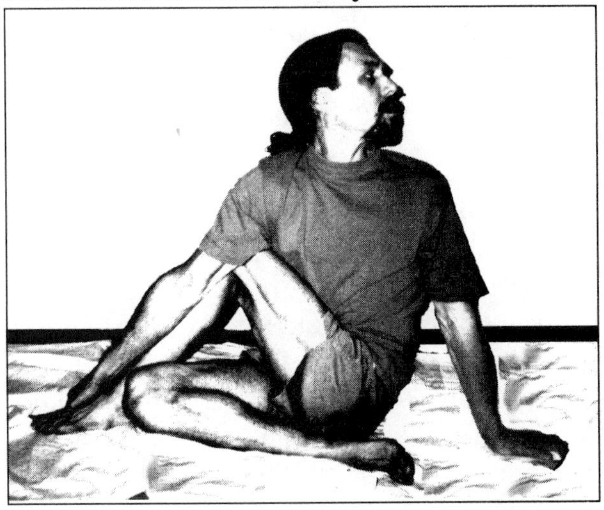

ARDHA MATSYENDRĀSANA

Method:
A) Bend the right foot by the side of the left buttock (i.e., left leg is crossed over the right knee). The right foot is in front of the left knee; the left knee is raised near the chest.
B) With the right hand grab the toes of the left foot, ankle, knee, or floor. Place the left hand around the back; or place the palm on the floor by the left side.
C) Inhale; gently and slowly rotate the spine and head to the left as far as is comfortable. The hands can hold the position, or the position can be held with the stomach and back muscles. Breathe naturally.
D) Exhale, gently and slowly un-twisting the torso to its original position.
E) Repeat the pose in the reverse direction.

Benefits: This pose channels *prāṇa* (*kuṇḍalinī*), awakening the *chakras* and the *suṣhumṇā nāḍī*. The posture also stimulates the navel or *manipūra chakra*. This maintains the body, harmonizes underactive or overactive functions, and removes sluggishness and diseases arising from this condition. The pose strengthens the digestive fire (*agni*) and improves nutrient absorption. It prevents the crown-moon nectar (neurohormones of the pituitary and pineal glands that activate the endocrine glands) from being burnt up by the navel-sun heat. Thus, diseases of old age and death are prevented or slowed. This nectar is associated with the *bindū* (semen/ovum). The navel or *manipūra chakra* is powered by *Samāna* Vāyu. This is responsible for nutrient and *prāṇa* absorption from food and air. This absorbs *Prāṇa Vāyu* as well. Through this pose *Apāna Vāyu* and *Prāṇa Vāyu* are made to meet at the *manipūra chakra*. They are combined, energized, and then moved into the *suṣhumṇā nāḍī*. The lower (animal) energies and the higher spiritual energies are united, and *kuṇḍalinī* is awakened.

This *āsana* relieves diabetes, constipation, indigestion, urinary problems, nerve and nervous conditions; lumbago, rheumatism, slipped discs.

Organs Helped: Pancreas, liver, spleen, stomach, ascending and descending colon; the pose tones nerve roots, adjusts and realigns the vertebral column; back muscles are pulled and stretched.

Doṣhas: All

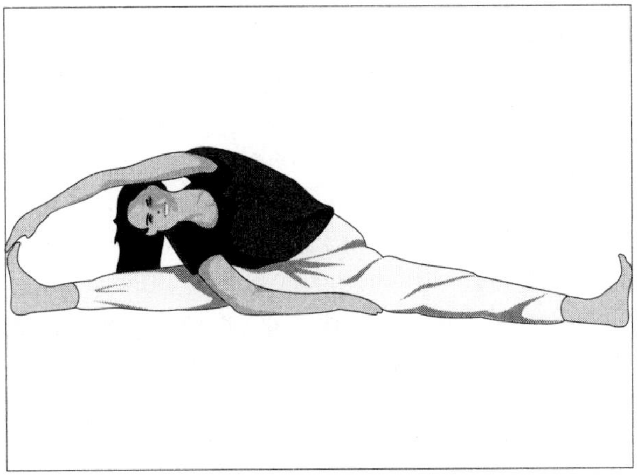

14. Gomukhāsana (Cow's Face Pose)

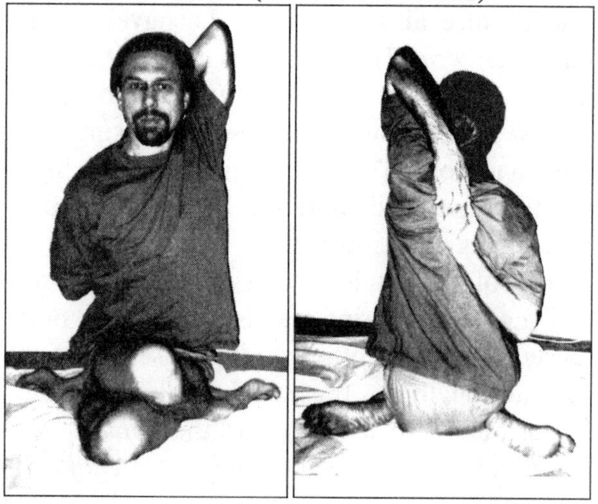

GOMUKHĀSANA (COW'S FACE POSE)

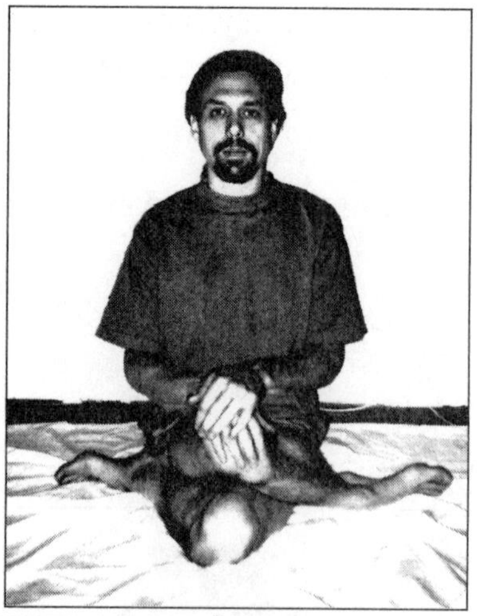

BEGINNER GOMUKHĀSANA (COW'S FACE POSE)

All the ancient texts agree on this posture—except the final arm position.

Method:
A) While seated, bend the legs so that the right heel touches the left buttock and the left heel touches the right buttock (the left leg is crossed over the right leg and the left knee is over the right knee).
B) Bring the left arm up behind the head and back. The right arm wraps around the side and back. The left elbow points straight up (towards the sky), and the right elbow points towards the ground. Clasp the hands behind the back.
C) Breathe naturally and hold the posture. The eyes can be open or closed, or practicing *śhaṃbhavī mudrā* (staring at the third eye).
D) Release and repeat, reversing the leg and arm positions.

Method: *Beginner*
A) After legs are positioned as above, palms may be placed on the upper knee, one hand on top of the other.
B) Some people press the hands on the knees to stretch the leg's muscles. Optionally, one can lean forward, the forehead, if possible, resting on the floor.

Benefits: This pose tones the shoulder muscles, nerves, and cardiac plexus (blood and lymphatic vessels in the heart region). *Nāḍīs* in the legs stimulate the reproductive organs and glands, and regulate hormone secretion. The *vajra nāḍī* is stimulated, preventing the outward flow of *prāṇa*. Thus, *prāṇa* accumulates at the *mūlādhāra* (first) *chakra*. The interlinking of the fingers prevents the *prāṇa* from escaping through the hands. This causes energy to flow through the spinal region. Persons will notice the arms forming an infinity sign that balances the higher and lower (positive and negative) *prāṇa*.

Organs Helped: Reproductive organs and glands, heart.

Doṣhas: All

15. Kūrmāsana (Tortoise Pose)

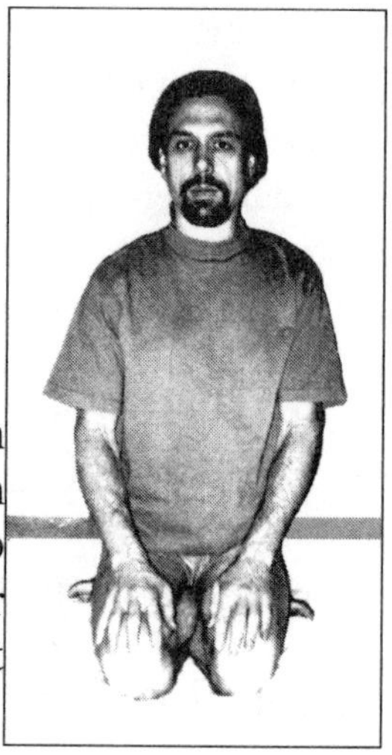

Method:
A) Cross the legs and sit on the ankles, pressing them firmly on the anus. Keep the knees as close together as comfortable. Toes point outward towards the sides.

B) Sit up straight; palms rest on their respective knees.
C) The body is balanced; weight is on the ankles, heels, and sides of feet.

Benefits: This pose straightens the curvature of the spine. The ankles or heels press the anus, closing the *vajra nāḍī*, preventing *kuṇḍalinī* energy from escaping. This pose is useful for both celibates and family members. It channels sexual energy to the higher *chakras*; it also regulates the sex glands, as well as the reproductive and excretory organs.

Organs Helped: Reproductive, excretory, visceral organs (*nāḍīs* in the side of the feet are stimulated—i.e., thorax, abdomen, heart, liver, intestines, and kidneys).

Doṣhas: All

16. Kukkutāsana (Cockerel Pose)

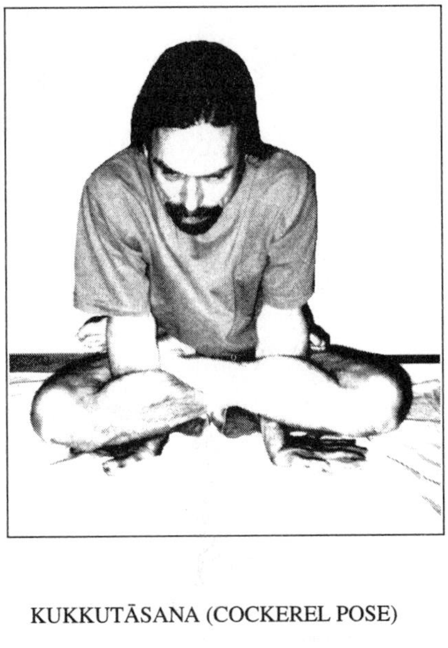

KUKKUTĀSANA (COCKEREL POSE)

Method:
A) Sit in *Padmāsana* (lotus pose) and insert hands between the thighs and knees (right hand between the right thigh and calf; left hand between the left thigh and calf).
B) Place the palms on the ground, fingers pointing forward.
C) Inhale, shifting the body weight to the hands and raising the body off the ground.
D) Hold the position and breathe normally. Focus the eyes on a fixed point in front of you.
E) Exhale, slowly returning to the ground.

Benefits: The pose awakens *kuṇḍalinī*, strengthens the wrists, arms, shoulder muscles, and abdominal walls.

Doṣhas: All

17. Back Bends

Various styles of back bends exist. Beginning poses are discussed below.

Kapotāsana (Pigeon Pose)

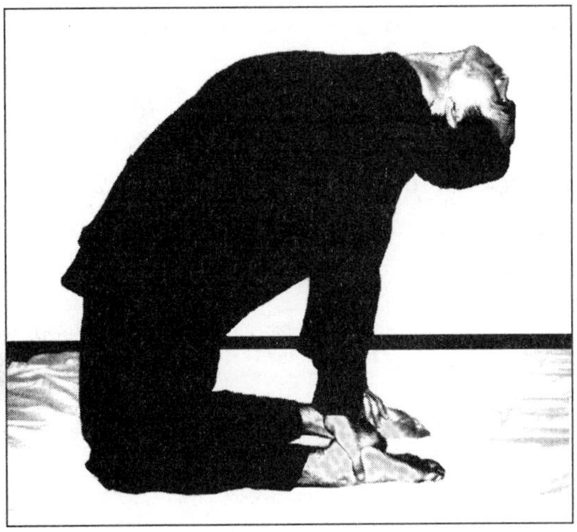

KAPOTĀSANA (PIGEON POSE)

Method: *Beginner-Advanced Beginner*
A) Place both hands and knees on the floor (i.e., like a cat).
B) Lift the hands and stand upright from the knees. Place the right big toe over the left big toe.
C) Move the arms behind the back, extended toward the heels.
D) Exhale, leaning the body backward until the

palms reach the heels. Then grab the heels (or touch them with the fingers).
E) Breathe normally and hold the posture.
F) Exhale, returning the torso to the upright position.

Precaution: Do not hurt the knees or spine.

Alternative:
A) Sit on the knees. Exhale, slowly lean backwards while resting on the elbows. Eventually you can rest your back on the floor.

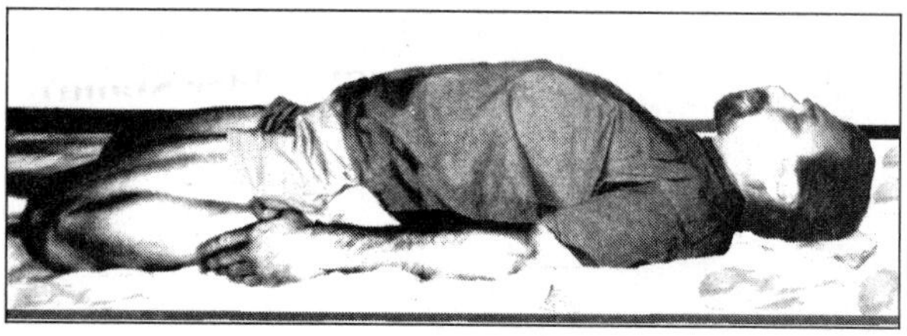

KAPOTĀSANA (PIGEON POSE) ALTERNATIVE

Benefits: These poses tone the spinal region, circulate blood around the spine, and stretch the pelvic region and lower back. The heart is massaged and healed; the diaphragm is lifted, and the chest is expanded. Kapha—diabetes, bronchitis; Vāyu—insomnia, rheumatoid arthritis, varicose veins, sciatica, reproductive organs, constipation, asthma, backache.

Organs Helped: Reproductive, diaphragm, heart.

Doṣhas: All; especially VK-

Standing Bow

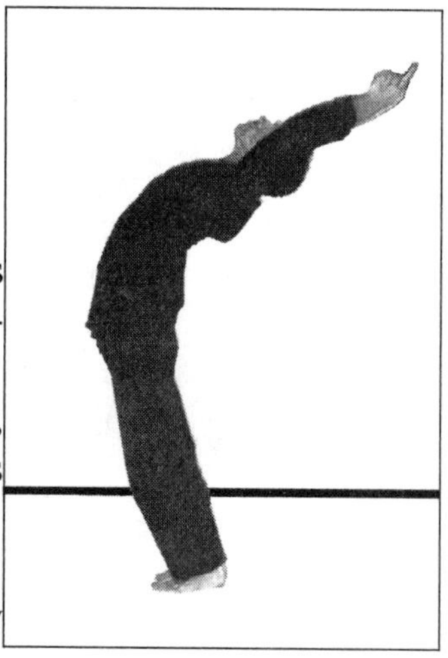

STANDING BOW

Method:
A) Stand erect, arms at sides; breathe easily.
B) Bend elbows, bringing the palms together at the chest in prayer position.
C) Slowly raise the hands up over the head (the arms cover the ears). Notice the rhythm of your breathing.
D) Inhale, slowly bending from the lower back; leaning backwards as far as is comfortable. Keep hands and arms in the same position at the head.
E) Exhale, slowly bringing the upper torso upright.
F) Slowly lower the "prayer hands" to the chest; then return the hands to the sides.

Precaution: Extreme care is required; especially if persons have a bad back or neck.

Benefits: This pose stretches the lower back and kidney area

Doṣhas: All

Ūrdhva Dhanurāsana (Upward Bow)

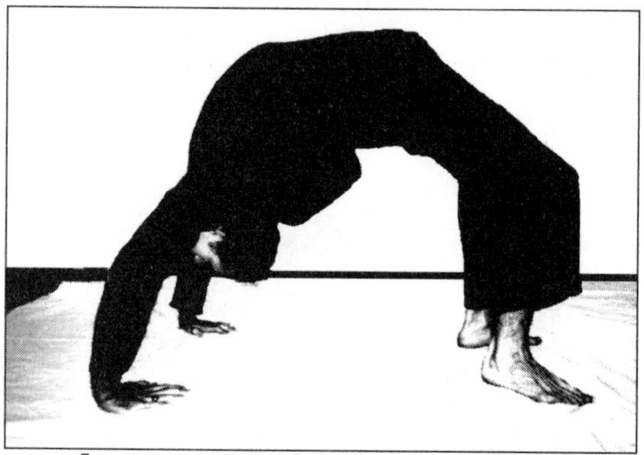

ŪRDHVA DHANURĀSANA (UPWARD BOW)

Method: *Advanced Beginner*
A) Lie on the back, bend knees. Soles of the feet are on the floor, and knees are together.
B) Arms are raised over the head with elbows facing the sky. The palms are on the ground, fingers facing the shoulders (hands are shoulder-width distance apart).
C) Exhale, raising the trunk and crown of the head off the floor.
D) Rest and breathe in this position.
E) Exhale, lifting the trunk and head further, arching the back so the weight is completely on the palms and soles (never put pressure on the

head and neck). Breathe naturally.
F) Stretch the arms from the shoulders and the legs from the thighs.
G) Eventually the elbows are straight and the thighs are stretched.
H) Exhale and stretch some more, pulling the thigh muscles by lifting the heels off the floor.
I) Extend the chest, stretching up the sacral region of the spine until the abdomen is taut; then lower the heels to the floor again. Hold the pose for some time.
J) Exhale, gently lowering the body to the floor again.

Benefits: This pose stretches and tones the spine, making the body alert and supple; strengthens the back, arms, and wrists; soothes the head, and promotes vitality, lightness, and energy.

Doṣhas: All

Setu Bandha Sarvāṅgāsana (Bridge Pose)

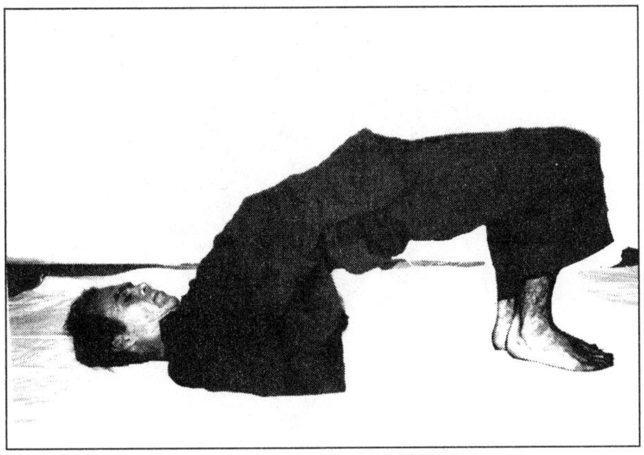

SETU BANDHA (BRIDGE POSE)

Method: *Setu means bridge*
A) Lie on the back with knees bent and the soles of the feet on the floor.
B) Exhale, raising the buttocks off the floor.
C) With elbows resting on the ground, place the palms on the small of the back, supporting the weight of the body. (A stretch should be felt in the small of the back.)
D) Optional—legs may then be extended straight out for further back-bending benefits.
E) Breathe easily while holding the position.
F) Inhale, lifting the buttocks. Remove the hands, exhale and gently lower the body to the ground.

Benefits: The spine flexes backwards and neck strain is removed. The result is a healthy, flexible spine and nervous system.

Doṣhas: All

18. Sālamba Sarvāṅgāsana (Shoulder Stand)

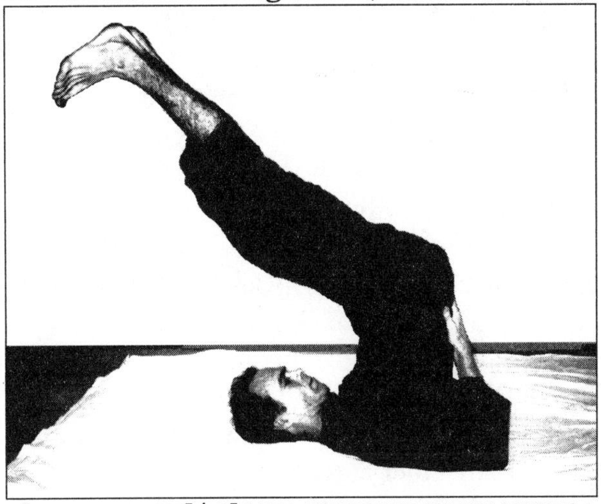

SĀLAMBHA SARVĀṄGĀSANA (SHOULDER STAND) FIGURE 1

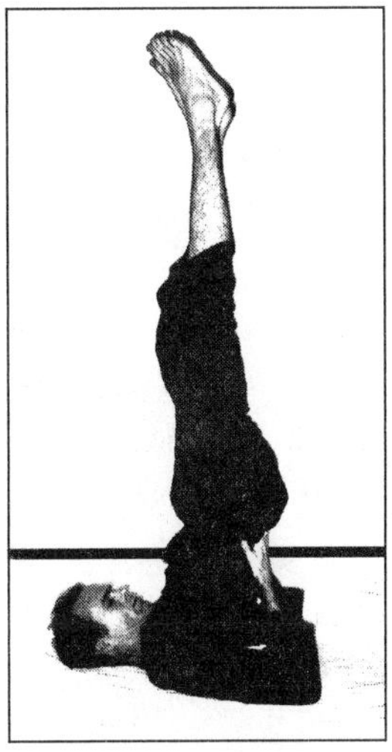

SĀLAMBHA SARVĀṄGĀSANA (SHOULDER STAND) FIGURE 2

Method:
A) Lie flat on the back, legs completely extended, knees together, hands at the sides, palms down.
B) Relax, take a few deep breaths; then inhale, raising the knees to the thighs.
C) Exhale, raising the hips from the floor. Brace the buttocks with your hands, while your elbows remain on the floor, supporting the buttocks. (Alternatively, cross legs and grab toes; then pull legs up to the head. This is an easy way to elevate the lower trunk. Then place the palms on the buttocks.)
D) Exhale, raising the lower trunk to a 45 angle with palms supporting the buttocks; or to a 90 degree angle (perpendicular) to the floor by walking the palms to the lower back.
E) Exhale, raising the legs and keeping them aligned with the trunk of the body; toes pointing to the sky.
F) The chin is locked into the chest.
G) Breathe naturally in this position.
H) Exhale, sliding the hands to the buttocks as the body begins to lower. Slowly return the body to the starting position.

Precaution: This pose must not be practiced by anybody with a heart problem, high blood pressure, or any other pressure (e.g., sinus, ear).

Immediately after this pose, practice the fish pose (*Matsyāsana*), or the serpent or cobra pose (*Bhujaṅgāsana*).

Always eat enough food daily, as this pose increases the digestive fire (*agni*); but do not eat for at least one hour before *āsanas*.

Elderly persons are advised not to perform this pose unless they have practiced it throughout adulthood.

Benefits: This pose bathes all the organs and brain in blood; increases absorption of nutrients, secretes hormones for balancing body and brain; heals anemia, asthma, breathlessness, palpitations, emphysema, bronchitis, throat problems, headaches, colds, sinuses, congestion, nasal disturbances, hypertension, irritation, constipation, urinary disorders, uterine displacement, menstrual troubles, hemorrhoids, hernia, arteriosclerosis, sexual debility, varicose veins, ulcers (stomach and intestinal), colitis, abdominal organ protrusion or pain; senility, dementia, epilepsy, anger, hate, irritability, short temper, insomnia; soothes nerves, frees the system of toxins, restores energy, hides gray hair and wrinkles after six months; develops vitality, happiness, confidence, joy, strengthens digestion, increases appetite, for convalescing.

Organs Helped: Endocrine organs or ductless glands, thyroid, parathyroid, pituitary, pineal... all organs of the brain and body.

Doṣhas: All

19. Halāsana (Plough)

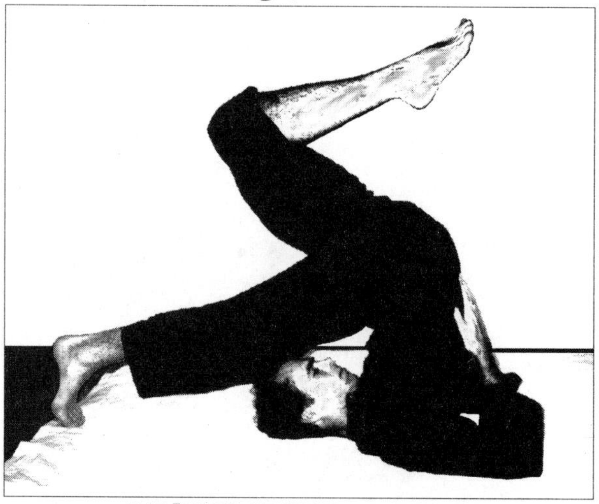

HALĀSANA (PLOUGH)—BEGINNERS

This is an advanced variation of the shoulder stand, but beginners can do a preparatory version of this pose.

Method: *Beginner*
A) Lie on the back, exhale, and bring knees to the chest.
B) Cross the ankles and grab toes with the opposite hands.
C) Exhale, pulling the feet over the head, taking care not to harm the spine.

D) Exhale, bringing the feet over the head, touching the ground (chin locked in the chest) if possible.
E) Hold this pose or fully extend the legs. One leg at a time may be extended to begin to stretch the back and leg muscles. Palms are pressed against the middle or upper back. Breathe naturally.
F) Inhale, slowly letting the hands and feet return to the original position.

Method: *Advanced*

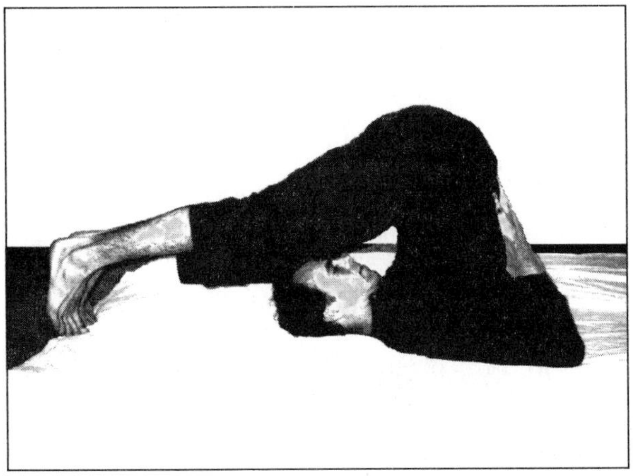

HALĀSANA (PLOUGH)—ADVANCED

A) From the shoulder stand, release the chin lock and gently lower the trunk slightly.
B) Move the arms and legs over the head (either with bent knees or straightened legs (most advanced).
C) Rest the toes on the floor. Breathe naturally.
D) Tighten the knees by pulling the hamstring muscles at the back of the thighs and raise the trunk.
E) Place palms in the middle of the back. Press the trunk to keep it perpendicular to the floor.
F) Extend the hands behind the back (opposite the leg position), palms on the ground.
G) Hook the thumbs and stretch the arms and legs.
H) Interlock the fingers and turn the wrists so the thumbs rest on the floor.
I) Stretch the palmsṄand fingers, tighten the arms at the elbows, and pull them from the shoulders. (Stretching the arms in the opposite directions fully stretches the spine).
J) Change the thumb that touches the ground from time to time; stretching the arms for an equal amount of time in each position. This develops harmonious elasticity of the shoulders.
K) After a comfortable amount of time, release the hands, raise the legs back to the shoulder stand, and gently slide the legs back to the floor.

Benefits: Same as the shoulder stand. Also, abdominal organs are rejuvenated, the spine receives extra blood to heal backache, hand cramps, stiff shoulders and elbows; arthritis, and lumbago. This pose creates lightness and mobility.

Vāyu—asthma, depression, sciatica, sexual debility, wrinkles, rheumatoid arthritis, headache, menstrual disorders, abdominal pain, and gas.

Doṣhas: All; especially V-

20. Matsyāsana (Fish Pose)

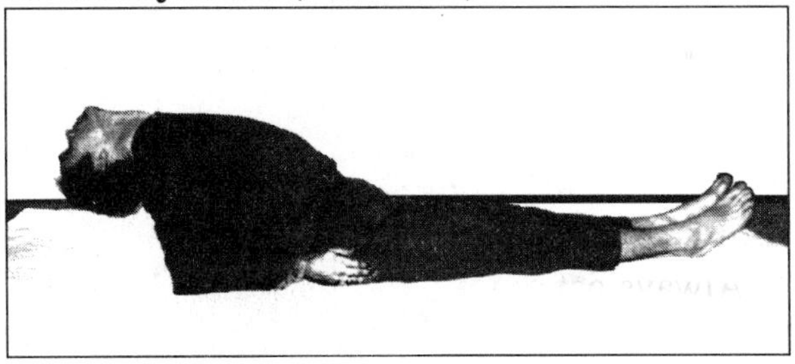

MATSYĀSANA (FISH POSE)

Method: *Beginner*
A) Lie on the back; inhale, raising the upper torso from the elbows (hands facing the feet, palms down).
B) Arch the back and lean the head backwards, but keep it off the floor.
C) Breathe easily and hold the posture, focusing on the lower back.
D) Exhale, gently lowering the head and torso to the ground.
Precaution: If the head is resting on the ground,

the neck and spine can become strained.

Method: *Advanced: Lotus-Fish*

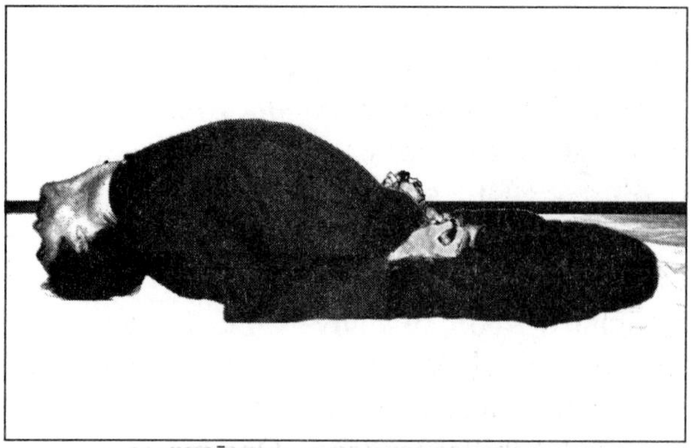

MATSYĀSANA (LOTUS-FISH POSE)

Start in lotus pose and lean on the elbows. Then arch the back and head.

Or, in the lotus position, grasp toes and roll onto the back and elbows. Then, lower the feet, lifting the torso, using the elbows, and arching the back and head.

Benefits: The chest is expanded, making breathing fuller and easier; stretches pelvic joints.
Pitta—absorption of nutrients, liver, thyroid, migraine.
Kapha—sinus congestion and headaches; gastrointestinal disorders, asthma.

Organs Helped: Liver, head, sinuses, gastrointestinal tract, thyroid.

Doṣhas: PK-

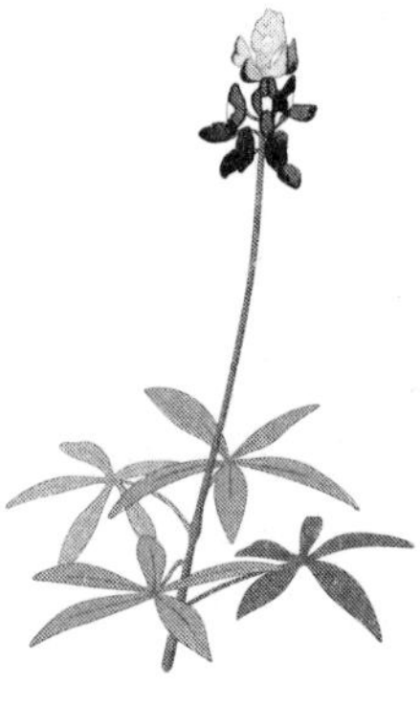

21. Jathara Parivartanāsana (Belly Roll)

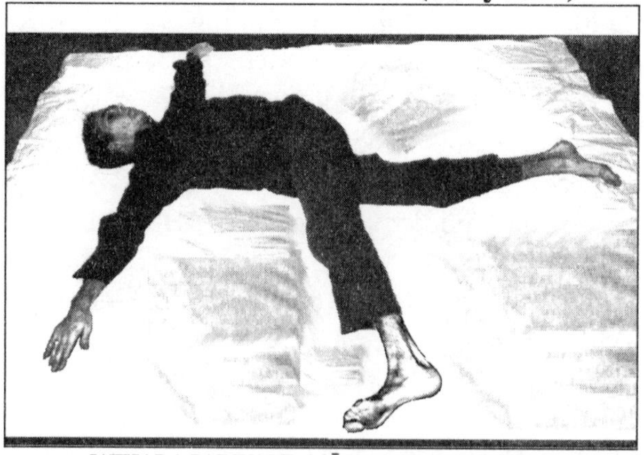

JATHARA PARIVARTAMĀSANA (BELLY ROLL)

Jathara means belly, and *parivartana* means roll or turn.

Method: *Beginner*
A) Lie flat on the back with arms stretched sideways (parallel to the shoulders, resembling a cross).
B) Inhale, lifting the left leg while keeping it straight, until it reaches 45 or 90 degrees above the floor. Breathe normally.
C) Exhale, slowly crossing and lowering the left leg over the right side, trying to touch the floor. Keep the leg straight. Also, try to keep the back and shoulder flat on the floor. Breathe normally.
D) Inhale, slowly lifting the leg back into the air. Hold, then exhale and slowly return to position A. Rest until breathing becomes normal again.
E) Repeat with the right leg.

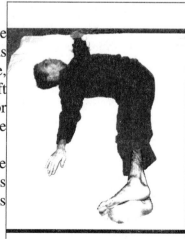

Advanced
A) Start in the same position as the beginners pose, only exhale and lift both legs to 45 or 90 degrees above the floor.
B) Follow the same instructions as in the beginner's pose.

Benefits: Reduces excess fat, tones liver, spleen, pancreas, and removes sluggishness; heals gastritis and strengthens the intestines, trims all the abdominal organs, relieves sprains, and loosens the hip and lower back region.

Doṣhas: PK-

22. Sūryāsana (Sun Pose)

The sun pose is a combination of poses designed to heal, tone, and rejuvenate all aspects of the mind, body, and spirit. It originally was practiced at sunrise, but can be done anytime of the day or night. It is a general pose that can be done by anyone.

Method:

Step 1

A) Stand erect, arms at sides; breathe easily.

B) Inhale, bending the elbows and bringing the palms together at the chest in prayer position.

C) Slowly raise hands over the head. The arms are covering the ears (notice a natural breath occurring in the lungs). Slowly bend from the lower back, leaning backwards as far as is comfortable. Keep hands and arms in the same position around the head. [Fig. 1]

D) Exhale, slowly bringing the upper torso upright. Slowly bring the hands back to the chest in the prayer pose; then return the hands to the sides. Slowly bend forward, letting the arms and head hang with the weight of gravity. Keep knees and legs straight (do not bend knees). If the fingers or hands touch the ground, fine, otherwise, allow the body to hang and relax. Breathe naturally. Feel gravity pulling the arms, hands, and face muscles; it releases all the tension from the face, shoulders, neck, arms, and hands. One may stay in this position as long as desirable. [Fig. 2]

Step 2

E) Exhale, bending the knees and squatting. Palms are placed outside the feet. One may hold this position as well.

F) Inhale, sliding the right foot backward and extending the leg until the knee is straight. The toes are bent and the heel is off the floor. The other foot is flat on the floor. The knee is parallel with the hands and the head directly over the bent knee, looking straight ahead. Arch the back with the chest closer to the ground. Hold this position and breathe naturally, feeling the stretch throughout the body, especially in the legs, back, and shoulders. [Fig. 3]

G) Inhale, sliding the left foot back, beside the right foot. Set both heels on the floor, raising the buttocks and feeling a greater stretch in the legs, feet, and Achilles tendons. One may remain in this position and breathe easily. [Fig. 4]

H) Inhale, bending the knees until they rest on the floor; then rest the chest on the ground. The shoulders are parallel to the fingers (for beginners).

I) Inhale, gently pushing the upper torso off the ground (cobra position). [Fig. 6]

Advanced option—inhale, lowering the head until it is parallel with the hands. Only the hands and feet touch the ground. Then arch the back. The chest is closer to the ground, the buttocks are in the air (a sort of ess shape) [Fig. 5]. Like a snake, slither or pull the head and body forward past the hands, winding up in the cobra position (the upper torso is almost perpendicular to the floor. The head looks forward).

J) Inhale, pushing the buttocks back into the air. The heels return to the floor as in position G.

Step 3

K) Inhale, sliding the right foot up to the chest. The toes are parallel with the fingers and the head faces forward. This is the reverse position from F, while the left heel comes off the floor. Arch the back (chest closer to the ground). Remain in this position and breath normally. [Fig. 7]

L) Inhale, sliding the left foot next to the right foot (returning to the squatting position). Remain in this position and breathe naturally.

M) Inhale, extending and raising the legs and

buttocks until the legs are straight. Simultaneously keep the upper torso bent forward (holding the feet and palms on the floor; or simply hanging, as mentioned before). Rest, breath, and let gravity pull the stress from the mind, face, and body. [Fig. 8]
N) Bring the palms together in prayer position. Inhale, extending the arms straight out and raising them. This pulls the upper torso back into the upright position.
O) Continue this motion, replicating the position of the arms and hands over the head (arms covering the ears), then leaning backwards again. [Fig. 9]
P) Exhale, slowly bringing the arms and torso upright again. Gently lower arms to the chest while the hands are still in prayer position. Release the hands and lower them to the sides of the body.

<u>Benefits</u>: All the benefits of each individual posture mentioned earlier are incorporated in this pose.

<u>*Doṣhas*</u>: All

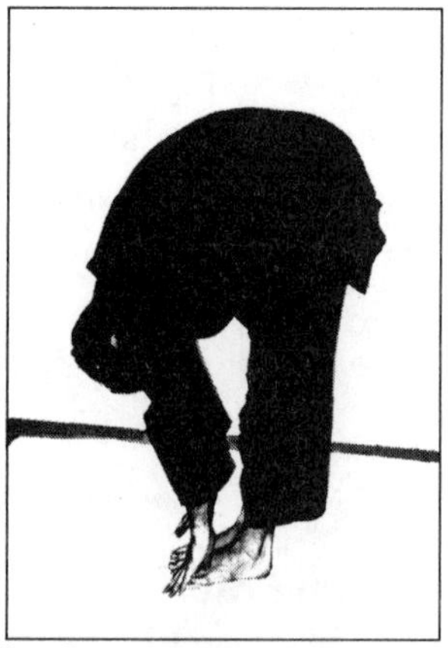

SŪRYĀSANA (SUN POSE)—FIG. 2

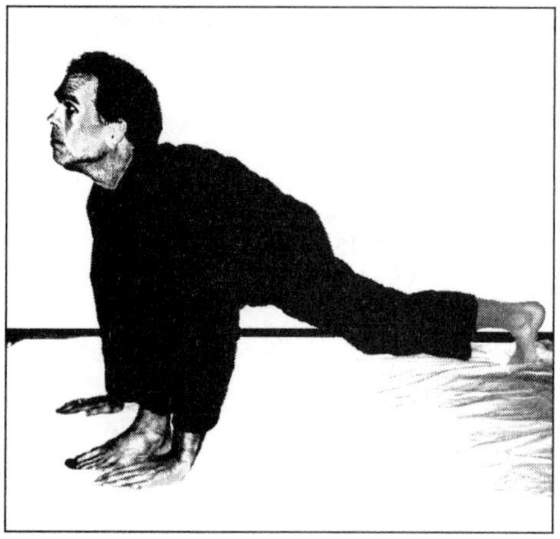

SŪRYĀSANA (SUN POSE)—FIG. 3

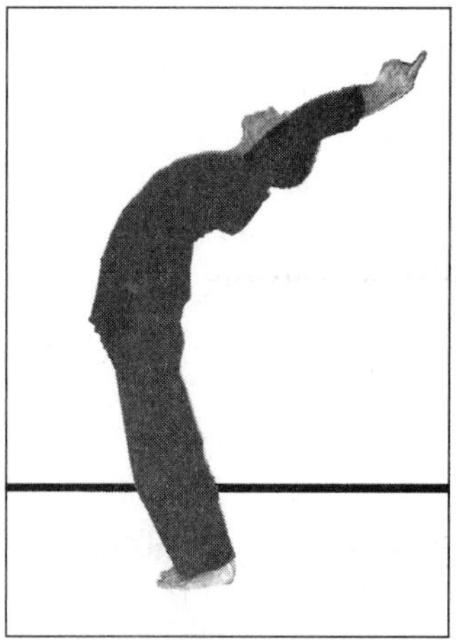

SŪRYĀSANA
(SUN POSE)—FIG. 1

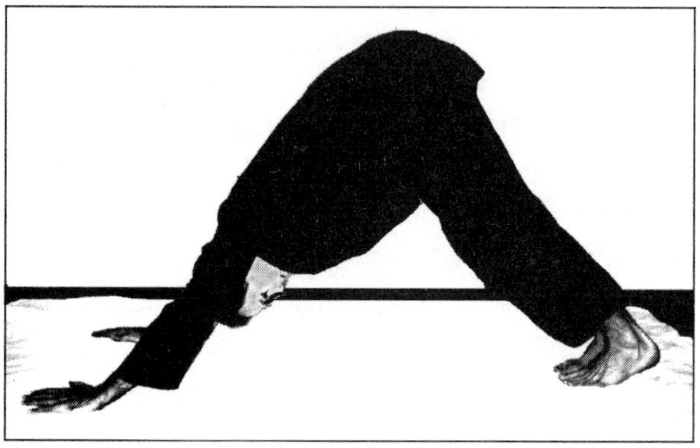

SŪRYĀSANA (SUN POSE)—FIG. 4

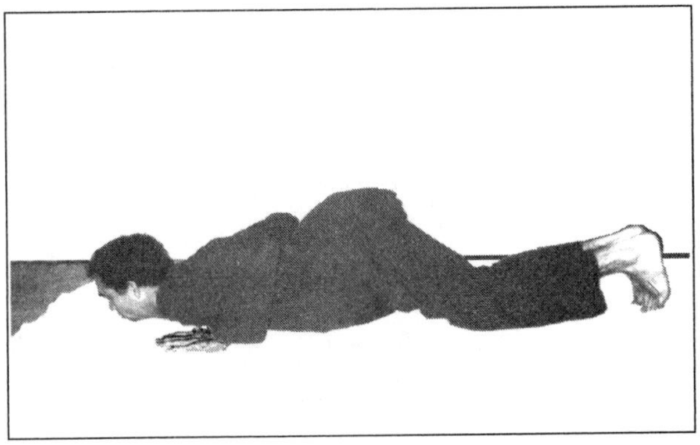
SŪRYĀSANA (SUN POSE)—FIG. 5

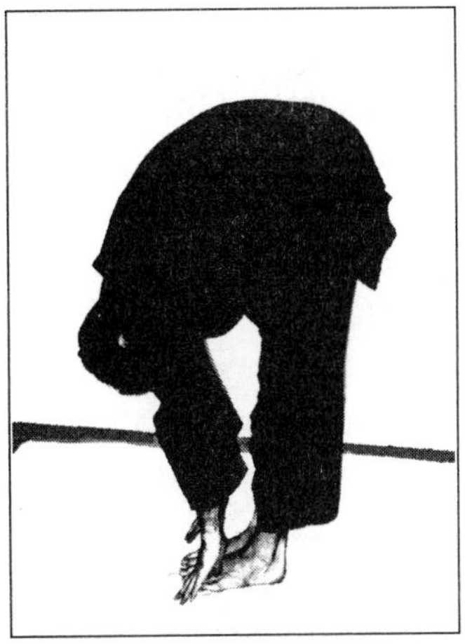
SŪRYĀSANA (SUN POSE)—FIG. 8

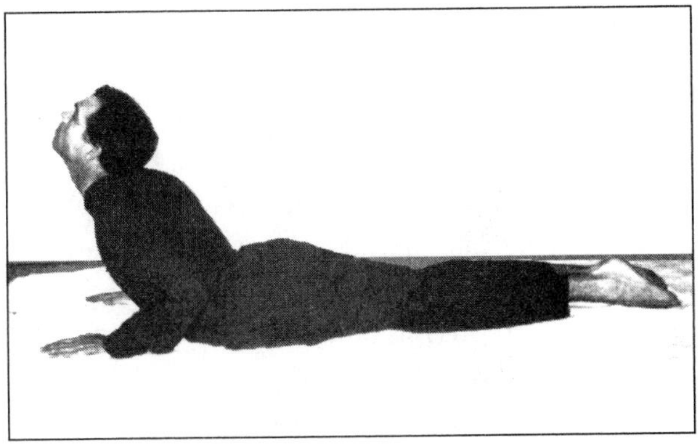
SŪRYĀSANA (SUN POSE)—FIG. 6

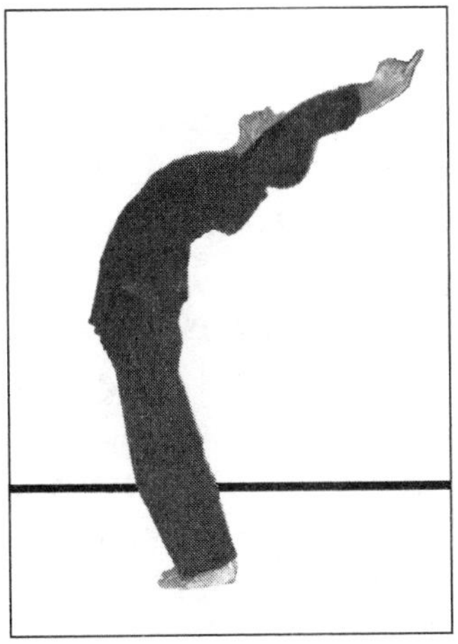
SŪRYĀSANA (SUN POSE)—FIG. 9

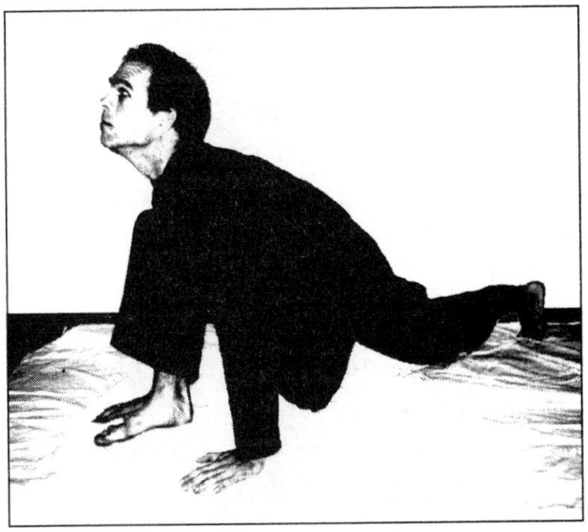
SŪRYĀSANA (SUN POSE)—FIG. 7

23. Śhavāsana (Corpse Pose)

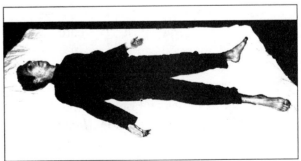

ŚHAVĀSANA (CORPSE POSE)

Method:
A) Lie on the back with hands at the sides (palms facing up). Feet are stretched out and are slightly

separated. The body should be aligned.
B) Slowly inhale through the nose. Feel the cool air entering the *mūlādhāra chakra* (base of spine). As it rises through the body, feel the air healing and sweeping away the toxins.
C) Slowly exhale and feel the air going out the crown of the head, releasing toxins and tensions from the face, head, mind, neck, and shoulders. Repeat this process several times.

Option
D) Slowly inhale as above; then during exhalation, chant the *mantra*, '*aum*'. Feel the voice vibrating through the entire body. Repeat several times, as the vibration creates a deeper relaxation.
E) Rest for 1 or more minutes, noticing your breath. Then let your mind drift where it may, or practice *sādhanā* (meditation).

Precaution: Although this seems like a simple pose, it is said to take 15 years to master the relaxation derived from it. Ending all *yoga* routines with this pose is imperative; otherwise, strain may occur while the body is adjusting to its new, healthier structure.

Benefits: This posture is to be practiced by everyone as the last pose of the routine. Y*oga āsanas* purify, heal, tone, and perform acupuncture on the body. Now the body must rest, restructure, and reorient itself to its new self. When this pose is completed, one will have developed a new mind, body, and spirit. The entire system is revitalized.

The pose develops physical awareness and *pratyāhāra* (withdrawal and liberation of the mind from the senses and objects—5th stage of *yoga*). This posture also develops *dhāraṇā* (concentration or visualization of one's deity—6th stage of meditation), and *dhyāna* (holding or meditation on that image—7th stage of meditation).

Śhavāsana is also useful when practiced between *āsanas*, and after a stressful day. This helps blood pressure, peptic ulcers, anxiety, hysteria, cancer, psychosomatic diseases, neuroses, realization of subconscious thoughts.

Vāyu—asthma, depression, varicose veins, insomnia. Pitta—anger or hatred.

Doṣhas: All

Part 2
Prāṇāyāma & Nāda

As discussed earlier, the life-breath (*prāṇ* or soul) saves the mind from the anxiety, nervousness, worry, fear, anger, impatience, hot temper, lethargy, agitation, and dullness. It improves concentration and memory, mental peace, and the delight of a silent, clear mind. The development of peace is synonymous with higher mental spiritual development.

This is because thoughts are a vibration of the life-breath. If the vibration is stopped, the mind is saved. As the mind becomes free from thought, it remains centered in the higher Self of eternity or Divine peace and bliss. One may wonder, if there are no thoughts, does one becomes a robot or brainwashed? Brainwashing is a state of imposing a certain philosophy on the mind and locking it in place. This keeps the mind locked into a 'specific-state' activity; not a state of freedom and peace. In this state of mental silence one feels clear-headed enough to make responsible decisions, while maintaining a peaceful mind.

Mental peace occurs when the life-breath ceases to flow in the *iḍā* and *piṅgalā*, and begins to flow in the *suṣhumṇā,* resulting in stillness. The *Vedic* texts or scriptures suggest that the best way for this to occur is through the practice of meditation, as instructed by a true *guru*. Four initial stages of mental development exist. The mind,

1) Is stuck in dullness, greed, and violence (*tamas*).
2) Seeks excess chatter or activity, or it seeks

empty fame and fortune (*tamas* and *rajas*).

3) Becomes conscientious, and wants knowedge, piety, and prosperity; realizing there is more to life than material possessions (*rajas*).
4) Becomes pure, kind, compassionate, clear, and happy. No trace of *rajas* exists (only *sattwa* exists). This fourth or *sattwic* state is the first stage of *samādhi* or peace. The quiet mind is now ready to hear the inner eternal calling. This eternal experience is even more alluring than happiness gained sensory pleasure. Then, the mind undergoes two more stages of the development of higher consciousness. The mind,
5) Becomes drawn towards the inner Divine attraction and becomes absorbed in eternal bliss. No awareness of thoughts of the outer world exist (second stage of *samādhi*).

5a) After this second stage of *samādhi*, one's awareness returns (i.e., getting up from meditation), but some of that inner peacefulness remains. This peace develops as one continues to meditate.

6) Full Self-Realization. This occurs when the second stage of *samādhi* remains, even when one is out of meditation. In this final stage of *samādhi* one sees the inner Self as Divine and eternal, and all people and things in life as that same Divine Self. One feels full compassion, peace, and eternal bliss. Activities and objects of the outer world no longer affect this eternal peace. One becomes the peace. Everything has become the peace. Thus, there is nothing that is 'non-peace'. The relative workings of the mind are fully stopped, and the life-breath flows permanently and quietly through the entire *suṣhumṇā*.

Prāṇāyām means stilling of the breath. Inhalation, exhalation, and breath retention, condition the breath to be still. Stillness of breath stills the mind. *Prāṇāyām* cleanses the channels (*nāḍīs*) and energy centers (*chakras*), just as a broom or vacuum clears the dirt from a house. Speaking in modern scientific terms, the breathing process is intimately linked to the brain and central nervous system. It is also related to the hypothalamus, which involves the emotions, body temperature, memory, and perceptions. Erratic thinking of the hypothalamus also leads to erratic breathing and eventually to asthma. So, a quiet breath keeps the body healthy and the mind at peace.

Prāṇāyām is related to the in and out breaths of the nose. Certain areas of the nose's mucus membrane are connected to the visceral organs (i.e., thorax, abdomen, heart, lungs, kidneys, and intestines). According to *yogic* thinking, when this nasal breathing becomes irregular, the visceral organs connected to the coccygeal plexus also become irregular. In turn, they send sporadic messages to the brain, causing further irregularities. When the breath is held, it allows for a longer assimilation time of the *prāṇa*. The result is the exchange of oxygen and carbon dioxide in the cells. Thus, the breath is intimately linked to physical and mental health.

Throughout *yogic* literature it is written that those who use fewer breaths will live longer. So, learning how to make the breath automatically stop, helps foster longevity. Spiritually, this stoppage of breath (i.e., the stopping of one's mind), allows one to delve more deeply into one's inner Self of peace, alertness, and harmony.

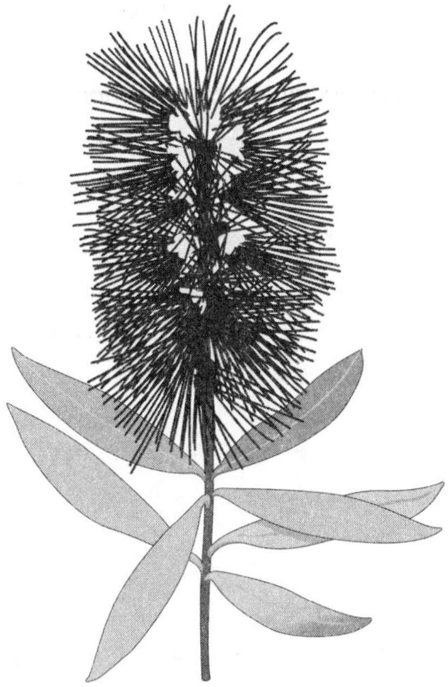

Five aspects of breath exist:

5 Breaths of Prāṇāyāma

Breath	Function	Direction	Organs
Prāṇ Vāyu	absorption	out	head, heart, lungs
Udān Vāyu	communication, will	up	throat & facial expression
Samān Vāyu	assimilation	omni-direction	small intestines
Vyān Vāyu	circulation	different directions	pervading the whole body
Apān Vāyu	elimination	down	urinary/ excretory, reproductive

According to some *yogis, samān* is the most important Vāyu sub-*dosha* because it is related to the *sushumṇā* channel or *nāḍī*. Through *yoga*, *prāṇ* and *apān* are united in the location of *samān*, and life-breath is suspended.

The *prāṇa* (life-breath, which is different from *Prāṇa* Vāyu) is made to flow through the *nāḍīs* (channels). *Prāṇa* cleanses the *nāḍīs* of impurities acquired from bad habits (e.g., junk food, fatigue, drugs, chemicals, radiation, pollution, etc.). *Prāṇ* naturally develops during *sādhanā* (meditation); and also cleanses *karmic* impurities (i.e., past life bad habits). The various *Vedic* scriptures say 72,000 to 350,000 *nāḍīs* exist in the human body.

The *prāṇa* that flows through the *nāḍīs* is stored in the energy centers (*chakras*) situated along the *sushumṇā* (tube) inside the spinal column. These centers, located in the subtle body, affect the physical body's nerve plexus. *Chakras* influence both the physical and causal bodies.

Six main *chakras* are generally recognized as having their own specific correlation to physical functioning (see table on next page).

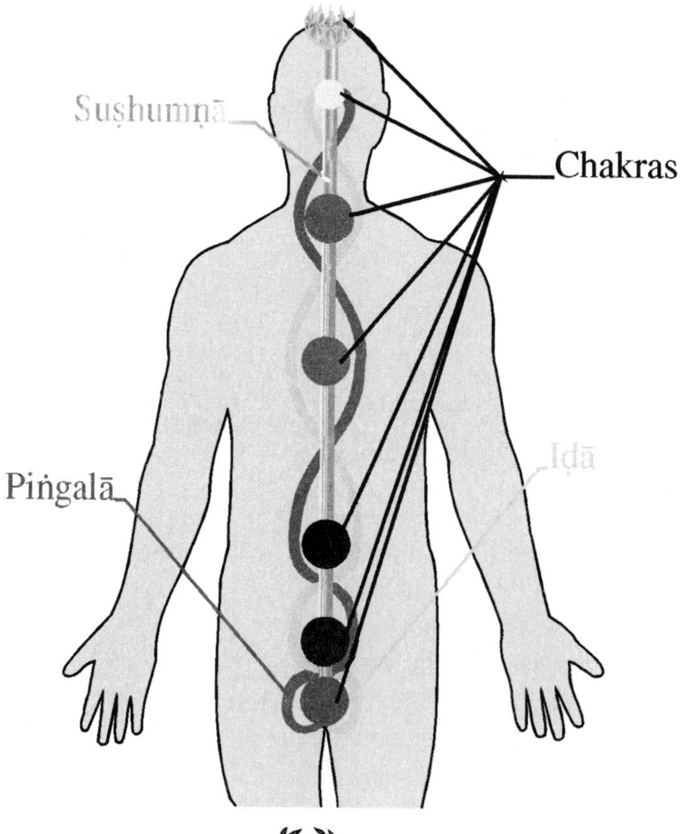

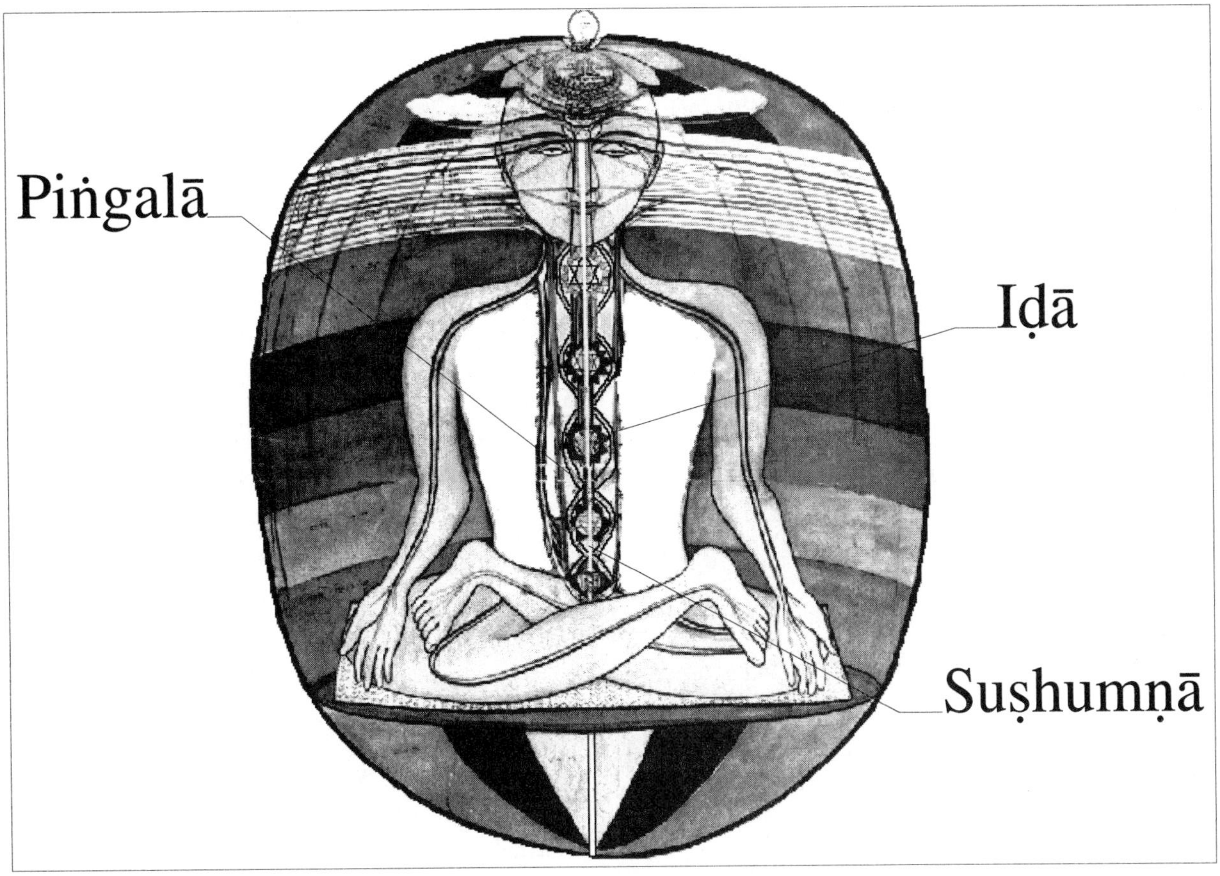

CHAKRAS, ORGANS AND SENSES THEY CONTROL

Chakra	Location	Organs	Sense
1. *Mūlādhāra*	perineum	urinary/excretory/ reproductive glands & hormones	nose/smell
2. *Swādhiṣhṭhāna*	two fingers above perineum	sacral plexus: urinary/reproductive glands & organs	tongue/taste
3. *Manipūra*	navel	digestive/ absorption	eyes/sight
4. *Anahāta*	heart	respiration, heart, lungs, thymus	hands/touch
5. *Viśhuddha*	throat	purifies mind and body, thyroid	ears/sound
6. *Ājñā*	third eye	medulla oblongata, pineal gland	intuition

The first five *chakras* have *nāḍīs* that extend to the various organs of sense and action. The sixth *chakra* relates to higher mental or spiritual activity. Beyond the sixth *chakra* one enters the realm of the "non-describable" and begins to merely "be" in the state of unbounded eternity or *Brahman*. This is the goal of life—*Brahman* or Self-Realization. It is for this reason that the *Vedic* sages do not put much emphasis even on the celestial experiences experienced through the sixth *chakra*.

The next chapter discusses the effects of *mantras* on the *chakras* and their corresponding health concerns. The chart below shows how the *chakras* relate to the various aspects of human personality.

Chakras	**Human Characteristics**
1. *Mūlādhāra*	animal instincts
2. *Svādhiṣhṭhāna*	selfish ego
3. *Manipūra*	sensuality, greed, ambition
4. *Anahāta*	emotions
5. *Viśhuddha*	accepting life's adversities, mental balance, sensitivity
6. *Ājñā*	gateway to Self-Realization

So we see that *prāṇa* cleanses the *nāḍīs,* and in turn the *chakras*. As they are cleansed, one's spiritual life-force is allowed to flow higher, developing or utilizing the benefits of the higher *chakras*. As one is able to live with their higher *chakras* opened, life becomes more peaceful, graceful, and Divine.

Yet, the *nāḍīs* and *chakras* must be cleansed gently and naturally; so that the sudden—and possibly harmful life-force—will not flow through the channels before they are ready. A clay pot must be baked in an oven to hold water properly; if it is not properly prepared, it will quickly disintegrate. Like the clay pot, the *nāḍīs* and *chakras* must be prepared to accept the flow of the life-force or they too will disintegrate. Medically speaking, *prāṇāyām* strengthens the sympathetic, parasympathetic, and the central nervous systems to accept the charge of life energy.

So, *prāṇa* is valuable from both the medical and spiritual viewpoints. Two ways of inducing *prāṇāyāma* exist: automatic or manual. The *Rig Veda Bhasyabhumika*, an ancient *Vedic* scripture, says that through proper *sādhanā* (meditation), *prāṇāyāma* occurs on its own, cleansing what is needed—when it is needed. The *Vedic* scriptures caution persons from trying to open their *chakras* on their own, for such an opening can cause great damage physically, psychologically, and spiritually.

Prāṇāyāma/Kumbhaka

Through *prāṇāyām* breathing exercises, one manually stimulates the *prāṇa* flow. Not only can this be dangerous without proper instruction, but it can also be considered unnecessary if one practices proper *sādhanā*. Then, should one care to do manual *prāṇāyām*, it is an option rather than a necessity.

Below are listed some of the more useful breathing exercises one may manually practice for the healing of specific diseases. They are also discussed to inform those who have these experiences occurring automatically in meditation, but who neither realize such experiences are normal nor understand their value.

Precautions: Do not hold the breath if suffering from high blood pressure. Inhaling, exhaling, and holding of breath should be gentle, slow, and comfortable at all times. Straining can cause harm.

Note:

1st Stage of practicing *prāṇāyām*: one may notice perspiration or warming sensation during the practice. This is due to increased sympathetic nervous system activity. Rub the body with this perspiration. It promotes steadiness and firmness (balancing and toning the nerves, muscles, and the entire system).

2nd Stage there may be quivering, trembling, or sensations in the spine; also twitching of the hands, face, or other muscles. This is normal as stresses are released; the mind and body reorient themselves to function in a more coordinated and efficient manner.

3rd Stage the mind becomes steady; the breath stops moving.

It is recommended to have milk and *ghee* added to one's diet when first beginning *prāṇāyām* practice. Persons should not eat at all for at least 1 hour before this practice. Foods should be based on one's Āyurvedic constitution.

General Benefits: Besides those benefits discussed earlier, *prāṇāyām* also removes hiccups, cough, headache (and migraine), eye and ear pains, respiratory and digestive problems (i.e., asthma, wheezing, indigestion, hyperacidity), mucus, fat, obesity. It helps with all diseases caused by the three *doṣhas*.

Discussed in the *Vedic* scripture, the *Yoga-śhikā Upanishad*, is a four-stage process of *Yoga* or Self-Realization: *Mantra*, *Haṭha* (and *prāṇāyāma*), *Laya,* and *Raja*. All stages develop or refine the breathing process until it ceases to flow. This is the goal of breathing exercises.

After one begins a natural form of *mantra sādhanā* (meditation), *haṭha yoga* begins automatically. *Prāṇāyāma* is related to *haṭha. Haṭha* means the unification of the upper and lower vital breaths of the body. By uniting the breath that flows through the thousands of channels, the breaths merge into the *suṣhumṇā,* or spiritual tube (inside the spine).

As previously discussed, the result of this unification is the stilling of the breath. The ceasing of inhalation and exhalation occurs spontaneously during the *Laya* stage of *yoga*. Here one is absorbed in their inner eternal, Divine Self. The senses do not perceive any outside objects or thoughts. This creates a great peace in the spirit that, healthwise, brings much mental and physical healing, alertness and calm.

Eventually this stillness of breath becomes permanent. This is called the final stage, or *Raja Yoga*, when a person remains permanently centered inside themselves. Their vital breath is ever still—unaffected—even when involved in activity.

So we see how spontaneously *prāṇāyām* is cultured through a natural process of *sādhanā* or meditation. It may now be understood more clearly why the *Vedic* scriptures say that *prāṇāyām* (that uses fingers to control the breath) are elementary methods of *yoga*. Still, when disease exists, *prāṇāyām* is recommended by the Āyurvedic practitioner for healing.

1. Śhītalī Kumbhaka (Cooling Breath)

Śhītala means cool. *Kumbhaka* means breath.

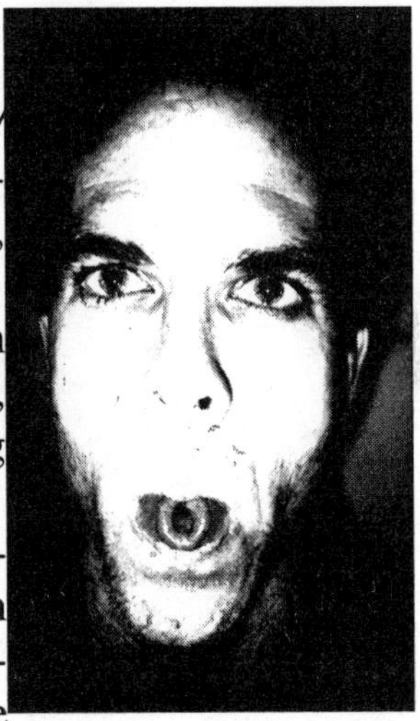

Method:

A) Sit in *Siddhāsana/ Siddha Yoni Āsana;* extend and curl the tongue, with its sides facing up.

B) Slowly inhale through the middle of the tongue, making a slight hissing sound.

C) *Options*: After inhalation, the chin may rest on the collar bone (*Jālandhara Bandha*); hold the breath if comfortable.

D) Slowly exhale through the nose. *Options*: one may make a humming sound during exhalation. This is 1 round.

E) Repeat for 5 to 10 minutes.

Alternative Slowly inhale through nose to accomplish the same effect.

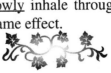

Alternative Curl tongue towards the back of the throat and slowly inhale.

Precautions: Do not use *śhītalī* with high blood pressure. Also, quick inhalation brings oxygen into the system and will increase heat; slow inhalation only allows nitrogen to enter the system.

Benefits: *Śhītalī* cools the entire system; soothes the eyes and ears, reduces fevers, bile, burning, heat sensations, indigestion, thirst, and removes phlegm.

Organs Helped: Liver, spleen, and all Pitta organs.

Doṣhas: PK-

2. **Nāḍī Śhodhana Prāṇāyāma**

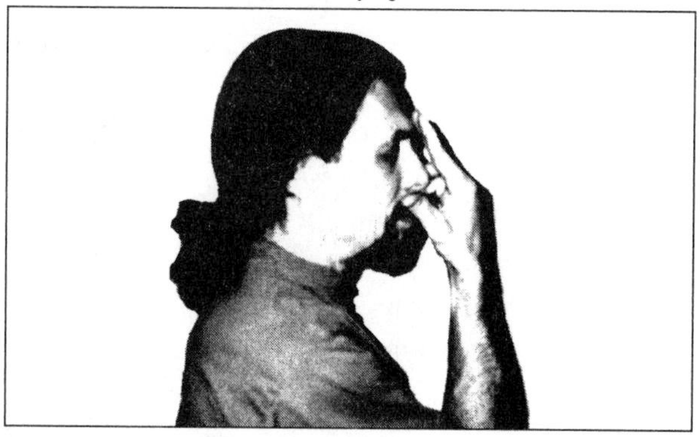

Method:
A) Sit in *Siddhāsana* or *Siddha Yoni Āsana*.
B) The right thumb closes the right nostril. The index and middle fingers rest on the third eye. The ring finger rests beside the left nostril.
C) Slowly inhale through the left nostril, breathing into the belly (the belly rises) until lungs are comfortably filled. Focus on the cooling, healing 'in breath'.
D) Close the left nostril with the ring finger. Remove the thumb from the right nostril and slowly exhale through the right nostril. Focus on the release of stress and tension with the 'out breath'.
E) Inhale through the right nostril; then exhale through the left nostril. This is 1 round. Repeat from step B for 9 more rounds.
Precaution: Those who do not have heart problems or high blood pressure, and who have practiced this method for some time, may begin to comfortably hold the breath before exhaling. Never strain to hold the breath—it may cause harm.

Benefits: This practice cleanses the solar and lunar channels (*piṅgalā* and *iḍā*), helping keep excess Kapha out of the body. This practice makes the mind silent and alert.

Doṣhas: VPK-

3. Sūryabheda Prāṇāyāma (Solar Breathing)

Method: (see previous photo)
A) Sit in *Siddhāsan/Siddha Yoni Āsana*. The right thumb is beside the right nostril. The index and middle finger rest on the third eye, and the ring finger is on the left nostril.
B) Slowly inhale through the right nostril, breathing into an expanding belly, until the lungs are comfortably full. Focus on the cooling, healing 'in-breath'.
C) Close the right nostril with the thumb. Open the left nostril and slowly exhale, focusing on the release of stress and tension. This is 1 round.
D) Close the right nostril and open the left nostril, and begin again with step B. Practice initially for 10 times. Later one can increase the time from 1 to 2 minutes.

Benefits: This improves energy, left brain, and sympathetic nervous system activity; it decreases parasympathetic functioning, and balances or promotes harmony between the two hemispheres of the brain. It balances Pitta and Kapha, removing dullness from the mind, reverses the aging process, and promotes longevity. Benefits result from the increased hormonal secretions of the pituitary gland and endocrine system (that cause aging). Some say this also removes excess Vāyu.

Doṣhas: VK-; this method increases the solar heat in the body. Breathing in the right nostril brings air through the *piṅgalā* or solar channel. *Sūrya* means sun. Some say not used by Pittas.

4. Chandrabheda Prāṇāyāma (Lunar Breathing)

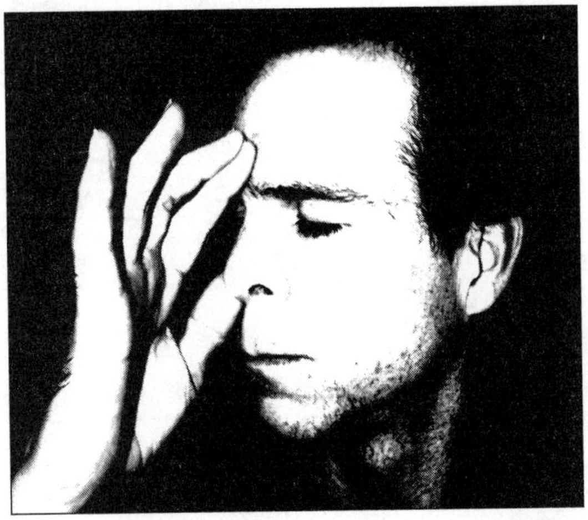

This is the reverse process of *Sūryabheda* (i.e., breathing through the left or *iḍā* nostril and exhaling through the right or *piṅgalā* nostril). Some say this is not recommended; however, when practiced by Pitta *doṣhas*, it can cool the system. Alternatively, a Pitta *doṣha* may practice *śhītalī* to cool the system instead.

5. Bhastra Kumbhaka (Bellows Breath)

This method gently forces the air in and out of the lungs with equal lung movement. The inhalation should be gentle enough so as not to cause the nostrils to be sucked closed. Air should only flow through the nose; not the throat. The body, shoulders, and chest remain unmoved throughout the practice. The lungs, diaphragm, and abdomen will move. Upon exhalation, the belly is to be pulled in; during inhalation release the belly muscles so the belly expands again.

Method:
A) Sit in lotus or *Siddhāsana/Siddha Yoni Āsana*. The body is aligned with hands on the knees.
B) Slowly and deeply inhale.
C) Breathe out quickly and forcefully through the nose (but without straining).
D) Immediately after the exhalation— just as forcefully—breathe in.
E) This can be practiced continually and rhythmically for 10 times (one round).
F) Rest and wait for breathing to return to normal; then practice again. Rest and repeat for three rounds).
As one acclimates oneself to this practice, speed will increase as rhythm is maintained.

Benefits: Awakens the life-force, removes excess mucus, pierces the psychic knots (*granthis*), stimulates the lungs, heart, and blood circulation; oxygenates the blood, and increases the sympathetic nerves in the respiratory center to release carbon dioxide. It improves oxygen absorption and visceral organs; the entire body is massaged, nasal and sinus passages are cleansed. It builds resistance to colds and respiratory diseases (e.g., asthma, sinusitis, bronchitis), helps arthritis, TB, constipation, sciatica, rheumatism, cancer, physical and mental tension. *Bhastra* improves clarity, sluggishness, increases appetite, vitality, and immune system functioning. It removes emotional insecurity, sexual tension, bile, obesity; and improves intuition. *Kuṇḍalinī* is stirred.

Doṣhas: All

6. Kapālbhāti Kumbhaka (Frontal Brain Cleanse)

Kapal means forehead, and *bhati* means light, splendor, or knowledge. Thus, this form of *prāṇāyām* invigorates the whole brain, awakening the dormant centers of subtle perception. Breathing should be like the pumping of a bellows. The exercise compresses the brain (slightly) and the fluid around it during inhalation. The brain and cerebrospinal fluid are decompressed during exhalation. Thus, the brain is massaged.

Method:
A) Sit comfortably and erect in *Siddhāsan/Siddha Yoni Āsana*; close the eyes and relax. Place hands in the *Jñyān* or *Chin Mudrā*.
B) Inhale deeply, then do 50 fast (shorter) inhale/exhales, with more emphasis on the exhalation and shorter inhales. Chin lock may be employed.
C) After the last exhalation, inhale deeply through the nose and exhale quickly through pursed lips.
D) Release the chin lock, raise the head slowly, and inhale slowly through the nose (1 round).
E) Practice 2 more rounds.
F) End by closing eyes and concentrating on the space between the eyebrows.

Precaution: Do not practice with bad lungs, eyes, ears, or high/low blood pressure. If dizziness or nosebleeds are experienced, breathing is too forceful. Stop and sit quietly until dizziness disappears, then try again less forcefully. If the nose bleeds, stop the practice for a few days.

Benefits: This method expels carbon dioxide and other waste gases from the cells and lungs; sinuses are drained, eyes are cooled. It invigorates the liver, spleen, pancreas, and abdominal muscles (thereby improving digestion); it also gives a sense of total exhilaration. This *kumbhaka* reverses the aging process, relaxes facial muscles and nerves, rejuvenates tired cells and nerves, and keeps the face young, shining and free from wrinkles.

Alternative Follow the same process, only breathe in one nostril, out the other, then in the latter and out the first.

Doṣhas: All

7. Bhramarī Kumbhaka (Humming Bee Breath)

It is best practiced in the early morning or late at night, when it is quiet, and one is better able to hear inner sounds. It is practiced after *āsanas* and active *prāṇāyāma,* and before meditation or sleep (on an empty stomach).

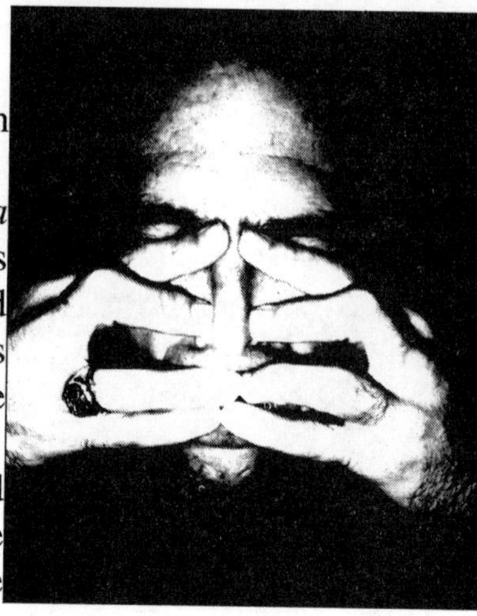

Method:
A) Sit in *Siddhāsana/Siddha Yoni Āsana* and relax. Eyes remain closed and the body is erect. Do the chin lock.
B) Slowly and deeply inhale through the nose, listening to the sound of the breath.
C) Close the ears with the index or middle fingers by pressing the outer part of the ear ligament into the ear hole.
D) Keeping the ears closed, exhale, making a soft, low pitched humming sound. Concentrate on the sound.
E) After fully exhaling, bring hands to the knees and breath slowly and naturally.
F) Practice this for 10 to 20 rounds.
G) When finished, keep eyes closed and listen for any subtle sounds.

Alternative: (See above photo) Close ears with thumbs, the eyes with the index fingers, the nostrils with the middle fingers, and the mouth with the ring and pinky fingers.

Hold the breathe and this position for as long as is comfortable, then exhale while keeping fingers in place. Be aware of any subtle sound vibrations or images that may appear while in this position.

Benefits: It awakens intuition and subtle or psychic sensitivity, relieves mental tension, anger,

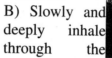

anxiety, and insomnia.

Doṣhas: All

8. Śhītkarī Kumbhaka (Hissing Breath)

The hissing sound, produced from inhaling through clenched teeth, makes a noise like the sound, 'seet'. *Karī* means produce. Thus, *śhītkarī* produces the sound of 'seet'. During hot weather, one can practice up to 10 minutes.

Method:
A) Sit comfortably in *Siddhāsana/Siddha Yoni Āsana*. Eyes are closed and the body is erect. Hands are on the knees in the *Jñyān Mudrā.* Do the chin lock.
B) Bring the teeth together (upper and lower) and separate the lips.
C) Slowly and deeply, inhale through the gaps in the teeth, listening to the sound it makes.
D) After inhaling, close the mouth and exhale through the nose.
E) Repeat 20 times.

Precaution: Practice only in the warm months as this exercise cools the body. Do not practice with chronic constipation. Some say not to practice when suffering from high blood pressure.

Benefits: One develops qualities of Divine love. It lowers blood pressure, cools the tongue, lungs, the entire body; and mind; it also harmonizes the endocrine system, and it regulates reproductive hormone secretion. It also creates charisma and develops purity.

Doṣhas: PK-

9. Ujjāyī Kumbhaka (Conquering Breath)

Ujjāyī means "to conquer." In this practice, the lungs swell up like one proud of victory.

Method:
A) Sit comfortably in *Siddhāsan/Siddha Yoni Āsana*, or lie in the corpse pose, and watch the breath.
B) Slightly contract the back of the throat (as when swallowing).
C) Inhale deeply and slowly through the nose. The contraction will cause a slight snoring sound, but do not use force. The sound will come from the throat, not the nose. Concentrate on the sound. Then exhale through the nostrils.
D) Practice for 1 to 5 minutes.

Alternative Curl the tip of the tongue to the back of the throat during the above practice.

Precaution: Do not practice with low blood pressure. Those with high blood pressure should practice while in the corpse pose.

Benefits: Dispels phlegm from the throat, increases digestion, cleanses *nāḍīs*; heals dropsy, insomnia, mental tension; aerates the lungs, soothes and tones the nerves and the entire body.

Doṣhas: All

10. Mūrchha Kumbhaka (Swooning Breath)

Mūrchha means to swoon or faint. This process develops the conscious experience of the unconscious.

Method:
A) Sit comfortably in *Siddhāsan/Siddha Yoni Āsana*, with chin lock. Palms are on the knees and eyes are closed.
B) Slowly and deeply inhale through the nose. Hold the breath.
C) Slightly release the chin lock and exhale slowly.
D) Wait for the breath to return to normal (1 to 2 minutes), then repeat.
E) Concentrate on the void sensation.

Precautions: Do not practice with high blood pressure, vertigo, or heart disease.

Benefits: Heart rate and pressure are adjusted, mind is silenced; anxiety, tension, anger, and lethargy are reduced.

Doṣhas: VK-

11. Bahya Kumbhaka
(Outer Breath Retention)
Method:
A) Sit comfortably in *siddhāsan/siddha yoni āsana*, with eyes closed and palms on the knees.
B) Slowly inhale through the nose; slowly and completely exhale.
C) The chin lock may now be used. Hold the breath without inhaling.
D) Release the chin lock and slowly inhale.
E) Rest and wait for the breath to return to normal (1 to 2 minutes), then repeat.

Precautions: Do not perform this exercise if suffering from high blood pressure.

Benefits: The life-breath is stabilized, absorption in *samādhi* (divine peace). *Kuṇḍalinī* penetrates the *chakras* as it rises up the *suṣhumṇā* and reaches the crown.

12. Kayvala Kumbhaka
(Automatic Still Breath)

This breathing is superior to all other forms of *kumbhaka*. This frequently takes place, when through the *guru's* grace, the *kuṇḍalinī* enters the *suṣhumṇā*. This is the automatic stabilization of breath, of its own accord. It produces indescribable comfort.

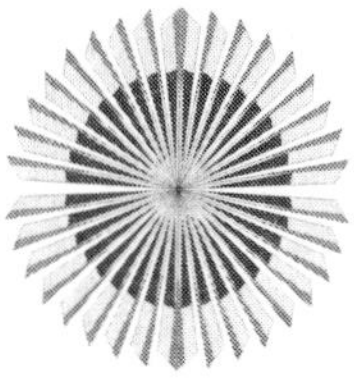

Nāda (Sound)

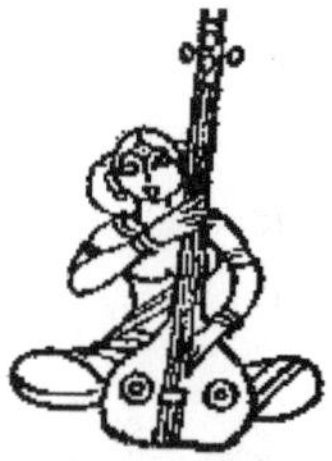

As with *āsanas*, *prāṇāyāma/kumbhaka*, *mudrās,* and *bandhas*—overlaps exist. *Nāda* is also briefly discussed at the end of part 3. *Nāda* occurs naturally during proper, natural *sādhanā* (meditation). Again, for those who may be naturally hearing these sounds, they should be secure in the knowledge that these are confirmations of spiritual development; they are not signs of trouble.

The practical benefits of developing *nāda* are that one's intuition and higher mental faculties are developed, along with more peace, concentration, clarity, and improved memory. It also improves hearing.

This is the value of sound or music therapy. Much insight can be gained from the expression, 'music soothes the savage beast'. In India, classical musicians know that certain scales, melodies, etc., produce certain moods and evoke various feelings. A whole science exists that prescribes certain forms of music for the various hours of the day, and for each season. Listening to the appropriate music at the right times balances the individual with time and nature.

Mantra therapy is also a part of sound. *Kuṇḍalinī* life-force is the essence of all *mantras* and all sounds. Traditionally, the *guru* enlivens the *mantra,* the life-force begins to awaken and rise up the *suṣhumṇā*, bringing peace and union to the individual. As the life-force rises it stills the mind. This is the value of *mantra* and all sound therapy. Through *sādhanā, Yoni Mudrā,* and *Brahmarī Kumbhaka, nāda* are developed.

Anahāta (unstruck sound) is the inner sound of 'chin-chin' heard in the distance, along with various other sounds. They are frictionless, so they are called unstruck. The *Vedic* scripture, *Haṅsopanishad,* says there are 10 different forms of *Aanahāta Nāda.* These are the unstruck sounds of the eternal, Divine. Through tracing them back to their source (the eternal), one begins to see the unification of all aspects of life, self, and environment as one integrated whole or eternal reality. That is, all sounds are subtler or grosser vibrations of eternity. The *Vedic* text, *Yogaśhikhopanishad,* says there is nothing (i.e., no *mantra* or incantation) that is superior to *nāda*, through which some obtain full Self-Realization.

In the book *Yoga Vani*, four stages of *nāda* are discussed:

1. *Parā*: *Nāda* evolves out of the *kuṇḍalinī* life-force at the *mūlādhāra* (first *chakra*), like a seed or a dot.
2. *Paśhyanti*: Only the most highly advanced spiritual adepts (*yogis*) can hear *nāda* at this stage. When one neither hears sounds nor feels with their ears, but hears sounds intuitively.
3. *Madhyama*: When *nāda* rises to the heart, it sounds like the rumbling of thunder. It is felt by the ears, but not heard; this is called *madhyama.*
4. *Baikhari*: When sound rises to the throat it produces voice or sound. *Nāda* heard by the ears is called *baikhari*.

All language comes from *nāda*. Thus, all sounds and language are grosser expressions of the life-force. *Nāda*, in turn is a subtle expression of the eternal, Divine. When one hears the unstruck sound, they are hearing the eternal itself.

Here was discussed *nāda* as it is developed through *mantras* guided by gurus. When a guru is not available one can use *mantras* for specific therapies; these are detailed in Chapter 10.

Part 3
Mudrās & Bandhas

Mudrās are specific body and hand positions that channel the energy created by *āsanas* and *prāṇāyām* into the *chakras* and *suṣhumṇā*; they stimulate higher mental functioning. Some *mudrās* are done with the *āsanas* and *prāṇāyām*, while others are done after these first two practices. As said earlier, merely by practicing *sādhanā* (meditation) instructed by a true *guru, āsana, prāṇāyām,* and *mudrā* occur spontaneously. However, for those who are interested, the specific exercises may be practiced separately. Various *mudrās* can be seen in performances by traditional Indian dancers.

Note that practicing these exercises can create problems if not taught or performed properly. Those who awaken their *kuṇḍalinī* without a *guru* can lose their direction in life. Without the knowledge of harmonizing or using these energies, they can become confused or mentally imbalanced. If the *kuṇḍalinī* rises through the *iḍā* or *piṅgalā*, instead of the *suṣhumṇā*, or if *chakras* are opened in an isolated manner, more harm than good can arise. Thus, *yoga* (*haṭha, kuṇḍalinī,* and *tantra*) need to be taught in a holistic or integrated manner.

Some *mudrās* and *bandhas* have briefly been discussed in part 1. Here, these same positions will be discussed without *āsanas*. Twenty-five major *mudrās* (and *bandhas*) are discussed in *Gheranda Saṃhitā*, and 10 in *Haṭha Yoga Pradīpikā*. These create longevity and reverse the aging process. Nine methods are outlined below.

Preparatory Bandhas

One first needs to learn three locks that are included in the *mudrā* positions. These have been discussed as automatic occurrences in various *āsanas* in section 1 of this chapter. *Bandhas,* or locks, cause the life-force to unite and rise towards the *suṣhumṇā* or inner spiritual tube of the spine. Some *bandhas* cause the life-force to rise through the *suṣhumṇā*. *Uḍḍīyāna Bandha* is one such lock. By locking, or binding, the opposite poles of energy or *śhakti* are united.

1. Uḍḍīyāna Bandha
(Abdominal Retraction Lock)

Uḍḍīyāna means to rise up. Thus, the contractions of the abdominal organs, which pull up, create a natural upward flow of energy. This is known as a stomach lift. Here, the *Apān* (downward moving air) is united with the *Prāṇ* (outward moving air) and the *samān* (equal moving air) at the navel center. It requires practice to accomplish this event, along with performing other *āsanas, prāṇāyām, mudrās, bandhas,* and *sādhanā.*

Uḍḍīyāna bandha involves the sucking in of the abdomen and stomach, and pulling it up (i.e., the belly is pulled towards the spine and upward). It may be done sitting, standing, or lying flat on the back.

It may be practiced with *āsanas, prāṇāyāma,* or afterwards. Practicing is easier after an inverted *āsana* (e.g., after a shoulder stand). Always practice the chin lock with this posture.

Precaution: Practice on an empty stomach.
Stool and urine should be evacuated first.
First learn the posture in the standing position.
Do not practice with stomach or intestinal ulcers, hernia, high blood pressure, heart disease, glaucoma, or raised intra-cranial pressure.

This position should be taught by a qualified teacher. This is an advanced practice; beginners may harm their bodies or minds. Simultaneously practicing the *vajrolī mudrā* (contraction of reproductive organs and lower urinary system) is even better.

Of all the bandhas, Uḍḍīyāna is the best
Haṭha Yoga Pradīpikā Ch 3; v 60

Method: *Uḍḍīyāna Bandha*
A) Stand with the feet separated, about two feet apart.
B) Bend the knees slightly, resting the palms on the knees. The thumbs face each other; fingers face outward.
C) Spine is straight, head is upright, eyes look forward.
D) Inhale deeply through the nose, then quickly exhale through slightly pursed lips (but do not force) until all air is expelled..

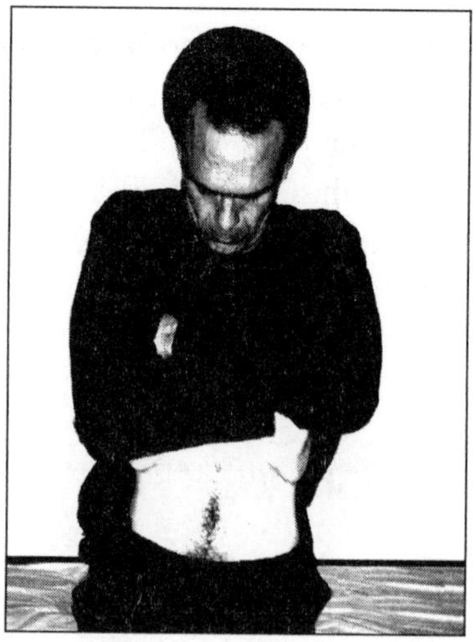

E) Engage the chin lock (to the chest) and raise shoulders.
F) Pull in the abdomen and stomach towards the spine, and then pull upward.
G) Hold for a few seconds (without discomfort). Concentrate on the throat or navel center. Inhale, relaxing the stomach and abdomen.
H) Release the chin lock, rest, and wait for breath to return to normal (1 to 2 minutes). This is 1 round.
I) Repeat another 2 rounds.

Alternate (Sitting) The instructions are the same, except one may sit in *Bhadrāsana, Padmāsana,* or *Siddhāsana/Siddhi Yoni Āsana.* (If seated in *siddhāsana/siddhi yoni āsana*, sit on a cushion to raise the buttocks.)

Benefits: This slows and reverses the aging process; it also develops vitality, tones heart region, muscles, nerves, and glands. It increases blood circulation and absorption of nutrients. The heart is gently massaged. Strength is developed in the autonomic nerves in the solar plexus, alimentary canal, diaphragm, and respiratory system. It removes gas and carbon dioxide; and increases oxygen absorption in the brain; raises the life-force into the *suṣhumṇā.*

Organs Helped: All

Doṣhas: All

2. Jālandhara Bandha (Throat Lock)

'*Jal*' means throat, '*jalam*' means water, and '*Dhārā*' means supporting tube. Thus *Jālandhara Bandha* is that which helps prevent the *bindū* (nectar) fluid from flowing down the throat and being consumed by the navel/sun. It is a very easy *bandha* to practice, but also very important. (Also discussed in part 1 on page 260).

This pose can be done sitting or standing, and can be used with *Uḍḍīyāna Bandha*. It is also done with *prāṇāyāma* and other *kriyās* involving breath retention.

Precaution: Do not practice with high blood pressure or heart disease. Do not practice without learning from a qualified teacher; the nerves in the path flowing to the brain may be impaired if performed improperly.

Method:
A) Sitting in *Siddhāsana/Siddha Yoni Āsana, Padmāsan, Śhukhāsan,* or *Vajrāsan*, place the palms on the knees and relax the whole body.
B) Inhale slowly and deeply through the nose and hold the breath.
C) Lower the chin as close to the collar bone as is comfortable; straighten the elbows and raise the shoulders. Hold the breath for as long as comfortable.
D) Slowly raise the chin and relax the shoulders.
E) Slowly exhale and rest until the breathing returns to normal (1 to 2 minutes). This is round 1.
F) Repeat for another 5 rounds.
G) Then do 5 rounds while holding the breath outside the body (i.e., holding the breath after exhaling all the air from the body).

Physical/Mental Benefits: Alleviates throat disorders (i.e., inflammation, stuttering, excess mucus in the throat, tonsillitis, etc.). It improves voice quality and the life-force in the thoracic region. Higher brain functioning is stimulated. The metabolism is balanced from the flow of pituitary hormonal secretions to the endocrine glands. This improves one's response to stress and develops instinctual abilities. Youthful vigor is maintained and restored. The throat mediates between the brain and digestive/assimilation processes. This gland secretes the hormone thyroxine (T4) that is responsible for the tissue metabolism rate, or tissue aging. The parathyroid glands properly regulate calcium metabolism and body density. Diseases of old age are reduced due to the enzymatic and oxidation of the cells. Mental clarity is improved.

Spiritual Benefits: *Kuṇḍalinī* ceases to flow in the *iḍā* and *piṅgalā*, and between the head and body. Thus the life-force is directed to flow through the *suṣhumṇā*.

Organs Helped: Pituitary, thyroid, parathyroid, brain, endocrine glands.

Doṣhas: All

3. Mūla Bandha
(Perineum/Cervix Retraction Lock)

When the muscles of the perineum are contracted, the whole pelvic region is pulled up. Contraction does not include the anus (*Aśhwinī Mudrā*). During initial practice, a tendency exists to contract this anal region as well, but it is not to be practiced here. *Mūla Bandha* occurs in the center of the body—not the front or back. In this way, the first *chakra* is directly stimulated, producing heat in the subtle body and awakening potential *kuṇḍalinī* (also see part 1).

This *bandha* is first to be perfected by itself, but then it may be used with *prāṇāyām*, breath retention (*kumbhaka*) chin lock (*Jālandhara*), and abdominal (*Uḍḍīyāna*) *bandhas.* [See page 260, 291-293]

Method: *Step 1—Preparatory*
A) Sit in any comfortable pose (preferably *Siddhāsan/Siddha Yoni Āsana* because it automatically contracts the *mūlādhāra* (1st) *chakra*.
B) Keep palms on the knees in *jñyān* or *chin*

mudrā; and eyes closed.
C) Keep the spine erect and the body relaxed.
D) Males need to contract just inside the perineum; so they need to concentrate on this area for a few minutes. Females should concentrate on the cervix because the cervix and vaginal muscles need to be contracted.
E) After concentration, gradually begin to contract and release the muscles of the perineum/cervix. (Contract for a few seconds and breathe normally.) Contract up to 20 times.

Method: *Step 2*
F) Follow step 1.
G) Contract the perineal/cervix muscles and hold for as long as possible, breathing naturally. Practice up to 20 times.

Method: *Step 3*
H) Contract gently and partially, and hold the contraction.
I) Contract a little more and hold. Continue, gradually increasing the tension 10 times until full contraction is achieved.
J) Hold the full contraction for as long as possible, attempting normal breathing.

Alternative: Mūla and *jālandhara bandha*; and internal and external breath retention.

A) Sit straight; inhale deeply through the nose.
B) Practice the above step 3.
C) Before exhaling, release *mūla,* then *jālandhara bandhas*. When the head is straight, exhale.
D) Practice 5 rounds of internal breath retention with step 2; then 5 rounds of external breath retention with step 3.
E) Practice 5 rounds with *Uḍḍīyāna Bandha*, using step 2; then 5 rounds of step 3.

It takes many months to become comfortable with *Mūla Bandha*, and many years to perfect it. Do not be discouraged if you cannot perfect it immediately. Like all processes of *yoga* and Self-Realization, it is a life process.

Physical Benefits: Pituitary hormone balance (testosterone and estrogen/progesterone) regulates the system and slows and reduces the aging process. Improved nutrient absorption, digestion, nervous system, blood circulation, mental functions (e.g., memory, concentration, alertness, less sleep, etc.).
Spiritual Benefits: *Prāṇ/Apān* and *bindū/nāda* are united. *Prāṇ* and *Apān* were discussed earlier. *Bindū* is the semen/ovum that has two parts: at the first and last *chakra*, these are united. Unification awakens the first *chakra*, and begins the spiritual awakening of the student. This transformation of *bindū* becomes *nāda,* or eternal, blissful seed-sound, that emanates within the brain.

By contracting the perineum, performing Uḍḍīyāna and locking iḍā and piṅgalā through Jālandhara, the suṣhumṇā becomes active. Through this...old age and sickness are reversed.
Haṭha Yoga Pradīpikā Ch 3 v74-75

4. Mahā Mudrā (Great Position)

This is to be performed after *āsanas* and *prāṇāyāma*, and before *sādhanā* (meditation). This *mudrā* is similar to the *Kriyā Yoga* practice.

Method: *[photo & alternate method—page 264]*
A) Press the left heel against the anus. The right leg is extended forward, and the back is straight.
B) The hands extend outward and reach the knee, calf, or big toe (keeping the back straight). Keep the eyes closed and relax.
C) Curl the tongue back towards the throat; slowly inhale, tilting the head slightly backwards (*Khecharī Mudrā*). Focus the eyes at the third eye (middle of the eyebrows—*Śhāṃbhavī Mudrā*).
D) Hold the breath for as long as is comfortable and contract the perineum or cervix (*mūla bandha*).
E) With breath held, rotate the awareness from

the third eye—to the throat—to the base of the spine. Mentally repeat the corresponding words, *ajñyā* (third eye), *viśhuddha* (throat), *mūlādhāra* (spine base) [or; *Śhāṃbhavī, Khecharī, Mūla*]. Repeat for as long as possible, comfortably holding the breath. Do not strain breathing!
F) Close eyes, release the perineum/cervix lock, bring the head upright, and exhale slowly.

Practice three times with the left leg folded, then 3 times with the right leg folded. Then keep both legs stretched in front and perform this method 3 more times.

Precaution: To prevent harm hold the breath only so long as it is comfortable. This *mudrā* should be taught and observed by a competent teacher.

Method 2: This method may be practiced in *Siddhāsan* or *Siddha Yoni Āsana* if it is more comfortable. Keep hands on the knees in *jñyān* or *chin mudrā* (finger position methods discussed on page 261). Sit upright.

Benefits: This method purifies all the bodily channels, balances the *iḍā* and *piṅgalā*, purifies *rasa dhātu* and *rasavaha srota* (plasma tissue and channels)—the basis of the entire body. It stimulates the flow of the *sushumṇā*, increases vitality, digestion, absorption of nutrients, abdominal disorders, constipation, skin diseases, and harmonizes all bodily functions. *Mahā Mudrā* improves clarity of thinking, removes depression, and stills the mind, preparing it for *sādhanā*. It creates a dynamic *prāṇic* and psychic vitality.

Doshas: All

5. Mahā Bandha (Great Lock)

This *bandha* is done between bellow-breath *prāṇāyāmas*. Each posture helps the breath retention of the other (see photo on page 264).

Method: Inner breath retention *(Antar Kumbhaka)*
A) Press the left heel against the anus; place the right foot on the left thigh.
B) Inhale through the left nostril and hold the breath. Perform the chin lock (*jālandhara bandha*). Squeeze the perineum or cervix (*mūla bandha*), and eyes gazing at third eye (*śhāṃbhavī mudrā*). Eyes may remain closed.
C) Hold the breath for so long as it is comfortable. Then, release the *bandhas* and *mudrā*, slowly exhaling through the right nostril.
D) Repeat B and C; only inhale through the right nostril and exhale through the left nostril.
E) Rest for 1 or 2 minute,s concentrating on the natural inhalation and exhalation of the breath. This completes 1 round.
F) Repeat for 2 more rounds.

Precautions: Do not practice if suffering from high or low blood pressure, hernia, stomach, or intestinal ulcer or heart ailments. Good health is necessary for this pose.

Alternative External breath retention
A) Sit in *siddhāsana* or *siddha yoni āsana*, with hands on the knees (in *chin* or *jñyān mudrā*). The spine is erect, the head is straight, the eyes are closed. Relax.
B) Slowly inhale through both nostrils. Then exhale forcefully and completely through pursed lips (drawing in the gut helps the expulsion of air). Retain the breath outside.
C) Do the *bandhas* and *mūla* as in the above method, keeping the breath outside for so long as it is comfortable.
D) Rotate the awareness from the spine base (*mūlādhāra*) to the navel (*manipūra*) to the throat (*viśhuddha*); mentally repeat the names of these *chakras* while concentrating on each of them.
E) When holding the breath is no longer comfortable, release the *bandhas* and *mūla* and slowly exhale.

F) Keep eyes closed and relax for 1 to 2 minutes. This is 1 round.
G) Repeat for 2 more rounds.

Precautions: Do not practice with high or low blood pressure, hernia, stomach or intestinal ulcer, or heart ailments. Good health is necessary for this pose.

Physical/Mental Benefits: Hormonal secretion is produced and regulated, halting the degeneration of the aging process.

Spiritual Benefits: One develops the spontaneous and natural ability of stopping the breath. It unites the *nāḍīs* in the *Āgñā chakra*, enabling higher meditation abilities. One experiences the silent witness. The individual merges with the universal.

Organs Helped: Pineal gland, endocrine system.

6. Mahā Bedha Mudrā
(Great Piercing Position)

The previous two exercises, *Mahā Mudrā* and *Mahā Bandha* begin to awaken the *kuṇḍalinī śhakti* (life-energy). This present *mudrā* releases and directs the *śhakti*. But doing the first two exercises without *Mahā Bedha Mudrā* is like purchasing a car without gasoline: you are prepared to travel but have no means to move. This position directs the *kuṇḍalinī* into the *sushumṇā* (inner central tube of the spine)—up to the *āgñā chakra*—by gently bouncing the buttocks on the floor.

This is not the same as the *Kriyā Yoga* practice, *Mahā Bedha Mudrā*, but it is similar. The *Kriyā* practice known as *Tadan Kriyā* is the same as this presently described position.

Method: *(Only for those who can sit in full lotus)*
A) Sit in full lotus, relax the body, keep the eyes closed. Place palms on the floor beside the thighs.
B) Slowly and deeply inhale through the nose. Hold the breath and do the chin lock (to the chest).
C) Raise the body off the floor by transferring the weight to the hands and gently bounce the buttocks against the floor from 3 to 7 times. Maintain awareness at the base of the spine (*mūlādhāra chakra*). [Buttocks and thighs should be touching the floor during the gentle bouncing, and the spine should be kept erect.]
D) Exhale slowly and deeply; then rest. Concentrate on the base of the spine, and wait for the breathing to return to normal (1 to 2 minutes). This is round 1.
E) Repeat for another 2 rounds.

[In the *Tadan Kriyā*, the breath is slowly inhaled through the mouth. The eyes are focused at the third eye (the chin lock is not done). Also, one bounces the buttocks gently on the floor. Then, one visualizes inhaling through a long thin pipe and exhales, visualizing the breath diffusing in all directions from the base of the spine. This is a more complex practice.]

Benefits: Restores youthfulness (slows the aging process), removes wrinkles, gray hair, and trembling of old age. Hormonal secretions are produced and balanced.

Organs Helped: Pineal and pituitary glands.

Doṣhas: All

Alternately: Sit in Mahā Bandha with breath retained; slowly and gently strike the lower armpits.

7. Yoni Mudrā

(See photo on page 288) [Different than yoni mudrā described on page 260]

Close the ears, eyes, nose, and mouth. A clear, distinct sound is heard in the purified suṣhumṇā
Haṭha Yoga Pradīpikā Ch. 4 v 68

This technique is discussed under the topic of mental peace, or *samādhi,* in *Haṭha Yoga Pradīpikā*. In *Gherand Saṃhitā* it is mentioned in the *mudrā* section.

We spoke earlier of the development from *mantra yoga* to spontaneous *haṭha* (and *prāṇāyām*), *laya,* and then to *raja*. After *raja yoga*, one attains Self-Realization or complete mental peace. This pose is related more to *laya yoga* than *haṭha yoga*, and directly awakens *raja yoga*. The awakening occurs through developing an awareness of inner sound (*nāda*).

Just as with all spiritual experiences that are out of the norm of supposed societal acceptance, the hearing of inner sounds or voices (*nāda*) has generally been associated with mental illness. Spiritual counseling reassures a person that their experiences and feelings are spiritual—not abnormal. Understanding *nāda* helps persons feel comfortable when hearing any inner sounds. As previously mentioned, all spiritual experiences are merely signs that progress is being made. One doesn't want to attempt to develop any particular experiences because, no matter how divine or blissful, they remain in the temporal field of relativity. One who goes beyond the limits of experience attains the limitless, eternal state of Self-Realization.

Method:
A) Sit in *Siddhāsana* or *Siddha Yoni Āsana*. Inhale slowly and deeply, and hold the breath.
B) Plug the ears with the thumbs.
C) Cover the eyes with the index fingers.
D) Close the nostrils with the middle fingers.
E) Cover the upper lip with the ring fingers.
F) Cover the lower lip with the pinkies.
G) Concentrate on any perceivable subtle sounds. If a sound is heard, listen to it. If many sounds exist, listen to those in the right ear. The first sound heard is to be followed. Then, the next sound heard is also to be followed.
H) When holding the breath is no longer comfortable, release this *mudrā*; then slowly exhale. This is 1 round. Practice 5 to 10 rounds.

Precautions: Be gentle with the fingers. Do not penetrate the ear too deeply or press too hard on the eyes.

Benefits: The mind is instantly silenced, mental bliss occurs, and spiritual 'unstruck' sound is heard. The Self-luminous soul is perceived; thus one becomes stainless from this sight.

Doṣhas: All

8. Nabho Mudrā
Method: Extend the head forward slightly, mouth open, and inhale into the esophagus.

Benefits: Reverses the aging process and destroys all diseases.

9. Bhujangini Mudrā
Method: The tongue is curled up inside the mouth and the breath is held. Do this all the time (whenever you think of it [*Gherand Saṃhitā*]).

Benefits: Removes stomach diseases and improves digestion.

10. Kaki Mudrā/Śhītalī
Method: Lips are pursed like a crow's beak; air is drawn in.

Benefits: Long life, purifies all Pitta concerns (e.g., fever, blood, spleen), tumors.

Final Note
Haṭha Yoga Āsanas, Bandhas and Mudrās

Rounds: All positions that require 3 rounds may slowly—over time, be increased to 10 rounds.

Part 4
Yoga for Pregnancy

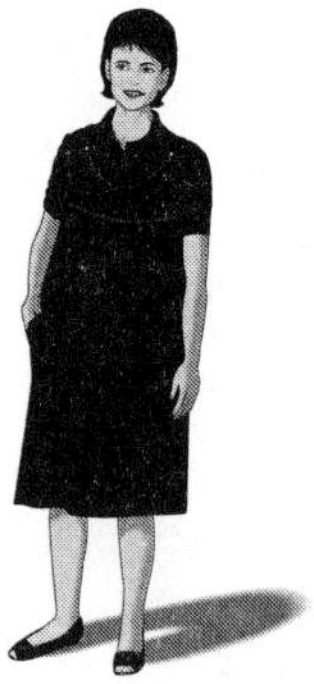

Practicing *āsanas* while pregnant can be a safe and very effective method to stay fit, and can ease pregnancy. Back, shoulder, and neck pain occur from carrying extra weight; abdominal muscles become stretched and unused, and leg muscles stiffen and swell. *Āsanas* help tone the body and keep it in shape and make the carrying time, labor, and recovery easier.

Although many *āsanas* are not recommended for the pregnant woman, various simple positions can help counteract the adverse physical effects of carrying a baby. Gentle *yoga* is often as important as strenuous *yoga*. The cervix should remain tight, and those with histories of miscarriages or cervical insufficiencies should take extra care when practicing *āsanas*. For nausea, fatigue, or dizziness, Āyurvedic herbs are available to balance these conditions (see Section 3, Chapter 23). Practice can last from 10 to 20 minutes daily, with rest after each posture.

This section is laid out in two parts, *āsanas* that can be done throughout the pregnancy; and *āsanas* that can be done after delivery. The poses are arranged in an easily followed order.

Precautions: Do not perform any postures that require lying on the stomach, that overly stretch the abdominal muscles, or that only twist from the rib cage up. Always bend from the hips (not the back). Keep the pelvis upright and the spine straight.

After the fourth month, practice only sitting and lying-on-the-side postures. As with all practices, always listen to your body. Do not hold any postures that cannot be practiced comfortably.

[See Chapter 23 for conception, delivery, postpartum herbs; *abhyañga*, and *mantras* for more details on Āyurvedic childbirth.]

1. **Correct Posture**

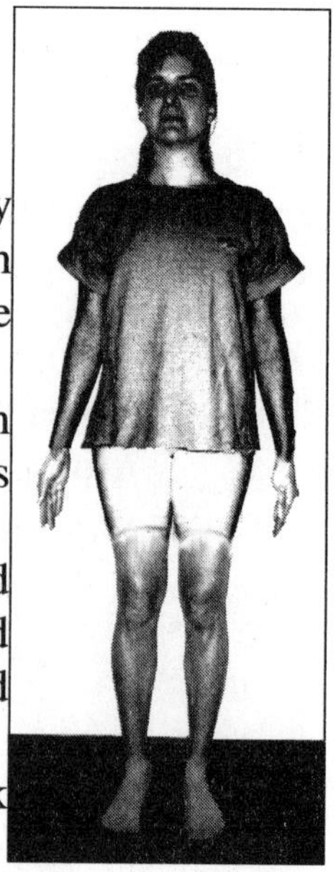

Method:
A) Stand erect, feet slightly apart—parallel with each other and directly under the shoulders.
B) Tighten the front thigh muscles to straighten the legs fully.
C) Set the shoulders back and the chest out (shoulders should relax and hang). Arms and hands are relaxed.
D) Extend the neck and look straight ahead.
E) Lower the tailbone to the floor and push the hip bones forward and up.

Benefits: Relieves lower back strain, aligns the vertebrae, improves breathing.

2. Thigh & Groin Stretch

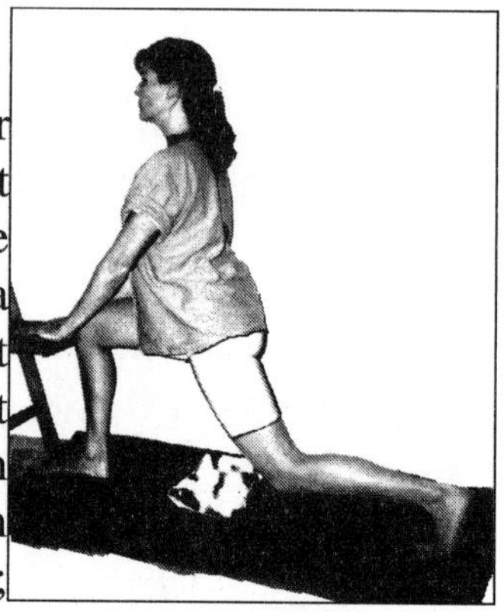

Method:
A) Place the chair (with its back) against the wall. Face the chair and kneel on a pillow. Lift the right knee, placing the right foot on the floor with the shin and thigh forming a right angle; toes under the chair. The back is straight.
B) Touch the right knee to the front of the chair. Place fingers on the top front of the chair.
C) Press the hands down and lift the chest to lengthen the spine; simultaneously push the tailbone down and lift the front hip bones up. The left knee is slightly back. Feel a gentle stretch in the center of the thigh muscles.
D) Repeat with the legs in the reverse position. Then rest by sitting comfortably on the floor in

Siddha Yoni Āsana (just cross the legs; do not lift the right leg up).

Benefits: Pelvic tilting stretches the spine, and the groin and thigh muscles.

3. Chest & Shoulder Stretch

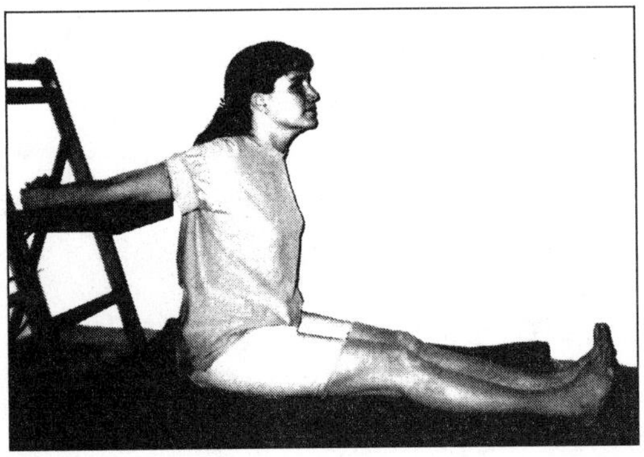

Method:
A) With the chair in the same position, sit on a mat or folded towel. One's back faces the front of the chair. Legs are extended straight forward and slightly apart.
B) Place the arms behind the back, resting them on the seat; interlace the fingers. (If this is difficult, put more blankets or pillows under the buttocks to raise the body higher, and/or hold the sides of the seat).
C) Tighten the thighs; slowly inhale and press the back of the legs and buttocks to the floor.
D) Slowly exhale, lifting the chest and rolling the shoulders back; breathe normally.
E) Remove arms from the seat, release hands, and sit comfortably.

Benefits: This pose stretches the chest and shoulder muscles, and relieves a rounded back and shoulders.

4. Wall Squatting Pose

Method:
A) Stand with the back against the wall. Separate the feet, bend the knees, and squat (while resting the back against the wall). *Alternate*—lean on a sturdy chair to achieve the squat.

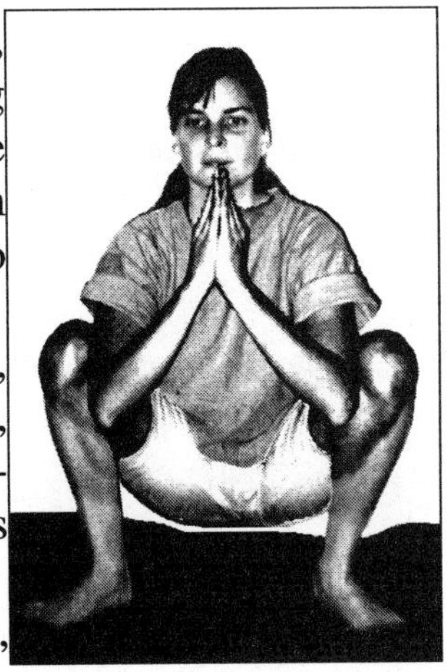

B) Spread the knees, turn the toes outward, and place the elbows inside the knees; press palms together.
C) Slowly inhale, spreading the knees apart with the elbows.
D) Exhale, pressing the back against the wall to stretch the spine, and moving the tailbone down. Relax the lower back muscles. Hold this position for 1 to 3 minutes.
E) Relax and sit on the floor. Lean the back against the wall and keep the feet straight out.

Benefits: Removes lower back pain; stretches the lower back, calf, and inner thigh muscles.

5. Bound Angle Pose

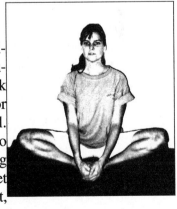

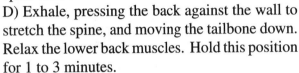

Method:
A) Sit on a small pillow or folded blanket. Keep the back against the wall or away from the wall. Bend the knees to the side and bring the soles of the feet together in front, holding the ankles.
B) Bring heels as close to the body as possible, then place palms on the floor.
C) Slowly inhale, gently lifting the spine.
E) Exhale and relax.
F) Place the palms on the inner thighs. Slowly inhale, then slowly exhale and gently press thighs to the floor.

G) If comfortable, gently lean forward from the hips and extend hands forward to the floor to straighten the spine and stretch the shoulders.
H) Relax, sit up, and extend both legs forward.

Benefits: This pose creates flexible hips and stretches the inner thigh muscles.

6. Wall—Single Leg Stretch

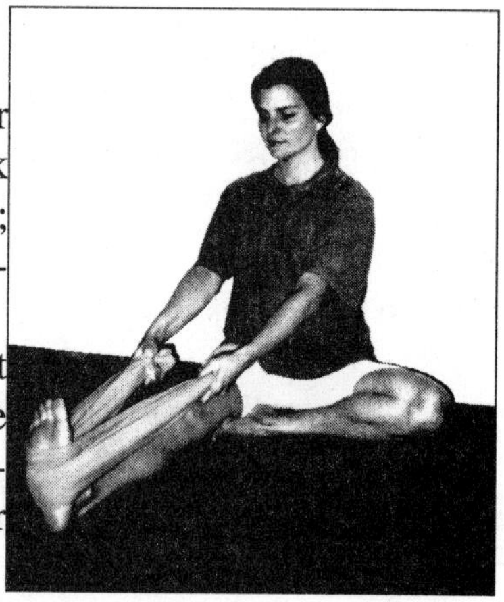

Method:
A) Sit on a rug or mat, with the back against the wall; extend the feet forward.
B) Bend the right knee, placing the sole against the inner left thigh or knee.
C) With palms on the ground, push the tailbone so that it touches the wall, then straighten the left leg. Place a towel or belt around the ball of the left foot, and hold the strap ends with both hands.
D) Slowly inhale, lift the chest, and press the entire back against the wall.
E) Slowly exhale, gently pulling the strap to tighten the front thigh muscle and flex the foot. The spine should remain against the wall while the back of the left leg is being stretched.
F) Repeat with the other leg
.
Benefits: Stretches the hamstring and calf muscles.

7. Wide Leg Spine Twist

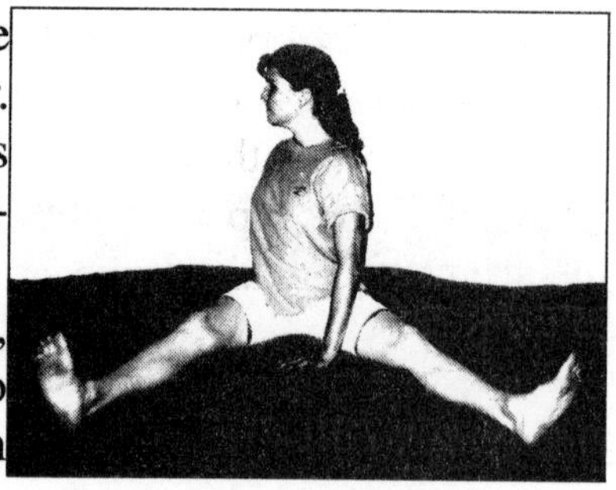

Method:
A) Sit on a rug or mat with legs spread and heels extended. Tighten the front thigh muscles; press the backs of the knees to the floor. Place the palms on the floor beside the hips.
B) Slowly inhale, pressing down to lift and lengthen the spine.
C) Gently twist or rotate to the right, placing the left hand in line with the navel and the right hand behind the right hip.
D) Slowly exhale. Gently lift the chest and twist to the right.
E) Bring both hands beside the hips, turn to face forward again and rest.
F) Bring the right hand in line with the navel. (The hand is on the floor.)
G) Exhale and gently twist to the left.
H) Repeat step F, gently bring legs together and rest.

Benefits: This pose stretches the spine and inner thigh muscles.

8. Hero's Pose

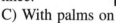

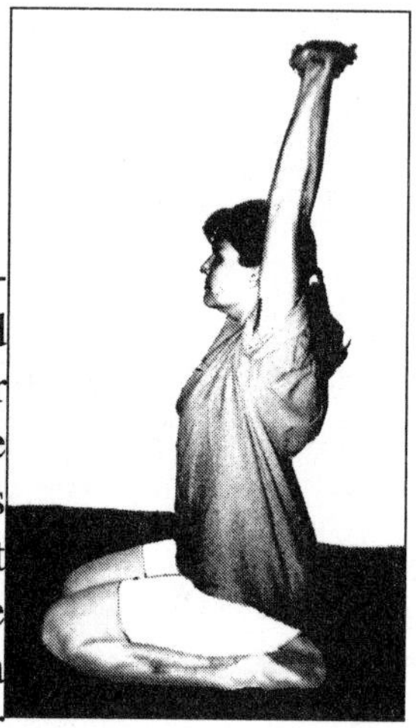

Method:
A) Kneel on a mat or blanket. Separate the feet and place hands on the floor for support. Gently lower the buttocks between the heels and sit on a folded blanket or small pillow. (Adjust the height for comfort; place a blanket on the ankles for comfort). The stretch should be in the thighs—not the knees.
B) Squeeze the knees together, pressing on the floor with the fingertips; and stretch the spine upward.
C) Place the palms on the knees, lifting and expanding the chest with each inhalation.

D) Interlace fingers and lift the chest. Slowly inhale, then slowly exhale—stretching the arms over the head, with palms facing the ceiling. Extend the arms up from the shoulder blades. Keep the spine straight and lift from the lower back.
E) Lower arms to the sides and widen the knees. Sit on the heels, bend forward from the hips and rest the head on the floor or pillow (do not press the belly on the floor). Arms are alongside the body.
E) Release and extend the legs; sit with the legs extended and rest.

Benefits: This pose may prevent varicose veins. Stretches the front of the thighs and the insteps. Relieves leg fatigue and indigestion.

9. Corpse Pose

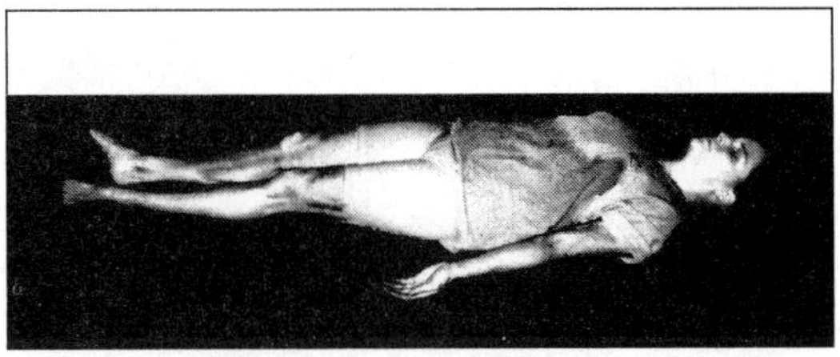

Method: Lie on back, arms at the side, palms up. Breathe normally and feel the mind and body relax.

Benefits: Body adjusts to its new tone, strength, and less stressful position.

Important: Always end all *āsana* routines with the corpse pose (*Śhavāsana*).

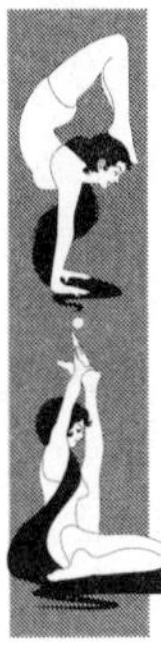

Part 5
Postpartum Āsanas

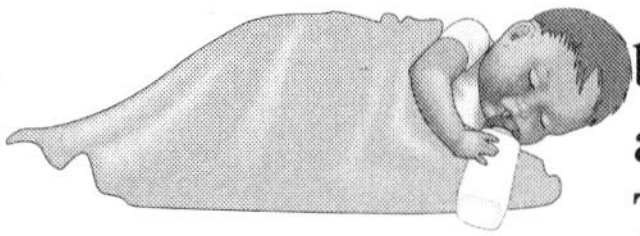

Once the baby is born, all postures are again safe to do. Those listed below are useful for strengthening abdominal muscles to help reduce stretches caused during pregnancy. Twisting poses re-shrink the uterus; relaxation poses help in recovering from fatigue. If there is no time to practice *yoga* with newborn babies around, postures may include them as part of the practice.

Immediately after birth it is prudent to avoid strenuous exercises to flatten the abdomen. With patience, the *āsanas*, along with other Āyurvedic herbs and *abhyañga* oils, help restore the belly to its original tone. Perform postures carefully and gently, as with all *yogic* practices. Do not practice *yoga* if a hernia or rupture occurs after birth (i.e., a small bulge in the abdomen).

To protect the spine, all abdominal tightening exercises should be done while lying on the back. For cesarean births, wait 6 to 8 weeks before beginning *āsanas*. Do not do shoulder stands until after postpartum discharge is completed.

1. Seated Wall-Leg Stretch - Adaptation

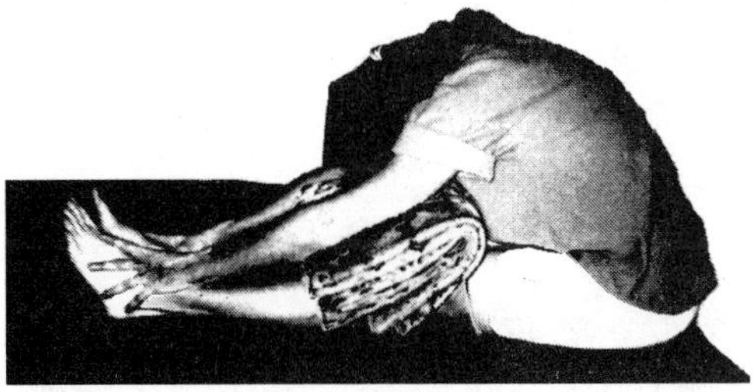

Method:
A) Sit and press the entire upper and lower back against the wall.
B) With blankets on the thighs, bend forward from the hips.
C) Slowly inhale, then slowly exhale, resting the forehead and chest on the blankets (use more

blankets to achieve a more comfortable height).

Benefits: Stretches calves and hamstrings, relieves back tension, massages the uterus and returns it to its normal size.

2. Seated Twist

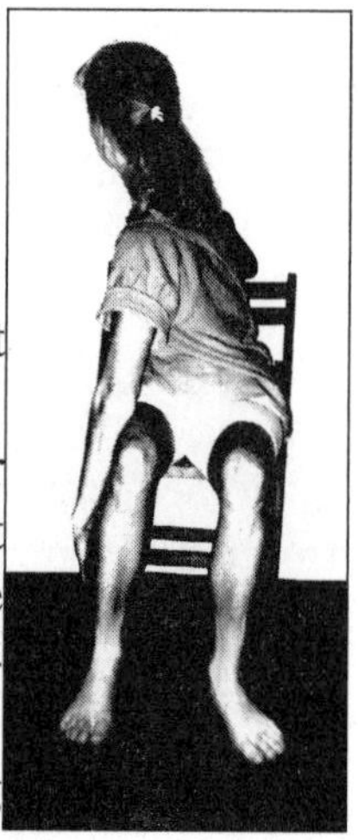

Method:
A) Sit on the front half of a seat or step, feet and knees together.
B) Place the back of the upper left elbow on the outer right thigh, and the right hand on the right side of the chair back, upper step, or wall.
C) Slowly inhale, squeezing knees together, lifting the chest.
D) Slowly exhale, pressing the left elbow into the right outer thigh and twist the torso to the right.
E) Reverse the hands and repeat in the opposite direction.

Benefits: This pose (and the forward bends) massages the uterus to return to its normal size; it also strengthens the oblique abdominal muscles.

3. Reclining Twist

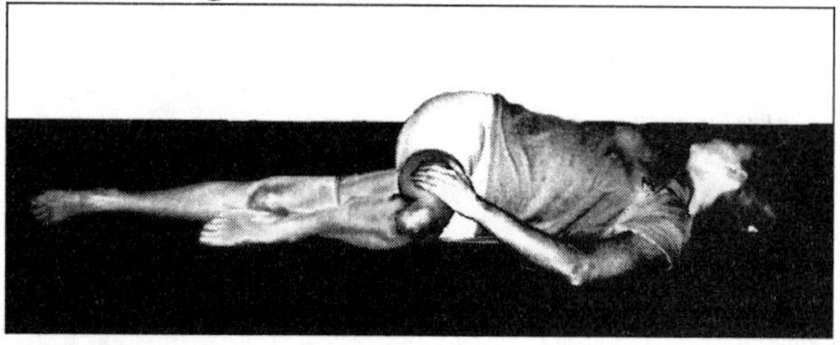

Method: A) Lie on the back on a thick rug or mat, legs extended.
B) Bend the right knee and rest the right foot on the floor (crossed over the left leg). Place the left palm on the right outer knee.
C) Slowly inhale; expand the chest.
D) Slowly exhale; twist the hips, spine, and shoulders to the left; press the knee to the floor.
E) Place the right arm on the rug and roll the right shoulder to the floor, turning the head to the right. Breathe normally.
F) Reverse the position and repeat in the opposite direction.

Benefits: This pose stretches the outer hip, back, and shoulder muscles. It counteracts soreness from nursing and carrying the baby.

4. Wall Relaxation Pose

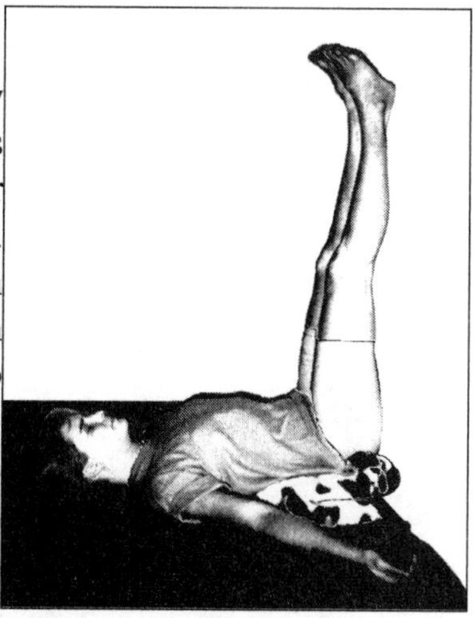

Method:
A) Place a few folded blankets on the floor against the wall. Sit sideways on the blankets with the right hip against the wall.
B) Bring the legs up against the wall as the back is lowered to a rug or mat. Slide the buttocks against or close to the wall, resting the hips and lower back on the blankets.
C) Breathe normally and feel the entire body relaxing. The baby may rest on the abdomen or can be held in the air over the chest.
D) Contract and relax the sphincter muscles around the generative organ.

Benefits: This pose relaxes the legs, relieves back fatigue, and shoulder tension caused by nursing. The contraction increases circulation, healing; restores lost sensation, tightens organ muscles, strengthens the pelvic floor muscles.

5. Wall-Boat

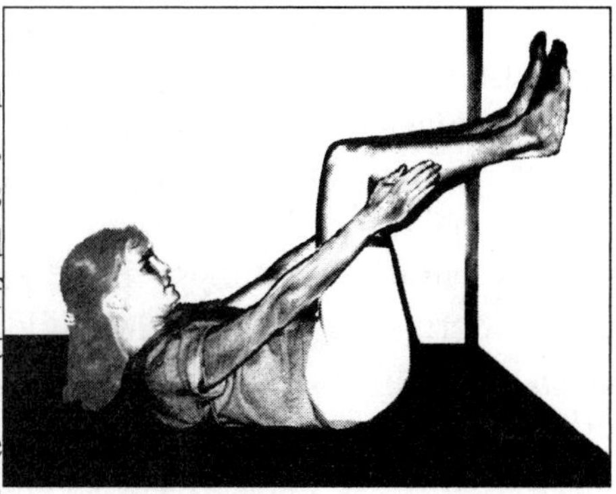

Method:
A) Lie on the back, with knees bent and the soles of the feet placed against the wall (shins parallel to the floor).
B) Slowly inhale and exhale while pressing the lower back firmly against the floor.
C) Contract and relax the sphincter muscles around the generative organ. Breathe normally.
D) Slowly exhale and slightly curl the head, shoulders, and upper back off the floor.
E) Slowly inhale and roll the spine back to the rug (or mat). Repeat the entire process from 2 to 10 times (as strength returns).

Benefits: This pose tones and strengthens the abdominal muscles; it also removes lower back pain. The contraction increases circulation and healing, restores lost sensation, tightens organ muscles, and strengthens the pelvic floor muscles.

6. Knee-To-Chest

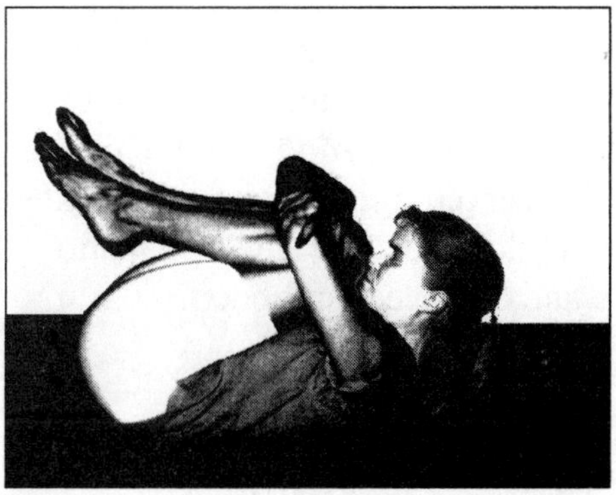

Method:
A) Lie on the mat or rug and bring the knees to the chest; wrap arms or hands around the knees.
B) Slowly inhale, expanding the chest. Slowly exhale and press the lower back to the rug, pulling the knees closer to the chest.
C) Bring the forehead towards the knees.
D) Muscles around the spine may be massaged by gently rolling from side to side. Breathe normally.
E) Contract and relax the sphincter muscles around the generative organ.

Benefits: This pose eases lower and upper back tension. The contraction increases circulation, healing, restores lost sensation, tightens organ muscles, and strengthens the pelvic floor muscles.

7. Easy Bridge Pose

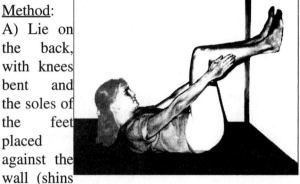

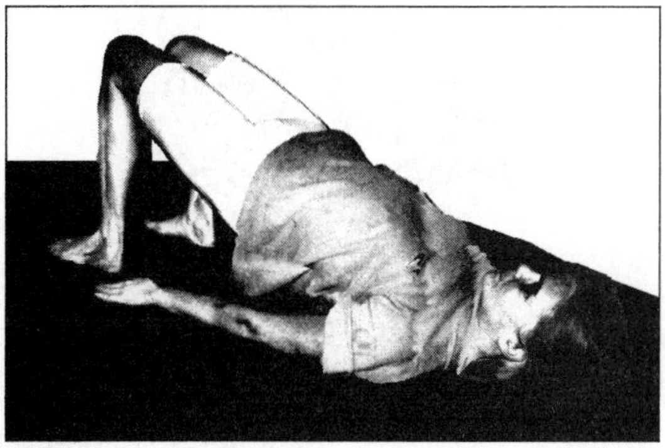

Method:
A) Lie on the back, knees bent, soles flat on the floor, arms by the side. Feet are 6 to 8 inches apart.
B) Contract and relax the sphincter muscles around the generative organ.
C) Slowly inhale and relax the back. Then slowly exhale and flatten the lower back to the floor.
D) While exhaling, lift the hips off the floor. The tailbone is curled upward (lift the pelvis higher than the abdomen) and squeeze the knees together (buttocks may also be squeezed).
E) Slowly inhale, relaxing and lowering the buttocks to the floor.
F) Repeat this pose again.

Benefits: This pose strengthens the knees, buttocks, and abdominal muscles. The contraction increases circulation, healing, restores lost sensation, tightens organ muscles, and strengthens the pelvic floor muscles.

9. Corpse Pose

Method: Lie on back, with arms at the side and palms facing up. Breathe normally and feel the mind and body relax.
Benefits: Body adjusts to its new tone, strength, and less stressful position.
Important: Always end all *āsana* routines with the corpse pose (*Śhavāsan*—see photo on page 301).

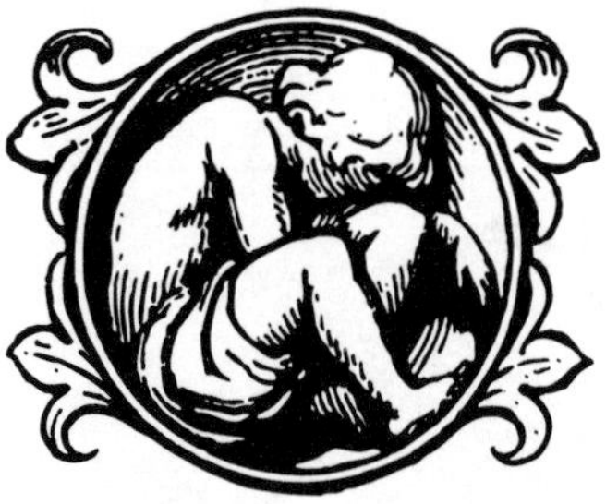

Part 6
Yoga for Children

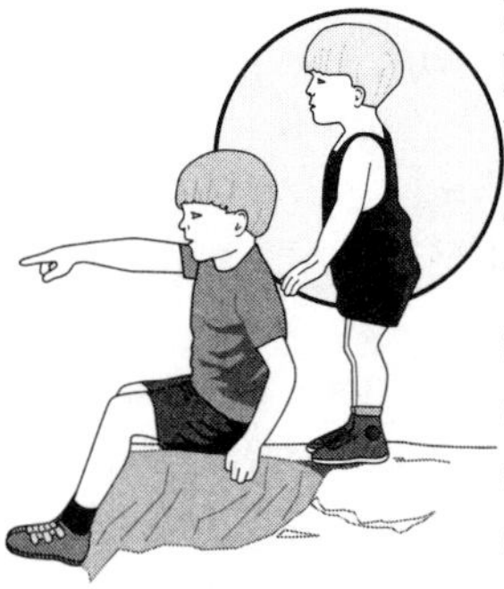

Children are naturally flexible, and generally have an innate sense of balance. Beginning *āsanas* during childhood will help maintain health and flexibility during adult and later years. The open spiritedness of children makes them naturally curious to try *āsanas*. Often they will want to follow along as parents practice their *āsanas*. With a little encouragement and education of physical, mental, and spiritual health, children will quickly take to the postures. Explain the benefits of *āsana* in terms they can understand, according to their age (teenagers can be told of the reduction of acne, improved concentration, and memory, etc.). Parents can help their youngsters attain these postures, making sure they do not strain or hurt themselves.

To make the child's *āsana* time more fun, parents can do two things. First, keep the sessions short, allowing for the child's attention span. Second, suggest that they pretend to be different animals, and give them the animal names of the *āsanas* (e.g., lion, snake, cat, etc.). They can also pretend to be objects—e.g., the bridge.

Prāṇāyām breathing exercises are also good for children to learn. As they learn to breathe during the *āsanas*, they will see how to take breaths from the lower abdominal cavity, rather than the chest.

Various forms of meditation can be introduced as well. Children can begin to understand that meditation means anything that makes the mind quiet and relaxed. Sunrises and sunsets, nature walks, and thinking of God are all helpful. If children understand the importance of setting aside a quiet time each day and making this a daily habit, they will retain this habit throughout their teenage and adult years.

Ethics and virtue are important principles that ensure sound health and longevity. If parents inculcate and exemplify these principles in daily life, children will better understand them and see these ideals in action.

Lastly, proper Āyurvedic diet, using herbs and incorporating aroma and color therapies, will round out the healing and balancing of the five senses. So *āsanas*, *prāṇāyām*, meditation, ethics, and Āyurvedic life habits are the keys to a healthy childhood, and the foundations of a healthy and balanced adulthood.

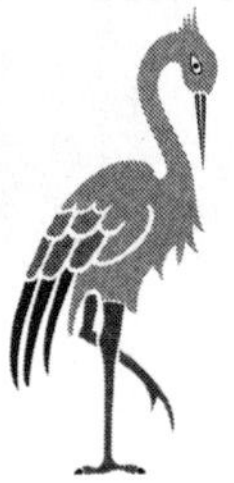

Part 7
Yoga for the Office

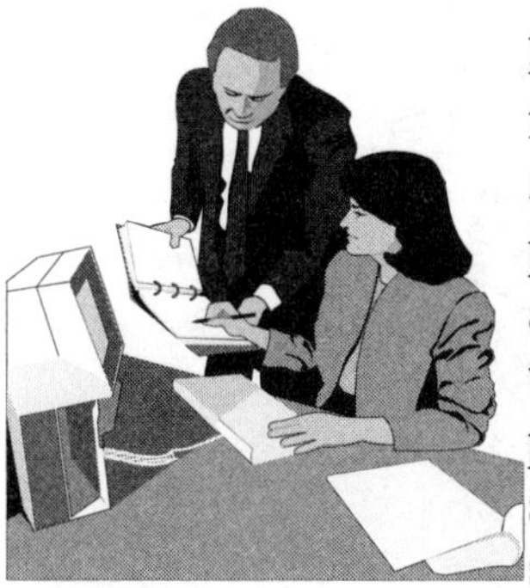

Unless a company has an exercise room, finding adequate space and acceptance for practicing *yoga āsanas* at work is unlikely. Yet, when stress becomes problematic, some stretching can be done surreptitiously.

To increase the sense of relaxation, aromatherapy can also be used. Place essential oils on the third eye or under the nose, or put a drop of oil on a light bulb to let the aroma mildly permeate the room (e.g., sandalwood for stress, frankincense for alertness). Aromas or fragrant flowers balance one's Āyurvedic mental constitution. The office can also host negative ion-producing herbs and plants (e.g., basil, corn plants, etc.). They promote clarity and freshen the air. Color therapy may also be used. Colors also balance one's emotional constitution. Paintings, rugs, flowers, wall paint, or other small items harmonize one's emotions.

Below are eight modified *āsanas* that can be practiced—without being noticed—in the office. Correct posture is always helpful. There are some general guidelines for preventing excess stress. Sit up straight in your chair. Get up and walk around from time to time to keep the blood circulating and the body loose. Open the window for fresh air. Breathe properly: slow inhalations and exhalations can help calm the mind and body, and make it more alert, and can be done without calling attention to yourself. Rubbing the neck, shoulders, back, legs, and face will also invigorate the mind and body; increase circulation, and remove muscle tension and mental stress. One can invent stretches as well. Lastly, persons can practice two *mudrās*: staring at the third eye, and a modified lion pose: 1) Staring at the third eye with the chin lock improves concentration and keeps the brain nectar from diminishing. The mind, neck, and upper back will release tension. 2) Sticking out the tongue (if it does not cause a scene), and/or making a yawning motion and facial contortions, will remove facial tension and keep wrinkles away.

Those who can remove the left shoe in the office may consider a modified *Siddhāsan/ Siddha Yoni Āsana*. Sit in your chair and place the left heel against the perineum or female generative organ. This will close the first *chakra* and keep your life-force from escaping. This will bring about increased energy, balance, and concentration.

1. Head/Neck Stretches

Method:

A) Lower the chin to the chest and rest for a few seconds, gently raise it, then gently lean it backwards. Hold for a few seconds and gently raise it upright.

B) Turn the face to the left shoulder and gently lower the chin. Hold it for a few seconds, lift the chin, turn to look at the right shoulder and lower the chin again. Hold for a few seconds, slowly lift the chin and face forward.

A-1

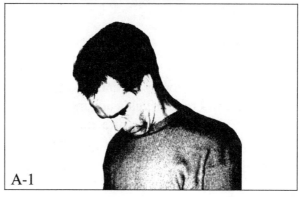

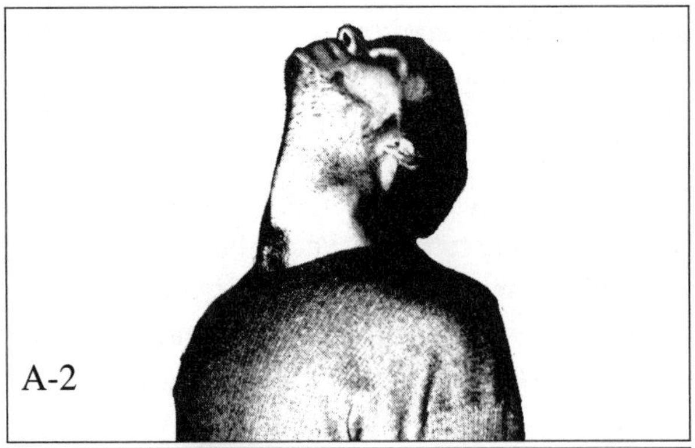

A-2

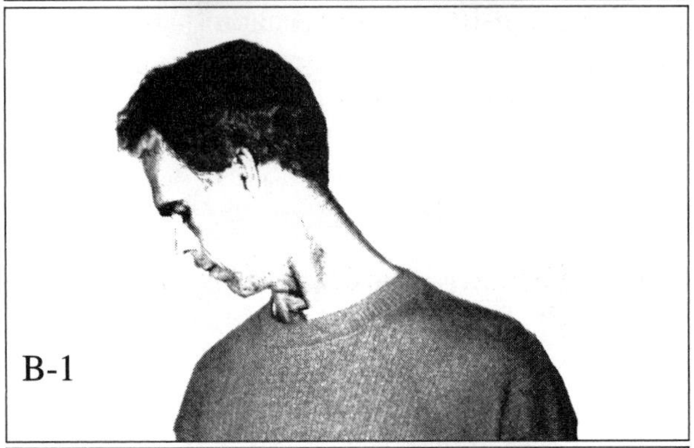

B-1

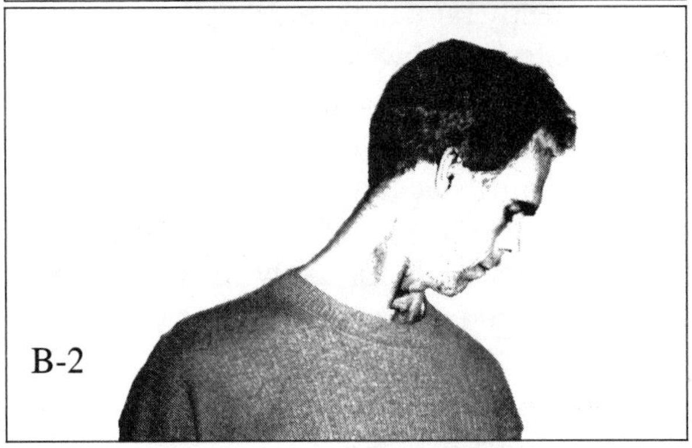

B-2

C) Face halfway between the front and left shoulder position, gently lower the chin and hold this position. Slowly raise the chin and then lean the head back in the opposite direction (midway between the back and the right shoulder). Hold and then return the head upright. Repeat in the opposite direction.
D) Repeat A.

Benefits: Removes neck and brain tension.

2. Chest Expansion (Modified Fish Pose)

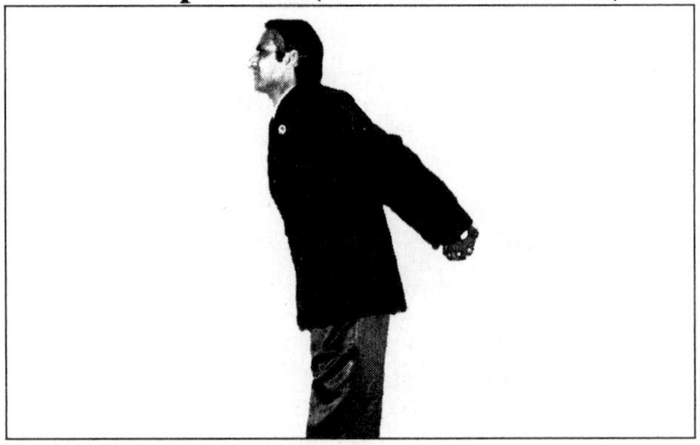

Method:
A) Sit on the edge of a desk or the arm of a couch with the arms behind the back and palms on the desk or the chair's arm.
B) Lean backwards and arch your chest outward, slowly breathing into the chest.

Benefits: This stretch increases oxygen needed for concentration and for the removal of stress from the upper torso, arms, and neck.

3. Spinal Twist

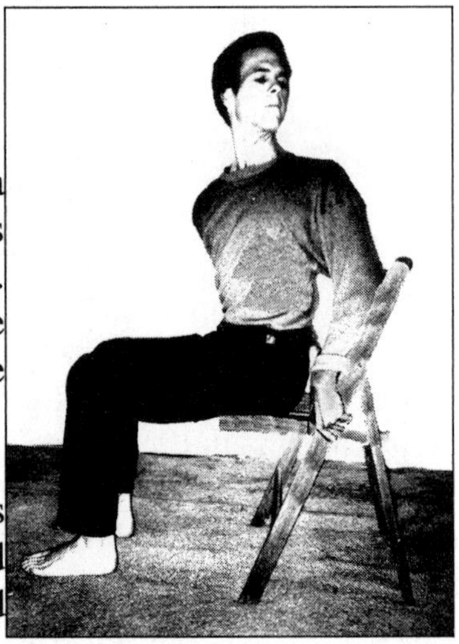

Method: Sit in a chair, with hands on the chair arms. Gently twist to one side, and then the other.

Benefits: Releases stress from bad posture, tones and loosens the spine, increases the flow of blood to the system; all this results in improved clarity and concentration.

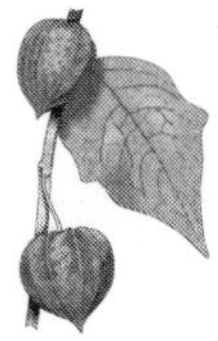

4. Lower Back Stretch

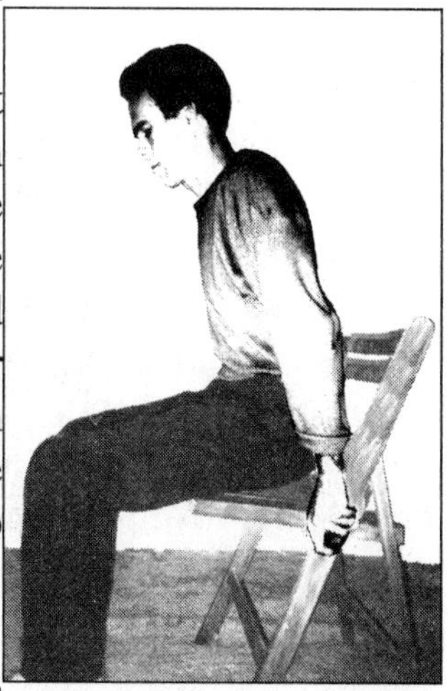

Method: Sit up straight in a chair with hands on the knees. Press the palms against the knees, arching and stretching the lower back. Concentrate on the lower back. (The chin lock can be also done.)

Benefits: This eases lower back pain and prevents the life energy from flowing out of the body. The result is more energy and flexibility, improved concentration and clarity.

5. Leg Stretches

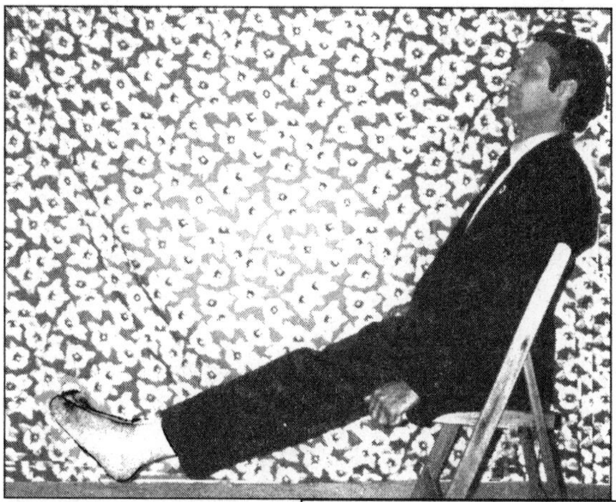

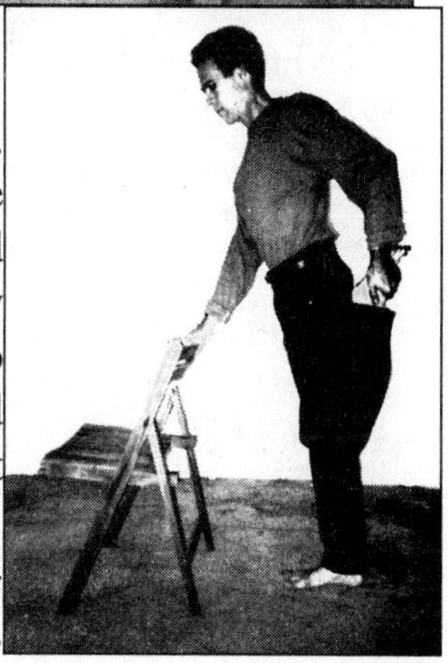

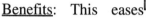

Method:
A) Stand up straight. Bend one leg until the ankle can be grabbed from behind. Gently pull the ankle close to the buttocks. Inhale and feel the stretch. Repeat with the other leg.
B) Sitting in a chair, extend one leg forward, parallel to the floor. Flex the toes up towards the ceiling and then downwards. Slowly inhale and feel the stretch in the calves. Repeat with other foot.
C) Slowly bend forward so long as you are comfortable, letting head and hands hang freely. Feel the release of stress from the face, arms, back, and shoulders. Also feel the stretch in the back of the thighs.

Benefits: Leg stretching increases flexibility and circulation in the legs, reducing stress caused by sitting and work-related tension.

6. ABC Stretch (Arm, Back, Chest)

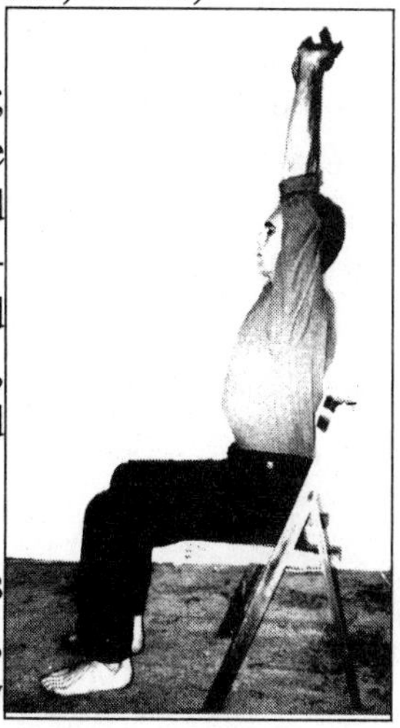

Method: Interlace fingers; slowly inhale while straightening arms and lifting them up to the ceiling (palms facing up) and expanding the chest (i.e., arching the back). Hold and breathe normally.

Benefits: Releases stress from the arms, shoulders, neck, and chest, caused by sitting, writing, poor posture, and work-related stress.

7. Isometrics

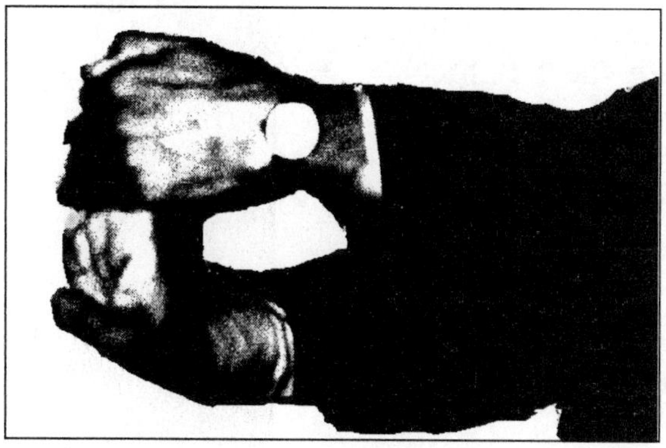

Hands: Place the left palm across the inside of the right-hand fingers (palm to palm). Inhale and gently pull the left palm towards the body, stretching the right hand fingers and wrist. Reverse the hand positions and repeat.

Benefits: This releases stress from writing, typing, and clenching of hands.

Arms: Interlace fingers and clasp hands together in front of the body. Push them together for several seconds, pull them apart (hands remain clasped). Try to lift one hand, then the other. Try to lower one hand, then the other. Stretch the arms outward and arch the back (caving in the chest) to stretch the pectorals and upper back. This can feel as though the body were yawning. (One may also keep the heel on the first *chakra* or, at least, contract the muscles in this area to prevent energy loss.)

Benefits: Releases stress, tones muscles.

Legs:

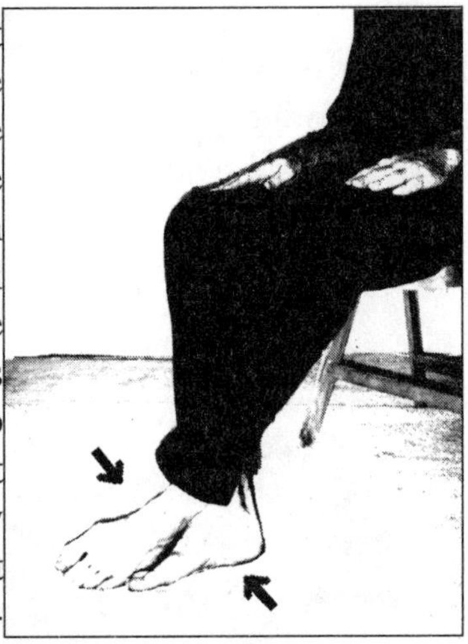

A) Cross the left ankle over the right. Try to lift the right foot up, as the left foot holds it in place. Try to pull the feet apart while keeping the ankles crossed. Try to push the left foot toward the body while the right foot stops the movement. Reverse the feet and repeat.

B) Place feet beside one another and press the feet and knees together.

Benefits: This stretch releases tension caused by sitting; improves flexibility and ease. Isometrics are also very helpful on long plane flights to relieve stiffness.

Foot massage rollers are available at many health food stores. A few seconds of rolling the feet on the wood will provide passive whole-body exercise, a release of stress, and help alleviate all digestive problems.

Part 8
Yoga for the Elderly & Handicapped

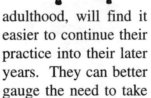

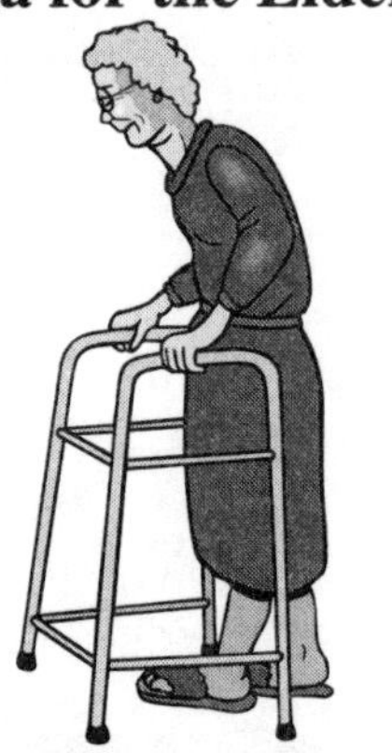

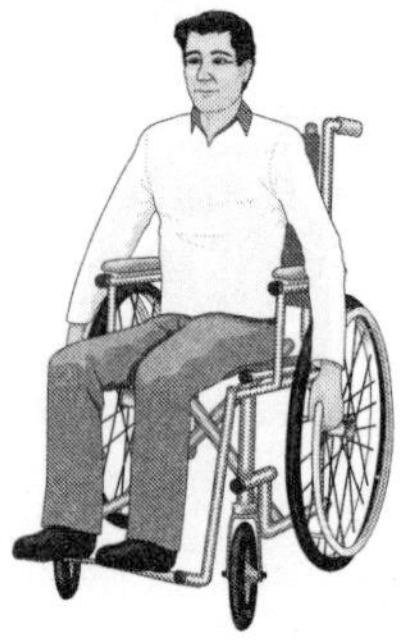

Those who have been practicing *āsanas* since childhood, teen years, or during their adulthood, will find it easier to continue their practice into their later years. They can better gauge the need to take the postures more gently. When people over 60 begin *āsanas* for the first time, they need to start slowly and gently. They need to do modified, less strenuous postures.

When people live for 60 or 70 years without using stress-reducing methods, their bodies become stiff and brittle. This is certainly not a description of the 'golden years.' Yet, with even a little *āsana* practice, symptoms of old age begin to disappear. The body has amazing healing powers, and *āsanas* quickly begin to improve flexibility and to increase the vitality of physical and mental powers. People also have an increased interest in their spiritual lives.

When first beginning the postures, the body feels very stiff. Massaging the body with oils and taking a warm bath with Epsom salt will loosen the muscles. Alternatively, one may want to practice the *āsanas* in the afternoon when the muscles are already loosened from the mornings activities.

Most of the postures discussed earlier will remove symptoms of old age. Should they seem too strenuous, *āsanas* can be modified for practice while sitting on a sturdy chair, leaning against a wall or on a sturdy table. People who have physical disabilities may work the parts of the body that are mobile, and even practice from a wheelchair. For muscles that may have become limited or even paralyzed, massage provides a passive form of exercise. The main rule for elders and physically challenged people is to be gentle; do not force any pose beyond comfort.

Prāṇāyām is also useful for improving the body and lungs, and mental and spiritual peace (including memory, concentration, and clarity). One's Āyurvedic life habits (e.g., nutrition, herbs, color, aromatherapy, etc.) will further remove the limiting experiences of old age while helping develop longevity. Particularly, oil applications (*abhyañgas*) help strengthen muscles and bones, improve circulation and heart strength, remove arthritis and other pains and diseases usually associated with old age; and regenerate the nerves and mental faculties.

Traditionally in India, age 60 was when people completed their responsibilities of raising a family and making a contribution to society. Then they were given the time to explore their inner spiritual life. By age 70, they would naturally begin to realize the illusory nature of life and wholeheartedly seek God as the only true and eternal experience worth having. So, meditation for persons over 60 will have a most profound experience. Retiring from a job may mean an end of one career, but by no means does it mean that life is over. Another phase of life, rich in spiritual development, is in the offing. Along with this is the ability for elder people to be counselors to the younger generations who need life-experience guidance.

Herbs that help slow and reverse the aging process include *aśhwagandhā, śhaṅka puṣhpī, brāhmī,* and *jaṭāmāñśhī.* These herbs increase memory, concentration, mind-body coordination, build brain and nerve cells and tissues, and prevent senility.

Ghee, sesame oil, *śhatāvarī*, and *aśhwagandhā*, build and strengthen the *ojas* (life sap), immune system; nourish and moisten bones, preventing brittleness. *Abhyañga, śhiro dhārā, śhiro basti,* and body massage with sesame oil provide passive exercise, increase circulation, and help remove arthritis and other pains and stiffness.

By beginning or continuing *āsanas*, *prāṇāyām*, Āyurvedic life habits, and *sādhanā* (meditation) during later years one will continue to heal, to avoid illness, to reduce the symptoms of old age, and to develop spirituality. Thus, Āyurveda helps make these years truly 'golden'.

Part 9
Yoga for Digestive Disorders

As discussed under the bow pose (p. 267), if the navel becomes displaced it creates all types of digestive disorders. To determine if the navel is displaced, one lies on their back with their legs extended straight out. Another person takes a string and measures from the navel to one big toe of the person lying down. Then, they measure from the navel to the other big toe. If the string differs in length then the navel is out of balance and can be helped by these specific *āsanas*.

Here, 3 postures are discussed that will properly center the navel. By practicing these three postures for 3 to 5 minutes daily, for 3 days, the navel will be returned to its normal position. Proper digestion will be noticed thereafter.

Bow (page 267)

The bow was discussed earlier. Parents can help babies and young children with the bow.

Method: *For babies*

A) The child is placed on their belly with arms stretched over their head and legs straight out.

B) Their wrists are gently pulled forward and upward so the upper torso is slightly off the ground (i.e., the navel is still on the ground). This position is held for 3 minutes—or until the child begins to feel uncomfortable.

Prone Half-Padmāsana

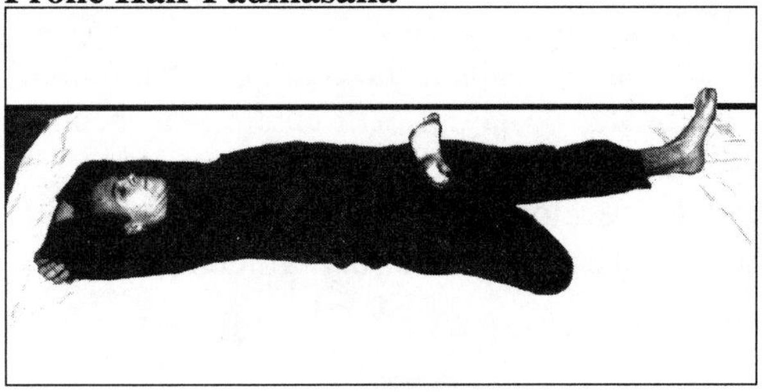

Method:

A) Lay on back with legs fully extended.

B) Bend one knee and place the foot across the upper thigh of the extended leg.

C) Gently press the bent knee to the ground and hold it for 3 to 5 minutes.

D) Release and extend the leg; repeat with the other leg.

Boat

This is perhaps the most difficult of the three postures; therefore, this pose is held only so long as it is comfortable. Make sure to breathe during the pose.

Method:

A) Lay on back with arms by the sides. Legs are fully extended and together.

B) Inhale, then exhale, slowly raising the head and upper chest off the ground. Simultaneously, lift the legs slightly off the floor (also keeping them together).

C) Exhale, slowly returning to the prone position again.

Part 10
Medical Definitions

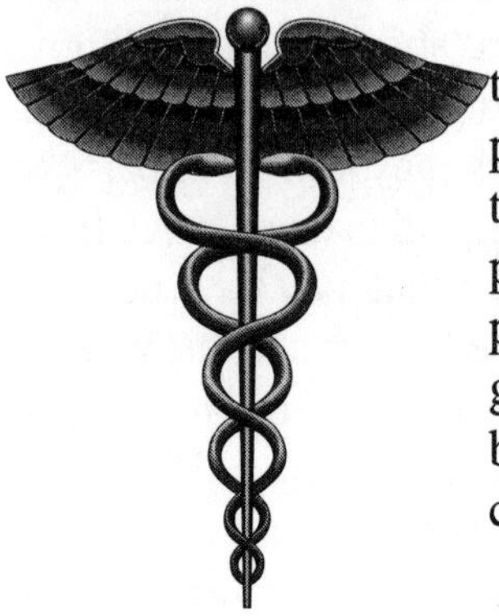

Throughout this section on *yoga āsanas*, physiological effects of the postures were explained. The more important systems and organs are further defined below in modern medical terminology.

Reticular Activating System: Controls the overall degree of central nervous system (CNS) activity. This relates to waking, sleeping, and clarity (alertness). This system influences the thalamus and hypothalamus.

Thalamus: Relays senses and connects with many brain areas including the cerebral cortex, basal ganglia, hypothalamus, and brain stem. It also senses pain, and is related to emotions and memory.

Hypothalamus:

Affects behavior—emotions, the subconscious, sensory-motor skills, intrinsic feelings of pleasure and pain, rage, fear.

Affects physical functions—body temperature, weight, blood pressure, water metabolism, the cardiac system, urinary output, kidneys, hunger, sodium, negative ions, thirst, communicates with the cerebral cortex, pupil dilation, shivering, GI tract stimulation, thirst, satiety, sexual drive, alertness, body temperature, uterine contraction, and breast milk ejection.

Thyroid: Secretes the two main hormones that regulate the metabolic rate and secretes a hormone for calcium metabolism. It affects proteins, cellular enzymes, growth, cholesterol, triglycerides, phospholipids, arteriosclerosis, muscles, sleep, sexual functions, blood flow, cardiac output, and body weight. It also affects liver/fat deposits, metabolic rate, respiration, carbohydrates, vitamin metabolism, gastrointestinal functions, and the CNS .

Autonomic Nervous System: Partially or wholly affects—psychosomatic conditions, visceral organs, blood pressure, urinary bladder, GI tract, sweat, body temperature, bronchi, and kidneys. It also affects skeletal motor nerves, blood, mind, nose, eyes, lungs, small intestine, colon, liver, gall bladder, and the pituitary gland.

Parasympathetic Nervous System: This system affects the iris/eyes, nose, lungs, liver, gall bladder, and the male generative organ.

Endocrine Glands: The glands secrete hormones that affect growth, thyroid, pancreas, ovaries, testes, parathyroid, placenta, RNA, gonads, antidiuretic, and the pituitary.

Pituitary Gland: This gland is connected to the hypothalamus. Most pituitary secretions are controlled by hormonal or nervous signals from the hypothalamus. Other secretions come from within the gland and release or inhibit secretions. It affects amino acids, carbohydrates, hair, gonads, breast milk, metabolism, anti-diuretic, thyroid, growth, proteins, mammary glands, glucose, insulin diabetes, water metabolism, and kidneys.

Suggested Reading

Gray H. *Gray's Anatomy*. Philadelphia, PA: Running Press; 1974

Guyton A. *Textbook of Medical Physiology.* Philadelphia, PA: Saunders Press; 1981.

Jordan S. *Yoga For Pregnancy*. New York, NY: St. Martin's Press; 1987.

Iyengar BKS. *Light On Yoga*. New York, NY: Shocken Books; 1976.

Saraswati Swami Mūktībodhāndana, (transl.) *Haṭha Yoga Pradīpikā*. Bihar, India: Bihar School of Yoga; 1985.

Shivananda Yoga Center. *Shivananda Companion To Yoga*. New York, NY: Fireside/Simon & Schuster; 1983.

Tirtha Swami Shankar Purushottam. *Yoga Vani*. Bayville, NY: Āyurveda Holistic Center Press; 1990.

Vasu RBSC. (transl.) *Gheranda Saṃhitā.* New Delhi, India: Oriental Books Reprint Corp.; 1980.

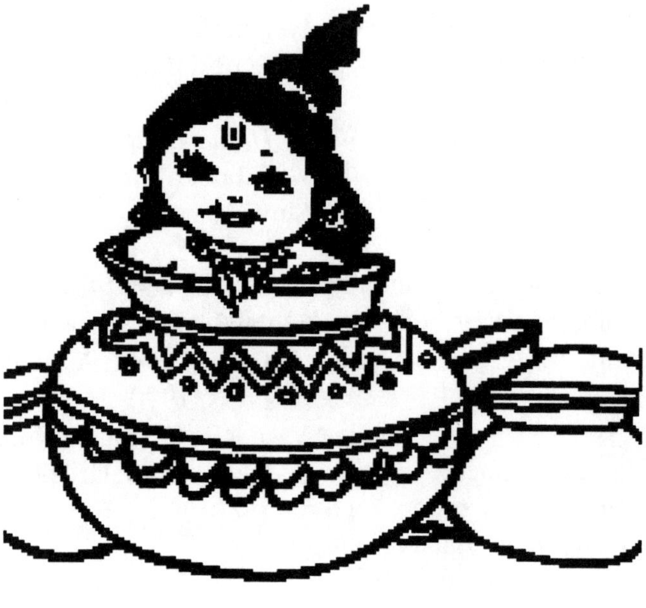

Like salt that is tasted in water
though we cannot see it,
so too, merging into Brahman
we are everywhere, but we cannot see it.
Vedic saying

Chapter 10
Sound Therapy: Mantras, Chakras & Music

In the last chapter, we briefly discussed sound (*nāda*). In the present chapter we investigate the entire realm of sound as a healing therapy for physical, mental, and spiritual disorders.

All of life is vibration: color, matter, energy particles; even love has a vibration or feeling. The *Vedas* state that creation arises from the first sound of the universe, the primordial sound *Aum*. The definition of *mantra* varies because there are so many types of *mantras*: Āyurvedic, astrological, deities, seed (*bīja*) *mantras*, and the like. Many books about *mantras* exist as well. A special group of *mantras* are *Guru mantras*. These are words enlivened by the spiritual teacher to awaken our inner *kuṇḍalinī śhakti* and develop our spiritual growth of Self-Realization. Different *Gurus* use different *mantras*; some use meaningless sounds, some use musical sounds, some use the *mantra aum*, *aum namaḥ śhivaya*, *haṅg saḥ*; and others use name-symbol or deity *mantras*. It is believed that any words the *Guru* speaks to a person are *mantras* or awakeners of *kuṇḍalinī*. If the *Guru* says, "eat an apple," that would be a *mantra* for that moment. Some *gurus* use only the playing of music to realize the Divine. Some meditate on the Divine as unmanifest, formless.

Sound itself belongs to the element of ether, the origin of all the other elements. By calming and awakening the inner self through sound, a person can calm, harmonize, and balance all the elements that are in his or her life.

ॐ ("AUM", THE 1ST SOUND OF THE UNIVERSE)

Guru Mantras

Mantra is that which saves us from the workings of the mind. Thought or meditation vanishes with the stopping of mental activities. With the stopping of mental activities, yoga is attained, which is nothing but self concentration or self centeredness.
Yoga Vani (Discourse 3)

Life-breath—or Soul (*Kuṇḍalinī Śhakti*)—is the *mantra*, the savior of the mind, because mind is a vibration of life-breath. When the life-breath flows through the *suṣhumṇā* (a mystical tube within the spine) to the crown of the head, the mind becomes fixed in the *Brahmarandhra*, within the *crown chakra* (*Sahasrārara*), and it disappears, becoming calm, peaceful, or inactive. Thus, the *mantra* is nothing but the breath of life.

This life-breath, when exhaled, makes the sound '*Hang,*' and when inhaled, makes the sound '*Sah*'. This *mantra* occurs in all creatures 21,600 times daily over the entire 24 hour period. Those of keen *yogic* awareness can actually hear this sound. This *Gāyatrī* or *mantra* is known as *ajapa*, and is the giver of salvation to *Yogis*. *Gāyatrī* originates at the *mūlādhāra*—or base *chakra,* has a dot-like appearance, and sustains the Self. *Nāda*—or sound—evolves from this imperceptible *kuṇḍalinī* sprout. *Yogis* perceive this sound as a sprout from an invisible seed. As it moves to the navel, it can *yogically* be perceived as visible rumbling, as if from the clouds. It then moves up to the heart as unstruck sound, and is finally heard in the throat so as to produce all sounds, alphabets, words, sentences, *mantras*, scriptures, etc. So all *mantras* emanate from *nāda*—or sound, originating at the first *chakra*.

Mantras, to be successful, must be enlivened or animated; this occurs by waking the *kuṇḍalinī śhakti*. Generally, it is believed that one needs a *Guru* to enliven the word or *mantra*. Otherwise, everyone could refer to a book or go to a religious service and feel the awakening of life within. Some rare individuals, who have developed much spiritual sincerity and earnestness, can enliven *mantras* for themselves, but this is rare.

In the book *Yoga Vani* there is a discussion of the benefits of name-symbol *mantras*. The importance of the *mantra* is the deity established by it. *Mantra* is the attribute and deity is the goal. Just as the term "sun" and its effulgence have a relationship, so the *mantra* and its deity have a connection. *Mantra* and its deity meditation, bring concentration through meditation, and the result is that the deity is revealed in the Soul.

Awakening Kuṇḍalinī

Like a double-tongued snake, *kuṇḍalinī* (the essential life force) has two mouths: internal and external. One mouth is stuck in the internal *suṣhumṇā* (a spiritual tube, running up the spine) that leads to Self-Realization. The other mouth is open to the external passage. This is why we are aware of the world and why we breathe; and this is why we see the diversity of life. When, through the grace of a *Guru*, the *kuṇḍalinī* is awakened, it may appear as a flash of lightning. Once awakened, the *kuṇḍalinī* gradually rises up the *suṣhumṇā*. It cleanses *karmic* sludge out of the spine and the *chakras*, just as a hot iron rod cleanses the dirt from a hookah pipe tube. Persons may have experienced quivering, shaking movements of the body, or suspension of breath during meditation. This is the experience of the *kuṇḍalinī śhakti* cleansing the inner tube and *chakras*.

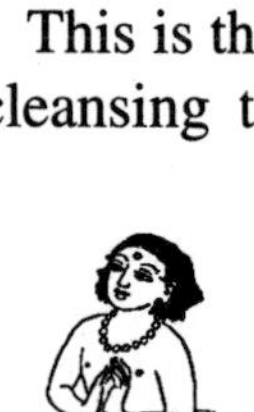

Āyurvedic Healing Mantras

Healing sounds balance both the mind and body, as well as the spirit. Practitioners find that imparting Āyurvedic *mantras* helps heal their clients. *Mantras* also help balance *prāṇa*, *tejas,* and *ojas*. They help harmonize nerve tissue, and they clear subtle impurities from the nerves and *nāḍīs* (subtle channels). These *mantras* also aid one's concentration and creative thinking.

Both practitioner and client use the *mantras* during a session. They empower all actions on a subtle level, infusing the cosmic life force into the healing process. Generally, *Vāyu doṣhas* mentally repeat *mantras*, while Pitta and Kapha *doṣhas* may also chant them. Kaphas do particularly well with chanting; it is suggested that they do so on a daily basis.

Aum: (long "ahh", then 'um' as in home) Most important, for it represents the Divine word, serving to energize or empower all things and processes. This is why all *mantras* begin and end with *aum.* Best for males.
Uses: It clears the mind, opens *nāḍīs*, and increases *ojas*. It awakens one's *prāṇa*—or positivity—needed for healing to occur.

Ram: ("a" sounds like the "a" in "calm")
Uses: Brings Divine protection (light and grace), giving strength, calm, rest, peace; good for mental disorders and high Vāyu (e.g., insomnia, bad dreams, nervousness, anxiety, excessive fear, and fright); it strengthens *ojas* and builds the immune system.

Hoom:
Uses: It wards off negative influences, which are manifested as diseases, negative emotions, or black magic. *Hoom* awakens *agni* and promotes digestive fire. It burns up *āma* and clears channels; it increases *tejas* and mental perception, and it is sacred to *Śhivā* as the sound of Divine wrath.

Aym:
Uses: Improves mental concentration, thinking, rational powers, and speech; awakens and in-

creases intelligence, mental and nervous disorders; restores speech, communication, control of senses and mind; is the sacred sound of *Saraswati*, the Goddess of Wisdom.

Śhrīm:
Uses: Promotes general health, beauty, creativity, prosperity, strengthens *rasa* (plasma) and *śhukra* (reproductive fluids), and overall health and harmony.

Hrīm:
Uses: Cleanses and purifies, giving energy, joy, and ecstasy. Although it initially causes atonement; it also aids detoxification.

Krīm:
Uses: Gives capacity for work and action; adds power and efficacy, good for chanting while making preparations.

Klīm: **K+**
Uses: Gives strength, sexual vitality, control of emotions, increases *śhukra* and *ojas*.

Śham: *Mantra* of peace (or '*Aum śhanti, śhanti, śhanti*')
Uses: Creates calmness, detachment, contentment; alleviates mental and nervous disorders, stress, anxiety, disturbed emotions, tremors, shaking, palpitations, and chronic degenerative nervous system disorders.

Śhum: (pronounced like "shoe" but with a shorter vowel sound)
Uses: Increases vitality, energy, fertility, sexual vigor, *mantra* for increasing *śhukra*.

Som: (as in home)
Uses: Increases energy, vitality, joy, delight, creativity, *ojas*; it strengthens mind, heart, nerves, and is good for rejuvenation and tonification therapies.

Mantras for the 5 Elements
One can strengthen the five elements through their *mantras*: *Lam*—Earth, *Vam*—Water, *Ram*—Fire, *Yam*—Air, *Ham*—Ether ("a" is a short sound, like the "e" in "the") and will strengthen the systems they govern.

Lam: Root *chakra*, excretory system, stabilizes *Apāna Vāyu*, grounds, stabilizes, calms, brings joy, happiness, and contentment.

Vam: Sex *chakra* and urogenital system; helps balance water metabolism, gives creativity, fertility, and imagination.

Ram: (pronounced like "but") *navel chakra* and solar plexus; increases *agni*, will, perception, energy, and motivation.

Yam: Heart *chakra* and circulatory system; gives energy and enthusiasm.

Ham: Throat *chakra* and respiratory system; gives breath and *prāṇa*.

Kṣham: Third eye *(ajña)* and mind; gives concentration, peace, stability, and calm to the mind.

Aum: Head center, awakens deeper consciousness, giving full expansion of consciousness.

Doṣha Mantras
Vāyu: *Mantras* need to be soft, warm, soothing, calming. They should not be chanted aloud or for too long, as this may deplete their energy. Chanting may be done for a few minutes, then continued mentally.
Precaution: *Aum* chanted in excess increases Vāyu (air and ether).
Best: *Ram, Hoom*

Pitta: *Mantras* must be cool, soothing, and calming.
Best: *Aum, Aim, Śhrīm, Śham*

Kapha: Does best with chanting or singing; needing warm, stimulating, and activating ones. Best: *Hoom, Aum, Aym*

Mantra Applications

For Practitioners:

1. During the session, purify healing room using *Aum* and *Hoom* .
2. Bring Divine light into room using *Aum* and *Ram.*
3. Chant mentally over the client to clear their psychic level using *Aum.*
4. Energize the healing power of herbs or medicines using *Krīm* or *Śhrīm.*

For Clients:

They can make use of these *mantras* at home to increase healing.

Mental or nervous disorders:

Śham—relieves pain and fever.

Hoom—restores nerve function and counters paralysis.

Som—rebuilds cerebro-spinal fluid

Round and round the circle
Completing the charm
So the knot be unknotted
The crossed be uncrossed
The crooked be made straight
And the curse be ended
T.S. Elliot

Part 2
The Life-Breath & Chakras

Life-breath is the main energy in the physical body. All 14 sense organ energies are manifestations (i.e., eye, ear, nose, etc.) of the life-breath. The life-breath has different names when doing different functions, just as one person can be an employee, a parent, or a child. For example, when the life-breath flows through the optic nerves in the eye, it has the function (energy) of vision. If the flow of life-breath is blocked, sight is impaired. Thus, the various sense organs are infused by the one life-breath.

When the life-breath, which is drawn in different directions through the different channels, is directed by *yoga* or union (devotional *sādhanā*) to flow through the *sușhumṇā*—or spiritual tube within the spine, Pure Knowledge is developed and one gains Self-Realization. All the other channels are for enjoyment. Deep inside the *sușhumṇā* lie the *chakras* (energy centers). They are visible only through the spiritual eye.

Some say there are 350,000 channels, some say 72,000 channels. There are 15 main channels; the 3 most important of which are discussed here: the *sușhumṇā*, *iḍā,* and *piṅgalā.*

Sușhumṇā is the most important channel, resting in the spine at the back of the body. It is experienced as brilliantly as the sun, moon, and fire; possessing *sattwa, rajas,* and *tamas.* It begins at the *chakra* at the base of the spine, the *mūlādhāra,* and extends to the *sahasrārar*—thousand-petaled lotus at the crown of the head. Inside the *sușhumṇā* is a finer *nāḍī*—or channel—called *bajra.* ***Bajra*** is seen like a blazing flame that enters from the *swādhișṭhān* lotus or sexual organ. Inside the *bajra nāḍī* is yet a finer *nāḍī* (channel) called *chitrini.* ***Chitrini*** is said to be as fine as a spider's web. Along this *nāḍī* run the six lotuses or *chakras*, extending from the base of the spine (*mūlādhāra*) to a little beyond the spiritual eye—or *ājñā chakra.* Devotees or *yogis* are said to be the only ones who see this *nāḍī.* Within the *chitrini nāḍī* is still another *nāḍī*, the white colored ***Brahmanāḍī.*** It is resplendent, running from *mūlādhāra* base *chakra* to the crown *chakra*, *sahasrāra.* This *nāḍī* is seen as a flash of lightning and is the fountain of pure knowledge and eternal delight.

The *iḍā nāḍī* (sometimes called the moon channel) begins from the *mūlādhāra* lotus. It is found on the left side of the spine and encircles the *chakras.* It ends above the *ājñā* or spiritual lotus, to the extremity of the left nostril. *Piṅgalā* (sometimes called sun channel) begins similarly on the right side. It goes on and ends similarly to the *iḍā,* ending above the extreme right nostril. Breath generally flows through the right or left channels; *rajas* or *tamas* prevail respectively. Through devotional *sādhanā*, life-breath flows through the *suṣhumṇā* (*sattwic* predominance), the mind becomes concentrated, and real meditation begins.

The remaining 12 major channels begin mostly at the navel:

Two channels go to the eyes.
Two channels go to the ears.
One channel goes to the extremity of the nose.
One channel goes to the stomach to digest four kinds of food (masticated, sucked, licked, drunk).
One (*Saraswati*) goes to the tip of tongue, resulting in perception of taste and expression of words.
One channel produces sneezing.
One channel moves from the throat, taking the essence of food to the brain. (From the navel, 3 channels go downwards as well).
One channels goes to the anus to purge.
Two channels go to the genitals to excrete urine and one to discharge semen.

Below is a discussion of the experiences of the *chakras* according to *Swāmī Śhaṅkar Puruṣhottam Tīrtha*, from his book, *Yoga Bani (Instructions for the Attainment of Siddhayoga).*

1st or Mūlādhāra Chakra: Experience of this *chakra* brings fulfillment of all desires, reveals the whole universe, makes one versed in the *Śhastras* (texts of wisdom), makes one pure and hale, and is considered great among people. It is seen as fresh lightning. It is found at the base of the spine, between the anus and genitals.

2nd or Swādhiṣhṭhān Chakra: Opening of this *chakra* annihilates passions such as pride. It is found at the root of the genitals.

3rd or Manipūra Chakra: Located at the root of the navel. Opening of this *chakra* gives one the ability to create, preserve, and destroy; speech never fails this person. Concentration on this *chakra* increases digestive power. It eases difficult breathing. Excess Kapha is removed from the body. One also can hear inner sound (*nāda*) by concentrating here.

4th or Anāhata Chakra: At the heart, when opened, grief and fear vanish through the grace of the Holy Preceptor. One also can hear the *Haṅgsaḥ mantra*, and the heart's desires are fulfilled. One gains command over speech, controls all senses and passions, can enter other bodies, and can create, preserve, and destroy this world.

5th or Viṣhuddha Chakra: Located in the throat, once opened, if the *yogi* is angered, the three worlds are shaken. One becomes a poet, a wise person, peaceful in mind, is free from disease and sorrow, and is long lived.

6th or Lalanā Chakra: Located in the palate, if concentration on this chakra occurs, fever, Pitta insanity, and the like are cured.

7th or Ājñā Chakra: Located in the middle of the brow, once opened, annihilation of desires occurs. One becomes equal to *Brahmā, Viṣhṇu,* and *Śhiva*. Food is taken in smaller quantities, and one passes less stool and urine. This *chakra* is also called the heart. Above the *ājñā* is the confluence of *iḍā, piṅgalā,* and *suṣhumṇā* (discussed above).

8th or Manas Chakra: Found a little above the *ājñā*. Here is the inner Soul, as knowledge and the knowable. One can see the letter *aum.*

9th or Soma Chakra: Located a little above *manas*, when open, a person gains patience, griefessness, stability, gravity, concentration, and other similar mental strengths.

Just above this *chakra* is the region of no support. Here air becomes stable without breathing or holding breath. Here all sense of physical existence vanishes. Perception of the eternal Self as most beautiful, pure and serene is then experienced. Everything is the Self and the Self is everything.

Sahasrāra Chakra: Beyond all chakras, the place of supreme perception, the site of Self-absorption (*Nirbikalpa Samādhi*), persons experience the stopping of all sensory functioning. The devotee is united with the One Universal Soul or *Brahmā*. Lassitude, decrepitude, and other diseases disappear, and one feels supreme delight. One experiences *Nirvana Śhakti*, mother of the three worlds. In utmost intimacy, She is thus experienced. No words can describe this experience. One experiences only vital force in various forms. Only new knowledge occurs, no physical attributes are noticed.

ॐ ॐ ॐ

Part 3
Music Therapy

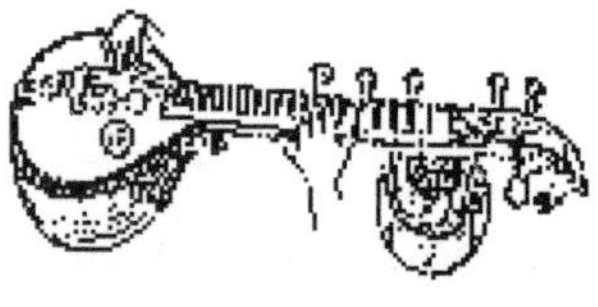

Our sages developed
music from time
immemorial for the
mind to take shelter
in that pure Being
which stands apart
as one's true Self.
Real music is not for
wealth, not for honors,
or not even for the joys of the mind-
it is one kind of yoga,
a path for realization and salvation,
to purify your mind and heart
and give you longevity
Ali Akbar Khan

From the earliest days in India, music was another form of attaining spiritual union, practiced by musicians without any thought of worldly gains. Music was found in the temples, sung as *bhajans* (devotional songs) in *āṣhrams,* and used by saints as a means of expression. Yet it was also found in the theater and the army tents. In short, music was a path for the musically inclined to reach God. The music teacher was the *guru*. By following the *guru's* musical instruction, the student or disciple also learned a spiritual lesson. The musical path towards Self-Realization was one lacking intellectual analysis or discussion. Merely by playing music, one would gradually merge with the eternal Divinity. The basic learning precept was, "*śhikṣha, dīkṣha, parīkṣha*": learning, dedicated practice, evaluation. Below is a discussion of classical North Indian music.

The traditional learning method was to live near the *guru's* home and spend each day in theory, vocal music classes, and so forth. Like all forms of *Vedic* learning, originally the teaching of music was an oral tradition, passed on from teacher to student. The teacher was always there to correct the student's performance or understanding of the music (*rags*—a melody base or form over which the musician may improvise). Students practiced small sections of the music until they gradually learned the entire song.

Today, unless one lives in India, finding such a teacher with whom to study is difficult. In the United States, although there are teachers with whom persons may study (usually for hourly classes), it is more likely that the aspiring musician will resort to books, audio tapes, and video cassettes that are available for self-instruction. An extremely devoted musician can study with some of the great Indian virtuosos who live in or visit the US.

The Indian music scale has certain similarities to Western music.

Sanskrit	English	Sanskrit	English
Sa	C	Ma	F#
ri	C#	Pa	G
Ri	D	dha	G#
ga	D#	Dha	A
Ga	E	ni	A#
ma	F	Ni	B

Classical Indian music (*rags*) has a great depth of healing and mind-balancing abilities. Each *rag* has its own mood, its own time of day, and its own season in which to be played.

Music is rhythm; in tune,
it gives you food for your soul
Ali Akbar Khan

About 75,000 *rags* exist, grouped under 10 parent scales, but each musician will have their own interpretation of the songs. The original treatises of classical Indian music are *Nātya-ṣhtāstra, Nāradakṣhiksa, Dattilam, Bridahhesi,* and *Sangītaratnākara.*

Each *rag* has a time of day or season associated with it. *Rags* are usually based on 3-hour intervals (*prahars* or watches).

Midnight - 3:00 a.m.	Noon - 3:00 p.m.
3:00 a.m. - 6:00 a.m.	3:00 p.m. - 6:00 p.m.
6:00 a.m. - 9:00 a.m.	6:00 p.m. - 9:00 p.m.
9:00 a.m. - Noon	9:00 p.m. - Midnight

Rag times are also adjusted for seasonal changes. Some *rags* are very specific. Some are played when the first ray of the sun is seen (i.e., *rag Ahir Bhairav*). Others are played when the sky first reddens in the late afternoon (i.e., *rag Purvi*). Still others are performed when the first candles are lit in the evening (i.e., *rag Bhimpalashri*). Some rags are played at different times of the day (during the morning, afternoon, evening, and night).

Rags emote many moods and effects: joy and love, pathos, compassion, or sadness. Other emotions include heroism, courage or valor, merriment and laughter, wonder or surprise, anger or rage, disgust, fear.

Today, many Indian and American musicians are blending the classical Indian music with jazz or new-age music, and developing unique new sounds. The serious musician should read *The Classical Music of North India*, by *Ali Akbar Khan*. Another source of Indian music training is the out-of-print collection of audio lessons, *Learning Indian Music*, by *Ravi Śhankar.*

Audiotapes and CD's of these classical *rags* are available through Indian grocery stores and through the *Ali Akbar* College in San Francisco, California. *Rags* are useful in helping attune oneself to the natural rhythms of the day and season, and enhance meditation and peace of mind.

Once King Akbar asked his court musician 'Tansen' to bring his teacher, Swami Haridass', to sing for him. The musician said that Akbar would have to visit the forest because Swāmijī did not visit anyone. Further, Akbar had to disguise himself as a servant. In the presence of the Swami, the musician intentionally sang a rag incorrectly, and the Swami sang it to show him his error. The musician then turned to the king and said, "I sing for men, but Swāmijī sings only for God."

Sample of Classical Indian Instruments

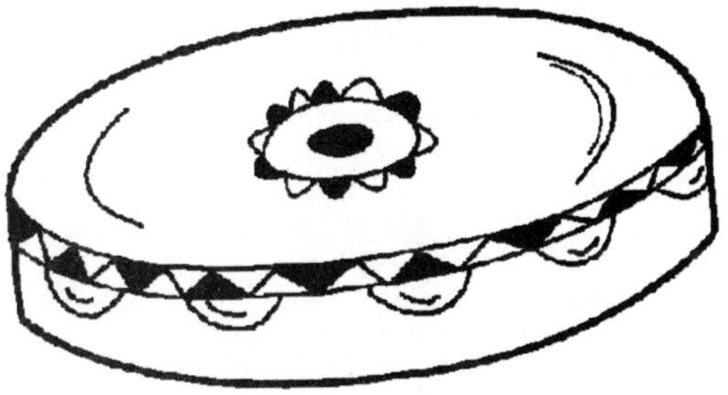

Dhapli

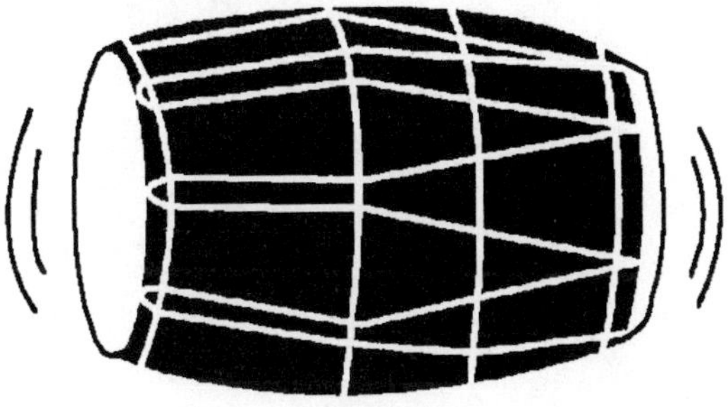

Dholak

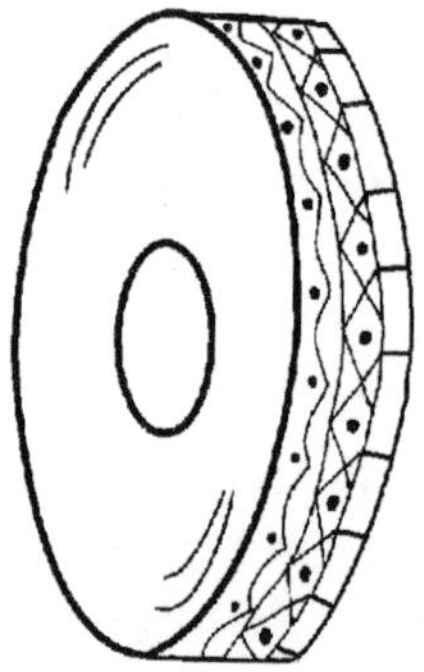

Duff

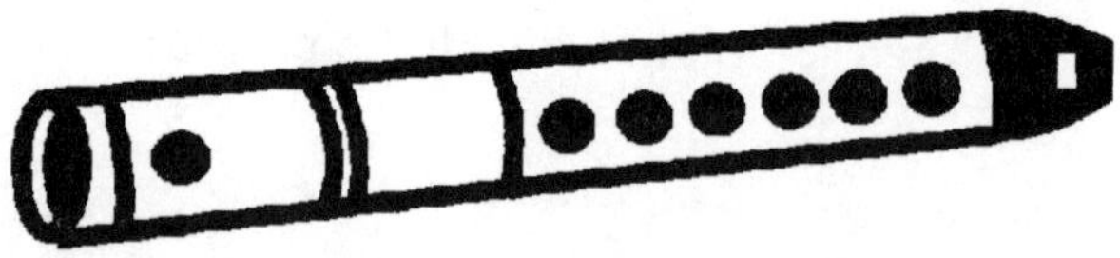

Flute

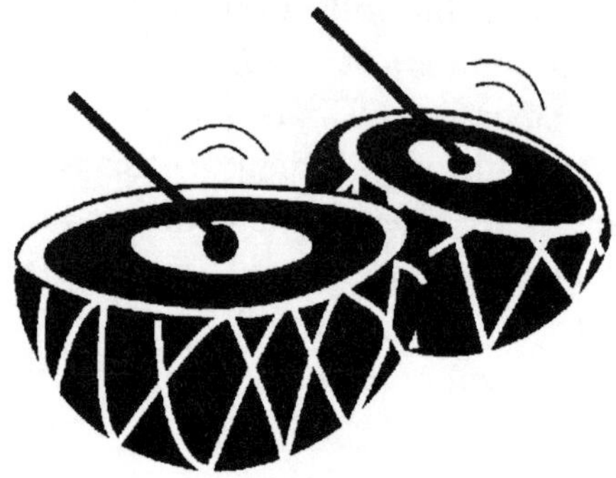

Nagada

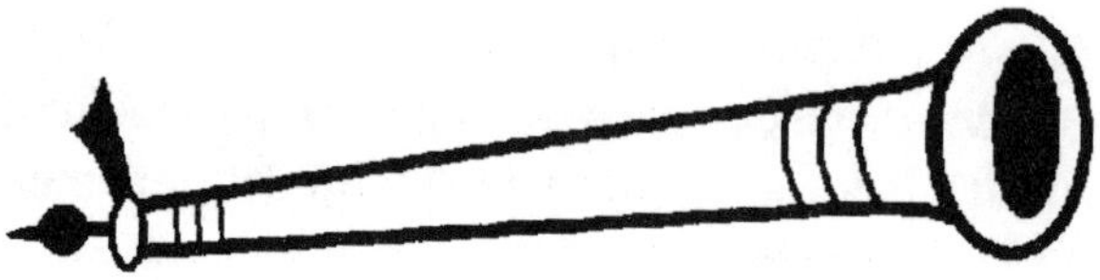

Shahnai

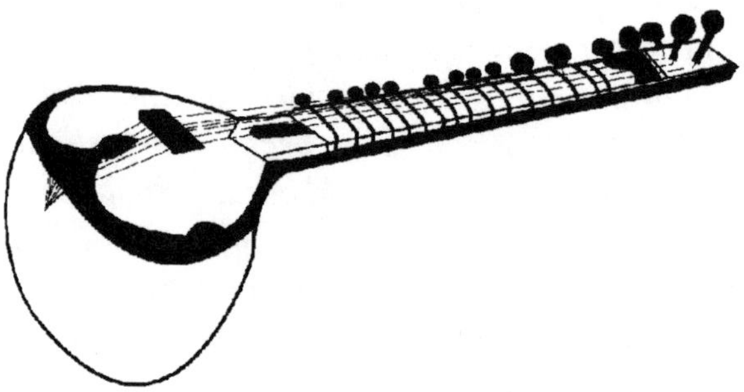

Sitar

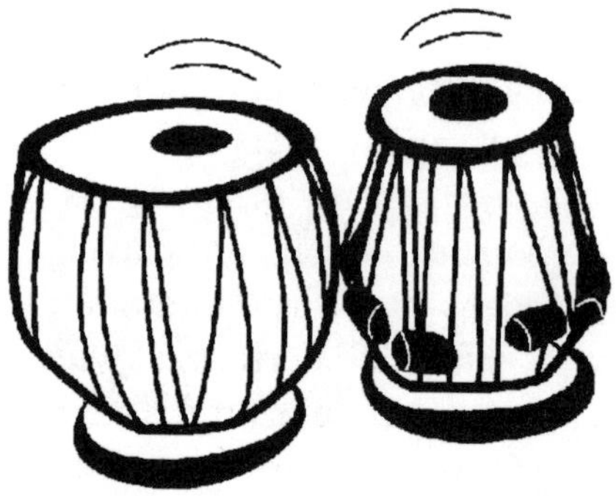

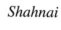

Tabla

(The Veena is shown on page 318)

People are bound by rites and freed by knowledge,
thus the sages have known this truth
do not perform rites.
Upaniṣhadic wisdom

Chapter 11
Color and Gem Therapies

Herbs and food bring balance through the sense of taste. *Abhyañga* achieves balance through the sense of touch. Aromatherapy heals through the sense of smell. Color therapy balances the *doṣhas* (mentally or psychically) through the sense of sight. Colors are absorbed primarily through the eyes or *Alochak* Pitta (and secondarily through the skin or *Bhrajak* Pitta). It is a crucial part of subtle mental and *praṇic* life-force nutrition as it energizes the nerves (which stimulate the mind). Besides absorbing colors, the mind and body produce them as well, adding the powers of digestion.

Tejas: Mental fire, or *tejas,* is the major realm that color therapy affects most. Bright colors increase *tejas*, and dark colors diminish it. However, if colors are too bright, *tejas* becomes burnt out (psychedelic drugs have this affect also), and disharmonious or clashing colors derange *tejas*. So *tejas* can be balanced by the right use of colors. To increase *tejas*, one meditates on a *ghee* flame or golden light. White or deep blue color reduces excess *tejas*, and green balances it.

Just as the choice of foods either balances or deranges the body's health, one's choice of colors acts similarly. Colors provide emotional strength and creativity. If misused, colors can cause a disturbance or depression (i.e., bright colors stimulate emotions and energy, dark colors suppress emotions and reduce energy—although they can also calm certain individuals). Healing psychological diseases is greatly assisted through color therapy.

Physically, color stimulates digestion, circulation, improves vitality, increases overall physical activity, and most of all, energizes blood (*Ranjak* Pitta). However, if colors inappropriate for the constitution are used, they weaken the circulation, depress the appetite, increase toxins in the blood, or cause mental hyperactivity. Colors act like gems; they strengthen the aura and astral body. This is the realm of pure color, and is suitable for subtle or spiritual healing.

Applied Color Therapy

The use of colors in one's daily life adds psychological harmony and peace of mind. Below are various methods of how color therapy is used.

Since color is so important,

-Use colored lamps, either by placing colored glass over light bulbs or by buying colored bulbs.

-Use soft lights instead of fluorescent or neon.

-Use full-spectrum lights in the winter (when there is less sunlight) to alleviate depression.

-Use mild and harmonious shades.

-Bathe the whole body or specific parts with various colored lights. For example, use dark blue light for inflammation, infection, or rheumatoid arthritis on the hands (use smaller bulbs for application on specific sites).

-Choose the colors of your surroundings—clothes, home furnishings, car, office, bedroom—with care.

-Note exposure to colors in nature: sky blue, ocean blue/green/ turquoise, white snow or moonlight, plush green trees, shrubs and grass; colorful flowers; meditate on colorful flowers such as a white lily, red rose or hibiscus, yellow chrysanthemum, or sunflower, blue iris.

-Meditate on stained glass, art, *mandalas*.
-Visualize colors in your mind.

Nature's own colors are the most beneficial, nourishing and strengthening

The Use of Colors

Color therapy affects the mind more than it affects the body. Thus, there is greater consideration of the *sattwic, rajasic,* and *tamasic* effects of colors, even more than their effect on the physical constitution.

Sattwa: All colors have shades that are *sattwic, rajasic,* or *tamasic*, so it is important to use only the *sattwic* shades—those shades that bring joy, harmony, and serenity. The best colors are white, gold, violet, and blue.

Rajas: Colors—bright, loud, flashy, artificial (i.e., neon signs), and *rajasic* shades—bright, metallic, penetrating, are sometimes useful when there is low or inert energy. Combinations of opposite colors can also be too stimulating and irritating (i.e., blue/yellow, red/green). *Rajasic* colors are yellow, orange, red, purple.

Tamas: Colors are dull, dark, turbid, and muddy (i.e., *stagnant green*). They cause the mind and senses to become heavy, inert, and congested. *Tamasic* colors are brown, black, and *gray*.

White and black are not really considered colors, but the polar opposites of light and dark, from which color is produced. Below is a list of colors. When healing, one should use primary colors in their most characteristic shades.

Color Therapy, Spirituality and Astrology

Vedic scriptures state that what is in the heavens and on the earth is also in humans. Furthermore, since humans, mother earth, and the universe are interrelated, they are linked together like strands of a web. Thus, it is natural to find a connection between colors, the heavens, and their effects on humankind.

In the *Vedic* texts on astrology (*Jyotiṣh*) and architecture (*Vāstu Śhāstra*), the colors are another name for different deities. The 7 colors of the spectrum (red, orange, yellow, green, blue, indigo, violet) are said to be the 7 rays, or deities, of the sun (*Sūrya*), only in the reverse order.

According to *Vāstu Śhāstra*, through proper positioning of one's house and building materials, the seen and unseen solar rays (i.e., colors) positively affect the dweller's health. It is a fascinating field of study in itself (see Chapter 27).

Gray	Uses: Gives objectivity, neutrality, reduces emotion and sensation
	Precautions: Can be depressing or devitalizing
Brown: Earthy	**Uses**: Grounds, stabilizes, neutralizes
	Precautions: May make one's personality coarser
Red K- V+ (in excess) Pitta/*Agni/ Tejas*+	**Uses**: Warm shades—energy, warmth, strengthens the heart, blood, circulation, will, energy
	Precautions: Promotes hostility, anger, violence, (the strongest of all colors), used with black, creates *rajasic* and tamasic effects
Orange: VK- P+	Uses: Energizing, intelligence, illumination, paralysis, thyroid, menstrual cramps
	Precautions: On a lower level, it can aggravate the second or sex *chakra*
Yellow: VK- P+	**Uses**: Motivation, energy, clarity, communication, nervous system, arthritis, brain
	Precautions: May make one superficial or hyperactive
Green: VP- K+ (in excess)	**Uses**: Harmonizes, life-giving, calms the mind, nerves, fever, acidity, headache; balances the metabolism, stabilizes weight, tones liver and spleen; pituitary
	Precautions: Increases Kapha when used in excess
Blue: V- (sky-blue) P- VK+ (in excess)	Spiritual Uses: Promotes solitude, meditation, independence
	Uses: Helps reduce tumors, congestion, fevers, and infections (natural antibiotic), neutralizes anger and hatred, cools the mind and eyes, sleep, pineal gland
	Precaution: Excess blue can make one overly cold-natured
Purple:	**Uses**: Gives authority, prestige, and distance, reduces heart pain, stiffness, cysts
	Precautions: May stagnate or suppress emotions—especially anger
Violet:	**Uses**: Detachment and devotion, antibiotic, builds white corpuscles in spleen
	Precautions: Same as purple
Gold: VK- P+	**Spiritual Uses**: Increases Self-consciousness
	Uses: Harmonizes the mind and strengthens the heart, *ojas,* immune, endocrine systems
White: VP- K+	**Spiritual Uses**: Promotes purity, virtue, spirituality
	Uses: Nurturing, heals fevers, infections and pain, calms the heart, mind, nerves and emotions, promotes vitality and supportive feelings
	Precaution: In excess causes passivity, lethargy, hypersensitivity, and inhibitions
Black: P- VK+	**Spiritual Uses**: Spiritual color for some religions/sign of death for others
	Uses: Promotes resistance, obstruction, opposition, enmity, hatred wards off and distances negative emotions
	Precaution: Increase fear and suspicion and paranoia
V = Vāyu, P = Pitta, K = Kapha '-' means reduces; '+' means increases	

Colors, Shapes and Doṣhas

Color therapy is applied in moderation as excess will disturb the humors.

Vāyu	**Use**: Gold, red, orange, yellow, white, emerald green, sky blue, pink
	Precaution: Overly bright, flashy colors (red, purple), overly dark colors
	Shapes: Round, soft, square, balanced
Pitta	Use: White, green, blue, mild, pastels
	Precaution: Reds, oranges, yellows, golds
	Shapes: Avoid angles, sharp, or penetrating forms
Kapha	Use: Reds, golds, yellows, oranges
	Precaution: Whites, pinks, other whitish colors
	Shapes: Pyramid, angular; avoid vertical round or square

All human activities are meant for the happiness of all living beings; such happiness is based on dharma, (righteousness). Hence, everyone is advised to always be righteous.

- Aṣhṭāñga Hṛidayam
Sū: Ch. 1; ver. 20

Part 2
Gem Therapy

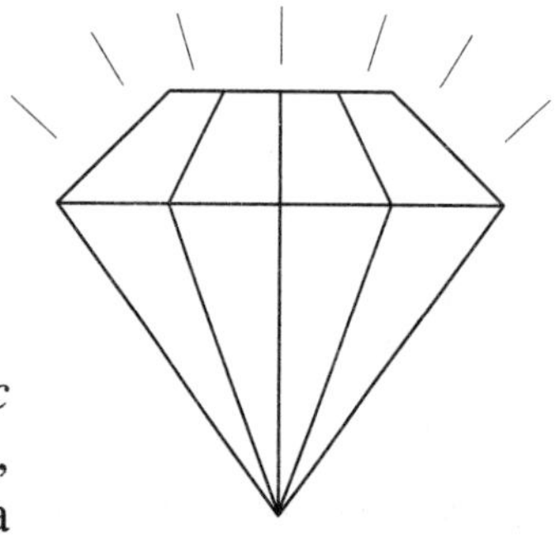

Astrological-Gem Therapies

Jyotiṣh is the *Vedic* astrological system, of which Āyurveda was once a part. This astrological system notes that gems are related to the various planets and produce a balancing effect to counter specific diseases. It is a primary method of a *Jyotiṣh* astrologer's therapeutic measures to heal physical, mental, and spiritual situations, based on one's astrology chart indicators. It is known that planets produce effects in humans. For example, the full moon not only causes high tides, but also affects the emotions of some people. The gemstones were studied and used to neutralize these effects.

The ancient Āyurvedic researchers studied healing properties of gems, and found that different stones created different effects in the human body. The planets were seen to have corresponding colors. The color or vibration of the gems affects the human body. They absorb and reflect (like a filter) the planetary rays or vibrations. Thus, gems relate to specific energy waves. It was found that the gems associated with each planet have varying wave lengths.

The planetary vibrations are negative, while the radiation of the stones is positive. When the positive and negative vibrations are combined, they are neutralized. Just as an umbrella or sun screen protects one from the sun, so gems protect one from the influence of the planets.

In ancient *Vedic* texts, like the *Brihat Samhitā*, the origin and healing powers of various gems are discussed. Persons may use substitute stones instead of the more expensive gems. Red garnet can replace ruby; moonstone can replace pearl; jade, peridot, or green tourmaline can replace emerald; and yellow topaz or citrine can replace yellow sapphire.

In the Āyurvedic tradition these stones are used to balance the three *doṣhas* and to heal specific diseases. The chart below shows the planetary stones, the *doṣhas,* and the diseases they balance.

Planet	Wave Length	Gem	Wave Length
Sun	65,000	Ruby	70,000
Moon	65,000	Pearl	70,000
Mars	85,000	Red Coral	65,000
Mercury	65,000	Emerald	75,000
Jupiter	130,000	Yellow Sapphire	50,000
Venus	130,000	Diamond (Clear Zircon)	60,000
Saturn	65,000	Blue Sapphire/Amethyst/Lapis	79,000
Rahu	35,000	*Gomedha* (Golden Hessonite Garnet)	70,000
Ketu	35,000	Cat's Eye (Chrysoberyl)	70,000

Precautions: The gems have been found to have side effects depending upon birth sign and planetary placement. This is especially true of blue sapphire. Different astrologers have different criteria to judge contraindications. Avoiding gem therapy, unless properly advised, may be best.

Jyotiṣh suggests wearing gems, and ingesting them internally (after a long heating process to make them safe), or as gem tinctures. Stones worn as rings and pendants are mounted so as to touch the skin. Pendants should touch the heart or throat *chakras*, and rings with different gem-stones should be worn on various fingers, as the elements dictate.

Planet	**Gem**	Helps	**Heals**
Sun	Ruby/Red Garnet	Vāyu/ Kapha	heart, spleen, hypertension, infections, fevers, bile, hot temper, impatience, brain, heart, acne, low energy, poor circulation, edema, eyesight, bones, arthritis
Moon	Moonstone/ Pearl	Vāyu/ Pitta	infertility, kidney, lung and mental disorders
Mars	Red Coral	Pitta	fevers, inflammations, ulcers, bleeding problems, weak muscles, liver, small intestines, vitality, accidents
Mercury	Green Gems	Pitta/ Mind	vertigo, giddy, lethargic, mental problems, stuttering, memory loss, anxiety, nervous indigestion
Jupiter	Yellow Gems	Vāyu/ Kapha	weak immune system, tumors, arterial circulation, weight, jaundice, liver, abscess, pancreas, nerve and gland dysfunction
Venus	Diamond/ Clear Zircon	Vāyu/ Kapha	reproductive and urinary system, kidneys, anemia, infertility, weak bones, weak immune system
Saturn	Blue Sapphire/ Amethyst/ Lapis	Vāyu/ Pitta	weak bones, nerves, vitality, constipation, epilepsy, paralysis, cancer, immune diseases
Rahu	*Gomedha*	All	nervousness, indigestion, loss of coordination, mental disorders
Ketu	Cat's Eye	All	poor digestion or circulation, bleeding, weak muscles, nervous system, cancer, paralysis, immune diseases

Each finger is related to one of the five elements. The pinky is earth, the ring finger is water, the middle finger is air, the index finger is ether, and the thumb is fire. The planets correspond to this system as well: Mercury—earth, the sun or moon—water, Saturn—air, Jupiter—ether. No specific planet rules the fire. Precious gems are worn as rings in 2-carat (minimum) and 5-carat pendants. Substitute stones are worn as rings in 4-carat (minimums) and 7-carat pendants. Determinations of planetary therapies are made differently than in Western Astrology.

Vedic Origin of Gems

The *Garuda Purana*, an ancient *Vedic* text, includes a discussion of the science of gemology. This mythologically-based story may have semantic parallels in modern scientific terminology, just as the seven deities of the sun are analogous to the seven colors of the spectrum (red, orange, yellow, green, blue, indigo, and violet) in *Vedic* Astrology. Thus, it is hoped that interested readers will seek out the parallels between these *Vedic* descriptions and modern science, rather than doubt its authenticity merely because of the use of words like "gods" and "demons."

Once, a very powerful demon, *Vala*, caused trouble for all the gods in the universe. After much hardship the gods developed a plan to capture *Vala* and kill him. Once dead, *Vala* was cut into pieces. His limbs were transformed into the seeds of precious gems. All the creatures of the universe rushed to gather the gem seeds. In the clamor some of the seeds fell to earth, dropping into rivers, oceans, forests, and mountains. There they developed into mother lodes.

Vala's blood became ruby seeds and fell over India, Burma, Afghanistan, Pakistan, Nepal, Tibet, Sri Lanka, and ancient Siam.

His teeth became pearl seeds that spread throughout the oceans of Sri Lanka, Bengal, Persia, Indonesia, and other bodies of water in the southern hemisphere.

The skin of *Vala* became yellow sapphire seeds, plummeting mainly to the Himalayas. *Vala's* fingernails became hessonite garnet seeds that fell into lotus ponds of Sri Lanka, India, and Burma.

His bile became emerald seeds and fell into the mountain ranges of modern day South Africa, South America, Afghanistan, and Pakistan. *Vala's* bones became diamond seeds. His war cry became the cat's-eye gem seeds. Blue sapphire seeds were transformed from *Vala's* eyes. Coral seed was transformed from his intestines. *Vala's* toenails became red garnet seeds. His body fat became jade seeds. Quartz crystal seeds were transformed from his semen. *Vala's* complexion was transformed into bloodstone coral seeds.

Gem tinctures are prepared like herb tinctures. Gems are soaked for some time in a 50% - 100% alcohol solution. Diamonds or sapphires (hard gems) are soaked from one full moon to the next full moon (one month). Opaque stones—pearls, coral (soft stones)— are soaked for shorter time periods or in weaker solutions.

Below is a list of gems, their related *doṣhas*, and their uses. Special Āyurvedic preparations exist in which gems are burnt into ash. This removes their harmful effects, enabling them to be ingested. Traditionally, gems were crushed and/or burnt in long processes to make ash. Sometimes they are taken alone, sometimes they are mixed with herbs. Gem ash (*bhasma*) is more costly than herbs, but healing is quicker. Currently, they are not imported into the United States due to the lack of understanding of their safety.

<u>Key to abbreviations:</u>
V = Vāyu; P = Pitta; K = Kapha.
'+' means increases the doṣha;
'-' means decreases the doṣha

Ruby VK- P++

Uses: Strengthens the heart and will, improves digestion, circulation, *agni* fire, and energy; promotes independence, insight, and power, Gem of the kings.

Worn: Usually set in gold and worn on the right-hand ring finger.

<u>Ash</u>: (*Manikya bhasma*)

Actions: Stimulant, nervine.

Uses: Heart tonic for weak heart, nerves, and general debility.

Pearl VP- K+

Uses: Gives the body fluid, nourishes tissues and nerves, strengthens female reproductive system, improves fertility, and calms emotions.

Worn: Usually set in silver and worn on the left-hand ring finger.

<u>Ash</u>: (*Moti bhasma*)

Actions: Tonic, alterative, sedative, nervine, antacid.

Uses: Hyperacidity, ulcers, nose bleeds, coughing blood, liver, kidney, nervous excitability, hysteria, general tonic for woman and infants.

Red Coral Harmonize P V- K+ in excess

Uses: Strengthens blood, reproductive system, gives energy, calms emotions, aphrodisiac, improves capacity for work, builds flesh and

muscle—especially for males; gives courage.
Worn: Set in silver and worn on either ring or index finger.
Ash: (*Pravāl bhasma*)
Actions: Alterative, antacids, tonic.
Uses: Cough, asthma, swollen glands, hyperacidity, impotence, bleeding from the lungs, anemia, sexual debility.

Emerald V= P- K+
Uses: Promotes healing, energizes breathing, strengthens lungs, increases mental flexibility and adaptability (calming agitation), regulates nervous system, helps stops nerve pain, improves speech and intelligence; cancer, degenerative diseases.
Worn: VK-set in gold; P-set in silver, worn on the middle or pinky finger of either hand.
Ash: (*Panna bhasma*)
Actions: Nervine, alterative, tonic.
Uses: Nervous and general debility, neurasthenia, heart tonic, asthma, ulcers, skin diseases, fevers, infections, children's tonic.

Yellow Sapphire VPK= V- P+ in excess
Uses: Best stone for promoting health, increases *ojas*; diabetes, all wasting diseases, convalescence, regulates hormones, energy, vitality.
Worn: Set in gold, and worn on the index finger.
Ash: None.

Diamond VP- K+
Uses: Strengthens the kidneys and reproductive system, enhances *ojas,* gives beauty, power charm, enhances creativity, protects life from diseases.
Worn: Set in white gold and worn in the middle or little finger.
Ash: (*Hīra bhasma*)
Actions: Tonic, nutritive, aphrodisiac.
Uses: Gives strength, firmness, protects life, increases sexual power and *ojas*; chronic and wasting diseases (i.e., diabetes, TB), preserves life in difficult diseases (e.g., cancer, AIDS).
Substitute: Zircon ash (*Vaikrant bhasma*).

Hessonite Garnet (Golden variety-Gomedha) VPK=
Uses: Good balancing stone, calms nerves, quiets mind, relieves depression, recommended for almost everyone as it is removes illusion (*maya*), and negative astral forces that are due to the dark age in which it is believed we live.
Worn: Set in gold, worn on the middle finger.
Ash: Not used.

Cat's-eye (Chrysoberyl)VK- P+
Actions: Nervine, stimulant.
Uses: Stimulates *tejas*, promotes psychic and spiritual perception, mental disorders, stone of seers and astrologers.
Worn: Set in gold, worn on the middle finger of the right hand.
Ash: Not used.

Quartz Crystal VP- K+
Action: Similar to diamond but much weaker.
Uses: It is considered a stone for Venus, and being cloudy or milky, a stone for the moon also.
Precautions: It amplifies the existing emotions, leaving one open to impressions, so purifying and energizing it is used regularly with *mantras* and *sādhanā* (meditation) is necessary.
Ash: Rock crystal (*Sphatika bhasma*)
Actions: Alterative, hemostatic, tonic.
Uses: Bleeding disorders, anemia, chronic fever, jaundice, asthma, constipation, general debility.

Mineral and Metallic Bhasmas

Many mineral and metal *bhasmas* also exist and are used for a variety of health disorders. They are more powerful than herbs and have a faster healing action. *Bhasmas* need to be obtained from only the most reliable pharmacies. If they are improperly burnt one can develop severe illnesses. Currently, the United States and a few other countries are not aware of the non-toxic healing properties of some of the *bhasmas* such as lead, tin, and mercury.

Herb-increasing Properties of Gems & Their Tinctures

Hot and spicy herbs: Properties increased by using ruby tincture, or along with wearing ruby gems or substitute stones.

Tonic and rejuvenative herbs: Properties increased with yellow sapphire or yellow topaz tinctures or along stones or substitutes.

Blood cleansers, cool, detox liver, remove tumors: Properties increased by taking blue sapphire tincture or along with wearing the stone or its substitutes (i.e., amethyst).

Nervines and harmonizing herbs: Properties increased by taking emerald tincture or also with wearing the stone or its substitutes.

Stimulants and aphrodisiacs: Properties increased by using with red coral tincture or with wearing the stone.

Emmenagogues and reproductive tonics: Properties increased by taking with diamond tincture or by wearing a diamond or its substitutes.

Demulcents and nutritive tonics: Properties increased by taking with pearl tincture or by wearing pearl or its substitute.

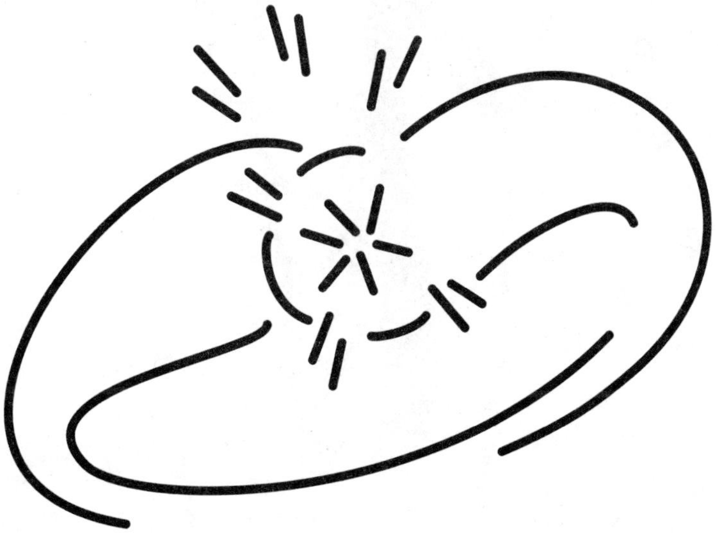

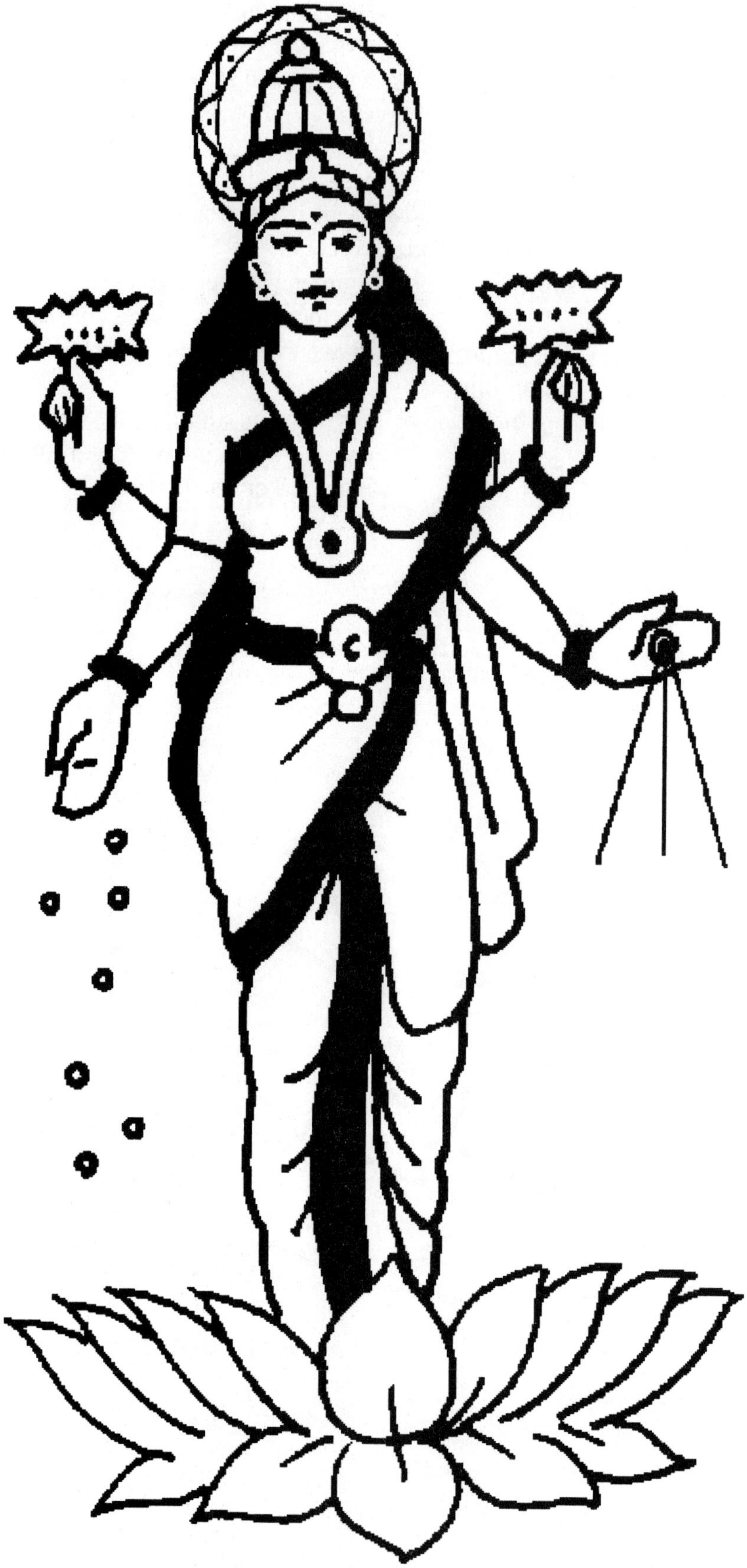

When one realizes Brahman,
what is there to realize,
and who is there to realize it?
Upaniṣhadic wisdom

Chapter 12
External Influences:
Lifestyles, Seasons, Exercise

Health prevention, in holistic terms, means balancing one's whole life. Thus, beyond considering one's physical, mental, and spiritual (inner) health, external situations of lifestyle and environment are also examined for their effects on health.

Morning & Evening Routine

'Cleanliness is next to Godliness,' as the saying goes. The ancient Āyurvedic texts placed great emphasis on the daily cleansing ritual. Below are some major suggestions.

Evacuation of bowels and urine is best done in the squatting position as the organs are aligned for the easiest release of waste (*malas*). This position also helps dispel gas.

Water (cool) instead of, or poured on toilet paper, is gentler to the anus. Oiling the anus after bathing is also healthy; it prevents drying.

Brushing with astringent, pungent, and bitter roots (or twigs made into brushes), twice a day, without injuring gums. Flossing is important and herbal tooth powders are also beneficial.

Scraping the root of the tongue with instruments of gold, silver, copper, tin, or brass. Curved U-shaped metal strips or spoons are used. Scraping removes obstructions in respiration. By scraping the whole tongue, one releases repressed emotions. Scraping the tongue is also done upon waking each morning.

Gargling with water or oil in the morning after brushing and scraping, improves voice, jaw, increases one's delight in eating; it also prevents a dry throat, cracked lips, and loose teeth (also see Chapter 19).

Eye Wash using cool to luke warm water improves vision and all eye disorders, and refreshes the mind (also see Chapter 7).

Oil Head *Abhyañga* using *brāhmī* oil (VPK=) or sesame oil (Vāyu), canola oil (Kapha) [ideally warmed], to avoid headaches, gray and falling hairs; it improves sense organs, promotes cheerfulness, and a pleasant glow. Sleep becomes sound and one feels happier. (Numerous oil *abhyañgas* are discussed in Chapter 7.)

Oil Ear *Abhyañga* A drop or two of vegetable glycerine, *brāhmī,* or canola oils rubbed into the ear holes heals and prevents Vāyu ear and hearing diseases, stiff back, neck, and jaw. This can be done several times a week (see Chapter 7).

Oil Body *Abhyañga* anointing the body with the same warmed oils used for the head, the body becomes firm, smooth-skinned, free from Vāyu, and tolerant of exertions and exercise. It is suggested especially to balance the sense of touch (Vāyu), as discussed in Chapter 16. Adding medicated oils such as *mahānārāyan* and *daśhmūl* to the base oil further nurtures tissues, and draws toxins out of the body. If digestion becomes sluggish due to oil application, the number of oil *abhyañgas* and the amount of oil used are reduced.

A Vāyu *abhyañga* includes the feet, lower back, colon area, neck, shoulders, and head.

A Pitta *abhyañga* includes the chest, the area of the back behind the heart, and head.

Kapha *abhyañga* covers the lower abdomen, chest, throat, and sinuses.

Foot *abhyañga* removes coarseness, stiffness,

roughness, fatigue, numbness, sciatica, vein and ligament constriction, cracks; it also improves vision and sleep. Since all the organs of the body have nerves extending to the feet, the entire body is exercised through foot *abhyañga*.

Marma abhyañgas Oil *abyañgas* described in Chapter 7 produce positive effects that heal and keep persons balanced. Heaviness, itching, dirt, anorexia, sweat, and odor are removed.

Bathing (or a shower) is purifying, an aphrodisiac, promotes life, removes fatigue, sweat, and dirt; rejuvenates, promotes *ojas*. Cleaning feet and excretory orifices daily promotes intelligence, purity, longevity, destroys inauspiciousness and dirt. Oil applied to the skin nourishes the tissue layers and draws toxins to the skin. Bathing after *abhyañga* removes these toxins, keeping the skin clean and healthy.

Clean clothes enhance one's charm, fame, and life span. They remove inauspiciousness and give pleasure, thus making it enjoyable to be around others.

Aroma Therapy oils, incense, scented soap, and flowers promote longevity, charm, nourishment, strength. They also enhance pleasing manners and destroy inauspiciousness (see Chapter 8).

Betel leaves chewed with certain fruits and cardamom aid in clarity and keep the mouth fresh.

Gem Therapy, colors, and ornaments promote wealth, auspiciousness, longevity, prosperity, happiness, charm, *ojas,* and destroy potential calamities in one's life (see Chapter 11).

Cutting hair, nails, beard/mustache is nutritive, life-promoting; beautifies and cleans.

An umbrella alleviates natural calamities, provides strength, protection, and guards one against the sun, wind, dust, and rains.

Carrying a stick gives support, strength, and longevity. It protects against enemies and destroys fears.

4:00 a.m. The *prāṇa* (vital air-force) is said to be purest at this time of day. Thus, it is good for a walk and for *sādhanā* (meditation).

Sunrise is a good time to have the eyes in the direction of the first rays of sunlight (though not looking directly at the sun). This exercise improves one's vision and vitality.

Sunlight is important to receive daily, if possible. Taking in sunlight in the winter is more difficult because it is colder and there is less sunlight. During summer the sunlight is best in the early morning or late evening, not in the intense heat between 11:00 a.m. and 2:00 p.m., when the sun is at its zenith and its rays are strongest. Sunlight is the only source of vitamin D4 and D5.

Find a livelihood that is not contradictory to one's *dharma* (God-given talents). Be civic-minded and care for the body: thus, happiness is brought about.

Wash hands before and after meals: cleanliness is next to Godliness.

Practicing *Sādhanā* (meditation) according to the instructions of one's *Guru* (spiritual teacher).

Snuff daily use for Vāyu, Kapha and Vāyu/Kapha *doṣhas* (see Chapter 7).

Seasonal Diet

It is recommended one's eating habits should depend primarily on one's *doṣha*, with a secondary consideration of the season. Āyurveda discerns six seasons in a year. The *Aṣhṭāñga Hṛidayam* also mentions transition periods between these seasons. Depending upon the country and geographical location one lives in, the seasonal experiences may vary.

The first three seasons are considered weakening because the sun takes away one's strength during the Northern Solstice. The sun and wind create a cooling, drying, and heating influence by removing the (nurturing) cool qualities of the earth, while the bitter, astringent, and pungent qualities develop. Thus, the tastes (qualities of the elements) of sharpness, dryness, and heat (Pitta or *agni*) gain predominance during this half of the year. It is the sun that burns up the *soma* (spiritual nectar) that weakens people. The tastes of bitter, astringent, and pungent are depleting in nature, so it is advised to eat foods having sweet, sour, and salty tastes to counteract the depleting effect.

The Six Seasons

Cool-Dewy (*Śhiṣhira*)	Mid-Jan. - Mid-March
Spring (*Vasant*)	Mid-March - Mid-May
Summer (*Grīṣhma*)	Mid-May - Mid-July
Rainy (*Varṣhā*)	Mid-July - Mid- Sept
Autumn (*Śharat*)	Mid-Sept - Mid-Nov.
Winter (*Hemanta*)	Mid-Nov. - Mid-Jan.

[Seasonal dates will vary according to country and geographical region. While the rainy season may not be literally experienced in some countries like the U.S., there may be subtler solar rays and gravitational influences that will still be applicable. Thus, some practitioners find the six seasons applicable even in countries outside of India.]

In the chart above the latter three seasons are considered a strength-giving time. The moon becomes more powerful, causing the sun to transfer his strength to the lunar orb. Heat is relieved by the moist and cool elements. In this Southern Solstice, where the moon predominates, the sour element is active during the rainy *Varṣhā* season; salt prevails in autumn and the sweet element grows in winter. These tastes gradually tone, or give strength to, humans. During *Varṣhā-Hemanta* (Rainy through Winter) the winds die down and the moon's cool rays produce *soma,* or nectar, that nourishes the spiritual energies of the people (and animals and nature). In these seasons, it is advised to eat foods of pungent, bitter, and astringent tastes to counterbalance the predominating tastes due to environmental effects. Traditional *pañcha karma* is not indicated at this time, but *Keralīya pañcha karma* is very helpful, especially for Vāyu *doṣhas* (see chart—page 40.)

Winter (Vāyu season) one avoids Vāyu-increasing, light foods, wind, cold drinks, and eats more steamed meals and dresses warmly. The digestive fire is much higher during this season, making heavier foods more easily digestible. If inadequate amounts of food are eaten, the *agni* fire will burn up the body's plasma *(rasa)*, vitiating Vāyu. Cane sugar, rice, oils, hot water, and milk products promote longevity, when taken during this season. Raw honey, sour and salty tastes are also suggested. Oil massage and heat (i.e., sauna, steam room etc.) are also suggested. During this season, physical expressions of love between married couples is healthy, according to Āyurveda. One's house is to be kept warm; drafts should be avoided.

Cool/Dewy (follow a program similar to Winter, only more intensely) The house needs to be wind-proof and amply heated. Sweet, sour, and salty foods are eaten, while pungent, bitter, astringent, light, cold, and Vāyu-increasing foods and drinks are avoided. Kapha accumulates in this season due to the cold and dampness of wind, clouds, and rain. This is the time that Pitta is balanced. This is the start of the Northern Solstice, whose winds begin to deplete human strength.

Spring is when the accumulated Kapha from the previous two seasons begins to melt or liquefy (i.e., Kapha becomes excessed), due to the gradual warming of the sun. This creates many Kapha diseases. Thus, evacuative measures like emesis are used, while heavy, sour, fatty, and sweet diet, and day naps are avoided because they increase Kapha. Exercise, oil massage, aroma therapy, smoking herbs, gargling, eye-washing and warm-water bathing are all suggested. Sandalwood paste is applied to body, and more barley (Pitta- and Kapha-reducing) and wheat (Vāyu and Pitta) products are eaten. Springtime is the season for amour (but not physical relations, as indicated during the winter season).

Summer is a hot and dry season (Kapha is normalized and Vāyu accumulates due to the dry or dehydrating effect of the heat). Thus, one eats more raw and lightly steamed vegetables, drinks cool juices, has more sweet things, *ghee*, milk, and rice. Sour, salted, pungent, and hot foods are avoided. It is suggested that there be little or no exercise at this time. One takes naps in a cool room during the day and sleeps in a well-ventilated room or on the roof (cooled by moon rays) by night. Sandalwood paste is also suggested for the body. Pearls and other cooling gems are suggested (depending on astrological indications). Fans, cool water, spending time in forests, and abstaining from sexual intercourse are suggested.

Mid-Jan. - Mid-July	eat more sweet, sour and salty tastes
Mid-July - Mid-Jan	eat more pungent, bitter and astringent tastes

Rainy The *agni* fire, already weakened from the dryness produced by the summer, is further diminished in the rainy season. During this season, the clouds are full of water; it is cold, windy, and in some places, snowy. These conditions continue to aggravate all three *doṣhas*. The water becomes muddy from the runoff caused by the rain, the warm earth creates sourness of water, while the *agni* digestive fire, as already mentioned, becomes even weaker. Pitta begins to accumulate due to weakened digestion and increased acidity in the atmospheric water. Vāyu, which had begun to accumulate in the dry or dehydrating summer heat, becomes aggravated due to weak digestion, acidic atmospheric conditions, and gas issuing from the earth. Kapha also becomes vitiated due to the acidity of the water.

Thus, in this season the three *doṣhas* start vitiating each other, causing many diseases of all three *doṣhas*. This is a troubling time for the mind and body, and all the *doṣhas* must be monitored very carefully. It is the transition season from the northern solstice (depleting), to southern solstice (strengthening). Depending upon the weather from day to day, one has to adjust their diet and lifestyle. Overall, one avoids cold drinks, day naps, dew, river water, exercise, sun, and intercourse. Foods and drinks are mixed with honey. On windy, cool, and rainy days sour, salty, and fatty foods are taken to pacify Vāyu. Also one takes wheat, rice, oils, soups, cooled Vāyu-reducing teas, oil massage, aroma therapy, baths, light clean clothes. A humidifier is used, if needed. *Pañcha karma*, purification therapies (see Chapter 7) are suggested as well (medicated emesis, purgation, enemas, and nasal oil therapy). Grain soups, medicated grape wines, or fermented foods are recommended.

Autumn The aggravated Pitta from the rainy season worsens as a result of the sudden warmth of the sun's rays. (In America, the equivalent is perhaps Indian summer— the transition between summer and fall.) Thus, Pitta reduction therapy is suggested. Medicated *ghee* (clarified butter with Pitta-reducing herbs), water, bitter, astringent, and sweet-tasting foods, easily digestible foods should be eaten, leaving room in the stomach (i.e., do not eat until satiated). Purgation therapy is also recommended. Lifestyle indications include sitting outside the house (on porches or balconies) in the evenings, wearing sandalwood oil or powder, drinking pearl water or wearing pearls, and moonlight bathing. It is advisable to avoid snow, ingesting alkalines, heavy meals, sour foods, excess or warm oils, fatty foods, exposure to the sun, alcohol or cigarettes, daytime naps, and eastern breezes.

Generally, persons should have a little of each of the six tastes (i.e., sweet, sour, salty, pungent, bitter, astringent) each day. However, during each month in which any of the tastes are environmentally predominant, one should reduce or avoid that taste to maintain balance. Since that taste is already excessed, consuming foods of that taste will only cause more imbalance. So each person must determine what constitutes a comfortable amount of each taste.

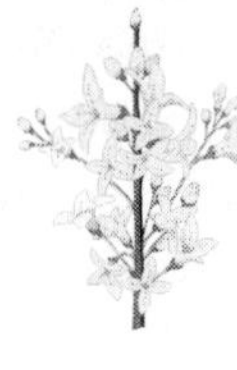

Seasonal Doṣha Balancing

Doṣha	**Slight Increase**	**Reduce *Doṣha***
Vāyu	Mid-May - Mid- July	Mid-July - Mid- August
Pitta	Mid-July - Mid- Sept.	Mid-Sept. - Mid- Nov.
Kapha	Mid-Sept. - Mid- Nov.	Mid-Dec. - Mid- Jan.

Transitional Periods are the seven days at the end and beginning of each season. Āyurveda advises slowly discontinuing the foods and lifestyle of the preceding season, and gradually adopting those suggested for the coming season. It is said that diseases are created by suddenly ending one habit, and just as suddenly beginning another. (*Aṣhṭāñga Hṛidayam- Sūtra*. Ch. 3. verses 58-591/2).

Exercise (Vyayama)

Another important lifestyle routine is exercise. It is a very important healing therapy for a balanced state of health. Exercise tones and balances all seven tissues (*dhātus*) and channels (*srotas*), improves blood circulation, muscle strength and tone, weight control, and the respiratory and digestive systems. Furthermore, it creates a harmonious state of mind. There are three levels of exercise: passive (e.g., massage), active (e.g., walking, skiing), and energy-balancing (e.g., yoga, Tai Chi). Yet, to prevent insufficient or excessive exercise, Āyurveda stresses an individual approach to exercise for each *doṣha* .

In the 1980's there was a popular saying, "no pain, no gain." However, this is only true for Kapha *doṣhas*. For Vāyu and Pitta constitutions, the saying is, "No pain, no pain." That is, exercise until one begins to perspire, then stop. Excess exercise will hurt and dehydrate Vāyu *doṣhas*, and it will overheat Pitta *doṣhas*. On the other hand, Kapha persons need a very active routine and are strongly advised to exercise a little past the point of fatigue. This improves mental alertness, digestion, and weight control. Professional and semi-professional athletes, and those who are on a program to build up their endurance, will need to perspire and feel some fatigue. These guidelines should always kept in mind and adapted as needed.

Vāyu *Doṣhas*: Though they prefer fast, exciting activities that will further raise their air element, they do better with slower, more grounding exercise. Active sports include walking (the best exercise), jumping on a trampoline, swimming, dancing, and cross-country skiing. To prevent drying out, it is best that Vāyu *doṣhas* oil their bodies as a warm-up. *Yoga* or stretching is also advised before and after exercising. Drinking Vāyu-reducing tea before exercise also prevents dehydration. Vāyu *doṣhas* tend to have joint and arthritic problems, so oil massage, stretching, and exercises that neither stress nor have high impact on the joints are useful. Varying exercises (cross-training) helps keep the Vāyu mind satisfied. Afterwards, eating a snack will restore energy. *Yoga* or stretching is suggested to remove stiffness. Five minutes in a steam bath or hot tub helps relax and offer moist, penetrating heat (but always keep the head out of the heat—see Chapter 7 on *pañcha karma*).

Active Sports

Doṣha	**Best Exercises**
Vāyu	walking (the best exercise), trampolining, swimming, dancing, and cross country skiing
Pitta	walking (the best exercise), down-hill skiing, water sports, team sports, hiking
Kapha	walking (best, especially after meals), active sports (e.g., basketball), jogging, water sports

Pitta *Doṣhas*: Have strong, athletic bodies. They love a challenge and competition, but need to maintain a sense of fun during their workout.

Team sports curb their tendency towards aggression and overly intense competitiveness, and develop their organization and leadership skills. Oil massage and *yoga* or stretching is advised before a workout. After exercising, *yoga* and relaxation are important. A cup of cooled herbal tea helps one to cool down. Enjoying a steam bath for 5 to 10 minutes is a good way to unwind (keeping the head out of the heat—see Chapter 7).

Kapha *Doṣhas*: Tend towards inactivity, yet need to exercise the most. They have the strongest constitution and require a strong workout, exercising a little past the point of fatigue. This improves their digestion, circulation, lymphatic system, controls weight and cellulite, and develops mental alertness. Having a dog as a pet takes advantage of their devoted nature to get Kapha *doṣhas* up and out on a walk. Jogging is excellent for the Kapha person (but not for Vāyu and Pitta *doṣhas*). They also do well in a structured exercise class.

Usually, persons are advised to breathe evenly during exercise to strengthen the lungs and digestive system; however, if there are respiratory, digestive, or inflammatory disorders, a workout is not advised.

Herbs

While many people take vitamins to enhance athletic performance, Āyurveda suggests that they may be difficult to digest and absorb. Herbs offer a more fundamental form of nutrition in their holistic or synergized form, which mother nature created—unlike vitamins, which may cause a potential for imbalance. Further, herbs are easily digested, assimilated, and work quickly. It is useful for the Vāyu *doṣha* athlete to drink some herbal tea or fruit juice before and after exercising to prevent dehydration.

The chart below lists herbs that athletes are advised to take between exercise sessions. They can be taken internally and applied externally as pastes.

Herb	Sports Benefits
Aśhwagandhā V- PK+ in excess	builds muscles and tissues, strengthens the mind and immune system; improves mind/body coordination and concentration; counters exhaustion and aging
Brāhmī VPK=	the best brain tonic; improves memory, concentration, intelligence and meditation; rejuvenates brain cells and nerves, the adrenals and immune system; purifies the blood skin and liver. When used with fo-ti it reverses the aging process
Chyavan Prāśh VPK= *	improves concentration and memory; an anti-oxidant; more vitamin C than oranges
Comfrey VP- K+	promotes tissue growth, heals sprains, wounds, and fractures
Fo-ti VP- K+	strengthens muscles, tendons, ligaments, and bones; rebuilds tissues, strengthens liver, kidneys, and the nervous system
Mañjiṣhṭhā PK- V+ **	heals damaged tissues and broken bones; cleanses and regulates liver, spleen, and kidney; the best blood purifier
Turmeric VPK=	stretches ligaments, heals strains, sprains, and bruises; one of the best antioxidants. Take 1 hour before exercise

** not recommended when congested*
***mix with cardamom or black pepper to balance Vāyu*

In all of life's activities, one should adopt
the middle course; avoid extremes.
Aṣhṭāñga Hṛidayam: Sū. Ch. 2; ver. 30

Chapter 13
Āyurvedic Psychology, Ethics and Spiritual Counseling

When reading the original Āyurvedic texts (i.e., *Charak Saṃhitā, Suṣhrut Saṃhitā, Aṣhṭhāñga Hṛidayam*), one sees that Āyurveda is truly a complete, or holistic, science. In these ancient writings, insights into the science of mind and body were seen as inter-dependent, and a complete system of psychological healing was laid out.

In Chapter 12, we discussed the role of the environment as one of several factors in creating imbalances. This also includes the external mental or psychological environment. Practically speaking, when a person cannot find any internal or physical causes for an illness, Āyurveda suggests looking to other factors (both mental and physical): for example, lifestyle plays a vital role in a balanced or healthy life. Environmental changes can balance a person as much as herbs, aromas, or other factors. Āyurveda emphasizes the natural restoration and development of harmony and health, in the home and surroundings. People are advised to do the following:

❶ Take in positive impressions.
❷ Release negative emotions (i.e., do not suppress them).
❸ Maintain and develop positive self-worth and self-esteem.
❹ Remember that the goal of life is Divine God Consciousness, or *mokṣha*.

Home:
❶ Insure surroundings of beauty and harmony.
❷ Gain rest and happiness.
❸ Use full-spectrum light bulbs in the winter if suffering from depression.

Make your dwelling, or at least some part of it, into a temple of sacred healing.

❺ Prepare an altar with photos of saints, sages, deities, sacred objects, statues, gems, *yantras*, incense, flowers, bells, and the like (according to your faith). When you use this space only for meditation and chanting, it will grow in spiritual peace and power, becoming magnetized by the constant devotion to Divinity.

Nature:
❶ Daily walks renew, revive, and refresh.
❷ Take hikes and nature walks; go camping.
❸ Visiting oceans, streams, waterfalls, and other natural bodies of water.
❹ Visit public gardens, or till and plant your own garden (with waterfall and pond if possible).
❺ Get adequate sun and fresh air daily.

Doṣhas and the Environment

Vāyu: Gains rest, relaxation, stability, peace and security from the environment.

Pitta: Needs relaxation, recreation, amusement, beauty, affection, and delight.

Kapha: Needs exercise, work, stimulation, motivation, exertion.

Love and Emotions

When a person is centered within themselves, there is a feeling that Mother Nature will provide all of one's essential needs, food, shelter, peace, contentment, grace, and Divinity. This faith in her will constantly grow. Faith emanates from within the individual, is automatically experienced, and is shared with others.

Faith, or Divine love, can be cultivated through *sādhanā* (meditation), proper diet, aromas, music, massage, *yoga*, and other therapies. These spiritual and healing methods allow persons to actively take positive control of their lives, clear their emotions, and enlarge their inner Divinity. These modalities help persons of different *doṣhas* in specific ways:

Vāyu: Releases fear and anxiety, and develops peace, faith, and courage.

Pitta: Releases anger, resentment, impatience, and develops love, compassion, and forgiveness.

Kapha: Releases greed, attachment, clinging, lethargy, and develops clarity and detachment from these emotions.

Developing Self-Worth

In the book *Yoga Vani; Instructions for the Attainment of Siddhayoga*, *Vedic* advice is offered for developing one's self-esteem. People are advised to try the following:

ॐ Test truth on the touchstone of their own heart.
ॐ Be aware that doubt can come even disguised as a friend, undermining one's desires and efforts for health and Self-Realization.
ॐ Realize that doubt is like a ghost trying to scare one from their *sādhanā* and spiritual life.

This *Vedic* advice provides methods to overcome doubts. A person learns what is true through a threefold process:

1) What one reads in the scriptures.
2) What one's *Guru* or teacher tells them.
3) What one experiences for themselves.

Only when all three situations come together will one have true knowledge. So one always makes sure they experience things for themselves before believing anyone or anything (i.e., does not follow blindly).

ॐ Have faith in one's *Guru* or and their meditation instructions.
ॐ The doubting or low self-esteem mind becomes peaceful through *sādhanā* and other Āyurvedic practices. A far-flying kite will easily come to hand when the string is wound around the stick. So too, the troubled mind comes under control through repeated repetitions (i.e., revolutions) of the *mantra*.
ॐ Practicing *sādhanā* daily forces the mind to work tirelessly, moving up and down the *suṣhumṇā* (the spiritual tube in the spine) until the mind tires and thoughts leave of their own accord. Then, the mind automatically becomes silent.

As one begins to feel and see this growing inner Divinity extend to others and the outer world, their sense of self-worth is strengthened. Thus, people are advised to notice and release negative attitudes and wishes (e.g., "I 'd rather be sick than confront this issue, I'm dumb and worthless, Nothing good ever happens to me.")

By contemplating, "*Who am I?*", one begins to feel inner Divine grace, thus instantly releasing negative thoughts, self-created or accepted from others. By not limiting oneself, one is able to accept their mistakes as a challenge—to alter the situation, and grow. Each mental *doṣha* has a specific exercise or focus to achieve balance:

Vāyu: Has to give up the negative self-idea that they are weak, afraid, isolated, agitated, or disturbed.

Pitta: Has to reduce the need to overachieve and take power (it makes the person appear domineering and others look worse).

Kapha: Has to practice atonement and give up the idea that they are defined by what they own, their family, culture, or job. They have to challenge a false sense of contentment.

Inner and Outer Worlds

As one releases negative ideas they hold about themselves and their life, they find that the outer world reflects how they feel within. People, animals, and nature are all a part of the same web of life; touch one area of the web and the whole web is affected. To help oneself, one must help others. As the realization of the interconnectedness or unboundedness of one's inner Divinity grows, the view of separateness between the inner and outer world diminishes. One begins to see that everyone and everything is a part of the same Divine essence. Conversely, when things are seen as separate from the Self, one longs for that which is believed to be other than the Self. This longing causes grief or suffering. However, as Self-Realization grows and one begins to see all things (i.e., themselves and others) as a part of the same Divine essence, then longing, grief, and suffering diminish. One begins to feel content because nothing is separate from themselves. Further, since the Self and others are seen as Divine, then the feelings of Divinity (i.e., eternal grace and bliss) replace the previously felt negative emotions and thoughts.

Another important way to develop this holy experience is by following one's *dharma* (one's life path or purpose; using one's innate or God-given talents). Working in a career one loves is another definition of following one's *dharma*. When persons work at something they love, it ceases to feel like work. When one uses their God-given talent, it creates a stronger connection between themselves and the Divine. Persons feel they are doing something meaningful and useful; life feels more purposeful.

Following one's *dharma* is not only uplifting for the individual, but by definition, is also beneficial for others. Thus, each *doṣha* begins to find a more positive social outlook.

Vāyu: The idea that the world is a harsh, unsupportive, clashing, chaotic, and unadjustable is reversed.

Pitta: Their idea that the world is a place to gain power and recognition is changed to a more harmonious and integrated view.

Kapha: A sense of greed and their need for outer security, clinging, and accumulation of material things is reversed.

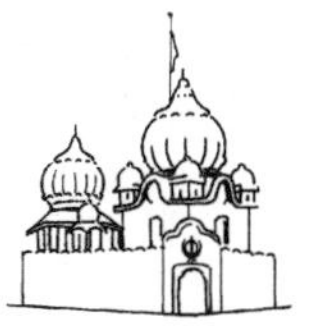

Āyurveda and Counseling

The ancient Āyurvedic texts were replete with information on how to live healthy and balanced:

❶ Lifestyle considerations based on physical constitution.

❷ Lifestyle considerations based on mental or emotional constitution.

❸ Psychological insights discuss personal, spiritual, career, relationship, and environmental issues.

❹ Maintenance, prevention, and longevity.

Charak Saṃhitā says that the practitioner who has even a basic knowledge of Āyurveda and practices out of love and caring for others will be a better practitioner than one who knows everything about the topic, yet is more concerned with fame and fortune. In short, to be completely effective, the essence of the practitioner must be able to touch the Soul of the client.

Practitioner/Client Exchange

The original Āyurvedic texts clearly state that counseling involves tact, diplomacy, and positivity on the part of the the practitioner. Respect for the client is paramount. Warmth, concern, and carefully listening to the client is better than having excess knowledge and skill while maintaining an impersonal or uncaring attitude. (Conversely, these ancient scriptures advise that the client also be respectful of the practitioner.)

Practitioners are advised not to become too intimate with clients (i.e., they should maintain a professional relationship), or else clients may begin to view the practitioner as a friend. Then, advice is only casually followed. A fine line exists between being sensitive and being casual or intimate.

Respect for the Divine within clients is urged because it allows them to listen to their own intuition and arrive at their own choices. As clients recognize the value and ability of their intuition, they find an increase in their own self-worth. Thus, it is important that clients understand the scope and potential that Āyurveda offers. In this way clients have more faith in the process and can more easily follow the Āyurvedic way. Clients must also feel their personal and spiritual life will be respected, knowing that consultations will be kept confidential.

Doṣha Personalities

The *Charak Saṃhitā* notes that each *doṣha* has a different personality; therefore, each *doṣha* requires a unique behavioral approach.

Vāyu: They are more fearful, and appear nervous, upset, or distracted. These *doṣhas* may feel hesitant, insecure, fidgety, unsettled, or doubtful about themselves or the therapy. Conversely, they may be overly enthusiastic and excited, expecting too much with no real motivation behind it. They tend to be ungrounded and hard to deal with (i.e., they need to have an 'into' body experience). These people may feel negative and worried about themselves and their condition, imagining things are worse than they really are (i.e., hypochondria).

Therapy: The practitioner attempts to get them to be more realistic about their situation and how to correct it; they need to bring them down to earth. They need to be treated delicately, like flowers. Vāyu *doṣhas* responsibly start their programs, then begin to slack off after a while.

Pitta: They think they know who they are and what they are doing. Probably, they will tell the practitioner what they should do for them. These people will analyze themselves and try to take over the consultation. They may have a critical, aggressive, or quarrelsome nature, asking for credentials or questioning the reliability of Āyurveda itself. Because they enjoy authority status and hierarchy, the practitioner needs to respond simply and objectively. This *doṣha* may expect the practitioner to heal them. They may judge the practitioner's qualifications or want the practitioner to tell them how they will be healed. However, the practitioner is advised not to be dragged into such game-playing. In short, *the more practitioners try to justify themselves, the more the Pitta doṣha will doubt them.* If the client is not happy with the credentials, then it is just as well; because with this client's frame of mind, the therapy could not work.

Therapy: First, the practitioner is advised to remain objective and rational, discussing the critical nature of the individual so they can learn to understand it as a cause of their imbalances. This process of awakening one's abilities to discriminate enables the client to control their lives as opposed to their trying to control life; they can change from having a critical nature to a discriminating disposition. Pitta *doṣhas* need to be treated in a friendly manner. These constitutions are cooled (balanced) by calm, pleasant circumstances and behavior. Only then will they feel the practitioner is on their side. This *doṣha* needs to feel they are seen in an authoritative light. When Pitta *doṣhas* understand what is entailed in self-responsible healing, they are very good at applying and following the therapies. However they must be cautioned not to become fanatical in the application of therapy; to avoid burnout, the practitioner should urge moderation. If the therapy does not go well, however, they are apt to become angry and critical. It is best for practitioners not to promise too much and to show that healing is the responsibility of the client.

Kapha: These persons need to be motivated, stimulated, or shocked into getting well. They are often lethargic, slow to act, or lazy; and find it hard to implement things. If left to themselves they will remain inert. They do not need comfort; although, they may seek it. Sentimentality is one cause of their health imbalances.

Therapy: Kapha *doṣhas* do not require much explanation; they need an extra a push. They need to be warned in order to make them respond and work on becoming healthy. This *doṣha* requires time and patience to implement information. They are more responsive to love and personal care, along with an insistence and firmness regarding the fundamentals of self-healing. If they slip back into their old habits, they return to their self-indulgent behavior. Thus, they may need more frequent visits and more interchange to stimulate them to get started. Once they start, they do well, with only an occasional need for motivation.

Vāyu/Pitta: This *doṣha* moves back and forth between fear to anger. They may only be looking for someone to dump their negative problems on. Usually their immune systems and energy levels are weak, and find it hard to undergo questioning or constructive criticism. Their fears and angers will often be suppressed.
Therapy: They need much nurturing, patience, consideration, and tact.

Pitta/Kapha: This dual *doṣha* is both energetic and stable; they are healthy and possess a strong immune system. Usually content, they approach holistic health for enhancement and improvement of energy. They lack the adaptability and flexibility of Vāyu energies. This *doṣha* prefers to dominate or control and to be possessive and conservative.
Therapy: They need movement, activity, creativity, and new challenges.

Vāyu/Kapha: These persons lack fire, energy, motivation, passion, and enthusiasm. They are generally weak, passive, dependent, and hypersensitive. They agree to everything they are told to do, but do not have the energy to carry through. Emotionally and mentally, they are nervous or easily disturbed. They can be chameleon-like in their personality, appearing as others want them to be.
Therapy: Delicate and sensitive questions are advised. These dual *doṣhas* respond to warmth and firmness, but it is hard to tell how well they are following the therapy. The practitioner is advised to see through them, helping them to become clearer and more practical in their lives.

Client's Attitude

First, the practitioner is urged to judge the sincerity of the client. Some people do not really want to be well, as they equate their lives with their illnesses. In this case, no one can help them heal. It is usually because one wants to be sick that they get sick. Being ill draws attention to themselves. The practitioner decides if a client wants help or merely attention.

The first questions addressed to the client are, "Do you want to be well? Do you have anything to gain by staying sick? Is your illness an escape? Will you spend the time needed to become well? Do you want to be healed or is this just a temporary amusement? Are you going to take responsibility for your health and heal yourself? Do you expect someone else to heal you?" The practitioner awakens the client's intelligence and waits to hear them make a commitment to heal themselves.

Yama and Niyama
Ethical Codes of Conduct

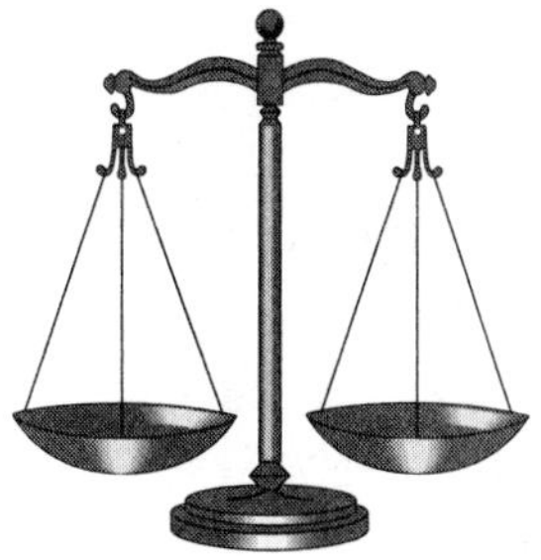

Good deeds done for reward bring heaven. Good deeds done without desire bring Liberation.

Upaniṣhadic Wisdom

Even the insects and ants should be treated with compassion and kindness, just as one's own self.
Aṣhṭāñga Hṛidayam: Sū: Ch. 2; ver. 23

To develop health and Self-Realization, *sādhanā* and Āyurvedic therapies are suggested. Further developments in spirituality and healing are gained by following the rules of virtuous behavior.

Yama

1. Ahimsa—not harming, not causing trouble to people, animals or the environment, or not feeling envy. One's job must be considered (i.e., this rule doesn't apply if one has a job that may require killing, like fishing or being a soldier. But even for the soldier, killing is to be only in self-defense or to protect the lives of the oppressed). Those whose job doesn't involve killing are advised not to kill.

2. Truth or saying what one means. Sincere words are meant to clarify one's ideas.

3. Non-Stealing—Not coveting other people's possessions; in thought, word, or action.

4. Brahmacharya—avoiding coition in thought, word, and action is applied to single persons. Married couples also have a form of *brahmacharya* as discussed in the *śhāstras*.

5. Aparigraha, or non-acceptance—to cease from wanting or chasing after material wealth or fame because it keeps one's mind attached or bound (i.e., not free or at peace).

Niyama

1. Purity (external) means pure food and cleanliness. (Internal) means a pure or *sattwic* mind attained through spiritual practices.

2. Contentedness with what is obtained through luck or the Grace of God.

3. Tapas, or rigor. Originally, tapas referred to being able to bear extremes of heat and cold, hunger, and thirst, etc. Today, many *gurus* say this sort of *tapas* is no longer needed. However, rigor may be seen in terms of personality. If a person offers excessive praise (warmth) or treats one in a very cold manner, persons are advised to ignore both and maintain their concentration on their inner Divine Self-Worth and the growth of their Self-Realization.

Wisdom sacrifice (spiritual inquiry from realized persons and meditation) is far superior to material sacrifice (austerities).
Bhagavad Gīta Ch 4 ver 25-34

Chapter 17 of the *Bhagavad Gīta* defines austerities as a threefold process involving the body, speech, and mind.

Body: Worship of God, holy persons, gurus, and the wise; act with purity, simplicity, continence, and non-injury.

Speech: That which doesn't cause harm or pain to others, is true, pleasant, and beneficial; and regular scriptural study.

Mind: Cheerfulness, kindness, silence, self-control, and purity of heart.

4. Study of Scriptures. Reading scriptures such as *Bhagavad Gīta, Yoga Vasiṣhta,* and *Upaniṣhads* is beneficial for developing a spiritual understanding or framework. Practicing *sādhanā,* as instructed by one's *guru,* is actually the deepest level of study because it is learned through direct experience within oneself.

5. Thinking of God as the Be-all and End-all. Credit all actions to the Supreme Soul. This helps eliminate the desire for the consequence of action, (e.g., I am not the doer, I am only the instrument. God is the doer) [of course this is not meant to be used as an excuse for living irresponsibly]. Thus, one becomes less attached to the material world and more devoted to the Divine Grace.

Faith

Faith develops Self-Worth. The highest form of Self-Worth is Self-Realization: seeing that the Self is Divine. It is an essential tool that keeps the mind from developing intellectual error. Intellectual error means to doubt one's true Self, and results in seeing objects as Eternal. So, faith in the growth of one's spiritual experiences (faith in what one experiences through their inner eye) is essential. Faith in the spiritual teacher and their instructions is needed.

Even well-meaning family and friends may cause one to doubt their inner spiritual feelings; others do not know what is in one's own spiritual heart. Thus, it is advised to hold onto what one knows from experience. Then, one's mind will continually maintain correct intellectual judgments for spiritual, mental, and physical health.

Yamas	**Results of Following Yama**
Ahimsa	no one feels enmity towards you
Truth	one's word becomes reality
Non-Stealing	wealth of gems is attained
Brahmacharya	power to infuse energy and knowledge unto the humbler ones grows
Non-acceptance	knowledge of previous births is gained
Niyamas	**Results of Following Niyama**
Purity	mind becomes *sattwic* (pure and holy)
Contentment	incomparable felicity is gained
Tapas	mental and physical impurities vanish

Spiritual Āyurveda

If money is lost, nothing is lost.
If health is lost, something is lost.
But if character is lost, everything is lost.
Smiles

As discussed earlier, the root cause of all illness is a lack of faith or connection with the Divine. Loss of love of one's inner, highest Self is the first stage in the development and cause of disease. Thus, if one devotes themselves to loving and thinking of themselves in the highest, most Divine sense, the root of illness is most easily eradicated.

To gain a deeper spiritual insight into Āyurveda, we look at the ancient *Vedic* scriptures that describe three bodies, or sheaths, that each human being has.

1) Physical Body: (*Sthula Śharīra*) is where the 3 humors, Vāyu, Pitta, and Kapha are the main energetic operating forces. Included in the physical body are 16 attributes, 5 sense organs, 5 organs of action, 5 elements and the mind (connected with the senses). There are two causes of lack of health, as discussed earlier, mind and body. Physical sorrow results in the loss of equilibrium of the *doṣhas*. Mental sorrow arises from anger, greed, desire, attachment, fear, melancholy, envy, and inability to attain desired objects. Troubles are also twofold, creatures and spirits. The first comes from the self and other people, animals, insects, and the like. The second comes from spirits (i.e., various forms of negativity) and weak planets found in one's *Jyotiṣh* astrology chart).

2) Astral Body: (*Sukṣhma Śharīra*) consists of 17 attributes:
Five senses of knowledge (attributes 1 through 5)
Five senses of action (attributes 6 through 10)
Five life-breaths (attributes 11 through 15)
Intellect, ego (attribute 16)
Mind, mind's heart (attribute 17)

It is not the physical organs (i.e., eyeball, nose, etc.), but the senses—sight, smell, vision, etc.—that provide information. Their physical limbs do not constitute actions, their essence does.

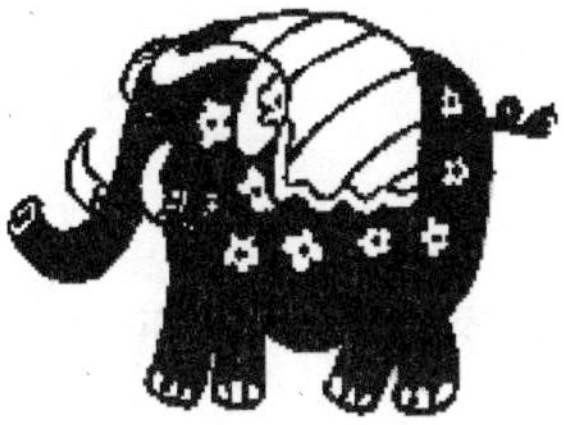

Senses of Knowledge

Sense	Ruler	Home
Sight	Sun	eyeball
Hearing	*Dik*	ear hole
Smell	*Aṣhvinī Kumar*	nostril
Taste	*Varuna*	tongue
Touch	*Vyān*	skin

Senses of Action

Sense	Ruler	Home
Speech *	*Agni*	organ of speech
Grasp	*Indra*	palm
Walk	*Upendra*	foot
Excrete	*Yama* **	anus
Urinate/pass semen	*Prajapati*	genitals

* *Speech produces sound from eight places: heart, throat, cerebellum, upper and lower lips, two palates, and tongue.*
** *He is different than* yama, *the codes of ethics discussed earlier.*

Senses of Life-Breaths

Vāyus	Direction/Property	Home
Prāṇ	out	heart
Apān	down	anus
Samān	digest food/equal	navel
Udān	up	throat
Vyān	distributes digested food	whole body

Life Breath Assistants

Ruler	Rules
Naga	hiccuping
Kūrme	opening the mouth
Krikara	sneezing
Devadatta	yawning
Dhananjaya	nutrition

Senses and Sub-Senses

Sense	**Mind**	**Ruler**
	Determination/ Irresolution	Moon
sub-sense	**Mind's Heart (Chitta)**	**Ruler**
	Inquisitiveness	*Achyuta*
Sense	**Intellect**	**Ruler**
	Coming to a conclusion	*Brahmā*
sub-sense	**Self (Ahamkara)**	**Ruler**
	Ego	*Saṃkara*

This subtle or astral body is also where the chakras exist.

3) Causal or Essential Body: (*Karana Śharīra*) surrounds the other two bodies in an oval or egg shape. It is the seed form of all attributes of the other two bodies. Yet, there are no attributes to it, just as an entire tree is contained in the seed but no tree is found at this level. The causal body consists of the five *tanmatras* (primal sensory energies, before they develop into the five senses) and the primal energies that develop into the elements (in the astral and physical bodies). Thirty-five astral potentials and 16 physical potentials exist here. Within this seed are the person's *karmic* impressions that motivate them through each birth. The causal body is located in the spiritual heart, situated just to the right of the center of the chest.

Creation itself emerges from this Supreme

energy, for it is the cause of causes. It is the knowledge of oneness of all things with the Creator (*Brahmā*). Being one, it causes many, yet 'the many' are essentially the one, just as a plate, a mug, and a pitcher are essentially all clay. It is called the delight cell due to its abundance of delight. One can experience delight through self-luminous experience. It is also called *pralaya*, or universal sound sleep, because the universe is annihilated in this body. Upon waking from sound sleep one may feel, "It was so peaceful, I was not aware of anything."

It is called a sheath because it conceals its true delight and properties. This sheath is the cause of ignorance. It has two energies, *abaran* and *bikṣhepa* (concealment and hallucination). A person may think the sun has become nonexistent when a cloud covers it. Similarly, a person may believe the causal body is nonexistent due to concealment by the causal sheath. It is the illusion that prevents persons from realizing their true inner nature. A piece of rope may appear to look like a snake. Similarly, the Soul may appear to be the actor. One may say, "I am a happy, a sad, or an infatuated person." This creates various illusions of life (*maya*). Properly stated, the reality of life is, "I am eternal and un-changing. Happiness or sadness is an ever-changing illusion."

Hairs grow of themselves, vegetables grow of themselves, so the first two bodies, the physical and astral, automatically grow from the causal body. The causal body grows by itself. No other reason exists for it to happen.

5 Delight Cells

The three bodies are divided into five cells, food, life, mind, knowledge, and delight.

Body	**Cell**	**Element**
Material	Food	Earth
Astral	Life, Mind, Knowledge	Water, Fire, Air
Causal	Delight	Ether

1. Food Cell (*Annamaya Koṣha*): The physical body is made up of food taken from the parents and transformed into semen and blood. Its cell or sheath hides the Soul, as a husk hides the grain. Thus, the Soul appears to be divided and troubled by birth, life, and death, when actually it is eternal —the creator of these processes.

2. Life Cell (*Prāṇmaya Koṣha*): This cell involves the fire organs of action and the 5 life breaths. The life sheath has concealed the true nature of the passionless Soul, making it seem full of passion. It makes the speechless Soul seem to be the orator and the desireless Soul seem to be full of desire.

3. Mind Cell (*Manomaya Koṣha*): This sheath includes the 5 senses of knowledge and mind, hiding the true nature of the Soul. The result is that the doubtless Soul appears as doubting, the sightless Soul appears to see, the sorrowless Soul seems full of sorrow, etc.

4. Knowledge Cell (*Vigñanamaya Koṣha*): This cell comprises the 5 senses of knowledge and the intellect. It conceals the true nature of the Soul by appearing as the doer or knower. It gives the Soul ego, action, name, fame, pride, etc.

5. Delight Cell (*Anandamaya Koṣha*): Delight constitutes love, delight, and enjoyment, concealing the true nature of the Soul which is beyond relative experiences of love, delight, etc. (i.e., these relative experiences have a beginning and end. The Soul is a never-ending experience of Divine love, etc.). This cell appears as the causal body of all beings.

Devotion:
The Best Āyurvedic Medicine

Through devotion or attention to the eternal Divine state of life, one heals and prevents disease and ultimately develops and attains Self-Realization, the goal of Āyurveda. For spiritual healing, a personal or devotional approach is crucial. Some people believe in *Kṛishṇa*, some in Jesus, others in Buddha, still others commune with their God through music. Devotion is considered the major healing practice of Āyurveda, for it is only through *sādhanā* (devotional meditations or prayer) prescribed by one's spiritual teacher or *guru* that *karmic* diseases can be erased and persons can merge with their beloved form of God.

In order to find a qualified teacher, or *guru*, one first must decide what one is looking for. Different *gurus* teach different subjects, much as is done in school. Many teach about powers, fame, and fortune. However, only a rare few teach simple, natural Self-Realization. A true *guru* is one who, at first sight, produces bliss or pleasure in a person. Also, they will charge students no fees for training.

Some people who have already been following a *guru* may feel they have learned all they can and need to move on to another *guru*. The *Vedic* scriptures not only validate this feeling, but suggest it is necessary for the student to make the change if and when the time comes. Specifically, the *Vedas* state that if a student has spent at least a year sincerely following a teacher's guidance and still does not have pleasant results, they have the right and obligation to change teachers. Thus, even the choosing of one's *guru* is very much along the Āyurvedic lines of taking control of one's health; self-responsibility. Persons are cautioned against blindly following teachers. The scriptures say that 3 aspects to knowing Truth exist: the words of the *guru*, the words of the scripture, and the experiences of the pupil. Only when all 3 are corroborated does one feel confidant that something is true.

In this state one embraces everyone and everything as the same (Divine) Self. One sees all as themselves; everything inside, outside, and in between is the same Divine eternal Self. The Divine Self is all that exists. Then, no separation can exist; no cause for wanting or longing can arise. When longing ceases to be, no suffering or disease can develop. Suffering only results from seeing something as separate from oneself and desiring to make it yours. Sadness develops because one misses that from which they believe they are separated. Once this illusion is seen through, the cause of suffering vanishes, just as the darkness cast by a cloud disappears once the sun shines unobstructed.

This is the *Vedantic* goal of life and the Āyurvedic goal as well. Thus, following one's personal spiritual path is the best Āyurvedic medicine.

While the importance of having a spiritual *guru* has been discussed, not everyone will find or desire a *guru*. In this case, one is advised to listen to their inner *guru*. The inner *guru* is the highest *guru*.

Origin of the Spiritual Body

The *Vedic* scriptures, the *Srutis*, discuss the spider that produces thread from within itself. The thread is woven into a web, and then withdrawn back into its own body. This is said to be analogous to the universe that is produced from Eternal Consciousness (*Chaitanya*) and then vanishes into itself. This is the only cause of creation. Further, it is said that from a mere 'glance' of the consciousness, its energy begins to move outward (with *tamas*—lethargy or destruction— as its main quality) and the sky (ether) is created. Consciousness then glances at the sky and air, or Vāyu is produced. Glancing at Vāyu, fire (*tejas*) is then created. From consciousness in-gazing at *tejas*, water (*ap*) is born. Lastly, earth (*pṛitivi*) is created from consciousness glancing at water. They are distinguishable because they are produced by *tamas*, the destroyer of the in-distinguishable. These 5 elements are essential or undivided. The spiritual and material bodies are created from them.

5 Senses of Knowledge	5 Essential Elements	5 Organs of Action
sattwa	elements	*rajas*
1. hearing (ear)	1. sky/ether	1. tongue
2. touch (skin)	2. air	2. hand
3. sight (eye)	3. fire	3. feet
4. taste (tongue)	4. water	4. genitals
5. smell (nose)	5. earth	5. anus
heart	all 5 essential elements	vital energy (life)

Five Senses of Knowledge (sense of hearing, sight, smell, taste, and touch) originate in the *sattwic* portions of the five elements. Five organs of action (tongue, hands, feet, anus, and genitals) originate in the *rajasic* (action) portions of the five elements.

The 5 senses of knowledge are *sattwic*, while the 5 organs are *rajasic*.

Sound is produced in the sky (*akaṣh*). The ears hear the sound and the tongue produces the sound.

Air can be felt (touched) on the skin, and the hands grasp through touch.

Fire's (*Tejas*) attributes are beauty and form. The eye appreciates this movement (seen as gracefulness) and comes from the feet that move.

Water's (*Ap*) attribute is taste. The tongue tastes, and the sexual organ is the main source of delightful sensation. For example, the sense of taste is on the tongue, producing delightful taste, and the action of delight is felt from the genitals.

Earth's (*Pṛitivi*) attribute is smell, and the anus is the primary discharging channel of malodorous smell, as stool.

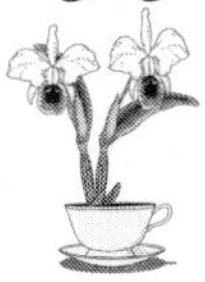

The heart has 4 aspects: mind, intellect, heart, and ego.	
Aspect	**Function**
Mind	resolution and irresolution
Intellect	decision making
Heart	inquisitiveness
Ego	self-existence
Vital energy has 5 aspects: *prāṇ, apān, samān, udān, vyān.*	
The spiritual body has 2 parts; individual and universal.	

Universal: Consciousness or Supreme Self, living in the universal spiritual body, is called *Sutrātma* (thread of the Self) because it is the common thread in every object, like a thread in beads. It is also called *Hiranyagarbha* and *prāṇ* because it possesses knowledge, will, and energy created by the 5 essential elements. This *Hiranyagarbha* is finer than the material elements. Within the body one feels as though in a state of half-sleep. Three cells—knowledge, mind and delight—exist here. Here the Soul possesses will, desire, etc., just as in the waking state; only it is not material. Thus, it is called the state of absorption of the material elements.

Individual: Consciousness (*Chaitanya*), living in the individual spiritual body, has a brilliant inner sense. It is finer than the individual material body; one feels the existence of the brilliance as the state of half-sleep. Three cells also exist in this state with will, desire, etc., and are also called the absorption of the material body. That is, the individual material body exists in seed form in the individual spiritual body.

Individual and universal spiritual bodies mentally experience the sounds concerning enjoyable objects (enjoying objects in secret).

Origin of the Physical Body

Hiranyagarbha or Supreme God, residing in the universal spiritual body, divides the 5 essential elements with 5 material elements. This happens with a 'glance', for revealing Himself in material form. The material world was created from these elements.

The 5 essential elements are divided into 2 parts (10). The first 5 parts are each divided into 4 equal parts. These smaller parts of each element are added to the other half of each element. These 4 equal parts combine with the half-elements, producing the material elements. Each material element is made up of 1/2 material element (i.e., water (*ap*) is 1/2 material water, 1/8 essential sky (*akaṣha*), 1/8 essential air (vāyu), 1/8 essential fire (*tejas*), and 1/8 essential earth (*pṛitivi*). [see diagram on next page]

From these 5 divided or material elements, the 14 worlds have been created (7 worlds above and 7 worlds below). In these 14 worlds the material bodies of 4 different kinds of beings are born (from the womb, egg, sweat, and earth). Their food and drinks are also produced in these worlds.

In addition to universal and individual spiritual bodies, individual and universal material bodies also exist. The individual material body arises from separate objects of knowledge (e.g., a tree, a drop of water, etc.). The universal material body is born of knowledge of objects in combination (e.g., forest, lake). The food cell and material body are products of foods arising from the transformation of edible fluids and material enjoyment respectively.

Consciousness in the universal material body is called *Vaiswanara* because it functions in all humans as a whole. It is also called *Virat* because it has various manifestations. This is the awakening of the universal material body.

Consciousness in the individual material body is called *Viswa* and functions as ego in different material bodies while maintaining the spiritual body. This is the awakening of the individual material body. In the waking state, these two material bodies perceive the material world through the senses (*Bahihpragña*).

Composition of the Five Elements

Material Element	Essential Elements			
1/2 Ether	1/8 Air	1/8 Fire	1/8 Water	1/8 Earth

Ether Material Element

Material Element	Essential Elements			
1/2 Air	1/8 Ether	1/8 Fire	1/8 Water	1/8 Earth

Air Material Element

Material Element	Essential Elements			
1/2 Fire	1/8 Ether	1/8 Air	1/8 Water	1/8 Earth

Fire Material Element

Material Element	Essential Elements			
1/2 Water	1/8 Ether	1/8 Air	1/8 Fire	1/8 Earth

Water Material Element

Material Element	Essential Elements			
1/2 Earth	1/8 Ether	1/8 Air	1/8 Fire	1/8 Water

Earth Material Element

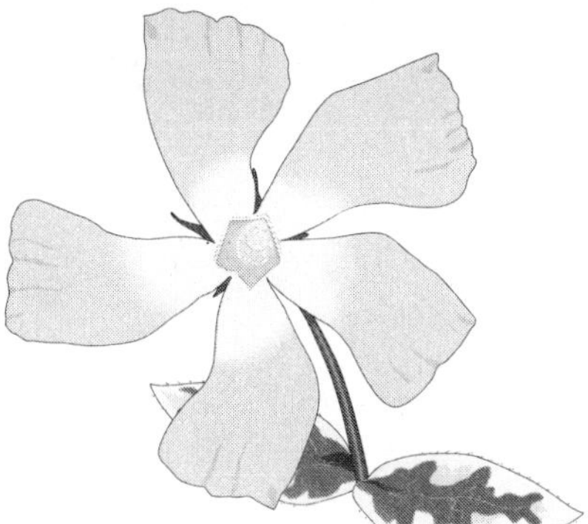

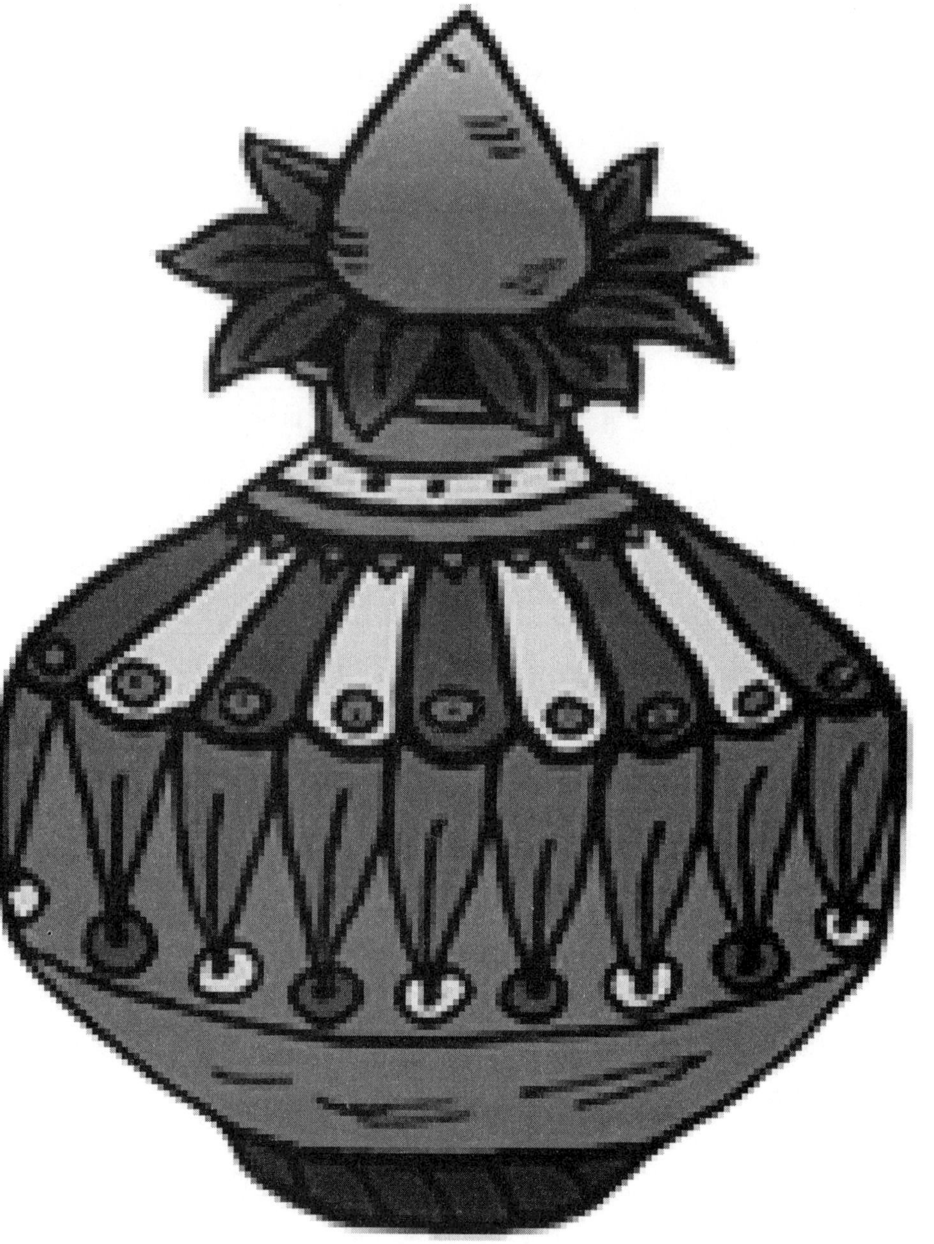

Section 4:

Specific Illnesses and Diseases; Signs and Symptoms, Cause, Development and Therapies

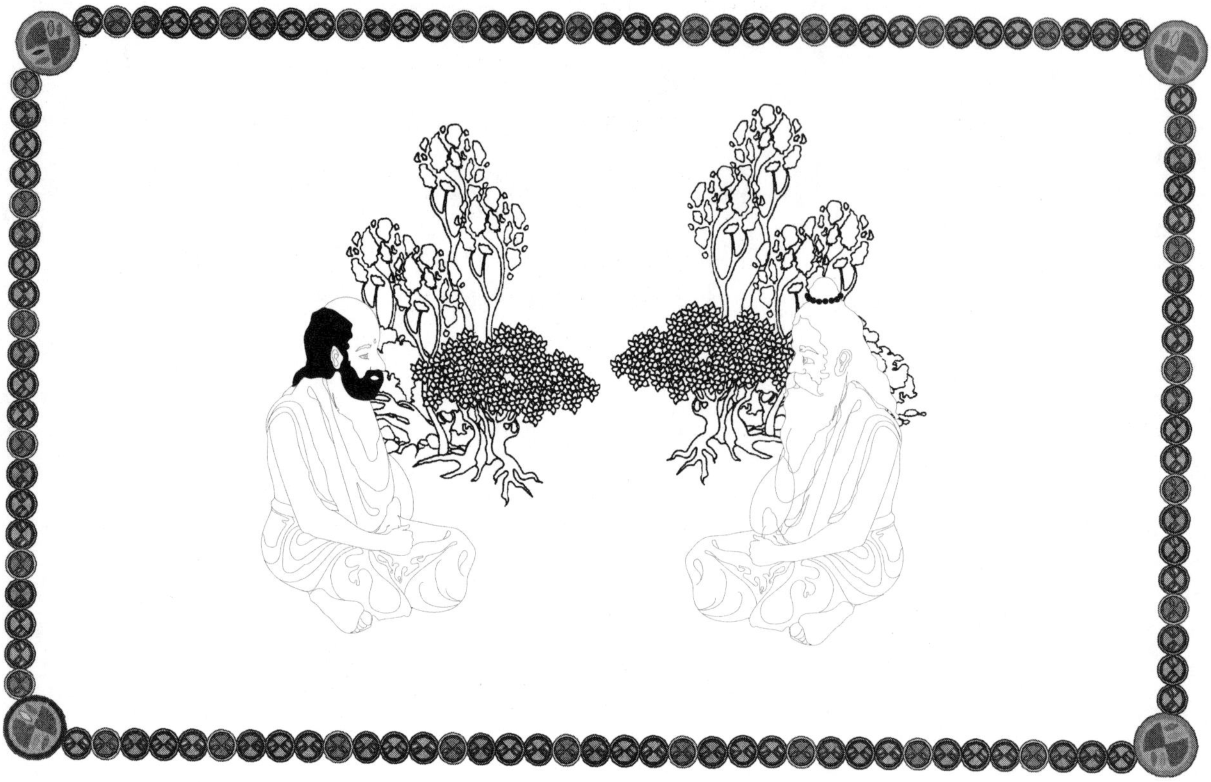

Chapter	System	Diseases, Conditions, Topics	Page
14	Circulatory	*Raktapitta*, anemia, heart diseases, blood pressure, arteriosclerosis, paraplegia	355
15	Digestive	Anorexia, vomiting, diarrhea/dysentery, digestive and abdominal disorders, jaundice, gall stones, dyspepsia, indigestion, gastroenteritis, colic, hyperacidity, gastritis, malabsorption, food allergies, parasites, constipation, hemorrhoids, obesity, candida, ulcers, toxin (*āma*)	363
16	Infections/ Wounds	Fever, abscess, sinus, wounds, ulcers, fractures/dislocations	393
17	Respiratory	Cough, breathing, hiccup, T.B., cold	409
18	Urinary	Stones, retention, gravel, obstruction, diabetes	419
19	Ear/Nose/ Throat	Ears, ear lobes, nose, throat, catarrh, hoarse throat, eyes, mouth disorders	429
20	Nervous	Nervous system, convulsions, sciatica, epilepsy, addictions, alcohol, fainting, coma, wasting, multiple sclerosis, Parkinson's, Alzheimer's	457
21	Skin	Warts, skin disorders, leukoderma, herpes zoster	479
22	Neoplasm	Scrotum, hernia, fistula, elephantiasis, tumors, cancer	493
23	Reproductive	Female reproductive, pregnancy/childbirth, *grahas* (planets afflicting newborns), male reproductive, prostate, venereal diseases	503
24	Immune	HIV/AIDS, epstein barr	527
25	Metabolic	Edema, meningitis, tonsillitis, gingivitis, dental abscess, goiter, hypo- hyperthyroid gout, thirst	531
26	Miscellaneous	3 vital *marmas* (heart, bladder, head), arthritis/rheumatism, dangerous spiritual practices, herbs for *dhātus* and organs, gland definitions, herb doses and times; recipes, mutually contradictory foods, herbal preparation, use, and mixing; acupuncture	541
27	External	Beauty Care, *Jyotiṣh - Vedic* Astrology, *Vedic* Architecture, Feng Shui, Scientific Research	557

With the understanding of Tridoṣha theory and the various therapies available in Āyurveda, this section looks at each individual illness and disease. Here, is described in detail, the cause, signs and symptoms (including the hidden symptoms), path of development, and therapeutic suggestions. When different *doṣhas* are responsible for various forms of an illness or disease, they are discussed individually.

The index above shows the disorders covered in this section, grouped according to the various bodily systems. In a few cases, some of the disorders can be related to two systems and so will be discussed at the end of one chapter and related to the next system (chapter) as well.

Blood Circulation
Principal Veins and Arteries

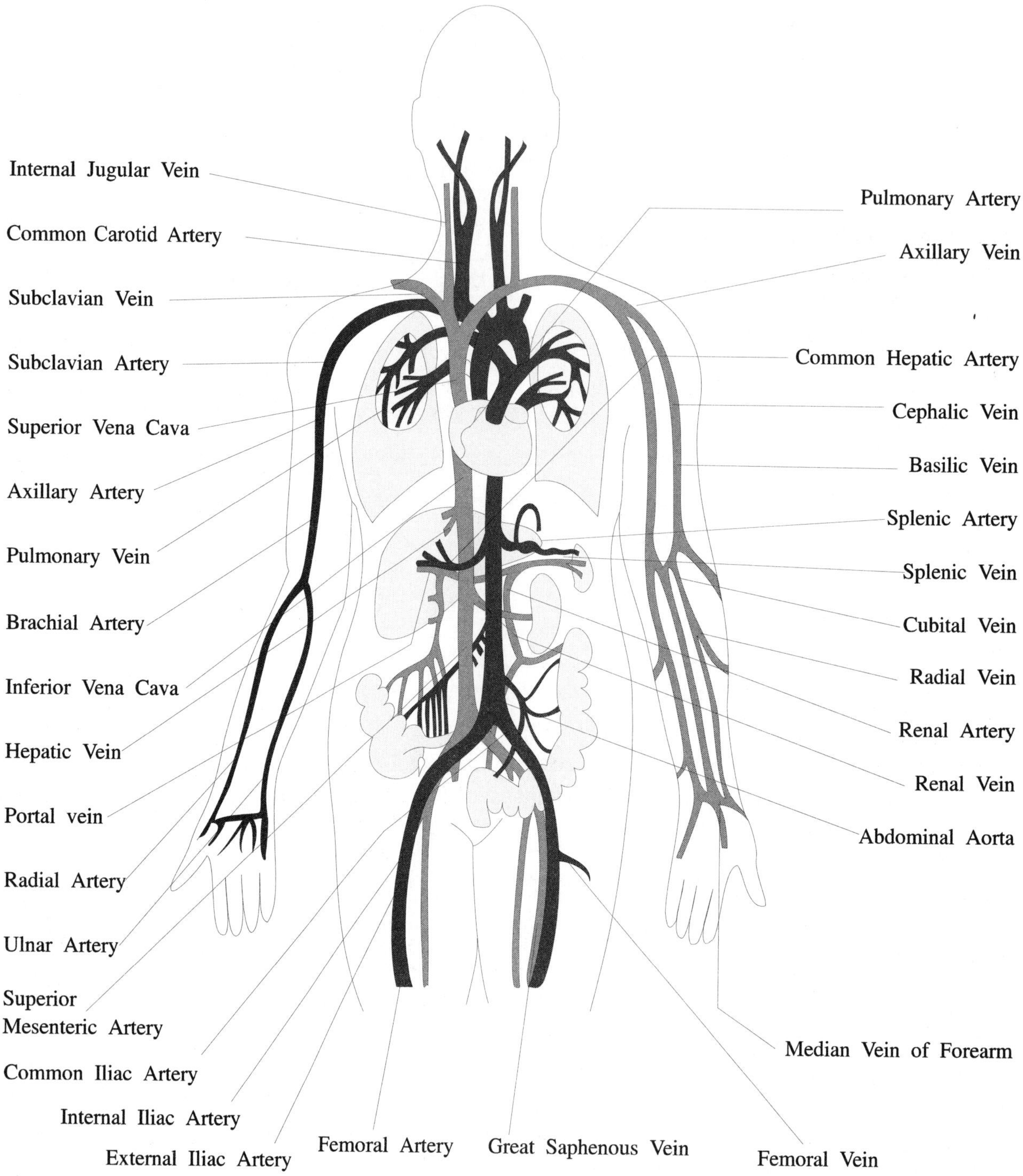
Internal Jugular Vein
Common Carotid Artery
Subclavian Vein
Subclavian Artery
Superior Vena Cava
Axillary Artery
Pulmonary Vein
Brachial Artery
Inferior Vena Cava
Hepatic Vein
Portal vein
Radial Artery
Ulnar Artery
Superior Mesenteric Artery
Common Iliac Artery
Internal Iliac Artery
External Iliac Artery
Femoral Artery
Great Saphenous Vein
Femoral Vein
Median Vein of Forearm
Pulmonary Artery
Axillary Vein
Common Hepatic Artery
Cephalic Vein
Basilic Vein
Splenic Artery
Splenic Vein
Cubital Vein
Radial Vein
Renal Artery
Renal Vein
Abdominal Aorta

Vāgabhata excels in sūtrasthāna.
Suṣhruta excels in sārīrasthāna.
Charak excels in chikitsā
preface in Charak Saṃhitā

Chapter 14
Circulatory System
Bleeding, Anemia, Heart, Blood Pressure, Arteriosclerosis, Paraplegia

Bleeding (Raktapitta)

Development: The causes of bleeding include overeating or drinking substances that increase Pitta, (e.g., red peppers, garlic, onions, alcohol; penetrating, pungent, sour, or salty tastes), animal products, dry vegetables; excess junk food or pastries after an excess of food. The excessed Pitta (blood or hemoglobin byproduct) opens the entrances of circulation channels. It then enters these channels and mixes with the blood, circulates throughout the body, and blocks the channels. The blood and Pitta vitiate or aggravate each other because they are both of a heating nature. As the heat increases, it becomes malodorous, and begins to penetrate vessel and tissue cell walls. Thus, it diminishes the clotting process and produces bleeding. The liver and spleen are the origin sites of bleeding. When Pitta is in liquid form, it is related to *ranjaka* and *pachaka* (which are in the stomach, liver, and spleen). Bleeding is due to Pitta associated with Kapha (and a little Vāyu). Examples of bleeding diseases are hemophilia, purplish skin patches (*purpura*), and an excess of red blood corpuscles (polycythemia vera).

Premonitory or Incubatory Signs: Heaviness of head, loss of appetite or taste causing burning sensations in the chest (which then produces indigestion), needing cold things and feeling hot, fumes coming from the stomach or mouth, increased acidity, vomiting or the fear of vomiting from seeing vomited materials, foul smelling vomit, cough, difficult breathing, dizziness, exhaustion, smelling or tasting iron, blood, and raw fish; burps of sour taste and vinegary smell, loss of voice, reddish, yellowish, or greenish eyes, skin, nails, urine, or feces; nose, mouth, ear and eye excretions; pimples, body ache, indistinguishability of blue, red, and yellow colors, seeing red, yellow, or blue colors in dreams.

Features: Bleeding from the facial orifices (nose, mouth, ears, eyes, throat), from the lower orifices (penis, urethra, vagina, genital tract, or rectum), from all channels, through hair follicles on the skin, or simultaneously through upper and lower orifices.

Pitta is the primary *doṣha* causing bleeding. Kapha is the secondary *doṣha* for upper orifice bleeding. Vāyu is the secondary *doṣha* for lower orifice bleeding. All three *doṣhas* are the secondary cause of simultaneous upper and lower orifice bleeding.

When vitiated blood (*Rakta* Pitta) becomes mixed with Kapha, it becomes dense, pale yellow, oily, and slimy. When *Rakta* Pitta is associated with Vāyu, it becomes gray, reddish, foamy, thin, and non-oily. If *Rakta* Pitta is further vitiated by Pitta, it becomes pale red and black. When two, or all three *doṣhas,* vitiate the blood, the signs and symptoms of the respective *doṣhas* occur. [Generally Pitta causes vitiated blood, but later it may mix with Kapha or Vāyu to cause what is referred to as Kapha-caused bleeding or Vāyu-caused bleeding. Secondary-*doṣha* rules are the same for other diseases (e.g., fevers that are mainly Pitta-caused or for tumors that are mainly Vāyu-caused). When the aforementioned primary *doṣhas* mix with the other *doṣhas,* they create fevers or tumors said to be caused by the other respective *doṣhas*.]

Upper Bleeding

This is indicated by bleeding from the nose, mouth, and ears. These diseases can be healed through purgation with Pitta-relieving herbs (bitters—e.g., *musta*, *chirāyatā*, *kuṭki*; and astringents—*mañjiṣhṭhā*, red raspberry, turmeric) that also relieve Kapha. After Kapha has been balanced, sweet herbs also can be used to balance Pitta. Upward bleeding mainly leads to association with Kapha.

Lower Bleeding

Places of lower bleeding include the rectum, urethra, and genitals. These diseases are controllable through emesis and sweet, moist, Vāyu-reducing herbs. Downward bleeding mainly leads to association with Vāyu.

Purgatives help reverse the direction of vomiting, whereas vomiting reverses the direction of lower orifice bleeding.

If bleeding is associated with only one *doṣha* it can be healed. If two *doṣhas* are associated with the bleeding, it cannot be healed, but it may be controlled. Simultaneous bleeding cannot be healed because no herb or therapy can produce simultaneous healing results. Tridoṣhic herbs are recommended (e.g., *gokṣhura*, gotu kola, *guḍūchī*, coriander, *bhṛiṅgarāj*, *triphalā*). Bleeding from both directions leads to association with Vāyu and Kapha.

Complications: Mainly hoarseness, but also weakness, anorexia, indigestion, difficult breathing, coughing, fever, diarrhea, edema, consumption, and anemia can develop.

Bleeding Therapies

After determining the cause, direction (and its main and secondary *doṣhas*), the strength of the person and the disease, the person's constitution, season and stage of disease, either reducing (purificatory) or toning (palliative) therapies are begun.

When a strong person has mild bleeding—produced by any one *doṣha* (without other complications), therapy is begun.

If bleeding is caused by overnourishment and the person is strong (and their muscles are strong), then it is not advised to stop the bleeding immediately because the *doṣhas* are mixed with *āma* and will have a natural tendency to be eliminated. Premature stoppage of bleeding can cause many problems such as throat obstructions, bad smell in the nose, fainting, anorexia, fever, benign tumors, enlarged spleen, constipation, skin diseases, difficult urination, hemorrhoids, abscesses, and poor complexion (but if the person is weak and the *doṣhas* are diminished, then it is necessary to stop the bleeding).

Fasting and Nourishing Therapies: Since Pitta and blood become aggravated due to *āma*, fasting is the first line of therapy. This holds true for upward bleeding, *āma*, aggravated Kapha, or if hot and oily factors caused the bleeding. For all other causes nourishing therapy is used.

The *Charak Saṃhitā* (*Chikitsāsthānam* Ch. 4 verses 31-35) suggest the following therapies,

Upper Bleeding During the earliest stage, a soothing tonic is given, boiling 12 grams of herbs [date palm sugar, grape juice, bitter herbs (e.g., *musta*, *āmalakī*, *bhṛiṅgarāj*, *gokṣhura*, *mañjiṣhṭhā*, jasmine), sandalwood and licorice] in 3.072 liters (approximately 3 quarts) of water until half the water is left. It is then cooled and taken with cane sugar (*tarpana*).

Downward Bleeding In the earliest stage, rice flour boiled with 11 parts water (*peyā*) is taken. This is a very good and time-tested remedy for hemorrhagic dysentery. Herbs appropriate for balancing the excessed *doṣha*(s) are used for both upward and downward bleeding. For one desiring sour tastes, *āmalakī* and pomegranate teas are used.

Sweet, nourishing liquids are useful in the earliest stage of bleeding, even when Kapha is involved, because they alleviate Pitta (the predominantly excessed *doṣha*.

Other Therapies

Cause	Overeating
Doṣha(s)	multiple *doṣhas*
Upper Bleeding	purgation therapy advised*
Lower Bleeding	emesis/and depending upon person's strength palliative or nourishing therapy*

** For purgation or emesis, one needs to have a strong digestion and constitution. Persons need to be prepared for the therapies, and should have no complications. These therapies are useful only when bleeding is caused by overnourishment and an excess of aggravated doṣhas. Muscle tissue also must be strong, and therapies should be practiced only during their appropriate times of day and seasons.*

Aṣhṭāñga Hṛidayam Therapies

Upper Bleeding	**Lower Bleeding**
1st: Corn flour with cold water, *ghee* and cane sugar	1st: Boiled, semi-watery rice (*peyā*)
2nd: Bitter/astringent herbs, teas can also include moistening herbs like sandalwood; fasting	2nd: Sweet nourishing herbs

Foods that alleviate bleeding disorders include rice, *mūngdal*, lentils, chick peas, kidney beans, neem, *chirāyatā*, steamed bitter vegetable soups, and *ghee*. When bleeding is associated with Kapha, more diuretic vegetables are used. Simple meals may be made from watery-cooked rice (*peyā*) with *ghee* and *balā*.

Should thirst be accompanied by bleeding, several therapies are useful: tea made with bitter herbs or fruit juices that are sweet or bitter (e.g., grape or cranberry). Should one have a strong digestion and constitution, they may drink water until satisfied. However, for all others, water is taken in small quantities.

For Vāyu-caused bleeding, demulcent herbs like comfrey, *balā*, and *vaṃśha lochana* are very helpful.

Anemia (Pāṇḍu-roga)

Development: When the *doṣhas* become aggravated, and Pitta is mostly excessed, the Pitta in the heart is forced into the arteries and veins attached to the heart. It is Vāyu that causes Pitta to move and then spread throughout the body. Pitta then vitiates Kapha, skin, blood, and muscles, causing them to turn yellowish white (most common color), deep yellow, or green. Five kinds of anemia exist: Vāyu, Pitta, Kapha, Tridoṣha, and a kind from eating mud.

Premonitory Signs: Heart palpitation, dry skin, loss of taste and appetite, yellowish urine, not sweating, poor digestion, weakness, and exertion.

Symptoms: The tissues become heavy and loose, *ojas* is burnt up; thus damaging the health of the blood and fat. Tissues become flabby, the heart rate increases, and eye sockets swell; there is debility, anger, and expectorating of phlegm. Other symptoms include loss of speech, dislike of food and cold things, hair loss, poor digestion, weak thighs, fever, difficult breathing, constant ear noise, dizziness, and exertion.

Vāyu: Body aches, piercing pain, tremors, blackish red complexion; discoloration of veins, nails, feces, urine, and eyes; edema, gas, astringent taste, dry feces, pain in the ribs and head, dry skin, anxiety, insomnia, and constipation.

Pitta: Veins, nails, feces, urine, and eyes are green and/or yellowish, fever, unconsciousness, thirst, perspiration, fainting, a desire for cold things, body odor, bad breath, bitter taste, loose bowels, yellow urine and stool, acidity, burning sensation.

Kapha: Veins, skin, face, eyes, urine, and stool are white; there is stupor, salty taste, hair standing on end, loss of voice, excess phlegm and salivation, cough and vomiting, edema, overweight, sleepiness, and heaviness of the limbs.

Tridoṣha: Symptoms of all *doṣhas* appear, and are difficult to bear.

Mud: Habitual eating of astringent mud aggravates Vāyu. Eating salty mud aggravates Pitta. Sweet mud aggravates Kapha. Plasma and other tissues are vitiated by the dryness of mud that further dries the tissue's channels. Mud does not get digested and fills and blocks the channels. This produces edema in the abdomen, legs, face, and genitals; parasites develop in the alimentary tract, feces are warm, watery, and mixed with blood and mucus, weakened sense organs, loss of physical strength, life sap (*ojas*) complexion, and digestion. Anemia develops thereafter.

Amoebic Dysentery: Yellow skin; wide, white eyes.

Therapies

General: After unction, strong emesis and purgation (using bitter herbs) are required. A wholesome diet is then followed (according to one's *doṣha*). Rice, barley, wheat, green gram (*mūng*) soup, lentils, and *ghee* are eaten along with herbs that balance one's *doṣha* and symptoms. Sesame seeds, pomegranates, black grapes, and cane sugar or molasses help build the blood. The Āyurvedic iron ash (*lauh bhasma*) quickly helps build blood. *Chyavan Prāśh, ghee,* and saffron in warm milk, taken twice daily; and turmeric *ghee* are very helpful. *Triphalā* and aloe vera gel cleanse the bowels and stimulate liver function. Other useful herbs include *mañjiṣhṭhā, śhatāvarī,* and *punarnavā.*

Vāyu: Organic yogurt, boiled milk, sesame oil, and *ghee*. Only steamed vegetables (i.e., not raw).

Pitta: Salads, sprouts, green leaf vegetables, dandelion leaf, and red raspberry leaf. Chlorophyll cleanses bile and blood. *Kaṭukā*, barberry, *chirāyatā* (king of the bitters), aloe, and the main liver herb, *bhūāmalakī.*

Kapha: Improves digestion and removes congestion with hot spices such as cinnamon, saffron, turmeric, or *tṛikatu*. *Harītakī* is another useful herb for Kapha *doṣhas*. As with Vāyu, steamed vegetables are required.

Traditional *Ghees (Ghṛita)*:

Dādimādya Ghṛita: 160 gms. pomegranate (*dāḍima*), 80 gms. coriander (*dhānyaka*), 40 gms. each of *chitraka* and ginger (*śhuṇṭhī*), 20 gms. of *pippalī*. All are combined into a paste and cooked with 800 gms. of *ghee* and 2.56 litters (@21/2 qts.). This *ghee* alleviates heart diseases, anemia, hemorrhoids, enlarged spleen, Kapha and Vāyu disorders, difficult breathing, cough, and difficult labor (it is even said to aid conception in a sterile woman).

Kaṭukādya Ghṛita: 41 gms. each of *Kaṭukā, musta*, turmeric, barberry, *kuṭaj*; 10 gms. each of *paṭola*, sandalwood, *trāymān*, *pippalī*, neem, cedar, *chirāyatā*. These herbs are pasted together and cooked with 640 gms. of *ghee* and 4 times as much organic milk. This recipe helps internal bleeding, fever, burning sensation, edema, fistula, hemorrhoids, menorrhegia, and skin eruptions.

In more serious cases and for Kapha-caused anemia, *harītakī ghee* is taken to alleviate anemia, followed by emesis. Emesis is brought about by drinking large amounts of milk with emetic herbs.

Sickle Cell Anemia (Yakrit Janya Raktalplata): Due to liver damage, red blood cells become sick and die earlier than normal. Iron supplements are not give in this case, although herbal irons such as *punarnavā* are useful. Purgatives are also useful.

Therapies: First, oil massage is applied, followed by strong emesis and purgation (if persons are strong enough). Wholesome foods and moderation of foods include *basmati* rice, barley, whole wheat, *ghee* soups, peas, lentils, and oils according to one's *doṣha*. Herbs include *triphalā*, turmeric, *guḍūchī*, *tṛikatu*, *musta*, *viḍaṅga*, *chitrak*, neem with honey; they are taken every morning with boiled milk and *ghee*. One-half cup yogurt with 1/2 cup water (Kapha takes 1/4 cup yogurt with 3/4 cup water) with *punarnavā* is advised. *Śhilājit* is also recommended. Black sesame seeds, pomegranates, black grapes, cane sugar, molasses, and *ghee*; herbs of aloe gel, *āmalakī*, *harītakī*, saffron (or safflower), *śhatāvarī*, *mañjiṣhṭhā*, and *punarnavā* are all blood builders.

Vāyu: Herbs include *chitrak*, coriander, *pippalī*, *triphalā*, *guḍūchī*, ginger, raisins, taken with boiled milk.

Pitta: Herbs include coriander, dandelion leaf, red raspberry leaf, nettles, chlorophyll, barberry, *kaṭukā*, aloe gel, *guḍūchī*, *musta*, *viḍaṅga*, neem, and grapes or raisins with boiled milk. Foods include leafy vegetables and sprouts.

Kapha: Herbs include *chitrak*, coriander, *pippalī*, *tṛikatu*, *viḍaṅga*, *musta*, turmeric, saffron or safflower, cinnamon, neem, and ginger, taken with honey. Foods include raisins and Kapha-reducing items.

Amoebic Dysentery: *Kuṭaj* and *musta*

Heart Disease (Hṛidroga)

Causes: Five causes of heart disease exist: Vāyu, Pitta, Kapha, Tridoṣha, and that caused by parasites or infections.

These disorders are caused by eating foods that are very hot, hard to digest, astringent, and bitter. They are also caused by excess fatigue, injury, reading aloud for many hours, excess worry, or suppression of natural urges.

Development: The causes listed above create *doṣha* excesses weakening plasma (*rasa*) tissue localizing themselves in the heart, causing pain.

Symptoms:

Vāyu: Severe pricking, piercing, bursting, constricting or splitting pain; dryness, immobility, emptiness, increased heart rate, unfounded helplessness, grief or fear, tremors, body contractions, dislike of noise, fainting or coma, obstructed breathing, tight chest, numbness, insomnia, difficult breathing, dry cough, dark rings around the eyes, hypersensitivity. Attacks occur after straining or from fear, anxiety, worry, etc.; and after fainting or nervous heart conditions.

Pitta: Thirst, dizziness, fainting, burning sensation, severe sweating, acidity, exhaustion, vomiting (sourness) bile, hot fumes; yellowish skin, eyes, and stool; fever, flushed or bloodshot eyes, dizziness, inflammatory heart conditions (e.g., myocarditis, endocarditis, pericarditis).

Kapha: Heart stiffness, heavy like a stone, coughing, poor digestion, expectorating mucus, excess sleep, lassitude, loss of taste and appetite, fever, congestive heart situations or cardiac edema.

Tridoṣha: Symptoms of all three *doṣhas*.

Parasites/infections: Eyes have black discoloration, fainting, heart feels oppressed or torn, dry, irritated skin, excess mucus expectoration.

Therapies:

General: Mental and physical rest; avoid worry, anger, etc. Persons need to meditate on what they truly would love to do with their lives. Gentle *yoga* or stretching is also useful to calm and integrate the mind and body. The main herb, *arjuna*, is useful for all forms of heart disease. It tones the heart and lungs, stimulates blood circulation, stops bleeding, promotes tissue healing, and strengthens the heart muscle. Additional therapies include *ghee*, *aśhwagandhā*, and saffron. For angina, *arjuna* and *kuṣhtha* (VPK=) or *hiṅg* and sage (VK-) are useful.

Vāyu: Ingesting Vāyu-reducing foods and

liquids; oily vitamins of A, E, and D, garlic, rest.

Pitta: The intake of Pitta-reducing foods and drinks, avoiding hot and pungent spices, salt, alcohol, garlic, onions, greasy foods, red meat. Herbs include *arjuna*, saffron, sandalwood, *śhatāvarī*, gotu kola, aloe vera gel, *kaṭukā,* and *chitrak.* Purgation is also useful.

Kapha: Avoiding dairy, sugar, eggs, fatty meat, salt, and other cholesterol-producing foods, and remaining on a diet of Kapha-reducing foods and liquids. Herbs include *arjuna*, *guggul*, calamus, cardamom, *ṭrikatu*.

Tridoṣha: Combinations of the above respective therapies.

Parasites: See Chapter 15 on parasites. Therapies include antiparasitical/anti-infection herbs. Dr. S. Sandhu's clinical experience finds that *arjuna chūrṇa* works better for the congestive cardiac diseases; *tamra bhasma* (copper ash/*yogendra rasa* is one such formulation) or wearing a copper bracelet is the best for obstructive cardiac heart conditions. Modern medicine also divides the heart conditions into these two main types (i.e., congestive and obstructive).

Other modern Āyurvedic authorities have found that constipation or diarrhea may be forcing air upwards, affecting the heart. Thus, just by regulating the stool, clients have found relief from some forms of heart disease.

Hypertension/High Blood Pressure

Its causes and therapies are similar to heart diseases.

Additional causes and development: First, excess mental stress (i.e., worry, anxiety, tension) can be caused by Vāyu. Second, certain hormonal imbalances (e.g., adrenal, thyroid, and reproductive hormones) can be caused by Pitta. Thus, obstruction of the blood or urinary channels (*srotas*) or kidney problems can be caused by Kapha. Should gas, constipation, or diarrhea be present, *Apāna Vāyu* (downward air) may be forced upward, putting pressure on the heart.

Symptoms:

Vāyu: Sudden changes in pressure, irregular or an erratic pulse—caused by worry, strain, overwork, nervousness, and insomnia.

Pitta: Flushed face, red eyes, violent headaches, sensitivity to light, nose bleeds, anger, irritability, burning, sometimes with liver complications.

Kapha: Constant high pressure, obesity, fatigue, edema, high cholesterol.

Therapies:

General: *Arjuna* strengthens the heart, especially if the pulse is weak.

Vāyu: Brain tonics such as gotu kola, *jaṭāmāṇshī, aśhwagandhā, śhaṅk puṣhpī, bhṛiṅgarāj,* garlic, and a Vāyu-reducing diet and lifestyle. *Śhirodhārā* (hot oil poured on the head for 7 to 14 sessions) also heal nerves and mental stress.

Pitta: Aloe vera gel, *chirāyatā, kaṭukā*, rhubarb, harmonizing herbs like *śhatāvarī, mañjiṣhṭhā, musta, triphalā, balā*, gotu kola, and a Pitta-reducing diet and lifestyle. Garlic, onions, and other hot, salty, and pungent items will aggravate the condition. *Śhirodhārā* is also very helpful.

Kapha: Myrrh, *ṭrikatu, arjuna*, hawthorn berries, diuretics like *gokṣhura,* and a Kapha-reducing diet and lifestyle. *Śhirodhārā* is also very helpful.

Long term use of blood-pressure medicine, or even herbs (i.e., *sarpagandha*), without balancing the underlying cause, will eventually cause side effects.

Arteriosclerosis

This condition relates to the blood vessels. The arteries thicken and harden because of deposits of cholesterol on the artery walls. This is one of the causes of hypertension: arteries loose their elasticity and cannot bear the pressure of blood flowing through them.

Causes: High cholesterol and clogged arteries.

Vāyu: Hardened arteries.

Pitta: Fat accumulation.

Kapha: Fat accumulation.

Therapies: similar to heart disease.

General: *Arjuna* strengthens the heart, especially if the pulse is weak.

Vāyu: Garlic, *yogaraj guggul*, myrrh, and saffron in boiled milk.

Pitta: *Kaiṣhore guggul*, turmeric, aloe vera gel, *kaṭuka.*

Kapha: Garlic and purified *guggul*, myrrh, saffron.

Hypotension/Low Blood Pressure

Causes: Usually a Vāyu disorder, it develops through debility, anemia, malnutrition, and other chronic diseases.

Vāyu: Caused by poor circulation.

Pitta: Hormone imbalance, anemia, damaged liver.

Kapha: Caused by congestion, phlegm, clogging, stagnation, blood flow reduction, dehydration, and edema.

Therapies:

General: *Arjuna* strengthens the heart, especially if the pulse is weak.

Vāyu: Garlic, turmeric, ginger, *pippalī*, cardamom.

Pitta: *Bhūmīāmalalī, mañjiṣhṭhā*, gotu kola, turmeric, and saffron in aloe vera gel.

Kapha: *Tṛikatu*, garlic, turmeric, ginger, *pippalī*, cardamom.

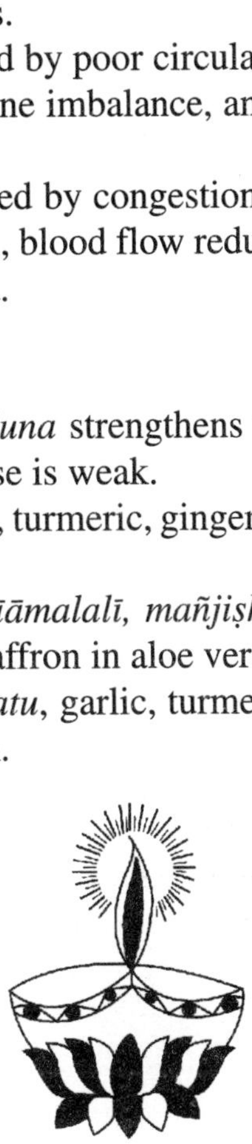

Paraplegia (Ūrustambha)

Definition: Excess Kapha and fat derange Vāyu and Pitta in the legs and stiffen them, causing immobility and coldness. Paraplegia is related to both the circulatory and digestive systems, so therapies need to address both systems.

Cause: This disorder can be caused by eating fatty, hot, light, and cold foods before digesting one's last meal, or by eating moist or dry foods, yogurt, milk, meat, or drinking bad wine. Other causes include excessive naps, staying up too late, under- or overeating, exertion, fear, suppression of the natural urges, or oiliness. Additional causes include toxins in the bowels (along with fat blocking any or all of the three *doṣhas*) that move to the legs and thighs through the blood vessels in the legs. This causes the buildup of excess fat to hamper leg coordination and restrict leg movement.

This excess Kapha in the thighs causes heaviness, exhaustion, burning, pain, numbness, tearing pain, contraction, quivering, and piercing, that may even be life threatening.

Premonitory Signs: Brooding, sleepiness, feeling excessively wet, anorexia, fever, hair standing on end, vomiting, and lassitude in the calves and thighs of the legs.

Symptoms: Excessive malaise of the legs, continuous burning and pain, feet ache when placed on the ground, no sensation to cold, unable to stand, feeling that the thighs are broken and carried by someone else. (If trembling, with burning and piercing pain, exists, the illness cannot be healed unless it has just developed.)

Precaution: Unction, emesis, purgation, and enema—although useful for all other diseases—will only aggravate this condition. With this condition, if the nervous system is weak and oil is applied to the legs, the symptoms are further aggravated, because unction and enema aggravate Kapha. Neither purgation nor emesis will remove Kapha in the legs (as it is well below the stomach, the seat of Kapha).

Therapies: Constant application of reducing and drying therapies removes the abundance of Kapha and toxins (*āma*). Foods include barley, warm, bitter and dry vegetables; herbs include neem, *triphalā*, *harītakī*, *pippalī*, *bilwa*, sandalwood, *musta*, *chitrak,* and calamus with honey water. Salts and sweets must be avoided.

If drying therapies cause excess dryness, then some *ghee* or canola oil with *gokṣhura*, calamus, *aśhwagandhā*, *pippalī*, *guggul*, *nirguṇḍī*, *chitrak,* and a small amount of rock salt are advised. These are all taken with honey and *basmati* rice.

External: Measures include Kapha-reducing therapies such as massaging the legs with sand from anthills, powder from bricks, honey, mustard, and *aśhwagandhā* paste, and sprinkling water with a decoction of neem*, bilwa, and gokṣhura*. Massage is also done with *mahānārāyan*, *pañchaguṇa,* and *viṣhgarbha* oil.

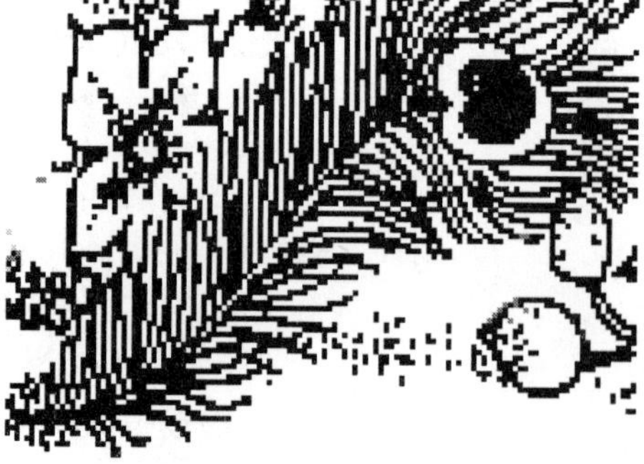

Physicians shouldn't feel shy if they don't know the nomenclature of the disease, for there is no rule, custom, or state that every disease has a name.

Aṣhṭhāñga Hṛidayam Sū. Ch. 12: ver. 64

Chapter 15
Digestive System
Anorexia, Vomiting, Diarrhea\Dysentery, Digestive and Abdominal Disorders, Jaundice, Gallstones, Dyspepsia, Indigestion, Gastroenteritis, Colic, Hyperacidity, Acid Gastritis, Malabsorption, Food Allergies, Parasites, Constipation, Hemorrhoids, Obesity, Candida, Ulcers, Āma

Anorexia (Arochaka)

Causes: There are 5 causes for loss of appetite, taste, or anorexia: Vāyu, Pitta, Kapha, Tridoṣha, and mental (e.g., grief, fear, anger). An excess of the *doṣhas* (individually or combined) or an apathetic mental state tends to block the heart region and the channels (*srotas*) that carry food (e.g., esophagus). This causes aversion to foods.

Symptoms: Continual vomiting may occur, leading to dehydration.

Vāyu: Overeating Kapha-increasing foods causes tingling gums, an astringent taste in the mouth, severe weight loss, loss of appetite, fear, anxiety, insomnia, chest and abdominal pains and cramps, palpitations, throat constriction, difficulty swallowing, and choking feelings.

Pitta: Bitter and sour taste, bad smell in the mouth, burning sensations in the heart region.

Kapha: Sweet or salty taste, Kapha-coated mouth, nausea, vomiting, exuding watery substance from the mouth or the nose, itching, heaviness of the body, water-brash, lethargy, and fatigue.

Tridoṣha: Abnormal taste or absence of taste.

Mental: Worry, anger, delusion, dullness, or other emotions, associated with a particular *doṣha* .

Therapies

General: Herbs

digestive herbs: cardamom, ginger

to stop vomiting: red raspberry, ginger

tonics: *chyavan prāśh, aśhwagandhā*

nervines: gotu kola, sandalwood, *jaṭāmāṇśhī, aśhwagandhā.*

Foods—bland rice and *mūng dal*. Avoid coffee, tea, drugs, stimulants.

Massage—sesame oil applied to the feet and head, and *śhiro dhārā.*

Aromas—sandalwood oil applied to the forehead.

General Regimen: Different types of foods are combined with the person's *doṣha*-balancing foods. Bathing cleanses the body from outside. Light emesis is done twice daily for internal cleansing (morning and evening). Oral hygiene—brushing, eating rock candy with *tulsī* herb.

Vāyu—first, emesis should be induced with a *vachā* decoction. This is followed by an herbal tea made with with *pippalī,* cardamom, and *viḍaṅga* powders. *Pippalī, viḍanga*, raisins, rock salt, ginger, and medicated wine can be ingested as an appetizer to stimulate hunger.

Pitta—persons are administered an emetic with *jaggery* (cane sugar) juice. Also, cane sugar, *ghee*, salt, and honey should be eaten.

Kapha—individuals are given an emetic with neem leaf decoction, *ajwan*, fennel, and alcohol mixed with honey.

Tridoṣha—all of the above measures are used.

Mind—herbs to calm the mind (e.g., *brāhmī, aśhwagandhā, jaṭāmāṇśhī*), providing consolation, sympathy, and cheerfulness, uncovering the cause of the trouble (e.g., disappointment with career), and planning strategies to change things for the better.

Vomiting (Chardi)

Causes: Vomiting is caused by the following: Vāyu, Pitta, Kapha, *Tridoṣha*, and unpleasant sensory experience. Upward moving Vāyu (*Udāna*) becomes abnormal and aggravates all the *doṣhas* causing them to move upward.

Premonitory Symptoms: Nausea, salty taste in mouth, excess salivation, loss of taste and appetite.

Symptoms:

Vāyu: Vomiting of food causes pain in the navel region, back, and ribs, regurgitating occurs a little at a time, with an astringent taste and frothy substance; it is blackish, thin, and is emitted only with difficulty and force. Other symptoms include belching, coughing, dry mouth, heart and head pain, hoarseness, and exhaustion. Vomiting caused by parasites, thirst, *āma*, and pregnancy are also caused by Vāyu.

Pitta: Vomit is ashen, brown, green, or yellow in color. It may be bloody, sour or bitter tasting, and hot. Thirst, fainting, heat, or burning sensations in the body may be felt.

Kapha: Substance is oily, thick, cold and thready, sweet or salty tasting, and comes out in a large, continuous quantity; hair stands on end, the face swells, one feels a stupor, nausea, and cough.

Tridoṣha: Symptoms of all the *doṣhas* appear.

Senses: Seeing, hearing, smelling, tasting, or touching unpleasant, dirty things, foul smells, disturb the mind, causing vomiting associated with heart region pain.

Therapies:

Only when vomiting is not associated with complications can it be healed. When severe vomiting occurs in persons who are weak, with bleeding or pus, or have a moon-like complexion, they cannot be healed.

General: All forms of vomiting are due to gastric irritation. Therapies of lightening (exercise, sunbathing), and for Vāyu-caused vomiting are used first. *Harītakī* with raw honey, or castor oil with boiled milk, reduces the upward motion of the *doṣhas*. An emetic is advised. Debilitated persons should use only pacifying measures.

Vāyu: *Bilwa*, barley, cardamom, cloves, coriander, ginger, raspberry, *vaṃśha lochana*, *pippalī*, black pepper, and garlic. If the person suffers heart palpitations, *ghee,* rock salt, yogurt, and pomegranate juice are recommended.

Pitta: Neem, *chirāyatā*, *bilwa*, coriander, raspberry, *vaṃśha lochana*, sugar cane. If Pitta is excessed in the stomach, an emetic with sweet herbs (e.g., licorice) is administered to cleanse the stomach. Afterwards, one drinks a mixture of cooked barley with raw honey and cane sugar, or *basmati* rice with green lentil soup. Grapes and coconut are also useful foods. *Āmalakī, pittapapra, balā,* and sandalwood may be mixed with food.

Kapha: An emetic made with a decoction of *pippalī*, neem, and rock salt cleanses the undigested food toxins (*āma*) from the stomach. Afterwards, (at meal time) barley may be eaten with neem and yogurt/water (1/4:3/4), green lentils. Herbs include cardamom, *bilwa*, cloves, ginger, *triphalā*, *musta*, and raspberry, which, when mixed with raw honey, stop vomiting.

Tridoṣha: Herbs, foods, and other therapies advised for each *doṣha* are used. Season, time of day, strength of the person, and their digestion, are all taken into consideration.

Psychological Stress: Pleasant conversation, consolation, exhilaration, stories, socializing with friends all help reduce the stress that causes vomiting. Additionally, pleasant aromas and flowers, fermented drinks, sour fruits and vegetables all contribute to healing.

If a person experiences any complications while vomiting, appropriate measures as described in the respective chapters are used. Long-term vomiting greatly aggravates Vāyu.

Thus, a Vāyu-reducing diet (i.e., bulk- and semen-promoting foods and herbs) is used to restore balance and strength.

Diarrhea (Atīsāra) and Dysentery (Pravāhika)

Cause: There are 6 forms of diarrhea: Vāyu, Pitta, Kapha, Tridoṣha, fear and grief, and undigested food (*āma*). Causes include drinking excessive amounts of water, eating very hot, dry, fatty, hard, cold, or unaccustomed foods, puddings, sesame seeds, sprouted grains, excess wines, over-eating, eating before the last meal is digested, and eating at unusual times. Further causes include improper oleation therapy, drinking bad water, excessive use of alcohol, overdoing water sports, suppression of natural urges, hemorrhoids, intestinal parasites, changes in lifestyle, and seasonal changes. As accumulating Vāyu becomes aggravated, it causes the Kapha (watery element) to move downward, dampening the digestive fire before entering the alimentary canal. This causes the feces to become watery and produce diarrhea.

There are 5 types of dysentery: Vāyu, Pitta, Kapha, Tridoṣha, and blood (*raktapitta*).

Premonitory Signs: Prickling pain in the heart region, rectum, and alimentary tract; weak body, constipation, gas, and indigestion.

Symptoms:

Vāyu: Watery feces, small quantity, expelled with noise, severe pain, and difficulty. It may be dry, frothy, thin, rough, or scaly, slightly brown and frequently expelled. Alternatively, it may seem gooey, burnt, and slimy. One may experience a dry mouth, prolapsed rectum, hair standing on end, and straining to expel stools.

Pitta: Yellow, black, algae green, blue, red, or deep yellow color, mixed with blood and foul smelling; thirst, fainting, perspiration, burning sensation, painful elimination, burning and ulcerated rectum.

Kapha: Solid, slimy, thready, white, mucus, fatty, frequent, heavy, foul smelling, difficult elimination followed by pain, sleepiness, laziness, dislike of food, mild straining to eliminate stools or frequent and urgent need to eliminate.

Tridoṣha: Symptoms of all three *doṣhas* simultaneously.

Fear/Grief: This situation can cause persons to eat very little. The heat of tears and secretions of the nose, mouth, and throat can increase and move to the alimentary tract to weaken digestion and blood tissue (*rakta dhātu*). Vitiated blood is then expelled, mixed with feces or by itself. It is very difficult to heal. Emotional causes increase Pitta and Vāyu, causing liquid feces and diarrhea; feces are quick, warm, fluid, and float on water. Symptoms are the same as Vāyu.

Undigested Food (Āma): Diarrhea is of two types: 1) with *āma* and without *āma*, and 2) mixed with blood and without blood. With *āma*, stools sink in the water, have a foul smell, are associated with intestinal gurgling; undigested food remains in the stomach, abdominal pain, excess salivation. Symptoms of "without *āma*" feces have the opposite qualities.

When food is not properly digested (*āma*), *doṣhas* combine with *āma* and become excessed. They then travel in the wrong channels, weakening tissues (*dhātus*), waste products (*malas*), and cause frequent, multicolored feces and abdominal pain.

If diarrhea is allowed to continue without being healed, it develops the disorders of the duodenum. This is discussed later.

Therapies:

General: Diarrhea caused by excess *doṣhas* (due to undigested food) needs to be eliminated. Initially, astringent herbs and foods are not used to stop diarrhea with *āma* (toxins) until the toxins are expelled with the stool. If the diarrhea is prematurely halted while *āma* is still in the body, it may cause various diseases (e.g., hemorrhoids, edema, anemia, tumors, fever, etc.). Rather, it is advised to allow initial *āma* diarrhea to come out, and even to induce it by taking *harītakī*. It is a part of the body's defense mechanism to expel toxins (*āma*). Thus, stopping diarrhea when it is still toxic goes against the body's natural healing process.

Persons with a moderate *doṣha* excess take decoctions to stimulate the appetite and strengthen the digestion. If *doṣhas* are greatly excessed, then lightening therapy (i.e., *pañcha karma*, etc.) is advised.

General: Herbs include *pippalī*, ginger, coriander, *harītakī*, calamus, *gokṣhura*, *bilwa*, fennel.

Vāyu: (the same as Kapha) *Balā*, *gokṣhura*, *bilwa*, ginger, coriander, calamus, *pippalī*, *chitrak*, sour pomegranate, *daśhmūl*, *āmalakī*, *ghee*, and rock salt are taken with foods and drinks to strengthen the digestion and the constitution.

Pain, gas retention, and the desire to pass urine or stool (but cannot): Are healed with *bilwa*, *pippalī*, ginger, cane sugar, and sesame oil.

Diarrhea with a dry mouth (dehydration): *Basmati* rice, barley soup, green lentils, sesame seeds, *bilwa*, *kuṭaj*, *īśhabgol* fried in *ghee*, and sesame oil/added with yogurt and pomegranate, cane sugar, ginger.

When Kapha is diminished, excessed Vāyu presents serious problems; therefore, this condition must be immediately healed.

Vāyu/Pitta: Enemas.

Pitta: *Kuṭaj*, *chirāyatā*, *kaṭukā*, *bilwa*, sandalwood, lotus seeds, ginger, pomegranate, sesame seeds, mango (taken with raw honey), *ghee*, and rice water.

If the appetite is good and digestion strong, goats' milk will heal Pitta diarrhea.

If pain recurs after cleansing, oil enemas should be administered immediately, using *ghee* to 1/4 the amount of sesame oil, with *śhatāvarī*, *bilwa*, and milk. If diarrhea continues, one receives a massage. Then, a *pichā basti* followed by bath is taken [the soft bark of silk cotton tree and *pawdar* mixed with oil and *ghee*]. Next, persons have meals of boiled milk and Pitta-reducing foods. If one eats Pitta-increasing foods in this condition, it may lead to bloody diarrhea and thirst, pain, burning, and rectal inflammation. Should this occur, boiled goats' milk with raw honey and cane sugar is ingested and used to wash the anus. Foods include boiled rice with this milk decoction, and *ghee*. If the person is strong, food (e.g., rice) should be eaten after milk is digested. Weak persons eat food just after the milk. Alternately, fresh butter mixed with honey and sugar is eaten before meals. The rice is soaked in water overnight, and crushed and rubbed the next morning. When the water from this rice is drunk, it heals bloody diarrhea.

Āma: Purgation is advised (i.e., see lightening therapies in *pañcha karma* chapter) if the person is strong. After lightening therapy, meals are to include barley gruel with *balā*, *śhatāvarī*, and *gokṣhura*. Green lentils improve digestion. If diarrhea continues, digestives like *ṭrikatu*, and astringents like comfrey, gentian, lotus seeds, red raspberry, and yellow dock may be used.

Thirst: Boiled water with *musta* and sandalwood.

Dysentery: One takes *bilwa*, sesame paste, yogurt, *āmalakī*, and *ghee*.

Amoebic dysentery: *Kuṭaj* along with immune-boosting herbs (e.g., *guḍūchī*). *Śhaṅk bhasma* (shell ash) reduces acid indigestion if present.

Bacillary Dysentery: See therapies for Pitta diarrhea.

Bleeding diarrhea: A diet of *śhatāvarī* or *ghee* cooked with milk (before or after passing stools) heals this disorder. Alternately, one may eat sandalwood mixed with sugar and honey, followed by rice water. For frequent movements with small amounts of blood, and associated with pain and Vāyu (i.e., difficulty in passing stools), *pichā basti*, or oil enema with *ghee* and the above mentioned herbs.

Upper/lower channel bleeding: If Pitta-increasing foods are continually eaten, severe rectal inflammation can develop, and is fatal. Herbs include lotus seeds, *dūrba*, and *nāgkeśhar.*

Chronic diarrhea: This causes a weak anus. Frequent, local application of *ghee* or oil can heal this condition.

Inflamed anus: This is caused by frequent movements. It is healed either by sprinkling a cold decoction of sugar cane, *ghee*, milk, and raw honey, or by applying the mixture as a paste on the inflammation. *Ghee* may also be applied first before sprinkling with *ghee,* neem oil, or sandalwood oil.

Kapha: Emesis (i.e., lightening therapy) and improved digestion are the first concerns. Ginger, coriander, *bilwa*, *musta*, *harītakī*, calamus, *pippalī*, *chitrak,* nutmeg, and sour pomegranate are used to strengthen the digestion. Later, *balā*, *gokṣhura*, *bilwa*, *viḍaṅga,* and rock salt are combined with foods and drinks to strengthen the constitution. One part yogurt mixed with 3 parts water (*lassi*) also promotes digestion. Alternately, either a mixture of *pippalī* with honey or a mixture of *chitrak* with *lassi* heals this condition.

When *āma* is digested persons may still suffer from diarrhea with small amounts of stool retention, pain, mucus, and the urge to pass stool or urine (but cannot). Therapy includes radish soup with *bākuchī*, yogurt, pomegranate, and *ghee.* (Other diuretic vegetables may be used.)

Should the above condition also have complications of passing blood and mucus with thirst, boiled milk with *ghee*, *bilwa,* or castor oil is used.

If rectum prolapse with pain exists after eliminating *āma*, first the inner rectum is oiled and fomented to soften it. Then herbs are taken including *āmalakī, ghee,* or oil enema (with *daśhmūl* and *bilwa*), or *ghee* cooked with dry ginger, sour yogurt, *triphalā,* and *śhatāvarī*.

Vāyu/Kapha: (or excessive diarrhea caused by Kapha or dysentery with pain), *pichā basti* is applied, followed by an enema with *pippalī*, *bilwa*, calamus, and black salt. Afterwards, one bathes, and then one eats. In the evening, one receives an oil enema made from the same herbs mixed in sesame oil.

Tridoṣhic: Herbs from each category are used. If all three are equally unbalanced, the order of healing is Vāyu first, Pitta second, and Kapha third. Otherwise, whichever is most unbalanced is treated first.

Fear/Grief: Vāyu-reducing therapies, psychotherapeutic measures that produce exhilaration and consolation.

Digestive Disorders (Grahanī) [related to duodenum; sprue/malabsorption]

Normal functioning of the digestive fire (*agni*) or enzymes, is responsible for proper digestion and metabolism. The digestive fire resides in the stomach, duodenum, small and large intestines, and directly affects complexion, strength, weight, immune strength, energy, vital breath, and life span. Digested food also nourishes the seven tissues (*dhātus*) and life sap (*ojas*). Thus, the whole body depends upon healthy digestion. Therefore, it is advised to eat fresh, organic, wholesome foods and liquids. This is done with a peaceful frame of mind, according to one's *doṣha*, the season, time of day, and in proper quantities.

Causes: Chronic diarrhea, ingesting foods and liquids that dampen and deplete the digestive fire (metabolism), fasting, eating before the last meal is digested, eating foods that are too heavy, cold, rough, stale, or contaminated. Other causes include misuse of *pañcha karma*, excessive oleation, emaciation, suppression of natural urges, and extreme mental stress.

Premonitory Signs: Weakness, taking a long time to digest foods, increasing acidity, salivation, bad taste in the mouth, loss of taste or appetite, thirst, exhaustion, dizziness, abdominal distention, vomiting, ear noise, intestinal gurgling, burning, heaviness.

Development: When feces are mixed with *āma* and food and are eliminated before, during or after digestion of the food, there may be no elimination at all, or elimination may sometimes be solid and sometimes liquid; or elimination occurs only after feces accumulate in the colon. This is said to be a serious illness. This cause of diarrhea differs because of excess elimination (with or without *āma*) only after digestion of food. Four types of gastrointestinal disorders exist: Vāyu, Pitta, Kapha, and Tridoṣha.

Air-Caused (*Vātaja Grahaṇiroga*): Vāyu is increased by eating foods that are pungent, bitter, and astringent; meals that are heavy, rough, or cold; fasting, excess travel, suppression of urges, excessive sexual intercourse, or extreme mental stress. This dampens the digestive fire, making digestion difficult or variable. Thus, food becomes fermented and many symptoms develop.

Fire-Caused (Pittaja Grahaṇiroga): Pitta is increased in the digestive tract by excessive eating of foods that are pungent, uncooked, sour, alkaline, and by foods that cause heartburn. This inactivates the gastric enzymes (like pouring hot water over a fire; or raises *agni* so hight it burns up nutrients).

Water-Caused (Kaphaja Grahaṇiroga): Excessive eating of foods that are very difficult to digest, fatty, cold; eating before the last meal is digested, and sleeping after lunch, cause Kapha excesses in digestion.

Tridoṣha *Grahaṇiroga*: Habits of all three *doṣhas* create this disorder.

Symptoms: Emaciation, heat, mouth fumes, difficult breathing, fever, fainting, headache, food remains stagnant in the stomach, swelling of hands and feet.

Vāyu: Palate dryness, difficult breathing, ear pain, pressure or noise; constant pain in the ribs, thighs, groin, and neck; simultaneous vomiting and diarrhea, desire for all tastes, increased hunger and thirst, cutting rectal pain, post-digestive gas, eating food brings comfort, abdominal tumor, hemorrhoids, splenic diseases, anemia, believing one has heart disease, difficult elimination occurs after long intervals, liquid feces are non-oily, thin, frothy, uncooked, cough, non-digesting of foods, headaches, fainting, giddiness, stiff back and waist, lower back pain, yawning, aches, thirst, fever, vomiting, griping, anorexia.

Hyperacidity causes dryness of throat, mouth, thirst, blurred vision, noises, thumping or ringing in the ears, pain, emaciation, debility, bad taste in the mouth, insatiable appetite for food, cough, difficult breathing.

Pitta: Food toxins, when mixed with Pitta, cause bluish-yellow—or yellow—liquid feces, body odor, sour belching, burning sensations in the heart and throat areas, loss of taste, appetite, and thirst.

Kapha: Poor digestion, vomiting, loss of taste and appetite, coated mouth, expectoration, cough, nausea, nasal mucus, heavy throat and abdomen, belching with bad smells and sweetness of taste, debility, loss of sexual desire, broken, uncooked, heavy, mucus-filled feces; large quantity of feces, weakness, and wasting (although persons are not emaciated).

Tridoṣha: Symptoms of all *doṣhas* are present.

To restore health, the digestive fire must be restored. Digestive illness is one of the 8 diseases said to be difficult to heal. The other 7 are diseases of the nervous system, urinary stones, leprosy, diabetes, enlarged abdomen, hemorrhoids, and fistula (abnormal passages from abscesses, cavities or hollow organs to the skin or other abscesses, cavities or hollow organs).

Therapies:

Poor digestion with āma (undigested food toxins): Symptoms include distention, salivation, discomfort, burning, anorexia, and heaviness. Therapies to eliminate these problems include drinking warm water or a decoction made of *pippalī* and black mustard seeds. [See also p. 391]

Vāyu: *Asafoetida*, ginger, black pepper, rock salt, herbal digestive wines.

Pitta: *Lodhra*, *āmalakī*, *nāgkeśhar*, *chirāyatā*, *viḍaṅga*.

Kapha: Nutmeg, rock salt, *ajwan*, *pippalī*.

Intestinal āma: Purgation and digestive stimulants such as castor oil and cardamom, respectively.

Rasa and āma: Lightening therapy (i.e., *pañcha karma*, exercise, foods that are light, hot, sharp, and dry, carminative/digestive herbs—[e.g., ginger and *musta*, *harītakī* and ginger, drunk with hot water]).

After the stomach is cleansed, persons eat light foods such as thin gruel and *kicharī*, followed by digestive stimulant herbs.

When the digestive fire begins to become stronger, but stool, urine, and gas retention continue, persons should be given oil massage and fomentation for 2 or 3 days, then followed by a non-oily enema.

After Vāyu is balanced and the toxins are loose, one takes castor oil purgation (2 tsp. in a cup of hot water before bed).

Should there be constipation, an oil enema is administered, along with digestive stimulants, sour herbs like *āmalakī,* and sour pomegranate, and other Vāyu-reducing herbs (i.e., cardamom, ginger, *balā*).

Vāyu: When *āma* is completely removed, one takes *ghee* with digestive stimulant herbs. Herbs like *daśhmūl*, ginger, *pippalī*, *triphalā*, *tṛikatu*, and *chitrak* reduce Vāyu and promote digestion. Black salt is also helpful. They are taken with warm water and also used for massage. One-half cup yogurt and 1/2 cup water (*lassi*) taken after meals also improves digestion.

Pitta: This *doṣha* is reduced by purgation or emesis. Afterwards, the digestive fire is stimulated by eating light, bitter, astringent, cool, and moist foods; cool liquids, *ghee,* and sour pomegranates. Herbs include sandalwood, *musta,* neem, ginger, *mañjiṣhṭhā*, *kaṭukā*, *kuṭaj,* and *bilwa*. *Tṛikatu* may also be taken for Pitta digestive problems, though its nature is heating. One-half cup yogurt and 1/2 cup water (*lassi*) taken after meals also improves digestion. Pungent and sour foods and black salt may be taken only when mixed with bitter and astringent foods. Cane sugar or rock sugar is also useful when mixed with the herbs.

Kapha: Pungent, hot, digestive, and bitter herbs include *viḍaṅga*, *chitrak*, *mañjiṣhṭhā*, cardamom, turmeric, *pippalī*, *tṛikatu*, *triphalā*, *musta*, calamus, *guḍūchī,* and neem. Kapha-reducing foods are taken as well, including barley.

Abdominal Diseases (Udara Roga)

Causes: All diseases, especially *udara roga*, are caused by deranged waste material in the body (*malas*—feces, urine, and sweat, and the three *doṣhas*), caused by poor digestion and metabolism. The main cause of abdominal disorders is constipation. Other causes include indigestion, contaminated food, and accumulation of *doṣhas* and wastes (*malas*).

When the digestive fire is weak and persons eat foods that are difficult to digest, indigestion develops. Other causes include unhealthy or unnatural habits like forcing the passing of stool. The result is an accumulation of the *doṣhas* that vitiates the *Prāṇa* Vāyu, *Agni,* and *Apāna Vāyu.* The excess of air obstructs the air circulating upward and downward. These excessed *doṣhas* become lodged between the skin and the muscle tissues. This causes abdominal distention, leading to all abdominal diseases, including the accumulation of fluid in the peritoneal cavity of the abdomen (ascites). This is caused by the simultaneous vitiation of all three *doṣhas*.

Different types of these diseases are caused by various situations, eating overly hot, salty, alkaline (laxatives), sour, and poisonous foods and liquids, and improper administration of *pañcha karma.* Other causes include improper food, liquids, and habits after *pañcha karma*; eating very dry, spoiled, or mutually adverse foods (e.g., fish and milk, milk and salt, hot and cold water). Further causes are emaciation from splenic diseases, hemorrhoids, and sprue (malabsorption, anemia, and gastrointestinal disorders).

Ignoring diseases by continually eating and drinking harmful food and liquids, and suppressing the natural urges will also cause abdominal disorders. Weakening of the channels of circulation, allowing undigested food toxins to remain in the body, and over- nourishment can also cause abdominal disorders. Other causes include the consumption of foods and liquids that irritate the mind and body; obstructions caused by hemorrhoids, hair, and hard stools; intestinal ulcerations or perforations; and excessive aggravation of the *doṣhas*. These are all related to excess Kapha and Vāyu; a deficiency of Pitta the and digestive fire.

Eight forms of abdominal distention exist: Vāyu, Pitta, Kapha, Tridoṣhic, enlarged spleen (and liver); rectum, intestines, and ascites (peritoneal).

Premonitory Signs: Loss of hunger, extended digestion time with burning, inability to tell whether food is digested (excess Vāyu), steady loss of strength, breathlessness after mild activity, increase of feces quantity but difficult elimination, slight leg and foot swelling, joint pain on the sides of the urinary bladder, distention with bursting pain (even with small quantities of easily digestible foods), with abdominal line marks and loss of abdominal folds. One may experience difficulty digesting sweet, oily, and heavy foods and liquids, indigestion arising from all foods and liquids, constant loss of strength, shortness of breath upon mild exertion, constipation due to dry foods and *Udāna* Vāyu (excess upward moving air), distention and pain in the lower belly, protruding vein networks, no folds in the abdomen.

Development: The three *doṣhas*, becoming aggravated, obstruct both the top and bottom channels of water metabolism, blocking the channels that carry sweat and water (*Svedavaha* and *udakavaha srotas*), and create abnormalities of outward and downward moving airs (*Prāṇa* and *Apāna* Vāyus) and the metabolism (*agni*). This causes water to accumulate between the skin, muscles, and joints, thus enlarging the abdomen. This causes abdominal disorders of a Vāyu, Pitta, Kapha, or Tridoṣhic nature (the first four of the eight forms of *udara roga*).

There are eight types: Vāyu, Pitta, Kapha, Tridoṣha, and those caused by enlarged spleen (or liver), intestinal obstruction, intestinal perforation, and fluid accumulation. Persons with this disease have dry palates and lips; swollen feet, hands and abdomen; inactivity, loss of strength and desire for food, emaciation, severe gas, and a deathly appearance.

Vāyu: Because of excess dry foods, insufficient water, exertion, suppression of the natural urges, upward movement of air, emaciation and fasting, excess Vāyu results. This excess moves through the abdominal sides, cardiac region, urinary bladder, and anus, weakening the digestion, and thereby increasing Kapha (due to undigested foods). Kapha then blocks the movement of Vāyu that then becomes stuck between the abdominal skin and muscle tissues, and causes swelling. Thus, Vāyu is the main *doṣha* responsible for poor digestion, while Kapha is a secondary factor.

Pitta: Caused by pungent, sour, salty, very hot and sharp foods, exposure to heat (fire and sun), eating foods that cause a burning sensation, and eating before the last meal is digested. When the excessed Pitta flows to locations of Vāyu and Kapha, it blocks them. Pitta then moves upwards to weaken the digestive fire.

Kapha: Due to a lack of exercise, taking naps, eating excess sweet and oily foods, eating yogurt, milk, meat, and living in marshy places. Thus, Kapha becomes excessed and blocks the circulatory channels, obstructing Vāyu in the outer intestines. Vāyu then puts pressure on Kapha, causing Kapha types of abdominal diseases.

Tridoṣhic: All three *doṣhas* simultaneously become excessed when a person with poor digestion eats unwholesome, raw, heavy, or mutually adverse foods. As a result, the three *doṣhas* slowly accumulate in the alimentary tract viscera, causing abdominal diseases.

Enlarged Spleen and Liver (Plīho-yakrddalu-

dara): Enlarged or displaced spleen is caused by overly irritating food, excess travel, strenuous exercise, lifting heavy objects, or walking long distance, overindulging in sexual activity, emaciation due to excess vomiting therapies, chronic illness, or excess blood (either due to an excess quantity of blood, fat, or muscle tissue). The spleen hardens as it becomes enlarged. When ignored, the spleen puts pressure on the abdomen and pancreas, causing this disorder. Five varieties of *plīho dara* exist: Vāyu, Pitta, Kapha, Tridoṣhic, and blood. The enlarged liver is identical to the spleen; however, it happens only on the right side of the abdomen.

Intestinal Obstruction (Baddha-gudo-dara): This is caused by Vāyu (as ruler of the rectum) becoming excessed from obstructions due to small hairs (e.g., eyelashes) in food, upward moving air in the abdomen, hemorrhoids, intestinal intrusion into its passage (lumen), and gas (obstructed *Apāna* Vāyu). This excessed Vāyu weakens digestive and metabolic enzyme power, obstructing the movement of feces, Pitta, and Kapha, and causes this disease.

Intestinal Perforation (Chidro dara): Caused by sand, grass, splinters, bones, or nails in food, deep yawns, or overeating. This intestinal wound begins to ooze and the food juices reach the exterior of the intestine. The rectum and intestine become filled with this liquid, which causes acute abdominal swelling.

Ascites (Udako dara): (Fluid accumulation in abdominal peritoneal cavity) Poor digestion develops from drinking excess water after oleation therapy, being emaciated by weak digestion, or worsening digestion caused by drinking excess water. From this, Vāyu within the lower left stomach and the duodenum (*kloman*) becomes blocked by Kapha. Also, the water circulatory channel (*udakavaha srota*) increases its water supply that obstructs the circulatory channels. Deranged Vāyu and Kapha further increase this water, causing ascites.

Symptoms:

General: Sides of the abdomen are distended, gurgling noises, leg and hand edema, poor digestion, smooth chin, and emaciation. One may experience stupor, debility, accumulation of feces, urine, and sweat (especially feces); poor digestion, burning, swelling, gas, and abdominal fluid during the most serious stages.

There is slight red color with veins appearing, gas and sounds, obstructions arising and subsiding in the navel region and intestines, pain in the heart, waist, navel, rectum and groin, expelling loud sounding gas, obstructed feces, insufficient urine.

Vāyu causes upward-moving air, pain, and gas. Pitta causes delusion, thirst, burning, and fever. Kapha causes heaviness, loss of taste and appetite, and abdominal hardness. The liver, situated on the right side, when enlarged and displaced, causes abdominal swelling similar to the spleen.

Vāyu: Swelling of hands and feet, scrotum, and pain in the central and upper abdomen, ribs, waist, legs, scrotum, and back. One may feel cutting pain in the joints, dry cough, body ache, heaviness of the lower body, waste accumulation, grayish or reddish skin, nails, eyes, urine, and feces; occasional increase and decrease of the abdomen, pricking and piercing pain, thick, black abdominal veins, hollow sounding abdomen (when tapped), gas moves all around the abdomen with pain and noise. Other symptoms include abdominal cracks, colic pain in the sides of the abdomen and chest, upward moving abdominal air, general weakness, emaciation, weakness, anorexia, indigestion, cracking pain in the fingers, lower abdominal heaviness, constipation, unable to pass gas or urine, Vāyu moving up, down, and sideways with colic pain and noise.

Pitta: Fever, fainting, burning, thirst, bitter taste, dizziness, diarrhea, yellow or greenish complexion, nails, eyes, urine, and feces; abdominal veins of yellow, blue, green, or coppery-red color; perspiration, heat, soft to the touch, quickly collects fluid. One may experience giddiness, pungent taste, sense of pain, smoke rising, and stickiness. These symptoms may indicate the development of ascites (*udako dara*).

Kapha: Physical debility, loss of the sensation of touch, swelling, heaviness, excess sleep, nausea, loss of taste and appetite, difficult breathing, cough, white complexion, eyes, nails, feces, and urine, smooth, unmoving abdomen with a whitish vein network, slowly increasing over time, becoming hard, cold, and heavy. One may also develop anorexia, indigestion, general weakness, numbness, hand, leg, thigh, and scrotal swellings, hard and heavy abdomen.

Tridoṣhic: Appearance of the signs of each *doṣha* listed above; nails, complexion, eyes, urine, and stool become afflicted with all the colors mentioned for each *doṣha*; a vein network with the colors of the *doṣhas* described above. Other symptoms include ingesting menstrual blood, wastes, etc., poisons. When *doṣhas* mixed with blood become aggravated and localized in the abdomen, it creates emaciation, fainting, dizziness, and produce an enlarged abdomen, symptoms of all the *doṣhas,* and quickly developing fluid. This is a serious condition, most troubling during cold, windy, and cloudy days.

Spleen /Liver (Plīho-yakrddalu dara): The spleen is displaced from the left side and becomes enlarged from habitually eating excessive amounts of food, exhaustion, excess travel, sex, exercise, heavy work, walking, vomiting, weakness due to diseases, increased blood, plasma, and other tissues. The enlarged spleen becomes hard like a stone, then as it increases, resembles a tortoise shell. This covers the whole abdomen, along with difficult breathing, cough, severe thirst, bad taste in mouth, pain, fever, yellowish-white complexion, fainting, vomiting, burning, delusion, slightly red or discolored, with blue or deep yellow lines. Other symptoms include weakness, anorexia, indigestion, constipation, urine and abdominal gas retention, fainting, thirst, vomiting, prostration, poor digestion, emaciation, finger joint or colic pain, alimentary tract distention caused by air, reddish or discolored abdomen, green, yellow, or blue vein network. The same symptoms develop for the liver as for the spleen.

Intestinal Obstruction (Baddha-gudo dara): Thirst, dry mouth and palate, burning sensation, fever, exhaustion in the thighs, cough, difficult breathing, weakness, anorexia, indigestion, constipation, not passing urine, abdominal distention, vomiting, sneezing, headache, colic pain in the heart, umbilical region, and anus, no peristaltic movement in the abdomen, reddish-blue vein network or a knotty vein network, elongated abdominal swellings looking like a cow's tail.

Intestinal Perforation (Chido dara): Eating bones or other sharp things can puncture or ulcerate the intestines. The undigested food flows out through that hole or ulcer in small quantities, collects in the rectum, gets mixed with feces, becomes foul smelling, slimy, yellowish-red, and gradually fills and enlarges the lower abdomen. Then fluid fills the abdomen, manifesting symptoms of the respective *doṣhas*, and being associated with difficult breathing, thirst, and dizziness.

Ascites (Udako dara): No appetite, thirst, colic pain, difficult breathing, cough, discharge from the anus, general debility, a multicolored vein network on the abdomen, hollow sounding abdomen (upon tapping).

Overall, this is considered a difficult disease to heal; therefore, before any water accumulates in the abdomen, the condition should be immediately attended to. If water is allowed to accumulate, the deranged *doṣhas* become displaced and liquefied. This will cause stickiness in the joints and circulatory channels, and divert sweat away from the external channels (moving the sweat sideways). This sideways movement further adds to the accumulated abdominal water. The sticky fluid makes the abdomen round, heavy, and numb; the sides of the abdomen become excessively enlarged. The vein networks then disappear and the navel area is mainly afflicted. Then the disease spreads to the rest of the abdomen and water begins to accumulate therein.

If the condition is still not corrected, persons experience complications of vomiting, diarrhea, *tamaka* (bronchial) asthma, thirst, and difficult breathing. Other complications include pain in the sides of the chest, hoarseness, anorexia, and suppression of urine. At this point, the disease can only be controlled but no longer healed unless strong medicines (i.e., with poisonous properties) are prescribed or surgery is performed.

After 14 to 15 days without treatment, abdominal swelling (*baddha-gudo dara*) cannot be healed (but can still be controlled). Ascites with water in the abdomen, and acute abdominal swelling due to intestinal perforation (*chidro dara*) can only be healed by poisonous medicines or surgery.

Although some illnesses are generally curable, there may be other complications that allow these illnesses to be controlled but not completely cured. Complications include swollen eyes, curved genitalia, sticky and thin skin, weakened strength, blood, muscle, and digestion.

Symptoms of swelling of the heart, difficult breathing, hiccup, anorexia, thirst, fainting, vomiting, and diarrhea are the most life-threatening complications.

Abdominal diseases may also exist without the accumulation of water (*ajā-todaka*). Its symptoms include almost no swelling (in the abdomen or legs), reddish abdomen, hollow sound upon tapping, not very heavy, gurgling sounds are always present. Persons may experience a vein network covering the abdomen, gas will move from the rectum to the navel, distending the navel area (distention releases after passing stool and gas). Other symptoms include colic pain around the heart, navel, groin, lumbar, and anus; forceful elimination of gas, moderate digestion. Excessive salivation causes a lack of taste in the mouth, scanty urine, and hard stools.

<u>Therapies</u>:

These diseases are the most difficult to heal unless the diseases are detected in early stages, there is no fluid, and the diseased person is still strong.

Therapy is suggested when there is no abdominal swelling, reddish, hollow sounding (upon tapping), not very heavy, and continual gurgling sounds. Other symptoms that require therapy include many vein networks, a distended navel (that subsides after passing the gas), pain in the heart, groin, waist, navel, and anus. Further symptoms include passing hard gas, moderate to strong digestion, mouth salivation causing tastelessness, scanty urine, or hard stools. All these signs indicate symptoms without fluid; they may undergo therapy for healing.

Persons having swollen eyes, crooked genitals, moist and thick skin, lack of strength, blood, digestion, and suffering from emaciation should not undergo therapy. Abdominal disorders, with complications of swollen vital organs, difficult breathing, hiccup, anorexia, thirst, fainting, vomiting, and diarrhea are considered fatal.

<u>General</u>: Since this illness is mostly caused by the contribution of all the *doṣhas*, therapies to alleviate all three *doṣhas* are used. Appetizing, light foods (e.g., *basmati* rice, barley, green lentils, *mūngdal*, barley gruel, vegetables).

Herbs include *pippalī*, *harītakī*, ginger, *chitrak*, and *viḍaṅga* with cane sugar, rock salt, and *ghee*. The watery residue of yogurt (whey—*muttadh/takra*) is useful in all abdominal diseases.

Persons should avoid animal products (especially fish), sesame seeds, pastries, foods that are hot, salty, sour, burning, and heavy; water, physical exercise, long walks, naps, long journeys.

<u>*Vāyu*</u>: When persons are strong, they first undergo oil massage and fomentation, followed by castor oil purgation. Once the *doṣha* is balanced and the abdomen no loner distended, a cloth bandage is wrapped around the abdomen to prevent Vāyu from distending it again; the cloth compresses space that can cause a pocket of gas. Purgation is done daily to remove accumulated *doṣhas* obstructing the digestive channels. After passing stool, one eats a Vāyu-reducing diet and drinks boiled milk (before meals or after food is digested) to develop strength. Once strong, the person gradually reduces intake of milk to prevent nausea.

If upward movement of Vāyu (*Udāna*/reverse peristalsis) occurs, the digestive fire is strengthened by vegetable soups with a bit of sour and salty tastes to it. Later, oil massage, fomentation, and dry enemas are given. Oil enemas are used for twitching, convulsions, pain in the joints, incases of twichings, convulsions, pain in joints, bones, sides, back, and sacrum. This enema is also useful for persons suffering from stool and gas retention, or for the strong person.

If persons are weak, old, or very young, or with only a slight increase of Vāyu, the only therapy suggested is pacification. Persons need a mild Vāyu-reducing diet. Examples include *ghee*, vegetables, soup, rice, boiled milk (alone), dry or oil enema, mild massage, yogurt/water drink (1:1) with *pippalī*, and black salt.

Nonoily enemas use *daśhmūl* with rhubarb or other strong purgatives, while oil enemas include castor or sesame oil cooked with Vāyu-reducing herbs (e.g., *triphalā*, cardamom), and sour herbs like *āmalakī*.

Vāyu: With side pain, stiffness, and constricted heart area, herbs include *bilwa and balā*. Oil laxatives like castor oil are useful. Afterwards, *tṛikatu*, *daśhmūl*, or *hiṅg* is taken.

Pitta: Strong persons use purgatives from the beginning of therapy, while weak persons are first cleansed by oil enemas, and then by milk enemas. When their physical and digestive strength returns, they receive an oil massage, followed by purgation with boiled milk and castor oil, yogurt/water (1:1) drink with cane sugar.

Kapha: First oil massage, then fomentation followed by evacuation through fomentation, sweat, and laxatives. After that, one takes Kapha-reducing foods, liquids, and herbs for pacification, 3/4 warm water with 1/4 fat-free yogurt (*lassi*) with *tṛikatu*.

Kapha/Vāyu: *Ghee* and sesame oil with ginger and *pippalī*.

Tridoṣha: The therapies used depend upon the most vitiated *doṣhas*. One quarter fat-free yogurt with 3/4 water (*lassi*), mixed with cane sugar, *tṛikatu*, and rock salt.

Enlarged Liver and Spleen: Aloe gel, *chirāyatā* (or gentian), saffron (or safflower), *punarnavā*, *bhūmīāmalakī,* and *bhṛiṅgarāj* with *ghee*. Light foods and vegetables are also eaten. Vāyu or Kapha forms may require cauterization. Pitta excesses require milk enemas, drinking boiled milk and bloodletting. Yogurt/water with honey, sesame oil, calamus, and ginger are other therapies.

Cirrhosis—*bhṛiṇgarāj* is the best herb; other herbs for enlarged liver.

Infected Hepatitis—*guḍūchī, sudarṣhan,* iron supplements; and enlarged liver herbs; *nila (isatis)*—antibiotic.

Chronic Liver Complaints—aloe gel, *guḍūchī* extract, *āmalakī, śhatāvarī;* olive, sesame, and avocado oils rebuild the liver.

Intestinal Obstruction: Fomentation followed by nonoily and oil enemas, irritant herbs (e.g., *chitrak*, pepper, ginger, *harītakī*), oil, and salt. Rhubarb, castor oil, or senna purge the system, healing reverse peristalsis and Vāyu. Yogurt water with rock salt and *pippalī* is also helpful. Boiled milk with ginger, *viḍaṅga*, *chitrak,* or *tṛikatu* is another useful remedy.

Intestinal Perforation: Kapha therapy is used (except for fomentation), and includes yogurt/water with *pippalī* and raw honey. If thirst, cough, fever, loss of weight (deteriorated in flesh), poor digestion, lack of hunger, difficult breathing, colic, or weakened senses exist, therapies cannot help the condition. [When the digestive fire (*pachak agni*) is reduced, food is not digested or absorbed. Thus, persons do not gain weight. Hot spices increase the digestive fire.]

Ascites: Kapha-reducing foods and few liquids. Herbs include *tṛikatu,* calamus, *triphalā,* and *chitrak*. Yogurt/water with raw honey and sesame oil are other useful therapies.

Complications: With edema, hard bowels, colic thirst, or fainting, herbs are used for debilitation after passing stools. Boiled milk is also helpful. *Aśhwagandhā* with *ghee* is spread on the abdomen, and water (with *punarnavā*, calamus, ginger, and coriander) is sprinkled over it (this herbal mixture is also ingested).

Vāyu with edema, distention, tumors and hemorrhoids: *Pippalī*, *chitrak*, ginger, and *daśhmūl.*

Jaundice (Kāmalā Roga)

Causes: Jaundice can develop either from anemia, or on its own. When it arises from anemia, it is caused by aggravated Pitta (from Pitta-increasing foods and lifestyle). The excessed Pitta then burns up the blood and muscles, producing jaundice in the alimentary tract (g.i.t.). The excessed *doṣha* then travels through the transportation channels (*srotas*) and produces jaundice in the different tissues. Its symptoms include deep yellow eyes, urine, skin, nails, mouth, and feces; burning, indigestion, thirst, greenish-brown complexion, and weakness of the sense organs.

When Vāyu and Pitta are excessed, there is greenish-bluish-yellow complexion with dizziness, no sexual desire, mild fever, stupor, physical weakness, and poor digestion.

Jaundice can occur simply from ignoring an aggravated Pitta condition. This leads to jaundice with edema and is hard to cure. Edema is the major secondary complication of anemia and jaundice.

Therapies: First, oil massage, then mild emesis and purgation with bitter herbs. Foods include *basmati* rice, barley, whole wheat, soups, peas, lentils, and oils that reduce Pitta; white radish, yellow squash, green leafy vegetables, chlorophyll, dandelion, and sugar cane. The best herbs include *bhūāmalakī*, *guḍūchī*, and *sudarṣhan chūrṇa* (will aggravate Vāyu symptoms). Other herbs include *triphalā*, neem, *balā*, *bhṛiṅgarāj*, *bilwa*, sandalwood, lemon grass, *kaṭukā*, barberry, vidārī kand, *āmalakī,* gotu kola, aloe gel, turmeric, barberry, *ṭrikatu*, dry ginger with boiled milk, cane sugar, and *ghee*.

Gallstones

Causes: Congestion obstructs the bile flow and inflames the gallbladder wall.

Symptoms:

General: Symptoms include acute pain in the liver and gallbladder, swelling, and tenderness.

Vāyu: Stones are black or brown, dry or rough; they cause severe pain but mild inflammation and fever.

Pitta: Stones are yellow, red, or green with sharp angles, painful and inflamed.

Kapha: Soft, round, whitish stones, rarely painful.

Therapies:

Purgation with aloe or rhubarb (mixed with fennel) is required in acute conditions. *Bhūāmalakī*, turmeric, and *mañjiṣhṭhā* are next used to cleanse the liver and blood.

Certain herbs break up stones. These include *gokṣhura*, *kaṭukā*, and *paṣhana bedha*. Taken with coriander or turmeric, the herb's actions are directed to the gall bladder.

Dyspepsia (Mandāgnī)

Four kinds of gastric fire or digestive activity (*jaṭharāgni*) exist: *Viṣhamāgni* (Vāyu-caused), *tīkṣhṇa* (Pitta-caused), *mandāgni* (Kapha-caused), and *samanāgni* (normal digestion). *Viṣhamāgni* is variable digestion. *Tīkṣhṇāgni* digests normal and excess quantities of food too quickly. *Mandāgni* cannot digest any food. *Samanāgni* digests normal quantities of food without causing any difficulties; this is the ideal state of digestion.

Indigestion (Ajīrṇa)

Three kinds of indigestion exist: *Āma* (Kapha-caused), *vidaghda* (Pitta-caused), and *viṣhṭabdha* (Vāyu-caused). [Some authorities suggest three other forms of indigestion: *Rasaeṣha* (indigestion of nutrients), *dinapāka* (food is digested the next day but without causing difficulty), and *prativāsara* (indigestion immediately after eating each meal).

Causes:

Drinking large quantities of water, eating insufficient or excess amounts of food at unusual times, eating unwholesome foods, suppression of natural urges, insomnia, and daytime naps. Mental causes include eating when angry, jealous, anxious, worried, frightened, grieing, miserable, or in pain.

Symptoms:

General: Weakness without exertion, heaviness of the body, not eliminating gas and stool, giddiness, constipation, or diarrhea.

Vāyu: Abdominal pain or distention, gas retention, delusion, and other Vāyu symptoms.

Pitta: Giddiness, thirst, fainting, sour and hot belchings, sweating, burning sensations (e.g., heartburn), and other Pitta symptoms.

Kapha: Abdominal and body heaviness, nausea, belching, swelling of the cheeks and eyes.

Nutrition: Aversion to food, abdominal heaviness, extreme belchings. Pain develops wherever *āma* resides in the body. Many diseases can develop because *doṣhas* travel in the body with *āma*.

Indigestion is the cause of many diseases. When it is healed, other diseases are healed automatically.

Complications:

Indigestion can lead to fainting, delirium, vomiting, excessive salivation, debility, giddiness, and even death. Insomnia, restlessness, tremors, suppression of urine, and fainting are the five most troubling complications. (Indigestion can cause three other diseases, *visūchikā, alasaka,* and *vilambikā*—see below).

Healthy Digestion:

Symptoms include belchings without bad smell or taste, enthusiasm, proper elimination of gas, stool, and urine; lightness of the body, natural hunger and thirst.

Therapies:

Vāyu: Moist heat (fomentation). Herbal combinations include *triphalā, yogaraj guggul, hiṅgwastock chūrṇa, sitopalādi, chūrṇa, laṣhunadi vaṭi,* and *lavaṇa bhāskar*. Other useful herbs include asafoetida, ginger, cumin, and rock salt.

Pitta: *Vamanna* (vomiting with warm salt water). Drinking cold water helps reduce acidic digestion. *Harītakī* and raw honey can be licked, or *harītakī* and *drākṣhā* ingested. Aloe vera, *musta, chirāyatā*, and *mahāsudarṣhan chūrṇa*.

Kapha: Fasting until one feels better. The same therapies as Vāyu, plus black pepper, *chitrak,* and *ṭrikatu* (i.e., hotter spices quickly raise the digestive fire).

Nutrition: Rest in bed, dry heat (fomentation); *harītakī,* and dry ginger. Cardamom, coriander, turmeric, and fennel can be taken with meals daily to maintain health and prevent indigestion.

Visūchikā (Gastro Enteritis)

Symptoms: When persons suffer from indigestion, mad food cravings, careless eating habits, and overeating, they may experience pricking pain (as if needles are sticking them). Other symptoms include fainting, diarrhea, vomiting, severe thirst, burning sensations all over, poor complexion, tremors, pain in the heart area and head, and twisting of the arms and legs. (Therapies below)

Alasaka

Symptoms: Severe abdominal distention, delusion, crying helplessly, upward-moving gas (i.e., blocked downward movement of the gas), not eliminating gas and stool; thirst, belching. (Therapies below)

Vilambikā

Excess Kapha and Vāyu remains in the body and cannot be expelled. This condition is very difficult to heal or cannot be healed.

Therapies:

If these 3 conditions can be healed, therapies

include dry heat (fomentation), strong emetics and purgatives, fasting, bathing, or sprinkling emetic or purgative decoction water, and nonoily enemas. Herbs include *vachā, hiṅg,* or *ativiṣhā* with tepid water. Rock salt, *ghee, triphalā, pippalī,* and *tṛikatu* are also useful. A mixture of *pippalī* and ginger in hot water is also effective.

Peyā (thin gruel), digestive and appetizing herbs (e.g., cardamom, cumin, coriander, fennel, etc.) are taken when hunger returns.

Anāha

This condition occurs when *āma* and/or feces accumulate in the digestive tract, obstructing normal movement. Accumulated *āma* produces thirst, runny nose, burning sensation in the head, stomach pain and heaviness, heart pain, stiff joints in the back and waist, obstructed feces and urine, fainting, vomiting of feces, difficult breathing, and other symptoms of *alasaka* (see above).

Therapies:

When *āma* obstructs the digestive tract

1) First, emetics are administered, then digestive herbs and foods.
2) If vomiting of feces does not occur, the body receives dry heat fomentation and digestive herbs are taken.
3) Purgative herb powders can be blown into the intestines with a tube (through the rectum).
4) Purgative herbal past suppositories (*vartis*) are then used.
5) Persons can take emetic or purgative decoctions.
6) Once *āma* is removed, nonoily enemas are used (purgative herbs, honey, and rock salt).
7) If needed, an oil enema can also be used.

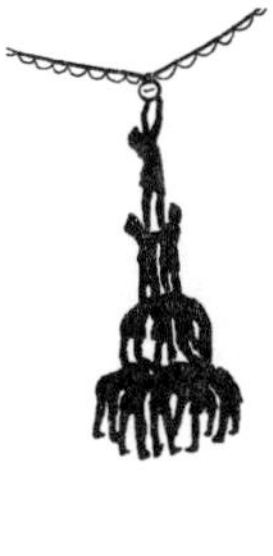

Colic (Śhūla)

Causes:

Vāyu: Excessive exercise, travel, or sexual intercourse; not sleeping at night, drinking very cold water, eating very dry foods (i.e., dry, astringent, and bitter items), overeating, injury, sprouted grains, incompatible foods (e.g., hot and cold items at the same meal), stale foods, suppression of natural urges, fasting, excessive laughing, or talking.

Pitta: Excessive intake of hot, pungent, sour, irritating, and fermented foods and liquids; anger, overheating, fatigue, overexposure to the sun, and sexual intercourse.

Kapha: Excessive intake of animal products, fatty substances, diary, sugar, nuts, and other Kapha-increasing items and habits.

Tridoṣha: Indulging in habits of each of the three *doṣhas* causes tridoṣhic colic.

Symptoms:

Vāyu: Pain in the heart, ribs, back, waist, and urinary bladder. The pain (pricking and tearing) becomes worse during or after digestion, in the evenings, in cloudy or cold weather. Other symptoms include gas, distention, insomnia, variable appetite, nervousness, and palpitations.

Pitta: Thirst, delusion, burning sensation near the navel, hyperacidity, heartburn, diarrhea, perspiration, irritability, fainting, and giddiness. Colic becomes more painful around noon and midnight during digestion and in rainy weather. Colic is relieved during cold weather and by eating and drinking sweet and cold items.

Kapha: Nausea, cough, debility, anorexia, salivation, stomach pain, white or clear phlegm, congestion, vomiting, feeling full after eating. These symptoms are worse at sunrise and in the spring and fall seasons.

Tridoṣha: Severe symptoms of all three *doṣhas* appear throughout the day and are difficult to heal. Practitioners do not attempt to heal incurable cases.

Therapies:

General: Since Vāyu is the underlying cause

of colic, air-reducing therapies are advised: fomentation (moist heat application), oil *abhyañga,* and *ghee.* Herbs include cardamom, ginger, and fennel for abdominal pain, dispelling gas, and digesting food and *āma. Hiṅg,* nutmeg, chamomile, and *jaṭāmāṇśhī* relieve colic pain. Light, simple meals are advised.

Vāyu: Herbs include rock salt, *viḍaṅga, chitrak, pippalī, hiṅg, lavaṇ bhāskar chūrṇa,* and *drākṣhā* (medicated grape wine). Small, light, and warm Vāyu-reducing foods and liquids are taken. An anti-*āma* diet is also useful for a few days.

Pitta: First, one drinks cold water and induces vomiting. Thereafter, cool foods, liquids, and lifestyles are advised (i.e., Pitta-reducing). Bitter herbs such as *chirāyatā* and *kaṭukā* are suggested. Carminative herbs like fennel, mint, coriander, cumin, and saffron are also helpful. *Avipattikar chūrṇa* with a little dry ginger is another useful mixture.

Kapha: This condition requires drinking an emetic decoction followed by vomiting. Dry fomentation (heat application) and heating herbs (e.g., *pippalī,* dry ginger, *vachā, tṛikatu, chitrak*) are used, as well as the Vāyu-reducing therapies discussed above.

Tridoṣha: The above therapies used depend upon the predominant symptoms.

Pārṣhva-śhūla

Causes, Development and Symptoms:

Excess Kapha in the sides of the body blocks Vāyu, causing abdominal distention and intestinal rumbling. Persons experience pricking pain in the ribs, heart, and bladder; insomnia, no appetite, difficult and painful breathing. This condition is caused by excess Vāyu and Kapha.

Therapies:

Hiṅg, rock salt, and *tumburu* are taken in a barley decoction. Castor oil and *drākṣhā* (medicated grape wine) are also effective.

Kukṣhi-śhūla

Causes, Development, and Symptoms:

Excess Vāyu affects digestion, and when located in the hips and abdomen, interferes with previously eaten meals. Thus, all foods remain undigested. Symptoms include heavy breathing due to accumulated feces. This causes the person to toss in agony, and to find no relief in any position or posture. This condition is caused by excess Vāyu.

Therapies:

Vomiting and fasting are advised if persons are strong. Acidic and appetizing herbs are taken to reduce Vāyu and *āma.* Dry ginger, *hiṅg, bṛihatī, kaṇṭkārī, vachā, kuśhṭā, ativiṣhā,* and *kuṭaj* are recommended. Purgatives, nonoily and oily enemas can reduce accumulated excesses. Oil *abhyañga* and sweating (hot poultices) are useful, as are fermented rice washes.

Cardiac Colic (Hirchula)

Causes, Development, and Symptoms:

Weakened plasma (*rasa*) causes excess Vāyu (which acts with Pitta and Kapha) in the heart area. This results in colic pain in the heart region. Symptoms include difficult breathing. The condition is caused by excess *rasa* and Vāyu.

Therapies:

Heart disease therapies are used (see Chapter 14), as well as those mentioned above for Vāyu.

Bladder Colic (Bāsti-śhūla)

Vāyu becomes excessed in the bladder because of suppression of urine and feces, causing pain in the bladder, groin, and navel. This causes further suppression of urine, stool, and gas. It is caused by excess Vāyu. Vāyu-reducing therapies mentioned above are used.

Urinary Colic (Mutra-śhūla)

Excess Vāyu causes piercing pain in the

genitals, intestines, hips, lower abdomen, and navel areas. This pain prevents the release of urine. Vāyu-reducing therapies are used.

Abdominal Colic (Vit-śhūla)

Vāyu becomes excessed when dry foods are eaten, weakening the digestive fire and preventing stool evacuation. This causes excruciating pain in the lower abdominal area. Pain begins on the right or left side, then eventually spreads to the whole abdomen. Other symptoms include rumbling sounds, unquenchable thirst, vertigo, and are followed by epileptic fits. Therapies include fomentation (moist heat application), emetics, nonoily and oily enemas, purgatives, and the Vāyu-reducing herbs mentioned above.

Annaja-śhūla

Overeating during weakened digestion aggravates Vāyu, preventing the digestive tract from digesting food. This causes intolerable colic pain. Symptoms include abdominal distention, epileptic fits, nausea, belching, *vilambikā* (see indigestion), shivering, vomiting, and fainting. Vāyu-reducing therapies mentioned above are used.

Gulma (benign abdominal tumor) therapies are used for all colic conditions.

Hyperacidity

Excessive gastric juice activity results in acidic or sour taste in the mouth.

Causes:

Vāyu: A variable digestion cannot always digest foods. When food is not digested, *āma* develops. These undigested food toxins begin to ferment, causing burning sensations.

Pitta: Eating too many hot, spicy, sour, greasy foods and spices (e.g., onions, garlic, red peppers); incompatible foods, alcohol, and overeat-

ing. Other causes include eating too many sweets, such as cakes, which ferment and produce acid in the stomach.

Kapha: Weak digestion allows *āma* to develop when food is not digested. Thus, toxins ferment and cause burning sensations.

Symptoms:

Heartburn, belching with sour taste or fluids, nausea, vomiting.

Therapies:

Vāyu: *Hiṅgwastock*, rock salt, *laṣhunadi vaṭi*, *drākṣhā*, along with antacids like *śhaṇk bhasma*, *avipattikar chūrṇa*, fennel, and *praval piṣhti*.

Pitta: Pitta-reducing foods and herbs, antacid foods like milk and *ghee*. Acidic and sour foods are avoided, including bananas (sour post-digestive taste), pickles, wine, and yogurt. Useful herbs include *śhatāvarī*, licorice, aloe gel, *chirāyatā*, and antacids like *śhāṇka bhasma* (conch shell ash) and *āvipattikar chūrṇa*.

Kapha: *Hiṅgwastāk*, rock salt, *laṣhunadi baṭi*, *drakṣha*; and antacids like *śhāṇka bhasma* (conch shell ash) and *āvipattikar chūrṇa*.

Acid Gastritis/Acid Reflux (Amlapitta)

This is an inflammation of the stomach and its lining.

Causes and Symptoms:

Eating incompatible food combinations, spoiled foods, and very sour or acidic foods or liquids increases Pitta in persons with already excessed Pitta. Symptoms include indigestion, exhaustion, nausea, belchings with bitter or sour taste, heaviness, loss of appetite, burning sensation in the chest and throat. Pitta symptoms are twofold, upward (*ūrdhvaga*) and downward (*adhoga*).

Downward Symptoms: Thirst, burning sensations, fainting, giddiness, delusion, diarrhea, nausea, skin rashes, poor digestion, hair standing on end, perspiration, yellowish skin.

Upward Symptoms: Vomiting green, yellow,

black, blue, red, sour, thin, and sticky materials, followed by mucus. Other symptoms include bitter or sour tastes from vomiting or belching, burning sensations in the throat, chest, upper abdomen, hands and feet; headache, loss of heat, loss of appetite, Kapha/Pitta fever, circular, itching, studded rashes with numerous pimples.

The longer a person has had gastritis, the more difficult it is to heal.

Vāyu-caused: Tremors, delirium, fainting, sensations of pins and needles, weakness, pain, darkened vision, giddiness, delusion, hair standing on end.

Kapha-caused: Expectorating thick phlegm, heaviness, fatigue, loss of appetite, coldness, weakness, vomiting, white coating on the tongue, burning sensation, itching, sleeping longer and more often.

Vāyu/Kapha-caused: Symptoms of both *doṣhas*.

Pitta/Kapha-caused: Belching with bitter, sour, and pungent tastes, burning sensation in the chest, upper abdomen, and throat; giddiness, fainting, loss of appetite, vomiting, fatigue, headache, salivation, sweet taste in mouth.

Therapies:

Therapies are the same as for hyperacidity. Milk is recommended for Vāyu and Pitta excesses.

Malabsorption (Sprue)

Causes: Environmental bacteria, poor eating habits, excessive eating or fasting, ingesting overly hot or cold items, eating canned, stale, or junk foods. It also develops from chronic diarrhea, constipation, or dysentery; excessive use of purgatives or colonics, antibiotics, and from excessive mental and physical stresses.

Symptoms:

Vāyu: Variable digestion, white spots or ridges on fingernails, teeth marks on the front arc of the tongue, constipation, abdominal distention, migrating pain, dry skin, cracked tongue, hemorrhoids, anal fissures, emaciation, weak muscles and bones, arthritis. Stools vary from watery to gaseous, hard, and dry movements. One may experience palpitations, anxiety, insomnia, depression, and faintness.

Pitta: Overly strong digestion, dysentery or diarrhea (yellow-colored), abdominal pain, low-grade fevers, infections, inflammation, ulceration, burning sensation, anemia, malodorous feces, white spots or ridges on finger nails, teeth marks on the front arc of the tongue. The tongue marks deepen when angry or irritable (i.e., Pitta-increasing emotional situations).

Kapha: Weak digestion, teeth marks on the front arc of the tongue, mucus in the stool, diarrhea and constipation, dull abdominal pain, congestion, edema, diabetes, white spots or ridges on fingernails.

Therapies:

General: Light, simple, easily digested meals depending upon one's *doṣha*. Yogurt-water (*lassi*) improves digestion. If persons are strong, they can tolerate a *lassi* fast for several days. *Kicharī* (*basmati* rice and *mūngdal*) should then be introduced into the diet. Absorption-promoting herbs include cardamom, fennel, cumin, *harītakī,* and *drākṣhā* wine.

Vāyu: Vāyu-reducing foods and *lassi* with fresh ginger are beneficial. Herbs taken with meals include cardamom, *pippalī,* fresh ginger, cinnamon, fennel, *hiṅgwastock*, cumin, *chitrak, harītakī, laṣhuṇa vati,* and *drākṣhā* wine. Useful foods include whole grains and steamed vegetables (i.e., not eaten raw).

Pitta: Pitta-reducing foods and *lassi* with cardamom are beneficial. Herbs taken with meals include cardamom, fresh ginger, fennel, cumin, *chitrak, harītakī, avipattikar chūrṇa,* and *drākṣhā* wine. Onions, garlic, red peppers, salty, fermented, fried and greasy foods increase Pitta, and therefore aggravate this condition.

Kapha: Kapha-reducing foods and *lassi* (1/4 cup lo-fat yogurt: 3/4 cup water) with dry ginger are beneficial. Herbs taken with meals include cardamom, *pippalī,* dry ginger, cinnamon, *hiṅgwastock,* cumin, *chitrak, harītakī, trikatu, laṣhuṇa vati,* and *drākṣhā* wine. Dairy, cold liquids, raw vegetables, salt, and sweets aggravate this condition.

Food Allergies

This condition is due to weak immune and nervous systems, and poor digestion—that creates toxins in the body. These systems are weakened through taking antibiotics, junk food and food additives, environmental pollution, anxiety, worry, and stressful lifestyle. Children born to mothers with weak immune systems and allergies may also exhibit these conditions; though breast-fed children are less likely to develop food allergies.

Vāyu *doṣhas*, having the most delicate nervous systems, are more likely to have food allergies. There may be a parallel emotion of not feeling nurtured. Kapha *doṣhas*, with weak digestive fire, may also exhibit food allergies.

Symptoms:

General: Gas, indigestion, bloating, diarrhea, constipation, congestion, skin rashes, headaches. Certain foods are more likely to cause allergic reactions such as milk and wheat (difficult to digest), corn, soy; nightshades (contain alkaloids) such as eggplant, tomato; strawberries, peaches.

Vāyu: Beans, soy, corn, and other Vāyu-increasing foods.

Pitta: Nightshades and sour fruits (e.g., strawberries, peaches, apricots).

Kapha: Dairy, wheat, and other Kapha-increasing foods.

Therapies:

General: Initially, persons need to avoid the foods that cause allergic reactions while taking herbs to improve the digestion (e.g., cardamom, coriander), calm the nerves (e.g., gotu kola), and improve the immune system (e.g., *guḍūchī*); follow one's *doṣha* food plan, exercise, and reduce stress.

Therapies listed under malabsorption are used here. Once the allergies are diminished, stronger immune-boosting herbs like *śhatāvarī* and *aśhwagandhā* can be taken.

Parasites (Krimi)

Causes: Both internal and external forms of parasites exist. Sweat, Kapha, blood, and feces are the 4 causes. There are 20 species of parasites.

External (Bāhya): Parasites are the result of poor hygiene; they are the size, shape, and color of sesame seeds, have many legs, and reside in the hair and clothes. Two types exist: head lice and body lice. Head lice are black, and hide in the roots of hair. Body lice are white and reside in the hairs of the pubis and armpit, and are also found in clothes, particularly in the seams. Both are passed from person to another on combs, brushes, clothes, and other personal belongings, or their eggs are transmitted on loose hairs. They produce rashes, eruptions, itching, and small tumors.

Internal (Abhyantara): Arise from aggravated *doṣhas* through unsuitable foods and lifestyles, harmful or unethical actions such as scolding, defaming, killing, robbing, or unethical past life actions. The aggravated *doṣhas* invade all the channels inside the body, vitiating the skin, lymph, blood, and muscles, making these areas welcome spots for parasites to live. They are also caused by too many sweets, molasses, milk, yogurt, grains, Kapha grains (Kapha parasites), leafy vegetables (that cause more feces), and green legumes (feces parasites).

Kapha: Parasites reside in the stomach and small intestine. When they increase in number, they move throughout the alimentary tract. Their size and shape vary. Seven species exist. They cause nausea, excess salivation, indigestion, loss of taste and appetite, fainting, vomiting, fever, gas, abdominal distention, emaciation, excess sneezing and nasal mucus.

Blood (Raktaja): Parasites reside in the blood vessels, are very small, without legs, round, copper colored, and are of six species. Symptoms include skin discoloration, burning, itching, pricking pain, raised patches, and symptoms of other skin diseases.

These parasites are related to malaria, filaria, bacilli (leprosy), and viruses in the blood, liver, and spleen. They come from mosquito, flea, and bedbug bites. Some parasites are carried in the alimentary tracts of people who help with health maintenance.

Feces (Purīṣhaja): Reside in the colon, usually moving downwards. When they increase in number they travel up to the stomach and small intestine. Then they cause the smell of feces in the mouth, belching, and exhalations. They are thick, round, thin, and threadlike, or thick, blue, yellow, white or black, and of five species. They cause diarrhea, dysentery, abdominal pain; they also cause food to remain undigested in the stomach, emaciation, poor digestion, and rectal itching when feces are expelled.

Sweet—causes growth of parasites: Kapha/feces—intestinal parasites (round-worms, hookworms, threadworms, tapeworms, amoebas, and eggs enter the body through infected water and food, when improperly cooked or cleaned. A strong digestion destroys the eggs and parasites, a weak digestion allows the eggs and parasites to grow and harm the person.

Therapies: Parasites are more common in Vāyu and Kapha *doṣhas*, usually associated with *āma* or undigested foods. Long-term infestation causes wasting of tissues and deranging Vāyu. Parasites are found in the three *doṣhas* in
Vāyu: Stool
Pitta: Blood
Kapha: Mucus or mucus membranes, stomach, or small intestine

General- Tridoṣhic:

1) First, a detoxification diet (*āma* reduction), avoiding sweets, meats, dairy, fried foods, and yeast products, while eating more lightly steamed vegetables.
2) Purgation first, then 3 to 5 days on antiparasitic herbs. For gentle purgation a cup of *triphalā* tea with two teaspoons of castor oil are be taken upon rising. By noon, three to five stools are passed. A stronger purgation involves making a rhubarb tea before bed (1 tsp. rhubarb powder). Rhubarb also has antiparasitical properties.
3) Immune-boosting formulas like *siddha makardhwaj, kutajahan vati* and *kutajariṣhta* help quickly overcome parasites.

Vāyu: Certain herbs cause *agni* (digestive fire) to burn up the parasites: *Hiṅg*, black pepper, cayenne, *triphalā*, *musta*. A Vāyu-reduction diet avoiding rich and sweet foods, and using hot spices and castor oil purgatives. If malnourished or weak, *aśhwagandhā*, *balā,* or ginseng are added.

Pitta: Bitter tastes cleanse and reduce worms. Herbs include *viḍaṅga* (the main Āyurvedic herb for worms), *kuṭaj* (the main herb for amebic parasites—especially for amoebic dysentery), *kaṭukā*, *tulsī*, *betel* nuts, *musta*, aloe gel, and *chitrak*. Pumpkin seeds may also be eaten freely throughout the day. Castor oil purgatives are also useful. A *Pitta*-reduction diet includes lots of raw foods, vegetable juices, and greens, and omits hot spices.

Kapha: Bitter tastes cleanse and reduce worms, *viḍaṅga* (the main Āyurvedic herb for worms), *kuṭaj* (main herb for parasites), *kaṭukā*, *tulsī*, *betel* nuts, *chirāyatā* and *musta*, *agni*- (digestive fire) promoting herbs to burn up the parasites: *hiṅg*, black pepper, *pippalī,* and ginger. Pumpkin seeds may also be eaten freely throughout the day. An anti-Kapha diet with lots of hot spices (consume until sweating begins), sugar, and dairy are avoided; rhubarb root is used as a purgative.

Constipation (Ānāha)

Signs of a Healthy Colon: No tongue coating, easy passing of stool immediately upon waking in the morning. Stools should float (not sink), two to three stools daily.

Signs of an Unhealthy Colon: The back third of the tongue is coated, stools sink, one or no stools passed daily.

Causes: Eating foods that are difficult to digest and/or are Vāyu-increasing; developing as a result of fever or infection, sleeping too much, suppressing the urge to defecate. Other causes include a hectic lifestyle, sexual intercourse in the morning (weakens the downward flow of air/*Apāna* Vāyu), coffee or tea in the morning (is drying), and a lack of exercise. Mental causes include excess emotions (e.g., worry, fear, anxiety, anger, impatience, nervousness.)

Symptoms:

Vāyu: Dry colon, gas (with or without pain), abdominal distention, brownish coating on the back of the tongue, bad breath, anxiety, headache (because air is pushed upward instead of down and out with the stool), urge to urinate but difficulty passing urine.

Pitta: Usually constipation occurs at the end of fevers because toxins collect in the small intestine and colon. Other causes include eating foods that are too greasy, fried, salty, spicy, pungent, and hot (i.e., Pitta-increasing items). Symptoms include anger, irritability, thirst, sweating, body odor, burning sensation, reddish tongue with yellow coating; bad breath, flushed complexion, headache, and violent dreams. The liver is usually in need of detoxification as well.

Kapha: Causes include sleeping too long, day naps, lack of exercise, and Kapha-increasing foods. Excess mucus develops and clogs the system, causing heaviness, lethargy, fatigue, mucus in the stool, a pale, fat tongue with white or mucus coating, abdominal bloating, dull pain, edema.

Therapies:

General: The best herb for the colon is *triphalā,* which draws toxins from the colon and promotes toning, rejuvenation, and the passage of stool. It is taken in the morning and evening (1/2 to 1 tsp. with 4 times as much water). *Triphalā* is a gentle and mild laxative made from three fruits, *āmalakī, bibhītakī,* and *harītakī*. To achieve a stronger effect, ginger is added to the mixture and *harītakī* is doubled in quantity. When passing stool, squatting is a more natural position for bowel movements.

Vāyu: Vāyu-reducing foods, liquids, and lifestyle are required. Ingesting *ghee* and sesame oil will moisten the colon, as will dairy and small quantities of oily foods like almonds and sesame tahini. Boiled milk with *ghee* and cinnamon are good to take before bed. Digestive herbs include ginger, cardamom, and fennel. *Triphalā* is excellent, but castor oil (2 tsp. in a cup of boiled water before bed) is stronger and may be required if *triphalā* is not effective. Castor oil doses need to be adjusted (more or less) according to individual needs. Herbs to boost digestion are also required; they include rock salt, *hiṅg, lavaṇ bhāskar chūrṇa*. *Īśhabgol* (2 tsp.) taken in 1 cup of warm water before bed also relieves constipation. Dry foods (e.g., cabbage family, chips, beans) increase gas and constipation. Nonoily and oily enemas are also useful (see Chapter 7).

Pitta: Pitta-reducing food, liquids, and lifestyle are required. *Triphalā,* aloe vera, and fennel cleanse the colon, small intestine, and liver (1/2 tsp. before bed). Warm milk and *ghee* before bed is beneficial. A rhubarb and fennel purgative is useful when constipation is not resolved by the therapies just mentioned. Before taking the rhubarb purgative, oil *abhyañga* and sweating therapies are required to move toxins in the body back to the small intestine where they first originated.

Kapha: Kapha-reducing foods, liquids, and lifestyle are required. Fasting, exercise, mental stimulation, and less sleep help heal this condition. Sweets, dairy, yeast products, salt, fried and fermented foods aggravate this disorder. *Triphalā*, aloe, and rhubarb are useful as a laxative and purgative. Hot spices are also needed to reduce fat, mucus, and toxins in the body (e.g., dry ginger, black pepper, *pippalī, trikatu*). One or 2 tsp. of herbs in a cup of hot water before sleep reverses this disorder. A nonoily enema with the above herbs cleanses the colon.

Hemorrhoids (Arṣhas)

Causes: Simultaneous vitiation of all three *doṣhas* weakens the skin, muscles, and fat, obstructing the veins in the muscles of the rectum. The predominating *doṣha* will determine the main cause and symptoms.

Varieties: Two types of hemorrhoids exist: those that are congenital or those acquired occurring during one's life. Their symptoms are either dry or bleeding.

Congenital (Sahaja): Due to improper or unhealthy activities of the parents or fate. This produces tridoṣhic hemorrhoids that can be checked, but not healed (as with all hereditary diseases). They are dry, face inward or outward; some are round, irregularly spread or matted together, yellowish-white, usually small, and accompanied by secondary diseases.

After Birth (Janmotta-raja): Five types of this disease can occur: Vāyu, Pitta, Kapha, Tridoṣhic, and blood-induced. Vāyu and Kapha cause dry (*śhuṣhka*) piles, while Pitta and blood cause bleeding hemorrhoids.

Congenital Symptoms: *Apāna* Vāyu, being obstructed from birth, moves the air upwards, aggravating the other 4 Vāyu sub-*doṣhas,* Pitta, and Kapha. This develops the following conditions. Persons are born thin, lean, emaciated, and weak, with excessive gas, urine, and feces that may be obstructed. Other symptoms include poor complexion, urinary tract stones, and gravel. Feces can vary, from constipation or dryness to diarrhea, or may be normal. Sometimes feces have toxins and mucus. They can be white, pale, green, yellow, reddish, thin, dense, and slimy. Severe pain may develop in the navel, urinary bladder, and pelvis areas. Other symptoms include dysentery, hair standing on end, urinary disorders, diabetes, intestinal gurgling, distention, a sensation of stickiness in the heart and sensory organs. Persons may experience excessive bitter and sour belching, poor digestion, irritability, weakness, and small amounts of semen. Additional symptoms include frequent coughs, difficult breathing, bronchial asthma, thirst, nausea, vomiting, anorexia, indigestion, chronic rhinitis, sneezing, fainting, and headaches. Persons may develop low, weak, hoarse, and broken voices; ear diseases, fevers, joint and bone pain associated with general weakness. Stiffness in the side of the chest and abdomen, urinary bladder, heart area, back and lumbar regions can occur. Mentally, one is very thoughtful, giddy, or lazy.

Acquired Hemorrhoids

Causes:

General: Hemorrhoids are caused by excess aggravation of the *doṣhas* through improper diet and lifestyle that weaken the digestive fire. They may be caused by excess sex, riding, straining, sitting for long periods on uneven or hard seats, or on one's heels. Other causes include enema nozzles, rough surfaces, washing with very cold water, straining during defecation, and suppression or early release of gas, urine, or feces. Emaciation caused by fever, abdominal tumors, diarrhea, excess *āma*, duodenal disorders, edema, anemia, and overexertion can also cause this disease. For women this disorder can be caused by abortion, miscarriage, and abnormal fetus development. This leads to an accumulation of undigested food (toxin waste or *āma*). Feces become lodged in the folds of the rectum, hardening and causing friction, thus developing hemorrhoids.

Premonitory Symptoms: Weak digestion, weak thighs, twisting pain in calves, dizziness, enfeeblement of parts of the body, swelling of eyes, diarrhea or constipation, gas with lower abdominal pain, cutting pain in the anus; feces are difficult to eliminate with accompanying noise. Other symptoms include intestinal gurgling, abdominal distention, emaciation, excess belching, excess urine, and insufficient feces, not feeling the need to defecate, hot fumes, acidity, pain in the head, back, and chest, exhaustion, skin discoloration, stupor, weakened sense organs, anger, and unhappiness.

Development:

General: Downward moving air (*Apāna* Vāyu) moves upward because of obstructions of the rectum. This aggravates the other four forms of Vāyu (*Prāṇ*, Udān, Vyān, Samān) in the body, as well as the urine, feces, Pitta, Kapha, the tissues (*dhātus*), and their sites. Thus, digestion is weakened, and *āma* and feces accumulate and sit in the folds of the rectum.

Poor digestion, accumulation of sweat, urine, and feces can develop by eating too many heavy, sweet, cold foods and liquids that block the channels of circulation and cause burning sensations. Also, eating mutually contradictory foods, eating before the last meal is digested, eating too small portions, junk food or stale food, animal products or excessive amounts of pastries can cause trouble. Other causes include dry or raw vegetables, vinegar, garlic, pickles, heavy fruits, fermented wines, polluted water. External causes include excessive oleation therapy, not eliminating toxins, wrong use of enema therapy, lack of exercise, excessive sexual acts, and day naps.

When *Apāna* Vāyu is excessive, it pushes feces to the anal sphincter and aggravates it, developing hemorrhoids. *Apāna* Vāyu is deranged from sitting on rough, hard, or uneven seats, bumpy rides, excessive sexual intercourse, enema nozzles improperly inserted, too much cold water, and scratching the anus. Other causes include straining in life and in passing feces, suppressing the natural urges, miscarriage, pressure of the uterus during pregnancy, and abnormal delivery.

Vāyu: Eating astringent, pungent, bitter, dry, cold, and light food, eating too little food or fasting, drinking sharp alcohol, sex, living in too cold an environment, hard exercise, grief, and exposure to the wind.

Pitta: Eating pungent, hot, salty, burning, and sharp foods (e.g., onions, garlic, cayenne), straining exercise, exposure to the sun and fire, living in very hot places, drinking alcohol, envy, anger, and impatience.

Kapha: Eating sweet, oily, cold, salty, sour, and heavy foods, eastern winds, living in cold climates, mental lethargy.

Tridoshic: Caused by combinations of foods and lifestyles mentioned above.

Symptoms:

General: Severe emaciation, lack of enthusiasm, helplessness, a weakened, broken voice, pale complexion, weakened tissues, and pain in the vital organs. Further symptoms include cough, thirst, bad taste in the mouth, difficult breathing, nasal mucus, exhaustion, faint body pains, vomiting, excessive sneezing, edema, fever, impotence, deafness, and blindness. Persons may develop urinary gravel or stones, worry, spitting, loss of appetite, pains in all the bones, joints, heart, navel, anus, and groin. Other symptoms include oozing from the rectum, hemorrhoids (either dry or bleeding—yellow, green, red, or slimy) may occur.

Vāyu: Dry, tingling, shriveled, bluish-red, uneven, coarse and hard, sharp, cracked, associated with pain, cramps and excessive itchiness, numbness, and tingling sensations. Other symptoms include severe pain in the head, ribs, shoulders, waist, thighs and groin, sneezing, and belching. Further disorders include food not moving through the digestive tract, sudden heart pain, loss of taste or appetite, cough or difficult breathing. Irregular digestion, ringing in the ears, dizziness, blackened skin, nails, feces, urine, eyes, and face may occur. Feces disorders include small quantity with noises and straining, or dysentery followed by painful release of frothy, slimy fluid. If this is not healed, it will lead to abdominal tumors, enlargement of the spleen, abdomen, and prostate. Oily and hot things relieve this condition.

Pitta: Thin, soft, flabby hemorrhoids are blue, red, yellow, blue, or black in complexion, exuding thin blood with a foul smell and burning sensation in the body. Other symptoms include asthma, ulceration, fever, perspiration, excessive sweating and discharge, thirst, fainting, and loss of taste and appetite. Further disorders are delusion, heavy stool, brown, green, yellow or deep yellow complexion, eyes, and nails. The stool becomes yellow or red, and bloody, burning, and itching. Colic or pricking pain, yellow or green loose stools or diarrhea develops. Copious, yellow and malodorous urine and stool develop. Cold things bring relief.

Kapha: Hemorrhoids are deeply rooted, large, swollen, thick, hard, round, white, and bulging. They may be oily, greasy, smooth, with dull pain (but painless to the touch), stiff, and rigid. Other symptoms include severe itching, cutting pain in the anus, urinary bladder, and navel region. Further developments include cough, difficult breathing, nausea, salivation, anorexia with mucus, and urinary disorders (e.g., dysuria, diabetes, stones, gravel). Persons may experience vomiting, excessive spitting, cough, cold, impotence, dull head pain, and fever with shivering. Feces symptoms include straining to eliminate, containing mucus and excess elimination. The stool can be reddish, white and sometimes with slimy discharge. The urine and stool are heavy, slimy, and white. Complexion becomes yellowish-white and greasy; there is constant edema, and the organs feel as though covered with sticky material. The mouth has a sweet taste. Tuberculosis and poor digestion associated with acute diseases caused by *āma* (undigested food toxins) can develop. This is a chronic condition. Dry and hot things bring relief.

Tridoṣha: Symptoms of all three *doṣhas* will appear simultaneously.

Blood: Hemorrhoids caused by blood aggravation have symptoms similar to Pitta and have the look of Vāyu. Feces are hard, and hemorrhoids may bleed suddenly. This bleeding can lead to a greenish or pale complexion and to other diseases associated with loss of blood, strength, enthusiasm, and sensory abilities.

The most serious secondary complication to arise along with hemorrhoids is constipation.

The most serious forms of hemorrhoids occur with cardiac and/or rib pain, limb pain, fainting, vomiting, thirst, and inflammation of the anus. Almost as serious are symptoms of hand, leg, face, navel, anal, or testicle edema. In these cases, hemorrhoids can only be controlled, but they cannot healed. Also in this category are hereditary symptoms due to tridoṣhic causes, when found in the internal anal sphincter.

If persons are strong and have good digestion, their hemorrhoids can be healed. Hemorrhoids may last for a long time when they are caused by the simultaneous imbalance of two *doṣhas*, when they are congenital, when they are tridoṣhic, or when they are found in the innermost folds of the rectum. However, they can be controlled if the digestive fire is adequately strengthened. Those hemorrhoids caused by two *doṣhas* found in the second rectal fold or those that have existed more than one year (chronic) are difficult to heal. Those caused by only one *doṣha,* found in the outer folds and that are non-chronic, are easily healed. Some suggest surgery or cauterization with alkalis.

There are 3 additional places where piles may occur: in the male organ (discussed later), at the navel (being slippery and soft), and on the skin as warts.

Therapies

General: Herbs of neem, *triphalā*, *guḍūchī*, licorice, *chitrak*, *viḍaṅga*, and *pittapapra* are most effective.

Hemorrhoids are classified into 2 main categories, dry and wet. Those caused by Vāyu and Kapha fall into the former category, those caused by Pitta and blood aggravation fall into the latter. Here blood is considered wet, and although Kapha hemorrhoids are oily, greasy, slimy, etc., they are considered dry.

Dry Symptoms and Therapies: With numbness, edema, and painful lumps, the mass is first smeared with *triphalā, bilwa,* or *chitrak* medicated oils. Afterwards, warm or oily compresses (fomentation) of barley, or sesame seed powder, lukewarm compresses of *vachā powder,* corn flour with sesame oil or *ghee*, dry radish pulp are applied.

Next, herbal water made from herbs of *bilwa, vāsāk, arka,* and castor oil may be sprinkled on the areas of the navel and anus. Persons may take sitz baths with water decoctions made from *triphalā, bilwa,* yogurt-water, whey, or radish leaves. One prepares for the sitz bath by smearing warm *triphalā* oil or *ghee* on the hemorrhoids.

Aromatherapy includes burning and inhaling *arka* root, *viḍaṅga,* barley, *aśhwagandhā,* or *pippalī* mixed with *ghee.* Ointments are also used, mixing sesame oil, *ghee,* or warm water with herbs until the mixture becomes a paste. The paste is smeared on the masses. Herbs used include *pippalī, chitrak,* turmeric, *triphalā,* and cane sugar. Ointments are specifically useful when there is edema, stiffness, itching, and pain.

Herbs that reduce the various *doṣha*-caused hemorrhoids are also used in the above therapies (i.e., cold, bitter herbs for Pitta; warm, oily herbs for Vāyu; bitter and warm herbs for Kapha). Bloodletting is administered (by qualified practitioners) when the above therapies do not work.

Herbal powder mixtures (*chūrṇas*) are also ingested; the mixture depends on the prevailing *doṣha* causing the hemorrhoids. *Triphalā* is a good general *chūrṇa.* Hot spices like ginger, *pippalī,* and black pepper (*ṭrikatu*) are used for Vāyu and Kapha conditions. These also help improve the digestive power, improve appetite, stimulate the downward movement of air (*Apāna* Vāyu), reduce swelling, itching and pain, promote strength and complexion. Barley, turmeric, *triphalā,* and *viḍaṅga* are useful for Pitta conditions.

Whe the patient suffers from both hemorrhoids and constipation, recipes include *triphalā* decoction, *triphalā* with yogurt-water (*lassi*), or just *harītakī* with *lassi*. *Lassi* (buttermilk) is considered the best medicine for healing hemorrhoids caused by Vāyu and Kapha (a teaspoon of *ghee* or sesame oil may be added for Vāyu conditions). Depending upon the person's strength and the season, they may take buttermilk (*lassi*) from 1 week to 1 month, gradually increasing and decreasing the number of glasses per day. [1 month example: 1 *lassi*—first day. 2 *lassis*—second day...adding 1 *lassi* per day until 15 *lassis* on the 15th day. On the 16th day—14 *lassis*, the 17th day—13 *lassis*...reducing the amount by 1 each day until 1 *lassi* on the 30th day.

If the person is weak, then *lassi* is given mornings and evenings. When persons are strong, they may mix fried barley flour with *lassi* for evening drinks. Rock salt (*saindav namak*), found in any Indian grocery store, may be added to the drink. Meals are eaten using foods that balance the person's *doṣha*. After meals *lassi* with *ghee* or oil, mixed with *basmati* rice is taken.

There are 3 types of *lassi*: (one for each *doṣha),* Vāyu's *lassi* is made with whole milk. Pitta's *lassi* is made with skim milk. Kapha's *lassi is* made with fat-free milk. *Lassi* cleanses the circulatory channels, enabling the plasma (*rasa*) to reach and nourish all 7 tissue layers (*dhātus*). It is said that hemorrhoids healed with *lassi* will not develop again.

<u>*Other useful foods and drinks*</u>:

1) Thin gruel (*peyā*)—rice flour, *pippalī, chitrak, bilwa, lassi*, fried in *ghee* or oil for Vāyu hemorrhoids. A *peyā* mix is 50 gms. (1.76 oz) *basmati* rice cooked with 8 times as much water.

2) Thick gruel (*yavāgū*)—*Basmati* rice with *pippalī, lassi*, black pepper for Vāyu and Kapha. A *yavāgū* mix is 50 gms. *basmati* rice cooked with 2 to 4 times as much water.

3) Vegetable soup—boiled and dry *paṣhana bedha*, dried radish, *bilwa, lassi*, any astringent herbs (e.g., raspberry) for Pitta.

4) For hemorrhoids with constipation—drinks consisting of cane sugar, *ghee*, barley, *gokṣhura,* and *lassi* are for all *doṣhas.*

Cane sugar, barley flour, pomegranate juice,

boiled water, and black salt for Vāyu.

Barley, honey, *pippalī*, dry ginger, black pepper, rock salt, and *lassi* for Kapha and Vāyu.

5) Green leafy vegetables are especially good for Pitta.

6) Fresh white unsalted butter with sugar and sesame seeds also heals this disease if taken for a long time.

Enemas:

1) For gastritis (upward moving air [*Upāna* Vāyu]—*chitrak*, *pippalī*, *bilwa*, licorice decoction). This is an *anuvāsana* enema.

2) Medicated enema for Vāyu—milk, decoction of *daśhmūl*, castor oil, and black salt. This is a *nirūha* enema.

Bleeding Hemorrhoid Therapy: Two types of this therapy exist: when Pitta is predominant, and when Kapha or Vāyu are secondarily aggravated.

Signs of Vāyu as a secondary cause—grayish color, hard and dry stool, not releasing gas through the anus, blood from hemorrhoids is thin, reddish, and foamy, pain in lumbar, thighs, and anus, great weakness. This is caused by drying foods and lifestyles. [Vāyu predominance—develops even in Pitta and Kapha excesses if bleeding is excessive.]

Therapies include oily and cold foods and lifestyles.

Signs of Kapha as a secondary cause—stool is loose, yellow, white, dry, heavy and cold; blood from hemorrhoids is dense, thready, pale yellow, and slimy. There is sliminess and numbness in the region of the anus. This is caused by heavy and dry foods and lifestyles.

Therapies include dry and warm foods and lifestyles. First, detoxifying or elimination therapies (e.g., fasting, purgation, emesis) are recommended, then herbs are taken.

Hemostatic Therapies (stopping bleeding): When toxic blood is exuded, continued bleeding is necessary to release the toxins. Should bleeding be stopped too soon, it can lead to various other diseases of *Rakta* Pitta. Examples include bleeding from other parts of the body, fever, morbid thirst, weakening digestion, anorexia and, jaundice. Other disorders include edema, colic pain in the anus and pelvic areas, skin diseases in the lumbar region and thighs, anemia, retention of gas, urine, and stool, headache, and heaviness.

Bitter drugs stimulate the digestion, metabolism, and stoppage of bleeding. If Vāyu is predominant even after the toxins are eliminated, then oily liquids, massage, and *anuvāsana* enemas are suggested. If Pitta is the only cause of the illness, and bleeding occurs in the summer, then hemostatic therapies are immediately given to stop the bleeding.

Hemostatic herbal decoctions: *Kuṭaj*, ginger (coagulates blood), sandalwood, neem, *musta*, *bilwa*, *nākeśhar*, *pittapapra*, red lotus, white lotus, *balā,* and cinnamon.

Recipes: Fried barley flour with any of the above herbs, onions taken alone or with barley and sugar (or with *lassi*, butter, and sesame seeds).

Sprinkling water, sitz baths, and ointments made from the above herbs also help stop bleeding. Water decoctions include licorice, *arjuna*, neem, and *vāsāk*. Bath herbs include sandalwood and licorice. Ointments include *ghee* with sandalwood and neem oils.

If rectum prolapse (determined by feeling a Pitta/Vāyu pulse) or burning or stickiness in the anus occurs, then it is rubbed with sesame oil or *ghee* and *mañjiṣhṭhā*, licorice, sandalwood and *neem*, honey, and *ghee*, red and white sandalwood.

Continuous Bleeding Therapy: Forehead paste and soup made of *dūrba* (the best blood coagulative), sandalwood, and *ghee*. Also, *anuvāsana* enemas with the luke warm upper portion of *ghee*, *dūrba,* and sandalwood.

Summary: Vāyu uses oily, sour and sweet therapies, Pitta uses bitter, dry and cool therapies, Kapha uses hot therapies.

Either hemorrhoids, diarrhea, and sprue (*grahanī*—malabsorption, anemia, and gastrointestinal disorders) can cause the development of the other 2 diseases. They develop from poor digestion and are healed by strengthening the digestive power. Generally hemorrhoids are healed by eating fried vegetables, thick barley gruel, vegetable/*ghee* soup, milk, and *lassi*.

Bloating
Due to Hemorrhoids (Udāvarta)

Causes: Vāyu is aggravated in the colon by eating air-increasing foods and drinks, i.e., foods that are bitter, astringent, and dry (e.g., broccoli, barley, apples, most beans, and dry cereals).

Developmental Symptoms: The accumulated air then becomes aggravated, blocking the downward movement of Vāyu (*Apāna*). This dries the moisture in these channels, obstructing the movement of feces, gas, and urine.

Following this, severe pain develops in the lower abdomen, ribs, back, and heart area, along with gripping abdominal pain, nausea, cutting pain in the rectum, severe and constant pain in the urinary bladder; cheeks may swell. Vāyu moves upward.

The next stage of symptoms includes vomiting, anorexia, fever, other Vāyu diseases of the heart, duodenum, and urine suppression. Other disorders include dysentery, deafness, blindness, difficult breathing, headache, cough, nasal mucus, mental anxiety, worry or fear, thirst, bleeding, abdominal tumors, and enlarged abdomen. Being secondary complications, these diseases—when associated with hemorrhoids—are difficult to heal. Therefore, constipation is the main complication to heal before these other symptoms appear.

Therapies:

Triphalā—Vāyu
Castor oil—Pitta, Pitta/Vāyu—2 teaspoons in a cup of hot water before bed.
Rhubarb—for stronger measures
Senna—the strongest therapy.

Therapies include oil massage (oleation) followed by sudation (sweating). Afterwards, oleation and sudation herbal suppositories are given, made of *pippalī, madanphal*, charcoal ash, mustard, and *jaggary.* In difficult cases castor oil purgation and *nirūha basti (enema)* (mainly using castor oil) are used.

Obesity

Causes: Generally, acceptable weight levels depend on cultural beliefs. Westerners aim at the slim, Pitta form. More ancient cultures praise Kapha forms (where physical activity is also more prevalent). Thus the definition of overweight may be determined by whether it causes health problems.

Causes of overweight include overeating, excessive eating of heavy or cold things, and oversleeping and lack of exercise. Other causes include hormone imbalance, emotional sentimentality, clinging, loss of love or low self-worth, insecurity, and poor digestion. Weight-reducing and appetite-suppressing drugs can weaken the digestion and increase air (thereby aggravating Vāyu). When overweight causes poor digestion, nutrients are not absorbed. Even after eating, the body does not receive the nutrients. So it sends a message to the brain to eat again. Even still, the digestive fire is unable to extract nutrients from the food. Thus, a vicious cycle of eating and overeating develops (absorbing little or no nutrition).

Vāyu: Sudden and fluctuating weight: (over, under, normal), variable hunger, eating lots of sugar to calm the nerves. Eating offers a feeling of security.

Vāyu/Kapha: This constitution reflects a nervous mind and weak digestion.

Pitta: Overeating is their main cause because appetite is strong. There may be addiction to sugar and red meat. Weight develops muscle and flabbiness.

Kapha: This is the most common *doṣha* that develops obesity, slow metabolism, easy weight gain, continuous appetite (addicted to eating), hypothyroid or other hormonal conditions that cause retention of weight, mainly water and fat retention, weak pancreas and kidneys, low pulse and energy, flabbiness, pallor, moist complexion and skin, excess phlegm or saliva, subcutaneous fat deposits and benign tumors may develop.

Therapies:

General: A mild, long-term reducing plan is more natural than crash diets. Winter is not a good time to begin dieting because the cold can lower one's resistance and body heat. Reducing or lightening therapy is needed, with a light diet, fasting, digestive (spicy) herbs, mild laxatives, and tonics like *guggul* (1 gram 3 times daily) or *śhilājit* (1/2 gram twice daily). This reduces obesity in a few months. *Brāhmī* calms the mind for conditions of excessive eating.

Vāyu: Vāyu-reducing herbs, diet, and lifestyle, complex carbohydrates (whole grains and starchy vegetables), avoidance of refined sugar, fewer hot spices and more sweet digestives like cardamom, coriander, *brāhmī, jaṭāmāṇśhī,* and *aśhwagandhā* calm the mind. *Guggul* helps cleanse and warm the body.

Pitta: Pitta-reducing foods, avoiding meat, fish, oily, greasy, or fried foods, sugars, and desserts. Raw salads, green herbs, and chlorophyll, digestive bitters and bitter laxatives are the best foods to reduce weight and counter sugar addiction. Herbs include aloe vera gel, *kaṭukā*, turmeric, *bhūāmalakī*.

Kapha: Kapha-reducing foods, avoiding refined sugars, salt, dairy, sweet fruit, bread, pastry, meat, fish, fruit juices, cold liquids, and oils. The best foods for digestion are sprouts: their enzymatic properties help digestion. Meals are eaten after 10:00 a.m. and before 6:00 p.m. Hot spices and fasting (if one is strong) help raise the metabolism. Spice teas, vegetable juices, steamed vegetables, beans, and whole grains are also advised. Suggestions include less sleep, no naps, and strong, aerobic exercise. Hot digestive herbs like black pepper, ginger, turmeric, and *tṛikatu* burn up fat and raise the digestive fire. Bitter herbs reduce fat and dry water. Bitters include *kaṭukā*, myrrh, *triphalā,* and *guggul. Gokṣhura* is a gentle diuretic. *Śhilājit* helps the kidneys. *brāhmī* is a useful nervine to calm the mind.

Candida (Yeast)

Cause: Usually starts in GI tract, then moves to the blood and other organs. Candida is generally caused by weak digestion due to *āma* (toxin). It is usually due to high Vāyu or Kapha, but it can also be caused by Pitta. Excessive use of sugars, drugs, antibiotics, frequent colds and flu, weak nervous system, worry, fear, grief, and anger can also cause candida.

Symptoms:

General: Chronic low energy, low-grade fevers, variable digestion, poor immune functioning, and food allergies.

Vāyu: Insomnia, lower back pain, dry skin, nervous, restless, light-headedness, ringing ears, depression, gas, bloating, constipation, and variable energy.

Pitta: Fever, thirst, burning, hyperacidity, and infections.

Kapha: Phlegm, frequent colds and flu, swollen glands, edema, heaviness, dullness, and excess sleeping.

Dual and Tridoṣha: Symptoms of 2 or all 3 *doṣhas*.

Therapies:

General: This condition is treated similarly to parasites. The goal is to destroy the yeast and boost the immune system. This is achieved through restoring digestive and immune strength.

Refined sugars, white bread, yeast products, dairy, sweet fruit, raw foods, and cold drinks are avoided.

Vāyu: Antifungal herbs include *asafoetida*, garlic, ginger, *pippalī, tṛikatu, triphalā, viḍaṅga, musta*. *Viḍaṅga* and *musta* are antifungal but deplete the immune system, so they are best used for only 1 or 2 weeks. Digestive herbs include

cardamom, cumin, ginger. Immune herbs include *brāhmī, guḍūchī, balā, yogaraj guggul*, and saffron. Later, *śhatāvarī and aśhwagandhā* are taken.
Pitta: *Viḍaṅga* and *musta* are used as antifungal herbs. Digestives include coriander, fennel, and turmeric. Immune herbs include *brāhmī, guḍūchī, balā, kaiṣhore guggul,* saffron, and *neem.* Later, *śhatāvarī* is used.
Kapha: *Viḍaṅga* and *musta* as antifungal herbs: cardamom, ginger, *asafoetida, tṛikatu,* and *triphalā* as digestive herbs. Immune-boosting herbs include *gokṣhura, brāhmī, guḍūchī, balā*, saffron. Also *guggul* and neem are used.

Lyme disease has been helped by Pitta-type candida therapies and antibacterial herbs. We have found this therapy to be helpful in all lyme disease cases at our center.

Ulcers

Inflamed ulcers are discussed in the next chapter. Here stomach ulcers are reviewed. When the mucus lining of the stomach becomes inflamed, one experiences pain, burning sensation, and eventual bleeding. The current Western view of ulcers is that they are caused by bacteria. Both viewpoints are discussed below.

Bacterial Therapies:

Āyurvedic therapies include antibacterial therapies.

Vāyu: Garlic, sandalwood, jasmine, turmeric.

Pitta: *Chirāyatā*, golden seal, aloe, sandalwood, jasmine, turmeric.

Kapha: Garlic, golden seal, aloe, sandalwood, turmeric.

Inflammation Therapies:

Usually these conditions develop from mental stress, worry, overwork, nervous sensitivity, etc. Foods also can play a part in this condition: for example, eating overly hot and spicy foods and drinking excessive amounts of alcohol.

General: It is best to follow a bland food plan with easily digestible items. A milk fast is beneficial. Alcohol and smoking aggravates ulcers, as do garlic, onions, pickles, vinegar, and salt. Bananas and the nightshade family of vegetables and fruit can also cause trouble. Therapies for hyperacidity are recommended here. Herbs to protect the mucus lining of the stomach are useful, and include aloe gel, *śhatāvarī*, and licorice.

Vāyu: Symptoms include more pain than burning, feeling cold, light-headedness, anxiety, with insomnia, gas, constipation, abdominal distention, and palpitations. Heat applied to the stomach brings relief. Excessive meals of dry and light foods can dry up the mucus secretions causing an ulcer. Thus a Vāyu-reducing diet is recommended. After a bland diet is followed for some time, spices can be safely used, such as *hiṅgwastock, lavaṇ bhāskar chūrṇa,* and *tṛikatu* (unless the tongue is dry, cracked or reddish). These herbs are taken with warm milk or *ghee.*

Pitta: Burning sensation is the predominant symptom. Anger and impatience are mental causes of Pitta ulcers. A Pitta-reduction diet is advised, along with bitter herbs like aloe, barberry, *chirāyatā, kaṭukā,* and *mahāsudarṣhan chūrṇa;* also demulcents like *śhatāvarī.*

Kapha: Ulcers are rare for this *doṣha.* Physical symptoms include white or clear phlegm, nausea, lack of appetite, dull pain, and heaviness. Mental causes include greediness, grief, or emotional attachment. Herbs to digest mucus are recommended (e.g., *tṛikatu, pippalī,* black pepper, and dry ginger).

Āma

Āma has been discussed throughout this book. When *āma* (undigested food toxin) is present it can cause many diseases. Thus, one can follow a special *āma*-reducing diet that mainly decreases excess Kapha (because foods that increase Kapha increase *āma*). An anti-*āma* diet is depleting, so the length of time persons should adhere to this diet depends upon their physical strength. Kapha *doṣhas* can stay on this plan for long periods of time. Pitta *doṣhas* eventually need to introduce rejuvenation therapies. Vāyu *doṣhas*, the weakest of the constitutions, are advised to stay on this diet for only 1 week before adding rejuvenating herbs and foods. The chart below lists *āma*-reducing foods. Foods are chosen from the *āma*-reducing column, according to one's *doṣha*.

Āma-Reducing Diet	
Āma Reducing	**Āma Increasing**
Lemon, lime, grapefruit, pomegranate, cranberry	Sweet fruits
Steamed Veges (Vāyu and Kapha) Raw for Pitta; best are sprouts, vegetable juices	Potatoes, mushrooms, carrot juice (alone is too sweet)
Whole grains (oats and wheat in moderation); *kicharī*	Breads, pastries, white flour
Mūng beans	All other beans
Pumpkin seeds in moderation	Nuts and seeds
Acidophilus, yogurt water (*lassi*)	Dairy
- - -	Pork, meat, fish, poultry, eggs, lard
Ghee (moderation), mustard, flax oils	Oils
Raw honey	Sugars
Spices	Salt
Warm liquids (tea, herb tea)	Cold liquids, coffee

Abdominal Digestive Organs

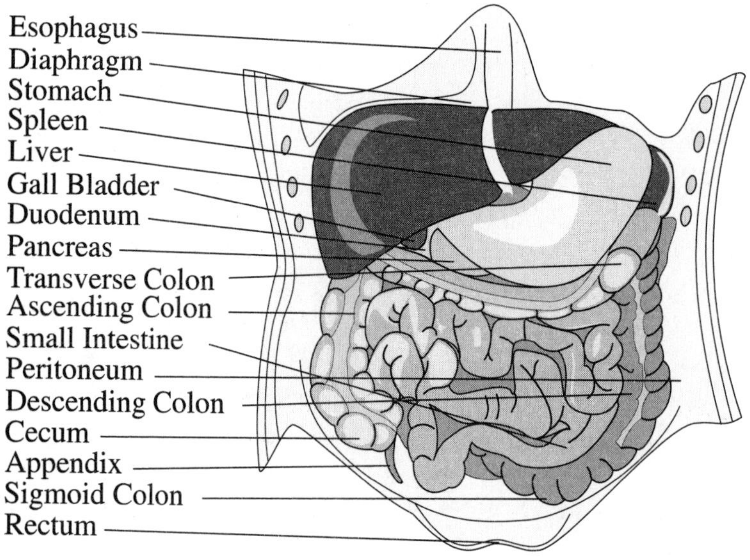

Thinking of sense objects causes attachment.
From attachment arises longing and from longing anger is born [anger causes fever].
From anger arises delusion; from delusion, loss of memory is caused. From loss of memory, the discriminative faculty is ruined, and from the ruin of discrimination, one perishes.
Bhagavad Gita Chapter 2; verse 62-63

It is desire, it is anger, born of Rajas Guṇa (passion); of unappeasable craving and great sin; know this as the foe in the world. - Bhagavad Gita Chapter 3; verse 37

Chapter 16
Infections or Wounds
Fever, Abscess, Sinus, Wounds, Inflamed Ulcers, Fractures/Dislocations

Fever (Jwara)

Fever, known as the lord of diseases, is said to be the most painful of all diseases. Its heat destroys the *ojas* (life sap) and afflicts the body, senses and the mind. It was the first disease of humans and is the first illness to develop among all diseases. Fevers afflict the entire mind and body. It is considered the most powerful of all diseases because it produces various forms of death and is also present during birth.

The *Vedic* mythology of fever states that it originated in *Lord Rudra* (*Śhiva*—the destroyer of ignorance) who unleashed his wrath on the *asuras* (demons). In the process, the gods (elements of nature) became afflicted with burning sensations and pain, and all creatures became unconscious. The gods propitiated *Śhiva* who restored them to health. He said that anger will take the form of fever, afflicting people at birth, death, and when they do not follow their prescribed Āyurvedic lifestyles. In short, people living virtuously will not suffer from fever. Fever causes emaciation, delusion, and heat discomfort, caused by unhealthy lifestyle habits and improper conduct.

In conventional medicine (allopathic) fever is also the predominant and common symptom of all illness. Fever is seen as the first warning the body gives in response to any imbalance or infection.

Eight Fever Types

There are 8 major forms of fever: Vāyu, Pitta, Kapha, Vāyu/Pitta, Vāyu/Kapha, Pitta/Kapha, Tridoṣha (*Sannipātika* 13 types), and external causes (five types). Both tridoṣha fevers and external causes can be provoked by one or two predominating *doṣhas*, and the blockage of life sap (*ojas*). Five varieties of recurring fevers (*viṣhamsa jwara*) also exist (malaria-related). Fevers have three stages, which will be detailed later.

Cause and Development of Fever

Improper or excessive use of oil, inflammation, over fatigue, wasting, indigestion, intake of bad, toxic or poisonous substances, poor diet, sudden change of diet or weather, poor conduct, grief, anger, passion, toxic fumes, malefic planets and stars at birth, spells, curses, or factors related to child birth (i.e., miscarriage, untimely delivery, improper self-care after delivery or during the first accumulation of breast milk after delivery).

Development: The *doṣhas* thus becoming vitiated and

1. Enter the stomach and intestines (*āmāṣhaya*) [each respective *doṣha*, Vāyu, Pitta, Kapha, when

entering the *āmāṣhaya* will aggravate and develop into its respective *doṣha* fever]

2. Mix with *āma* (undigested food toxins)

3. Lodge in the plasma or lymph chyle (*rasa*) due to their inherent heat.

4. Then, they mix with the plasma, obstructing the plasma (*rasa*), hemoglobin (*rakta*), muscle (*māmsa*) and sweat channels (*sweda srotas*).

5. Next, it pushes the *agni* digestive fire enzymes out of the GI tract. The *agni* then spreads throughout the body (i.e., into all of the tissues, organs, etc.), pushing the heat to the skin. This raises the body's temperature and stops perspiration. The parallel of this process in modern science is known as the increase of metabolic activity. This in turn increases body temperature.

To learn all necessary information about fever, the Āyurvedic practitioner (*vaidya*) must analyze the,

1. Nature of the disease	9. Symptoms and signs
2. Precipitating factors	10. *Doṣhas* involved
3. Origin	11. Features
4. Cause	12. Healing signs and symptoms
5. Premonitory or incubatory signs and symptoms	13. Preventing relapse
6. Location	14. Reasons for relapse
7. Strength of the disease	15. Healing the relapse
8. Time of occurrence	

Further, the *vaidya* needs to have an understanding of fever caused by alcohol, the seven *dhātus*, knowledge of the first and later stages of fever and chronic fevers.

Causes of Fever

mental/physical
cold/heat
internal/external
seasonal/unseasonal
curable/incurable

Either the mind or the body can be the cause of a fever. Mythologically, it is said that the *Soma* god causes cold fevers and the *Agni* god causes hot fevers. Fevers occurring in their respective season are healed in their respective season. Fevers are easily healed, difficult to heal, or incurable.

Incubatory or Premonitory Signs and Symptoms

listless	indifference	sluggish
heaviness	lassitude	fainting
low	spirit	distaste
no appetite	teary eyes	body aches
tires easily	indigestion	low strength
excess sleep	drooping	great thirst
tingling teeth	calf pain	forgetfulness
depression	dark vision	moody
hair stands on end	pale complexion	excess yawning
desire hot/ cold things alternately	desire pungent, sour and salty tastes	impatience for good advice
strongly dislike sweets, music, children, cold water, shade and sun		

Premonitory Doṣha Symptoms

Vāyu	constant yawning
Pitta	burning eyes
Kapha	loss of hunger
Tridoṣha	all symptom
Dual-*Doṣha*	symptoms of both

Causes Aggravating Air Fevers (Vāyu Jwara)

snuff	assault	fasting
anxiety	grief	excess exercise
suppression of natural urges	staying up late	poor posture
excess emesis, purgation or drying enemas		excess sex
Over indulgence of oily, light, cold foods		excess blood- letting

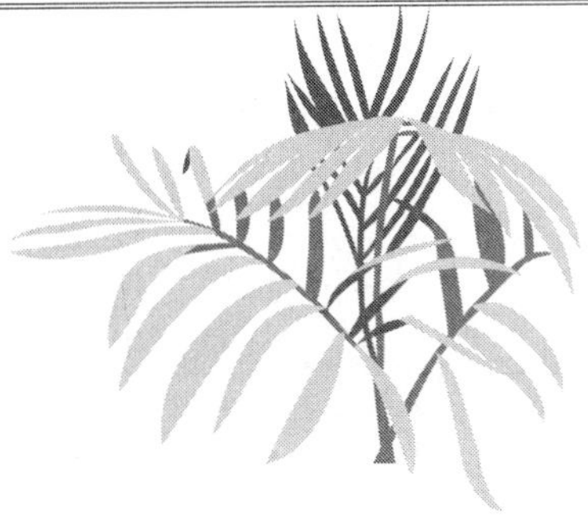

Symptoms of Air Caused Fevers (Vāyu Jwara)

twisting calf pain	loss of sensation and rigidity of the feet	contracting abdominal or shoulder pain
loose joints	weak thighs	ringing ears
no elimination of sweat, feces or urine	sharp, cutting pain in upper body	reddish face, eyes, nails, urine, throat, lips, skin, feces
splitting back or bone (and rib) pain, dry skin	astringent or bad taste in the mouth	loss of taste and lack of hunger
chest pain	anorexia	desiring sun
headache	dizziness	insomnia
dry cough or dry heaves	hair stands on end	dry lips, mouth, throat
sorrow	dry skin	indigestion
drooping body parts	intermittent temple pain	rambling speech
desiring hot things	irregular temperature	irregularity- acute/mild
shivering	stiff jaw	tingling teeth
irregularity in onset and alleviation	occuring after digestion in the afternoon, dawn, end of summer	

The general words to describe Vāyu fever symptoms are sharp, cutting, shifting pain, coldness, and dryness.

Causes Aggravating Fire Fevers (Pitta Jwara)

irregular diet	eating with indigestion	exposure to hot sun and fires
exhaustion	excessive hot, salty, sour and pungent foods	

Symptoms of Fire Caused Fevers (Pitta Jwara)

dizzy	fainting	toxicity
diarrhea	acidity	great thirst
red skin rashes	burning sensations	rambling speech
perspiration	high fever	bile in vomit
expectorating blood	desiring cold things	malodorous breath
delirium	restlessness	naps
hives	giddiness	intoxication
occurs during digestion	occurs at noon, midnight, autumn	
pungent taste	green/yellow skin, nails, eyes, urine, stool	liking cold things

In short, the key words for Pitta fevers include, heat, sweat, red, yellow, or green, blood, bile, impatience.

Causes Aggravating Kapha Fevers

lack of discipline	lack of exercise	naps
excess intake of oily, heavy, sweet, slimy, cold, sour and salty foods		

Symptoms of Water Caused Fevers (Kapha Jwara)

lassitude	nausea	mild fever
sweet taste	running nose	heaviness
glassy/white eyes	cold swellings	no hunger or taste
drowsiness	slight heat	acid belching
obstructed channels (*srotas*)	no assimilation of foods	obstructed feces, urine, sweat
difficult breathing	fever after eating	desiring hot things
goose bumps	cough	shivering
fainting	stupor	heart coating
slight limb pain	increased salivation	cold skin eruptions
heavy chest	vomiting	poor digestion
whitish skin, nails, mucus, urine, stool	fever during morning, evening, spring	desiring hot things

The key words for Kapha fevers are white, cold, slow minded.

Causes of Multiple Doṣha Fevers

Four types of multiple fevers exist.

1. Vāyu/Pitta
2. Vāyu/Kapha
3. Pitta/Kapha
4. Vāyu/Pitta/Kapha

Again, these fevers have 12 subdivisions, when one, two or all three *doṣhas* are predominant (e.g., Vāyu/Pitta equal predominance, Vāyu/Pitta with Vāyu predominance, Vāyu/Pitta/Kapha with Pitta and Kapha predominance, etc.)

Fevers of all three *doṣhas* begin during their respective times of day (or night), season, and digestion (as discussed earlier). The rainy season (mid July- mid September) is most likely to cause Vāyu fevers. The autumn season (mid September- mid November) is most likely to produce Pitta fevers. The spring season (mid March- mid May) is when Kapha fevers are most likely to occur. When *doṣha* fevers arise outside their respective season they are more difficult to heal, unseasonal Vāyu fevers are the most difficult. All Vāyu fevers are usually difficult to heal.

During the seasonal fevers, food may be taken (i.e., fasting is not necessary). Fasting is advised when persons are strong and the Sun is weak (rainy, autumn and winter seasons). It is also necessary for practitioners to remember that Vāyu and Pitta are weak at the beginning of spring. They are moderately strong in the middle of the season and strong at the end of this time. Similarly, Kapha is weak at the beginning of autumn, moderate in the middle and strong at the end of this season. Thus, the strength of the patient with fever is known at these times.

Other causes include combinations of these factors, or due to,

<table>
<tr><td>irregular diet</td><td>fast</td><td>poison intake</td></tr>
<tr><td colspan="3">improper oleation, fomentation, emesis, purgation, or enema; improper diet or lifestyle after pañcha karma</td></tr>
<tr><td colspan="3">improper child deliver or poor diet after delivery</td></tr>
<tr><td colspan="3">sudden change in diettoxic fumes or materials</td></tr>
</table>

Two Doṣha Fevers (Dwandvaja Jwara)

Fevers caused by two *doṣhas* exhibit symptoms of both *doṣhas*. Vāyu/Pitta fevers cause a desire for cold things (i.e., Pitta heat predominates). Vāyu/Kapha fevers cause a desire for hot things.

Tridoṣha Fevers (Sannipāta Jwara)

Sannipāta Jwaras are caused by the same actions described above for each *doṣha*. Thus, fevers caused by all three *doṣhas* exhibit symptoms of all three *doṣhas*.

During dual or tridoṣha fevers, one *doṣha* is predominant. Thus, the predominant *doṣha* is mainly focused on when healing the illness.

Difficult to Heal or Incurable Sannipāta

Doṣha obstruction or non-elimination, destroyed *agni* enzymes, fully manifested signs and symptoms.

Externally Caused Fevers (*Āgantu*)

Four types of externally caused fevers exist.

1. Trauma or Injuries are associated with Vāyu within vitiated blood (*rakta*) [and sometimes the other tissues (*dhātus*)]. Symptoms include pain, swelling and discoloration. According to modern science, these symptoms are explained as inflamations caused by infections or injuries.

2. Emotions, Infections (e.g., bacteria, virus, poisons), Evil Spirits

Emotions are caused by vitiated Vāyu and Pitta. They first occur in the mind, then fever develops during the times and seasons of the respective *doṣhas*. Modern Psychology calls these events psychosomatic; the mind affects the health of the body.

Anger is due to excess Pitta (and sometimes the other *doṣhas*). Its symptoms include wrath, tremors, and headache.

Fear is aggravated by Vāyu. Its symptoms are delirium and apprehension.

Grief is aggravated by Vāyu. Its symptoms are excessive crying or heavy breathing.

Lust is caused by excess Pitta, and produces loss of appetite, burning sensations, frequent breaths, absence of shame, sleep, intelligence and courage.

Pollen, Dust causes fainting, headaches, vomiting, intoxicating, wetness and sneezing, and is caused by all *doṣhas*. This is easily healed.

Poison symptoms include blackened face, burning sensations, diarrhea, heart pain, disliking food, thirst, limb pain, extreme weakness, wetness, epilepsy, caused by all *doṣhas*. This is easily healed with their antidotes.

Evil spirit's symptoms include laughing or crying without reason, and are caused by all three *doṣhas*. These occur rarely, but are hard to heal.

3. Curses (are caused by all three *doṣhas*).

4. Sorcery or Witchcraft (are caused by all three *doṣhas*).

The last two types of spells rarely occur. Their symptoms include thirst and fainting, all signs of tridoṣhic fever and are hard to bear. The Āyurvedic practitioner (*vaidya*) determines these last two fevers by,

1. Observing the deed
2. Hearing about the deed
3. Through inference
4. By healing the fever

Sometimes eternal fevers remain exogenous. Sometimes they later become associated with the *doṣhas*. Its premonitory symptom is pain. Fever may occur first, then the symptoms, or vice versa.

External Fever Therapies

Spiritual therapies are used for externally caused fevers. These therapies include rites, rituals, good deeds, fasting, light meals, and herbal decoctions.

Three Stages of Fever

Three stages of a fever include,

1. Association with *āma* (undigested foods)
2. Metabolic transformation
3. Non-association with *āma*.

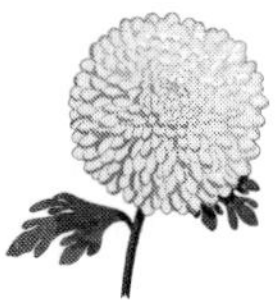

First Stage Fever Symptoms (With Āma)

emaciation	indigestion	drowsiness
body and abdominal heaviness	heart feels impure/heavy	constant temperature
laziness	salivation	nausea
acute attack	rigidity	numbness
no hunger/tastelessness	unformed stool	heavy stomach
excessive urine	no elimination of wastes, *doṣhas*, sweat	

During this stage, one is not to take naps, bath, massage, heavy foods, sexual intercourse, anger, wind, exercise,or astringent tastes.

Second Stage Fever Symptoms (Pachyamāna)

excess fever/thirst	mucus in feces	difficult breathing
delirium	giddiness	

Third Stage Fever Symptoms (Nirāma)

reduced temperature	appetite
elimination of *doṣhas* and wastes	lightness

These symptoms will generally appear by the eighth day

Recovery From Fever

Healing from fevers is easy when persons are strong, the *doṣha* is mildly increased and there are no secondary complications (*āma* fevers). Symptoms of fevers with *āma* include excess urine, constipation or diarrhea, and loss of hunger. Fever, thirst, delirium, difficult breathing, dizziness, and nausea are symptoms of fever with heated *doṣhas*. Fevers that are long lasting, recurring after seven days or appear after fasts are fevers without *āma*.

Remittent/Intermittent Fevers (Vishama Jwara)

Doṣhas and Dhātu Fevers - Malarial Fevers

Fevers are generally caused by all three *doṣhas*. However, due to one's *doṣha*, the fevers may manifest as described above in the various tissues (*dhātus*). After tridoṣhic fevers subside a slight residue of the deranged *doṣhas* and weakness exists. Through improper healing measures and poor diet, Vāyu becomes vitiated and re-aggravated. Further, this can cause five fevers lodged in any or all of the five Kapha sites (stomach and intestines, the chest, throat, head, and joints).

Modern medicine sees remittent fevers as different types of malarias caused by mosquitos (various species of plasmodium). The mosquitos infect the blood and act upon the red blood cells. These blood infections affect the various supporting elements of the tissues (*dhātus*). Malaria is considered a bacterial infection, while typhoid is classified as a parasitic infection.

Fevers of plasma, hemoglobin, muscle and fat are easy to heal. Bone and marrow fevers are more difficult to heal. The six fevers are

1. *Santata Jwara*/Plasma (*Rasa*) Fevers: This fever starts in the plasma (and sometimes in the other *dhātus*), quickly spreading to the three *doṣhas*, seven *dhātus*, urine and feces. The fever is continuous and hard to tolerate. They are caused by *rasa* spreading the aggravated *doṣhas* throughout the body and are difficult to bear. If purified, Vāyu fevers last for 7 or 14 days, Pitta fevers last for 9 or 10 days and Kapha fevers last for 11 or 12 days. This fever is continuous due to the vitiated *rasa* spreading throughout the body. For all fevers of plasma origin, fasting is the first healing therapy. Various forms of this fever disappear for a day or two, then recur during their aggravating time of day and season. They last for another seven or 14 days. Recurrence is caused by improper convalescing and diet.

Symptoms include heaviness, misery, anxiety, prostration, vomiting, anorexia, malaise, and yawning.

2. *Satata Jwara*/Hemoglobin (*Rakta*) Fevers: Vitiated *doṣhas* reside in the blood or hemoglobin, deranging the blood. These fevers are caused and develop according to the time of day or season. They appear twice within 24 hours; they can develop and become healed merely by the time of day or season, or by attending to the aggravated *dhātu* or one's *prakṛiti* (constitution) with appropriate therapies. (Sometimes called *Santataka Jwara*)

Symptoms include blood, pimples, thirst, burning, discoloration, giddiness, intoxication, delirium.

3. *Anyeduṣhka Jwara*/Muscle (*Māṃsa*) Fevers: One's *prakṛiti*, *dhātus*, the *doṣhas*, or seasons can cause the muscle channel (*māṃsavaha srota*) obstructions. These fevers occur once a day.

Symptoms include burning thirst, unconsciousness, wetness, diarrhea, foul smell, body spasms.

4. *Tṛtīyaka Jwara*/Fat (*Medas*) Fevers: These are Vāyu-caused fevers, which manifest every other day. (Symptoms of Vāyu/Pitta predominant—sudden head pain, Vāyu/Kapha predominant—sudden pain in the entire back, Kapha/Pitta predominant—sudden pain in the upper back or lumbo-sacral joint).

Symptoms include excess sweat, thirst, delirium, frequent vomiting, dislike of one's own body odor, wetness, anorexia.

5. *Chaturthaka Jwara*/Marrow (*Majjā*), Bone (*Asthi*) and Fat (*Medas*): When the *doṣhas* are in the fat, marrow, and bones, fever occurs every fourth day, manifesting either with Vāyu excess (beginning in the head), or Kapha excess (beginning in the calves). Some say only when *doṣhas* are in the marrow does fever occur every fourth day.

Fevers caused by *doṣhas* simultaneously in bone and marrow are called *Viparyaya Jwara*, which is of three kinds (one for each *doṣha*). These fevers last for 2 days, disappear for a day and then reappear, continuing this cycle.

Some authorities believe these three fevers are caused by afflictions of the previous alternate *dhātus* (i.e., afflicted *rakta dhātu* causes *anyedyuṣhka* (fat) *jwara*; muscle afflictions cause *tṛitīyaka* (bone fevers); *doṣhas* in the fat (*med*as) tissue cause *chaturthaka* (marrow) fever.

Symptoms of bone fevers include diarrhea and vomiting, bone pains, unusual sounds, and body spasms. Symptoms of marrow fever include hiccup, asthma, bronchitis, dark vision, vital organ pains, outer coldness, and internal burning.

6. Ojas Nirodhaja: The life sap or *ojas* tissue (*śhukra dhātu*) may also be blocked by Vāyu and Pitta. Symptoms include shivering, numbness, unconsciousness, drowsiness, delirium, slight pain, and ejaculation. Vāyu fevers appear every 7 days, Pitta fevers arise every 10 days, Kapha excess fevers appear every 12 days.

Symptoms of Relief From Fever

When fevers begin to be relieved, the *doṣhas* in the *dhātus* (tissues) create abnormalities and become liquefied. Persons begin to breathe heavily, sweat profusely, moan, vomit, and shake. They become delirious, have unusual body movements, experience heat and cold, become angry, have noisy, malodorous diarrhea, become pale, and lose consciousness. Fevers may leave suddenly or gradually. Certain fevers can produce anxiety, so persons must be treated with care. After the fever is healed the person gradually returns to a normal state of health.

Fevers that heal suddenly are termed "healed by crises" in modern medicine. When persons take antibiotics to kill bacterias, viruses, etc., these pathogens are suddenly killed. When they die, they release various toxins into the bodily systems. The body reacts to this sudden release of toxins, and develops various disorders. (When fever is healed gradually the toxins are slowly released into the body, giving it time to adapt and excrete them).

Symptoms of Healed Fever

Lightness, normal functioning of the mind and senses, normal sweating, appetite, itching head, absence of exhaustion, delusion and heat, mouth ulcers, and discomfort.

Therapies

Remedy for All Fevers:

Sudarṣhan Chūrṇa

The Āyurvedic seers have created this formula for all fevers (intermittent and other *doṣha* and *dhātu* fevers). This formula is a combination of 48 herbs (the main herb used is *chirāyatā*). *Sudarṣhan chūrṇa* is taken with cold water. On the right index finger of Lord Viṣhnu resides a powerful discus that destroys all kinds of enemies. It is called *Sudarṣhan Chakra*. Because this herbal remedy destroys all kinds of fevers, it was named after this discus or *chakra*. *Sudarṣhan chūrṇa* can even be used during the first stages of fevers. According to the experience of some modern Āyurvedic doctors, *sudarṣhan chūrṇa* works best for the malarial (remittent) fevers; others prefer *sitopaladi*.

Sitopaladi Chūrṇa

For fevers associated with flus and respiratory disorders, *sitopaladi chūrṇa* works best. It is up to each modern practitioner to decide whether *sudarṣhan* or *sitopaladi chūrṇa* works better for the client. A recipe for typhoid or malaria (recurring fevers) is 1/2 tsp/ *sitopaladi chūrṇa* with warm water—3 times daily for 8 weeks. The first 10 days one follows a liquid fast. Within 3 to 4 days, persons should feel better. After the 8-week program the fever will not occur.

Thus, regardless of the type of fever (i.e., Vāyu, Pitta, remittant, etc.), *sudarṣhan* and *sitopaladi chūrṇas* are the only herbal therapies needed. Depending on the *doṣha*(s) causing the fever, persons are advised to follow the corresponding food and lifestyle guidelines that balance and maintain their health.

Abscesses (Vidradhi)

Causes: Eating stale, very hot, and dry foods, (causing burning during digestion); lying on an uneven bed, foods and lifestyles that vitiate the blood. The *doṣhas* become aggravated and weaken the skin, muscles, fat, bones, ligaments, blood, and tendons, producing swelling in any one or several of them. This occurs either inside the body (with severe pain) or on the outer body. Abscesses are either round or wide. Six forms of abscesses exist: Vāyu, Pitta, Kapha, Tridoṣha, blood, or trauma caused.

Symptoms:

External: Forming anywhere on the body, being difficult to bear, they are hard and raised.

Internal: More difficult to bear, deep seated, hard, growing upwards (like an anthill), near the navel, urinary bladder, liver, spleen, heart, abdomen, groin, kidneys, or rectum. It is very serious.

Vāyu: Severe pain, blackish-red, takes a long time to grow, forming and discharging pus, irregularly placed, unevenly shaped, painful, cutting, rotating, spreading easily, gaseous, throbbing, and producing sounds.

Pitta: Red, coppery or black, causing thirst, delusion, fever, burning, quick to grow, form, and discharge pus.

Kapha: White, itching, with nausea, cold, stiffness of the body, excessive yawning, loss of taste, heaviness of the body, slow to grow, form, and discharge pus.

Tridoṣha: Symptoms of all the *doṣhas* simultaneously.

Blood: Surrounded by black eruptions, blue colored, severe burning, pain, fever, and other symptoms of aggravated Pitta. It is external in all cases except those developing in the uterus.

Trauma: Vāyu becomes aggravated from the force of assault, unsuitable foods or lifestyle. It displaces the heat at the trauma site, aggravating Pitta, and causing symptoms of Pitta and blood. This causes the severest secondary complications.

Depending upon the site of the abscess will determine the secondary symptoms.

Abscess	Complication
near navel	hiccup
in bladder	difficulty eliminating/foul smell
in liver	difficult breathing
in spleen	difficulty exhaling
in pancreas	thirst
all over body	sharp pain/ rigidity
in heart	great delusion, unconsciousness, cough, friction/pain in the heart
on front/top of stomach	pain/gurgling in upper abdomen, pain in ribs and shoulders
in groin	stiff thighs
in kidneys	sharp pain in waist and back, rib pain
in rectum	obstruction of gas

The early, middle, and advanced stages of abscess development are similar to inflammatory edema. In the advanced stages of abscesses localized above the navel, they expel pus or blood through the mouth, and when present below the navel, discharges are through the rectum.

The features of the *doṣhas* and of that which is exuded is similar to ulcers (rather than from trauma). Tridoṣhic abscesses in the heart, navel, urinary bladder and those that have burst after maturing (either inside or outside), are unable to be healed. Also, those that burst inside and expel their contents, those arising in debilitated persons, and those that have secondary complications cannot be healed.

Therapies: These therapies are the same as for sinus (next section).

Sinus (Nāḍī-Vraṇa)

If persons neglect abscesses or swellings sinus problems can develop. Five forms of *nāḍī* exist: Vāyu, Pitta, Kapha, Tridoṣha, and *Śhalyaja*.

Causes and Symptoms:

Vāyu: Rough, short-mouthed size, aching pain within the sinus, secreting a frothy matter, increasing by night with aching pain, thirst.

Pitta: Lethargy, heat, piercing pain. Fever occurs at the beginning and there are large amounts of hot, yellow sinus secretions. Secretions develop more frequently during the night.

Kapha: The sinus is hard, itching, and slightly painful or numb. An excess of thick, shiny, white colored pus secretions exist, and is expelled more at night.

Dual and Tridoṣha: Symptoms of two or three *doṣhas*. Tridoṣhic symptoms are considered severe.

Śhlayaja: Foreign matter (e.g., dirt, bone, splinter, etc.) becoming fixed in a body part and still visible, opens the skin and creates a form of a sinus. Symptoms include constant pain, instant secretion of a sort of hot, bloody, frothy liquid matter.

Therapies:

General: In each case the therapy is three-fold. First antiseptics are used to wash the wound, then antibiotics cleanse and balance the *doṣhas* and finally healing measures are applied.

Vāyu: Constantly wash the ulcer with an herbal decoction of *daśhmūl* (i.e., an antiseptic). Sesame oil cooked with turmeric, *kaṭukā, balā,* rock salt, myrrh, and *bilwa* are used to purify the ulcer by filling it with the medicated oil (i.e., antibiotic and *doṣha* balancing). The lesion is constantly washed with a decoction of *triphalā, amaltas,* and milk. Finally oil cooked in neem, *viḍaṅga, chitrak, pippalī, vachā*, and mustard are applied to promote healing. [*Aṣhṭāñga Hṛidayam* therapy]

Charak first uses herb poultices including garlic, cloves, *chitrak,* and *pañchmūla*. Then the channels with pus are cut opened with a knife and bandaged with sesame paste and turmeric. A poultice is then applied of licorice, sesame, salt, and *devdaru, daśhmūl*, garlic, cloves, and *chitrak.*

Pitta: According to *Aṣhṭāñga*, first the sinus is washed with herbal decoction of *mañjiṣhṭhā, arjuna,* mango, and licorice for antiseptic purposes. Then a poultice of *guḍūchī*, licorice, and sesame paste is applied as an antibiotic and to heal the excess *doṣha*. Finally, healing is effected by medicated *ghee* cooked in milk with herbs of *mañjiṣhṭhā*, poppy seeds, *vidārī kand*, turmeric *triphalā,* and licorice. [16 parts milk, to 4 parts *ghee*, to 1 part herbs (all combined)]

Kapha: First, antiseptics are used in a decoction form. Herbs include neem, *guḍūchī*, mango leaves, and *chitrak*. Next, antibiotic therapy includes barley flour, turmeric, and sesame paste applied as a poultice. This purifies or balances the *doṣhas*. Finally, healing is achieved through a medicated oil of myrrh, *chirāyatā, danti*, black or sea salt, and *trivṛit*.

Tridoṣha: Will not respond to therapies.

Shlayaja: First the foreign matter is removed, then the sinus is cleansed and purified with a plaster of sesame paste, raw honey, and *ghee*. Herbs are cooked into the oil (*bilwa*, *musta*, and other herbs used in the above Pitta therapy).

Breast Abscess (Stana Vidradhi)

In the same manner as described above, the *doṣhas* enter the open channels of the female breast during pregnancy or after delivery. They produce a hard swelling in the breasts (having features of external abscesses). This generally does not happen in young girls because the channels in their breasts are still small.

Therapies are treated like *vraṇa* (ulcer), but without applying the warm poultice. Incision may be applied by qualified persons, being careful not to injure the milk ducts.

Wounds (Vraṇa)

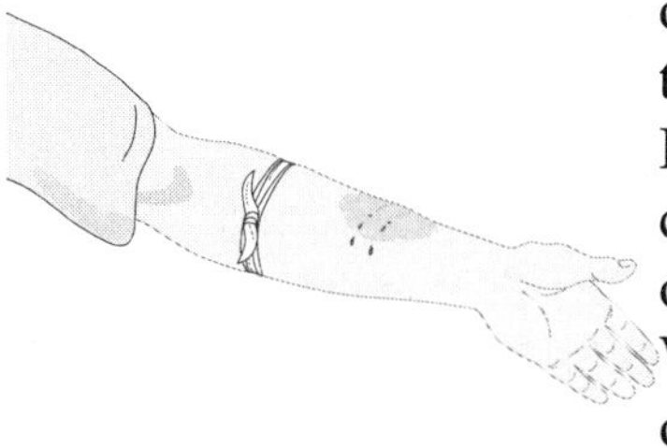

Causes: Two types of wounds exist: internal and external. Internal wounds are caused by excesses of the *doṣhas*. When Vāyu, Pitta or Kapha becomes excessed and move to the external passages, they cause innate wounds. When external wounds are not able to be healed and have internal symptoms the same therapies as innate wounds are applied.

Symptoms:
Vāyu: These wounds cause stiffness, are hard to the touch, slow to develop pus, have great and piercing pain, throbbing, and are black in color.
Pitta: Thirst, confusion, fever, sweating, burning, impurity, tearing, malodorous, and pus-filled.
Kapha: Slimy, heavy, oily, wet, with mild pain, pale, with slight fluid, and chronic.

These two forms of wounds have 20 varieties, incisable/unincisable, defective/undefective, in vital parts/not in vital parts, open/closed, severe/mild, oozing/non-oozing, poisoned/non-poisoned, even/uneven location, with/without pouch, and raised/depressed.

Five variations of wounds exist:
Defective wounds: Twelve types exist: white, narrow or depressed passages, very wide passages, grayish, blue, black, red, numerous boils, difficult to heal, bottleneck shaped, and malodorous.
Locations: Eight types, in the skin, blood vessels, flesh, fat, bone, ligaments, vital parts, and viscera.
Discharges: Fourteen types, lymph, water, pus, blood, yellow oozing, reddish, brownish, ochre, blue, green, oily, rough, black, and white.
Complications: Sixteen types, *visarpa* (erysipelas), paralysis, blood vessel blockages, tetanus, confusion, insanity, wound pain, fever, thirst, lockjaw, cough, vomiting, diarrhea, hiccup, difficult breathing, and trembling.
Defects: Twenty types, preventing healing, moist ligaments, excess blood vessel fluid, deepness, with maggots, bone cracking, with foreign bodies, toxic, spreading, and scratches that produce tearing. Other types include, skin friction, hair friction, faulty bandage, over oiling, and emaciation from excess reduction therapy. Further types are, indigestion, over eating, eating incompatible foods, unsuitable foods, grief, anger, naps, excess exercise, insufficient exercise, and sex.

Examination falls into three categories,
Inspection: Noticing client's age, complexion, body parts, sense organs, and touch.
Questions: Asking about the cause of wounds, development, pain, and digestive power.
Touch: Noting softness/hardness and coldness/warmth.

Healing is possible if the wound is in the skin or muscle when in an easy place to treat, when young, without complications, due to a wise patient, and if it is immediately tended to. Herbs include licorice, *tagar*, red sandalwood, *jaṭāmāṇśhi,* turmeric, barberry, and *kūt*.

Therapies:
General: First, emesis, purgation, enema, and surgery are used depending upon the *doṣhas* involved and the strength of the person. Wounds become quickly healed from these cleansing measures.
Thirty-six Measures: These measures include anti-swelling, six surgeries, pressing, cooling, uniting, fomenting, pacifying, probing, cleansing, healing, detox paste, healing paste, cleaning oil, healing oil, leaves, bandages, diet, elevation/depression, cauterization, hard and soft aromas, hard and soft pastes, powders, colors, and healing.

Inflammation—when seen as an initial sign, blood-letting prevents the wound from developing. Toxins are cleansed first (except Vāyu caused wounds, which one needs to eat *ghee* and Vāyu- reducing decoctions) using the appropriate *pañcha karma* therapy. Paste of *śhatāvarī*, sandalwood, parched barley flour mixed with *ghee* are useful to cool inflammations. If this is ineffective then the herbs are applied as a warm poultice (of parched barley flour and *ghee*), that ripens the wound. When it is ripe, it is pierced. If one has a delicate condition, then instead of piercing, linseed oil and *guggul* are applied to the wound to allow it to open on its own.

Operations—Six types of operations exist: incisions, puncturing, excision, scraping, scarification, and suturing. Incisions are used for sinuses, ripened inflammations, intestinal wounds or obstructions, swellings with foreign bodies inside. Puncture is useful for ascites, ripe and blood tumors, blood disorders, boils. Excision is applied to protruded wounds with thick margins, raised and hard, hemorrhoids. Scraping is done on leucoderma and other skin diseases. Scarification is performed on Vāyu blood disorders, glands, pimples, urticarial rashes (i.e., burning, itching, stinging, smooth patches), red patches, skin diseases, injured parts, and swellings. Suturing is needed for bowels, abdomen, and other deep or invasive surgery.

Pressing—any wound with a pouch or small opening is pressed with a paste of wheat flour and peas. Herbs include onion, *archu*, turmeric, *guggul*, and licorice.

Cooling—*balā* paste or *balā*—water sprinkling is used when heat is present. For blood-related wounds, cold *ghee* or cold milk is applied.

Long Wounds—paste of honey and *ghee* is evenly applied. Then *mañjiṣhṭhā*, turmeric, neem, *tulsī* (holy basil), *harītakī* bark, and *guggul* are placed over this. A bandage is then wrapped over the wound.

Small Wounds, Much Oozing, Pouchy—(not within vital parts), soft or hard probing is advised. Soft probes are soft plant stalks, hard probes are iron rods. Deep muscle probing also needs hot iron rods for cauterization.

Odorous, Discolored, Much Oozing & Pain—These are said to be caused by uncleanliness. They need to be cleansed and kept clean with decoctions of *triphalā*, *balā* and neem. Paste of sesame, salt, turmeric, and neem are also good cleansers. [Black, pale, painful, raised, and protruded (and not very red) wounds are considered already clean and not in need of cleansing.]

Leaves & Bandages—*arjuna*, neem, and *pippalī* leaves or sterile bandages are used to cover wounds.

Depressed Wounds—galactagogues, vitalizers, and bulk promoting herbs (e.g., *śhatāvarī*, *aśhwagandhā*, and *śhweta musali*) are used to raise depressions. To depress raised wounds *guggul*, *triphalā,* and castor oil are used.

Excess Hemorrhaging—(after excision) tumors, Kapha nodules, glands, stiffness and Vāyu disorders, wounds with pus or lymph, deep and firm, cauterization is needed.

Fractured Bones/Dislocated Joints—after the bone or joint is set, herbs of aloe, *guggul*, and *lodhra* are applied as a paste and bandaged (dipped in *ghee*). Then the bone or joint is immobilized with splints, casts, etc. Pitta-reducing foods are eaten. Other complications are also to be tended to.

Vāyu (Dry, Pain, Stiff): Massage, fomentation, bolus, poultices, and ointments with ghee, milk, and *balā*, *guḍūchī*, and *śhatāvarī*, sprinkling with *daśhmūl*, ingesting *ghee and* sesame oil.

Vāyu with Burning and Pain: Warm paste of linseed and sesame oil, dipped in milk, roasted barley flour. Herbs used include *mañjiṣhṭhā*, neem, and onion.

Pitta: Oils, paste and water sprinkling using cold, sweet and bitter herbs (sandalwood, licorice, *balā, viḍaṅga, kuṭaj, triphalā*, *musta*, cardamom), sesame oil and *ghee*, ingesting *ghee* and purgation. A Pitta-reduction diet (i.e., no salt, hot, sour, pungent, heavy or burning foods or drinks) and no sexual intercourse, in order to heal these disorders. Cool foods and drinks, naps, and rest are also useful healers.

Kapha: Oil and water sprinkling with astringent, pungent, hot, and rough herbs; emesis and other reduction therapies, digestive herbs.

Inflammed Ulcers (Dvivraniya)

Causes: Ulcers fall under two categories, internal and external.

Internal: Causes may be due to excesses of blood, Vāyu, Pitta, Kapha, or Tridoṣha.

External: Causes are due to bites from animals, accidents, and injuries, poisons, etc. Cooling therapies are immediately used to cool the expanding heat of the ulcer. This heat is Pitta related and may be pacified with a mixture of honey and *ghee* applied directly on the wound for 1 week. After that, the appropriate internal therapies are followed.

Symptoms: Sixteen forms of ulcers exist. Pain is associated with each, while specific symptoms vary from form to form.

Vāyu: Brown or bright red, cold, thin, and slimy secretions, tension, throbbing, pricking, and piercing pain inside the ulcer, and feeling of expansion.

Pitta: Bluish-yellow, grows quickly, burning, oozing, redness, and surrounded by small yellow pustule eruptions.

Kapha: Gray, extended, raised around the circumference, itching, thick, compact, covered by vessels and membranes, slightly painful, hard, cold, thick, white, and slimy secretions.

Blood: Looks like a lump of red coral, surrounded by black vesicles and pustules, malodorous, painful, feels like fumes rise from it, bleeding, and other Pitta symptoms.

Vāyu/Pitta: Red or bright red, pricking and burning pain, feels like fumes rise from it, bright red or bluish yellow secretions.

Vāyu/Kapha: Itching, piercing pain, heavy, hard or calloused, constant exuding of cold, slimy secretions.

Pitta/Kapha: Heavy, hot, yellow, burning, pale, or yellow secretion.

Vāyu/Blood: Dry, thin, piercing pain, loss of sensation, blood, or bright red secretions.

Pitta/Blood: The color of the surface cream of *ghee*, fishy smell, spreads, hot, and blackish secretions.

Kapha/Blood: Red, heavy, slimy, glossy, hard or calloused, itching, or bloody yellow secretions.

Vāyu/Pitta/Blood: Throbbing, pricking and burning pain, thin yellowish bloody secretions, with sensation, and feeling like fumes arise.

Vāyu/Kapha/Blood: Itching, throbbing, tingling, thick, gray, and blood-streaked secretions.

Pitta/Kapha/Blood: Redness, itching, pus forming, burning, thick, gray, and bloody secretions.

Tridoṣha: Various pains, secretions, and colors associated with all three *doṣhas*.

Vāyu/Pitta/Kapha/Blood: Burning and piercing pains, throbbing, itching, complete loss of sensation, redness, pus forming, various colors, pains, and secretions common to all *doṣhas* and the blood.

Shuddha-vrana: (clean ulcer) Ulcers that are the same color as the back of the tongue, smooth, painless, soft, shiny, well shaped, and without secretions.

Therapies: Sixty therapies and surgical methods exist, including fasting and light meals, plastering, irrigation or spraying, anointing, fomentation, massage, large and small poultices, inducing oozing, draining. Other therapies are internal intake of oils and *ghee*, emesis, and purgatives. Surgical methods include excision, opening abscesses, bursting, scraping, extraction, probing, vein puncturing, inducing discharge, suturing adhesion, and pressing. Further methods include stopping bleeding, cooling, suturing, decoction washes, plugs, pastes, external *ghee* and oils, internal herbal use, dusting and rubbing with herbs. Other methods are, growing hairs, fumigation, raisings, destroying, softening, hardening, caustics, cauterization, blackening, and healing with scars. Additional methods include burning (cauterization), enemas, urethral and vaginal injections, bandaging, leaf application, vermifuges, rejuvenatives, disinfectants, and *śhiro virechana* (nasal evacuation). Further therapies are, snuff, gargling or holding herbs in the mouth, smoking, honey/*ghee*, *yantras* (physical therapy machines), nutrition, and protection from malicious spirits.

Discussed here are the more common internal

ulcers that inflame the stomach's tissue lining. Usually they are Pitta disorders causing pain, burning, or bleeding. They are most commonly caused by stress, worry, working too hard, spicy and sour foods, alcohol, and smoking.

General: Bland diet, whole grains, digestible foods, milk fast (if one is strong). Nightshades (e.g., tomatoes, eggplants, white potatoes), citrus fruit (lemons, limes and grapefruits), and bananas are avoided. Herbs to soothe the mucus lining include aloe gel, *śhatāvarī*, and *balā*. Also useful is *praval piṣhti, śhaṅkh bhasma* (conch shell ash), and *sūktī bhasma* (sea shell ash).
Vāyu: Vāyu-reducing foods, liquids, herbs and spices.
Pitta: Pitta-reducing foods, aloe, barberry, *kaṭukā*, *āmalakī*, and *chirāyatā*.
Kapha: These conditions may be caused by emotional issues like sadness, greediness, or attachment. Herbs include hot and pungents like *tṛikatu* and cloves.

Bone Fractures and Joint Dislocations (Bhagnam and Sandhi Mukti)

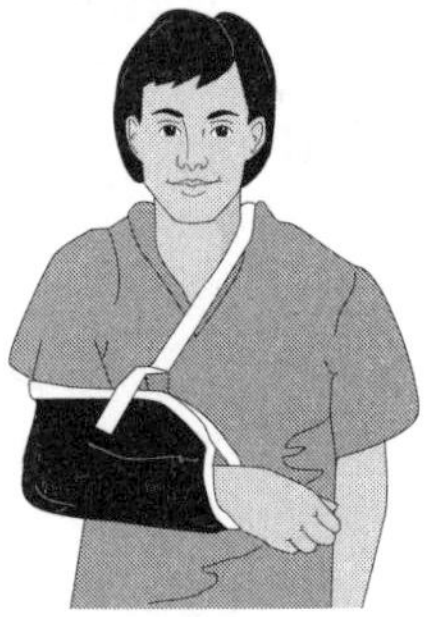

Causes: This is due to falling, pressure, blow, violent jerking, or bites. Six forms of dislocations exist: friction, looseness, abnormal projection, lateral and oblique dislocation. Twelve types of fractures exist.

Dislocation Symptoms:
General: Persons experience loss of movement, extension, flexibility, rotation, and painful when moved or touched.
Joint Friction: (*utpliṣhtam*) This is due to two joint extremities causing swelling on either side of the joint. Various pains are felt at night.
Looseness: (*viśhliṣhtam*) Symptoms include slight swelling with constant pain, and poor functioning of the joint.
Lateral displacement: (*vivartitam*) Symptoms are pain and uneven joint setting.
Dislodged Bone: (*adha-kṣhiptam*) Excruciating pain, dislocated bone looseness, and hanging from the joint can develop.
Abnormal Projection: (*ati-kṣhiptam*) The dislocated bone moves away from the joint and is very painful.
Oblique Dislocation: (*tiryak-kṣhiptam*) Projection or displacement of bone on one side causes unbearable pain.

Fracture Symptoms: (*Kānda-bhagnam*)
General: Symptoms include violent swelling around the seat of the fracture, throbbing, pulsation, abnormal position of the fractured limb with unbearable pain when touched. Other experiences include cracking sounds when pressure is applied, looseness of limb, various pains, and discomfort in all positions.

The most difficult to heal are impacted, drooping, severed, and shattered fractures. Also, displacement or looseness in children or in very old or weak persons, those suffering from asthma, skin problems, or *kṣhata-kṣhīṇa* (lung abscess or injury) are difficult to heal.

Symptoms that cannot be healed include pelvic bone fracture or dislocation, compound fracture of thigh or skull flat bones. Other unhealable symptoms include frontal bone fractures (into small pieces) or dislocation, simple breast bone, back bone, temporal and cranial bone fractures.
Bulging: (*Karkatam*) Pressing or bending the fractured bone at its two joint extremities causes bulging at the middle of the fracture, resembling a knot.
Upward Projection: (*aśhvakarṇam*) Symptoms include an upward protrusion and looks like the ear of a horse.
Shattered Fragments: (*churnitam*) Palpitations and cracking sounds develop.
Smashed Bones: (*pichitam*) Large swellings appear.

Splintered: (*asthi-challitam*) The bone covering or skin (periosteum) is splintered off.

Compound Fracture: (*kānda-bhagnam*) Bones that are completely broken, broken in several places, or several bones projecting through the skin are these symptoms.

Impacted Fracture: (*majjānugatam*) A fragment or broken bone pierces the bone, digging out the marrow.

Drooping: (*ati-pātitam*) The fractured bone droops or hangs.

Arched: (*vakram*) The unloosened bone is bent, forming an arch.

Severed: (*chinnam*) One joint extremity of the bone is severed.

Holes: (*pātitam*) A slight fracture is pierced with many holes with excruciating pain.

Greenstick Fracture: (*sphutitam*) Cracked, swollen, pain, and prickliness develop.

Bending of gristle or cartilage is called a fracture, long bones are usually severed, skull bones are generally cracked, teeth are usually splintered off.

Therapies:

All dislocations or fractures are manually manipulated to replace bones in their proper position and then bandaged.

Bandaging: Fractures are dressed and bandaged weekly during the winter, every fifth day during spring and autumn, and every fourth day in the summer. The affected area is first covered with a piece of linen soaked in *ghee*, then the splint is applied and properly bandaged. Bandages are made neither too loose nor too tight.

Healing fractures or dislocations is difficult when they occur in Vāyu *doṣhas*, in the over-indulging person and in one who eats too little. Fractures are also difficult to heal in those who have fever, abdominal distention, suppress urine or stool (and similar disorders). Fractures in young persons, those with only slight imbalances of the *doṣhas* or in the winter are easily healed within 1 month. Healing in mid-life takes 2 months, while elderly people require 3 months to heal.

Salt, acidic, pungent and alkaline foods and spices need to be avoided. Rest, shade oily foods and drinks, and other Vāyu-increasing foods and habits need to be followed. Foods include rice, *ghee*, or boiled milk. Herbs include *mañjiṣhṭhā*, red sandalwood, *śhatāvarī*, flaxseed, horsetail, solomon's seal, and comfrey, and may be taken internally (every morning with *ghee*) and used as an external plaster.

Herbs of the *nyagrodhādi* group are used for bandaging and washing. Herbs in this group include licorice, *lodhra*, *pīpal* tree, *guggul* (*salai* tree), Indian persimmon *(tinduka/temru)*, mango, *arjuna,* and *harītakī*. The tree bark of each of these herbs is used.

Washing: A cold decoction of the above herbs is used to wash the fractured part. When pain is great, *daśhmūl* or *mahānārāyan* oil (oil is warmed in the winter) are applied to the fracture. If the fracture has ulcerated complications, astringent herbs mixed with honey and *ghee* are also used (such as raspberry, *āmalakī*, *arjuna*, and *musta*). Crushed or dislocated joints are not shaken. Cold washes, plasters and oils are used.

Ghee: Is first used on fractures and dislocations before they are reset.

Discrimination, courage, strong will and knowledge of the soul etc.
are the ideal therapies for the mind.
Aṣhṭāñga Hṛidayam Sū. Ch. 1: ver. 26

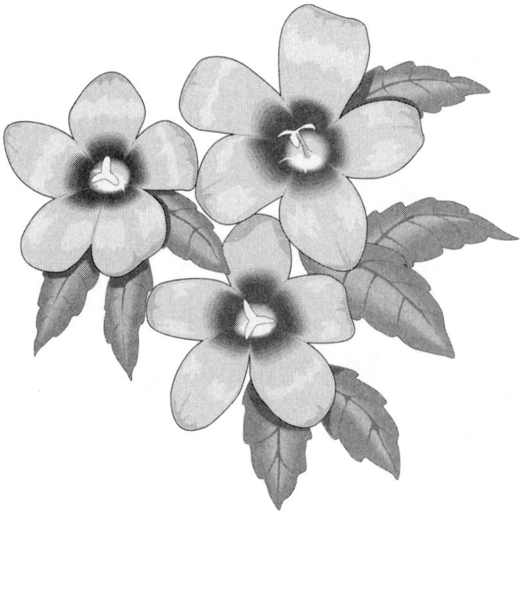

Modern science is based on the study of physical principles to conquer nature.

Āyurveda requires deep spiritual insight in order to live in harmony with nature.
Anonymous

Chapter 17: Respiratory System
Cough, Breathing, Cold, TB, Hiccup

Cough (Kāsa)

Introduction:

There are 5 kinds of coughs: Vāyu, Pitta, Kapha, those caused by lung injury, and those caused by wasting (i.e., pulmonary tuberculosis).

Premonitory Signs: Throat irritation, loss of taste or appetite, thorny feeling in the throat.

Development: When the downward movement of Vāyu (*Apāna*) is obstructed, it begins to move upward to the chest and throat, and eventually to the head. This affects the eyes, back, chest, ribs, and eventually comes out the mouth as a cough.

Vāyu Cough: As the accumulation of Vāyu increases into aggravation, dryness is produced in the chest, throat, mouth, ribs, heart, and head. The dry air also causes delusion, mental agitation, loss of voice, and results in a dry cough with violent bouts, great pain, noise, and hair standing on end. A dry spit may be coughed out, which reduces the coughing fits.

Pitta Cough: Yellow color in the eyes and mucus, a bitter taste in the mouth, fever, dizziness, vomiting of bile and blood, thirst, hoarseness, fumes emitted from the mouth, acidity, and continuous coughing that makes persons stare upwards.

Kapha Cough: Mild pain in the chest, head, and heart region; heaviness, throat coating, debility, runny nose, vomiting, loss of appetite and taste, hair standing on end; thick, sticky, white, or clear mucus is expelled.

Lung Injury Cough: From trauma caused by fighting, or strenuous activities. Vāyu becomes increased, mixes with Pitta, and produces coughs. Symptoms include large amounts of yellow or black blood mixed with mucus. It is dry, nodular, and foul smelling. Severe pain is present in the throat, chest (i.e., feeling like pricking needles), joints, and ribs. Other symptoms include fever, difficult breathing, thirst, hoarseness, tremors, and cooing sounds. Strength or vigor steadily diminishes. One's digestion and desire for eating is reduced, and poor complexion develops. Persons become emaciated, and there is blood in the urine, with sharp back and waist pains.

Wasting Cough: This is caused by all the *doṣhas*, but mainly Vāyu. Mucus is putrefied, pus-like, yellow, foul smelling, and is green or red. The ribs and heart feel as though sliding and falling down, and an unreasonable desire for hot or cold comforts develops. Persons overeat but still lose strength. The face is oily, yet has a pleasing radiant look and glittering eyes. Once this symptom appears, tuberculosis gradually begins to develop. If a person is emaciated, or if tuberculosis (*kśhayaja*) lingers for a long time, it is considered harmful. If aggressively treated with all the appropriate measures during the early stages, a person can be completely cured.

If one *doṣha* is the cause of any of these 3 types of coughs, the illness can be healed. If two *doṣhas* cause any of these coughs, the illness can be controlled. If unattended, *doṣha*-caused coughs lead to lung injury resulting in TB.

Therapies

Vāyu: When persons are undernourished, excess Vāyu is reduced with *ghee*, oil enemas, a wholesome diet including *basmati* rice, whole wheat, barley gruel (with *bilwa*, ginger, *daśhmūl*, *chitrak, jaggery,* and black salt), warm and moist vegetables, and sesame oil. Persons should drink boiled milk, *lassi* (1/2 yogurt to 1/2 water), or sour fruit juices—all mixed with sugar cane.

Ghee should be mixed with Vāyu-reducing herbs including *aśhwagandhā*, ginger, *pippalī*, licorice, calamus, *viḍaṅga*, black salt, *chitrak*, *daśhmūl*, *kapikachū*, *balā*, *guḍūchī*, *triphalā*, *ṭrikatu*, *gokṣhura,* and *śhatāvarī*. These herbs promote digestion and reduce coughs. Raw honey and cane sugar can also be mixed with the herbs and barley. [Traditional texts speak of barley as reducing Vāyu; however, modern experience indicates most Vāyu *doṣhas* find that barley causes gas. If needed white *basmati* rice is an easily digested and nutritious substitute.]

Other therapies include massage, water sprinkling, oil fomentations, snuff, and smoking Vāyu- and Kapha-reducing herbs. For constipation and gas retention, enemas should be administered. *Ghee* should be taken before meals if there is upper body dryness.

Smoking(Herbs): Relieves coughs that cannot be helped by ingesting herbs and foods. Herbal smoke includes *musta*, *balā*, black pepper, cardamom, *vaṃśha lochana*, ginger, *aśhwagandhā*, and *harītakī*. This also relieves Kapha-caused coughs.

Vāyu with phlegm: *Viḍaṅga*, ginger, *pippalī*, *asafoetida*, black salt, barley powder, with *ghee*.

Pitta: Castor oil purgation is useful.

Pitta with phlegm: Emesis with *ghee*, licorice, and sugar cane. After the *doṣhas* are cleansed and balanced, one takes Pitta-reducing foods and liquids (cold and sweet properties).

Thin phlegm: Sugar cane is mixed with emesis formula. Foods and liquids are oily and cold, including barley, green *dal,* and *ghee*. Herbs include lotus seeds, *pippalī*, *musta*, licorice, fresh ginger, dry ginger, *āmalakī*, sandalwood, *bibhītakī*, *vaṃśha lochana*, *gokṣhura*, mixed with *ghee*, sugar cane, and honey.

Thick phlegm: Bitter herbs and vegetables are mixed with emesis formula. Dry and cold foods and drinks are recommended. Neem and raw honey are added to the above herbs. Grape juice mixed with sugar cane, sugar cane water, and milk, should be drunk.

Chest Wound and Wasting Cough with burning and fever: Boiled milk with *śhatāvarī*, *balā*, and licorice.

Chest Wound, Wasting: *Ghee* with boiled milk, *śhatāvarī*, cane sugar, *pippalī*, *vaṃśha lochana*, black pepper, turmeric, *karkata śhringi,* and *chabchini*.

Kapha: First, administer an emetic (if persons are strong) with barley and pungent herbs like *pippalī*; then, a castor oil purgation. Foods should be light, including vegetable soup, radish, and *pippalī*, and a little *ghee*, sesame oil, mustard oil, and *bilwa* fruit. After eating, drink raw honey, sour drinks (e.g., *āmalakī* juice), hot water, or *lassi* (1/4 yogurt to 3/4 water). Herbs should include sugar cane, sandalwood, *vāsāk, tulsī, apāmārga, āmalakī*, *musta*, *harītakī*, calamus, *balā*, *ṭrikatu*, *viḍaṅga*, *chitrak*, *punarnavā*, *āmlavetasa*, *gokṣhura*, ginger, and black pepper mixed with raw honey.

Another recipe includes 10 gms. (.35 oz.) of *pippalī* fried in canola oil mixed with cane sugar or rock candy.

Smoking: Herbs are the same as for Vāyu (*musta*, *balā*, black pepper, cardamom, *vaṃśha lochana*, ginger, *aśhwagandhā*, *harītakī, chakramarda*).

Kapha/Vāyu: *Pippalī*, ginger, *musta*, *harītakī*, *āmalakī,* and rock candy, made with honey and *ghee.* (Sesame oil can be used for Pitta *cough.*) Dry and oily foods and drinks are used for wet and dry symptoms, respectively, to balance these conditions.

Kapha/Pitta: Pitta-reducing herbs (i.e., bitters) and *vāsāk*, turmeric, *vaṃśha lochana*, cardamom, and honey are recommended.

Chest Wounds: Sweet and vitalizing herbs such as *śhatāvarī* and sugar cane. Also *pippalī*, boiled milk, barley and wheat flours, *āmalakī*, sesame oil, *ghee*, and honey are helpful. Therapies for chest wounds generally follow the Pitta-pacifying regime.

If physical pain from Vāyu and Pitta exists, *ghee* massage is useful. The chest is warmed with a hot, dry cloth, and massaged with medicated oil.

Should Vāyu cause the spitting of blood with burning sensation, along with heart or side pain, *ghee,* mixed with rejuvenatives (e.g., *śhatāvarī*), *vāsāk*, and *dūrba,* is recommended. For any bleeding complications, *ghee* is ingested and used as nasal oil (Tuberculosis is usually accompanied by bleeding.).

When the wound is healed but Kapha remains in the chest and head, causing coughing fits, one smokes *aśhwagandhā*, *balā,* and ginger with sugar cane juice.

Emaciation: Wholesome, restorative foods (e.g., *basmati* rice gruel) and herbs include *triphalā*, *chitrak*, *pippalī*, ginger, *guḍūchī*, calamus, *śhatāvarī*, with black salt, and *ghee*. Grape juice is also advised. Herbs like cardamom are also used to strengthen digestion. When one is strong, but still has excesses of the *doṣhas,* mild oil purgation is useful (*triphalā* and *ghee,* or castor oil).

Other recipes: *Ghee* cooked in grape juice with *harītakī*, *musta*, ginger, black pepper, and *pippalī*; *ghee* and *āmalakī* boiled in milk, and pomegranate juice with cane sugar.

For thirst, boiled milk is given. With diminished Pitta and Kapha, *ghee*, boiled milk, and *balā* are used. For dysuria or urine discoloration, boiled milk with *ghee*, *vidārī kand,* and *gokṣhura* are used. For pain and swelling in the penis, anus, hip, and groin, oil enemas with a little *ghee* are used.

The ashes of metals and gems (*bhasmas*) are widely used in India for rapid healing. Iron ash (*lauh bhasma*) is suggested to regain strength from wasting and emaciation quickly. *Abhrak*, *pravāl* and *maukta bhasmas* are also useful.

As with all diseases, therapy depends upon the aggravating *doṣha* .

Difficult Breathing (Śhvāsa) [including asthma]

Causes: Difficult breathing arises from many factors, from increases of cough, *doṣha* aggravation, diarrhea owing to indigestion, vomiting, poisons, anemia, fever, allergies, smoke, breeze, injury to vital organs, and drinking very cold or ice water. There are five types of difficult breathing.

Development: When movement of Vāyu is obstructed by Kapha, it spreads in all directions and vitiates the channels of respiration (*prāṇa*), water (*udaka*), and food (*anna*). The obstruction rises from the stomach (i.e., the origin site of Kapha) into the chest, causing difficult breathing.

Premonitory Signs: Pain in the heart and ribs, upward respiratory movement (of *prāṇa*), gas, splitting temple pain, heaviness in the throat and chest, astringent taste in the mouth, and abdominal rumbling.

Symptoms of the Five Types:

1. Exertion (kṣhudrā śhvāsa): Caused by exertion or overeating. It is not serious, subsiding after rest or digestion.

2. Bronchial Asthma (tamaka śhvāsa): Aggravated Vāyu begins to move upwards in the respiratory channel (*Prāṇavaha srotas*), aggravating Kapha, making it difficult to breathe. Sharp pains in the head, neck, chest, and ribs appear. Coughs may be experienced with cracking sounds, delusion, loss of taste or appetite, runny nose, and thirst. Heaviness or forced breathing may develop, causing distress and loss of consciousness. Expectorants bring temporary comfort, but there is difficulty breathing when lying down (or sitting). Eyes are wide and gaze upward, sweating develops on the forehead, and the mouth becomes dry. Persons desire hot things, and develop tremors or shivering. Breathing becomes more difficult on cloudy days, after drinking cold water, from cold breezes or direct wind, when eating Kapha-increasing foods. (Another form of this asthma is associated with fever and fainting. It is resolved by cold foods, drinks, and air.) Overall, bronchial asthma may be healed if treated when it first arises, otherwise it is only controllable.

The latter 3 types may also be healed if treated in the early stages

3. Cheyne-stokes (chinna śhvāsa): When interrupted breathing with sharp pain develops (i.e., extreme pain similar to the pain of injury to vital points (*marma*), vital organ pain occurs along with sweating, fainting, gas, burning sensations, and urinary stones. Eyes gaze downward, are unsteady and teary; one eye is red. Coma, dry mouth, erratic speech, feeling of helplessness, and loss of complexion can also develop.

4. Mahā śhvāsa: Heavy breathing, feeling helpless, breathing noises, continuous high-pitched sounds, loss of common sense and intelligence, unsteady eyes and face, constricted chest, blocked urine and stool, broken voice, dry throat, frequent delusions, severe pain in ears, temples, and head.

5. Ūrdhva śhvāsa: Prolonged exhalations with inability to inhale, mucus lines the mouth and throat, eyes gaze upward, rolling and terrified, severe pain, inability to speak (owing to the pain in the vital organ).

Specific *Doṣha* Symptoms

Vāyu: Dry cough, wheezing, dry skin, dry mouth, thirst, constipation, desiring warm liquids, anxiety. Attacks happen mainly at dawn or dusk.

Pitta: Wheezing and coughing with yellow phlegm, sweating, irritability, fever, desiring cold air. Attacks happen mainly at noon or midnight.

Kapha: Wheezing and coughing with excess clear or white phlegm, lung fluid, rattling sounds. Attacks mainly develop in the morning and evening.

Therapies:

General: Bronchodilators, such as lobelia and ephedra, quickly open breathing passages. Long-term use can be depleting for Pitta and Kapha, and immediately weakening for Vāyu. Tridoṣhic herbs include *harītakī, balā,* and saffron. Each person must follow their appropriate *doṣha* diet.

After attacks, the lungs must be strengthened with tonics like *chyavan prāśh, balā, aśhwagandhā, harītakī,* and *brāhmī.* Rebuilding the lungs in this way can help prevent future attacks.

For difficult breathing associated with

Vāyu: *Ghee* and *pippalī*, *vaṃśha lochana*, and *guggul*; lemon or lime juice.

Vāyu/Pitta: Milk, *ghee*, rice water, *bibhītakī*, *vāsāk*, and *trikatu.*

Pitta: *Ghee, vāsāk, vaṃśha lochana*, ginger, *pippalī, brāhmī, and kaiṣhore guggul.*

Pitta/Kapha: *Vāsāk*, *pippalī, guggul, kaiṣhore guggul,* and honey.

Kapha: *Vāsāk*, *pippalī, aśhwagandhā, guggul,* and honey. Apply a mustard paste to the chest.

Kapha/Vāyu: Emesis and purgation, including herbs that reduce these *doṣhas*.

Hiccup (Hikkā)

There are 5 kinds of hiccup. Their causes, premonitory symptoms, kinds, and development are the same as diseases of difficult breathing.

Type 1. Food-caused (annajā hikkā): Vāyu becomes aggravated by eating too quickly and improperly, or eating and drinking dry, penetrating, rough, and unaccustomed foods. This produces a painless hiccup. It is quiet, then followed by sneezing. It ceases when foods and drinks that one may be accustomed to are ingested.

Type 2. Exertion-caused (kṣhudrā hikkā): Vāyu becomes mildly increased from exertion. This causes a slight hiccup from the base of the shoulders. It ceases after eating food.

Type 3. Indigestion-caused (yamalā kihhā): This type arises when one hasn't eaten for many hours or when digestion is not working properly. These hiccups come in pairs, causing tremors in the head and neck, gas, severe thirst, nonsensical speech, vomiting, diarrhea, unsteady eyes, and yawning.

Type 4. (*mahatī hikkā*): Rigidity develops in the eyebrows and sides of neck, eyes become red and teary, there is loss of body movements, speech, memory, and awareness. Food is obstructed from moving, causing the vital organs to feel like they have been hit. The body bends backwards and emaciation develops. These types of hiccups arise from deep inside the body, forcefully, with great sounds.

Type 5 (gambhīrā hikkā): This hiccup begins either in the colon or in the navel region. Symptoms are similar to Type 4, but with more yawning, body expansion, and vibrating sounds.

Hiccups caused by food and exertion are most easily healed. Severe hiccups should be taken seriously.

Therapies: For both difficult breathing and hiccup oil and sweat (*nāḍī*, bolus or steam tent—see Chapter 7) are required. First, persons undergo an oil massage with black salt (with Pitta constitution) When there are Pitta problems, such as burning, excessive bleeding or sweating, weakness and tissue depletion, or pregnancy, black salt should not be used. Oil loosens and dissolves the thick phlegm blocking the breathing channels, softening them, and re-balancing Vāyu.

Afterwards, a light diet of *basmati* rice and *ghee* or sesame oil is taken to increase Kapha. Then one is ready for emesis with *pippalī*, rock salt, and honey (reducing Kapha and Vāyu). After emesis releases the excess Kapha, the channels are cleared, and the Vāyu begins to flow properly. Should there be any remaining Kapha, turmeric and barley grain are mixed with *ghee* and smoked.

When either of these illnesses are associated with a weak voice, diarrhea, internal bleeding, or burning, one eats foods that are sweet, oily, and cold.

Short periods of fomentation are applied to the chest and throat. Warm oil is mixed with cane sugar, or poultices are made with sesame and whole wheat, Vāyu-reducing herbs, foods, sour herbs (e.g., *āmalakī*), and milk are ingested. Other herbs include *daśhmūl, pippalī, ṭrikatu, balā, chitrak,* dry ginger, *gokṣhura, guḍūchī,* black salt; along with yogurt, *ghee*, dry radish, *ghee*, rice, and barley. *Daśhmūl* also removes complications of thirst.

A general herbal recipe includes *bilwa, gokṣhura, guḍūchī, balā, ṭrikatu, chitrak, pippalī,* ginger decoction with *ghee*, black pepper, and black salt.

If a strong fever with toxins (*āma*) develops, reduction therapy (*laṅgan*) is used (i.e., *pañcha karma*, exercise, sun bathing, etc.). Emesis with salt water is especially useful.

Should these therapies cause a Vāyu excess, balanced can be regained through Vāyu-reducing foods and warm massage.

If gas, distention, and constipation develop owing to Vāyu, foods with black salt, *āmlavetasa,* or *hiṅgwastock* are recommended.

Hiccup is predominated by Kapha, and is healed through emesis, purgation, a wholesome diet, and pacification therapy, using herbal smoking (for strong persons only).

When weak children or elderly persons develop excess Vāyu, oil therapies are used to reduce excess air. It is important not to use laxatives when there is not an excess of Kapha. To do so may dry up the vital organs and threaten the person.

See difficult breathing section (page 411) for specific *doṣha* therapies.

For hiccup, *ghee* mixed with *triphalā,* or castor oil quickly stops the situation. Suddenly sprinkling cold water on persons with hiccups is helpful. Slowly drinking water nonstop for 30 seconds or until the hiccups cease is another option. Other therapies include frightening or causing surprise, anger, exhilaration, or separation from loved ones.

All foods and herbs should simultaneously reduce excess Kapha and Vāyu. *Ghee* is used in all situations.

Pulmonary Tuberculosis (Rājā-yakṣhmā) [and other wasting diseases]

Mythology: *Chandra*, the moon, was married to the 28 daughters of *Dakṣha Prajapati*, but he favored only one of the daughters, *Rohinī*. Having exhausted and emaciated himself by depleting his *ojas* (life sap) through sensual pleasures with this one woman, he had no strength to satisfy the remaining ladies. Their father, *Dakṣha* became angry and caused the moon to develop tuberculosis. The moon soon apologized and was forgiven by *Dakṣha*, who sent the two celestial physicians (*Ashwins*) to heal him with *soma* nectar (restoring his *ojas*).

Causes: The Sanskrit word, *Rājā yakṣhmādi*, means king of the diseases. There are four causes of *Rājā yakṣhmādi*: 1) sudden or excessive exertion or chest wound, 2) suppression of any of the 13 natural urges (e.g., urine, feces, flatulence, etc.), 3) excessive loss of semen (*śhukra*), life sap/tissue essence (*ojas*), or tissue lubrication (*sneha*) [*pratilomak* diabetes—depletion of *dhātus*] 4) improper nutrition [*anulomak* diabetes—depletion of *dhātus*]. All forms of TB are caused by the simultaneous excess of all three *doṣhas*.

Development: Owing to any of the above causes, Vāyu overwhelms the chest, deranging Kapha and Pitta. This vitiated Vāyu then spreads throughout the body to all the body joints, veins, and plasma channels. These increases spread in all directions (i.e., up, down, sideways), excessively constricting or dilating their channels. Thus, disease is created.

1) Vāyu in the joints causes yawning, malaise, and fever. Vāyu in the stomach and small intestine produce anorexia, palpitations, cardiac pain, and other chest disorders. When Vāyu aggravates the throat, irritations and hoarseness develop. When the channels through which vital air flows through are affected, breathing is difficult and persons feel cold. When the head is affected, head disorders develop. Constant coughing causes chest injury, irregular Vāyu movement, and throat irritation. If coughing continues, the chest can be further injured. This weakens the person even more. These complications cause emaciation, developing weight loss, wasting of muscles, loss of appetite, and debility.

2) By suppressing natural urges of gas, urine, and feces (owing to bashfulness, disgust, or fear), Vāyu becomes superabundant, and while mixed with Pitta and Kapha, move in all directions. As Vāyu moves to the bones, stomach, etc. (as described above), it causes many disorders. Tridoṣhic symptoms include coryza, cough, frequent vomiting and diarrhea, dry stool, rib and shoulder pain, anorexia, panting, head disorders, coughing, difficult breathing, fever, hoarseness, and colds. These develop emaciation that leads to weight loss, wasting of muscles, loss of appetite, and debility.

3) Excessive weight loss can be caused by great grief and worry, envy, terror, jealousy, anxiety, fear anger, excessive sexual intercourse, excess oily diet when emaciated, fasting, or insufficient sizes of meals when weak.

Should one continue having sexual intercourse after the depletion of semen, Vāyu then enters the blood vessels and is ejaculated. This causes loose, dry joints, and further excesses Vāyu and weakens the body. This deranged Vāyu spreads throughout the body and further deranges Kapha and Pitta (i.e., reduces them). Other symptoms include reduction of muscle tissue and blood, rib pain, grinding shoulder pain, throat irritation, head congestion (owing to excessive Vāyu vitiating Kapha), malaise, anorexia, and indigestion. These symptoms can develop into fever, cough, difficult breathing, hoarseness, and excess mucus. This can lead to consumption that will develop into TB if not corrected.

4) From poor eating habits, the three *doṣhas* can become imbalanced and spread throughout the body, obstructing the entrances of the circulatory channels. This results in most foods becoming converted into feces and urine instead of

tissue elements. Persons become depleted and emaciated. Vāyu causes colic, malaise, throat irritations and hoarseness, rib and shoulder pain, and excessive mucus. Pitta causes fever, diarrhea, and burning. Kapha causes excessive mucus, anorexia, coughing, and heaviness of the head. Excessive coughing injures the lungs, resulting in spitting blood, which further weakens the person. This develops into TB.

Premonitory Signs: Nasal mucus, excessive sneezing, salivation, sweet taste in the mouth, poor digestion, physical weakness, imagining objects (e.g., dirt, flies, grass, hairs) in food and drinks, nausea and vomiting (even during meals), loss of appetite or taste, weakness or tiredness when eating, fault finding, staring at hands, swelling of the feet and face, excessive showing of the whites of the eyes, denying one's emaciation, imagining one's looks are disgusting, excessive desire for sexual intercourse, wine and meat; miserliness, excessive passion, cruelty, covering the head with clothes, nails and hair grows at an unusually rapid rate, unusual dreams (e.g., being defeated by small animals and insects, climbing on piles of hair, bones, and ash; visions of deserted villages, empty places, dry wells, stars, and mountains falling, trees burning).

Symptoms: Symptoms of tuberculosis include heaviness of the head, coughing, difficult breathing, hoarseness, vomiting phlegm, spitting blood, rib pain, shoulder pain, fever, diarrhea, loss of appetite and taste, coughing up mucus with sticky, thick odorous, green, white, or yellowish phlegm.

Vaghabāta (*Aṣhṭāñga Hṛidaya*) states that, depending where in the body the *doṣhas* are found, different symptoms will manifest.

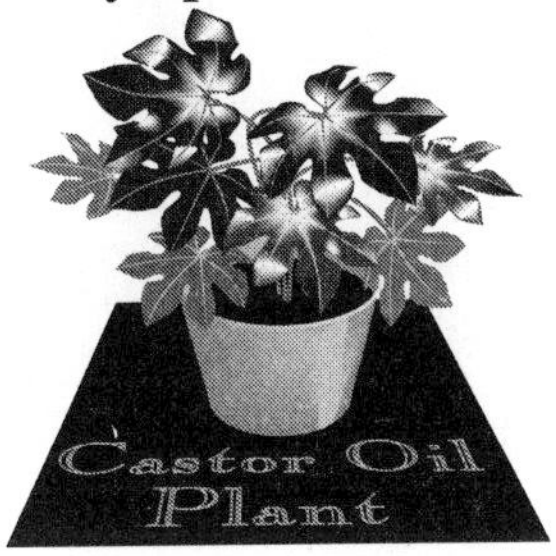

Pulmonary TB	
Location	**Symptoms**
Upper body	nasal mucus, difficult breathing, cough, pain in shoulders and head, hoarseness, loss of appetite and taste
Lower body	diarrhea or constipation. Digestive tract vomiting
Sides of the body	rib pain
Joints	fever

The signs and symptoms vary according to the site of development of tuberculosis (e.g., pulmonary, intestinal, bone, kidney, adrenals, etc.). Main symptoms according to modern medicine include weight loss (despite proper diet, low-grade fever, and pain.

Secondary diseases include chest pain, excess yawning, body aches, expectoration of mucus, weak digestion, bad breath, and throat problems.

Vāyu causes pain in the head and ribs, shoulder and body aches, hoarseness and other throat problems.

Pitta causes burning sensations on the soles, shoulders and palms, diarrhea, vomiting blood, bad breath, fever, and toxins.

Kapha produces loss of taste and appetite, vomiting, cough, heaviness of head and body, excess salivation, mucus, difficult breathing, weak voice, poor digestion. When Kapha is predominant, the digestive fire is weakened owing to excessive coating of the plasma channel (*rasa dhātu*). This causes the channel to become obstructed, preventing plasma from going into other tissues (*dhātus*). Blood is forced upward and expectorated with mucus. Further, the undigested food, which becomes toxic (*āma*), does not allow for proper absorption of nutrients, preventing the nourishment of the other tissues. As a result, weakness occurs. If one is strong and not emaciated, therapy is recommended. Tuberculosis can be healed in persons who are still strong or who have regained strength.

Therapies:

Pacificatory Therapies:

Coryza: Sudation, massage, smoking, pastes, sprinkling, whole baths. Ingesting barley, rock salt, sour, pungent herbs, and foods mixed with *ghee* or oil. Herbs include *pippalī*, ginger, and *āmalakī*. Foods include pomegranates, radish sour, wheat, rice, tea of *daśhmūl,* coriander, ginger, or *bhūmīāmalakī.*

The throat, sides, chest, and head are fomented using a bolus (see Chapter 7). The head is sprinkled with a lukewarm water decoction of *balā* and *guḍūchī*. *Nāḍī sweda* (tube steam) can also be applied to these areas. Steam water is mixed with Vāyu-reducing herbs.

Headaches and pain in the sides and shoulders receive poultices of *balā, vachā, vidārī kanda, ghee,* and sesame oil. A paste of *kuṣhṭhā, tagara,* and sandalwood mixed with *ghee* also relieve these symptoms.

When these symptoms include secondary *doṣha* complications, *balā*, cedar, sandalwood, *nāgakeṣhar, punarnavā, vidārī kanda, śhatāvarī*, sesame oil, and *ghee* are used according to the *doṣha s*they reduce (as an external ointment).

Toxic blood may require blood-letting. *Abhyañga* with sandalwood oil or *ghee* is helpful. Snuff and smoke are also useful. Sprinkling milk or sandalwood decoction is also advised (see Chapter 7 for various therapies).

If the person is strong, emesis and purgation are advised. They are given with *ghee* or oil to prevent drying and debilitation.

Cough, difficult breathing, hoarseness, head, side, and shoulder pain: After stool evacuation, a snuff is made with *ghee, balā, vidārī kanda,* and mixed with rock salt. Frequent ingesting of *ghee, balā, daśhmūla,* and milk after meals (and/or *balā* and *ghee* during the middle of the meal) alleviates these symptoms.

Fever, difficult breathing, cough, hoarseness: Eating *ghee* mixed with dates, cane sugar, raw honey, and *pippalī* heals these conditions.

Therapies for other symptoms are discussed in their respective chapters.

Wasting and emaciation: Vāyu-reducing herbs and foods. Other therapies include *abhyañga* followed by bathing in oil and milk. This removes the blocks in the channels (*srotas*) and heals the person. After bathing, the person receives another *abhyañga*. Ingredients for this *abhyañga* include *śhatāvarī, mañjiṣhṭhā, punarnavā, aśhwagandhā, apāmārga, balā, vidārī kanda, kuśhtā*, rice, linseed, sesame, and yeast, barley powder in a mixture of 3 to 1 with the preceding ingredients is added, then, honey and yogurt. This mixture anointed on the body promotes nourishment, complexion, and strength.

Next, persons dress in special clothes offered in worship and place essential oils on themselves. A wholesome diet according to their *doṣha* is taken, including light whole grains. Meditation music, celibacy, pleasant company, company of elders, meditation, prayer, ethics, and nonviolence are other aspects required to restore good health.

Cold (Pratiṣhyāya)

Causes:

When the head or nasal passages are filled with excess Kapha or Pitta they may move towards the Vāyu location in the head (*prati).* This causes a serious form of cold (coryza) and develops emaciation of the body.

Signs and symptoms are headaches, stuffy nose, cough, mucus, nausea, hoarseness, heaviness, fever, fatigue, anorexia, and poor mind/body coordination. This develops into tuberculosis.

Therapies:

Kapha: If mucus is abundant, white, or clear, take Kapha- and *āma*-reducing foods and herbs.

Light, warm, simple foods. Dairy, sweets, fried foods, herbal tonics, and breads (with yeast) must be avoided because they increase Kapha. If a person is strong, a short fast is useful. Tea with lemon juice, fresh ginger, and raw honey reduces Kapha.

Sweat therapy is advised, using diaphoretic anti-cough and expectorant herbs prepared as a tea (e.g., cinnamon. ginger, *pippalī, tulsī,* licorice, *sitopaladi* mix). Steam tents or sleeping under many blankets to promote sweat are also useful.

Pitta: (Yellow or green mucus, high fever, sore throat, flushed face) *Gokṣhura, punarnavā,* coriander, fennel, spearmint, and other cooling diaphoretics used for Pitta *doṣha*. *Sitopaladi* or *sudarṣhan* mixture is especially useful for fever.

Vāyu: (Little mucus, dry cough, hoarseness, insomnia) For a dry nose, 3 drops of sesame oil can be placed in each nostril. Warming diaphoretics used for Kapha are mixed with a smaller dose of demulcent herbs like *aśhwagandhā, śhatāvarī,* and licorice. Here, too, *sitopaladi* is an excellent mixture, and can be mixed into warm milk.

The Lungs and Chest Cavity

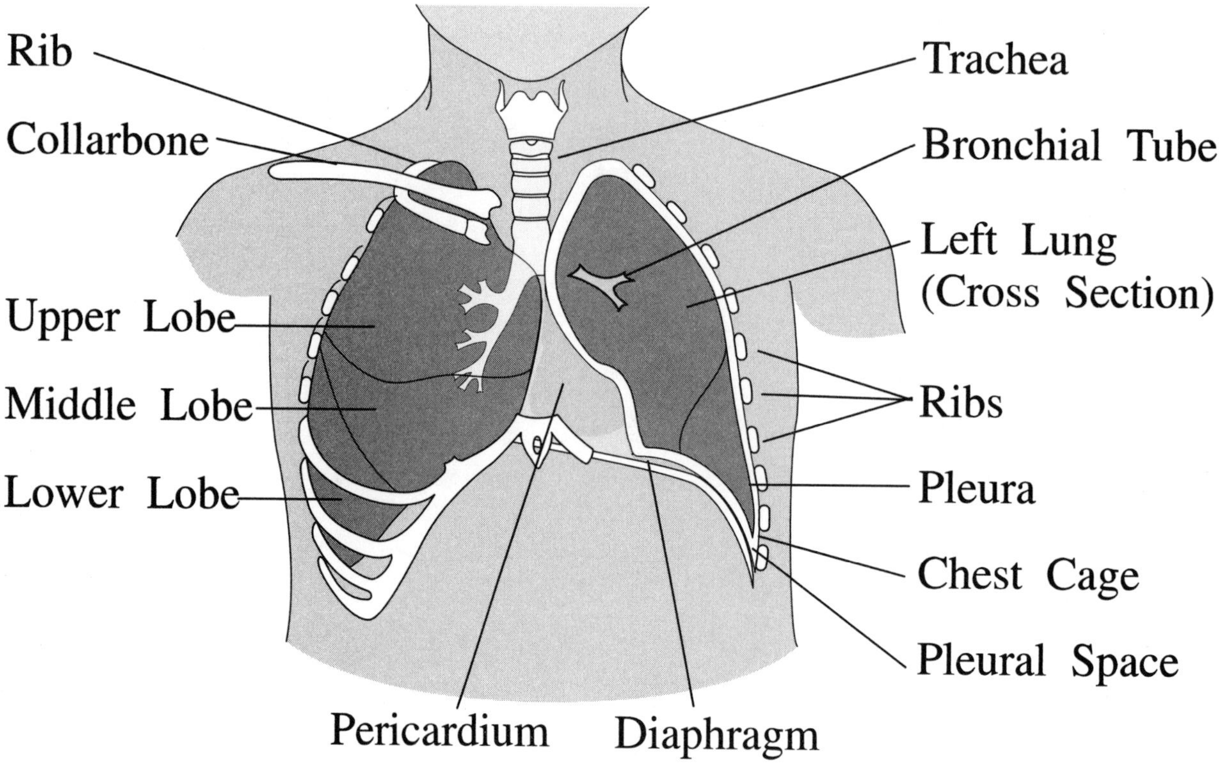

Nothing in this universe is non-medicinal;
all substances can be used for various healing purposes.
Aṣhṭāñga Hṛidayam Sū. Ch. 9: ver. 10.

Chapter 18
Urinary System
Urinary Diseases, Gravel, Obstructions, Diabetes

Urinary Diseases (Mūtrā-ghāta)

Definition and Causes: Although the bladder is full, urine will not pass. The area involved includes the urinary bladder, ureters (which connect the kidneys with the bladder), and urethral passage. Urine is secreted into the urinary bladder through minute channels. Excessed *doṣhas* enter the bladder through these channels to produce 20 variations of urinary diseases.

Dysuria (Mūtrā-kṛichra)
Difficult or painful urination

There are 4 types of dysuria: Vāyu, Pitta, Kapha, and Tridoṣha. [It's symptoms can be early signs of urinary stones—see below]

Vāyu: Pain in the bladder, groin, and urethral passage; small quantities of urine are frequently emitted.

Pitta: Yellow urine is discharged with burning sensation, or blood may be voided.

Kapha: Heaviness, edema of the bladder, and urethral passage; disrupted flow, slimy urine.

Tridoṣha: Symptoms of all three *doṣhas* are present.

Therapies:

General: For all urinary retention disorders licorice, *harītakī*, and cedar are taken as powder in milk or water.

Vāyu: Oleation and sudation are applied, especially on the lower abdomen. Medicated oil is made of *ghee*, cooked with *daśhmūl*, castor oil, barley, *śhatāvarī*, *punarnavā*, and rock salt; mixed in equal parts. One tsp. of the medicated oil is taken internally. Also, *daśhmūl* with sesame oil, vinegar, and *ghee* can be used in equal amounts—1 tsp. total

Pitta: Cooling measures are used to alleviate Pitta. A decoction of *śhatāvarī, gokṣhura, vidārī kand*; with honey and sugar (equal amounts to make 1 tsp.) Also, the seeds of cucumber, licorice, and turmeric; with grape juice and rice water can be taken (equal amounts—4 gms. or .14 oz. per dose).

Kapha : Emesis, sudation, an anti-Kapha diet, and *lassi* are advised. The powder of small cardamom with the juice of *āmalakī* is also recommended. Another remedy includes *gokṣhura*, small cardamom, and *tṛikatu* with honey. Lastly, *pravāl piṣhti* with rice water is useful.

Tridoṣha: The above therapies are used depending upon the predominant *doṣha*.

Urinary Stones (Mūtrā-Āṣhmarī)

Causes: Vāyu covers the mouth of the bladder, drying up the urine inside. The urine then mixes with Pitta, Kapha, or semen, causing stones. Three types of this disorder develop: Vāyu, Pitta, and Kapha.

Premonitory Signs: Urinary bladder distention, severe pain in and around the stone, urine smells like a goat, difficult elimination of urine, fever, or loss of appetite.

Symptoms:

General: Pain in the navel area, and in the seam and head of the bladder; urine flow is interrupted when stones obstruct the path/easy flow when there is no obstruction, clear, golden-yellow urine, pain if straining to pass urine, blood in urine if stones cause internal wounds.

Vāyu: Severe pain causes persons to grind teeth, shiver, squeezing penis, rub the navel, cry constantly, passing feces with gas, frequent urination, and in drops; stones are black, rough, and thorny.

Pitta: Burning sensation in the bladder, the color of the stones are red, yellow, or black.

Kapha: Pricking pain in the bladder, and feeling cold and heavy; stones are big, smooth, golden, or white.

Therapies:

General: This is considered a serious disease that can even lead to death if it is not healed. At the early stages, herbal therapy can heal the condition. However, at later stages, surgery is required. The best herb for all urinary disorders is *gokṣhura*.

Vāyu: *Gokṣhura ghee,* or *gokṣhura* taken alone or with *lassi,* also produces good results.

Pitta: Medicated *ghee* prepared with a decoction of *gokṣhura, kuśha, vidārī kand*, red and white *punarnavā*. *Śhilājit* is also useful.

Kapha: Medicated *ghee* made with a decoction of *gokṣhura, elā, guggul*, black pepper, *chitrak, hiṅg*, myrrh, and rock salt. *Śhilājit* is also useful.

Urine Retention (Mŭtrā-ghātādi)

All the therapies mentioned above are useful for urine retention. Purgations, *basti,* and *uttara basti* (urinary bladder enema) are also suggested if needed.

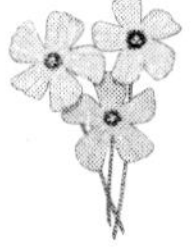

Seminal Stones (Śhukrā-śhmarī)

Causes:

These stones occur in adults due to preventing ejaculation of the semen, once leaving its origin site. By withholding the semen, it becomes dried by Vāyu inside the scrotum.

Symptoms:

Bladder, pelvis, or genital pain; difficult urination, scrotum swelling, stiffness or pain; semen begins to flow but stops in the middle, coming out only when squeezed; urine mixed with semen.

Therapies:

Strong enemas, especially urinary bladder enemas (*uttara basti*) are taken to purify the semen receptacle. Aphrodisiac herbs are then taken (e.g., *śhatāvarī, aśhwagandhā*).

Urinary Gravel (Mūtrā-śharkarā)

Causes:

Urinary gravel is a collection of small sand-like urinary stones caused by Vāyu. According to modern science, urinary gravel combines to form urinary stones. Both systems are saying the same thing in different ways. The gravel is expelled with the urine when Vāyu is moving downward, and it is obstructed when Vāyu is moving upward.

Today, modern science breaks the urinary stones with lithotripsy (a sonic vibration), turning them into gravel. Then, they are expelled through the urinary system.

Therapies:

Powder of *gokṣhura* taken with water and cane sugar expels gravel. *Tumburu, apāmārga*, and barley are good for both stones and gravel.

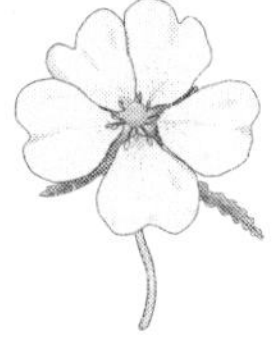

13 Urine Obstruction Disorders (Mūtraghāta)

Below are discussed various other urinary obstructions. In all cases the therapy involves *basti* and *urethra basti*.

Vātabasti - Obstruction Due to Suppressing the Urine Urge

Habitual suppression of the urge to urinate aggravates Vāyu and Pitta. This causes the urine to dry up and block the mouth of the urinary bladder. Thus, red or yellow urine is passed with pain, irritation, and may distend the bladder. This can also cause burning, throbbing, twisting, urine expelled in drops, or in a continuous flow if the bladder is pressed. There are 2 forms of *Vātabasti*: difficult and very difficult (to bear and to heal). These symptoms are similar to benign hypertrophy of the prostate (BPH).

Vāta Kundalikā - Radiating Bladder Pain

Due to urine retention, *Apāna* Vāyu (upward moving air) becomes excessed. Aggravated Vāyu, moving circularly in the bladder, causes severe, radiating bladder pain, circular moving of urine in the bladder, obstructed flow, heaviness, urine is released little by little, accompanied with expelling feces. One may also experience stiffness, heaviness, and cramps.

Mūtrā-tīta -
Obstruction Due to Slow Elimination

When trying to expel urine after suppressing the urge for a long time, it fails to come out or flows with mild pain.

Mūtro-tsaṅga -
Obstruction Due to Narrow Urethral Duct

Either urethral blockages or aggravated Vāyu can cause some urine to remain in the bladder, urethra, or urethral passage. Urine thus becomes obstructed, flowing slowly (without pain). The remaining urine produces heaviness in the urethral passage.

Mūtrā-granthi -
Obstruction Due to Bladder Tumor

Pain similar to that of a urinary stone is experienced from round, immovable, hard, and small tumors that may suddenly develop inside the cavity of the urinary bladder. Blood affected by Vāyu and Kapha cause the hard nodular mass at the urinary bladder opening.

Mūtrā-śhukra - Obstruction Due to Semen

Performing sexual intercourse when there is a strong urge to urinate causes the displacement of semen, and is obstructed. Semen will then be expelled just before or after urination.

Viḍghāta -
Obstruction Due to Impacted Feces in Rectum

(Fistula in between urinary bladder and rectum)

Persons who are excessively dry, thin, and debilitated may experience Vāyu moving upwards, bringing a small amount of feces into the urinary bladder and urethra. This results in urination with the odor of feces.

Uṣhṇa-Vāta - Obstruction Due to Bladder Inflammation or Cystitis

(Hematuria-blood in the urine)

Aggravated Pitta, due to excess exercise, hot, penetrating foods, long distance walking, and excessive sun-bathing, overflows into the bladder because of aggravated Vāyu. This causes pain, burning, or inflammation in the bladder and urethral passage (cystitis), and yellow urine. It may be mixed with blood, or only blood flowing alone; urine is warm or comes out repeatedly with difficulty.

Mūtrā-saṃkṣhaya - Due to Diminished Urine

Dry, debilitated persons may experience Vāyu and Pitta depositing into the urinary bladder, diminishing urine, causing pain, and burning.

Mūtrā-sāda - Obstruction Due to Bladder Inflammation or Cystitis

If Vāyu aggravates Pitta and Kapha (alone or together), difficult urination is produced. Urine is yellow, red, white (or all colors mixed), thick, accompanied with pain, and is dry.

Therapies: Kapha- and Pitta-reducing measures are used to heal this condition, in addition to the common therapies for all these 13 urinary conditions.

Vātāṣhṭhīlā - Obstruction Due to Enlarged Prostate (or prostate tumor)

When aggravated Vāyu becomes trapped between the rectum and urinary bladder, it results in an enlarged prostate, or a hard, elevated, immovable tumor. It causes abdominal distention and blockages of urine, feces, and gas.

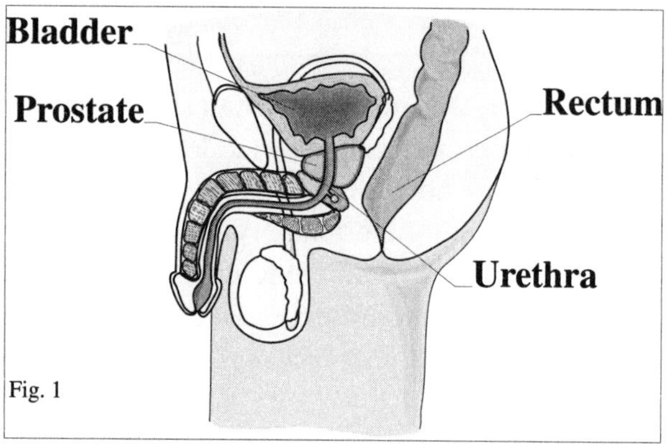

Fig. 1

The prostate is situated below the bladder and in front of the rectum. The urethra tube runs from the bladder to the penis or vulva. The prostate surrounds the urethra.

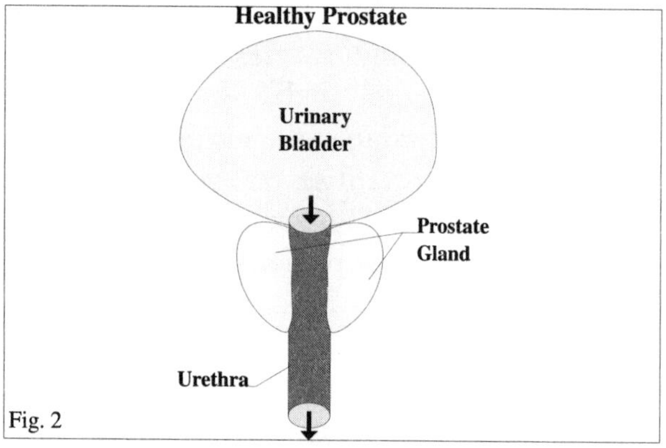

Fig. 2

Prostate and Ureter

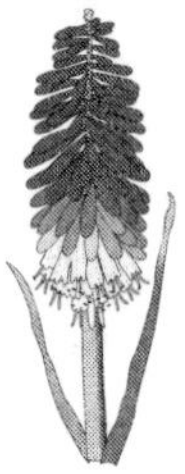

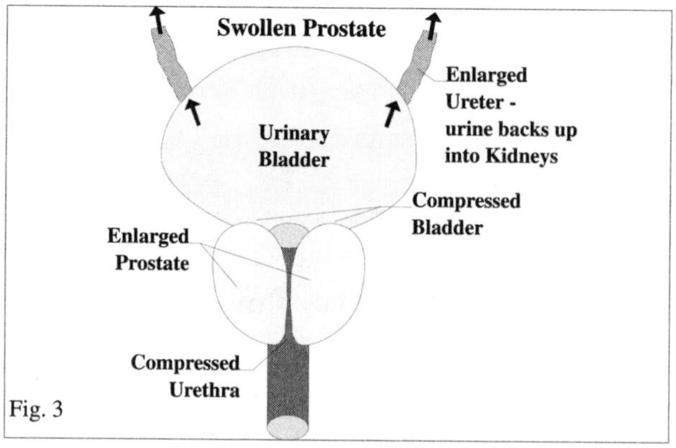

Fig. 3

An enlarged prostate compresses the lower ureter, obstructing the passage of urine. This dilates the bladder and thus weakens it. The backed-up urine in the bladder enlarges and weakens the upper ureters that run to the kidneys. The kidney pelvis becomes damaged. Continued pressure on the kidneys causes damage to kidney tissue.

Therapies for this disorder are covered under cancer and tumors, Chapter 22 page 501.

Mūtrā Jaṭhara - Obstruction Due to Enlarged Bladder

Habitual suppression of urine causes Vāyu to become obstructed and move upward. A full bladder results in abdominal distention below the navel, severe pain, indigestion, and accumulation of feces.

Therapy: Diuretics (e.g., *gokṣhura*) are used to heal this condition (in addition to the common therapies for all these 13 urinary conditions).

Basti Kuṇḍala - Obstruction Due to Bladder Displacement

This condition is similar to *Vātabasti*.

Vāyu: Due to fast travel, jumping, exertion, injury, or pressure on the urinary bladder it may shift out of place and remain expanded. This will cause pain, shaking, and burning. Urine will pass in drops, or if pressed, will come out in a stream. One can experience stiffening, cramping, and distress. It is a severe condition.

Pitta: One feels burning, pain, and abnormal urine color.

Kapha: Persons experience heaviness, swelling and oiliness; whitish and precipitant urine.

Pitta and Kapha forms can only be controlled

but not healed.

Obstinate Urinary Diseases (Prameha)

(Excessive Urination, Diabetes, etc.)

Causes: There are 24 forms of this disease: 4 are due to Vāyu, 6 result from Pitta, and 10 are caused by Kapa. The main causes of these diseases are fat, urine, and Kapha buildups due to;

1) Foods (e.g., sweets, sours, salts, hard to digest, slimy, cold, raw grain; marsh, domesticated, and aquatic animal meats).

2) Liquids (e.g., beer, sugarcane juice, molasses, and milk).

3) Lifestyles (e.g., sedentary, sleeping while sitting).

4) Other things causing an increase of Kapha, fat and urine.

Development:

Kapha prameha: Excessed Kapha overflows into the body channels and becomes mixed with the *dhātus* (i.e., tissues of fat (*medas*), plasma/lymph (*rasa*), muscle (*māṃsa*), and sweat (Kapha *mala*). This situation weakens the *dhātus* and brings them into the urinary system, causing the 10 types of Kapha *prameha.*

Pitta prameha: Aggravated Pitta and blood also can vitiate the urinary bladder when the watery tissues are depleted. If fat (*medas*), muscle (*māṃsa*), and plasma (*rasa*) are already weak or depleted, then this Pitta excess in the blood produces the 6 types of Pitta *prameha*.

Vāyu prameha: Vāyu may also weaken the bladder by drawing the depleted tissues into the bladder. Vāyu diabetes is due to vitiated *ojas*, marrow, and lymph. When Kapha and Pitta *doṣhas* become decreased Vāyu becomes excessed, bringing fat (*medas*), muscle (*māṃsa*), marrow (*Majjā*), and *life sap (ojas)* to the urinary system. This produces 4 types of Vāyu *prameha.*

Kapha *prameha* involves *rasa, māṃsa*, and *medas.* They are similar in nature. Thus, the herbs to heal this *prameha* will not imbalance the other *doṣhas*. Pitta *prameha* involves plasma (*rasa*), muscle (*māṃsa*), and fat (*medas*) *dhātus* that are opposite in nature to Pitta-reducing herbs (i.e., Pitta reducing herbs are cool). These herbs will increase plasma, muscle, and fat tissues. Still, Pitta diabetes (*prameha*) can be helped with special herbs (e.g., *śhilājit* and *guḍmar*) if *dhātu* depletion is not extensive. On the other hand, when Vāyu *prameha* involves muscle (*māṃsa*) and fat (*medas*) *dhātus,* it is very difficult to treat because all the therapies for reducing Vāyu will further increase the already excessed fat and muscle tissues. In this case, Vāyu becomes aggravated either due to depletion of the reproductive (*śhukra*) and life sap (*ojas*) tissues (*dhātus*), or from obstruction of the channels due to excess fat (*medas*) and muscle (*māṃsa*) tissue.

Premonitory Signs:

Common to all forms of diabetes is an excess of perspiration, body odor, looseness of body parts, desiring rest, thickening heart, eyes, tongue, and ears; stoutness of body, fast growth of hair and nails, wanting cold things, dry throat and palate, always having a sweet taste in the mouth, numbness and burning of the hands and feet (and other organs), sweet urine, matted hair, sticky excreta from orifices, ants and insects attracted to the body and urine, abnormalities of the urine, urine smells of raw flesh.

Analysis Cautions

1) If the urine is yellowish or expelling blood without the aforesaid premonitory signs of *prameha*, a person is not to be said to have *prameha*, but rather a disease of *Rakta* Pitta. Since the signs and symptoms of these two diseases are similar, being sure of the disease is important.

2) If persons with *prameha* expel sweet, slimy, and honey-like urine, it is caused by the depletion of *doṣhas* (a Vāyu-caused disease), or from over nourishment (a Kapha disease).

If Vāyu, Pitta, or Kapha *prameha* is left untreated after their premonitory signs and symptoms, they are not able to be healed. Generally, Pitta *prameha* is controllable. If the adipose tissue (fat/*medas*) is not depleted, then Pitta *prameha* can be healed. Kapha *prameha* is usually able to be healed.

Symptoms:

General: Common to all forms of diabetes is the increased quantity and turbidity of the urine.

Kapha: Excess Kapha weakens the body fluids, muscle, and fat; and are drawn into the urinary bladder and kidneys. This results in 10 forms of Kapha *prameha.*

1) *Udaka*—large quantities of clear urine, white, cold, odorless, watery, sometimes slightly murky and slimy.

2) *Ikṣhumeha*—urine is sweet, cold, slightly salty, and muddy.

3) *Sāndra*—urine becomes thick when kept overnight.

4) *Surā*—urine looks like beer (clear on top and thick on the bottom) when kept overnight.

5) *Piṣhta*—hair stands on end, urine is thick and white.

6) *Śhukra*—urine looks like semen or is mixed with semen.

7) *Sikatā*—urine has dirty particles, like sand, frequently cold, sweet urination.

8) *Śhītā*—urine contains small hard things (because the weakened *doṣhas* pass through).

9) *Śhanair*—urine passes very slowly, with little force.

10) *Lāla*—urine is thready (like saliva) and slimy.

Pitta: Aggravation of fire is caused by

a) Excess of hot, sour, salty, alkaline, and pungent food.

b) Eating before the previous meal is digested.

c) Exposure to sun, fire, physical exertion, and anger.

d) Eating mutually contradictory foods (e.g., fish and milk, hot and cold thigs; see page 551).

Manifestation of Pitta forms of diabetes is quicker than that of those caused by Kapha. The 6 Pitta forms are only able to be controlled because it is a different element (fire) than the watery elements. Bitter and pungent herbs heal Kapha. Bitters help Pitta, but the pungents will cause aggravation. The stomach, small intestine, fat, and the abdominal wall membrane (which connects the stomach with the other abdominal organs) are involved here. The 6 forms are;

1) *Kṣhāra*—urine smells, looks tastes and feels salty.

2) *Nīla*—urine is blue.

3) *Kāla*—urine is ink black.

4) *Hāridra*—urine is pungent or bitter, yellowish, and burns when expelled.

5) *Mañjiṣhṭhā*—urine smells like raw flesh and has a slight red color.

6) *Rakta*—urine smells bad, is hot, slightly salty and reddish.

Vāyu: These 4 forms of diabetes immediately become aggravated due to;

a) Overeating of astringent, pungent, bitter, rough, light, and cold things.

b) Over indulgence in sexual acts and exercise.

c) Over use of emesis, purgation, dry enemas, head evacuation.

d) Suppressing natural urges, fasting, physical accident, excess sun, anxiety, grief, blood-letting, staying up late at night, poor posture.

The excessed Vāyu then overflows, along with muscle fat (*vāsā*) and enters the channels (*srotas*) with urine, causing the development of fat in the urine (lipuria). It may also carry marrow to the urinary bladder (via the *mūtravaha srota*), deranging the marrow (*majjā*) as myelouria. Marrow may be expelled with urine as Vāyu pushes the marrow out. Should there be an excess of lymph entering the bladder (due to deficient insulin), large amounts of urine are produced, with a need for constant urination (without pressure). Vāyu converts the sweetness of life sap (*ojas*) into an astringent taste and brings it to the bladder. This causes roughness, which develops Diabetes mellitus [Either (a) an insufficient production of insulin that causes abnormal metabolism of carbohydrates, fats and proteins. Sugar levels are increased in the blood and urine causing great thirst, frequent urination, wasting, and acidity.

This can occur in childhood or early adolescence, or (b) A mild form appears in adulthood aggravated by obesity and an inactive lifestyle. Few symptoms exist, and insulin may not be needed].

The 4 Vāyu-caused diseases are serious because of the risk of secondary diseases developing due to the loss of all the tissues. Vāyu-diabetic urine is grayish, reddish, and painful.

1) *Vasā*—urine is expelled with muscle fat or fat may be passed alone and frequently (fat-lipid-like urine).

2) *Majjā*—urine is frequently expelled with marrow, or marrow may be passed alone (marrow-like urine).

3) *Hasti*—urine passes continuously and without force, mixed with lymph, and without difficulty (urinary incontinence/diabetes tuniflues).

4) *Madhu*—sweet and astringent urine, which is pale and oily (diabetes mellitus).

This is caused either by aggravated Vāyu depleting the tissues, or by obstructing the movement of the *doṣhas* covering it. In the latter case, Vāyu shows signs of the *doṣha* covering it, without any other reason, occasionally, and thus the bladder is sometimes empty, sometimes full. These diseases cannot be healed.

Any form of diabetes not tended to eventually develops into *Madhu* (honey-like) diabetes. All the sweet forms of *diabetes* (i.e., sweet-tasting urine and sweet-smelling body) are called *Madhu*.

Sweet, slimy urine may be confused as being caused by either Kapha (excess nutrition) or Vāyu (malnutrition). Should Kapha and Pitta forms be experienced with all the premonitory signs (and Vāyu forms, after lasting for a long time) cannot be healed. The 4 Vāyu types are unable to be healed because they afflict the deepest tissue layers (marrow and semen). The Pitta forms which last for a long time are controllable. Forms where the fat tissue is not greatly excessed are healable.

Secondary Complications:

Kapha Forms: Poor digestion, anorexia, vomiting, excess sleep, cough, nasal mucus.

Pitta Forms: Pricking pain in the bladder and passage, oozing from the scrotum, fever, burning, and loose stools.

Vāyu Forms (upward moving air): Tremors, sharp abdominal pain, insomnia, dry mouth and throat, cough, difficult breathing.

Hereditary and genetic diabetes (like all hereditary and genetic-caused diseases) cannot be completely healed due to the dysfunctional genes. However, these forms of diabetes can be controlled; persons can live symptom-free as long as they remain on the proper herbs and diet..

The 7 types of diabetic carbuncles (skin or subcutaneous tissue bacterial infections that exude pus) require surgery.

Diabetes involves the imbalance of carbohydrate metabolism that is controlled by the insulin secretion of pancreas. The blood level of sugar/glucose rises beyond the normal limits in the system that is excreted by the urinary system.

General Therapies:

There are 2 general categories of urinary diseases: persons who are strong and obese, and those who are weak and emaciated. The former category of people use elimination therapies, while the latter follows nourishing therapies. After oleation, the strong and obese person follows Kapha-reducing therapies to eliminate the excesses through the upward and downward channels. Once the toxins are eliminated (and digestive power is strong) one follows refreshing therapy (*santarpana*) [e.g., barley with honey] instead of fasting. Fasting immediately after elimination may cause cystic tumors; wasting, kidney, urinary bladder, and genital disorders. Alleviation therapy is used for people not strong enough for elimination therapy.

Diet: The most important herbs for all *doṣhas* are *śhilājit, guḍmar,* turmeric, neem, *āmalakī*, *gug-*

gul, and *arjuna*. Turmeric with aloe vera gel (1 to 3 gms./.035 to .1 oz) is best used during the early stages of diabetes for regulating pancreas and liver functions. Other therapies include roasted or fried barley, corn flour, light, bitter vegetables, barley porridge, *ghee*, rice, and herbs like *gokṣhura*, *guḍmar*, *triphalā*, *musta*, cardamom, fenugreek, or coriander, mixed with honey. *Triphalā* with *āmalakī* juice can also be used to heal *prameha*. Barley is the main food to heal urinary diseases. Other methods to heal *prameha* include strenuous exercises, oil massage, steam, sitz or waist bath, and sprinkling of water and ointment. Herbs of dry ginger, cardamom, and sandalwood are used in baths, and taken orally. *Guḍmar* is the best herb for digesting sugar in the pancreas. *Guḍmar* and *śhilājit* are an excellent herbal combination used by modern Āyurvedic practitioners.

Simultaneously, the foods and life habits that caused the disease are avoided.

Kapha Therapies:

1) Emesis and fasting.

2) Food: Barley soaked in a *triphalā* decoction overnight, then mixed with honey and eaten several times a day (cane sugar may also be used).

3) Herbs: Include decoctions of *triphalā*, fenugreek, *musta*, *arjuna*, sandalwood, *lodhra, ajwan, gokṣhura, viḍaṅga, guḍūchī, harītakī*, and *chitrak*. These may be taken with a small amount of *ghee*. *Guḍmar* and *śhilājit* are excellent.

Pitta Therapies: Only when muscle tissue (*medas dhātu*) is excessively aggravated is Pitta *prameha* unable to be healed.

1) Purgation is the best therapy for healing.

2) Herbal decoctions include sandalwood, *musta*, *āmalakī*, neem, *kuṭaj, turmeric,* blue lotus, and *arjuna*. These are taken with *ghee* or sesame oil. *Guḍmar* and *śhilājit* are excellent.

Vāyu Therapies:

1) *Guḍmar* and *śhilājit, triphalā*, fenugreek, *musta,* turmeric, *harītakī*, and *āmalakī* mixed with raw honey and *āmalakī* juice. They may be added to a drink of roasted corn flour mixed with raw honey.

2) Medicated oils and *ghees*.

Pitta/Kapha Therapies:

1) For either Pitta or Kapha urinary diseases, herbs of *gokṣhura*, *bibhītakī,* and *kuṭaj* are mixed in *āmalakī* juice. After digesting this drink rice and soup (with *ghee*) may be taken.

2) For Vāyu secondary excess with Pitta *prameha*, medicated *ghee* and Pitta-reducing herbs.

3) For Vāyu secondary excess with Kapha *prameha*, medicated oil (canola or mustard) is used with the same herbs to reduce Kapha.

4) For *Tridoṣhic* symptoms, both the *ghee* and oils are used with the same herbs.

Diabetic Ulcer, Pimple, Pustule, etc. (Prameha Piḍakā)

Causes:

If *madhumeha* (diabetes mellitius) is not treated, 10 forms of eruptions can develop on the joints, vital spots, and muscular areas during diabetes. All three *doṣhas* are aggravated.

Symptoms:

1) *Śharā-vikā*: Raised edges, depressed centers, black, oozing, painful, saucer-sized and shaped.

2) *Kacha-pikā*: Deep continuous or intermittent pain, extending over large areas, smooth, and tortoise shell-like.

3) *Jālinī*: Stable, vein networks, oily, oozing, with a large inner cavity, severe, intermittent pain, minute openings.

4) *Vinatā*: Large, found on the back or abdomen, blue, deep pain, oozing, bending downwards.

5) *Alajī*: Burning, raised, hard to bear, spreading, reddish-black, severe thirst, boils, delusion, fever.

6) *Masū-rikā: Lentil sized and shaped.*

7) *Sarṣha-pikā*: The size and shape of a mustard seed, severe pain, surrounded by similar eruptions.

8) *Putriṇī*: A large eruption surrounded by many smaller eruptions.

9) *Vidā-rikā*: Round and hard shaped.

10) *Vidhradi*: Abscesses (discussed in the next section).

The first 3 ulcers are caused by fat and are difficult to bear and heal. The rest are bearable and easy to heal. Aggravated symptoms of these eruptions are similar to diabetes. These symptoms may occur even without diabetes as they are caused by vitiated fat tissue.

Symptoms of deep yellow or red urine, without experiencing any premonitory signs of diabetes, are classified under bleeding disorders (*Rakta Pitta*—Chapter 14) and require the same therapies.

Piḍakā Therapies:

General: Early stages of all 10 eruptions (*piḍakā*) use inflammatory edema (*śhotha*) therapies (Chapter 25). Advanced stages of eruptions use therapies according to ulcers (Chapter 16).

Small eruptions that appear only on the skin, are soft to the touch, slightly painful, easily form pus and then burst, and develop on persons who are strong, can be healed. When symptoms include eruptions in the rectum, heart region, head, shoulders, back vital parts, and joints, associated with complications, and who have poor digestion, no therapy is available.

Medicated oil herbs for ulcers include cardamom (*elā*), saffron or safflower, sandalwood, and *kaiṣhore guggul.*

Massage herbs include neem, *guḍūchī, bhū-āmalakī*, and *paṭola.*

Sprinkling (*pariṣheka*) water requires herbs of *kaṭukā,* neem, *viḍaṅga, mañjiṣhṭhā, guḍmar,* and *guggul.*

Liquids and foods include herbs of *kaṭukā,* black pepper, cardamom, *vachā, hiṅg,* and *viḍaṅga.*

Charak suggests surgical procedures.

Incontinence

Useful herbs are cardamom, *bākuchī, yogaraj guggul*, nutmeg, skullcap, cinnamon.

Renal Failure

Punarnavā is the recommended herb to use until the kidneys begin to function again.

Urinary System

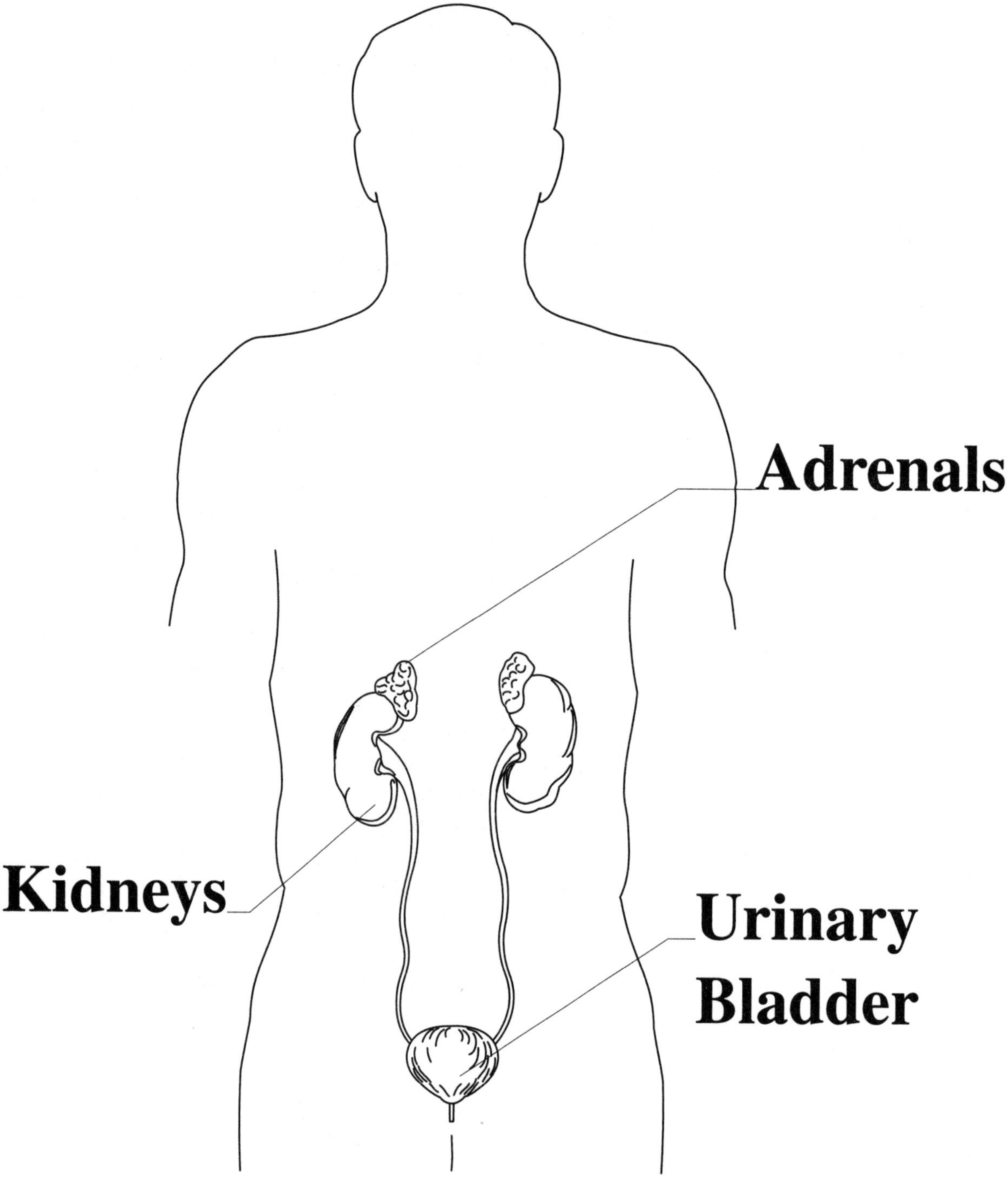

Pouring warm water over the body bestows strength,
but the same over the head, makes for loss of strength of hair and eyes.
Ashṭāñga Hṛidayam - Sū. Ch. 2: ver. 17

Chapter 19
Ears, Nose, Throat, Catarrh, Hoarse Throat, Eyes, Mouth

Diseases of the Ear
Karṇa-gata-Roga-Vijnāniya

Twenty-eight different types of ear disorders exist: ear (*karna*) diseases, earache (*karna-ṣhula*), ringing/noise (*pra-nāda*), deafness (*vādhirya*), windpipe sounds (*karna-kṣhveda*), secretions (*karna-srāva*), itching (*karna-kandu*), *karna-guntha*, parasites (*krimi-karna*), *prati-nāha*, two forms of local abscess (*vidradhi*), boil/pus formation (*karna-pāka*), pus and malodor (*puti-karna*), four kinds of cysts, seven forms of tumor, four types of swelling (*śhopha*).

Causes and Symptoms:

Earache (karṇa-śhula): Great aching pain in the ear region and inside the middle ear (*tympanum*) from local Vāyu excess that becomes aggravated and obstructed by the other imbalanced *doṣhas*.

Ringing/noise (karṇa-nāda): Ringing and other sounds resulting from excess local Vāyu entering the ear the wrong way and becoming blocked in the sound channels.

Deafness (vādhirya): When excess Vāyu remains in the sound channels along with Kapha imbalances and is not healed or balanced.

Wind-Pipe Sounds (karṇa-kṣhveḍa): Results from cold object or exposure to nasal purgatives for the head, or continual derangement of Vāyu in the sound channel and aggravated by excess work, any wasting process in the system, or by ingesting astringent or dry items. The sound is caused by excess of Pitta, Kapha, and blood.

Secretion (karṇa-srāva): Caused by excess Vāyu in the ear cavity, resulting from head injury, remaining underwater for a long time, or a spontaneous formation and bursting of an inner ear abscess.

Itching (Karṇa Kaṇḍū): Excess itching from local Kapha.

Excess Ear Wax (Karṇa Gūthaka): Accumulated mucus in the ear dries and is hardened by local Pitta heat.

Inner Ear Fistula (karṇa-prati-nāha): When dried ear accumulations caused by secretions become liquefied and seep from the nose (and/or the mouth) and head, diseases (and certain forms of headaches) may develop.

Parasites (krimi-karṇa): These vermin, collecting in the ear impair the hearing.

Abscesses (karṇa-vidradhi): These are caused by ear ulcer, external injury to the ear, or other unknown causes. Symptoms include choking and burning sensations, piercing and sucking pain, yellow, red, or bloody secretions.

Pus-Boil- Ulcer Formation (karṇa-pāka): When pus forms in the boils of the ear from excess Pitta, a blockage and consequent malodor in passageway of the ear occurs.

Pus and Malodor (puti-karṇa): When the pus, with or without accumulation of mucus in the ear passage is secreted after being heated by excess Pitta, it may cause swelling (*śhopha*—Chapter 25), tumors (*arbuda*—Chapter 22) and multiple growths (polypoid—*arśhas*—Chapter 15).

Therapies:

General: Therapy includes ingesting *ghee* after meals, rejuvenative herbs such as *śhatāvarī* and *balā*, refraining from exercise and sex, avoiding wetting the ear, and less talking.

Vāyu: For all Vāyu-related ear diseases (earache,

ringing, wind sounds, and deafness), oil is first used internally and externally (in the ear too) in addition to emulsive purgatives (e.g., licorice/*viḍaṅga*). Then the ear is fomented with Vāyu-reducing herbs by means of steam (*nāḍī sveda*) that is applied to the ear through a tube. Ringing in the ear is helped by placing three drops of clove oil in the ear.

Vāyu/Kapha earache: These are helped by smoke fomentation. Herbs include *bilwa*, castor oil root, *aśhwagandhā*, barley, and *vaṃśha lochana*, boiled in fermented rice, It is applied via tube fomentation (*nāḍī sveda*). Warm oil (*mahānārāyan*, *daśhmūl*, sesame, *guggul-ghee*) is dropped into the ear for instant relief (one or two drops). Ingesting *ghee* after meals and *śhirobasti* are also useful. Rice should not be eaten at the dinnertime meal, but replaced with milk and *ghee* . The same herbal oils can also be used as nasal therapies, sprinkling and ingested. Three drops of garlic oil may be placed in the ear for V/K earaches.

Vāyu earache: Three drops of warm garlic oil are applied to the ear.

Pitta earache: *Ghee* cooked with licorice, *musta*, *mañjiṣhṭhā*, sandalwood and milk, used as ear drops (three drops per ear).

Kapha earache: Three drops of mustard or garlic oil are placed in each ear. Strong nasal evacuatives and gargling with *guggul*, *pippalī* and ginger are also useful.

Blood earache: Pitta therapies are followed.

Deafness (vādhirya): Sesame oil cooked with milk, water, *bilwa*, licorice, *mahānārāyan,* and *daśhmūl* oils is applied (3 drops per ear).

Itching (karṇa kaṇḍū): Local steam (*nāḍī sweda*) to the ear; herbal emetics, smoke, and head purgatives may also be taken.

Pus/Malodor (puti-kaṇna), Secretion (kaṇnasrāva) and Parasites (krimi-karṇa):

General therapies: These include ear-drop therapy as discussed above, nasal therapy, smoke, medicated washing herbs (see below).

Secretion (karṇa-srāva): Ear drops made from cane sugar, licorice, and *bilwa (Bilwadi Tail)* are made into a paste and mixed with goat's milk and sesame oil.

Pus/Malodor (puti-karṇa): Ear drops made from milk, honey and herbs of licorice, *āmalakī, patta, dhātakī, mañjiṣhṭhā, lodhra,* and *prīyaṅgu*. The herbs are boiled in milk and sesame oil, and are either dropped into the ear or ingested.

Parasites (krimi-karṇa): This includes *viḍaṅga, kuṭaj, musta, guggul* taken internally, and mixed with warmed mustard oil to be applied to the ear canal. Smoke of *guggul* destroys the odor. Emetics and gargling are also useful.

Wind Pipe Sounds (karṇa-kṣhveḍa): Mustard oil ear drops are useful (3 drops per ear).

Abscess (karṇa-vidrahi) is the same as ordinary abscesses. The ear is fomented after being filled with oil (to soften the deposit). Discharges can then be removed with a probe.

Inner Ear Fistula (karṇa-pratināha): Therapies include oil and sweat, followed by nasal evacuatives. Diet and lifestyle changes that reduce the imbalance causing this disease are recommended.

Ear Inflammation - pus - boils (karṇa-pāka): Therapies include lightening (see *pañcha karma*: Chapter 7), vomiting, and bitter herbs (e.g., *chirāyatā, kuṭki,* neem, aloe vera, gentian, barberry). Blood-letting and purgation are also employed. Dirt, parasites, or other foreign objects stuck in the ear cavity should be removed with a probe.

Ear Lobes (Karnapālī Rog)

There are 5 main diseases of the ear lobes.

Inflammatory Swelling (Paripota): The lobe is suddenly pulled and held for a long time in this position, it becomes numb, painful, swollen, blackish-red, and may spontaneously burst or crack as a result of excess Vāyu.

Traumatic Swelling (Utpāta): This condition results from friction and the weight of earrings. Painful swelling, burning, and pus develops in the ear lobe and may be brown or red-colored,

owing to toxic blood and Pitta.
Piercing/Pulling (Unmantha): Pulling the ear-lobes creates excess Vāyu and Kapha at this site, causing painful swelling, itching. The color of the lobe depends upon which *doṣha* is present in excess.
Ulceration (Duhka-vardhana): Swollen, painful, burning, itching lobes result from being pulled and lengthened, leading to pus formation.
Pustules (Parilehi): Small oozing pimples, painful, burning, and itching may cover the lobes. These result from toxic blood, excess Kapha, or parasites. This disease quickly spreads. Inflammation and fever may develop. The lobe may be destroyed.

Ear Lobe Therapy
General: These five diseases are considered very dangerous and may eventually destroy the lobe if not quickly attended to. The first line of therapy includes a wholesome diet of foods, drinks, and lifestyle habits. Oils and sweat, ointments, washes, plasters, poultices, and blood-letting are used for all five disorders. Vāyu does best with oils, poultices, and enemas. Pitta does best with purgatives. Kapha does best with emetics.
Inflammatory Swelling (Pari-potaka): Licorice, *apāmārg, devadaru, bākuchī,* and *mañjiṣhṭhā* are pasted together and cooked with milk, *ghee*, sesame oil, and are applied to the lobe.
Traumatic Swelling (Utpāta): *Mañjiṣhṭhā*, sesame oil, licorice, *śhatāvarī*, *musta*, turmeric, and mango are cooked together and applied to the lobe.
Piercing or pulling (Unmantha): A medicated oil of *bākuchī, guggul, mañjiṣhṭhā, viḍaṅga, turmeric, musta*, and ginger is applied to the lobe.
Ulceration (Duhka-vardhana): *Ghee* and sesame oil are mixed with milk (10 times the weight of the *ghee* and oil) and are cooked with *aśhwagandhā* and *apāmārga*. The finished recipe is then filtered before application to the ear lobe. Constant application and fomentation helps the regrowth of the lobe, making it soft, healthy, smooth, painless, evenly developed, and able to bear the weight of earrings.
Pustules (Parilehi): The lobe is oiled with warm *ghee*, sesame or sunflower, cooked with *bākuchī, guggul, mañjiṣhṭhā, viḍaṅga*, ginger, and turmeric. A powder of these herbs is also dusted on the lobe. The use of medicated oil on ear lobes preserves their health.

Diseases of the Nose
Nāsā-gata-roga-Vijñāniya

There are 31 forms of nasal (*nāsā*) diseases: obstruction (*apīnasa*); malodor (*pūti-nāsā*); inflammation/pus pimples (*nāsā-pāka*); bloody pus in the nose (*puya-rakta*); hemorrhage (*śhonita-pitta*); sneezing (*kṣhavathu*); mucus sneezes (*bhramṣhathu*); vapors (*dīpta*); stuffiness (*nāsā pratināha*); cold/ mucus/coryza (*nāsā-parisrāva*); dryness (*nāsā- ṣhoṣha*); four types of *arṣhas* (nasal hemorrhoids); four forms of swelling (*śhopha*); seven types of tumors; and five forms of *prati-śhyāya*.

Causes, Symptoms, and Therapies
1. Obstruction—Wasting or Atrophic Rhinitis (*apīnasa*)—excesses of Vāyu and Kapha cause symptoms of choked and burning nostrils with dryness and dirty and slimy mucus in the passage. This deadens the faculty of smell and taste. [This is identical to the type of mucus (*pratiṣhyāya*) block discussed in the next section.]

Therapies include applying oil and steam to the nasal passage, emetics, and purgation, taking light and moderate meals, drinking boiled water, and nasal inhalation of the smoke from *viḍaṅga, pippalī*, and *apāmārga*. Nasal oil is made from mustard oil and herbs of *trikatu, hiṅgwastock*, calamus, *kuśhtā, viḍaṅga*, and applied daily.

2. Malodor (*pūti-nāsā*)—Excess Vāyu mixed with other *doṣhas* in the throat and palate roof causes a malodorous smell in the nostrils and mouth. The same therapies are used as described for obstructions.

3. Inflammation/Pus/Pimples (*nāsā-pāka*)—Excess Pitta causes sliminess, malodorous ulceration inside the nose, secretion, putrification. Internal and external Pitta-reducing therapies are required. *Ghee* is mixed with *āmalakī, guḍūchī, dūrba, elā*, and *dhātakī* flowers. This is applied as a wash and a plaster in the nasal passages after bleeding.

4. Bloody Pus/Ulcers (*pūya-rakta*)—resulting from trauma to the head. Pitta and Kapha become very heated, causing a discharge of blood or blood-streaked pus. For Pitta reduction, a porridge made of milk, *ghee, dūrba, mañjiṣhṭhā,* and *nāgkeśhar* is used as a poultice. Then the sinus is cut open with a knife and a plaster of licorice, *dūrba, nāgkeśhar, mañjiṣhṭhā*, turmeric, and *kuṭaj* is applied. Neem and turmeric are used to wash the ulcer daily. Medicated *ghee* of *triphalā*, turmeric, *kuṭaj, dūrba, nāgkeśhar,* and *balā* are used to lubricate the sinus. For Kapha reduction, poultices of white mustard seeds, *dūrba, nāgkeśhar,* and *mañjiṣhṭhā* are used daily until softened.

The sinus is then cut open with a knife and plastered with neem, *dūrba, nagheśhar*, *mañjiṣhṭhā,* and sesame paste. A decoction of neem, *guḍūchī*, and *mañjiṣhṭhā* is used to wash the ulcer. Sesame oil is cooked with myrrh, *chitrak*, neem, *guḍūchī,* and *mañjiṣhṭhā,* can be applied to the ulcer. Nasal therapy using a few drops of herb juice or medicated oil is also useful. Another useful therapy is smoke inhalation of *Śhadbindū oil* (*endrojo, pippalī, black pepper, dry ginger, calamus (vachā), kūt, kuṭaj,* and *tulsī* seed). After the blood and pus are reduced, purifying herbs are used.

5. Hemorrhage (*śhonita-pitta* or *nasā pūyarakta*) decoctions and snuffs are discussed under bleeding (*Raktapitta*) in Chapter 14.

6. Excessive Sneezing (*kṣhavathu*)—the nasal *marma* results from *doṣha* imbalance or trauma, causing Vāyu and Kapha to flow from the nose while sneezing. If something touches the nose hairs, a trickling sensation develops. This sensation can also develop from eating or smelling any pungent aromas or from looking at the sun. Therapies include evacuative herb nose drops, such as *pippalī, kayphal,* dry ginger, *kūt, viḍaṅga, bilwa, munuka* (dry grapes), and ginger. Inhaling smoke is also advised. The head is fomented with Vāyu reducing herbs (e.g., *aśhwagandhā, balā*), and oily snuff, including turmeric, *balā, kaṭukā,* and *bilwa.*

7. Mucus Sneezes (*bhramṣhathu*)—Excess thick and salty Kapha accumulations in the head become liquefied from the heat of Pitta and are expelled through sneezing. The same therapies used for sneezing may also be used here.

8. Burning Sensation/Vapor (*dīpta*)—Vapor breaths of Vāyu emit from the nostrils with a great burning sensation. Pitta-reducing therapies are used to heal *dīpta.*

9. Stuffiness/Deviated Septum (*nāsā-pratināha*)—Upward moving Vāyu (*Udān*) becomes excessive as a result of Kapha and blocks the nasal passages. Therapies include applying blowing powders of *viḍaṅga*, millet seed, *vachā, kūt, kayphal,* frankincense, sage, and *tulsī* to the nose. *Talisadi chorine* with honey or *śhṛiṅgyādi chūrṇa* may be taken internally. Vāyu-reducing herbs such as *aśhwagandhā, bilwa bark, gokṣhura, kaṇṭkārī, punarnavā* will provide relief. *Balā or nārāyan* oil is also useful.

10. Cold and Mucus/Coryza (*nāsā-parisrāva*)—Constant clear or white watery secretion of Kapha will emit from the nostrils (especially at night). Therapies include powdered herbs of *musta, kuṭki, pippalī*, turmeric, *chitrak*, rock salt, and *kayphal* inhaled through the nose. Fresh herb juice poured in the nose is also useful. Inhaling aromas of *chitrak* and cedar may also be taken.

11. Dryness (*nāsā-pariṣhoṣha*)—Excess Vāyu and Pitta causes difficult breathing owing to dry-

ing, hardening, and accumulation of the mucus (Kapha). Therapies include *ghee* and sesame oil used as a nasal lubricant.

* Excess Mucus (*Nāsā-srāva*)—Vāyu and Kapha block the passages of respiration (similar to pratināha). Consequently, a continuous discharge of yellow or white fluid runs from the nose. Vāyu/Kapha therapies are used.

* Dry Frontal Sinus (*Srotaḥ śhṛiṅgāṭa-śhoṣha*)—Nose oil drops of *aṇu taila* [sesame oil, goat's milk, *madhuka, daśhmūl* decoction and rock salt] may be used.

The four nasal hemorrhoids or polyps (*arṣhas* —Chapter 15) [*Guggul, triphalā* and *pippalī* are used.] and four swellings (*ṣhophas*—Chapter 25) result from the three deranged *doṣhas*, either separately or in combination. Therapies are the same as those discussed in their respective chapters.

Seven different nasal tumors (*arbuda*) exist, (Vāyu, Pitta, Kapha, Vāyu/Pitta, Vāyu/Kapha, Pitta/Kapha, Tridoṣha).

General Therapies: *Triphalā,* antiseptic and germicidal herbs are taken internally, as snuff and oil drops.

Vāyu: Comfrey, ginger, licorice, sandalwood, turmeric, *asafoetida, bhṛiṅgarāj, brāhmī.*

Pitta: Barberry, dandelion, sandalwood, turmeric, jasmine, *mañjiṣhṭhā,* neem, *bhṛiṅgarāj, brāhmī.*

Kapha: Barberry, dandelion, sandalwood, turmeric, jasmine, *mañjiṣhṭhā,* neem, *asafoetida, bhṛiṅgarāj, brāhmī.*

Rhinitis (Pīnasa)

It is caused by all *doṣhas*. Two stages of rhinitis can occur: early and advanced.

General Symptoms: Intense pain and distress occurring in all three *doṣhas*.

Early Symptoms: Heaviness of the head, no appetite, discharge of thin fluid from the nose, feeble voice, and frequent expectoration of mucus and saliva.

Advanced Symptoms (*Pakva*): Mucus becomes thicker, staying in the nasal passages; voice returns, mucus returns to its normal color. If this condition is neglected, it can develop deafness, blindness, loss of smell, eye diseases, body swellings, poor digestion, and cough.

Pīnasa Therapies:

(also see next section—Hoarse Voice)

When symptoms of one *doṣha* dominates, the following therapies are used.

Vāyu: Unction followed by nonunctuous enema. A light, Vāyu-reducing diet using, oily, sour, and hot foods. Hot water is also used for drinking and bathing. Homes should be draft-free. Anxiety, exertion, excessive talking, and sexual intercourse should be avoided.

Pitta: *Ghee* should be taken with bitter herbs and milk boiled with ginger to help dispel the toxins. This is followed by nasal evacuatives, such as *viḍaṅga, apāmārga,* and *pippalī* (with turmeric). Pitta-reducing foods and liquids can also be taken.

Kapha: Lightening therapy (emesis) is used with symptoms of heaviness or anorexia. To improve digestion, *ghee* is applied to the head, followed by fomentation and water sprinkling (*pariṣheka*). Sesame seed paste is eaten, followed by emetic and pungent herbs (e.g., garlic, *kuṣhṭhā, vachā, pippalī*), with green gram powder, rock salt, and *ghee* boiled in milk. This drink causes emesis. The herbs can also be made into a medicated mustard oil and applied to the nasal passages. Kapha-reducing foods and liquids are taken.

For all nose and head disorders, śhadbindu, bilwa and nārāyan oils are useful.

Catarrh
Inflamed Mucus Membranes of the Nose and Throat (Pratiśhyāya-Pratiśhedha)

Causes:

Overindulgence in sexual intercourse, heating of the head, inhaling dust or smoke through the nose, excessive heat or cold, suppression of stool and urine, eating raw foods, or excessive talking can instantly cause nasal catarrh. Excesses of Vāyu, Pitta, Kapha, Tridoṣha or blood may cause catarrh (*pratiśhyāya*).

Premonitory Signs:

Heavy head, sneezing, aching limbs, goose bumps.

Symptoms:

Vāyu: Hoarseness, stuffiness, thin mucus secretions, dry throat, palate and lips, pricking and piercing pain in the temples, excessive sneezing, bad taste in the mouth.

Pitta: Hot, yellow, hot smoky mucus secretions, heated skin, thirst, emaciation, yellow skin.

Kapha: Constant runny nose, cold, white or clear mucus, swollen eyes, heavy head, tickling and itching in the head, throat, lips and palate.

Tridoṣha: Spontaneous appearance or disappearance of symptoms of all three *doṣhas*.

Blood: Bloody secretions from the nose, red eyes, bruised pain in chest, bad breath and smell, loss of smell, small white or black worms in the nose.

Chronic Coryza (duṣhṭha pratiśhyāya): Neglect of coryza and poor eating habits, causes this condition to worsen. Serious conditions are noted by constant alternation between dry and slimy nostrils, and between contracted and expanded nostrils, foul smell and loss of smell. Nasal diseases previously discussed can also develop. Other symptoms include ear, eye, head disorders, graying or baldness, whitening of body hairs, thirst, difficult breathing, cough, fever, intestinal bleeding, swellings (*śhopha*), hoarse voice, and consumption. Chronic coryza symptoms are difficult to heal. Inhaling smoke of roasted gram flour and *ghee* is advised.

Therapies:

General: *Ghee* emetics and fomentation are useful except during the beginning and acute stages of catarrh. Fresh herb juice (according to *doṣha*) is applied as nasal drops (for blood conditions such as bloody secretions from the nose) add sugar cane and milk). Acidic foods should be lukewarm and taken with ginger, fresh or dried. Sugar cane juice and pungent tastes may help thicken mucus secretions.

When mucus is too thick, it can be loosened and secreted by using nasal head purgatives, non oily enemas, inhaling warm aroma smoke, and medicinal gargles.

Persons should rest in draftless rooms, with their heads covered to protect them from the temperature. White *basmati* rice, *harītakī* and other herbs related to the excessed *doṣha* are eaten. Wine, cold liquids and baths, sexual intercourse, anxiety, grief, suppression of stool and urine, and eating very dry foods should be avoided.

Fasting (if one is strong) or light meals with digestive and appetite-increasing herbs are used when catarrh is accompanied by vomiting, aching, heavy limbs, fever, lack of hunger, apathy, and diarrhea. Adults with a Vāyu/Kapha-caused illness should drink a large quantity of liquids and them vomit.

Vāyu: *Ghee* cooked with *vidārī-kand, balā, vāsāk*, licorice, *triphalā, tṛikatu, chitrak*, and rock salt. Snuff of warm and moist herbs and oils may also be used.

Pitta and Blood: *Ghee* cooked with bitter herbs is ingested. Decoctions of bitter herbs are used to wash and plaster the affected area. Red sandalwood, *guḍūchī*, licorice, *śhatāvarī, triphalā*, honey, and cane sugar are boiled in milk and/or oil and used as a gargle and nasal purgative.

Kapha: *Ghee* is applied to the affected area. Persons should eat barley gruel and sesame seeds or paste, followed by vomiting. Then Kapha-reducing measures are used. Oil cooked with *balā, viḍaṅga, pippalī, tulsī, kūt, vāsāk, elā* and black pepper are used as nasal drops. Herbs of chamomile, *aśhwagandhā, vāsāk, viḍaṅga and harītakī* are smoked.

Tridoṣha: *Ghee* cooked with bitter and pungent herbs is ingested; herbal smoke (*dhūma*), as for Kapha catarrh (e.g., *viḍaṅga, vāsāk*) is used; pungent foods are eaten. Nasal therapy and gargling use sesame oil cooked with *musta, brāhmī*, cardamom, *pippalī, vachā, kaṭukā, pippalī*, myrrh. Vāyu-reducing herbs are cooked in milk and water (twice as much water as milk) and cooked to half the amount. Then *ghee*, cane sugar, licorice, and red sandalwood are added. This mixture is also used as a nasal therapy—4, 6, or 8 drops are put into each nostril.

Chronic Coryza (Duṣhṭha Pratiśhyāya): The smoke of roasted gram flour and *ghee* is inhaled. When the nose is dry, an oil snuff is made from sesame oil, goat's milk (made into paste), *daśhmūl* decoction and 10 times as much licorice and rock salt. *Anu Taila* is another good oil for the this condition. Therapies to reduce all *doṣhas* are required.

Hoarse Voice (Svara-bedha)

Cause Hoarseness may result from Vāyu, Pitta, Kapha, Tridoṣha, TB, or excess weight.

Symptoms:

Vāyu: The throat is dry, harsh, unsteady and thorny. Relief comes from oily and warm foods and liquids.

Pitta: Burning sensation and dryness of the palate and throat, inability to speak.

Kapha: The throat feels coated, voice is slow, husky, and obstructed.

Tridoṣha: All three *doṣha* symptoms are experienced.

TB: Painful upon speaking; hot fumes emit from the mouth. There is no therapy for this type of hoarseness.

Over Weight: Kapha symptoms, some difficulty speaking. There is no therapy for this type of hoarseness.

Therapies:

All forms of TB are caused by simultaneous derangement of all three *doṣhas*. Depending upon one's strength, the predominant *doṣha* aggravating the condition, and the stage of development, the appropriate therapies are applied. There a two general therapeutic categories: the specific and general. Specific disorders include colds, headache, and difficulty breathing. All seven of the weakened tissue elements must be balanced to promote general healing.

Alleviation Therapies These therapies include *ghee*, sesame oil, lemon and lime, *pippalī, vāsāk, dūrba, nākeśhar*, black salt, and *āmalakī* eaten hot, with foods such as thick or thin gruel (barley, rice, or wheat, depending upon *doṣha* and strength). External therapies include fomentation, massage, aromatherapy, sprinkling, bath,) and blood-letting.

Colds/Rhinitis (*Pīnasa*) are healed *with chitrak, harītakī,* and *triphalā.*

Fomentation: Applied over the throat, chest (and the sides of the chest), and head, using thick gruel or pudding made with boiled milk, barley, *daśhmūl*, oil, and *ghee*. For headache or pain in the chest, sides, or shoulders, a thick hot ointment is applied using calamus, *guggul, punarnavā, śhatāvarī*, sandalwood, *vidārī kand, balā, vāsāk, cardamom, ghee,* and oil. For these conditions, aromatherapy, *sneha*—sandalwood oil massage, and medicated enemas are useful after meals.

Water Sprinkling (Ekānga dhara or Pariṣheka sveda): Water boiled with *balā, guḍūchī, aśhwagandhā, śhatāvarī*, sandalwood, barley, and honey are poured over the head when the mixture becomes lukewarm.

Elimination Therapies: First, oleation and fomentation therapies are undergone, then mild emetics and purgation. As with all therapies, physical strength and health must be considered.

Therapies should neither deplete nor causing diarrhea.

Persons who have extensive depletion of the *dhātus* must not undergo elimination therapy. Solely the heat-producing properties of the feces (*purīsha mala*) sustains life. All the digestive fires of the *dhātus* are weakened; only the main digestive fire is active.

General: *Ghee* boiled with *balā*, *daśhmūl*, turmeric, milk, *sitopaladi*, and eating after meals. These therapies are useful for cough, throat disorders, difficult breathing, and pain in the shoulders and sides of the chest, and headache.

Cough: Nasal oils and aromatherapy herbs include *balā*, *vidārī kand, vāsāk, aśhwagandhā*, and *chyavan prāśh.*

Throat: Aromatherapy with *ghee*, *pippalī*, *balā, kaychant*, licorice, small cardamom seeds, and milk.

Burning, fever, upper body bleeding: *Vāsāk*, *śhatāvarī, dūrba, nāgkeśhar,* and *ghee*, grapes. Care should be taken to follow therapies for the appropriate stage of fever (see Chapter 14 for fevers).

Excess Phlegm: If persons are not too weak, and predominantly of Kapha constitution, therapies may include boiled milk with *pippalī*, *apāmārga*, cardamom, *tulsī*, and *vāsāk*. Another useful therapy is thick barley gruel boiled with emetic herbs and *ghee*.

Vāyu causes excessive phlegm, so oily and hot therapies are necessary.

Vomiting: When phlegm results from excess Vāyu and Kapha, Vāyu-reducing foods and herbs (e.g., black pepper, *ajwan*, ginger, honey), and *arjuna* for the heart are taken.

Diarrhea: People with TB have weak digestive fire, causing diarrhea, mucus, bad taste in the mouth, and loss of appetite. Therapies include thick barley gruel with *bilwa*, *kuṭaj*, ginger, *īśhabgol*, or *āmalakī*, *arjuna*, *gokṣhura*, *ghee,* and *mūng* flour, mixed as a drink.

Bad Taste in Mouth: Brush teeth morning and evening. Chew herbs of cardamom, turmeric, *musta*, *āmalakī*, *pippalī*, and coriander to remove bad tastes. They may be mixed with sesame oil, *ghee*, honey milk, and sugar cane, and kept in the mouth as a thin paste. Herbs include cardamom, *khadir*, and *majuphal*.

Miscellaneous Therapies: Oil massage, wearing new clothes, taking medicated baths, medicated enema, using pleasant aromas, soothing music, good company, meditation, prayer, donating, celibacy, truthfulness, having good conduct, and nonviolent activities, words, and thoughts. Other therapies include drinking goat's milk and staying in a pine forest. A parallel in Western medicine was the use of sanitariums for healing and recuperation.

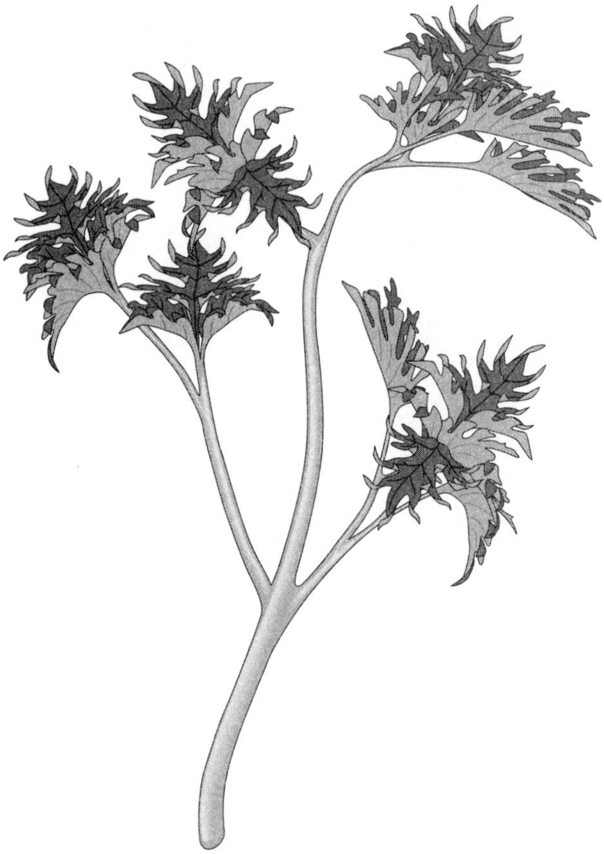

Eye Diseases

(Aupadravikam Adhyayam)

Eyeball (Nayana-Budbuda):

The eyeball consists of all five elements. Earth (*bhu*) forms the muscles. Fire (*tejas*) forms the blood in the veins and arteries. Air (*Vāyu*) forms the iris and the pupil. Water (*jala*) forms the cornea. Ether (*akāṣha*) forms the ducts or sacs that discharge secretions.

Rasa and *alochaka* Pitta support the anterior coat (retina). Muscle (*māṃsa*) supports the chorid or second coat. Fat tissue (*medas*) supports the third or scleroid coat and cornea. There are many divisions and subdivisions of these coats.

Blood vessels, muscles, vitreous body and the choroid hold together the various parts of the eyeball. The eyeball itself is held by a watery substance, the capsule of tenon, which is supported by various vessels. When excessed *doṣhas* pass upward into the eyes through the veins and nerves, many diseases are caused.

DIAGRAM 1: EYE

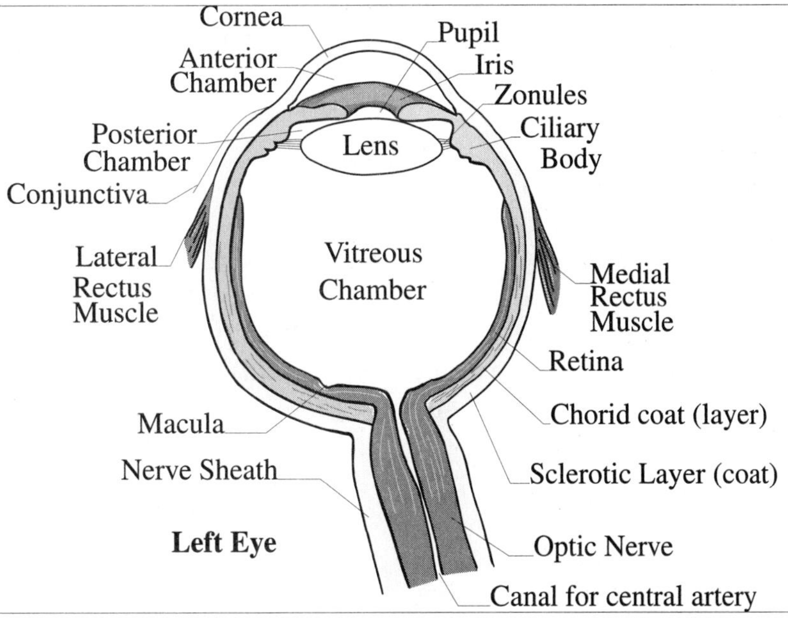

DIAGRAM 2: EYE

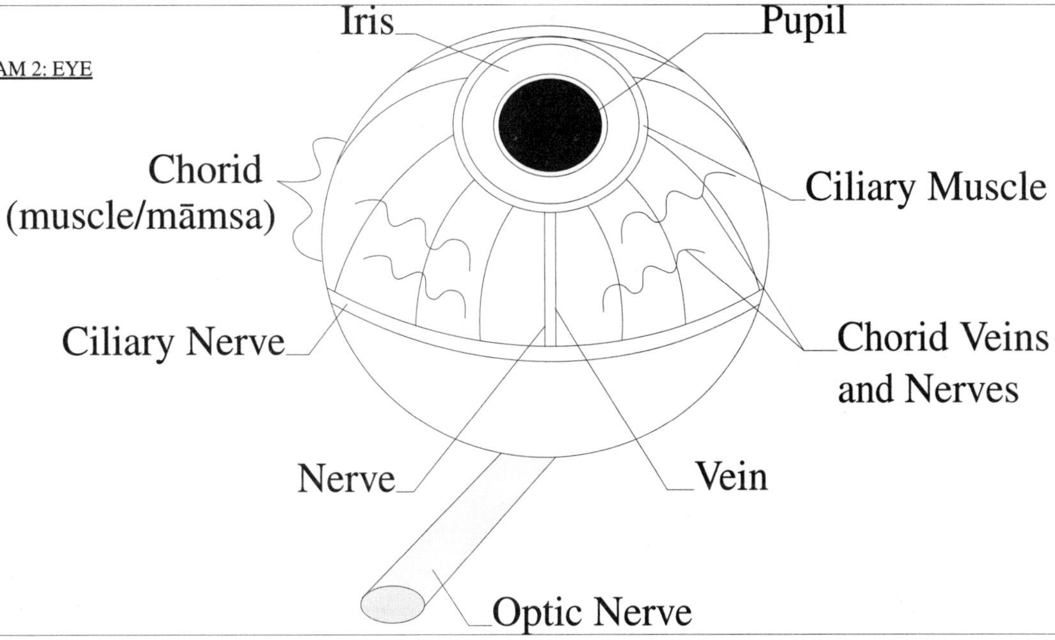

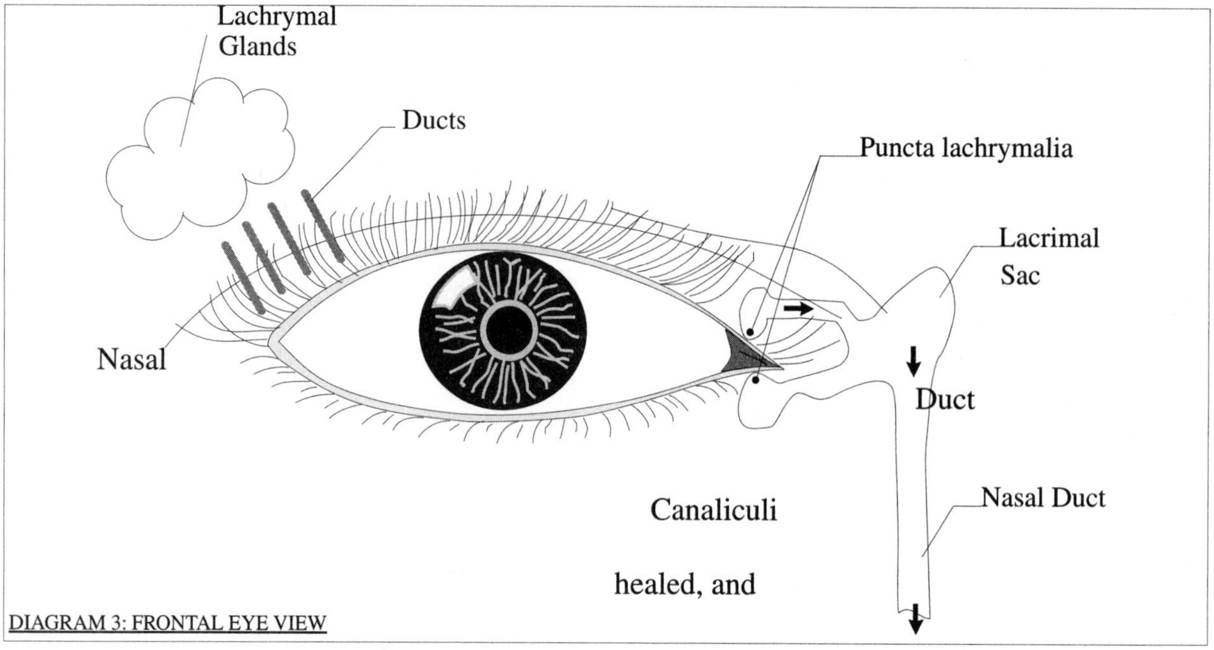

DIAGRAM 3: FRONTAL EYE VIEW

Premonitory Signs: Cloudy vision, slight inflammation, tear secretion, accumulated mucus, heaviness, burning, aching, and red eyes.

Eyelid inflammation causes feelings of bristles studded in the eyes, pricking pain, and impaired sight (seeing colors with the eyes opened or closed).

Causes: Local *doṣhas* become imbalanced from submerging the head in water immediately after exposure to heat and constant glaring at the sun, straining to see objects far away, taking naps, staying up late, forced staring, excessive crying, grief, worry, fatigue, being hit or bumped, excessive sex, overeating or drinking, suppressing the natural urges, smoke, dust or sweat entering the eyes, excessive or blocked vomiting (i.e., pressure), and constant squinting to see tiny objects.

There are 76 forms of eye disease: 10 Vāyu, 12 Pitta and 13 Kapha, 16 forms related to excesses or toxic blood, 25 from tridoṣhic causes, and 2 resulting from external trauma.

Development and Symptoms:

Vāyu: Five Vāyu disorders are healable, *anyato*-Vāyu, ophthalmia (*adhi-mantha*), *śhuṣhkākṣhi-pāka*, *abhiṣhyanda*, and *maruta-paryaya*. Vāyu cataracts can only be temporarily healed, and four diseases cannot be healed. Three disorders affect vision (*hatā-dhimantha, nimiṣha, gambhirikā*), and one afflicts the sclerotic coat (*Vāyu-hatavartma*).

Pitta: Seven Pitta eye diseases can be healed (*abhiṣhynda*, ophthalmia/*adhi-mantha, amlādhy-uṣhita, sūktikā, Pitta-vidagdha-driṣhti, pothaki*, also known as gramulocyte tracoma, and *lagana*). Three can only be prevented from getting worse (*kācha, parimlāyi, nila*). Two disorders cannot be healed (*hrasva-jādya, jala-srāva*).

Kapha: Eleven disorders can be healed (conjunctivitis (*abhiṣhyanda*), cataracts (*adhi-mantha*), *balāsa-granthita, śhleshma-vidagdha-driṣhti, pothaki, lagana, krimi-granthi, pariklinna-vartma, śhuklārma, piṣhtaka, śhleṣhmo-panāha* (healed by excision). Only Kapha cataracts (*Kapha Kācha*) are containable. *Srāva-roga* is incurable.

Blood: Twelve forms are healable (cataract/*adhi-mantha, abiṣhyanda, kliṣhta-vartma, sirahar- ṣha* and *siropāta, anjana, sira-jāla, parvani,* non-ulcerated *avrana, ṣhukra-roga* (corneal calcification)*, śhonitārma, arjuna*). *Kācha* cataracts are only pacifiable. Five are incurable (*raktasrāva, ajakājata*, pendent/*avalambita, śhoni-tārṣhas, śhukra-roga* [If the third sclerotic layer is affected then it is incurable]. When the first and second sclerotic layer are affected, they are difficult to heal.

Tridosha: Eighteen diseases cannot be healed (*vartmāvabandha, sirāja-pidakā, prastāryarma, adhi-mānsārma, snayvarma, utsangini, puyālasa, arvuda, śhyāva-vartma, kardama-vartma, arṣhovartma, śhukrāṣhas, śharkarā-vartma*, two inflammations without local swelling/ *saṣhopha-pāka* and *aṣhopha-pāka, bahala-vartma, kumbhikā*, and *visa-vartma*). Two disorders are controllable (*kācha*-cataract [palliative] and *pakṣhma-kopa*). Four diseases cannot be healed (*puya- srāva, nakulāndhya, akṣhipākā- tyaya, alaji*).

External: Both forms are incurable; *sanimitta*/external blow, and *animitta*/seeing the sudden light of a celestial being.

Locations: Of the 26 diseases, 9 affect the joints, 21 the eyelids, 11 the vitreous humor, 4 the choroid, 17 the entire eyeball region, and 12 the pupil or crystalline lens. The two external diseases affect the entire eyeball.

General Therapies: All types of eye disease discussed in this chapter can be helped with any of the following;

1. *Triphalā*, sarsaparilla and turmeric
2. Barberry and raw honey, or just raw honey
3. *Punarnavā* decoction with rose water
4. *Chandrodaya varti*
5. *Triphalā ghee*
6. *Pravāl piṣhti*
7. *Saptamrita lauh* (iron ash)

Joint and Binding Membrane (Sandhigata- Roga -Vijñaniya)

Development, Symptoms, Therapies: There are 9 related diseases. These include symptoms of Vāyu, Pitta and Kapha diseases, and are the premonitory symptoms of eye diseases.

1. Puyālasa: A pus-filled swelling that develops at any joint and is malodorous and dense (some say it is painful and without pus). It is treated with blood-letting. After oil and fomentation around the affected area, blood-letting is performed, followed by a poultice of myrrh.

2. Upangha: A large painless cyst at the union of the pupil and choroid (*Kṛiṣhṇa-mandala*) [see diagram 2], with itching and a little pus. This is caused by Kapha. The affected area is opened and rubbed with *pippalī* and honey. Then the surrounding area is scraped. Before pus forms, oil and light fomentation therapy is used.

3-6. Srāva: Deranged Pitta, Kapha or blood, passing through the lachrymal ducts into the binding tissues of the four joints produces a painless secretion with symptoms of the excessed *doṣha*. Four forms exist:

a) *Puyā-srāva*—A pus-filled swelling at any eye joint where the pus is secreted. This results from Kapha, Pitta, and blood. Rock salt and honey heal this disease.

b) *Śhleshmā-srāva*—A thick, slimy, white secretion of mucus and pus, without pain. Rock salt and honey heal this disorder.

c) *Raktā-srāva*—A copious, thin, warm and blood-streaked secretion. It results from toxic blood at that location. Rock salt and honey heal this condition.

d) *Pitta-srāva*—A warm, watery, yellow-blue (or reddish yellow) secretion from the middle part of the joint results from excess Pitta. Rock salt and honey heal this malady.

7) Parvani: A small, round coppery swelling at the joint of the choroid (*Kṛiṣhṇa-mandala*) and sclerotic coat (*śhukla-mandala*) due to deranged local blood, with burning and aching. Rock salt and honey heals this disorder.

8) Alaki: A similar swelling that occurs at the same place, but it is larger. Rock salt and honey or rose water are used to heal this ailment.

9) Krimi-granthi: A cyst or swelling with itching, appearing where the the eyelids and lashes meet, resulting from parasitical germination. The parasites infect the inner lining of the eyelid where it is connected with the sclerotic coat, invading and weakening the eyeball. After fomentation and incision, a decoction of *triphalā* and myrrh is used on the affected area.

Eyelids (Vartmagata-Roga-Vijñāniya)

Development, Symptoms, Therapies: The *doṣhas*, either alone or in combination, expand through the nerves and veins of the eyelids (*vartma*), causing excess blood and fleshy growth. This causes excess fleshy growth that is responsible for 21 diseases of the eyelids.

1. *Utsangini* (conjunctival cyst): A rolled or indented boil or pimple appears on the outer lower eyelid, with its head pointed inward. Therapy includes *amritahwardivarti (guḍūchī,* lotus stem, *bilwa, paṭola,* licorice, *prapaundarīka,* cedar, and sarsaparilla. A quantity of 320 gms of these herbs is made into a decoction, then strained and reheated until thick. Then 10 gms of white pepper and 40 gms fresh jasmine flowers are added until the decoction becomes sticky. Then one drop is placed in the eye. It can also be treated with scarification.

2. *Kumbhika* (internal stye-hordeolum cyst): Resulting from all three *doṣhas*, many boils or pimples develop on the joint of the eyelids and lashes, burst and then become inflamed. This is healed with *chitranjan* (1.25 gms black pepper, 5 gms *samudraphena* (cuttle-fish bone) and 1.25 gms lead sulfide are pounded finely during *Citra* constellation (a *Vedic* astrology/*Jyotiṣh* mystical star) It can also be treated by scarification. A general treatment includes placing one drop of honey in the eye.

3. *Pothaki* (trachoma/granular conjunctivitis): Many red, hard boils or pimples (such as red mustard seeds), that are painful, itchy, and secreting. Honey or barberry is used to heal this condition. It can also be treated by scarification.

4. *Vartma-śharkarā* (infection of meibomian gland/trachoma): Rough large pimples surrounded by very small and thick pustules (that cover the entire length of the eyelid). *Chandrodaya varti* is used to heal this disorder. Scarification may also be used.

5. *Arṣho-vartma* (papillary trachoma): Small, soft, rough pimples on the eyelid, with little pain. *Chandrodaya varti (śhaṅk bhasma* (conch shell ash), *bibhītakī, harītakī, lead sulfate, black pepper,* all mixed in equal quantities). Then goat's milk is mixed with the *chandrodaya varti* until it becomes a paste. The paste is then rolled into a cylindrical form with a diameter of about 1/12 of an inch. This rod is dipped in water briefly, then applied to the eye. It can also be treated by scarification.

6. *Śhuṣhkārṣhas* (chronic papillary trachoma or a form of tumors): Long, rough, hard numb pimples on the eyelid. *Rasāñjana* (Berberis aristata DC extract) is used to heal this malady. Scarification can also be used.

7. *Anjana* (external stye-hordeolum cyst): Small soft, coppery pimples on the eyelid, with burning, pricking, and slight pain. It is treated by excision. After fomentation, a spontaneous bursting may occur. This requires pressing and rubbing with a plaster of jasmine, cardamom, and myrrh mixed with honey.

8. *Bahala-vartma* (multiple chalazion): Equal-sized pimples that are hard, along the eyelid, and of similar shape and color. *Nīlathotha* (crude copper sulfate), lead sulfite, small *elā* and *pawchi* with honey. It can also be treated by scarification.

9. *Vartma-bandha*: Eyelid edema with itching and slight pain, preventing opening of the lids. *Nīlathotha* (crude copper sulfate or copper acetate, or basic copper acetate), lead sulfite, small *elā,* and *pawchi* with honey.

10. *Kliṣhta-vartma* (angio-neurotic edema): Mild, coppery inflamed swellings of both eyelids (simultaneously), with slight pain, suddenly becoming red or discharging blood. *Punarnavā, triphalā,* and rock salt mixed with honey are recommended. Scarification may also be used.

11. *Kardama-vartma* (non-ulcerative blepharitis): When the previous disorder (*kliṣhta*) is affected by Pitta. Inflammation of the lid margin with redness develops. Further, the area can become thick, forming scales and crust, shallow marginal ulcers or discharge dirty blood and mucus. Honey or barberry heals this condition. Alternatively, it is treated by scarification.

12. *Śhyāva-vartma* (ulcerative blepharitis): A dark brown coloration of the eyelids, both internally and externally, with swelling, pus secretion,

and itching. Therapy includes red *sphatik* (alum), *elā,* and barberry with rose water. It can also be treated by scarification.

13. Praklinna-vartma: The outer eyelid swells (edema) with mucus deposits in the inner surface, with little pain, secretion, itching, and pricking. Surgery is contraindicated. Oil, fomentation, venesection, purgation, nasal evacuatives and non oil enemas are required to cleanse the system. Then eye washes, salves, drops, snuffs, and aromatherapies are used. Herbs include *musta*, turmeric, licorice, *punarnavā*, *triphalā*, *vaṃśha lochana,* with honey. Myrrh and white pepper applied as a slave alleviates itching of the eye.

Itching: One application of an eye salve of black salt, white pepper, red sandalwood, sugar cane root, barberry, cedar, white salt, and *chamellī* leaf in equal parts.

Swelling (śhopha): *Musta*, cedar, *triphalā, punarnavā, lodhra*, are pasted together as an eye salve.

14.Aklinna-vartma (ankylo belpharon): The eyelids stick together without any pus or secretion (even if the eyes are constantly washed with water. Surgery is contraindicated.

15. Vātāhata-vartma (lagophthalmos): Drooping or inactivity of the eyelids, with or without pain, obstructing the opening of the eye lashes. The lids seem to be out of joint. It is treated by scarification. Pitta causes this disorder. Therapies include *triphalā* pasted with water and applied on the eyelids, or *pippalī* and olive oil paste on the eyelids.

16. Arvuda (eyelid tumor or angiomas): An uneven, red, knotty swelling or shape which quickly grows on the inside of the eyelid, with little pain. Herbal therapies include *pippalī* and olive oil paste on the eyelids. *Triphalā* pasted with water can also be used. It is also treated by incision.

17. Nimeṣha (ptosis): Wrinkling of the eyelids due to excess Vāyu in the nerves or veins.

18. Shonitārṣhas (internal hemorrhage): Soft, fleshy growths on the eyelids, which reappear even after they are surgically removed. Pain and burning are also present, resulting from excess blood. Useful herbs include *triphalā*, *guḍūchī*, *āmalakī*, turmeric, and licorice.

19. Lagaṇa or Nagana (chalazion cyst): A thick, hard, slimy, painless nodular swelling on the eyelid, with itching and no pus or secretion. It is treated by excision.

After incision, *vaṃśha lochana* or *pippalī* are mixed with honey and applied to the incised area. *Harītakī*, ginger, black pepper, neem, *vāsāk,* and *lodhra* mixed together are also useful. Larger incisions require cauterization with alkali or fire. This is caused by Kapha.

20. *Visa-vartma*: An inflamed swelling of the eyelid, dotted with tiny punctures or pores. It is treated by excision. Useful herbs include red sandalwood, rose water, *guḍūchī, punarnavā,* and *mamīrā*. It is caused by an excess of Kapha.

21. Pakṣhma-kopa (Eye Lashes—trichiasis districhisis and entropion): Excessed *doṣhas* accumulate around the eye lash, causing them to become rough and sharp pointed. This develops eye pain, which is relieved when the lash is pulled off. The eye is sensitive to wind, heat, or the light of a fire. Therapy can be palliative or provide temporary relief, if persons still have their sight. This disease cannot be healed, but it can be controlled. Herbs, including *bilwa, śhyonaka, patluppu, gambhari, arni, kaṇṭkārī,* and the entire castor oil plant are made into a decoction and used to wash the eyes. Surgery may also be indicated.

Sclerotic Coat (Śhuklagata-Roga-Vijñāniya)

Development and Symptoms: Eleven diseases of the sclerotic coat exist. These are all caused by Kapha. All these conditions are helped by rock salt, *triphalā*, ginger, black pepper, and white coral. The first five are known as pterygium.

1. Prastāīyarma: A thin, extended, reddish-blue glandular swelling on the sclerotic coat. This is treated by incision.

2. Śhuklārma: A group of soft, white growths, developing over the entire sclerotic coat. This is treated with incision.

3. Lohitārma: A reddish fleshy growth on the

cornea. This is treated with incision.

4. Adhi-mānsārma: A soft, thick, dark brown, and extended fleshy growth on the cornea. This is treated by incision.

5. Snāyvarma: A rough, yellowish or white fleshy growth on the white coat that slowly grows larger. This is treated with incision.

6. Śhuktikā (xerosis/xerotic Keratitis): Dark brown, fleshy or oyster colored specks on the white area of the eyeball). Surgery is contraindicated.

7. Arjuna (ecchymosis kerato-conjunctivitis): A single dot or speck on the cornea that is blood red. Surgery is contraindicated. The same therapies apply as for Pitta *abiṣhyanda*. Sugar cane juice, honey, milk, turmeric, *punarnavā,* and licorice are used as an eye wash or salve. *A triphalā* decoction may also be used as eye drops. Turmeric, barberry, *guḍūchī*, *bilwa,* and licorice may also be used to wash the eyes.

8. Piṣhtaka (pinguecula): A white or transparent, elevated, circular dot or speck on the white coat. Surgery is contraindicated. A thin plaster of ginger, *pippalī*, *musta*, black and white pepper may be pasted together and used as a salve.

9. Sirā-jala (scleritis): Large red patches of a hardened network of veins spreading over the sclerotic coat. It is also treated by incision.

10. Sirā-Pidakā (deep scleritis): A group of white pimples on the white coat, near the edge of the iris, covered with shreds of veins. Therapy includes *rasāñjan* with honey. It is also treated by incision.

11. Balāsa Grathita (conjunctivitis): A metal-colored speck, covered with veins on the white coat. (Some say the speck appears like a drop of water.) Surgery is contraindicated. The eye is cleansed by blood-letting or by using herbs. The herbs include *triphalā, punarnavā, nirguṇḍī, chamellī,* barberry, *banyan* tree (*Vata-ala* or ginger) bark (or juice), and rock salt. This is followed with the same therapies as Kapha ophthalmia.

Black part of the chorid and iris (Krishna-Gata- Roga-Vijñāniya)

Development and Symptoms: Four diseases related to this area exist. These are all forms of calcifications of the cornea.

Savrana-Śhukra (keratitis/corneal ulcer): A puncture-like dip in the area, pricking sensation, great pain, hot secretion. If the seat of the disorder is far from the pupil (marginal keratolysis), the entire retina has no pain or discharge, if it is not deep-seated or without double spots, it can be healed.

A-vrana-Śhukra (corneal opacity): A whitish film overlays the choroid region, including the iris, like a speck of transparent cloud in the sky, tear secretion, slight pain due to ophthalmia (secretion). This is easily healed. When a non ulcerated form of this disease is thick, deep seated, and chronic, is difficult to heal. If it is a chronic situation which is mobile, covered with fleshy shreds, full of veins or stretching down to the second skin layer in the eye, it cannot be healed. Other unhealable symptoms are obstructed vision, severed in the middle and with a reddish tint in the extremities. Some authorities also say if spots are on the iris, with pimples, and hot tear secretions, it also cannot be healed. This is a Kapha disorder.

Therapies- (for this milk-white fleshy growth in the eye): The non ulcerated form (*a-vrana*) follows the above blood caused ophthalmia. Should these therapies not work, then scarifying is used. The ulcerated form (*sa-vrana*), be it in the first or second layers, or rough, one follows the same therapies. Scarifying (rubbing) myrrh, black pepper, *pippalī* powders on the affected area, and used as a salve is useful.

Eyelid inflammation (Akṣhi-Pākātyaya): A milky white film over the black part of the eye, slowly covering it completely, (and some say) with great pain. It is treated with venesection.

Akṣhi pākātyaya (Akshi-Pākā, Netra-pāka): (Inflammation of the entire eye.) Oil and fomentation is done for both swelling (*sa-śhopha*) and non swelling (*a-ṣhopha*) forms. Venesection is then done. *A triphalā* decoction is used as eye wash and eye drops, nasal evacuatives, and *Puta-pāka* are also applied.

Puta-pāka: *Triphalā* and water are first mixed into a paste. The paste is then pasted on the bottom side of two leaves of *Jamum* or *Vat*, and left in the sun to dry. After the eyes are cleansed, myrrh, ginger, *pippalī*, black pepper, *viḍaṅga*, *ghee*, honey, and milk are used as an eye salve.

Ajakā (anterior staphyloma): A reddish painful growth rising from below the surface of the black area, with red, slimy secretions. The watery accumulation in the eye is drained by a needle puncture on either side of the cornea, and the hole filled with *ghee*. *Chandrodaya varti* with honey is used for this condition. Scarifying or rubbing is frequently done if the punctured area becomes elevated.

Disease Affecting the Entire Eye (Sarva-gata-Roga-Abhiṣhyandha/ Conjunctivitis)

Development, Symptoms and Therapies: Seventeen forms of eye diseases affect the eye as a whole. Herbal therapies are useful when these diseases are not severe. Only when conditions are serious is venesection required.

1-4. Ophthalmia (Abiṣhyanda): Eye inflammation (four types)

a) Vāyu—causes pricking eye pain, numbness, irritation, roughness, dryness, restricted movement, cold tears, lack of secretions, and headache. First, a few drops of *ghee* are applied in the eye. Then the forehead, over the eye is fomented. Next, local venesection is done. Other useful therapies include, oil enema for cleansing, eye drops of *triphalā*, raw honey, *ghee* (tepid in winter, cold in summer). Eight drops are used for scarifying, 10 drops for lubricating, and 12 drops for healing. Aromatherapy (frankincense and sandalwood), eye washes (*triphalā*), and nasal evacuative oils using *āmalakī,* and *śhatāvarī* are also useful. Plasters of *triphalā* and licorice with milk are used as a collyrium for acute Vāyu ophthalmia. *Punarnavā* is also useful for all Vāyu eye diseases. Another recommendation is the mixture of *pippalī*, *dhātakī* flowers, rock salt, and 10-year-old *ghee*. This is applied in the eye.

b) Pitta—burning, inflammatory secretions, needing coldness in the eyes, excess hot secretions, cloudy vision, yellow eyes. It is treated with venesection. Blood-letting, purgatives (rhubarb, castor oil, *triphalā*), eye washes, plasters (around eyes), medicated nasal oils, eye salves, and Pitta-*Visarpa* (erysipelas) therapies. Herbs include cardamom, *lodhra, musta,* cane sugar, *dūrba, ghee*, raw honey, red sandalwood, licorice, milk, turmeric, *punarnavā*, *viḍaṅga*, cardamom. Depending upon the consistency, liquid or paste, they may be used as plasters, washes, salves, eye drops, or taken internally.

c) Kapha—desiring warmth, heaviness, itching, swelling, excess whiteness, constant deposit and discharge of slimy mucus. It is treated with venesection. During acute aggravation when fomentation does not help, the local vein is opened. Nasal drops using fresh herbs (*avapida nasya*), eye salves, aromatherapy, washes, plasters, gargles, *putapāka rukṣha*. Persons fast every 4 days on *ghee* cooked with *arjuna, triphalā, musta*, sandalwood, turmeric, *śhatāvarī,* and calamus taken in the morning. Lunch and dinner meals should not aggravate Kapha. Mild fomentation with *bilwa* and *triphalā* is applied around the eye. A thin plaster of *triphalā,* ginger, cedar, *lodhra*, barberry root, and *elā* (cardamom) is applied over the eyelid or entire eye. *Triphalā*, licorice, *asafoetida*, turmeric, licorice, ginger, *pippalī*, black pepper, *harītakī*, *viḍaṅga, punarnavā, tṛikatu, musta,* and white pepper are mixed with water into a paste and applied in the eye as a salve.

d) Blood—red eyes, coppery tears, deep red stripes, Pitta symptoms. It is treated with venesection. *Ghee* is taken internally and externally, therapies for blood/Pitta and Pitta *visarpa* are followed, and a Pitta-reduction diet is required.

5-9. Adhimantha (acute glaucoma): All chronic types must be quickly treated or excruciating eye pain (as if the eye is being torn out) will develop. The pain extends upward to half the head, feeling as though it is crushing the head. Specific *doṣha* symptoms also exist.

a) Vāyu—cloudy eye, feeling as though it is being torn out and stirred, is irritating, piercing and painful, with local fleshy swelling. The side of the head with the affected eye develops symptoms of twisting, cracking, swelling, and shivering. It is treated with venesection (also see Vāyu ophthalmia therapies).

b) Pitta—blood-streaked eye, secretions, burning sensation in the eye and head, swelling, perspiration, eye secretion, yellowed vision, fainting, liver-colored eyes and feeling ulcerated. It is treated with venesection (also see Pitta ophthalmia).

c) Kapha—swollen eyes, slight congestion (inflammation), cold, itching heavy secretions, slimy deposits of mucus, slight clouding, dilated nostrils, headaches, objects are seen as dusty. It is treated with venesection. See Kapha ophthalmia therapies.

d) Blood—pricking pain and blood-streaked secretions of the eye, bright red eyes, unbearable to touch, objects seem as if on fire, eye extremities become red, cornea (white coat of the eye) looks as if it is submerged in blood. It is treated with venesection. See blood ophthalmia therapies.

If one does not follow a wholesome diet (according to the excessed *doṣha*) blindness may occur (within 3 days for Pitta, 6 days for Vāyu, 5 days for blood, and 7 days for Kapha).

10. Netra-pāka:

a) Swelling (Sa-śhopha)—itching, mucus deposits in the eye, teary secretions, redness, burning, coppery colored, heavy, pricking pain, swelling, constantly secreting cold or hot slimy discharges, eventually forming pus. It can only be treated with venesection.

b) Nonswelling (A-śhopha)—the same symptoms except swelling. It is treated with venesection. Blood-purifying herbs and diuretics, such as *mañjiṣhṭhā* and *gokṣhura*, respectively are useful.

11. Blinding Eye Inflammation (Hatādhimantha): Excessed Vāyu becomes caught in the optic nerve. This is incurable.

12. Vāyu-Paryāya: Shifting pain in the eye lashes (or just the eyebrows and eyes). The same measures as Vāyu ophthalmia are used, including, ingesting large amounts of *ghee* before the meal with *daśhmūl, tṛikatu, tagar, mañjiṣhṭhā*, barberry, *figs, kaṇṭkārī*, and *musta*. It may also be treated with venesection.

13. Śhuṣhkā-kaṣhi-pāka: Eyelids become dry, hard, remain closed. Vision is cloudy and hazy vision. Great pain is experienced when opening the eyelids. Surgery is contraindicated. Cedar, powered ginger, milk, and *ghee* are mixed and used as a collyrium. Ingesting *ghee* with *balā, śhatāvarī* and licorice, and dropping this liquid in the eye is also useful. Alternatively, dry ginger and rock salt can be used internally or as eye drops. Nasal oil of *brāhmī* and *triphalā ghee* is helpful, as are eye washes of milk with black salt or milk cooked with cedar.

14. Anyato-vāyu: excessed Vāyu in the head, ears, cheek bones, back of the neck, the nerves on either side of the neck (the *manyā marmas*) causes great pain in the eyes or eye brows. It is treated with venesection. The same measures as Vāyu ophthalmia are used, including ingesting large amounts of *ghee* before the meal with a decoction of *bilwa, gāmbhārī, sonapatta, paṭola, ajwan,* and sarsaparilla. This decoction is also used as an ointment.

15. Amlādhyushita-Drishti: Eating excessive amounts of acidic foods (or from acid indigestion) causes the eyes to swell and develop a bluish red tint. Surgery is contraindicated. The same therapies as Pitta ophthalmia are used, and *triphalā ghee*.

16. Sirotpāta (hyperemia conjunctivitis): The veins throughout the eye become coppery, with or without pain. If not quickly attended to, copious discharges of transparent and coppery color develop, leading to complete blindness. *Rasāñjan* is advised, i.e., barberry, *vaṃśha lochana*, white pepper, *sāmudra phena* (os sepiae or cuttlefish bone), and *phitkārī* (alum, sulfate of alumina and potash or of aluminum and ammonium; aluminous sulfate) mixed with honey. Additional therapies include honey and *ghee* as an eye salve. It is also treated with venesection.

17. Sirā-harṣha (orbital cellulitis): If *sirotpāta* is not quickly teated, large amounts of transparent and coppery eye secretions develop and cause blindness. Therapies include rhubarb, *musta,* and *amalatas* mixed with honey, and used as an eye salve. It is also treated with venesection.

Pupil Diseases (Driṣhti-gata-Roga-Vijnāñiya)

Development and Symptoms: There are 12 diseases of the pupils. One disease affects the coating over the entire pupil.

1st Pupil Coat (Patala): When the excessed *doṣhas* pass into the eye's innermost coat through the veins, objects appear dim and hazy.

2nd Pupil Coat: When excessed *doṣhas* are found in the second coat, false images appear before the eyes (of bugs, hair, nets, cobwebs, circular patches, flags, and earrings), objects appear covered in mist, haze, as if underwater, or seen through colored droplets falling in all directions.

3rd Pupil Coat: When the excessed *doṣhas* reach the third coat, one only sees higher placed objects, and cannot see objects below a certain level. If the crystalline lens is affected, objects reflect the colors of the lens. Objects seem covered with cloth. One does not see ears, eyes, noses etc. on other people. When the *doṣhas* affect the lower area of the crystalline lens blocks near vision, affecting the upper area causes distant blocking, and excessed *doṣhas* in the lateral areas blocks lateral vision. When the *doṣhas* affect the entire lens, objects are seen as dim and confused. If the middle part of the lens is affected, objects appear to be cut in two. When the *doṣhas* are in two places, there is triple vision. A multi-image of objects develops when the *doṣhas* are all over the lens.

4th Pupil Coat: Loss of vision (*timira*) results from excessed *doṣhas* being trapped in this area. Superficial excesses only allow for the vision of bright objects, whereas deep-seated excesses cause blindness.

Six Healable Diseases

All six healable diseases of the pupil and lens, the local veins, loss of vision (*timira*), cataracts (*kācha*), *linga-nāṣha,* Vāyu, Pitta, Kapha, blood (*rakta*), *tridoṣha,* and *parimlāyi* are bled, persons are duly purged using *ghee* mixed with herbal purgatives.

Vāyu symptoms of all six diseases: Castor oil with boiled milk is used as a purgative.

Pitta/blood symptoms of all six diseases: *Triphalā ghee* is used as a purgative.

1. Blindness (*Timira*):

Triphalā ghee is useful in all types of *timira*. Nasal evacuatives with sesame oil are also goo for all forms of this disease.

Vāyu-caused blindness requires *triphalā* mixed with sesame oil. Kapha-caused *Timira* needs *triphalā* mixed with honey. Pitta-caused therapy involves goat's milk boiled with *kākolī, kṣhīr kākolī*, honey, licorice, and *saraswat*. Vāyu *doṣhas* use a decoction of *aśhwagandhā, bilwa,* and *śhatāvarī*. Kapha *doṣhas* inhale smoke of *viḍaṅga, patta (corchorus capsularis), apāmārga* seed, and *hingot* bark powders. Also, an ointment of *vat, pippalī, kākolī*, turmeric, and fig tree bark (*anjīr*) is useful.

An eye salve using *ghee*, honey, salt, licorice is useful. Ingestibles for all causes of blindness include *ghee, triphalā, śhatāvarī, āmalakī,* and barley. Blood-letting is never used for this disease if the eye is red as it will aggravate the condition.

If a lack of redness exists, and the disease in only in the first coat, the disease is healable. When redness develops, and the second coat is affected, it is very difficult to heal. Should the third coat be affected, showing redness on the first coat, it is only controllable.

Vāyu Blindness—objects appear cloudy, moving, crooked and red. This cannot be healed. Therapies include *triphalā, śhatāvarī,* and sesame oil paste is eaten. Another therapy is *āmalakī, rock salt, pippalī* (in equal amounts), and a little black pepper. All these herbs are mixed and taken with honey. Yogurt water may be taken as well.

Pitta Blindness—objects seem to be rainbow-colored, like a flash of lightning, the feathers of a peacock or with a dark blue-black tint. Therapies include *triphalā ghee* paste is eaten. Sarsaparilla, licorice, cane sugar, and honey are applied as an ointment. *Lodhra*, *elā*, *punarnavā* mixed with honey can also be used as an ointment.

Kapha Blindness—objects appear with a thick cloud-white coating in a dull, oily, hazy, or as though looking through water. This is a progressively developing cataract. *Triphalā* and honey are eaten. Sarsaparilla, dry ginger and dry molasses cakes are applied to the eyes.

Blood Blindness—objects appear red, gray, black, or multicolored, or enveloped in gloom. *Lodhra, triphalā, punarnavā*, rose water applied as a collyrium (black powder). Another therapy is sandalwood, *śhilājit, kesar*, neem gum, and white lotus, made into a collyrium.

Tridoṣha Blindness—objects seem variegated and confused with double or triple vision, with stars and planets appearing broken, or with additional armatures, and floating. *Chandrodaya varti* can probably heal this condition. Otherwise, it cannot be healed.

Pitta/Blood: (*Parimlāyi*) The corners of the sky seem yellow and bright like a sunrise, trees appear to sparkle with lights like fireflies. The same therapies as Pitta cataracts are used here. Should this not balance the *doṣhas*, salves and nasal oils are also applied.

Cataract (*Kācha*) Therapy: This is a corneal calcification preventing persons from seeing.

Vāyu: *Ghee*, milk, and *triphalā* as an eye salve.

Pitta: *Ghee* is used as nose oil and as a meal. *Triphalā* is ingested. *Puta-pāka* and an eye salve of *paṭola patra, punarnavā*, red sandalwood, barberry, *āmalakī,* and *lodhra.*

Kapha: *Triphalā* and sesame oil are cooked together and used as a nasal oil, aromatherapy using *viḍaṅga, paṭola patra, punarnavā,* turmeric, red sandalwood, *āmalakī,* and *lodhra. Ghee* and honey are mixed with these honey. This mixture is applied to the eye as *puta-pāka.*

Tridoṣha: *Triphalā* decoction and licorice are used as a salve, *in puta-pāka* and as food.

Linga-nāṣha (cataract): Surgery is required. Sometimes, therapies of barberry with honey, or *chandrodaya varti* with honey may be helpful.

Vāyu—reddish-looking pupils, circular patches that move around, and are rough to the touch. This cannot be healed.

Pitta—blue, yellow-blue or metal-colored circular patches and pupils. This cannot be healed.

Kapha—whitish pupils circular patches are thick, oily and white, looking like a drop of water. It moves when the eye is rubbed. This cannot be healed.

Blood—blood-red pupils.

Tridoṣha—pupils are multicolored with symptoms of the different *doṣhas*. This cannot be healed.

Pitta/Blood—a blue or yellow blue circular patch, looking like a blade of grass on the pupil. Occasional glimpses of light are possible.

Two forms of *linga-nāṣha* due to trauma also exist. Surgery is contraindicated for these diseases.

1. *Sa-nimitta* (determined origin): Loss of sight resulting from overheating of the brain (causes include inhaled poisons) and toxicity in the blood. The pupil is sunken, pierced, or impaired. *Triphalā ghee* is advised in this condition.

2. *A-nimitta* (undetermined origin): Loss of vision resulting from excessively bright lights, including that of celestial beings. The eye is not outwardly affected. *Triphalā ghee* or *gāmbhārī* flower, licorice, *lodhra,* and barberry are suggested.

Pupil and Crystalline Lens Therapies: Three of these diseases can be healed, three are incurable, and six can only be controlled. The general therapies are again suggested.

<u>Pitta-*Vidaghda-Drishti*</u>: Pupils and objects appear yellowish, persons only have night vision. It is caused by excess Pitta in the third coat. Surgery is contraindicated. All the therapies for Pitta (except surgery) are used here. *Triphalā ghee* is also very good for this condition. *Gāmbhārī* flowers, *licorice*, *lodhra,* and barberry are also suggested.

<u>Kapha-*vidagha-drishti*</u>: Kapha appearing over the three parts of the lens, causing objects to be seen whitish and night blindness. Surgery is contraindicated. All the therapies for Kapha (except surgical operations) are used here. *Traivrita ghee* is very good for this condition. Also, *nirguṇḍī* seed, *elā,* and *pippalī*, mixed with goat's milk is suggested.
For Pitta and Kapha *vidagdha-drishtis*, eye salves are used with myrrh, *pippalī*, pepper, *ashok, triphalā,* and *kapikachhū* mixed with honey.

<u>*Kapha Vidhagha* (night blindness)</u>: Myrrh, *pippalī*, ginger, licorice, *triphalā*, and *balā* are used on the eye and also ingested. A salve consisting of *triphalā*, myrrh, *pippalī*, and cardamom mixed with honey is also useful.

<u>*Dhūma-drishti* or *Dhūma-darshin*</u>
(<u>Smoky vision</u>): Objects seem dusty or smoky resulting from grief, high and prolonged fevers, straining, excessive physical exercise, or head injuries. Surgery is contraindicated. The same healing therapies as Pitta ophthalmia are suggested. *Ghee* is taken internally and externally, therapies for blood/Pitta and Pitta *visarpa* are followed. A Pitta reduction diet is required.

<u>*Hrasva-Jatya* (Day blindness)</u>: Cold weather causes a loss of Pitta that creates difficulty with seeing small objects in the daytime that may easily be seen at night. A combination of myrrh, licorice, *triphalā*, *ghee,* and honey is used as an eye salve.

<u>*Nakulandhyatā*</u>: The pupil seems to emit luminous flashes and day vision appears multicolor. This is treated similarly to night-blindness.

<u>*Gambhirikā* (paralysis of the carrial nerve)</u>: Excess Vāyu contracts the pupil and deforms it, causing it to sink in its socket . It is associated with extreme pain.

<u>Scarifying/Rubbing (*Lekhana*)</u>:
This therapy requires licensed medical care, and will not be discussed in detail here. *Vartmāvabandha, klishta-vartma, bahala-vartma, pothaki* eye diseases are gently scraped, then scarified. *Śhyāva-vartma* and *kardama-vartma* diseases are moderately rubbed (neither too light nor too deep). Small, hard coppery pus pimples that may arise from rubbing are cut. Small and slightly swollen pimples on the exterior eyelid surface are fomented and plastered.

<u>Incisions</u>:
<u>*General*</u>: Before pus develops, oil and light fomentation are administered to the eye. Once pus has developed, therapies for healing an ulcer are used.

<u>*Visha-granthi*</u>: First fomentation is conducted, then holes are cut to remove swelling. This is followed by dusting with myrrh and cardamom powder. *Ghee* and honey are applied over the dust and a loose bandage is applied.

<u>*Upanāha*</u>: The area is opened and rubbed with *pippalī* and myrrh powders mixed with honey. It is then scraped, and the surrounding area is also gently scratched.

<u>Excisions</u>: Only surgeons are qualified to perform exicsions. Diseases requiring excision include *arman, sirā-jāla, sirā-pidakā, parvanikā,* and the inner eyelid.
<u>*Śhukti-pāka*</u>: (Inflammatory diseases, such as blepharitis, styes, conjunctivitis, etc.) The same therapies as Pitta ophthalmia are used, and *triphalā ghee*. An eye salve with cooling herbs (e.g., *musta, viḍaṅga*) is useful for lower eye

disorders.

Arjun and Sulel: General therapies are used.

Eye Therapy Glossary

Triphalā may be ingested and used as an eyewash (after straining). Depending upon the *doṣha* responsible for the illness, herbs are used to reduce the *doṣha* excess.

Soothing (*tarpana*):

These remedies are used in the morning or afternoon after nasal purgation, elimination of stool and digestion of the previous meal. (Technically, the planets should be auspiciously situated.) Persons lie on a bed in a clean, draftless room where the sun does not get in their eyes.

The eyelids are thickly coated with a paste of black *gram* and water and built as a circular wall to surround the eye. *Ghee* and tepid water are poured within the wall, in the eye, up to the eye lashes (see *Netra Basti* in Chapter 7 page 244). Healthy Kapha-, Pitta-, and Vāyu-imbalanced persons should allow the *ghee* to remain in their eyes for 3 periods of time: 8 minutes/20 seconds, 10 minutes, and 16 minutes/20 seconds respectively. Other authorities suggest the length of retention varies according to what part of the eye is affected: *sandhi—-five minutes, vartman*—eight minutes/20 seconds, white (*śhukla*)—11 minutes/45 seconds, black (*kṛiṣhṇa*)—16 minutes/45 seconds. For diseases affecting the entire eye—13 minutes/20 seconds. Still, others say that such eye diseases require 16 minutes/45 seconds, and diseases affecting the puplis require 30 minutes.

The *ghee* is then released through the inner corner of the eye. Kapha becomes excessed in this area and is then relieved by inhaling Kapha-reducing aromas such as cedar, frankincense, or myrrh. This continues for 1, 3, or 5 days for Vāyu, Pitta, and Kapha, respectively, or some say for mild, moderate, and severe symptoms, respectively.

Tarpana is used for symptoms of shriveling or debilitation of the eyelashes, cloudy and dark vision, arched vision, no tears, parched eye, hard eyelids, and severe diseases of the eye.

Precautions: *Tarpana* is not used on cloudy, very hot or very cold days. Persons who are anxious or fearful should not use *tarpana*. Nor should it be used before major symptoms have cleared up.

Puta-pāka:

Three forms exist:

1. Emulsives (*snehana*)—used in very dry conditions.
2. Scraping (*lekhana*)—used when oil is frequently applied to the eye.
3. Healing (*ropana*)—used when eye diseases are healed.

Preparation:

1. Emulsives—*ghee* with *śhatāvarī, balā* and licorice, are held in the eye for 3 minutes/20 seconds.
2. Scraping—*ghee* with *pravāl piṣhti* or salt (scraping properties), and are used for 1 minute/45 seconds.
3. Healing—*ghee*, milk, raw honey, and herbs such as *mañjiṣhṭhā*, barberry, turmeric, neem, *cham-ellī*, sandalwood, *bilwa, ajwan,* and onion. These herbs are kept in the eye for 5 minutes.

Puta-pāka is done from 1 to 3 days, 1 day for Kapha disorders or for scraping measures, 2 days for Pitta eye diseases or emulsive therapy, 3 days for Vāyu eye disorders or healing *puta-pāka*.

Oil, fomentation and aromas are used for emulsives and scraping *puta-pāka*, but not for the healing version. Persons must carefully follow their diets and lifestyles (according to their *doṣha*) for twice as long as the therapy lasts.

Proper use of *tarpana* and *puta-pāka* results in clearing of the symptoms involved, whereas improper use will result in a worsening of vision, pain and other unhealthy symptoms.

Precautions: Follow all the precautions of *tarpana*, nasal evacuatives, and internal oils. After the *doṣhas* are rebalanced, all precautions are met and *tarpana* is applied, *puta-pāka* is then used.

Upon completion of *tarpana*, one should not stare at bright lights, including the sun, a fire, or any luminous object. Further, one is required to prevent wind gusts from hitting the eye. If these precautions are not followed and the eyes are hurt, or if they are hurt from improper *puta-pāka* and *tarpana* remedies, eye salves, drops, nasal evacuatives, aromatherapy, and fomentation can alleviate the troubles.

Procedure: General herbal therapies are used.

Sprinkling (śheka) and Eye drops (āschyotana):

(See Chapter 7- *Pañcha Karma* page 243 for more details). Eye drops are used for mild diseases of the eye, and sprinkling is used for severe symptoms. Three forms of these therapies exist, just like *puta-pāka*,

Scraping (*lekhana*)—7 to 8 drops
Emulsive (*sehana*)—10 drops
Healing (*ropana*)—12 drops

Some say eyedrops are held as long as *puta-pāka*, and sprinkling is held in the eye for twice as long. Others say that both are held in the eye twice as long as *puta-pāka*. Both therapies are applied in the morning, afternoon, or evening (depending upon the *doṣha* imbalanced), or whenever there is eye pain. Again, proper application results in feeling better, whereas improper application results in feeling worse. (This is stated because there is a belief in many holistic circles that detoxification causes one to feel worse before they feel better. This is not so with Āyurvedic therapies, except for some skin conditions).

Head Bladders (*śhiro-basti*): (See Chapter 7—*Pañcha Karma* page 240). This is used for various head disorders. After receiving purgatives and emetics (depending upon the *doṣha* imbalance), and having eaten according to the *doṣhas* imbalanced, persons are ready for *śhiro basti*. In the evening, sitting erect, a bladder or cone that will not leak from oil placed inside it, is placed on the head, and firmly tied around the forehead. Emulsive oil is poured inside the cone, to allow the head to soak in the oil. (Some authorities use various pastes between the cone and the forehead to prevent leaks.) The head is soaked for 10 times or as long as the time the *tarpana* is held in the eye.

Eye salves (*añjana*): There are three forms of eye salves:

1. Scraping (*lekhana*)—herbs used may be of one or more taste, except sweet (i.e., sour, salty, pungent, bitter, astringent). The tastes used will depend upon the *doṣha* imbalanced.

Vāyu: sour and salty
Pitta: astringent
Kapha: pungent, bitter, astringent
Blood: astringent

Dual/Tri-*Doṣhas*—combinations of the tastes

When an excess of the *doṣhas* exists in the eye, eyelids, in the eyeball, its passages and capillaries, and in the nose gristle, they are secreted through the mouth, nostrils, and corners of the eye through the application of scraping salves.

2. Healing (*ropana*)—Herbs used contain bitter and astringent tastes, mixed with a little *ghee*. This cooling therapy brings color and strength to the eye.

3. Invigorating (*prasādana*)—Sweet herbs are used with a large amount of *ghee*. This tones and invigorates the vision.

Punarnavā or *chandrodaya* salves are used in the morning for Kapha disorders, afternoon for Pitta imbalances, and evening with deranged Vāyu. Other authorities say scraping is done in the morning, healing in the afternoon, and invigorating at night. A third opinion to sue them according to the seasonal *doṣhas*.

Salves may be in pill, liquid and powder form, and may be used for serious, moderate, and mild symptoms. A typical dose is 4 to 6 gms

Procedure: The eyelids are made to slant with the left-hand fingers while the salve is applied with the right hand. The salve is applied from the cornea to the *apañga* (corners) and back again (along the inner eyelid). It is repeated two or three times. A rod is used for the inside eyelid, and the finger is used on the outer eyelid. The salve is only thinly pasted in the corners of the eye (from the cornea to the corner) so as not to hurt the area. Only after the *doṣhas* are reduced is the eye to be washed, otherwise the symptoms might be further aggravated. First the eye is washed with water. *Pratyanjana* [sarsaparilla, honey, sugar, licorice, and *relegar mainṣhil* (antimony sulfide) mixed with water] is then used depending upon the *doṣha* imbalanced or one's constitution.

Herbs: *Triphalā*, myrrh, *punarnavā*, *kuṣhṭhā*, sandalwood, cardamom, licorice, *pippalī*, black pepper, *jaṭāmāṇśhī*, *mañjiṣhṭhā*, cedar, *lodhra*, barberry, and *tālīspatra*.

Precautions: *Anjana* is not used when there is fever, *udāvarta*, with head diseases, during anger, grief, fear, crying, intoxication, constipation, or urine retention because it might cause tears, pain, redness, blindness, swelling, or giddiness. It is not to be used with insomnia as it may cause blindness. *Anjana* is not to be used on windy days, as it may cause impairment to the sight. When the eyes have dust or smoke in them, *anjana* may cause redness, ophthalmia, or tears. It is not used after nasal therapies as it may cause aching and eye swelling. Any head disease will be further aggravated by using *anjana*. It is not used before sunrise, after bathing, on very cold days, or with indigestion. When the *doṣhas* are imbalanced, *anjana* should not be used. This is especially true for scraping *anjana*. Instead, these symptoms are treated with washing the eyes with water, drops, plasters, smoke, nasal therapies, and gargles, depending upon the symptoms of the imbalanced *doṣhas*.

As with other therapies, proper application of scraping *anjana* results in improved conditions, whereas improper application (excess or deficient application) results in increased troubles. For improper application, the *anjana* is completely removed through using nasal therapies, *anjana,* and steam therapy.

Invigorating and healing salves are applied properly when the symptoms are soothed. Excess or deficient application results in aggravation of symptoms. To heal excess and deficient application, *puta-pāka*, aromas, and nasal therapies are used.

External Eye Injury
Nayanā-bhighāta- Pratiṣhedha

Causes and Symptoms: Violent, unbearable eye pain with redness and swelling, caused by injury to the eye, or resulting from excess fomentation, smoke, glare, fear. or agony, is healed by nasal therapies, plasters, sprinkling (*seka*), soothing (*tarpana*) measures, *puta-pāka*, and all therapies for Pitta and blood conjunctivitis (*abiṣhyanda*). Cool, sweet, and bulk-promoting herbs are also useful. For excess fomentation, smoke, glare, fear, agony, pain, or injury, these therapies are used during the first week of the disease. Afterwards, therapies identical to those used for conjunctivitis (depending upon the excessed *doṣha*) are employed. Mild conditions may be immediately relieved by applying warm breath fomentation (steam in the mouth).

If ulceration is on only one coating of the eye, it is easily healed. When two coats are affected healing it is difficult. If three coats are affected it cannot be healed. When eye looseness, dislocation, sunkeness, deep impressions, or loss of vision exist, the situation is only containable. Poor vision with pupil dilation, without extreme redness or eyeball dislocation, and good vision are signs that therapies will be helpful.

To raise a sunken eye, holding one's breath, causing vomiting, sneezing, or choking the windpipe is useful. If the eyes are hanging from the sockets, it is reinstalled without damaging the nerves, and gently pressed with the palms (with a lotus leaf between the pupil and the palm). The eye is then filled with a *tarpana* of milk, and medicated *ghee*. This liquid is also used as a nasal therapy. Long breaths of air are taken through the nostrils, and cold water is poured on the head.

Infant Inner Eyelid Disorder (*Kukunaka*-opthalmia): Vāyu, Pitta, Kapha, and blood may become imbalanced owing to poor quality of breast milk. Symptoms include excess itching of the eyes, frequently rubbing the eyes, nose, and forehead with fists. Tears are constant, and sunlight is unbearable.

Therapies first involve blood-letting (with leeches), scraping with rough leaves, and then rubbing with *ṭrikatu* and honey paste. The mother follows therapies described earlier for improving the quality of breast milk. The child should be given black salt, honey, *pippalī*, *jamun* (a black, sweet fruit in India), *āmalakī*, mango leaves and bark, neem, *guḍūchī,* and *ghee* as an emetic. Therapy is stopped when the child begins to vomit.

If the child is drinking breast milk and solid foods, the emetic is given with calamus. For older children no longer drinking breast milk, the emetic is given with rock salt, *apāmārga* (*kapikachhū*) seed, *pippalī*, *mainsphal,* and milk. The eyes are washed and sprinkled, and eye drops of *triphalā* and *guḍūchī ghee* are applied. Salves of black pepper, myrrh, *ṭrikatu*, onion, licorice, neem, turmeric, *lodhra,* and *punarnavā,* pasted with honey and water are useful.

Mouth Cavity (Mukha Roga)

These diseases include the lips (*ūsth*), gums (*dantmūl*), teeth (*dantaka*), tongue (*jihvā*), palate (*tālu-gata*) i.e., tonsillitis, throat/larynx (*kaṇṭa roga*), entire mouth cavity (*savra-sara*).

Diseases covered under this section include gingivitis, tartar, tooth abscess, and laryngitis.

Causes: There are 65 diseases of the mouth cavity: 8 lip disorders, 15 gum problems, 8 tooth ills, 5 tongue concerns, 9 palate complaints, 17 throat conditions, and 3 maladies of the entire cavity.

Two forms of healing are available for all disorders:

Gandūsha: One sits in a darkened room with no draft, while the neck and shoulders are massaged and sudated. The mouth is filled with liquid and held, until there is no room for movement, or until the nose and eyes begin to tear.

Kavala (gargling): The directions are the same as *gandūṣha*, only half the mouth is filled with the liquids, so there is room to gargle. All the herbs and discussed below are used here as well. Either approach can be used, *gandūṣha* or *kavala*.

Therapies*:* Tingling or pains associated with the teeth (*Vāyu excesses*): sesame oil, warm water. (Perhaps the calcium in sesame oil heals tooth and gum problems.) *Triphalā* decoction is one of the best general remedies for oral diseases. It can be used for either *kavala* or *gandūṣha*.

Incurable Mouth Diseases

Mouth: Caused by imbalanced muscle, blood, or tridoṣhic causes:

Gums: Tridoṣhic sinus in the gums (*nāḍī vraṇa*) and tridoṣhic *śhauṣhira* (gingivitis with cavity).

Teeth: *Ṣhyāva-dantaka* (black or blue discoloration on teeth), *dālana* (toothache), and *bhanjana* (chipped tooth).

Tongue: *Alāsa*.

Palate: *Arvuda* (palate cancer).

Throat: *Valaya* (*tumor*), *vṛinda* (large tumor), *balāsa* (sarcoma), *śhataghni* (malignant growths), inflammatory swelling (*vidārī*), tridoṣhic inflammatory swelling (*māṃsatāna*), *rohini.*

Tumors and palate cancer require surgery as well as detoxifying herbs (see Chapter 22). For impacted teeth (*adhimāmsakā*) additional herbs of *vachā, pippalī,* and neem are used, followed by *śhirovirechana*, snuff and inhaling smoke.

For throat edema, tonsillitis, palatal abscess, acute superficial glossitis, gingivitis, dental abscess, goiter, and hyperthyroidism, see the Metabolic System; Chapter 25.

Mouth, and Tooth Disorders (Mukha Roga)

Causes: Over-eating animal products, milk, and yogurt causes gum and tooth disorders, as well as an excess of all three *doṣhas* with a predominance of Kapha.

Lips:

Vāyu causes lips to become rough, hard, immovable, painful, and to develop cracks and fissures.

Pitta excesses cause painful inflammatory elevations with burning. Ulcers and are yellowish.

Kapha increases cause the lips to develop slightly painful elevations (papules). Lips are unctuous, cold, and heavy.

Tridoṣhic excesses cause black, yellow, or white lips, with a bumpy appearance or having several elevations.

Blood (*rakta*) excesses cause red elevations that discharge blood.

Muscle (*māṃsa*) excesses cause lips to become heavy, thick, lumpy, with discharges from the corners of the mouth that contain worms.

Fat (*medas*) excesses cause lips to appear shiny like *ghee*, develop heaviness, and exude large quantities of a clear fluid. Ulcers can form and not heal. Lips do not return to their normal softness.

External injury can cause bleeding, swelling, or itching.

Gum Disorders (Dantamūla Roga)

Bleeding, Spongy Gums (*śhitāda*) with foul smell, blackening, oozing, soft, tearing muscle, and pus formation result from excess Kapha and blood (*rakta*).

Gum Swelling/Gingivitis(*dantapupputaka*) [of 2 or 3 teeth] is also caused by Kapha and *rakta*. See the Metabolic System Chapter (25).

Pus, Blood, Shaky Teeth /Bleeding Gingivitis/Pyorrhea (*dantaveṣhṭa*) are caused by bad blood.

Swelling at the root of a tooth (*śhauṣhira*) causes excess saliva. This is caused by Kapha and *rakta*.

Loose Teeth, Palate Fissure and *śhauṣhira* symptoms (*mahāśhauṣhira*) are caused by all three *doṣhas*. Herbal therapies are not useful for this condition.

Gum Decay and Bleeding (*paridara*) result from excess Pitta, *rakta,* and Kapha.

Burning Gums, Ulcers, Shaky Teeth (*upakuśha*) result from excess Pitta and *rakta*.

Gum Chaffing, Burning, Ulcers, Shaky Teeth (*vaidarbha*) result from trauma.

Extra Tooth [growing over an existing tooth] causes severe pain during growth (*khalivardhana*) results from excess Vāyu.

Irregular or Ugly Teeth (*karāla*) result from excess Vāyu. No therapy exists for this condition.

Large Swelling at Last Molar causes great pain and dribbling saliva (*adhimāṃsaka*) is caused by excess Kapha.

Gum Sinus Ulcers (*nāḍī vraṇa*) [five kinds] are similar to those discussed in Chapter 16, page 405.

Tooth Disorders (Danta Roga)

Toothache (*dālana*) results from excess Vāyu.

Black Holes in Teeth, Bleeding, Swollen, Painful (*krimidantaka*) is caused by excess Vāyu.

Irregular Shape of Face and Teeth (*bhañjanaka*) is caused by excess Vāyu and Kapha.

Sensitive Teeth (*dantaharṣha*) results from excess Pitta and Vāyu.

Tooth Tartar (*dantśharkarā*) results from Pitta and Vāyu. In addition to herbal therapies, scraping, dusting and snuff are required.

Excess Tartar, Flakes and Decay (*kapālikā*). This is very difficult to heal.

Black or Blue Teeth (*śhyāvadantaka*) results from Pitta and *rakta*. Herbal therapies are not useful for this condition.

Gum Abscess (with pus and blood, burning and pain) (*dantavidradhi*) is discussed under Metabolic System, Chapter 25.

Tongue Disorders (Jihwā Roga)

Vāyu excesses cause fissures, loss of sensation, and are leaf-like in appearance.

Pitta excesses cause burning sensations with studded elevations and reddish thorny lesions.

Kapha excesses cause thickness, swelling, and muscular sprouts.

Large Swelling (*alāsa*) has symptoms of excess Kapha and rakta, making it difficult to move the tongue. An ulcer develops at the root of the tongue. This condition cannot be helped with herbs.

Salivary Cyst (*upajihvā*) is a severe swelling under the tip of the tongue caused by Kapha and *rakta*. Symptoms include excess salivation, itching and localized burning sensation. This is discussed in Chapter 25, page 533.

Palate Disorders (Tālugata Roga)

Enlarged uvula (*kaṇṭa śhuṇḍi*) is caused by excess Kapha and *rakta*. Symptoms include thirst, cough, and difficulty swallowing. Herbs are used after surgery.

Hard Swelling (*tuṇḍikerī*) is an advanced stage of enlarged uvula. Symptoms include burning sensation and pus or ulcer.

Soft Swelling (*adhruṣha*) is caused by excess *rakta* with fever and severe pain.

Palatal Tumor (*kachapa*) is caused by excess Kapha. It develops slowly and is painless. See Chapter 22 for cancer therapies.

Palate Cancer (*tāluarbuda*) is a swelling at the palate center caused by excess *rakta*. This condition is painless. Herbs are used after surgery (see Chapter 22).

Benign Tumor (*māṃsa sanghata*) is caused by Kapha it is called *māṃsa-saṅghāta*. This swelling is painless. Herbs are used after surgery (see Chapter 22).

Fatty Cysts (*tālu pupputa*) is caused by Kapha and fat. Small papule sized, it is painless and does not move.

Dryness (*tāluśhoṣha*) results from excess Vāyu. Symptoms include difficulty breathing.

Ulcer (*tālu pāka*) results from excess Pitta.

Throat Disorders (Kaṇṭha Roga)

Rohini : All three *doṣhas* become excessed and invade the muscle tissue (*māṃsa dhātu*) and blood (*rakta*), causing sprouts in the throat that obstruct the throat and may lead to death. Any of the the *doṣhas* can predominate.

—Vāyu excesses cause severe pain over the surface of the tongue (and other symptoms of Vāyu abscess—see Chapter 16)

—Pitta excesses cause sprouts that quickly appear, develop pus and ulcer. These are accompanied by a high fever and other symptoms of Pitta abscess.

—Kapha excesses cause large, hard, immovable sprouts that totally block the throat.

—Tridoṣha (equal strength of the *doṣhas*) cause deeply rooted sprouts. This condition is incurable.

—Rakta sprouts are small, with red papules and symptoms of Pitta abscess.

Small Tumors (*kaṇṭa śhālūka*) are caused by excess Kapha. They are hard, immovable and can only be healed by surgery. Detoxifying herbs are used thereafter for prevention of further growths (see Chapter 22).

Swollen adenoids (*adhijihvā*) is caused by excess Kapha and *rakta,* causing a swelling at the back of the tongue. If pus or ulcer develop, herbal therapy is not useful. Detoxifying herbs are following surgery for prevention of further growths (see Chapter 22).

Tumor (*valaya*) results from excess Kapha and obstructs the passage of food. This condition can not be healed with herbs. Detoxifying herbs are used after surgery for prevention of further growths (see Chapter 22).

Sarcoma (*balāsa*) is caused by excess Kapha and Vāyu causing swelling, difficulty breathing, pain, and vital organ pain. This condition cannot be healed with herbs. Detoxifying herbs are used after surgery for prevention of further growths (see Chapter 22).

Tumor (*ekavrinda*) is a round, elevated swelling with burning sensations, itching, hardness. It does not develop pus or ulcer. It is caused by Kapha and *rakta*. This condition cannot be healed with herbs. Detoxifying herbs are used after surgery for prevention of further growths (see Chapter 22).

Large Tumor (*vrinda*) is caused by Pitta and blood. It is an elevated, round swelling with severe burning sensation and high fever. If Vāyu is involved it is also painful. This condition cannot be healed with herbs. Detoxifying herbs are used after surgery for prevention of further growths (see Chapter 22).

Malignant Growth (*śhataghni*) is a swelling studded with muscle-sprout spikes, causing different kinds of pain and is life-threatening. This condition cannot be healed with herbs. Detoxifying herbs are used after surgery for prevention of further growths (see Chapter 22).

Tonsillitis (*galāyu*) See the Metabolic System—Chapter (25).

Pharyngeal abscess (*gala vidradhi*) is caused by all three *doṣhas* and is associated with swelling and different kinds of pains.

Sore Throat (*galaugha*) is a swelling that obstructs the swallowing of food, water, and breathing, and is accompanied with fever. It is caused by excess Kapha and *rakta*.

Laryngitis (*svaraghna*) symptoms include difficult breathing, darkness of vision, dryness, hoarseness, loss of movement of the throat. The air passage is obstructed by Kapha (saliva). It is caused by Vāyu.

Inflammatory Swelling (*māṃsatāna*) is wide, severely painful, and can become life-threatening as the swelling begins to expand into the throat. It is caused by all three *doṣhas*.

Inflammatory Swelling (*vidārī*)
—Vāyu symptoms include painful papules that cover the throat.
—Pitta symptoms include burning sensation, pricking pain, coppery colored, with muscle decay. Papules are red or yellow, and thin.
—Kapha symptoms include painless papules and itching.

Sense Organs : Hearing

external ear

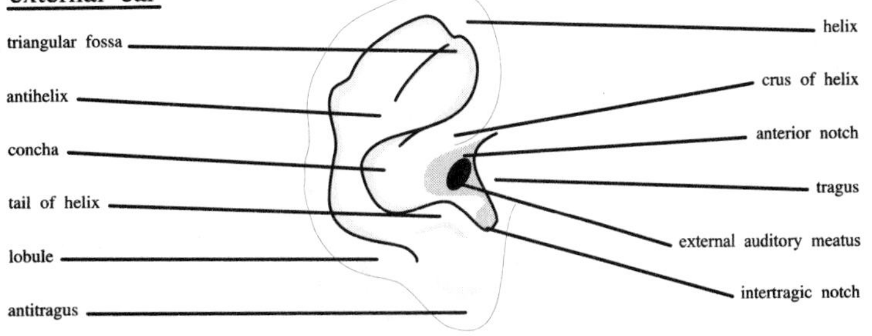

internal and middle ear

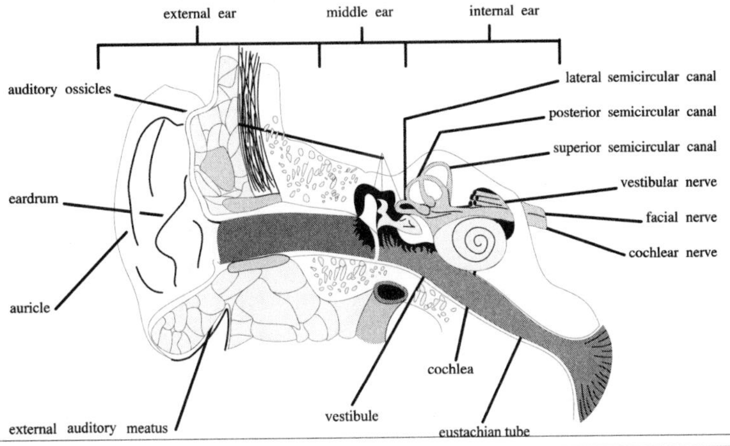

Sense Organs: Smell

External Nose

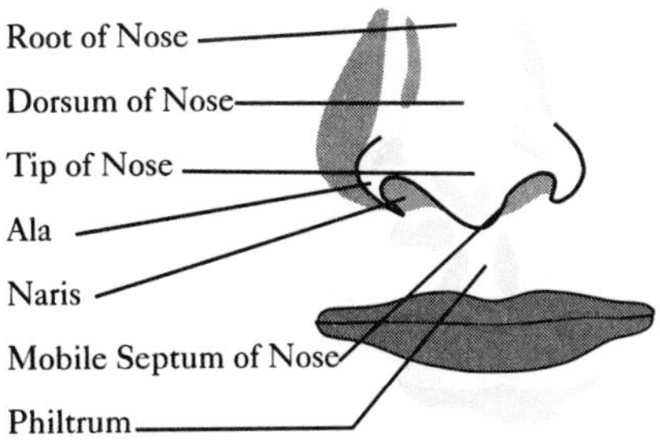

Nasal Fossae

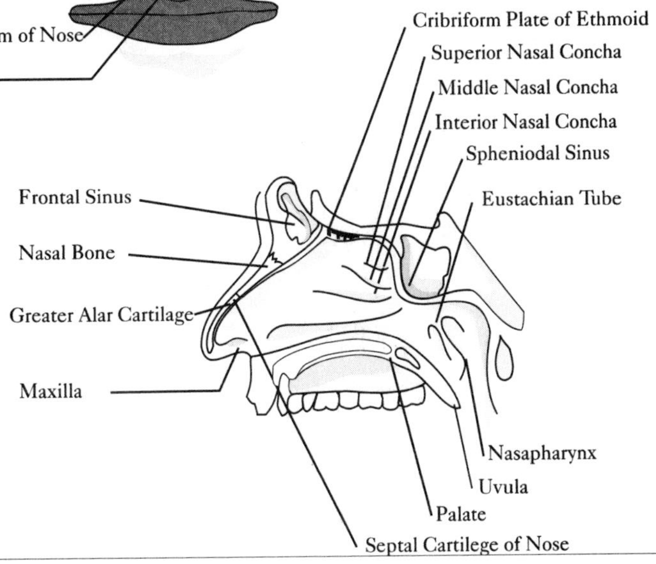

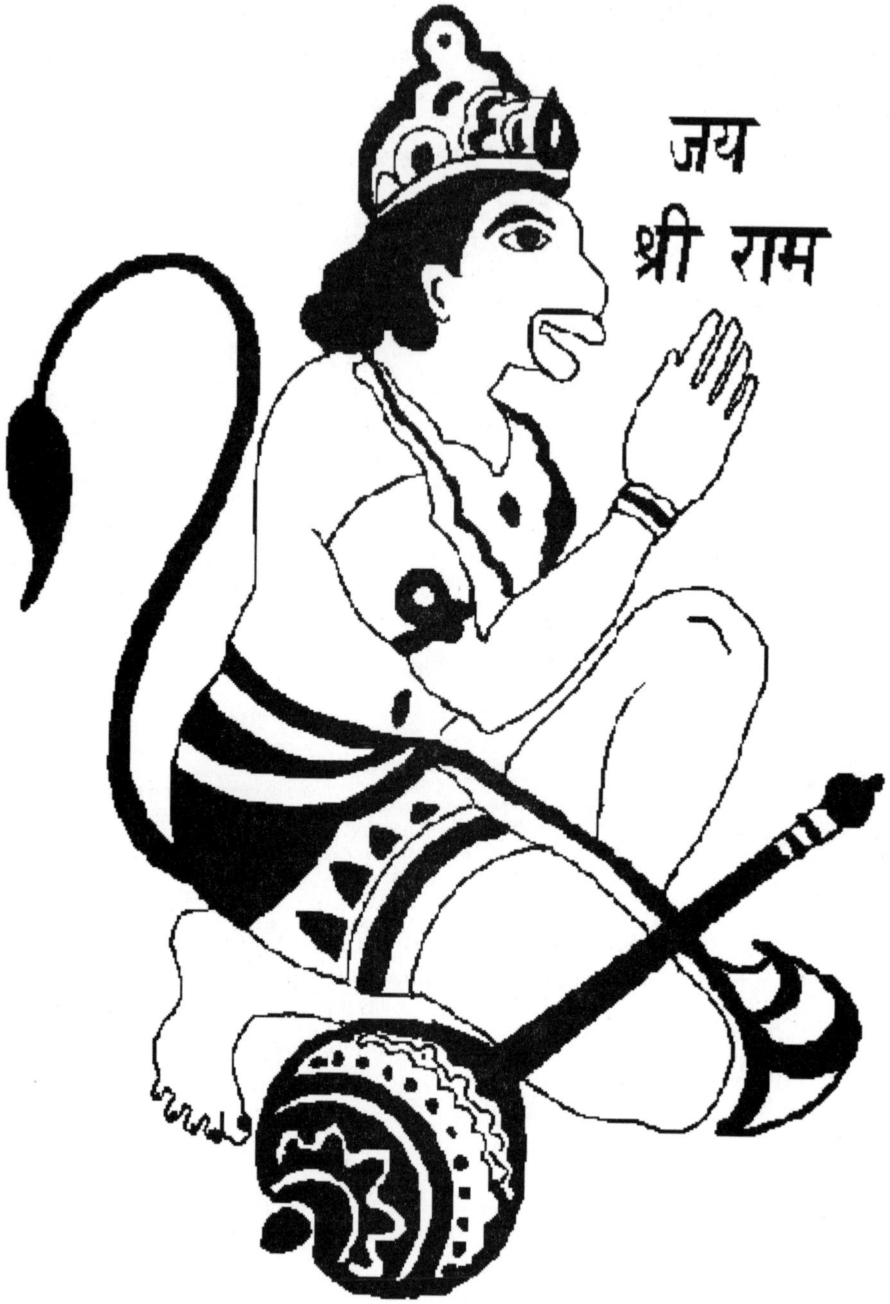
जय
श्री राम

Persons whose Vāyu is in balance live 100 years without disease.
Mādhava Nidānam - Ch. 22; ver. 80

Chapter 20
Nervous System (Vāta-vyādhi)
Convulsions, Sciatica, Insanity, Epilepsy, Addictions, Alcohol, Fainting, Coma, Wasting, Multiple Sclerosis, Parkinsons, Alzheimers

As Vāyu is the sustainer of life, those whose Vāyu flows properly will live a long and healthy life. The five forms of Vāyu governing the various physical and mental movement of air have been previously discussed. They are repeated here, to show how the Vāyu sub-*doṣhas* can afflict the nervous system.

Vāyu	Location	Controls
Prāṇa	head, chest, throat, tongue, mouth, nose	digestion, breathing, belching, sneezing spitting, heart function
Udāna	navel, chest, throat	speech, effort, energy, complexion, aspiration, memory
Samāna	sweat, *doṣhas*, fluid, small intestine	digestion
Vyāna	entire body	circulation, muscle and joint movement, blinking, secretions
Apāna	colon, genitals, urinary bladder, navel, thighs, anus	semen, urine, stool, menses, fetus

If any of the Vāyus is imbalanced, or moves to the wrong channel, the body becomes afflicted with various disorders that can be life-threatening.

Cause: Vāyu is the vital nerve-force that pervades the entire body. It is considered identical to Divine eternal energy and is, therefore, self-generating. Vāyu is at the root of all nervous disorders. Causes include cold, roughness, lightness, little or no food, excessive sex, talking or staying up late; or excessive release of toxins and blood. Other causes are leaping, jumping, traveling, or exercise in excess, wasting of the tissues, excessive emaciation from anxiety, grief, fear, or illness. Further causes are uncomfortable beds and chairs, anger, naps, fear, suppressing natural urges, *āma* (toxins), injury, fasting, injuring vital organs, or accidents. Vāyu becomes excessed, filling the body channels, causing disorders associated with those body parts.

As tissues become depleted, Vāyu fills the channels with air, or become mixed with the other *doṣhas* that have filled the channels. A second way Vāyu becomes excessed is by increasing the functioning of the channels. When Vāyu is the only cause of vitiation, the result is more severe; when it is mixed with Pitta or Kapha, it is not as powerful.

Development: Vāyu accumulates in its home site, the colon, causing colic, gas, gurgling, feces obstruction, urinary stones, herniated scrotum, hemorrhoids, sharp pain the back and waist, and other difficult diseases related to the lower body parts.

Symptoms: Excess Vāyu causes contraction, stiff joints, hands, back, or head; tearing of bones or joints, hair standing on end, delirium, limping, crippling, humpback, organ dryness, and insomnia. It also causes organ numbness, crookedness of the head, nose, eyes, neck, and clavicular area; miscarriage, destruction of sperm or ovum, pulsation, tearing or piercing pain, distress, convulsions, confusion, and exhaustion.

When Vāyu becomes aggravated

In the Whole Body (Sarvānga): Symptoms include tremors, twitching, pulsating, cutting pain, joint pain

In the Abdomen/Alimentary Tract/ Bowels (Koṣhṭhā-ṡhrita): Symptoms include obstruction to the passage of urine and feces; abdominal tumor, heart disease, hemorrhoids, and rib pain.

In Rectum (Gudāṡhrita): Urine, stool, and gas retention; colic, urinary stones or gravel, abdominal distention, pain and emaciation in legs, calves, thighs, pelvis, sacrum, feet, and back can develop.

In Stomach and Small Intestine (Āmāṡhaya): Person's experience pain in the heart, navel, ribs, and abdomen; thirst, belching, cough, dry throat and mouth, difficult breathing, vomiting, vertigo, and epilepsy.

In Colon (Pakvāṡhaya): Experiences include intestinal gurgling, colic, meteorism, difficulty passing stool and urine, bowel hardness, piercing pain in the navel area and sharp pain in waist and back. Other experiences include hemorrhoids, cough, indigestion with vomiting and diarrhea simultaneously; herniated scrotum, thirst, vomiting, and difficult breathing. Further symptoms include throat obstruction, scanty and painful urination and stool (or complete stoppage); excess belching, coccyx, pain and diseases related to the body above the navel.

In Sense Organs (Indriyagata): Loss of sensation (e.g., ears, eyes)

In Skin (Twak): Symptoms include rough, cracked, numb, and thin skin; redness, joint pain, dryness, discoloration, and twitching. This leads to tingling and piercing skin pain, with cracks and fissures.

In Blood (Raktagata): Persons experience severe pain and heat, poor complexion, thinness, anorexia, body pimples, indigestion, loss of sensation, redness, ulceration, loss of appetite, emaciation, and dizziness.

In Muscles (Māṃsagata): Symptoms include nodes and tumors with severe pain and hardness, exertion, heaviness, and rigidity.

In Fat (Medogata): Persons develop painless tumors with ulcers.

In Marrow (Majjāgata): Symptoms include drying of bones, causing constant pain throughout the body and insomnia.

In Bones (Asthigata): Experiences include thigh, bone, and joint breaking pain; loss of strength, wasting, cracking, and bursting.

In Semen/Ovum (Ṡhukragata): One experiences premature ejaculation or retention of semen and fetus (including abnormal fetus).

In Tendons: Symptoms include sciatica, tetanus, and hunch back.

In Ligaments (Snāyu): Cramps, humpbacked, neck, torso, and back problems (opisthotonus, emprosthotonus) are symptoms of this disorder.

In Veins/Arteries - Blood vessels (Sirāgata): Persons experience mild pain, dry swellings, emptiness, tremors, stiffness or constriction, and neuralgia.

In Joints (Sandhigata): One experiences air-filled swellings and pain when moving limbs.

Convulsions (Ākshe-paka)

Vāyu excesses cause convulsions, drying of hands, feet, blood vessels, ligaments, tendons, and hips. Symptoms include frequent jerky movements of the body. This disease cannot be healed if it lasts longer than one year. All convulsive disorders are experienced intermittently.

In Half the Body: When excess Vāyu is in one half of the body, it dries up the blood, hands, legs, and knees. The limbs and tissues are also contracted. This results in the face, nose, eyebrows, forehead, eyes, and jaw becoming crooked. The tongue is raised; the voice is hoarse, weak, and speech is hindered. It causes loose teeth, impaired hearing, pains in the foot, eye, leg, temple, ear, and cheek. These symptoms occur in either half of the body or the face (facial paralysis).

Throughout Body: The lower body is first affected, then, the upper extremities and head, or the whole body are affected; deranging all the tissues. Persons experience numbness or paralysis, limb convulsions and contractions, pricking, splitting, throbbing, cutting pain, stiffness, convulsions, tremors, and swelling.

In the Neck Carotid Arteries/Nerves - Stiff Neck (Manyāsthambha): Vāyu can become excessed alone or with Kapha from day naps, irregular posture or looking in an upward direction for a long time.

—*Āñtarāyāma*: *Stiff arteries/nerves at the side of the neck (manyā dhamanis)*. Experiences include neck bending inwards, stiff carotid arteries throughout the body; shoulder constriction, grinding of teeth, salivation, the back bending inward like a bow, stiff head, yawning, and lockjaw. It also causes convulsions, loss of eye movement, vomiting of mucus, rib pain, and difficulty speaking.

In the Back - Opisthotonos (Vahirāyāma): When excess Vāyu dries up the external vessels of the back and carotid arteries, it causes back stiffness that results in one bending outward or downward. The head leans backwards. The chest is pushed upwards. Carotid arteries are stiff, and the neck is bent downward. There is grinding teeth, discoloration of teeth and mouth, yawning, salivation, loss of speech, excess sweating, physical debility, restlessness. It may be life-threatening.

Convulsions and Unconsciousness (Apatantraka): When aggravated Vāyu becomes obstructed in its downward movement, it starts moving upwards, causing pain in the heart, head, and temples, making the body bend like a bow. One experiences convulsions and loss of consciousness. Other symptoms include difficult breathing, wide-eyed (without blinking) or eyes completely closed, and cooing sounds. Causes include abortion, heavy bleeding, and trauma. Healing is difficult. Long-term conditions cannot be healed.

Convulsions and Consciousness (Apatānaka): This is a similar condition to *apatantraka*. Symptoms include eyes having a fixed gaze, unconsciousness, cooing, intermittent relief. Healing is difficult. Long-term conditions cannot be healed.

Vāyu/Kapha Body Paralysis (Dandaka): When excess Vāyu further develops an excess of Kapha, both *doṣhas* overflow into all the body's channels, filled with undigested food toxins (*āma*), it makes the body stiff (like a wood log) with paralysis. A major symptom is jaw bone paralysis. Healing is very difficult, if not impossible.

Tetanus (Dhanustambha): Excessed Vāyu causes the body to bend in a bow shape.

—*Inner-Bending Bow* (*Abhyanthrāyāma*); When the excessed Vāyu affects the nerves and tendons located in the toes, heels, abdomen, heart area, chest, and throat, it causes severe convulsive movements. Other symptoms include fixed gaze, stiff lower jaw, withdrawn ribs, vomiting mucus, and the body bending inwards.

—*Outer-Bending Bow* (*Bāhyāyāma*); When Vāyu affects the tendons and nerves of the external body parts, persons develop outward bending (of the front portion of the body), degeneration (dystrophy) of the chest, waist, and thighs. This cannot be healed.

Trauma/Hemorrhage (Vraṇāyāma): When the *doṣhas* become aggravated in wounds on vital organs by Vāyu, they spread throughout the body and produce convulsions. Symptoms include thirst and a yellowish-white complexion. This is a very serious condition. Any or all of the *doṣhas* can become excessed.

Convulsions caused by abortion, trauma, or excessive bleeding cannot be healed.

Tongue Difficulties (Jihvā-sthambha): When Vāyu is caught in the tendons, nerves, and veins, near the vocal cords, it causes paralysis of the tongue with consequent inability to swallow and speak.

Lock-Jaw (Hanusramsa): Loose jaw or lockjaw. Owing to excess tongue scraping, eating dry foods and trauma, Vāyu becomes localized and excessed at the lower jaw. This displaces the lower jaw, making it stay open or closed, causes chewing and speaking difficulties. Healing is difficult. Long-term conditions are incurable.

Facial Paralysis (Ardita): Vāyu becomes excessed and localized in the upper body from carrying heavy loads on the head, excess laughing, speaking, facial exertion (e.g., mimicking), sneezing, physical strain, sleeping on uneven or hard pillows, and chewing very hard foods. Symptoms include irregularities in half of the face (especially during laughing and with sight). The head begins to shake. Premonitory symptoms include speech obstructions, loss of eye movement, tremors, teeth shaking, hoarseness, deafness, blocked sneezing, loss of smell and memory, delusions, exhaustion during sleep, saliva coming out of the mouth during sleep, one eye becomes closed, severe pain above the shoulders, half of the body, or in lower body. When this disorder exists in emaciated persons for over 3 years, who can not wink and slur their speech, it is incurable.

In Blood and Veins (Sirāgraha): Vāyu becomes excessed in the blood and veins of the head, causing them to shrink, become hard, painful, and black. This disorder is difficult to heal or may not be healed.

Hemiplegia - Half of the Body Veins and Tendons (Pakṣhavadha or Ekāṅgaroga): Vāyu becomes excessed in half of the body, drying the veins and tendons by loosening the joints. The result is the loss of function and tactile sensation.

—*Whole Body Paralysis (Sarvāñgaroga)*: As above, when Vāyu affects the entire body, the disorder is difficult to heal. The involvement of excess Pitta and Kapha render this condition incurable.

Pitta symptoms include burning sensation, increased temperature of the affected body parts, and fainting. Kapha symptoms include cold, swelling and heaviness of the affected body parts.

Pakṣhavadha caused by Vāyu is difficult to heal. When it is caused by Vāyu and other *doṣhas*, it is easy to heal. Symptoms of emaciation or wasting cannot be healed. When *Pakṣhavadha* is found in pregnant women, women who have just given birth, the elderly, emaciated person, caused by excessive bleeding, or experiencing no sensation at all in the affected limb, treatment should not be attempted.

Shoulder Caused Arm Paralysis (Apabā-huka): Vāyu situated at the shoulder's roots constrict the tendons, nerves, and veins, and cause emaciation of the local muscles. Loss of arm movement develops.

Hand Caused Arm Paralysis (Vishvā-chī): Tendon constriction in the palms and fingers and back of the arm, leads to loss of arm functioning.

Leg Paralysis (Khañja/Paṅgu): Vāyu localized in the thighs and waist constricts these tendons causing lameness to either one (*khañga*) or both (*paṅgu*) legs.

Leg Obstructions (Kalā-vakhañja): Symptoms include trembling legs and pain when beginning to walk, as well as limping and loose joints. This is caused by eating peas or lentils.

Stiff Thighs (Ūru-sthambha): Excesses of Vāyu, Kapha, fat, and undigested food toxins are caused by overeating cold, hot, moist, dry, heavy, fatty, cooked or raw foods, overexertion, debility, not sleeping, or oversleeping. This results in the accumulation of *doṣhas* and toxins in the thighs, filling the interior of the thigh bone with Kapha. The thigh becomes stiff and inactive, cold, senseless, heavy, and with severe pain. Symptoms include, excessive belching, worry, body aches, inactivity, stupor, vomiting, loss of appetite and taste, fever, weakness in the feet, difficulty lifting, and loss of the sense of touch.

Knee Swelling (Kroshṭuka Śhīrṣha): Vāyu and blood becoming excessed, produces a swelling in the middle of the knee that is very painful and large.

Ankle Pain (Vāta-kaṇṭaka): Vāyu accumulates in the ankle joint or heel owing to walking improperly or by overexertion, causing severe heel or ankle pain.

Finger/Toe Contraction (Khalli): The legs, thighs, calves, chest, and arm contraction and pain.

Foot Sleeping (Pāda-harṣha): Experiences include tingling sensations in the feet (i.e., loss of tactile sensations or it feels like pins and needles.) This is caused by Kapha and Vāyu.

Burning Soles (Pāda-dāha): Vāyu, Pitta, and blood cause burning sensations in the soles of one involved in excess walking.

Nasal/Stammering (Minminatwa/Gadgadatwa): Excess Vāyu and Kapha invade the vessels of the voice box, causing muteness, talking through the nose, or stammering.

Cutting Pain in Rectum, Bladder, Groin (Tūnī): When excess Vāyu moves in a downward direction, severe cutting pain is experienced in these areas.

Cutting Colon Pain (Pratitūni): When excess Vāyu moves in an upward direction, the pain is felt in the colon.

Lower Abdominal Distention (Adhmāna): Excess Vāyu causes obstructed gas that develops intestinal gurgling, severe pain, and distention of the lower abdomen.

Upper Abdominal Distention (Pratādhmāna): When excess Vāyu and Kapha are involved the above symptoms are felt in the stomach (but not in the heart or rib area).

Prostate Tumor/No Pain (Aṣhṭila): A tumor obstructs the passage of feces and urine. Also see Chapter 18.

Prostate Tumor/Pain (Pratyaṣhṭila): A tumor obstructs the passage of gas, feces, and urine, and causes pain. Also see Chapter 18.

Tremors (Vepathu): Vāyu excesses throughout the body cause tremors (including tremors of the head).

Should any of these diseases not subside within 5 years, they cannot be healed.

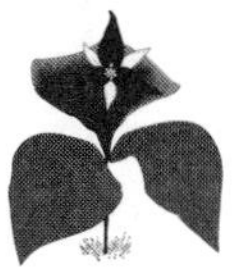

Sciatica (Gṛidhrasī)

Excesses of Vāyu either alone or with Kapha cause difficulty and severe pain in the lumbar region down through the thighs, knees, calves, and feet. Vāyu causes rigidity, throbbing, pricking pain, intermittent symptoms, irregular shape of body parts, and severe stiffness of the knee and waist. Kapha symptoms include stupor, heaviness, poor digestion, salivation, and aversion to food.

Dual Doṣhas

When Vāyu enters the origin sites of Pitta and Kapha (small intestine or stomach), mixed symptoms occur.

Vāyu/Pitta: Burning, heat, thirst, fainting, and other Vāyu diseases related to that part of the body can develop.

Vāyu/Kapha: Symptoms include coldness, swelling, heaviness in the associated area of the body.

Vāyu/Blood: Pricking pain that is unbearable to touch, or numbness, and other Pitta symptoms occur.

Prāṇa Vāyu/Pitta: Vomiting, burning, and other Pitta symptoms develop.

Prāṇa Vāyu/Kapha: Symptoms include weakness, lassitude, skin discoloration, loss of taste, and appetite.

Udāna Vāyu/Pitta: Burning, fainting, epileptic fit, giddiness, vertigo, or fatigues develops.

Udāna Vāyu/Kapha: Symptoms include lack of perspiration, goose bumps, poor digestion, coldness, and numbness in the related body parts.

Samāna Vāyu/Pitta: Excess perspiration, heat, burning, or epilepsy develops.

Samāna Vāyu/Kapha: Experiences include excess mucus, urine and feces, hair standing on end.

Apāna Vāyu/Pitta: Heat, burning, and menorrhagia can develop.

Apāna Vāyu/Kapha: Heaviness of lower limbs can occur.

Vyāna Vāyu/Pitta: Symptoms include limbs burning and jerking, and fatigue.

Vyāna Vāyu/Kapha: Persons can develop heaviness of limbs, stiff or numb bone joints, and can find it difficult to move or walk.

Vertigo: This is caused by constipation. Vāyu presses bile into the heart and the heart presses air into the head. Thus, it is a disease of Vāyu and Pitta.

Vāyu—loss of hearing, suffocating, dry nose, and tongue. *Brāhmī* (gotu kola) is helpful.

Pitta—burning eyes. *Brāhmī, śhankh puṣhpī, and śhatāvarī* are useful.

Other therapies: *Śhiro basti* and *urd dal* for brain and semen building/balancing are advised. *Shad bindu* oil is used in the nose.

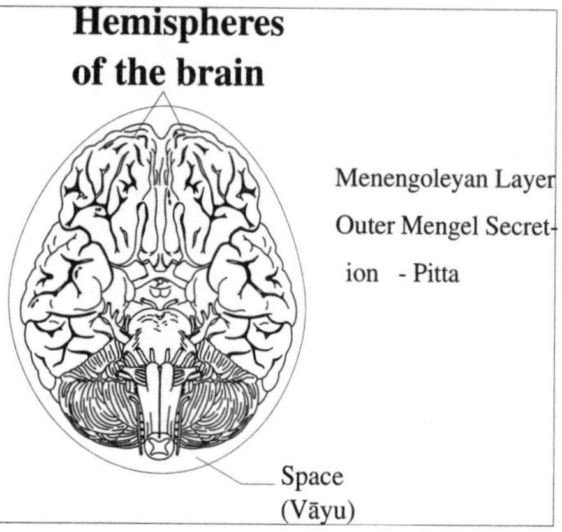

Figure 1

Vāyu causes excesses of Pitta and Kapha and result in dual *doṣha* disorders.

Vāyu/Pitta: Symptoms include burning, thirst, pain, giddiness, darkness, desire for cold things; burning is exacerbated by eating and drinking hot, pungent, sour, and salty things.

Vāyu/Blood: Persons experience burning, distress, and the area between the skin and muscles become red, swollen, and rashes develop.

Vāyu/Kapha: The above symptoms are experienced along with drowsiness, heaviness, and anorexia.

Vāyu/Muscle: Symptoms include hard, discolored boils, swelling, hair standing on end, a feeling like ants are crawling on the body.

Vāyu/Fat: Persons experience anorexia, shifting, oiliness, softness and cold swellings of body parts. This is difficult to heal.

Vāyu/Bone: One desires hot compresses and massage and experiences breaking and piercing pain, sickliness.

Vāyu/Marrow: Bending, yawning, cramps, and pains (eased when pressed) develop.

Vāyu/Semen-Ovum: Semen is either excessive or not emitted; sterility occurs.

Vāyu/Food: One experiences abdominal pain when eating; pain disappears when stomach is empty.

Vāyu/Urine: Urinary retention, bladder bursting.

Vāyu/Stool: Symptoms include constipation, anal/rectal cutting pain. Oily items are quickly digested; hard bowels occur after meals; pain occurs in hip, groin, and back; Vāyu moves backwards; the heart becomes weak.

Therapies: Certain symptoms can be healed if they have recently developed or if persons are strong. Symptoms include joint displacement, lockjaw, contraction, humped-back, paralysis of one or both sides of the body; wasting of limbs, marrow and bone disorders, stiffness. Depending upon how deeply they are located will determine how easy or difficult they are to heal.

When Vāyu is excessed without Pitta or Kapha and is easily reached, *ghee* and oil (internally and externally) soothe the nervous system. Unction quickly nourishes the dried body tissues, promoting strength, digestion, weight gain, and vital breath. Unction is given until one feels they have had enough, then some time is allowed to pass without taking unction. Unction is again taken, this time, with boiled milk, vegetable soup, rice, and milk (cooked with *āmalakī* and black salt), oil enema, snuff, and moist foods. When persons are well-saturated, they then begin fomentation. After massage, oil fomentation is taken. These measures are said to make even crooked or stiff limbs pliable again. This has been seen to occur in persons afflicted with Parkinsonism. Piercing pain, distress, dilation, swelling, seizures, hair standing on end, and other nerve-caused disorders (e.g., worry-caused dysuria) are quickly pacified. Unction and sudation are frequently administered. Once bowels are softened from unction, Vāyu disorders are quickly resolved.

Impurities develop from undigested fatty, sour, salty, and hot foods, that block Vāyu in the channels. If excess impurity exists and the disorder is not healed by the above therapies, persons should take mild, oil purgatives (e.g., castor oil) to assist the evacuation process. Warm carminative herbs, such as cardamom, ginger, cinnamon, cloves, and turmeric, help dispel gas, improve digestion, and assist absorption of undigested foods that cause impurities. Weak persons use non-oil enemas and digestive herbs, and foods instead of purgatives.

General: Therapies include *ghee*, sesame oil, Vāyu-reducing foods and lifestyle, aromatherapy using sandalwood oil on the forehead, hot-oil head massages (*śhiro dhārā/śhiro basti*); gotu kola oil (3 drops) in the nose, then gently massaged; baths and sprinklings (on the afflicted body part and after massage) with decoctions of the herbs listed below. Poultices made from the herbs and foods listed below, may be wrapped around the affected body part.

Herbs: *Vaṃśha lochana*, *guggul*, *harītakī*, *brāhmī*, *gokṣhura*, *aśhwagandhā*, *bibhītakī*, *bhṛiṅgarāj*, *balā*, cedar, *daśhmūl*, *tṛikatu*, and *brāhmī ghee* are useful.

Foods: Almonds (soaked overnight and peel the skin), sesame tahini, *ghee*, sesame oil, boiled milk, black *dal*, whole wheat, and barley are suggested. Yogurt/water (*lassi*) mixed with *tṛikatu* is also useful in soothing nerves.

In Belly: Suggestions include *āmalakī* and *triphalā* (sours and laxatives) mixed with carminative herbs to reduce malnutrition.

In Anus, Rectum and Colon: Herbs to reverse excess upward moving air are used. This includes *hiṅg*, *ajwan*, black salt, *chitrak*, ginger, and black pepper. A castor oil purgative and basti are advised.

In Stomach: If strong, emesis is first done. Vāyu-reducing herbs and foods are used. *Chitrak* and *kaṭukā* are also advised.

Throughout Body: Massage, and non-oil and oil enemas are used.

In Skin: Sudation, massage, bath, and delicious foods reduce Vāyu in the skin.

In Blood: Cold applications, purgation, and blood-letting are useful.

In Muscle and Fat (or with Āma): Fomentation, *abhyañga*, poultice, non-oil enema, milk, *ghee*, and pacifying therapies are used.

In Bone and Marrow: Internal and external unction are needed. Bones may need to be bound.

In Semen/Ovum: Foods and herbs to promote semen (e.g., almonds, tahini, boiled milk, *śhatāvarī*, *aśhwagandhā*) are required. However, if blocks in the seminal passage occur, purgatives are first used to remove the obstruction. Sitting in baths or sprinkled with water—both include Vāyu-reducing herbs—is advised.

For Dry Fetus Or Child: Boiled milk with cane sugar are suggested.

In Urine/Bladder: Diuretics like *gokṣhura* and steamed vegetables are helpful; urethral douche, oiling the body, poultices with Vāyu-reducing herbs, *abhyañga*, plasters, and fomentation are advised.

In Stool: Castor oil purgative, foods, and herbs to reduce Vāyu are used.

In Heart: Boiled milk with *arjuna*, *chitrak*, *pippalī*, *triphalā*, and black salt.

In Navel Area: *Bilwa*, *chitrak*, and *ajamodā* are advised.

For Twisting: Poultices with Vāyu-reducing herbs are pressed on the twisted body parts.

For Contractions: Sesame oil cooked with black *dal*, sesame oil, and rock salt are massaged into the disorder.

In Arms and Head: Snuff and ingesting *ghee* after meals is helpful.

Below the Navel: Juice enemas and snuff alleviate these conditions. Herbs include ginger and *nirguṇḍī* decoctions.

For Facial Paralysis: Snuff, head oil massage (*śhiro dhārā/śhiro basti*—around 16 minutes), tube fomentation and poultices with *ghee*, *aśhwagandhā*, ginger, *tṛikatu*, *nirguṇḍī*, *guggul*, *kuṭki*, *kūt*, and *brāhmī* are used.

For Paralysis of One Side: Sudation, unction, and purgation are recommended.

For Cramps: Hot poultices of boiled rice-milk, or cooked rice-bean, with oil or *ghee* are advised.

For Sciatica: *Haṭha yoga* leg and back stretches (see Chapter 9), and herbs of *pippalī*, *gokṣhura*, and *balā* are taken.

For Lock-Jaw: Open mouth—foment the jaw,

then press jaw with thumbs and lift the chin up to close the mouth. Displaced—adjust to proper placement. Stiffness—foment, then bend.

Vāyu/Pitta: Cold and hot measures are alternately applied; purgation, and licorice are added to the general therapies listed above.

Vāyu/Kapha: Barley, sudation, strong, dry enemas, purgation, and mustard oil are used along with Kapha-reducing therapies listed above. When this excess is in the head, snuff and herbal smoking is advised.

Tridoṣhic: Pitta is pacified before Kapha. When Pitta spreads over the entire body, purgation is used. When Kapha moves to the stomach, emesis is advised. Enemas are used after Kapha becomes liquefied through fomentation, and once Pitta symptoms appear. When Pitta and Kapha are removed, yet Vāyu remains in the respiratory channels, the above Vāyu-reducing therapies are used.

Afflictions of the Five Vāyus

Each of the five Vāyus may afflict the other four, creating 20 different symptoms.

For heart diseases and painful stomach: *Ghee* with *chitrak*, *tṛikatu*, *triphalā,* and *hiṅg* are beneficial.

Prāṇ covers Vyāna: Symptoms include vacant senses, weakened intellect, memory, and strength; senselessness, and loss of speaking. *Balā* oil and *amridadya* are used.

Vyāna covers Prāṇ: Symptoms include excess sweating, skin diseases, numb body parts, hair standing on end. Castor oil purgatives are advised.

Samāna covers Prāṇ: Symptoms include abdominal pain, digestive disorder (*grahanī*), rib, heart, and stomach pain disorders. *Ghee* with appetizing herbs (e.g., cardamom and cinnamon) are suggested.

Prāṇ covers Samāna: Persons experience feeling stunned, stammering, and dumbness. Unction is used internally for massage and in snuff; and enemas are recommended. When acute headaches, respiratory problems, heart disease, and a dry mouth develop, smoking herb and consoling the patient are advised.

Prāṇ covers Udāna: Symptoms include a stiff head, cold, and mucus, difficult breathing, heart disorders, dry mouth, sweating, skin diseases, and the organs seem dead. For these conditions, therapies include oily laxatives (e.g., *ghee* or castor oil).

Udāna covers Prāṇ: One experiences a loss of immunity, strength, activity, complexion; this may be life threatening. Sprinkling with cold water, consolation, and giving all comforts desired are the therapies used.

Prāṇ covers Apān: Experiences include vomiting and difficult breathing. Enemas with raspberry; carminative herbs with *harītakī* for vomiting and breathing, respectively, are advised.

Apān covers Prāṇ: Symptoms include confusion, weakened digestion, diarrhea. Emesis and appetizing and astringent foods and herbs are best.

Vyāna covers Apān: Persons experience vomiting, abdominal distention, tumors, distress, cutting pain. Unction is the best remedy.

Apān covers Vyāna: Experiences include excessive stool, urine, and semen. Astringent herbs and foods are required.

Samāna covers Vyāna: Symptoms include fainting drowsiness, delirium, illness, poor digestion, immunity, and strength. Physical exercise and light foods are needed.

Udāna covers Vyāna: Experiences include stiffness, poor digestion, no sweating, less activity, inability to keep the eyes opened. Wholesome, moderate-sized, light meals are most useful.

In the "*Chikitsā-sthānam*" section of *Charak Saṃhitā*, these 12 combinations are listed to illustrate how the five Vāyus combine and what therapies are used. Based on this, *Charak* suggests one carefully consider the symptoms and therapy for the remaining combinations. One needs to remember is that *Prāṇ* should be carefully protected owing to its delicate location. *Udāna* is led upwards, *apān* downwards, *samāna* in the middle, and, *vyāna* in all directions.

Pitta covers Prāṇ: Symptoms include fasting, burning in the body parts or organs, giddiness, pain, desiring cold things, and vomiting partially digested foods.

Kapha covers Prāṇ: Symptoms include spitting, sneezing, belching, respiratory problems, anorexia, and vomiting.

Pitta covers Udāna: Experiences are, fainting, burning in the navel and chest areas, exhaustion, depletion of *ojas*, sickliness.

Kapha covers Udāna: Symptoms include a poor complexion, speech problems, debility, heaviness, anorexia.

Pitta covers Samāna: Experiences include excess sweating, thirst, burning, fainting, restless, and heat disorders.

Kapha covers Samāna: Lack of sweat, poor digestion, hair standing on end, and very cold body limbs can develop.

Pitta covers Vyāna: Burning throughout the body, exhaustion, restricted movements, pyrexia, and pain can occur.

Kapha covers Vyāna: Symptoms include heaviness, joint and bone pain; movement is greatly restricted.

Pitta covers Apān: Experiences include deep yellow urine and stool; heat in the anus and genitals; excess menstrual discharge.

Kapha covers Apān: Persons experience stools passed in pieces with *āma,* mucus, and heaviness.

Kapha covering *Prāṇ* and *Udāna* are serious conditions, as life depends upon *Prāṇ*, and strength relies on *Udāna*. If improperly analyzed and the situation continues unchecked beyond a year, or if improper therapies are used, it will not be curable.

The results of neglect are heart disorders, abscesses, enlarged spleen, tumors, diarrhea. If all five Vāyus are excessed, carminatives are immediately used with oils (that cleanse the channels rather than block them), yet do not aggravate Pitta and Kapha. Thus one takes sweet, rejuvenative enemas, and oil enemas until strength returns. Then, mild purgatives are given. The best rejuvenatives are *śhilājit* or *guggul* with boiled milk. Other herbs include *āmalakī* and *harītakī*, taken with a wholesome or *sattwic* diet.

Apān covers other Vāyus: The only remedy is eating appetizing, astringent and carminative herbs and foods that cleanse the bowels and dispel gas.

Pitta covers Vāyus: Herbs and foods that reduce both Pitta and Vāyu are used.

Kapha covers Vāyus: Kapha-reducing and carminative herbs are used.

Insanity (Unmāda)

Causes: *Charak* defines insanity as, "the perversion of the mind, intellect, consciousness, knowledge, memory, desire, manners, behavior, and conduct." Five types of insanity exist: Vāyu, Pitta, Kapha, Tridoṣha, and externally caused insanity. It is the main disease of Vāyu *doṣha*. The main causes of insanity, as we will see, result from personal misdeeds. When any of the three *doṣhas* cause insanity, symptoms quickly develop in persons with certain conditions. These characteristics include timidness, an agitated (*rajasic*) or lethargic (*tamas*) mind, or an imbalance in the physical *doṣhas* . Other conditions include following an unwholesome diet or lifestyle, when other health concerns are present, or if the mind is constantly afflicted by emotions (e.g., fear, anger, greed). Further characteristics include physical assault, trauma, or injury. From these situations the mind becomes greatly imbalanced.

Vāyu: Caused by fasting or an excessive intake of dry or cold foods. This affects the heart and mind with worry, passion, and anger; which results in distortion of memory and perceptions.

Pitta: Resulting from indigestion, excess of hot, pungent, sour, or burning foods and liquids, excessed Pitta afflicts the heart of a person lacking self-control.

Kapha: This is caused by overeating and an excessive use of oily foods. This aggravated Kapha afflicts the heart, troubling the mind and memory.

Tridoṣha: Caused by the excessed condition of all three *doṣhas*. It is considered serious because the therapies will aggravate one or more of the *doṣhas*. Therefore, this condition is incurable.
External: This results from a lack of following ethics and virtues in this life, or in past lives, causing problems by the dogs, sages, demons.

Development: The above causes weaken the *doṣhas* that afflict the (mind's) heart when there is less *sattwa* (purity) in one's life and mind. The disease develops through the *mānovaha srota* (mental channels) that sends psychic energy to the mind.

Premonitory Signs: Empty feeling in head, congested eyes, ear noises, excessive heavy breathing, excessive salivation, no desire to eat, anorexia and indigestion, cardiac spasms, fatigue, fainting, and anxiety at the wrong time and place. Other signs include hair standing on end continuously, frequent and quickly rising fevers in children that produces convulsions, fickle mindedness, upper body pains, facial paralysis on one half of the face, frequent dreams relating to (1) inauspicious objects that are wandering, moving, or unstable; (2) the two hemispheres of the brain; (3) being churned by whirlwinds; and (4) retraction of the eyes. Unlike other diseases, insanity develops immediately after premonitory symptoms. This includes a variety of mental problems, such as schizophrenia and manic-depression.

Symptoms:

General symptoms include, impatience, fickleness, unsteady vision, a sensation of a vacuum in the heart, loss of peace, memory, and intellect.
Vāyu: Constantly wandering, spasms of the eyes, eyebrows, lips, shoulders, jaws, forearms, legs; constant incoherent speech, frothing of the mouth, always smiling, laughing, dancing, singing, and playing with musical instruments at the wrong time or place. Other symptoms include loudly imitating a flute, conch, or cymbals; riding in dangerous vehicles, desiring excessive jewelry and ornaments, longing for foods that cannot be obtained; emaciation and rough, reddish skin; reddish, projected eyes; shock, depression, symptoms worsen by continuing to follow Vāyu-increasing lifestyles and foods.
Pitta: Irritation and anger, excitement at the wrong time, place, or for the wrong reasons; causing injury to others; fleeing; need for shade, cold water, and cooling foods; overly daring, intimidating; constant anguish, anger, impatience, passion, intolerance; going naked; yellow complexion; ferocious eyes that are coppery, green, or yellow. Symptoms worsen by continuing to follow Pitta-increasing lifestyles and foods.
Kapha: (with Pitta) Staying in one place and observing silence; sluggishness in speech and activity, occasional movement, discharging saliva and nasal excretions, lack of hunger and longing for solitude, excessive sexual desire, frightening appearance, aversion to cleanliness, anorexia, depression, greed, always sleepy, whitish nails, facial edema, eyes are white, timid and contain excreta. Symptoms worsen by continuing to follow Kapha-increasing lifestyles and foods.
Tridoṣha: The combined imbalance of all three *doṣhas* causes symptoms of all three *doṣhas*. This form of insanity is incurable.

Therapies: Oleation, fomentation, emesis, purgation, medicated and cleansing enemas, detoxification, fumigation (burning *jaṭāmāṇśhī* and inhaling the smoke), eye wash, aromatherapy, eye salves, medicated snuffs (*brāhmī nasya*), massage, sprinkling, unction, tying, confinement, frightening, inducing astonishment and forgetfulness, depletion, surgery, appropriate *doṣha* foods and lifestyles.
Vāyu: First, oil and *ghee* therapies (*sneha*) are used, if the air passages are not blocked. If they are blocked, laxatives are given with the oils and *ghee* to remove the blocks.
Pitta or Kapha: First, oleation and fomentation therapies are used, then purgatives, followed by emetics, are given. After that, one begins to eat

from thinner and lighter, to thicker and heavier foods (according to post *pañcha karma* food regimes—Chapter 7). Lastly, medicated enemas with oil or *ghee* are given, along with *doṣha* evacuation from the head (via the nose—*śhiro virechana*), using the herbs *jaṭāmāṇśhī* and gotu kola (*brāhmī*).

If the *doṣhas* are extremely excessed, these therapies are taken several times. The result of these therapies is the cleansing of the heart, head, senses, gastrointestinal tract. The mind gains alertness; memory and consciousness improve. Head evacuation is useful after cleansing if the person's personality still shows signs of imbalance.

Psychology: Therapeutic methods depend upon the symptoms. Methods include shouting, giving gifts, consoling, scaring. In this way, the cause of the illness is confronted and dealt with. In serious cases, hitting and shocking. are advised. If insanity is caused by fear, grief, anger, passion, exhilaration, jealousy, or greed, approaching person's with the opposite emotions will heal them.

Miscellaneous therapies include, *abhyañga,* ingesting *ghee* to stimulate the mind, intellect, memory, and consciousness and applying thick ointments.

General herbs to use include, *tṛikatu* with *ghee*; *triphalā*, *viḍaṅga*, sandalwood, *mañjiṣhṭhā*, *arjuna*, *daśhmūl*, *ghee*.

External: This is defined as signs and symptoms, different from those described above. These result from inappropriate past and present life deeds (intellectual blasphemy, or the disregarding of or malicious dealings with deities, spiritual people, parents and grandparents, teachers).

Premonitory external symptoms: Desire to cause injury to deities, cows, holy people, religious places; anger, delinquent behavior, disliking things and habits that reduce one's *ojas*, complexion, and strength; abuse and incitement by the gods, spirits, teachers.

External Causes: Deities, preceptors, elders, holy people's curses; appearance of the spirits of the deceased, demonic possession, or harassment.

External Symptoms: Superhuman strength, energy, enthusiasm, charisma, memory; artistic, oration, and spiritual abilities in the person.

Symptoms occur at the beginning of the above-mentioned deviant actions, when past *karmas* manifest in this life, when one is home alone or alone at a crossroad; sexual intercourse at sunset or on new or full moon days; intercourse during menstrual cycles, when reciting scriptures, or performing rites improperly; breaking one's vows during battle, when performing destructive deeds, during inauspicious planetary positions, during child delivery (for women); contact with unclean or inauspicious creatures during emesis, purgation, and bleeding; when visiting sacred places when unclean and not following the prescribed rules; when eating remnants of meat, honey, oil, candy, and alcohol; when unclothed, visiting cities, towns, gardens, cremation grounds, cross roads, or slaughter houses at night; when insulting holy people, teachers, gods; when misinterpreting scriptures, or when beginning any other inauspicious or harmful activity.

External Causative Goals: The causing of insanity has three aims: to inflict injury, to play or to offer prayers. Playing or prayer forms of insanity can be healed. Inflicting injury includes burning, drowning, falling, or harming oneself (including suicide).

Therapies: Herbs, such as musk and frankincense, chanting *mantras*/prayers (e.g., *"Aum Namaḥ Śhivaya"*), wearing talismans and jewelry, performing auspicious rites, religious sacrifices, oblations, taking vows, fulfilling religious duties, atonement, fasting, receiving blessings, obeisance and pilgrimages. Following wholesome foods and lifestyles is also necessary. *Ghee* may be eaten as often as desired. One should sleep in a draft-free room.

Brāhmī Ghee- (4 days worth)
brāhmī—50 gms., *Śhaṅkha puṣhpī*—50 gms., *aśhwagandhā*—50 gms., *jaṭāmāṇśhī*—50 gms., *Ghee—100 gms.*
Dose: 1 tsp. 2 times daily
Preparation: Make a paste from the herbs and roll into a ball, boil the *ghee* and add the paste and cook for 1/2 hour, filter.

(May be used for any mental disorders)

Insanity may also be caused by both internal and external factors. Thus, their signs and symptoms will be combined. When curable and incurable varieties of insanity appear together they all become incurable. For combinations of curable internal and external varieties, a combination of both therapies is suggested. Blood-letting is also advised for insanity.

Signs or Recovery:

When one's clarity and sense of normalcy reappear, it is a sign that the symptoms are removed.

Epilepsy (Apasmāra)

Causes: Epilepsy is defined as occasional unconsciousness with the vomiting of froth and abnormal body movements related to the distortion of memory, intellect, and other mental abilities.

Four types of epilepsy exist: Vāyu, Pitta, Kapha, and Tridoṣha. Sometimes external situations combine with internal *doṣhas* to cause this disease, but external events can never be the sole cause.

Epilepsy will develop quickly in five instances: (1) when one's mind has excess *rajas* and *tamas*; (2) when the *doṣhas* are excessed and imbalanced; (3) by eating unclean and unwholesome foods, eating mutually contradictory properties, eating foods contaminated by one having contagious diseases, or not eating according to one's *doṣha*; (4) not living according to one's *doṣha*; (5) when one is excessively debilitated.

These situations aggravate the *doṣhas* that affect the mind full of *rajas* and *tamas*. The excessed *doṣhas* then spread to the heart (home of the soul and sense organs). This aggravates passion, anger, fear, greed, attachment, excitement, grief, anxiety, and leads to epilepsy.

Premonitory Symptoms: Eyebrow contraction, constant, irregular eye movements, hearing non-existing sounds, excessive discharge of saliva and mucus, lack of hunger, anorexia, and indigestion; cardiac spasms, lower abdominal distention with gurgling sounds, weakness, cracking bone pain and debility, unconsciousness, entering darkness, fainting and giddiness, frequently dreaming of intoxication, dancing, murdering, aching, shivering, and falling.

Symptoms:
Vāyu: Losing and regaining consciousness rapidly, projected eye balls, speaking incoherently, vomiting froth, excessive heaviness and a rigid neck, bending the head to the side, twisted fingers, unstableness of arms and legs. Other symptoms include reddish, dry, and brownish nails, eyes, face, and skin; objects appear as unstable, coarse, and dry (before losing consciousness). Symptoms increase from Vāyu-increasing foods and lifestyles.
Pitta: Losing and gaining consciousness instantly, breathing with snoring sounds, rubbing the earth; green, yellow, or coppery nails, eyes, and complexion; objects appear as bleeding, terrifying, burning, and angry (before losing consciousness). Symptoms increase from Pitta-increasing foods and lifestyles.
Kapha: Slow to regain consciousness, falling, little distortion of activities, dribbling saliva, white nails, eyes, and complexion; objects appear as white, heavy, and oily (before losing consciousness). Symptoms increase from Kapha-increasing foods and lifestyles.
Tridoṣha: Symptoms of all three *doṣhas*. This condition is incurable.

If any disease spreads sideways, it will become chronic.

Therapies: First, oleation and fomentation are applied.

Internally-Caused: Next, for internally-caused epilepsy, the appropriate *pañcha karma* measures are used to cleanse and balance the heart, circulatory channels, and the mind that contain excess *doṣhas*.

-Vāyu epilepsy requires medicated enemas.

-Pitta calls for purgation.

-Kapha needs emetics.

As with all diseases, the strength of the person afflicted with the illness must be considered. Then foods are given, beginning with light meals, then moving gradually to heavier ones.

Externally-Caused: For epilepsy causes associated with external situations, *mantras,* prayers, rituals are suggested. Therapies include musk, chanting *mantras*/prayers (e.g., *"Aum Namaḥ Śhivaya"*), wearing talismans and jewelry, performing auspicious rites, religious sacrifices, oblations, and rites. Other therapies include taking vows, fulfilling religious duties, atonement, fasting, receiving blessings, obeisance, and pilgrimages. Following wholesome foods and lifestyles is also necessary. *Ghee* may be taken as often as desired. Sleep should be taken in a draft-free room.

Friends and spiritual leaders are advised to encourage understanding, patience, memory, and meditation.

General Herbal Therapies: After purification, the person is strengthened, then alleviation therapies begin to heal the epilepsy. *Ghee* mixed with *brāhmī, bilwa*, *gokṣhura*, *triphalā*, turmeric, sandalwood, *hiṅg*, rock salt, *pippalī*, calamus (*vachā*), and *kuṭaj* are useful. Mustard or sesame oil may also be added to these formulas. *Brāhmī ghee* is also effective. *Abhyañga* is useful for both internal and external conditions. The above mentioned herbs are burned as aromatherapy (*Śhatāvarī* and *jaṭāmāṇśhī* are added for inhalation).

Medicated oils may also be placed in the nostrils (2 to 3 drops). Along with the above herbs, *triphalā*, black pepper, ginger, *pippalī*, *jaṭāmāṇśhī*, *śhatāvarī*, gotu kola and *musta* may be added to the oil.

Vāyu/Kapha: *Guḍūchī*, calamus, and *guggul* may be added to *brāhmī ghee*.

Chronic Epilepsy: If the disease is not healed through the above remedies, then one takes garlic with sesame or mustard oil, *śhatāvarī* with boiled milk, *brāhmī* with raw honey, or calamus with raw honey.

Addictions

Symptoms:

Vāyu: All addictions increase Vāyu by causing a nervous dependency on them, resulting in a loss of objectivity. Vāyu *doṣhas* can give up addictions for a while, but will begin them again or switch to another habit.

Pitta: Unless these persons are convinced that a habit is bad for them, it will be very difficult to give up addictions.

Kapha: These persons have the most difficult time giving up their bad habits due to attachment and because their constitution is strong enough to take more abuse.

Smoking: Can be caused by any of the *doṣhas*.

Vāyu—These persons smoke to calm anxiety and worry. Symptoms include dry cough, constipation, and lung weakness.

Pitta—These persons smoke to feel the fire and power. Symptoms include lung, liver, and blood infections.

Kapha—These people smoke to feel clearer and stimulated. Symptoms include congestion.

Alcohol: Increases fire in the body and damages the blood, liver, and causes other Pitta diseases. Because it contains sugar, alcohol may also be a substitute for sugar addiction (in Kapha and Vāyu *doṣhas* mainly).

Drugs: Damage the holy or *sattwic* mental

nature, dulling the mind and nerves. Hallucinogens raise the mental fire (*tejas*), artificially creating clearer perception and an experience of higher consciousness. However, they burn up the life sap (*ojas*), weakening one's overall vitality. Sleep-promoting drugs eventually cause insomnia. Smoking marijuana poisons the liver and brain. It also causes liver and lung cancer.

Vāyu—becomes greatly imbalanced from long-term drug use (prescription, nonprescription, and recreational). Drugs are also usually diuretics, causing constipation, dryness, weakening to the kidneys, and reduces life sap (*ojas*). Stimulants overly aggravate Vāyu.

Pitta—short-term use of stimulants aggravates Pitta, causing burnout, eye damage.

Kapha—sedatives overly increase dullness (*tamas*). All drugs increase dullness, inertia, and poor perception (for all *doṣhas*).

General Therapies:

General: Brain tonics help reduce emotional needs for addictive items, tissue-healing herbs for the liver, lungs, brain, and immune system are also needed. Wholesome foods and lifestyles according to one's *doṣha* are important. Understanding the nature of dependencies is also needed. Spiritual counseling helps to clarify the true nature of a person's higher Self by transferring unhealthy addictions to addiction to devotion of the Divine. (This is a natural, gradual process that slowly fills the person with inner worth).

Smoking:

Vāyu—*aśhwagandhā*, *brāhmī*, milk, almonds, sesame seeds, *balā*, and *śhatāvarī* return moisture to the lungs.

Pitta—*brāhmī*, chamomile, aloe vera gel, bayberry, and *śhatāvarī* are good detoxing and toning herbs.

Kapha—*brāhmī,* herbal cigarettes, and hot spices will clear up congestion after a person gives up smoking.

Alcoholism: (see section specific for alcohol)

Vāyu—*brāhmī* is best for detoxifying the brain tissues.

Pitta—aloe vera gel is best for balancing the functioning of the liver. Other good liver and blood herbs include *brāhmī, kaṭukā, bhūmī-āmalakī, and mañjiṣhṭhā.* Turmeric and barberry together clear congested emotions due to liver toxins.

Kapha—turmeric and barberry together clear congested emotions due to liver toxins.

Drugs:

Drinking fresh juice of grapes, dates, and pomegranates is excellent for reducing addiction.

Generally, the best diet is a Vāyu-Pitta-reducing diet. *Ghee* nourishes the nerves. *jaṭāmāṇśhī* is an excellent sleep-promoting herb. *Yogaraj guggul* cleanses the deeper tissues. *Brāhmī* cleanses hallucinogens from the liver and brain.

Vāyu—*aśhwagandhā* rebuilds the nervous system. Calamus restores mental faculties and clears toxins from the liver and brain caused by marijuana.

Alcohol Recovery (Madāt-yaya)

Whereas improper use of foods can lead to disease or even death, drinking also leads to loss of self-worth, life path, wealth, true pleasure, intelligence, and courage.

Aṣhṭāñga Hṛidayam:
Nidānasthāna; Ch.6/ver. 11

Properties of Wine and Alcohol: The properties of alcohol are the opposite of life sap *(ojas),* and similar to poisons. The only difference is that alcohol is less potent than poison, so it does not kill the person. Alcohol penetrates deeply into the tissues. It is dry and causes drying, sourness; spreads throughout the body, and is heating. Alcohol loosens bone joints, dries life sap, and causes mental disorders. There are 3 stages to addiction.

First stage: Causes a loss of life sap and begins mental imbalances.

Second stage: Persons are at a critical point in choosing harmful activities and enjoying thinking about them. They begin to think they will receive true happiness from these choices. The mind is primarily in a state of *rajas* (agitation-/irritation-promoting) and *tamas* (slowing, clouding, dulling) during this stage. Persons may go on wild rampages of harmful activity. This is where vices and self-destruction begin.

Of all thy ways to bring self-destruction, drinking (i.e., alcohol and wine) is the most harmful.
Aṣhṭāñga Hṛidayam: Nidān; Ch. 6, verse 6

Third stage: A person lies lifeless on the ground. The experience is one of being poisoned.

Hazards: Loss of understanding right from wrong, happiness or unhappiness, beneficial or harmful, suitable or unsuitable. Drinking causes delusion, fear, grief, anger, insanity, infatuation, fainting, epilepsy, convulsions, and death. Further, loss of memory, awareness, and common sense occur.

[Strong mental and physical Kapha persons who come from families that drinks with meals as a daily habit and have strong digestion do not become greatly intoxicated or addicted.]

Causes:

Vāyu: When one is emaciated as a result of sex, grief, fear, travel, carrying overly heavy objects, eating rough or too little amounts of food, and then drinking rough, old wine in large amounts in the night, will disturb sleep. It causes Vāyu alcoholism.

Pitta: When one takes large quantities of hot, sour, and sharp wines, while eating hot and sharp foods, it burns the plasma and lymph, transforming their character into alkaline. The result is internal symptoms of burning, fever, thirst, mental confusion, giddiness, and narcosis. This leads to Pitta alcoholism

Kapha: When one takes large amounts of fresh, sweet wine, while eating sweet, oily, and heavy foods and takes frequent naps, and no exercise, Kapha alcoholism is caused.

Symptoms:

General: Profound delusion, heart discomfort, diarrhea, constant thirst, mild or severe fever, loss of taste and appetite, pain in the head, ribs, and bones; tremors, twitching, sharp pain in the vital organs and upper back, constricted chest, blindness, coma, cough, hiccup, swelling, ear, eye, and mouth disorders; mental disorders and confusion, unintelligent speech, vomiting, nausea, anorexia, thirst, severe yawning, dizziness, giddiness delusion, delirium, hallucination, nightmares.

Vāyu: Insomnia, hiccup, difficult breathing, tremors, headache, dreams of wandering, pain in the sides, falling, and talking with demons. Speech becomes impaired, talking becomes fast, delirious, slurred, and unsteady; activity is hindered, complexion becomes dry and blackish-red.

Pitta: Burning sensation, fever, perspiration, fainting, giddiness delusion, diarrhea, thirst, dizziness, green or reddish-yellow complexion, reddish eyes and cheeks, quick to anger, argumentative.

Kapha: Vomiting, excess sleep, skin rashes, anorexia, nausea, heaviness. One talks less, slurred speech, worry, laziness and lack of enthusiasm, yellowish-white complexion, cold feeling.

Tridoṣha: Symptoms of all three *doṣhas*.

Miscellaneous: Suddenly starting drinking after stopping for a long time creates two types of diseases of Vāyu origin that are difficult to heal and one type of Pitta origin.

Type 1—expectorating mucus, dry throat, excess sleep, irritated by noise, stupor.

Type 2—severe pain in the head and body, heart and throat disorders, delusion, cough, thirst, vomiting, fevers.

Type 3—When one sees blood or develops an increased volume of blood, the body becomes stiff, eyes are fixed in a gaze, other Pitta symptoms occur.

Alcoholism leads to fainting, and develops into a loss of consciousness. The channels of plasma, blood, and consciousness become obstructed.

Therapies: All forms of alcoholism are tridoṣha, so one first attends to the most excessed *doṣha* (although generally Kapha is the most excessed). If all three *doṣhas* are simultaneously imbalanced, one begins healing Kapha, then Pitta, and lastly Vāyu.

Vāyu: When wine causes the air to block the channels, it causes head, bone, and joint pain. To moisten Vāyu (i.e., restore balance), Vāyu-reducing foods are taken, followed by salty wine (made from flour) with *āmalakī* and ginger. This improves absorption, sharpness, and hotness. This dissipates the obstructions, dispels wind, and increases appetite. Foods include sours (e.g., pickles, yogurt), barley, wheat, *basmati* rice, vegetables, hot baths, ointments, enemas, *ghee*, milk, oil massage.

Vāyu/Pitta: When these *doṣhas* are in excess, if one feels great thirst, cold grape juice removes the imbalances. After food is digested, persons drink yogurt/water (*lassi*) with cane sugar, followed by cold water boiled with *musta* and *āmalakī*, to quench thirst. A paste of *āmalakī*, barley flour, and *ghee* may also be placed in the mouth to quench thirst.

Pitta: Alcoholism caused by excess intake of sharp, hot, sour, and burning wine is healed by cold, sour, grape wine with sugar, pomegranate, and roasted barley flour, having secondary tastes of sweet, pungent, bitter, and astringent. The acid and wine combination neutralizes the alkali. Foods include *ghee*, cane sugar and *āmalakī* mixed with *basmati* rice, peas, green lentils, *āmalakī* water.

Cold water boiled with *musta* and *āmalakī*, quenches thirst. A paste of *āmalakī*, barley flour, and *ghee* may also be placed in the mouth for alleviating thirst. Other therapies include, cold drinks and foods, sandalwood water, or drinking cool water from gold, silver, or bronze vessels. External therapies include cool rooms and breezes, moonlight walks, wearing clothes made of flax, and being near lotus and lily flowers. Green gems (e.g., emerald, jade), pearls, and moonstones further reduce Pitta alcoholism.

For burning sensations, sandalwood, lotus, or lily water is sprinkled on the body; cold baths or showers. Further, beautiful scenery, melodious music, jokes, and peaceful conversation balance this disease.

Pitta/Kapha: When both are excessed in the stomach, it causes burning and thirst. Grape juice or water is taken, then vomiting is induced to heal this illness quickly. Whenever the desire for alcohol appears, grape juice or water is immediately taken. This stimulates the digestion, which in turn digests the undigested food toxins.

If there is bleeding cough, pain in the breasts and sides, thirst, burning, excess *doṣhas* in the heart and chest, one takes *guḍūchī, vāsāk, dūrba, musta,* ginger, *ghee,* and sugar cane juice.

Kapha: If alcoholism is caused by faulty or excess drinking, it is merely healed by moderation. First, fasting and emesis are used. Later, herbs are used to remove *āma*, improve appetite, and return one's lightness.

When thirst and fever develop, persons drink warm water boiled with *balā*, or cooled water boiled with *balā*, *musta,* and ginger, to help digest the alcohol excesses. When *āma* is removed and appetite returns, cold wine with water, rock salt, and fresh ginger and honey is taken in moderation.

Small portions of food, including barley or wheat with ginger; thin vegetable soup with dried radish and pungents like ginger, sours like *āmalakī*, and a little *ghee*.

To promote appetite, white seedless grape juice, pomegranate juice, pungent herbs, cardamom, turmeric, and black pepper are mixed with raw honey.

Foods include hot foods and drinks. External therapies include hot baths and steam, physical exercise, staying up late and waking early, no naps, dry-body massage (promotes strength and complexion), and wearing rough heavy garments. Inhaling warm aromas, such as frankincense and cedar, is also helpful.

If the above measures are not effective, wines should not be drunk, but substituted with boiled milk with cinnamon, *ghee,* and honey. Gradually return to small amounts of wine.

Fainting (Mūrchā)

When drinking continues and one's health becomes more seriously impaired, fainting occurs as a second, more serious stage of this illness.

Symptoms:

Vāyu: One sees the surrounding space as light red, black, or blue; enters darkness or unconsciousness, then shortly regains awareness. Symptoms include heart pain, tremors, dizziness, emaciation, and a blackish-red complexion.

Pitta: Surrounding space is red or yellow. The person becomes unconscious, then soon after regains consciousness. One feels sweat, burning sensation, thirst, increased heat, diarrhea, blue or yellow feces, reddish or yellow eyes, and an unsteady gaze.

Kapha: One's surrounding awareness is cloudy, resulting in fainting. Persons return to consciousness after a long time. The heart is oppressed and one develops increased salivation. The body feels heavy and restricted, as if walking in soaking wet clothes.

Tridoṣha: Includes symptoms of all three *doṣhas* and falling to the ground in a faint.

Therapies:

General: Constant sprinkling or spraying of water over the body, plunging one into a cold bath, contact with cold gems and flower garlands, cold compresses and plasters, cold breeze and fanning, cold-scented drinks (i.e., all cooling measures).

Drākṣhā (medicated grape wine), pomegranate juice, rice, and barley are suggested foods and drinks. Herbs include *nāgakeśhar* and black pepper; *pippalī* and raw honey, *harītakī* decoction and *ghee*, *āmalakī* and *ghee*.

Comas (Saṃnyāsa)

When drinking continues, one's health becomes most seriously impaired. The coma is the third and most dangerous stage of drinking. Therefore, before persons decide to drink, they must think about many factors.

Alcohol Factors Considered for Avoiding Comas

Alcohol Factors Considered for Avoiding Comas			
physical strength	drink potency	season	time of day
place	*doṣha*	age	quantity used to drinking

As the accumulation of all three *doṣhas* become aggravated together and get localized in the mind and intellect, speech, body and mind become impaired. Persons become stiff as a log, and therapy must be given immediately.

Therapies include strong snuff, strong collyrium, passive snuffing (i.e., someone else blowing snuff into the client's nose), pricking needles under the nails, pulling hairs, touching the person with a hot object, or putting sour and bitter tastes in the mouth. Once persons regain consciousness, they are given juices of fresh garlic and lemon, with saffron, *tṛikatu,* and salt. A light, easily digestible meal is also taken.

Atrophy (Kṣhaya)

Cause: *Ātrea* discusses atrophy (phthisis) after epilepsy because after falling during a seizure, the chest may become injured. Atrophy is listed in this book under nervous system disorders. It is this injury to the chest that can cause atrophy or emaciation. Internally, it is caused by a deficiency of semen (*śhukra*) and life sap (*ojas*). These deficiencies result from an overindulgence in sex and other life-sap-depleting habits, such as fasting, eating dry foods, and eating small quantities of food. Other causes include eating at the wrong time or season, eating foods of only one taste (i.e., either sweet, or salty, or sour, or pungent, or bitter, or astringent).

Since *ojas* originates in the heart, injury to the chest will also deplete this life sap. Other causes include excessive straining during sports or work (e.g., lifting weights that are too heavy, singing scriptures at the top of one's voice, hard jolts to the body). Thus, it is a disease of Vāyu *doṣha*.

Development and Premonitory Signs: As a result of any of these causes, the chest becomes broken, cracked, or perforated, the chest thus becomes squashed. This causes emaciation and tremors that slowly lead to the loss of strength, complexion, appetite, and digestive fire (*agni*). Fever, pain, depression, and diarrhea develop (although Pitta is deficient, the suppression of digestive power can cause diarrhea). Symptoms include, coughing up malodorous, grayish, yellow, and knotty phlegm with large amounts blood. When semen and *ojas* are diminished from the above causes, emaciation also becomes worse.

Symptoms: The main signs of chest injury are vomiting, bleeding, and coughing. The main symptoms of semen and *ojas* deficiency is blood in the urine, and torso stiffness.

When the signs and symptoms are mild, when the patient is strong, or if the situation has just occurred, then the person can be healed. If the disease has lasted for more than 1 year, then it can only be controlled (i.e., the symptoms can diminish but may return if not careful). Should all the signs and symptoms simultaneously present themselves, the disease is incurable.

Therapy:

New injury: Coagulative herbs (astringents) like raspberry and *nāgkeśhar (*stop bleeding), taken with boiled milk and raw honey.

Chest and rib or urinary bladder pain: (with poor digestion) Herbs include *guggul*, *vāsāk*, neem, *chopchinī*, turmeric, with boiled milk, and raw honey or cane sugar.

Diarrhea: *Īśhabgol* (and *musta* if Vāyu is not excessed)

Strong digestion: Herbs include coagulatives with boiled milk, *ghee*, and raw honey or cane sugar.

To heal injuries: (same therapies as chest/rib).

Fever and burning sensation: (same therapies as chest/rib).

Cough, and rib and bone pain: Herbs include *pippalī*, *balā*, *ghee*, and raw honey.

Limping: *Ghee* with rock salt are suggested.

Weakness, emaciation, chest injury, insomnia, excess Vāyu: Herbs include turmeric, *śhatāvarī*, *aśhwagandhā*, *balā*, *ghee*, and raw honey or cane sugar.

Weightloss, muscle emaciation, no appetite, debility: Therapies include cane sugar, barley, wheat, raw honey; and afterwards, boiled milk, *aśhwagandhā*, *dūrbā*, *pippalī*, turmeric, and honey, with *ghee*—to promote blood, tissues, and muscle development.

Chest injury with semen loss: *Śhatāvarī*, *aśhwagandhā*, *aṣhoka*, and *vāsāk* are suggested.

Chest injury: Boil *brāhmī ghee* (page 468) with equal amounts of milk. As an option, a decoction of 4 times as much licorice as *ghee* may be added to the *brāhmī ghee*.

Muscle and Blood Builder: 1/4 to 1/2 tsp. *pippalī* and the remainder of the teaspoon with raw honey, taken for a week. Then for 2 to 3 days, this mixture is not taken. This regimen is continued as described.

Fever and cough: *Sitopaldi* and cane sugar are advised.

Emaciated women: *Vidārī kand*, *āmalakī*, and

sesame seed tahini are advised.

Debility and loss of body weight: Therapies include *aśhwagandhā*, *śhatāvarī*, *āmalakī*, *ghee*, and wheat flour.

Urinary bladder, uterus or kidney problems, or loss of semen or ovum, due to excess sexual indulgence: *Ghee* with *aśhwagandhā*, *śhatāvarī*, and *daśhmūl* are suggested. When persons are strong, a medicated enema is also useful.

Poor digestion: Therapies include barley powder, raw honey, and *brāhmī ghee*.

Dendrite Heads

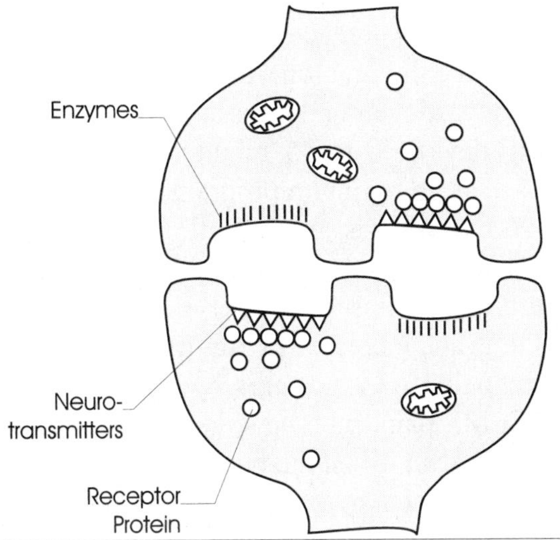

Multiple Sclerosis

In the nerve cell, axons and dendrites (see diagram below) are covered by cells that contain myelin (a fatty substance needed for normal conduction of electrical impulses). Certain diseases attack myelin and the cells that produce it. The cells are stripped of myelin or scarring (plaque) is caused. This causes the nerves to partially or completely stop normal nerve impulse conduction.

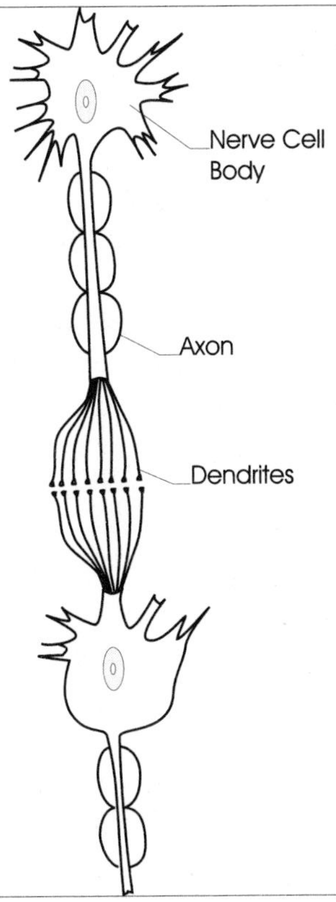

Multiple sclerosis (MS) is the most common of these demyelinating diseases. However, it is not equally present throughout the world. Although it is prevalent in the U.S., it is not equally distributed within the country. MS is mainly concentrated in temperate climates (and rarely found in tropical or arctic regions). Thus, western science feels there may be a geographic or climactic influence. MS is a disease involving the central nervous system.

From the Āyurvedic standpoint, MS results from Vāyu and Pitta excesses, caused by anxiety (Vāyu) that leads to hypertension. An inability to withstand heat can develop.

Therapies

Herbs that calm and strengthen the nerves and immune system are very useful. A special gold ash preparation (*Survana Vasant Malti*) work best but is more costly than plain herbs [1 pill daily—in the morning—with 1/2 tsp. raw honey].

Females—After age 50 Pitta is affected. Herbs include *jaṭāmāṇśhī, śhatāvarī, aśhwagandhā, yogaraj guggul, triphalā, brāhmī*. The healing process is longer after age 40.

Males—The healing process is longer after age 50. Herbs include *vachā, śhatāvarī, aśhwa-*

gandhā, yogaraj guggul, triphalā, and *brāhmī.*

Other important therapies include *śhiro dhārā* (hot oil head drips) and *śhiro bhyañga* (head-oil baths), as they reduce the excess Vāyu in the head, and calm and tone the nerves of the brain and body. Seven or 14 sessions (daily or alternating days), 30 to 45 minutes per session, is advised as an optimum program.

Haṭha yoga is another effective therapy to slow and reduce the effects of MS. Mind-body coordination, muscle and nerve toning, immune building, and increased flexibility are the benefits of practicing *yoga* postures.

For MS pain, rubbing sesame oil mixed with *mahānārāyan* oil on the body has been found to be very effective; people report that pain is stopped for several hours at a time.

Following a food plan according to one's *doṣha* is also required. Lifestyle changes may be necessary to reduce undue stress in one's life.

Nasya with medicated brain oils like śhad bindu are also very helpful—3-6 drops per .

Parkinson's Disease

This is a condition that develops from a loss of dopamine-producing cells in the substantia nigra area of the basal ganglia. Although it usually affects persons after age 50, it sometimes is found in persons as young as age 35.

Symptoms:

Early stages are slight shaking of hands during fine hand movement. Advanced symptoms include shaking or tremor, stiffness or rigidity, hindered walking and stooped posture.

Therapies:

Generally this is a Vayu or Vayu/Pitta condition (sometimes Vayu/Kapha). All therapies for MS are advised here, especially *kapikachhū, abhyañga, śhiro dhārā, nasya* (e.g., *śhad bindu* oil), *basti, yoga* postures

Alzheimer's Disease

The exact cause of Alzheimer's disease is not yet known to Western medicine. However, it is considered a function of the nervous system. Nerve cells in the memory region of the brain are found to be greatly reduced in size and number as compared with those of a healthy person.

Tourette's syndrome, ataxia, aphasia, stuttering, dyslexia, and other diseases of the brain and nervous system are modern names for conditions that have not been found in ancient India. Thus, their therapies have not been specifically discussed.

For all nervous system disorders one can follow therapies for MS and other previously discussed diseases based on similar symptoms. *Kapikachhū* has been found to be especially effective in Parkinson's research.

One who is ever mindful of their life purpose
and how they are living,
their life will never become sad.
Aṣhṭāñga Hṛidayam Sū. Ch. 2 : ver. 47

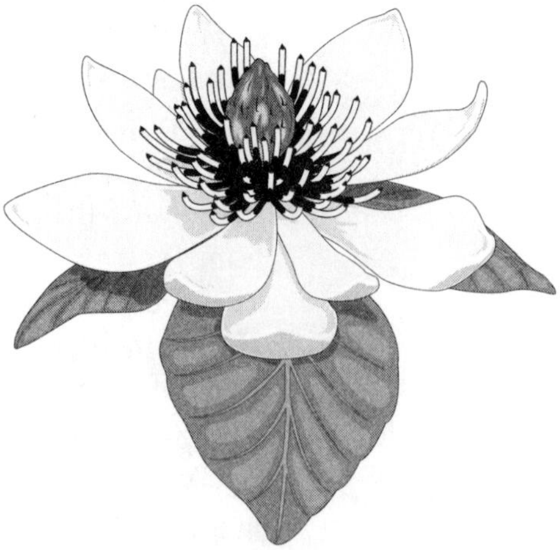

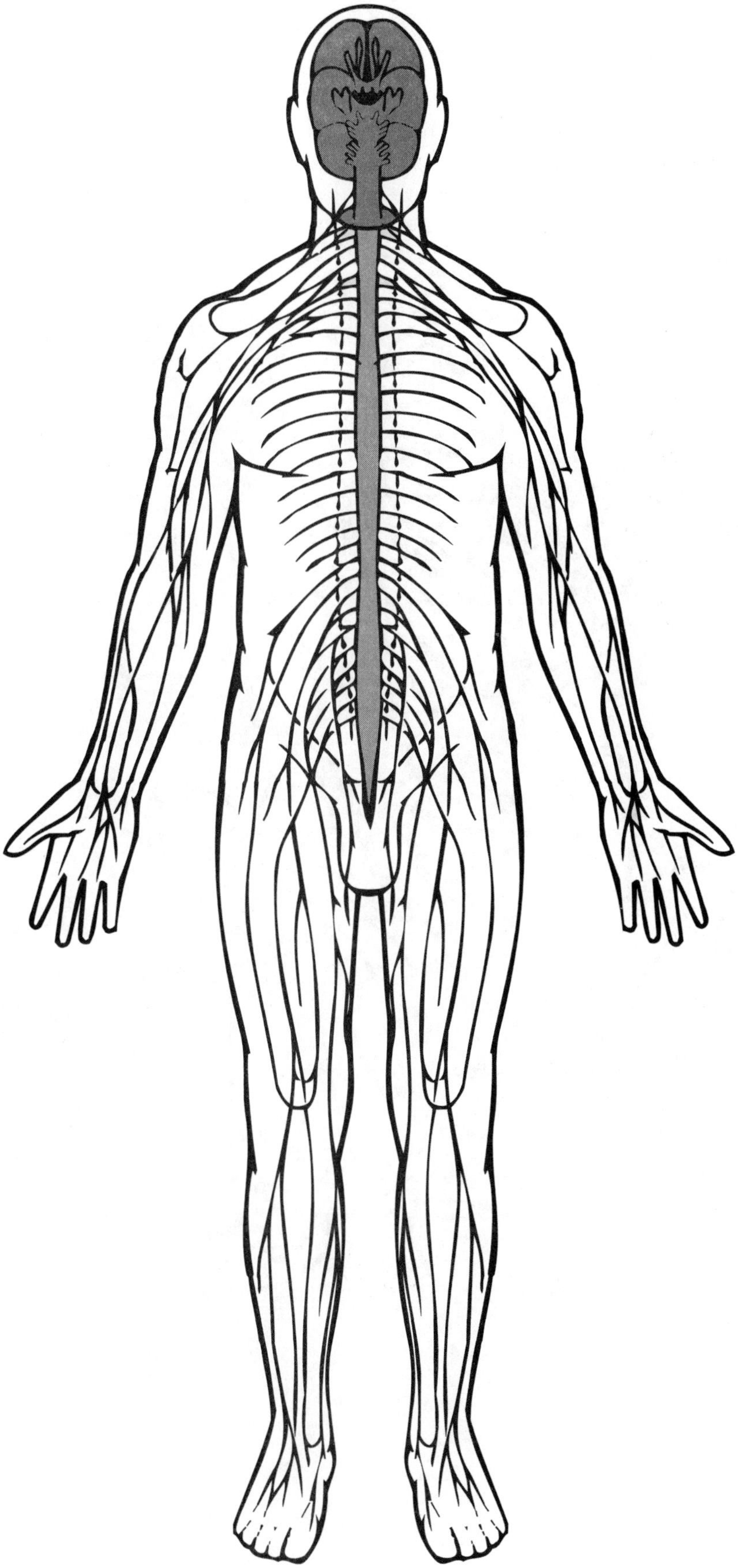

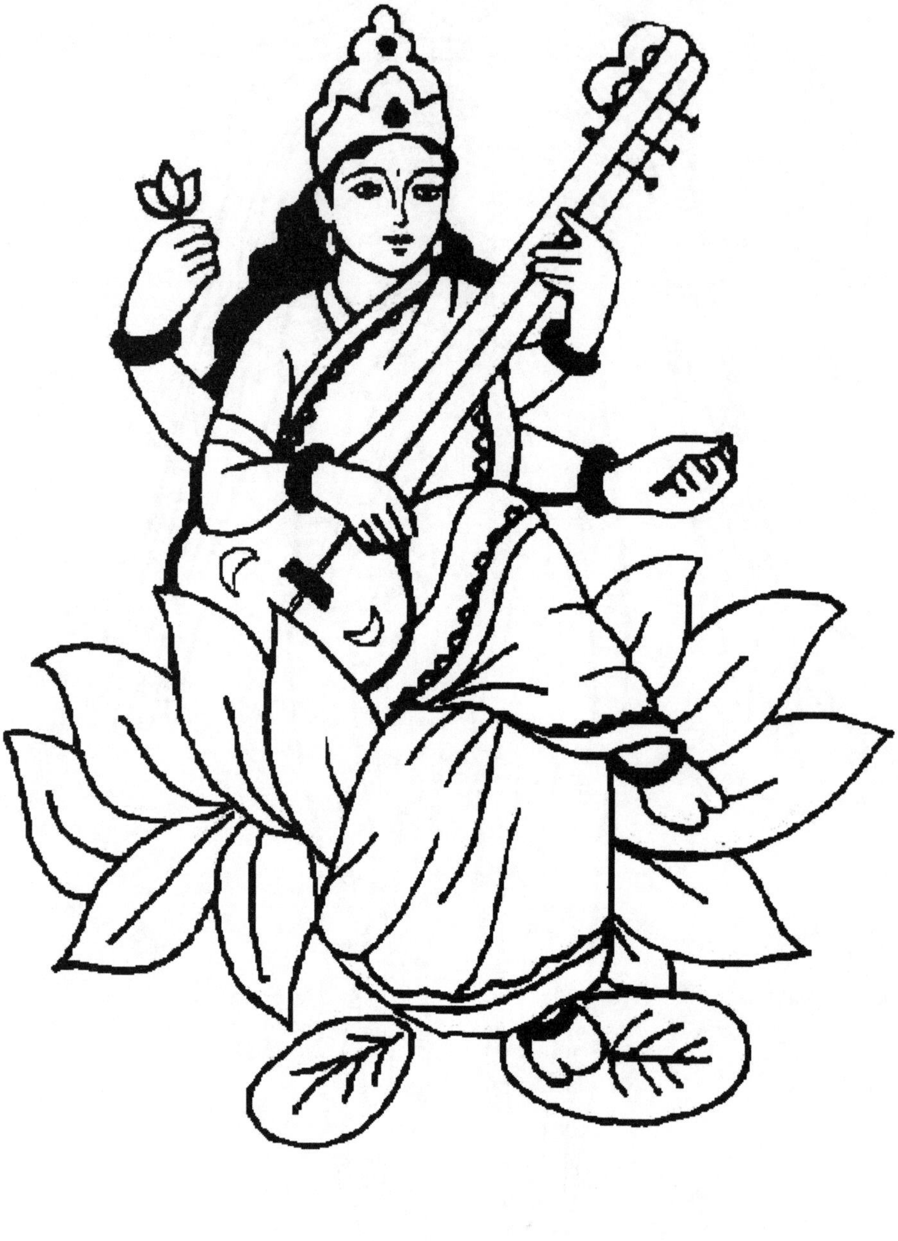

Education is a development from within, not an accretion from without; it comes through the workings of natural instincts and not in response to external force; it is an expansion of natural powers, not an acquisition of information; it is life itself, not a preparation for a future state remote in interests and characteristics from the life of childhood. *Rousseau*

Chapter 21
Skin Disorders
Warts, Skin, Leukoderma, Herpes Zoster

Warts

When Vāyu and Kapha combine on the skin, they are nail-like in appearance, hard, rough, and immovable. When Vāyu predominates, pain and roughness develop. With Pitta predominance they look blackish-red. Should Kapha predominate they are greasy, knotty, and the same color as the skin.

Kapha creates soft skin. Pitta causes hard skin. They combine when following incompatible therapies (e.g., ingesting milk and salt together), and cause warts.

Therapies: Externally, lemon juice or tea-tree oil applied to the warts (daily, for several weeks).

Warts are similar to hemorrhoids in their development and appearance. Thus, therapies are the same as for hemorrhoids.

Obstinate Skin Diseases (Kuṣhṭha)

Causes: These arise from aggravated Vāyu, Pitta, and Kapha that become deranged by four tissues (*dhātus*): skin-plasma/lymph (*rasa/lasīkā*), muscle (*māṃsa*), and blood (*rakta*). Then, they spread throughout the body.

The beginning stages of skin diseases are caused only by the four *dhātus*, but eventually spread to the other *dhātus*. All skin disorders involve the three *doṣhas* and four *dhātus* (i.e., plasma, lymph, blood, and muscle). The various types of disorders depend upon the combinations of the *doṣhas* and their physical locations. The combinations of *doṣha* and locations cause various pains, colors, shapes, and manifestations; although they are produced by the same causes. For example, in some cases the quality of dryness of Vāyu is excessed, while at other times the coldness of Vāyu is predominant.

Skin diseases are caused by ingesting mutually contradictory foods and drinks (e.g., fish [hot] and milk [cold]). They can also be caused by suppressing any of the natural urges, exercise after meals or under very hot weather conditions; fasting, and eating heavy meals. Other causes include drinking cold water just after being in the hot sun, fright, raw foods, eating before the last meal is digested. Improper use of *pañcha karma* and its follow-up therapies also can cause skin diseases. Further causes include excessive eating of yogurt, salt, fish, radish, pastries, sesame seeds, milk and sugar, and sour foods. External causes include, sex after meals, naps, insulting holy people, Gurus, and other sinful actions.

Some say there are many skin disease classifications. Others say 18 (major and minor) skin disorders occur. Still others say only 7 types exist. Discussed below, are the 7 major classifications.

Premonitory Signs: Lack of, or excess perspiration; discoloration, itching, pricking pain, numbness, tingling, burning, hair standing on end, rough or excessively smooth skin, coarseness, heaviness, frequent development of edema, spreading severely, sticky excreta in body orifices, excessive pain from oozing, wounds are difficult to hear. After these signs, the individual symptoms appear.

Seven Major Skin Diseases (Mahā-Kuṣhṭhas)

Depending upon the degree of excess, many permutations of skin disorders exist. *Charak* and *Suṣhrut* have different listings of major and minor skin diseases. This is due to the differences of surgical and medicinal therapies. Below are 7 major skin diseases.

Kaphāla: (*macula caelulum*/azure colored spots) due to excess Vāyu—dry, reddish, rough, and with rough edges; uneven, thin, slightly elevated on the edges, excessive numbness, bristly hairs and great pain, burning, pus, black or azure in color. They develop instantly, and are difficult to heal.

Udumbara: Due to Pitta—coppery, and covered with coppery colored hair; thick with copious, thick pus, blood, and oozing; itching, sticky oozing, burning, and hot. The manifestation and ulceration happen instantly.

Mandala: Due to Kapha—oily, heavy, swollen, smooth and yellow borders; white and red colored, and covered with many white hairs; excessive, thick, slimy, white, sticking oozing, itching, round; they develop slowly, are difficult to heal. [*Charak Saṃhitā*]

[*Aruna*: Caused by Vāyu, is light vermilion colored, thin, spreading, pricking and piercing pain, numb to the touch—listed in *Suṣhrut Saṃhitā* as one of the seven instead of *Mandala*.]

Risyajihva: Due to Vāyu/Pitta—rough, reddish with dark brown centers and edges; they can be blue, yellow, and coppery shaded; excessive burning, cutting, piercing pain and pus, elevated centers and thin edges, rough pimples, elongated and round, and they develop instantly.

Pundarīka: Due to Kapha/Pitta—white and red with red edges and covered with red lines and blood vessels, swelling, thick excessive discharge of blood and pus, itching, circular, raised, burning, and develop slowly.

Sidhma (macule atrophica): Due to Kapha/Vāyu—rough, reddish, fissured edges with thin centers, smooth, dusty, white and red shaded; there are many of them; they are generally found on the chest, and they develop slowly. [*Ātreya* says it is a major illness, while *Suṣhrut* considers it a minor one].

Dadru (ringworm): Faint blue or coppery, spreading, pimples, itching, circular, slow to develop, raised. [*Ātreya* lists as a minor illness. He sees it being caused by all three *doṣhas*. *Suṣhrut* considers it minor, based on surgical measures. Further, he sees it being caused by Vāyu and Kapha].

Kākanaka: *Ātreya* says it is due to Tridoṣhic symptoms; all forms of skin diseases are experienced, many colors yet mostly red, and cannot be healed due to the vitiation of all three *doṣhas* (all other forms of disorders are healable). *Suṣhrut* says it is due to Pitta, black, sucking or burning pain, emitting hot fumes, developing pus and break rapidly, eventually they develop parasites.

Tridoṣhic: Simultaneous aggravation of all three *doṣhas* are caused by

1) Eating cold and hot foods, and nourishing and depleting diets.
2) Excess and long term use of honey, fish, radish while there is indigestion.
3) Excessive sexual intercourse, exercise, and heat exposure before digesting meals.
4) Suppressing the urge for emesis.
5) Excessive oleation.
6) Entering cold water just after developing fear, grief, and exhaustion.

These habits aggravate the *doṣhas* in the four *dhātus*, and weaken them. Due to this weakening, the tissues (*dhātus*) cause skin disorders.

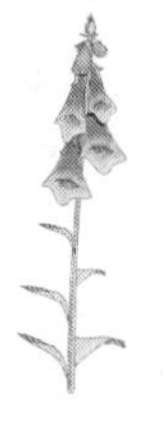

11 Minor Symptoms (Kṣhudra Kuṣhṭhas)

Eka (ichthyosis): Vāyu/Kapha—no perspiration, vast, localized groupings, scaly (like a fish), reddish color, not healable.

Charma (hypertrophy): Vāyu/Kapha—thick skin patches (like elephant skin), burning, restlessness, pus, piercing pain, epileptic fits and loss of consciousness, sucking, drawing pain in the palms and soles (with itching).

Kitima (keloid tumors): Vāyu/Kapha—blackish-brown, rough (excessive scar tissue), hard to the touched.

Charmandala: Pitta/Kapha—redness, itching, pustules, pain, skin cracks, and tender.

Pāmā (eczema): Pitta/Kapha—great itching, white, red, or blackish/brown small pimples, itching, burning secretion.

Vicarchikā (psoriasis): Kapha—blackish-brown, itching, copious oozing, great pain, dry cracks on hands, feet and body.

Vipādikā (lower psoriasis): Vāyu/Kapha—cracks in palms and soles, great pain, burning, found only in the lower extremities.

Sphota: Pitta/Kapha—thin, white or reddish pustules.

Śhatāru: Pitta/Kapha—red or blackish-brown ulcerated patches, burning and pain.

Alasaka: Vāyu/Kapha—nodular growth with great itching and redness.

[All skin diseases (*Kuṣhṭhas*) are the same causes as Erysipelas (*Visarpa*)—an acute disease of the subcutaneous tissues—only *Kuṣhṭha* develops gradually, while *Visarpa* spreads very quickly.]

[*Parisarpa, Visarpa, Kachus, Rakasā, Mahā Kuṣhṭham, Sthulāruṣhka, Kilāsam*; *Suṣhrut* sees these as minor diseases.]

Sthulāruṣhka: Kapha—pimples around the joints that are very thick at their base, difficult to heal, with hard pimples on the surface.

Mahā-kuṣhtham: Kapha—contracted skin bursts, causing piercing pain, loss of sensation and general lassitude.

Visarpa: (discussed in its own section) Pitta—pimples in the skin, blood and fat, quickly spread over the entire body, with burning, restlessness, pus, piercing pain, and epileptic fits leading to fainting.

Parisarpa: Vāyu—oozing pimples that slowly spread over the entire body.

Kachus (localized eczema): *Pāmā* symptoms with burning are found only on the legs, hands, and buttocks.

Rakasā (dry erythema/abnormal red skin due to irritation and dilation of capillaries): Kapha—dry, non- oozing pimples, intense itching, all over the body.

Complications: If skin disorders are not tended to properly, germs in the skin, muscles, blood, oozings, and sweat further weaken the *doṣhas* and cause secondary disorders.

Vāyu: Blackish brown or reddish in color, rough, dry, piercing or pricking pain, emaciation, trembling, hair standing on end, stiffness, numbness, exhaustion, ulcerations, and fissures.

Pitta: Burning, sweating, tissue softening, putrefaction, oozing, pus, and redness.

Kapha: Whiteness, coldness, itching, steadiness, heaviness, swelling, oiliness, and stickiness.

Four Dhātus: Germs eat away at the skin, muscles, blood, plasma, vessels, ligaments, bones, and cartilage, causing oozings, ulcerated organs, thirst, fever, diarrhea, burning, weakness, anorexia, and indigestion.

The simultaneous excesses of all three *doṣhas* are the cause of all forms of skin diseases, yet some *doṣhas* are predominant for each variety. The predominant *doṣha* and the causes of the illness are learned from the specific form of the disease, and vice versa. Thus, after analyzing the signs and symptoms, the *doṣha* that is predominant is balanced first, then the other *doṣhas* are healed later.

Vāyu Symptoms and Therapies: Rough, dry, hard, scaly skin, coarse, hair standing on edge, brown and red, itching, constipation, distention, increased by wind and dryness; oils are soothing. Therapies include Vāyu-reducing foods, liquids and lifestyles; castor oil laxatives, enemas, sesame oil massage, *triphalā*, *guggul*, myrrh, *śhatāvarī*, and cardamom.

Pitta Symptoms and Therapies: Burning, redness, oozing, malodor, stickiness of limbs, swelling, infection, fever, irritability; increased by heat; oil make them worse. Therapies include Pitta-reducing foods, drinks, and lifestyle; avoiding nightshades (eggplants, peppers, tomatoes, potatoes, peaches, strawberries), sour, and hot things. Helpful therapies include coconut juice, aloe vera gel, cilantro juice, gotu kola, and *bhṛiṅgarāj* oils (internally and externally); herbs include gotu kola, burdock, red clover, *chirāyatā*, aloe, rhubarb, *mañjiṣhṭhā*, *bhūmīāmalakī*.

Kapha Symptoms and Therapies: White complexion, cold, localized, raised, heavy, sticky, unsightly, oozing, congestion, edema, itching; increased by damp and cold weather, and oil. Therapies include Kapha-reducing foods, drinks, and lifestyle; avoiding heavy, greasy, and oily foods including cheese and yogurt, and external oil massage. Helpful herbs include burdock, *gokṣhura*, *guggul*, *triphalā*, *mañjiṣhṭhā*, ginger, *bhūmīāmalakī*, and gotu kola.

Therapies: It is said that the skin condition is not able to be healed if, tridoṣhic symptoms exist; symptoms develop in weak persons, while experiencing great thirst and burning sensations, poor digestion, and if the patches have bugs in them.

Preliminary Therapies

Vāyu: First—enema using oils and *ghee*.

Pitta: First—purgation (and blood-letting) using *triphalā*.

Kapha: First—emetic therapy when the *doṣhas* are excessed in the heart or center of the body, and are not stuck or rooted in the upper part of the body. Emetics include *kuṭaj*, neem, and honey.

When the *doṣhas* are greatly excessed, these preliminary therapies are repeated several times, always monitoring one's health and strength, as these therapies may weaken the patient and their Vāyu.

Secondary Therapies

Only after the *doṣhas* are significantly reduced, oleation therapy is given repeatedly. After the therapies, one begins a food diet that balances their *doṣhas*. [Beginning with thin gruel-thick gruel, vegetable soup, etc. as describe in the *pañcha karma* section of Chapter 7. Thin gruel is taken for three meals, then for two meals, and then for one meal.] Medicated enemas are also taken, using barley and *musta* ,with *ghee* or oil (e.g., sesame, canola, sunflower).

If excess Vāyu still exists even after these therapies, food plan, and enema, one takes an *anuvāsana* medicated enema of oil mixed with *harītakī* and *triphalā* (depending upon their strength).

Inhalation Therapy: Rock salt, black pepper, *pippalī*, *jaṭāmāṇśhī*, and gotu kola are inhaled to heal skin diseases (and parasitic infections and Kapha diseases).

Medicated *ghee* may be used internally and externally to heal skin conditions of the three *doṣhas*. Pitta-, blood-, and Kapha-caused imbalances use bitter and astringent herbs (e.g., *musta*, raspberry).

Kapha skin disorders are healed with *chitrak*, *guḍūchī*, cardamom, *chakramarda*, sarsaparilla, *kuśhtā*, and *punarnavā*.

Vāyu—*triphalā, musta*, raspberry, *mañjiṣhṭhā*, *gokṣhura*, *chitrak*, neem, *guḍūchī*, cardamom, *punarnavā,* and calamus are useful for Vāyu.

Vāyu or Kapha:_Decoctions of *ṭrikatu*, *triphalā*, cane sugar, and sesame oil, taken for 1 month. Herbs are mixed in equal amounts. These decoctions are also applied externally to the skin. Massaging the decoctions (mixed with oil) into the skin also promotes healing. Vāyu uses sesame oil, Pitta, sunflower or coconut oil, Kapha uses mustard or canola oil. Sesame or mustard oil decoctions of *bākuchī*, *ṭrikatu*, *kuṭaj*, and *viḍaṅga* are massaged into the skin quickly prevents the bursting of mandala skin diseases and itching.

Sidhma and newly occurring *likāsa* leukoderma can be healed. Herbs include *bākuchī*, *kuśhtā*, and *mañjiṣhṭhā*.

Charma, *eka*, *kitima* and *alasaka* skin disorders are healed with medicated *ghee* and oil, boiled with *mañjiṣhṭhā*, sarsaparilla, an equal quantity of milk, and bees' wax.

Mandala herbs include *viḍaṅga*, *vachā*, neem, *arka*, *chitrak*, *musta*, *kuṭaj*, castor oil, and *tṛikatu*. The skin is massaged with sesame or mustard oil.

Vāyu and Kapha skin disorders are healed with *chitrak*, *guḍūchī*, cardamom, and *punarnavā*, mixed with 1/4 yogurt and 3/4 water. *Vatsaka*, sandalwood/barley decoction for Pitta. Pitta and Kapha herbs include sandalwood, *kuṣhṭha*, and *kuṭki*.

Vāyu/Pitta: Herbs include *khair*, sandalwood, neem, red sandalwood, *triphalā*, and *ghee*.

For burning patches, or skin diseases in general, massage with a *triphalā* decoction mixed with sandalwood, *pippalī*, turmeric, *musta*, red sandalwood, *khair*, turmeric, licorice, *vatsaka*, and *ghee*. These herbs are also for *Charmadala* skin disorder, stickiness, scaling, shedding skin disjointing, or burning, along with water dripped on the skin.

Sidhma: Herbs include *kuṭaj* bark, *nilotpalam, and satyanasha* (yellow thistle).

When skin disorders are predominantly blood and Pitta excessed, *vāsāk*, *bākuchī*, *guḍūchī*, *mañjiṣhṭhā*, neem, and *ghee* are used.

When disjointedness, serious exudation, or maggots appear, persons take a neem and *viḍaṅga* bath. After the blood is purified, *pañcha karma* therapies are used. The skin is washed with neem and *viḍaṅga* as antiseptic wash externally to prevent and check the infection, and then *pañcha karma* internally to help recovery.

Dadru (ringworm): Plaster of mustard seeds, turmeric, *tṛikatu* with yogurt/water (*lassi*) is applied to area affected by the ringworm. Internally, the same herbs, and, *viḍaṅga*, neem, sarsaparilla, *chakramarda*, *khadir*, *chitrak*, ginger, *triphalā* may be taken. In viral ringworm, baths with a decoction of the above herbs are also useful.

Minor Skin Disorders: Drinking tepid decoctions of turmeric, *mañjiṣhṭhā*, *gokṣhura*, *triphalā*, *bhṛiṅgarāj*, gotu kola, sandalwood, aloe vera gel. Blisters can develop on the patches. After blisters burst, a plaster of turmeric, *mañjiṣhṭhā*, *viḍaṅga*, neem, *harītakī*, and aloe vera gel is applied to the skin.

Foods are light and wholesome, mixed with *ghee*, and bitter leafy vegetables are advised. Herbs include *tṛikatu* and *kaiṣhore guggul*. One simultaneously avoids eating sour foods, milk, yogurt, meat, cane, sugar and sesame seeds (except as remedies). Baths (i.e., soaking the problem skin) with herbs of *musta* and *triphalā* are useful as well.

Leukoderma (Śhvitra) [Vitiligo] Pigmentation Loss/White Skin Patches

Causes: It arises from the aggravation of Vāyu, Pitta, Kapha, blood, muscle, and fat. Vāyu forms are easiest to heal, becoming increasingly more difficult to subdue, with fat as the most difficult to heal. Generally it is caused by excesses of all three *doṣhas*, but sometimes it is caused by one or two *doṣhas*.

Symptoms:

Vāyu: Dry, light red skin

Pitta: Coppery red, burning, and destroys the hair in the infected area.

Kapha: White, thick, heavy, and itching skin.

Blood, Muscle, Fat: These tissues have the same respective colors as the three *doṣhas*.

Recovery: Symptoms of black hairs, mild skin patches; not joined, of recent onset, and not caused by burning fire can be healed. The remainder, including those found on the genitals, palms, soles, and lips are difficult or unable to be healed.

Therapies: First oleation, then elimination therapies (depending on one's strength) are suggested. Afterwards, *bākuchī*, *mañjiṣhṭhā*, neem, turmeric, *āmalakī*, *makoy*, *khadir*, *bilwa* bark, and *chakramarda* are taken with cane sugar. Following this, persons sun bathe to cause purgation. This will cause thirst, for that thin gruel (*peyā*) is taken for 3 days.

All therapies for skin disorders, are also useful for internal and external Leukoderma disorders (including *bākuchī* and rock salt for external application—2:1 proportion).

Pustule eruptions: When they occur on the Leukoderma are first punctured to remove the fluids. For the next 15 mornings one takes *bākuchī*, *mañjiṣhṭhā*, neem, turmeric, *āmalakī*, *makoy*, *khadir*, *bilwa* bark, and *chakramarda*.

Varieties: The three forms, *dāruna*, *chāruna,* and *kilāsa*, are all caused by the simultaneous excess of all three *doṣhas*. When it is found in the blood, it is red; in the muscle it is coppery; and if in the fat, it is white. When it is in the blood, it is the mildest form; in the fat, it is the most serious.

This disorder cannot be healed if patches are overlapping, several patches exist, red hair grows through the patches, and diseases last for several years.

Leukoderma is caused by sinful acts in this life or previous lives; eating mutually contradictory foods, disrespect and lying to people and deities.

Minor Ailments (Kṣhudrarogam)

Causes: There are 44 forms of minor ailments. All the different writers give different views of this section. Thus, there is no generally accepted number of ailments or sequence of the diseases.

Symptoms:

Pimples and Swellings

Ajagallikā: Vāyu and Kapha—pimples that are shiny, knotty, painless, the same color as the surrounding skin, and is found in infants.

Yāvā-prakṣhyā: Vāyu and Kapha—barley-corn-shaped eruptions, very hard, thick in the middle, knotty, and confined to the flesh.

Andhālaji: Vāyu and Kapha—pimples are dense, raised, slender at the top, in circular patches, exuding some pus.

Vivritā: Pitta—pimples are the color of ripe figs; flat at the top, in circular patches, unbearable burning.

Kachapikā: Vāyu and Kapha—pimples are in groups of five or six; hard, raised, nodular, tortoise shell-shaped, appearing anywhere on the body.

Valmīka: All three *doṣhas*—knotty, undurated, pimples that slowly develop on the soles and palm joints, neck and above the collar bone, ant hill shaped.

Indra-vriddhā: Vāyu and Pitta—pimples on the skin, arranged circularly.

Panasika: Kapha and Vāyu—very painful pimples/ abscess in or around the ears.

Pāṣhāna-Garddabha (mumps): Kapha and Vāyu—slightly painful, non shifting, hard swelling, appearing on the jawbone joint.

Jāla-Garddabha: Pitta—thin, superficial swelling, shifts position, fever, burning, but does not form pus. [Some say when they are circular, raised, studded with pouches, red, painful, and caused by Vāyu and Pitta.]

Kakṣhā: Pitta—black, painful pimples on the back, sides and armpit area.

Agni-Rohini: All three *doṣhas*—blisters around the waist, bursts the local flesh, fever, burning inside the affected area; this cannot be healed. (Some say death occurs seven, 10 or 15 days from its onset.)

Chippam: Vāyu and Pitta—fingernail flesh develops pain, burning and pus.

Kunakham: Fingernails are rough, dry, black, due to being hit (e.g., with a hammer).

Anusayi: Kapha—small swelling on the body, the same color as the skin, but is deep-seated, and forms pus in the deeper levels.

Vidārikā: All three *doṣhas*—gourd-shaped round, red swelling on the groin region; symptoms related to each respective *doṣha*.

Śharkarār-budam: Vāyu and Kapha—flesh, veins, ligaments, and fat develop cysts that burst with a large quantity of honey-like secretion. Excessive secretion creates excess Vāyu, drying the area of the skin in the shape of many gravel-like pimples. Malodorous, multi colored secretion from the veins can develop. The veins may suddenly bleed. The three forms are eczema, psoriasis, and *rakasā* (dry erythema/abnormal red skin due to irritation and dilation of capillaries), and have been previously discussed under *Kuṣhṭhas* (Skin Disorders).

Yauvana-pidakā or Mukhaduṣhikā (acne): Vāyu and Kapha—thorny pimples on the face of young people, due to blood.

Padmini-Kantaka (skin papilloma): Vāyu and Kapha—circular, gray patches or rash-like pimples with thorny pimples, with itching.

Jatumani (mole): Blood and Pitta—reddish, shiny, circular, painless, congenital, level with the skin.

Maśhaka (lichen): Vāyu—hard, painless, black, raised pimples on the skin.

Tilakālaka (freckles): Any of the *doṣhas* —painless black spots (sesame seed sized) on the skin (non elevated). Some call this *Nilikam* if it is black and arise anywhere but on the face.

Nyacham: Painless, congenital, circular, white, or brown skin patches contained to small areas of the body.

Charmakila (skin hypertrophy/non-tumorous enlargement): Discussed in the skin disorder section.

Vyañga: Thin, circular, painless, brown patches or stains. Vāyu becomes excessed due to anger, over exertion, and fatigue; associated with Pitta cause this disorder to appear on the face. (Some say it is due to absorption of blood by Vāyu and Pitta).

Romāntikā (measles): Pitta and Kapha—when small eruptions appear all over the body, along with fever, burning, anorexia, and excess salivation. Herbs to reduce Vāyu, Kapha, and Pitta, are advised.

Viṣhphoṭaka (small pox)

Causes and Development: Overeating hot, pungent and sour foods causes burning sensation during digestion. Any heat-increasing activity (e.g., sun-bathing, summer heat) causes all three *doṣhas* to become excessed. The excessed *doṣhas* invade the skin, blood, muscles, and bones. Fever develops then blisters appear on the skin—on the whole body, or any part of it. Symptoms of blood and Pitta appear.

Eight forms of small pox exist: Vāyu, Pitta, Kapha, Vāyu/Pitta, Vāyu/Kapha, Pitta/Kapha, Tridoṣha, and blood. Conditions caused by one *doṣha* are easily healed. Dual-*doṣha* disorders are healed with difficulty. Tridoṣha conditions cannot be healed.

Symptoms:

Vāyu: Headache, severe pain, fever, thirst, joint pain; pimples are black.

Pitta: Fever, burning, pain, pus exudation, thirst; pimples are yellow or red.

Kapha: Vomiting, loss of appetite, lassitude; pimples are itching, hard, white, with no pain. Pus forms very slowly.

Vāyu/Pitta: Severe pain.

Vāyu/Kapha: Itching, hardness, and tightness

Pitta/Kapha: Itching, burning, fever, vomiting.

Tridoṣha: Pimples have depressions at their center and elevated edges; are hard, little pus, burning sensation, redness, thirst, delusion, vomiting, fainting, pain, fever, delirium, chills, and stupor.

Blood: Red pimples and symptoms of Pitta. No therapies exist for this condition.

Masūrikā (chicken pox)

Cause and Development:

Overeating sour, salty, and alkaline foods, incompatible foods, excess amounts of food, eating before the last meal is digested, excess fasting, eating contaminated foods and liquids, malefic planetary influences on certain communities of a country; all cause an excess of the *doṣhas* and bad blood. This develops lentil-sized eruptions all over the body. Five *doṣha* forms exist, and 7 tissue *(dhātu)* forms exist.

Premonitory Symptoms:

Fever, itching, pain all over the body, restlessness, giddiness, swelling and discolored skin, reddish eyes.

Symptoms:

Vāyu: Black or crimson eruptions, rough, very painful, hard, slowly forming pus; joint pain, cough, shivering, restlessness, exhaustion, dry lips, throat, and tongue; loss of appetite.

Pitta: Red, yellowish-white eruptions with severe burning and pain; quickly forming pus; diarrhea, pain all over the body, thirst, loss of appetite, mouth ulcers, red eyes, very high fevers, and great distress.

Blood: Similar to Pitta conditions.

Kapha: Watery discharge from the mouth nose and eyes; inactivity, headache, heaviness, nausea, loss of appetite, sleep, stupor, lassitude; white, soft large, itching eruptions that are slightly painful and slow to form pus.

Tridoṣha: Blue eruptions, flat, broad (depressed in the center and elevated at the edges), very painful, slow to form pus, copious exuding of malodorous pus, throat obstruction, loss of appetite, body stiffness, delirium, and restlessness. This condition is difficult to heal.

Localization Symptoms:

Plasma/Skin (*rasa/twak*): Eruptions are like bubbles of water, exuding thin watery fluid upon pricking; symptoms of mildly increased *doṣhas*.

In Blood (*rakta*): Red eruptions, quickly forming pus; thin skin, eruptions bleed heavily when pricked; symptoms of medium-increased *doṣhas*. This condition is difficult to heal.

Muscle (*māṃsa*): Hard, greasy eruptions, quickly forming pus; thick skin, pain all over the body, thirst, itching, fever, and restlessness.

Fat (*medas*): Eruptions are round, soft, slightly elevated, large, greasy, painful; high fever, delusion, restlessness, and distress. This is difficult to heal.

Marrow (*majjā*): Small, flat, rough eruptions, slightly elevated or at skin level; severe delusion, pain, and restlessness.

Bone (*asthi*): Cutting pain in the vital organs (thus endangering life) and bone pain.

Reproductive Fluid (*śhukra*): Ripe, waxy, small, very painful eruptions; stiff body, restlessness, delusion, burning, toxicity. This is a life-threatening condition.

Any of the above seven tissue conditions may also have one or more of the excessed *doṣha* symptoms present.

Easily Healed: Residing in the skin, caused by blood, Pitta or Kapha separately, or Kapha/Pitta.

Difficult to Heal: Vāyu, Vāyu/Pitta, Vāyu/Kapha.

Cannot be Healed: Tridoṣha whose symptoms include coral-colored eruptions or colors of all three *doṣhas*.

No herbal therapies are available when symptoms include hiccup, cough, frequent urination, high fever, severe delirium, restlessness, fainting, thirst, burning sensation, body curvatures, bleeding through mouth, nose or eyes; cooing, or difficulty breathing. Also for yellow or coppery pimples with pain, fever, burning all over the body, face, and inside the mouth.

Herpes Zoster (Visarpa)

Seven types of herpes exist: Vāyu, Pitta, Kapha, Vāyu/Pitta, Vāyu/Kapha, Pitta/Kapha, Tridoṣha, and trauma. It is found externally, internally, or both. External herpes is easiest to heal. The internal/external form is the most difficult to subdue.

Cause and Development: Its development is identical to edema. The *doṣhas* become aggravated due to their own causes, with the main development being the eating of salty, sour, pungent, and hot foods. Aggravated *doṣhas* quickly spread to all the internal parts (lymph, blood, skin, and muscles). When excessed *doṣhas* are outside, they spread to all the external parts. When the *doṣhas* are excessed in both the inside and outside, they spread in all places.

Inner herpes arises due to diseases of the vital organs (i.e., heart, head, urinary bladder, etc.), loss of consciousness, severe injury due to the sense organs, extreme thirst, sudden poor digestion, and physical weakness, forcing of the physical urges. Outer herpes arises from infections.

Symptoms

Vāyu: Similar to Vāyu fevers, and edema, pain that is throbbing, intermittent, piercing dilating, cutting, and tingling.

Pitta: Similar to Pitta fevers, and is quick spreading, with red swelling, miscellaneous eruptions of small and medium size.

Kapha: Similar to Kapha fevers, and itching, herpes are greasy.

When herpes are not tended to, all forms of herpes develop eruptions with symptoms of each *doṣha*, and eventually burst. This leads to ulcers with symptoms according to each *doṣha*.

Vāyu/Pitta (Agni Herpes): Fever, vomiting, fainting, diarrhea, thirst, dizziness, splitting bone pain, poor digestion, blindness, loss of taste and appetite. Burning, blackish, blue, or red skin eruptions look as though burnt by fire, and spread quickly in a line diagonally along the torso from the left shoulder to the bottom right side of the chest (and around the back to the left shoulder (due to Vāyu). This form of herpes attacks the vital organs, causing them severe pain, creates loss of consciousness and sleep, difficult breathing, and hiccup. At this stage, there is little comfort, difficulty moving, and a sort of coma-type of sleep.

Vāyu/Kapha (Granthi Herpes): Vāyu is obstructed by Kapha and breaks into many parts; or it vitiates the blood in the skin, veins, tendons, and muscles in persons with aggravated blood. This causes a chain of blood tumors that are either long, small, round, thick, or rough. It is associated with severe pain, fever, difficult breathing cough, diarrhea, dry mouth, hiccup, vomiting, dizziness, delusion, discoloration, fainting, cutting pain, and poor digestion.

Pitta/Kapha (Kardama Herpes): Fever, stiffness, excess sleep, stupor, headache, physical debility, tremors, irrelevant speech, loss of taste or appetite, dizziness, fainting, poor digestion, splitting bone pain, severe thirst, heaviness, mucus in feces, excess toxic coating in the plasma channels. Generally, it begins in the stomach and then spreads elsewhere. Eruptions are mildly painful, deep yellow, red, or yellowish-white, or black in color, and greasy. They can be dirty, swollen, heavy, undergoing ulceration from deep within; with excess heat and moisture in the muscles. Other symptoms include being slushy to the touch, exposed bundles of tendons and veins, gangrene, and foul odors.

Tridoṣha: Symptoms of all three *doṣhas* simultaneously, quickly spreading to all the tissues.

Kṣhataja (Trauma): Pitta and blood are aggravated producing herpes studded with boils. Other symptoms include fevers, severe swelling, pain, burning, and is blackish-red.

Herpes caused by any one *doṣha*, or by two *doṣhas* without secondary complications is easy to heal. Several causes of herpes make it difficult to heal, or cannot be healed. These causes include trauma, *tridoṣha*, invading the vital organs, loss of tendons, veins, and muscles; and those that are extremely moist and malodorous.

Modern science associates these infectious diseases with erysipelas, cellulitis, herpes zoster, gangrene, eczema, some forms of dermatitis, and skin cancer.

Therapies

The following herbs are taken internally and applied externally as a poultice.

Vāyu and Pitta: *Mañjiṣhṭhā, chandan, sārivā,* neem

Kapha: *Dāruharidrā*, turmeric, *chop chini*

Dual and Tridoṣha: Combine the required herbs

Trauma: Black pepper, *chandan, mañjiṣhṭhā, kākamāchī*

Foot-Skin Disorders

Pādadārikā: People who walk a lot find their soles becoming dry with painful cracks, caused by Vāyu in the feet. Burning soles are due to eating hot spices.

Kadara (corns): Knotty painful, hard growth; raised in the middle or sunken around the sides; secretions, appearing at the soles and maybe palms, due to blood and fat in the palms or soles. It is due to external causes such as shoes, gravel, thorns etc.

Alasa (athletes foot): Wetness (e.g., dampness, mud, etc.) causes burning, pains, itching, and secretions in between toes.

Head-Skin Disorders

Indralupta (balding), [also called *Rujya* or *Khālitya* (alopecia)]: Vāyu and Pitta cause hair to fall from their roots. Blood and Kapha fill these pores, preventing fresh hair growth.

Dāruṇaka: The roots of the body hairs become hard, dry and itchy, caused by Kapha and Vāyu.

Arunśhikā: Ulcers containing mucus and pus, and having many openings, appearing on the scalp str due to parasites, blood, and Kapha in the scalp.

Palitam (premature graying): Due to overworking, fatigue, stress, grief, anger, heat; Pitta become excessed and causes the hair to gray prematurely.

Genitals-Skin Disorders

Parivartikā (phimosis): *Vyāna* Vāyu becomes excessed due to masturbation; pressure or injury to the penis, forming a knot-like structure or constriction to the foreskin, prevents it from drawing back to uncover the head of the penis. Symptoms include pain, burning, occasionally forming pus; when the knot hardens, it is caused by Kapha and is itchy.

Avapātikā (paraphimosis): It occurs in young girls before they develop menses or the rupture of the hymen. When the outer covering of the *glans clitoridis* (prepuce) is abnormally turned back through such conditions as excited coition or other forcible entry.

Niruddha-prakāṣha: Vāyu causes the foreskin to cover up the urethra orifice, preventing the release of urine, causing great pain. Partial closure causes a thin release of urine with some pain.

Sanniruddha-guda or Niruddhaguda (narrow rectum): By obstructing the natural urge to pass stools, the rectum becomes clogged with feces, deranging *Apāna* Vāyu. This causes constriction of the passage, resulting in difficulty in passing stools. This is very difficult to heal.

Ahiputana: Itchy pimples around the anus of children are caused by not cleaning urine, perspiration, feces, etc. from their diaper. The eruptions are caused by deranged blood and Kapha, becoming eczema-like, and oozing a malodorous discharge with constant scratching. Eventually it spreads, and is difficult to heal.

Vriṣhana-kachu: When persons do not wash their genitals, or do not dry them after washing, local perspiration causes itching and eczema, resulting in constant scratching. It is due to Kapha and blood.

Guda-Bhranṣha (anus prolapse): In weak and thin persons, Vāyu is excessed through straining or urging the passage of stools, or from dysentery.

Therapies

General: In all disorders, most of the external herbal therapies may also be taken internally to heal the cause of the imbalances.

Aja-gallikā: Blood-letting with leeches when there is no pus formation and bursting of pimples; then, plasters of oyster shell powder or rhubarb. When pus and bursting pimples develop, ulcer therapies are used. [A Vāyu/Kapha disorder]

Yava-prakhyā, Antrālaji (Anhālaji), Panasi, Kachapi and Pāṣhāna-gardabha (mumps- non pus stages): Plastered with *kuṣhṭā*, *kūt*, *lavaṇ bhaksar*, cedar, *vaṃśha lochana*, and *ghee*. When pus sets in, pimples are cut by incision and then ulcer therapies are used.

Visphoṭaka (small pox), *Indra-vriddhā, Kakṣhā, Jāla-gardabha, Irivelli, Gandhanāmni, Gardabhi, and Vivritā*: Therapies for the Pitta-form of Visarpa are used—lightening (see *pañcha karma* section), bitter herbs (e.g., *chirāyatā*, *kuṭki*, neem, aloe vera, gentian, barberry), blood-letting, and purgation are also used. Foods include barley and *ghee* with *balā*, lotus root, sandalwood, *basmati* rice, peas, lentils, green lentils, *triphalā*, and pomegranates. Hot, burning spicy foods are to be avoided (e.g., onions, garlic, red peppers). It is also recommended to avoid nightshades (eggplants, potatoes, tomatoes, peaches, strawberries), naps, anger, exercise, sun, fire and wind.

Externally, *ghee* cooked with bitter herbs and sandalwood are applied to pimples when pus forms or bursts.

Chippam and Kunakham: First, washing the affected area with hot water is required, and the pus drained by cutting with a knife. Then, medicated oil is applied to the area using coriander, neem, sandalwood, aloe, turmeric, *mañjiṣhṭhā*, onion, black pepper, rhubarb, and *ghee* in a sunflower oil decoction.

Vidārikā: First, oil and fomentation are used; then, the area is rubbed with the fingers. A plaster of *bilwa*, *gambhari* bark, *peyu padal* bark, *archu*, and *śhyonaka* are applied to the swelling. The toxic blood is let out by scarification or leech/blood-letting. This is followed by applying a plaster of *musta*, *mañjiṣhṭhā*, turmeric, rose petals, neem, sarsaparilla, *bhṛiṅgarāj*, gotu kola, and sandalwood in sunflower or coconut oil. As soon as it becomes ulcerated, alterative and disinfecting therapies including *musta*, *mañjiṣhṭhā*, turmeric, *bhṛiṅgarāj*, gotu kola, sandalwood, *bibhītakī*, golden seal, neem, *guggul*, burdock, and gotu kola in sunflower or coconut oil are used. When ulcers are fully manifested, lancing followed by plastering with *guḍūchī*, *ghee*, and sesame oil, and then bandaging are required. The ulcer is washed frequently with antibiotic and antiseptic herbs like echinacea, golden seal, turmeric, neem, *guggul*, *bibhītakī*, gotu kola, *mañjiṣhṭhā*, and sarsaparilla.

Śharkarār-buda: This is treated like Kapha tumors (see Chapter 22), [or eczema, psoriasis, and *rakasā*; three diseases discussed under *kuṣhṭha*].

Kachu, Vicharchikā, Pāmā: These disorders are treated like obstinate skin diseases. A paste of white mustard seeds, calamus, turmeric, or an oil decoction of *kaṭuka*, aloe vera gel, *mañjiṣhṭhā*, neem, or sandalwood is applied to the affected skin area.

Pāda-dārikā: The vein affecting the disorder is opened, and the troubled area is treated with sesame oil or *ghee*, *mañjiṣhṭhā*, sarsaparilla, and musk.

Alasa (athletes foot): A plaster of sesame, neem, *harītakī*, and *kaṇṭkārī* is applied to the affected parts. Blood-letting is also useful. In less serious cases, only sandalwood powder need be applied to the area.

Kadara (corns): The corns are scraped off with a knife and cauterized by applying heated sesame oil.

Indra-lupta (balding): The bald area is oiled and fomented; then, constantly scraped and covered with a paste of black pepper, *chitrak*, cedar, *kaner*, wild licorice, Spanish jasmine, and *tagar* (Ceylon jasmine). Internally, *bhṛiṅgarāj*, gotu kola, *āmalakī*, *chitrak*, and *śhatāvarī* are useful.

Arunṣhikā: The affected scalp area undergoes blood-letting (by venesection or with leeches), then a neem decoction is poured over it. Next plasters are applied using herbs like turmeric, neem, licorice, and castor oil.

Dārunaka: Oil and foment the diseased hair roots. Then, herbs are applied (and ingested) that reduce Kapha and Vāyu, such as turmeric, *pippalī*, *aśhwagandhā*, *khadir*, *kākolī*, and ginger.

Palitam (premature graying): An oil decoction of *bhṛiṅgarāj*, *triphalā*, *mañjiṣhṭhā*, and licorice are used as nasal oil, head oil, and face oil to help cure baldness, wrinkles, and improve sensory organs.

Masūrikā and Romāntikā: Therapies for *visarpa* are used. Also helpful is internal and external use of turmeric, *mañjiṣhṭhā*, sandalwood, aloe vera gel, *bhṛiṅgarāj*, gotu kola, *musta*, *guggul*, and *harītakī*.

Jatumani (moles), *Maśhaka* (lichen), *Tila-kālaka* (freckles): The areas are scraped with a knife, then gradually cauterized with alkali when superficial, and with heat when deep seated.

Nyacha, Vyañga, Nilikā: Opening of local veins

in the temporal region, etc. is useful. Then, the areas involved with the disorder are rubbed with plaster of *balā*, licorice, *atibalā*, *bhūmīāmalakī*, *kṣhira kākolī*, bark, with milk, honey, or *ghee*.

Charak's therapy for *Vyanga* is turmeric, *mañjiṣhṭhā*, calamus, red and white sandalwood, and lotus filaments; pasted together with milk and *ghee*, and cooked. This helps remove wrinkles, tans, specks, moles, pimples, and improves the complexion.

Yuvāna-Pidakā (acne): Emetics are useful therapies. Herbs are ingested and applied to the face, include sandalwood, *mañjiṣhṭhā*, *lodhra*, calamus, and white *musta* seeds. Turmeric creme is also good to apply topically.

Padmini-Kantaka: A neem, *ghee* and honey decoction is taken as an emetic and is also applied to the diseased area.

Parivartikā (turned-back foreskin): *Ghee* is rubbed on the area and fomented, and plasters are applied for 3 to 5 days. Then, after lubricating the area with *ghee*, the glans penis is gently pressed and the foreskin is smoothly drawn over the head, entirely covering it. Lastly, the foreskin is fomented with warm poultices; Vāyu-reducing foods, including *ghee* and sesame oil are ingested. Poultices are made from barberry, wheat flour, onion, and cane sugar. They are made into a decoction and used as an ointment.

Avapātikā (paraphimosis): The same therapy is used for girls, as above.

Niruddha-Prakaṣha (urethra blockage): A tube that is open at both ends is lubricated with *ghee* and gently entered into the urethra. *Ghee* and sesame oil, mixed with Vāyu-reducing herbs such as *śhatāvarī*, licorice, *balā*, etc., are sprinkled over (or poured into) the area as a decoction or plaster. Every third day, thicker tubes are placed in the urethra. In this way the urethra passage is made to dilate. Emollient foods are eaten to help heal the condition.

The *doṣha* causing the below three disorders is first determined; remembering that these disorders cannot be healed. However, they may be controlled.

Agni-Rohini: This is treated like *visarpa* (see *visarpa* section).

Sanniruddha-Guda (narrowed rectum): This disorder is treated like *niruddha-prakaṣha* (urethra blockage).

Valmīka: This is treated as abscesses. Surgical procedures involve scraping off diseased patches, and cauterizing them with alkali or fire. Afterwards, purifying and healing the area is similar to tumors. If the disorder is not on a *marma* point (see *marmas* in Chapter 7), and not very large, purgatives, emetics, and enemas (depending upon the *doṣha* involved), followed by venesection, are used for purification. Plaster of *guḍūchī*, *kalaparni*, *arakvadam*, black salt, sesame seed paste, *ghee*, horsegram (*kulattha*), and barley flour is applied. When pus is involved, a poultice with the same ingredients is applied at a lukewarm temperature. When the pus is at its zenith, they are opened with a knife, cauterized, cleansed, and then recauterized with an alkali (*bhasin kchhar*). Healing therapies are next used, including neem oil cooked with cardamom, red sandalwood, *mañjiṣhṭhā*, *khadir*, and sarsaparilla. For symptoms appearing on the hands or feet, with complications of swelling and many cavities, no therapies exist.

Ahi-putanā, Vrishana-Kachu: When infants contract these diseases, first the mother's breast-milk is purified (see female reproductive section). The area affected is washed with *triphalā ghee*. Then, a paste of rock salt is applied. Sandalwood powder is frequently used to keep the area dry.

Guda-Bhranṣha (prolapsed anus): The protruding part is fomented and lubricated with *ghee*, then gently reinserted. Next, it is bandaged, leaving a small opening directly under the anus for passage of stools. The anus is frequently fomented; boiled milk with *ghee*, *śhatāvarī*, cardamom, *balā*, cinnamon, and *guggul* are taken as drink. It is said that even the most difficult prolapses can be normalized by this measure.

Subcutaneous Layers

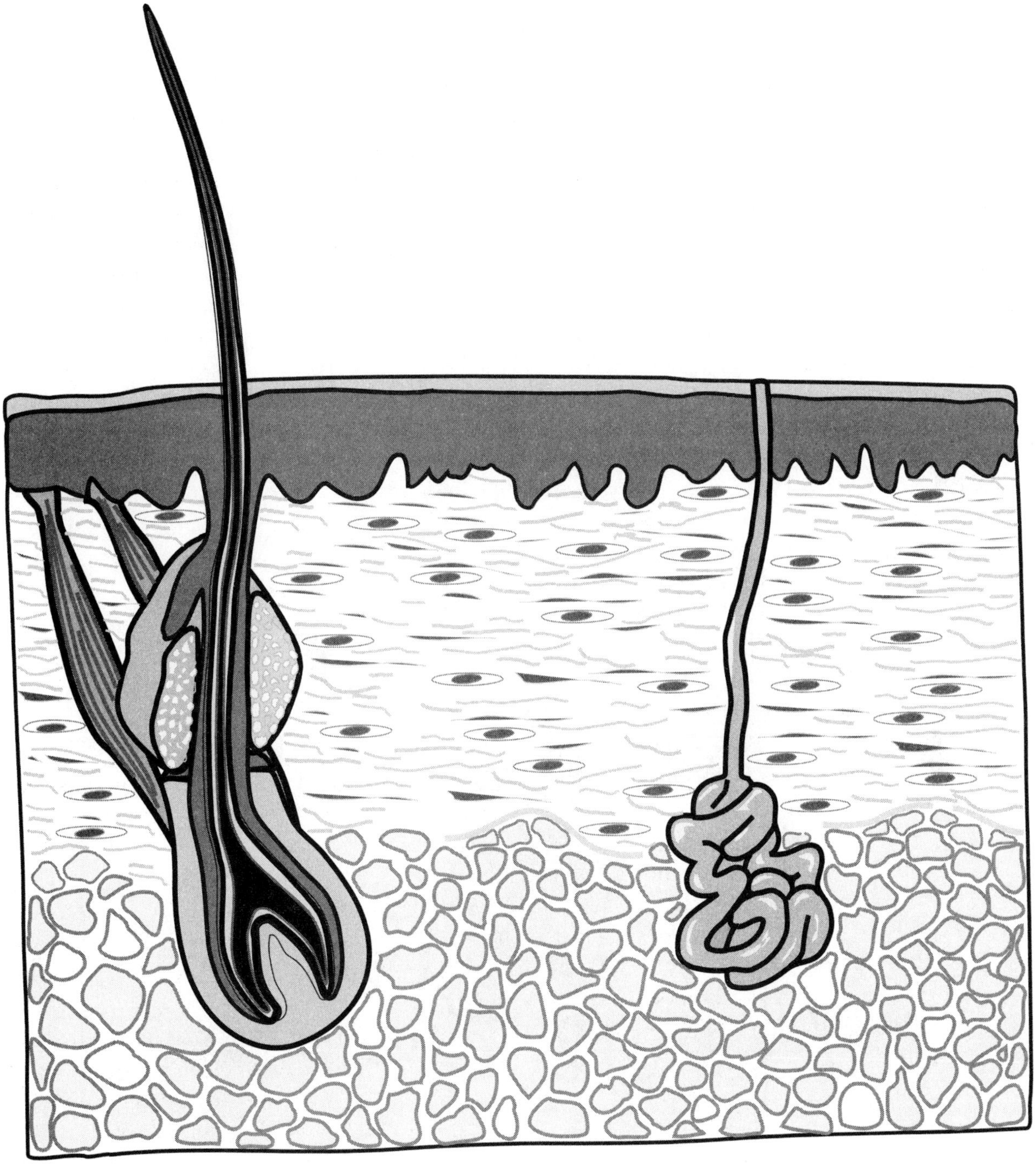

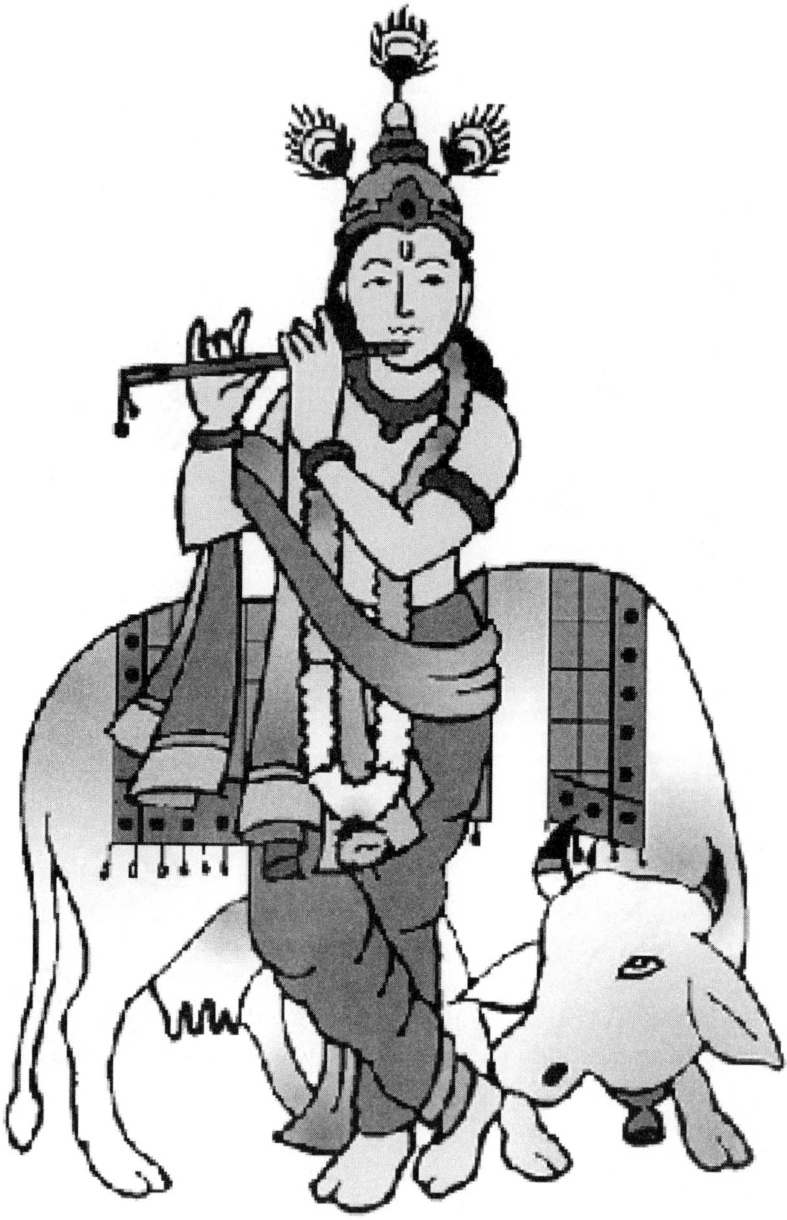

For an intelligent person, the whole world is a teacher,
so one should imitate the world after carefully considering
their meaning and effects of such actions
Aṣhṭāñga Hṛidayam Sū. Ch. 2: ver. 45

Chapter 22
Abnormal Growths/Neoplasm

Scrotum, Hernia, Fistula, Elephantiasis, Tumors, Cancer

Enlarged Scrotum (Vṛiddhi)

Causes: When Vāyu becomes aggravated owing to obstructed movement, it begins to move from the groin to the scrotum. This produces swelling and pain, then a pulling downward, and finally a swelling of the blood vessels. There are seven origins of this disease: Vāyu, Pitta, Kapha, blood, fat, urine, and intestines. Enlargements related to urine and the intestines are caused by Vāyu; however, these are separately categorized according to the organs involved. *Bradhna* is the swelling of the scrotal region caused by any of the *doṣhas*.

Symptoms:

Vāyu: Scrotum looks like a leather bag filled with air; is dry and painful.

Pitta: Scrotum is brownish-red and small, with burning, heat and the forming and discharging of pus.

Kapha: Scrotum is heavy, cold, oily, itching, hard, with slight pain.

Blood: Scrotum is studded with black boils and has other Pitta symptoms.

Fat: Soft, swollen scrotum, which is large, blackish-blue, oily, and hard to the touch.

Fluid in Scrotum
Hydrocele (Mūtra Vṛiddhi)

By habitual suppression of urine, the scrotum resembles a leather bag filled with water. It is painful, soft, with round rings underneath, and is accompanied by difficult urination.

Inguinal Hernia (Antraja Vṛiddhi)

Causes: Eating Vāyu-increasing foods, bathing in cold water, suppressing Vāyu, or premature release of urges (e.g., urine, feces), carrying heavy loads, walking long distances, improper movements of the body. All these increase Vāyu and pull down the weakened small intestine, producing an inguinal hernia. If the hernia is neglected, the small intestine then drops into the scrotum, causing swelling. Vāyu then causes an enlarged scrotum with gas, abdominal pain, and rigidity. Hiatal hernias occur near the navel, usually in weak children.

Symptoms: Scrotal pain, hollow sounding, recedes but comes back again on the release of pressure. It has all the symptoms of Vāyu *vṛiddhi*.

Swelling Therapies

Purgation, massage, medicated enema (*nirūha*), neem paste applied externally to the swelling. Recommended herbs to be taken internally include neem, turmeric, *mañjiṣhṭhā*, and *guggul.* For all swellings caused by Kapha, the swellings should be cut and cleansed first.

Fistula-in-Ano (Bhagandara)

[Anal abscesses on the sides of anus]

A pimple develops on either side of the anus within a 1-1/2 inch rads. It is painful and exudes. There are 5 forms of this condition:

Causes:

1. Vāyu (*śhataponāka*): Eating foods that

are astringent and dry causes excess Vāyu that produces an anus pimple (papule). If neglect, the pimple develops pus, then bursts, creating many small ulcers. Urine, feces, and semen may come out frothy, crimson colored, and painfully.

2. Pitta (*uṣhṭraśhirodara*): Excessed Pitta causes red pimples in the anal region that quickly develop pus. When the pus discharges it is hot and malodorous.

3. Kapha (*parisrāvī*): Itching, thick, oozing, hard, slightly painful, white colored.

4. Tridoṣha (*śhambūkavārtā*): Different colored pimples, oozes, looks like cows hoofs, and is spiral (like a seashell).

5. External Causes (*unmārgī*): Minor injury (such as one caused by thorns) at the anus will lead to sinus formation if neglected. Later, small ulcers form.

Pitta/Kapha-reducing therapies are suggested.

Therapies

Therapies appropriate for each respective *doṣha* are required. Purgation, probing, cleansing the site, cutting, cauterizing with oil, and suturing with alkaline thread.

Śhlīpada (Filariasis/Elephantiasis)

Mādhavakara, author of the *Mādhava Nidānam* defines this disease as a parasitic worm infestation in the tissues. If neglected it develops into elephantiasis. This condition is generally prevalent in areas where water stagnates for a long time and remains continually cold.

Cause and Development: Deranged muscle, blood, and Kapha causes swelling of the calves and lower legs, beginning in the front of the leg.

Symptoms: Swelling of the groin, gradually involving the legs, lips, nose, neck, ears, and hands. It is accompanied by fever and severe pain.

Vāyu: Black, rough swelling, cracks, or ulcers between the skin and mucus membrane, severe pain, and fever without apparent cause.

Pitta: Yellow-colored, swelling, burning sensation, soft to the touch, fever.

Kapha: White, smooth, heavy, and hard swelling.

Therapies

Swellings that grow upwards (like an anthill) with many sprouts; swellings that have grown for over 1 year, and swellings that are very large, with conditions that are caused by food and lifestyle habits that increase Kapha. In Kapha doṣhas, when swellings have exudation, when severe itching is present or when all symptoms are present should not be treated. Therapies that reduce the appropriate *doṣha* are advised. Antiparasitical and antiworm herbs are also useful (e.g., *kuṭaj, viḍaṅga* (see Chapter 15). Mustard paste is applied over the swelling (except in Pitta conditions).

Abdominal Tumors (Gulma)

General Causes: There are 8 types of *gulma*: Vāyu, Pitta, Kapha, Vāyu/Pitta, Vāyu/Kapha, Pitta/Kapha, Tridoṣha, and (in women only), tumors related to menstrual blood/ovum.

These occur when weak from fever, vomiting, diarrhea, and other debilitating diseases, or from excessive or improper therapies of emesis, purgation, and enema; eating an excess of Vāyu increasing foods; drinking cold water when hungry. Other causes include excess jumping, swimming, or other strenuous activities just after eating; forcing vomiting, suppressing the natural urges (e.g., passing gas and urination), undergoing purificatory therapies without oleation and sudation, not following the recommended eating and lifestyle habits after pañcha karma (purificatory therapies).

From these conditions the *doṣhas*, with Vāyu predominant, become increased individually or in combination (two or three *doṣhas* or with blood), invade the alimentary tract, spreading both upward and downward, causing abdominal pain, and then a perceivable, elevated, hard mass (tumor).

General Premonitory Signs: Loss of appetite, poor, irregular digestion, indigestion, anorexia, vomiting, loss of natural urges, colic, intestinal gurgling, hair standing on end, belching.

Vāyu Tumors: For Vāyu *doṣhas* or others who have been greatly emaciated by fever, emesis, purgation, or diarrhea; tumors are caused by eating an excess of Vāyu-increasing foods, cold food, drink and habits, non-oily emetic or purgative therapies, forcing vomiting, suppressing the urges to pass gas, urine, and stool, excessively drinking water after heavy food, excess bumpy travel, excess amounts of sex, exercise, drinking, anxiety; accidents, irregular postures during sitting, sleeping, standing, or walking.

Premonitory Signs: Excessive belching, constipation, gruesome feeling of contentment, intolerance, intestinal gurgling, air moving in the intestines, gas, poor digestion.

Vāyu Causes: These tumors are caused by weakness from tissue depletion or loss in the colon, passage obstruction by Kapha, feces, or Pitta. Vāyu becomes aggravated, localized in the alimentary tract, and forms into a hard mass by causing dryness. The tumor is called primary if it develops in the colon (the primary site of its origin), and secondary if it develops in the small intestine or stomach. Secondary tumors have branches or cause similar kinds of growth at a distant organ or area (metastasis). Usually, these tumors are found in the urinary bladder, navel, heart, or rib area.

Vāyu Pathology: Aggravated Vāyu enters the alimentary tract or *mahā srotas,* causing it to become dry and hard. Vāyu then relocates and manifests in the heart, bladder, sides of the chest or navel area. It causes colic and nodules.

Vāyu Symptoms: Tumors change in size and intensity of pain alternating between experiencing and not experiencing piercing and throbbing, expansion and contraction, numbness and hair standing on end. There may be a feeling of ants crawling on one's limbs, afternoon fever, dry mouth, difficult breathing, and hair standing on end at the onset of pain.

One experiences pain in the sides of the neck, headache, fever, enlarged spleen, gurgling intestinal sound, pricking pain, constipation, difficulty breathing, stiff body, dry mouth, emaciation, irregular digestion, dry, black skin, nails, eyes, urine, and feces; its shape is indefinite, found in various places, changes location, and size. The nature of pain may range from throbbing and cutting pain to a feeling that the tumor is being swarmed by ants.

Vāyu Complications: These include spleen problems, intestinal gurgling, poor digestion, malaise, head pain, swollen lymph glands of the groin, black, red or rough skin, nails, eyes, feces, urine, and stool; hardening of the alimentary tract.

Vāyu Tumor Therapies

1. Oleation is first administered through foods, massage, drinks, and *nirūha* and *anuvāsana* medicated enemas (see Chapter 7).

a. Oily drinks are especially useful for tumors above the navel area.

b. Both enemas are used for tumors in the colon or abdomen.

c. When there are also obstructions blocking gas and stool, oily, hot, and nourishing foods and liquids are taken (after the digestion is improved).

Medicated ghee and sesame oil are suggested for drinking, for massage, and both forms of medicated enemas. They are taken very frequently (ensuring that Pitta and Kapha do not become aggravated). Medicated ghee includes boiled herbs of ginger, *balā, kaṭukā, viḍaṅga,* and *triphalā.* Should Pitta, Kapha, or blood become excessed, then standard therapies to reduce these *doṣhas* are applied, ensuring Vāyu does not become further deranged.

Ingesting ghee boiled with the herbs of *triphalā,* coriander, *viḍaṅga, chitrak*, and milk (4 times the amount of the ghee) heals Vāyu tumors. A decoction of daśhmūl may be added to increase the efficacy of therapy. *Hiṅgwastock* paste, coriander, *chitrak,* calamus, cardamom, and yogurt boiled in *ghee* alleviates colic pain, and abdominal distention.

Alternatively, *śhilājit* (mineral pitch) with daśhmūl and barley is another way to heal tumors.

2) Fomentation therapy is next used to soften the circulatory channels, reduce excess Vāyu, colic pain, abdominal distention, and constipation, which results in healing the tumor.

If Vāyu tumors are not healed by the above therapies, then blood-letting will heal the illness.

Pitta Tumors

Pitta Causes: Pitta becomes deranged along with Vāyu in persons emaciated from fever, emesis, purgation, or diarrhea. This is caused by excess hot or burning foods (i.e., salty, pungent, sour, alkaline, sharp, and fermented), old wine, salads, eating before digesting the previous meal, emesis with a dry stomach, habitually suppressing natural urges, excessive sun, and wind exposure.

Pitta Pathology: Deranged Vāyu manifests in the stomach and small intestine, producing similar pains as in Vāyu tumors. Traveling through the *raktavaha srota* (blood/circulatory system) produces burning in the areas of the pelvis, heart, chest, and throat as a result of vitiated Pitta. This causes sour burps with smoke, burning sensation in tumor with pain, sweating, soft, loose, tender, or with slight raising of the hair in this region.

Pitta Symptoms: Persons experience acidity, fainting, diarrhea, sweating, thirst, fever, green or deep yellow skin, nails, eyes, urine, and feces; tender to the touch and burning, giddiness, throbbing pain, dry throat, palate, and mouth.

Pitta Tumor Therapies

1) When caused by oily and hot foods, laxatives like rhubarb or senna are used.

2) When caused by dry and hot foods, ingesting *ghee* is useful.

3) When the Pitta tumor is in the colon, an enema is given with bitter herbs and milk; or a purgative with lukewarm milk boiled with bitter herbs and *ghee* (if there is strong digestion and physical strength).

4) If the illness is associated with thirst, fever, excessive burning, colic pain, sweating, weak digestion, and anorexia, then blood-letting is employed. To restore strength after blood-letting, nourishing soups with *ghee* and sesame oil are used.

5) Pus-Free Tumors (*apakva*): A tumor that has not developed pus will be heavy, hard, fixed, raised, and located deep in muscle tissue without causing a change in skin color.

6) Pus-Forming Tumors (*pachya-māna*): One experiences a burning sensation, fever, colic, and sawing pain; irritation, insomnia, general distaste for things. Hot medicated oils (e.g., sunflower oil with brāhmī, turmeric, and cardamom) are used to heal this type of tumor.

7) Pus Tumors: When the Pitta tumor is also associated with vitiated blood (*rakta*) and Pitta, the tumor may develop pus. Surgery is required for Pitta tumors.

Symptoms of external tumors that are suppurated include the exfoliation of skin, protrusion, grayish color with a red outline, feeling that it is full of water. After pressing down on the tumor, it immediately rises to its original position; pain occurs when the sides of the tumor are pressed together.

When the tumors are internal or there is swelling in the region of the heart, signs and symptoms are the same. External tumors will protrude towards the sides of the abdomen.

The ancient Āyurvedic physician, Suṣhrut and the ancient author *Ātreya* (*Charak*) have delineated between pus-filled and non-pus-filled tumors. *Suṣhrut* stated that tumors do not develop pus, whereas *Ātreya* notes that pus develops in tumors embedded in the tissues, creating abscesses. Being an experienced surgeon, *Sushrut* refers to the neoplastic growths, whereas *Charak* refers only to infectious swellings.

Some scholars differentiate between internal and external tumors. All tumors develop in the gastrointestinal tract. Should they develop pus there, they are called internal tumors. If the tumors rise to the surface and then develop pus, they are called external tumors.

Self-Healing Pus Tumors: When this tumor has softened the passageway, it moves up or down (interior tumors), that is, the aggravated *doṣhas* are eliminating their excesses without need of therapy. At these times, persons need not resort to herbal or surgical therapies, but focus only on the proper diet for 10 to 12 days. Afterwards, more *ghee* is taken to help eliminate the *doṣhas.* When the *doṣhas* have regained balance (excesses are eliminated), persons ingest *ghee* boiled with bitter herbs and raw honey.

To reduce the burning sensations of Pitta tumors, the tumor is massaged using sandalwood oil or *ghee*.

Kapha Tumors

Cause: Kapha tumors (with Vāyu) occur in emaciated persons from fevers, diarrhea, excess or improper emesis or purgation. They result from overeating, excessive eating of oily, heavy, sweet, and cold foods; overindulging in pastries, sugar, milk, sesame seeds, candy, salads, animal products; excessive amounts of immature yogurt and wine, suppressing natural urges, drinking too much water when not thirsty, and physical trauma.

Kapha Symptoms: This causes the excessed Vāyu to settle and develop in the stomach and small intestines, producing pains similar to that experienced with Vāyu tumors. Excessed Kapha then causes fevers that start as a cold, anorexia, indigestion, malaise, hair standing on end, and heart disease. Other initial symptoms include vomiting, oversleeping, laziness, timidness, heaviness and pain in the head, loss of taste or appetite, weakness, and fibroids. Tumors remain stationary (i.e., not moving), heavy, hard, deep seated, with numbness. When the tumor is overly aggravated, one experiences cough, difficult breathing, mucus, TB, whitish skin, nails, eyes, urine and feces.

Tumors caused from each *doṣha* generally develop in their original site and produce pain at times specific to the *doṣha* involved.

Kapha Tumor Therapies

1) Tumors caused by ingesting cold, heavy, and oily foods require fasting if one is not strong enough for emetics (vomiting) and has weak digestion.

2) With poor digestion, minimal pain, heaviness, sluggish gastrointestinal tract, nausea, and anorexia, emetics are advised.

3) After emetics and fasting, persons are counseled to eat hot, pungent, and bitter foods and herbs. When digestive strength is restored from these three therapies, persons take *ghee* boiled with laxatives and pungents, such as *triphalā* and *pippalī* respectively.

4) For tumors that are hard and raised, accompanied with distention and constipation, fomentation is first used; later the tumor is massaged to help dissolve it.

5) When the tumor becomes dislodged from its manifestation site, purgatives, such as castor oil, are suggested. Oil or *daśhmūl* enemas may also be used.

6) Once the GI tract is well oiled, if pus is in the tumor and one experiences weakened digestion or retention of wind, then herbal powders or decoctions are used to relieve these conditions. Herbs include *triphalā,* cardamom, and coriander to remove gas; and *pippalī* for strengthening the digestion.

Should the tumor be well-rooted, large, hard, immovable, and heavy, then persons are given laxatives, medicated herbal wines (*ariṣhṭas*), and cauterization.

Laxatives are repeated every 1 to 3 days to

develop physical strength. Kapha purgatives are taken at double the strength used by Vāyu *doṣhas*. *Ariṣhṭas* (medicated herbal wines) are used to improve digestion, remove anorexia, and clear the circulatory channels. Cauterization is used if all of the above therapies prove ineffective. Cauterization is useful for both Kapha and Vāyu tumors. For Kapha tumors, surgery is recommended.

Dual and Tridoṣha: Symptoms are of both *doṣhas* or all three *doṣhas*. Tridoṣha tumors also provoke severe pain, burning, quickly forming and secreting pus, hardness, and greatly elevated tumors. Tridoṣha tumors cannot be healed.

Vāyu/Kapha Therapies (*Dvandvaja* Tumors)

1) Symptoms include poor digestion, anorexia, nausea, heaviness, and drowsiness. The main therapy is emetics (*vamana*). [See Chapter 7]

2) With colic pain, abdominal distention, and constipation, suppositories are useful, along with herbs that reduce Vāyu and Kapha (e.g., *triphalā*, ginger, and cardamom).

Vāyu/Pitta Therapies: If Vāyu tumors develop Pitta complications with fever and burning sensations, then mild purgation (so as not to aggravate Vāyu), such as castor oil (2 teaspoons in one cup of hot water before bed), is useful to help stimulate downward moving air (*Apāna* Vāyu).

Dual/Tridoṣhic Therapies: The above mentioned therapies for the appropriate *doṣhas* are practiced.

Medicated enemas are the best for healing tumors. It balances Vāyu in the site of origin, thereby removing the cause of the tumor, and eventually, the tumor itself. Both *nirūha* (non-oil-based) and *anuvāsana* (oil-based) medicated enemas are frequently used to heal tumors for Vāyu, Pitta, and Kapha tumors.

After undergoing fasting for any of the three *doṣhas* experiencing undigested toxins (*āma*), thick barley gruel and herbal soup is eaten.

Anti-tumor Herbs for Specific Conditions

All Tumors: *Mañjiṣhṭhā, guggul,* aloe, *kuṣhtha, harītakī, balā, mamīrā,* neem, garlic, and *lavan bhaskar* mixture.
Abdominal Tumors: *Pippalī*
Glandular Tumors: Yellow dock
Brain Tumors: *Brāhmī*
Breast Tumors: *Musta*
TB Tumors: *Kañchanar* bark with ginger paste
Vāyu Tumors: *Paṣhana Bedha*

Blood (Raktaja Gulma) (Uterine/ovarian tumors and cysts)

Causes: These conditions develops during a woman's menstrual period, soon after delivery (or miscarriage), with uterineor vaginal diseases, and from partaking in Vāyu-increasing foods and lifestyles (e.g., fear, worry) immediately after delivery or menstrual period. Other causes include fasting during menstruation or pregnancy and suppressing natural urges. These activities aggravate Vāyu, causing it to enter the cervix and obstruct the monthly menstrual blood in the uterus. [Blood tumors occur in men only if there is vitiation of the blood; see Chapter 13.]

Symptoms: Experiences include pregnancy-caused symptoms (i.e., nausea, longings, breast-milk disorders, emaciation, distention), colic, diarrhea, anorexia, cough, malaise, oversleeping, laziness, timidity, excessive salivation, fainting, darkening of the lips and breasts, eye strain, swollen feet, growth of small hairs, and pulsation of round tumors (usually during pregnancy only a portion of the fetus pulsates). Gradually the blood, associated with Vāyu and Pitta, cause symptoms of pain, stiffness, burning, diarrhea, thirst, fever, severe uterine pain (from accumulated vitiated blood), oozing, foul smell, and tearing and pulsating pain in the vagina. Sometimes the tumor moves around the uterus causing pain, but only the tumor grows (i.e., not the abdominal cavity, as in pregnancy). These tumors are treated only after a span of 10 months.

Tumors grow and seep pus after a long time, or not at all, because they are caused by *doṣhas*. Abscesses quickly grow and seep pus because they are caused by vitiated blood.

Tumors in the alimentary tract cause pain in the urinary bladder, upper abdomen, heart, and spleen; weaken digestive activity; cause loss of complexion and strength, and urinary and gaseous retention, and constipation and restraint of other natural urges. Tumors in the abdominal organs and outside the alimentary tract cause the opposite symptoms (i.e., mild pain, discoloration at the tumor site and greater outward growth).

Blood Tumor Therapies

After 10 months of this illness, one undergoes oleation (oil), fomentation (sweat), and purgation with oily ingredients (*sneha virechana*). See Chapter 7.

To dissolve the blood tumor, the powder of *clerodendron siphonanthus* (*bhargi*), *ghee, jaggery, pippalī, pippalī* root, *devdaru*, and *tṛikatu* are eaten with a decoction of sesame plant stems.

Another excellent herb for this condition is *aṣhoka*.

Gas (*Ānāha*): Due to obstructed upward and downward Vāyu, severe abdominal pain with gurgling, great enlarged abdomen occurs.

Aṣhṭhīlā and *Pratyā-ṣhṭhīla*:

Raised, hard stone-like tumors with gas are called *aṣhthīlā*. When these tumors are elevated sideways they are called *pratyāṣhthīla*. Tumor (*gulma*) therapies are followed.

Tūonī and *Prati-tūnī*: Vāyu-causing severe radiating pain from the colon to the rectum and urethral passage is called *tūnī*. When the pain radiates in the reverse direction it is called *pratitūnī*. *Pippalī* and *hiṅg* are taken with *ghee*. Medicated enemas are also indicated.

Cancer (Arbuda)

Causes: Āyurveda sees cancer as an emotional disease. Usually persons who feel a lack of meaning or purpose in life are afraid or unaware of what to do with their lives. These people develop something internally instead of creating something meaningful in their lives. Another view is that the aura is disrupted, allowing negative astral forces to enter the body. Cancer may be caused by environmental pollution, junk food, lethargy, lack of spiritual purpose, suppressed emotions or stagnation. Past-life *karma* also plays a role in this disease. Therefore, beyond physical healing, emotional healing requires meditation and psychic cleansing.

Although one humor is the main cause of a cancer, there are usually imbalances of all three *doṣhas*. Poor digestion allows for a buildup of toxins in the body. Downward moving air (*Apāna* Vāyu) excesses develop negative life-force, which may mean that distention, constipation, and diarrhea may be the first physical causes of cancer. There is also a lack of oxygen (*prāṇa*) in the cells. Brain tumors are mainly Kapha, secondarily Pitta.

Symptoms:

Vāyu: Fear, anxiety, depression, and insomnia; dry, hard tumors of varying size, gray or brown complexion, distention, constipation, and other Vāyu diseases. Colon cancer is usually a form of Vāyu cancer.

Pitta: Anger, impatience, irritability, hatred, resentment, inflamed, infected burning or bleeding tumors. Skin, eye, and liver cancers are usually Pitta-related.

Kapha: Tumors are caused by any of the constitutions, but more often found in Kapha *doṣhas*. Symptoms include fatigue, excess sleeping, congestion, and salivation. First tumors are usually benign (not hard or well-defined to the touch) and are accumulations of mucus or subcutaneous fat; swollen, with dampness, and congestion. Later, they may turn malignant. Hot and bitter herbs help reduce fat, such as ginger, black pepper, turmeric, and *kaṭukā* and barberry. *Tṛikatu*, *triphalā,* and honey is a useful combination. Tumor-reducing herbs include saffron, turmeric, safflower, dandelion. Surgery is useful if canceris found early enough. Lung or breast cancer is usually Kapha-related.

Blood (*Raktārbuda*): Excessed doṣhas invade the blood, causing large, exuding muscle tumors that are studded, fast-growing, and discharge large amounts of blood. This condition causes anemia to develop resulting from the loss of blood.

Muscle (*Māṃsārbuda*): External blows to the body can derange the muscle tissue, causing painless, smooth, stone-like, and skin-colored tumors on the skin. These more commonly occur among nonvegetarians, and cannot be healed.

Any cancer tumor that heavily exudes, develops on vital organs or channels, and those that are immovable, cannot be healed.

Adhyarbuda: A secondary cancer developing from the first cancer. This cannot be healed.

Dvirarbuda: A secondary cancer developing simultaneously with the first cancer. This cannot be healed.

Therapies

General Overview:

4 Step Cancer Healing Process

Four cancer healing therapies are required:

1) Cleansing Therapies: (For advanced cases)

a) Castor oil for 40 days. 1 to 2 teaspoons of castor oil are mixed in 1 cup of hot water and ingested before bed. If one has more or less than three stools the next morning, the dose should be adjusted until persons have only three stools in the morning. Castor oil therapy is an excellent, gentle cleansing process.

b) *Harītakī* for 1 year. One-quarter tsp. of *harītakī* is ingested 3 times daily. Depending on the season, add 1/4 teaspoon of sweets or spices to the *harītakī*.

Summer/Fall: Mix with *jaggery* (when humid also add rock salt)

Winter: Mix with ginger (when extremely cold use pippalī).

Spring: Mix with raw, uncooked honey

c) Avoid meats, dairy (except *lassi*) and other protein-rich foods (although some protein is needed) because cancer is believed to be caused by excess protein.

d) For Pitta- or Kapha-related cancers antitoxin herbs (bitters and pungents) like *kaṭukā* and peppers are needed for cleansing the blood and improving circulation.

[For less severe conditions, see additional therapies below.]

2) Immune-Boosting Herbs:

The immune system must strong to fight off the illness. For those undergoing chemotherapy, the need for immune-boosting herbs becomes even greater.

a) One or 2 teaspoons *of chyavan prāśh* is taken once or twice a day.

b) Several herbs help boost the immune system without aggravating one's *doṣha* (e.g., *śhatāvarī, aśhwagandhā, vidārī kand*). The dose taken is between 3 grams to 1 ounce daily.

3) Music Therapy:

Soothing meditation music harmonizes and heals the mind, thoughts, and nervous system. Classical Indian *ragas* (songs) and devotional chants can be listened to throughout the day and night. Certain *ragas* are designed to create harmony for specific times of the day and night. Chants like *Aum Namah Śhivaya* are especially useful. [See Chapter 10 on music therapy for more details.]

4) Jyotiṣh Astrology:

A wider range of causes can exist when considering a serious illness. Ancient India has understood and successfully used the fields of medical astrology, life-purpose or *dharma*; and *karma* (past life actions that affect one's present life).

These early spiritual astrologers(*Jyotiṣhis*) found a correlation between certain planets and corresponding diseases. Saturn and the north and south nodes of the Moon (*Rahu* and *Ketu*) were particularly related to mysterious diseases like cancer. From one's astrology chart, the disease-causing planets were recognized, and the appropriate therapies suggested.

As discussed earlier, Āyurveda believes when a person does not know or live the life they were meant to live, they feel a lack of purpose or emptiness. Life-purpose is also called God-given talent, or simply, doing what you love to do. In short, if one does not do what they love to do, an emptiness develops that can lead to longing and suffering, eventually developing into (physical) cancer.

Whenever persons develop serious illness, a wide range of complications, or a sudden onset of a health concern, *Vedic* belief suggests that it is related to harmful actions performed by the person in previous lives. Although the idea of reincarnation is certainly not scientific in the modern sense of the word, astrologers have successfully helped people understand and heal such disorders from the standpoint of *karmic* causes. It is presented here in brief only as an option available to those wishing to consider this field of cause and therapy.

Even if one chooses not to investigate *Jyotiṣh* astrology, considering a career that one loves is still a useful therapy to follow.

Thus, the *Jyotiṣh/Vedic* astrology chart becomes a useful tool to gain deeper insight into medical astrology, *dharma* or life-purpose, and *karma*. For the skeptical mind, these therapeutic approaches may be considered when other options fail.

Additional Therapies

Vāyu: Immune-strengthening herbs are best used when persons are very weak or undergoing surgery or chemotherapy. Herbs include *aśhwagandhā, yogaraj guggul* (Vāyu-/Kapha-reducing), *kapikachū* (Vāyu-reducing), *śhatāvarī* (Vāyu-/Pitta-reducing), *guḍūchī, balā, śhilājit, triphalā* (tridoṣhic), taking 1 or more ounces daily.

Pitta and Kapha: (Lymph or skin cancer) blood cleansers like *manjiṣhṭhā,* saffron, *brāhmī,* red clover, burdock, jasmine, and sarsaparilla are used, 1 to 3 ounces daily with meals. They are best used fresh, if possible.

Vāyu/Kapha: (Thyroid, neck or lymph cancer) these phlegm-reducing herbs include kelp, seaweed, Irish moss, *pippalī*, ginger, black pepper, *yogaraj guggul,* jasmine, myrrh, turmeric, *tṛikatu.* Doses may be 1/2 teaspoon, 3 times daily after meals.

Tridoṣhic: (Breast, uterine, liver, pancreatic cancer) strong circulation-improving herbs break stagnation, reduce masses, and aid tissue healing. These include turmeric, saffron, safflower, myrrh, *mañjiṣhṭhā, bhūmīāmalakī* (liver cleanser), *yogaraj guggul.* Doses can be about 1/2 teaspoon, 3 times daily.

Foods: Meat, dairy, and excess protein are not advised since cancer cells are basically protein (though some protein is needed for digestive enzyme secretion). Raw vegetables and juices like wheat or barley grass, dandelion, celery, alfalfa and sunflower sprouts are best for Pitta and other strong persons, but should be taken with spices like ginger and garlic to keep the digestion strong. The green juices have much positive life-force (prāṇa), cleansing negative life-energies. Weak persons need to take immune-boosting herbs listed above.

Brain tumors (brain)Tumors: *Mañjiṣhṭhā* and *brāhmī* (internally and as nasal snuff), *śhiro dhara,* and *pañcha karma* therapies appropriate to each doṣha are very useful if persons are strong.

Prostate Cancer: *Chandraprabha vati* 1,000 mg twice daily; *shilājit* 500 mg. twice daily; *kaṇchnar* 500 mg. twice daily; *punarnavā* 500 mg. twice daily; *aśhwagandhā* 500 mg twice daily; carrot juice 4 oz every morning. Herbs for Pitta and Kapha are also useful (see above).

Jasmine is also useful for bone cancer. Tumors, goiter, and scrofula are discussed under the Metabolic System (Chapter 25).

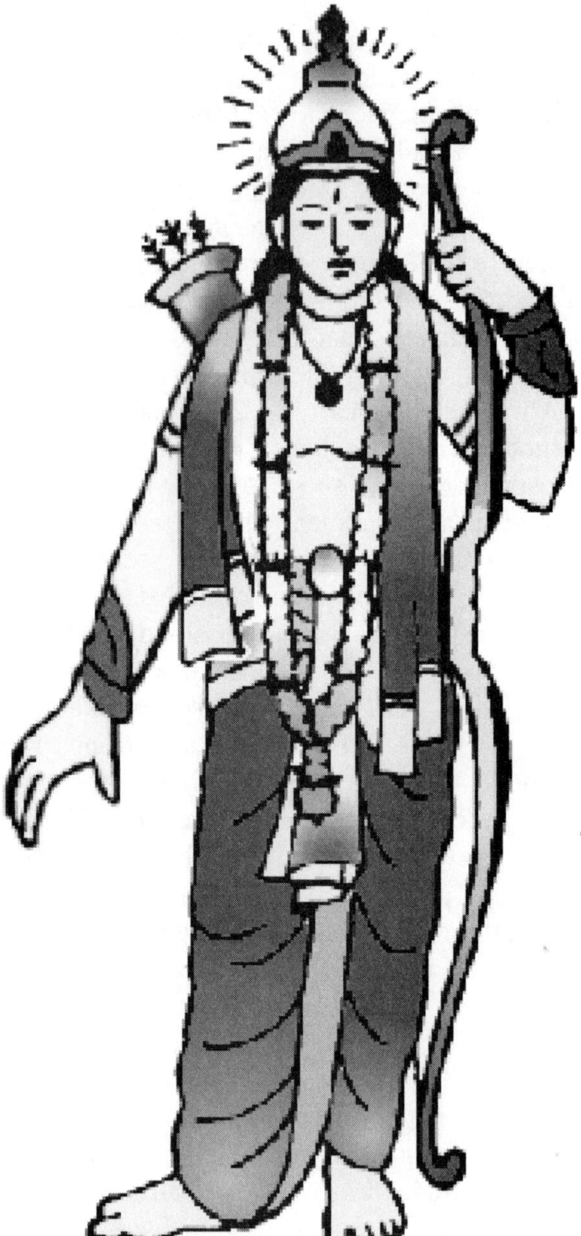

Tradition, ethics, knowldege, humility;
these are the four doors to a good mind.
Mahabharata

Chapter 23
Reproductive System
Female Reproduction, Childbirth, Planets and Newborns, Male Reproduction (including prostate), Venereal Diseases

Female Reproductive Tract (Yonivyāpat)

Causes: Twenty disorders of the female reproductive tract exist, caused by poor diet and lifestyle, imbalanced menstrual flow, defective ovum and ovary, and past *karma*. This results in an inability to conceive and other health concerns (e.g., tumors, hemorrhoids, menorrhagia).

Specific Causes, Development and Symptoms:
1. *Vāyu*: Causes include excessive ingesting of foods and liquid, and lifestyles that increase air. The excessed Vāyu moves to the genital tract producing many types of pain, vaginal numbness, exhaustion, and other Vāyu diseases. Menstrual discharge is painful, frothy, thin, rough, and with sounds.
2. *Pitta*: Causes include excessive ingesting of foods and liquids (e.g., sour, pungent, salty), and lifestyles that increase fire. The excessed Pitta moves to the genital tract and produces burning, inflammation, fever, and heat. The menstrual flow is blue, yellow, or black with excessive hot discharges and foul odor.
3. *Kapha*: Excessive watery foods, liquids, and lifestyles create excess Kapha, forcing it to move to the female tract. This causes experiences that are slimy, cold, itching, pale, with mild pain. The menstrual flow is pale and slimy.
4. *Tridoṣha*: Symptoms include excessive use of air, fire, and water foods, liquids, and lifestyles. This causes the three *doṣhas* to move to the genital tract and uterus, causing symptoms of all three *doṣhas* (i.e., burning and pain with slimy, white discharges).
5. *Sāsṛijā (Menstrual Blood)*: Pitta excesses afflicting the blood move to the female tract, causing excess bleeding.
6. *Arajaskā (Uterus, Tract and Blood)*: Excess Pitta in theses areas causes leanness and a poor complexion.
7. *Acharaṇā*: Not washing the genitalia causes itching and excessive desires for men. It is caused by Vāyu excesses.
8. *Aticharaṇā*: Excessive sex aggravates Vāyu, producing swelling, numbness, and pain in the genital tract.
9. *Prāk-charaṇā*: Young women having sexual relations at too early an age causing Vāyu to afflict the female tract. This results in back, waist, thigh, and groin pain. It is caused by Vāyu excesses.
10. *Upa-plutā*: Taking Kapha-increasing foods in excess while pregnant or suppressing the urge to vomit or breathe causes Vāyu excesses to carry Kapha to the female tract. This produces pale fluid discharges with piercing pain, white mucus, and Vāyu and Kapha disorders during orgasm.
11. *Pari-plutā*: Pitta *doṣha* females who suppress the urges to sneeze and belch during sex cause Vāyu and Pitta to afflict the female tract. This produces premature orgasm.
12. *Udā-vartānī (dysmenorrhea)*: Suppressing natural urges causes Vāyu to move upward in the genital tract, causing painful and difficult menstrual discharges. After the discharge, relief is immediately felt. See page 508 for more details.

13. *Karṇinī*: Untimely straining during labor causes Vāyu to become blocked by the fetus and combines with Kapha and blood. This produces growths (polyps) that block the menstrual flow.
14. *Putra-ghnī*: Morbidity of menstrual fluid or ovum may produce Vāyu (roughness) that results in the death of the fetus.
15. *Antar-mukhī*: Sex after overeating and lying in unhealthful positions causes Vāyu to press against the food. Vāyu and food become blocked in the genital tract and cause vaginal curves and Vāyu bone and muscle disorders. The vagina becomes very painful; sex becomes intolerable.
16. *Sūchī-mukhī*: Symptoms of roughness of Vāyu in the mother's genital tract affects the genital tract of the fetus (if female) and creates a decreased vaginal opening.
17. *Śhuṣhkā Yoni*: Suppressing natural urges during sex excesses Vāyu. This results in painful feces, urine retention, and dryness of the vaginal opening.
18. *Vāminī*: When semen stays in the uterus and is expelled after 6 or 7 days, it is not accepted, and may be discharged with or without pain. It is caused by Vāyu excesses.
19. *Ṣhaṇḍhī*: When Vāyu genetic defects destroy the fetus's ovaries, a female child will be born with no breasts.
20. *Mahā-yoni*: Uncomfortable positions during sex on an uncomfortable bed, causes Vāyu to become excessed. This dilates the uterus opening and the genital tract. Symptoms include pain, roughness with frothy discharge, fleshy growth, and joint and groin pain.

For each *doṣha*, general symptoms can be identified by the *doṣha* responsible for the imbalance.

Vāyu: Disorders include scanty menstrual fluid that is dark red or brown, dry, or old. Symptoms include, menstrual cramping with lower back pain, headache, depression, nervousness, fear, anxiety, and loss of strength and resistance. Other symptoms include vaginal dryness, gas, constipation, distention; menses lasts 3 to 5 days; irregular and variable menses.

Pitta: Disorders include excess menstrual flow, dark red or purple blood, warmth, clotting, fever, burning, flushed, red eyes, skin rashes, acne, anger, irritability, impatience, diarrhea, yellow stools; menses lasts 5 to 7 days.

Kapha: One experiences a moderate flow, pale or light red blood, sometimes with mucus, heaviness, tiredness, nausea, vomiting, excess phlegm and saliva, swelling breasts, edema, and sentimentality.

Therapies:

General: All female tract disorders are affected by Vāyu. Thus for all female tract disorders, Vāyu-reducing foods, drinks, and lifestyles are used. First, Vāyu is balanced, then the other *doṣhas* are treated. All disorders include therapies of unction (oil), sudation (sweat), and mild use of the five *pañcha karma* measures. Herbal tampon, pouring water and oil *abhyañga* (massage-like) can always be done, using *chitrak*, *guḍūchī*, *balā* with boiled milk and sesame oil.

1. *Vāyu*: Oil, fomentation (moist heat), enema, and Vāyu-reducing habits, such as *ghee*, sesame seeds, and Vāyu-reducing herbs, such as *triphalā*, *punarnavā*, turmeric, *śhatāvarī*, *balā*, *pippalī, chitrak,* and *guḍūchī*. First, *abhyañga* with sesame oil and black salt is advised. Next, tube fomentation (*nāḍī sveda*) and bolus fomentation is applied. Lastly, warm water is poured over the forehead, lower abdomen, and genitals; herbal tampons and *abhyañga* are also used. *Śhatāvarī* or *aśhwagandhā* is boiled in sesame oil and used as a vaginal douche.

Stiff, Hard Tract—Sesame (V-), mustard (K-) oil, or *ghee* (P-) is applied locally to soften the tract.

2. *Vāyu/Pitta*: A good tonic includes *śhatāvarī*, *balā*, *pippalī*, *guḍūchī,* and *punarnavā* with *ghee* in boiled milk.

Tract Pain—Boiled milk with *gokṣhura*, *guḍūchī*, and *triphalā,* are helpful.

Pain In Genital Tract Sides—Herbs include *pippalī*, black salt, calamus, *chitrak*, and *ghee*.

3. *Pitta*: Cold, blood-pacifying measures, and Pitta-reducing herbs are suggested. *Ghee* is used

in pouring water, *abhyañga*, and herbal tampons. Herbs include *śhatāvarī* and *pippalī* boiled in milk. Foods include grapes, cane sugar, and raw honey.
Uterine inflammation—Red raspberry is useful.
Endometritis/PID (pelvic inflammatory disease)—Both are Pitta conditions resulting from accumulated heat and stagnant blood, with infection and inflammation. Additionally, liver therapies are needed. Pitta-reducing herbs are needed, including *śhatāvarī*, aloe vera gel, gotu kola, dandelion, *kaṭukā, bhūmiāmalakī*, and *mañjiṣhṭhā*.

4. Kapha: Rough and hot therapies and Kapha-reducing habits are suggested. Cleansing suppositories are frequently used that are made of cloth, barley powder, black salt, *pippalī,* and black pepper. (They are followed by a warm water wash). It is also used for cleansing the genital tract.
Swollen slimy discharge, *Upaplutā*, flat, painful, with eruptions—Tampons of neem, *āmalakī*, mango, and pomegranate, with boiled milk and sesame oil are used. This is followed by massaging the waste, back, and sacral region and administering an oil enema. *Balā*, *aśhwagandhā*, ginger, and *pippalī* are boiled in sesame oil and used as a vaginal douche.
Pale/white discharges—Herbs include *āmalakī* paste (i.e., made with water), cane sugar, and raw honey. First oil is placed in the vagina. Then licorice, *lodhra*, and *prīyaṅgu* powder are mixed with honey, and made into a big, round tablet. This tablet is then placed in the vagina at bedtime. It is washed out at dawn with hot water. Suppositories made of red raspberry, bayberry, *bibhītakī* (astringents), and raw honey are placed in the vagina to remove the discharge. Vaginal fumigation is done with *guggul*, barley, sesame oil, and *ghee*.
Endometriosis—This is usually a Kapha disorder with extra uterine membrane growth. Kapha-reducing habits are required, including herbs such as *aśhoka*, *guggul*, myrrh, turmeric, dandelion, black pepper, *kaṭukā,* and honey. These herbs reduce tumors, fibroids, and Kapha.
5. Dual/Tridoṣha: Combination therapies
6. *Sārijā (Uterine Bleeding/Raktayoni)*: Sesame seeds, yogurt, *ghee*, honey, red raspberry, *mañjiṣhṭhā, musta,* and turmeric. Vaginal douche with *kuṭaj* is used.
7. *Arajaskā* (*amenorrhea—delayed or no menses*): A vaginal douche with *dalchīnī*, aloe gel, small cardamom, ginger, *gulkand*, *kuṭaj* bark, and old jaggery are used. Another douche includes, yogurt, sour fruit, *āmalakī*, *aśhwagandhā*, *śhatāvarī*, *ghee,* and boiled milk. It is generally a Vāyu condition, but sometimes Pitta or Kapha will be the cause.
Vāyu: (Due to coldness and other Vāyu excesses). Aloe vera gel, myrrh, turmeric, ginger, cinnamon, Vāyu-reducing foods, drinks, and lifestyle are advised. Warm sesame oil sprinkled over the lower abdomen or as a douche is useful. Herbal iron supplements, laxatives like *triphalā*, aloe vera gel or castor oil are used. Rejuvenatives include *aśhwagandhā*, *śhatāvarī*, *kapikachhū*, and *musta*.
Pitta: (mild symptoms) Turmeric or saffron in boiled milk; rose, *musta*, and dandelion are advised.
Kapha: (Resulting from congestion and sluggishness) Recommended herbs include ginger, cinnamon, *pippalī*, myrrh, safflower, turmeric, cinnamon, and *jaṭāmāṇśhī*.
8. *Acharaṇā*: Wash and remove discharges with neem, *vāsāk*, *pippalī*, grapes, and vinegar; or *triphalā* and yogurt/water. *Śhatāvarī* and *aśhwagandhā* boiled in sesame oil may also be used as a vaginal douche.
9.) *Aticharaṇā*: Sesame oil enemas and Vāyu-reducing foods and drinks; with *śhatāvarī*, *aśhwagandhā*. Barley, wheat, yeast, *kūt*, *prīyaṅgu*, and *balā* are placed in the vagina.
10. *Prāk-charaṇā*: *Śhatāvarī* and *aśhwagandhā* boiled in sesame oil are used as a vaginal douche. Sesame oil enemas and Vāyu-reducing foods and drinks; with *śhatāvarī*, *aśhwagandhā* are used. Barley, wheat, yeast, *balā*, *kūt*, and *prīyaṅgu* are placed in the vagina.
11. *Upa-plutā* (or *pari-plutā*): Unction, fomenta-

tion, and sudation are followed by oil tampons and medicated oil drops that are placed in the vagina for lubrication. Herbs include *kūt*, *prīyaṅgu,* and *balā.*

12. Udā-vartānī (dysmenorrhea): Unction with *ghee* and oil; fomentation, boiled milk, sesame oil, *ghee,* and *daśhmūl* enema are taken for enemas and vaginal douches. See page 508 for further information.

13. Karṇinī: *Śhatāvarī* and *aśhwagandhā* are boiled in sesame oil and used as a vaginal douche. Suppositories with *kuśhtā*, *pippalī*, *triphalā,* and black salt may be mixed into a semi-solid paste. Therapies include *lodhra*, *prīyaṅgu*, and soft *arka* leaves with rice vinegar (*kañji*).

14. Putraghnī: Vaginal douche with *kuṭaj* is used. *Kuṭaj* and *gambhārī* barks boiled with *ghee* are ingested.

15. Antar-mukhī: Vāyu-reducing therapies are used.

16. Sūchī-mukhī: Vāyu-reducing herbs are used with surgical repair.

17. Śhuṣhka Yoni: *Śhatāvarī* or *aśhwagandhā* is boiled in sesame oil and used as a vaginal douche. Unction with *ghee* and oil; fomentation, boiled milk, sesame oil, *ghee*, and *daśhmūl* is taken as enemas and vaginal douches. *Ghee* boiled with *śhatāvarī* is poured into the vagina and held there for 2 hours. This procedure is continued for a month or until healed.

18. Vāminī: Unction, fomentation and sudation are used followed by oil tampons, and lastly Vāyu-reducing medicated oil (e.g., *śhatāvarī* and *ghee*)(see above).

19. Ṣhaṇḍhī:

Conception: Therapies include *ghee* with *triphalā*, *punarnavā*, turmeric, *śhatāvarī*, *chitrak*, *lodhra*, *aśhoka*, bayberry bark, and *guḍūchī*.

Miscarriage Cleansing: *Musta*, *triphalā*, neem, *guḍūchī*, aloe gel, turmeric, *mañjiṣhṭhā*, and myrrh with honey are taken for 1 to 2 weeks. Tone with *śhatāvarī*, *aśhwagandhā*, aloe gel, *mañjiṣhṭhā*, gotu kola, red raspberry.

20. Mahāyoni: Unction with *ghee* and oil; fomentation, boiled milk, sesame oil, *ghee,* and *daśhmūl* is taken for enemas and vaginal douches. *Ghee* boiled with *śhatāvarī* is poured into the vagina and held there for 2 hours.

Prasrastā Yoni (Genital Tract Displacement): After unction and fomentation the tract is replaced. Covered tracts are pressed with the hand; contracted tracts are dilated; bulged tracts are pushed inside; dilated ones are manipulated. *Abhyañga* (massage-like) is done with *ghee* and added to the milk for fomenting. *Āmalakī*, licorice, ginger, *salum*, *kṣhīr kākolī*, and *mahā medā* are boiled with *ghee*, then poured into the vagina. It is retained until the urge for urination occurs.

Menorrhagia (Asṛigdara or Pradara)

Excess menses or spotting is usually due to Pitta excesses. It is caused by eating excess salty, sour, heavy, pungent, burning, and fatty foods and animal products. The Vāyu and blood thus becomes excessed and move into the menses channels, increasing the menstrual flow. There are 4 types of *pradara* : Vāyu, Pitta, Kapha, and Tridoṣhic. Normal menses is known by its monthly regularity without symptoms. It is normal in color, lasts for 5 days, and is moderate in quantity.

Symptoms

General: Aches all over the body, pain in the abdomen during menstruation.

Vāyu: Frothy, thin, rough, blackish or reddish, with or without pain; intense pain in the waist, groin, heart, ribs, back, and pelvic areas.

Pitta: Bluish, black, deep red or yellow, very hot, frequent and painful with burning, redness, thirst, mental confusion, fever, and giddiness.

Kapha: Symptoms include slimy, pale, heavy, oily, cold, and viscous discharge, with mild pain; associated with vomiting, anorexia, nausea, difficult breathing, and cough.

Tridoṣha: Symptoms of all three *doṣhas* are seen.

Therapies: Are the same as those listed above for

the three *doṣhas* related to female tract disorders. Generally, herbs include red raspberry and *mañjiṣhṭhā* to help stop bleeding. Then tonics can be given such as *aśhwagandhā*, *aśhoka*, *śhatāvarī*, aloe vera gel, and *āmalakī*.

General: Warm water or sesame oil is poured over the lower abdomen and genitalia and used as a douche. Foods, drinks, and lifestyles appropriate to the implicated *doṣha* are followed.

Vāyu—Therapies include sesame powder yogurt, *ghee*, and honey.

Pitta—Therapies include lotus root, *musta*, boiled milk, cane sugar, and honey.

Kapha—Therapies include mustard oil, licorice, *lotus, āmalakī* leaves, and alum.

Malodor: A decoction or paste of aromatic herbs *guḍūchī*, neem, *dhātakī* flower, *chitrak*, and *nāgkeśhar* are applied to remove odors.

Miscellaneous: For genital tract defects, menses, and white, blue, yellow, red, and black discharges, mango, *kuṭaj*, *bilwa*, *musta*, black pepper, ginger, red sandalwood, *arjuna*, and honey, followed by rice water are helpful.

Miscellaneous Disorders and Therapies

Menstrual regulators: Turmeric and saffron (or safflower) are used.

Spasm regulators: Herbs include fennel, *asafoetida*, and *jaṭāmāṇśhī*.

Rejuvenatives/tonics: Herbs include *śhatāvarī*, red raspberry, saffron, aloe vera gel, turmeric (with ginger, fennel, and cardamom).

Tumors/Cysts/Fibroids: They are most common in Kapha *doṣhas* and are usually benign. Symptoms include swelling, dampness, and congestion. Large tumors or cysts are safe to remove through surgical measures. The best herb is *aśhoka*. Additional herbs include *guggul*, saffron, *musta*, *mañjiṣhṭhā*, *pippalī*, turmeric, *kaṭukā*, and barberry with honey.

Vāyu: Symptoms include pain, dryness, varying in size and location. Herbs include *musta*, *guggul*, *mañjiṣhṭhā*, aloe vera gel, myrrh, red raspberry, and *jaṭāmāṇśhī*.

Pitta: Inflammation, infection, swelling, and heat. Herbs used are *aśhoka*, *mañjiṣhṭhā*, *musta*, red raspberry, *mañjiṣhṭhā*, chamomile, aloe vera gel, *guggul,* turmeric, and saffron.

PMS

Vāyu Symptoms: Anxiety, depression, insomnia, constipation, headache, severe cramping, spacey, dizziness, fainting, rapid mood shifts, being hard to please, feeling abandoned, chills, thirst, dry skin, and feeling suicidal.

Pitta Symptoms: Anger, irritability, argumentative, diarrhea, fever, sweating, warmth, acne and skin rashes, abundant menstrual flow, possibly with clots, early onset of menses, spotting.

Kapha Symptoms: Fatigue, heaviness, crying, sentimentality, longing for love, mild emotions, cold or flu, mucus, lack of hunger, nausea, swollen breasts, edema, late onset, white or pale menses with clots or mucus.

Therapies:

General: Herbs include turmeric, saffron, *musta*, and angelica.

Vāyu: Herbs include turmeric or saffron to promote menses; fennel or *jaṭāmāṇśhī* to reduce spasms; *śhiro dhārā* or oil poured over the genitalia or lower abdomen; vaginal douche with *aśhwagandhā* and *śhatāvarī* is recommended. Coffee, tea, tobacco, alcohol, and drugs should be avoided. Vāyu-reducing foods, drinks, and lifestyle are advised.

Pitta: Herbs include turmeric, saffron (as above), *śhatāvarī*, *musta*, *mañjiṣhṭhā*, gotu kola, aloe vera gel, and *bhṛiṅgarāj*. Pitta-reducing foods, drinks, and lifestyle are advised.

Kapha: Herbs include aloe vera gel, turmeric, *musta*, cinnamon, *pippalī*, and ginger. Avoiding heavy or oily foods is advised. Kapha-reducing foods, drinks, and lifestyle are advised.

Menopause

Hormonal and emotional balancing and reproductive tract rejuvenation are essential. It is generally related to Vāyu symptoms of nervousness, insomnia, depression, and anxiety. Vāyu-reducing foods, drinks, and lifestyle are required, along with aloe vera gel, myrrh, *śhatāvarī*, saffron, *kapikachhū*, and *aśhwagandhā* in boiled milk. *Chyavan prāśh* is another good tonic.

Pitta: Symptoms include anger, irritability, impatience, hot flashes. Pitta-reducing habits are followed, along with aloe vera gel, *śhatāvarī*, and saffron in boiled milk.

Kapha: Symptoms include heaviness, fatigue, lethargy, tendency towards overweight and water retention. Herbs include *pippalī*, ginger, and *guggul*.

Dysmenorrhea

(Difficult menses, often with cramping)

This is generally a Vāyu condition.

Vāyu: Symptoms include spasms, uterine dryness, bloating, gas, or constipation. Suggested herbs include *musta*, *śhatāvarī, guggul*, aloe vera gel, myrrh, red raspberry, turmeric, and *jaṭāmāṇśhī*. Warm sesame oil is poured over or applied to the lower abdomen. Sesame oil and *śhatāvarī* are used as a douche.

Pitta: Congestion develops from stagnant blood obstructions, with burning and diarrhea. Herbs include *brāhmī, musta,* turmeric, and saffron. The latter two can be boiled in milk.

Kapha: Congestion develops from stagnant blood obstructions, with edema or phlegm (congestion). Hot herbs are used, such as *pippalī vachā, guggul,* myrrh, and ginger.

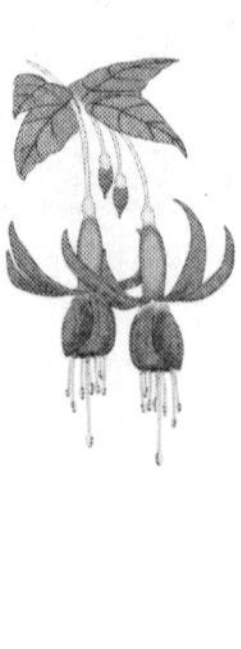

Leukorrhea/prolapse

(Abnormal vaginal discharges)

When the natural acidic nature of the vagina is not healthy, bacteria, fungi, or protozoa will develop. It usually results from Kapha-excess mucus, antibiotics, excess sex, infections, venereal diseases, and lack of cleanliness. Therapies focus on the excess, not the bacteria. Sour douches of vinegar or yogurt are most useful, along with acidophilus tablets.

Kapha: Herbs include aloe powder, ginger, and *pippalī* taken with honey. Other useful herbs are red raspberry, *śhatāvarī*, lotus seeds, and *guggul*.

Pitta: Symptoms include yellow color, foul odor, bloodiness, and burning. Herbs include aloe powder, *kaṭukā*, and *bhūmīāmalakī*. For internal use only, aloe vera gel, turmeric, and *mañjiṣhṭhā* are advised.

Vāyu: Symptoms include brown color, stickiness, dryness, and severe pain.

Hysterectomy

The removal of the uterus creates hormone imbalances, devitalization, imbalanced metabolism (leading to weight gain), emotional imbalance, and insecurity.

Vāyu: Air increases, causing ungroundedness and anxiety.

Pitta: Symptoms include anger, irritability, and heat.

Kapha: Symptoms of fatigue, sentimentality, weight gain, and congestion can develop.

Immediately after surgery, turmeric and *arjuna* are taken to promote healing. Therapies include reproductive and hormonal tonics like *śhatāvarī*, aloe vera gel, saffron, *chyavan prāśh*; brain tonics, such as *brāhmī* (or *brāhmī ghee*), *bhṛiṅgarāj*, and *jaṭāmāṇśhī* are recommended.

Note: Most of the conditions pertaining to the female reproductive system are related to hormones. The main cause of hormone-related diseases is life style and diet. In our modern society, food is produced in larger quantities in the shortest possible time. To achieve this end, a variety of growth hormones and chemicals are used to develop these products. Processed foods that are loaded with hormones and chemicals create a serious imbalance in the body's own rate of growth and hormonal system. A large number of the hormones and chemicals used to fatten animals are female hormones. Thus, when foods containing these chemicals are ingested, they wreak havoc with hormonal balance in the female body.

Many of the problems caused by eating animal products can be solved if organic animal products are taken. However, Āyurveda still cautions about the subtler *karmic* implications from eating animals.

Āyurvedic Obstetrics (Childbirth)

Discussed in this section are the Āyurvedic principles of conception, pregnancy, embryology (the development of the fetus), and delivery. Scientifically minded readers will see some amazing parallels between what is known today through modern medicine and technology and what was known intuitively more than 5,000 years ago. Procedures for pregnancy, *mantras*, foods, and *abhyañga* (a type of massage) are also discussed.

Embryology

The Soul (*ātma*), based on past life actions (*karma*), enters healthy semen (*śhukra*) and and ovum (*ārtava*), forming an embryo. The embryo is formed by the subtle elements ether (*ākāsha*), air (*vāyu*), fire (*tejas*), water (*ap*), and earth (*pritvi*). All five elements are contained in both the semen and ovum. Later, the soul or *ātman* enters the embryo.

Males are developed when there is more semen (a Y chromosome, thus producing XY chromosomes). A female fetus is created when there is more ovum present (X chromosome, thus producing XX chromosomes). Vāyu divides the semen and ovum into many parts, giving rise to many embryos (i.e., fertilization of more than one ovum). The best chance for healthy offspring will occur when the female, 16-years-old or over, mates with a male who is over 20- to 25-years-old, and both people are healthy (i.e., none of the three *doṣhas* are vitiated).

The *Charak Saṃhitā* notes that the child receives from the ovum, their skin, blood, flesh, fat, umbilicus, heart, liver, spleen, kidneys, bladder, rectum, stomach, colon, anus, small intestine, and organ membranes. Derived from the semen are the hair, nails, teeth, bones, veins, ligaments, arteries, and reproductive fluid. Factors derived from the ātman (soul) are the taking of birth, life span, Self-realization, mind, senses, intake and excretion, stimulation and essence of the senses. Other factors include shape, voice, complexion, desire for happiness and sorrow, likes and dislikes, consciousness, courage, intellect, memory, egoism, and efforts. Wholesome food and lifestyle form a healthy fetus. This produces healthy *rasa* (plasma) in the women that is necessary for both her life and the production of the fetus' growth, strength, satisfaction, plumpness, and enthusiasm. The wholesomeness of the mind is also essential, since the mind connects the soul to the physical body. The factors that the mind gives the embryo are conduct, likes and dislikes, purity, memory, attachment, and detachment. Other factors include valor, fear, anger, fatigue, enthusiasm, sharpness, softness, seriousness, and stability or instability. The more *sattwic* the mind, the more predominant the positive qualities. Thus, the embryo is formed from various factors. (*Charak Saṃhitā*: *Sharīrasthāna*, Ch 4, verse 6,7,10-13)

Doṣhas are healed with herbs described earlier (e.g., *aśhwagandhā*, *śhatāvarī*, and *ghee*, which build the semen and ovum (*śhukra dhātu*). Additionally, the female organ is cleansed using herbal *uttarabastis* (vaginal douches). Healthy semen is white, heavy, unctuous, sweet, copious, and thick like honey or *ghee*. Healthy menstrual blood is noted by its not staining a cloth after it has been washed.

Preparation and Conception

When a couple desires to conceive, the following procedures are followed. At the first sign of menstruation, for three days, the woman is advised to think only good thoughts, avoid bathing and dressing up, reduce her weight, and avoid sexual activity. She is also advised to sleep on a hard bed and take meals (in small portions) consisting solely of milk and small barley for purification of the alimentary tract. On the fourth day, she bathes, and along with her husband, dresses in white. They adorn themselves with flower garlands and should feel attracted towards one another. A woman becomes fertile following menstruation and fresh blood is formed in the uterus. It is said that if a couple wants a male offspring, to conceive on an even day; and for a female child, on an odd day. These days are counted from the first day of menstruation. (Additionally, there are many sacred rites that can assure conception of a healthy male child with good qualities. (See *Charak: Śhārīrasthāna* Chapter 8 Verse 10-14; and *Aṣhṭāñga Hṛidayam: Śhārīrasthāna* Ch 1, verse 37-38)

"The couple who have pure śhukra and ārtava (semen/ovum) are healthy and in love with each other...indulge in oleation, purificatory therapies, and nourishing enemas. The male uses milk and ghee with sweet, ojas-building herbs. The woman uses sesame oil, black gram, ovum building, and Pitta-increasing herbs." (*Aṣhṭāñga Hṛidayam: Śhārīrasthāna Ch 1, verse 18a-20a*)

The bedroom should be clean and filled with pleasant aromas. The man ascends the bed with his right leg first; and the woman with her left leg. A woman is advised to lie on her back to keep the three *doṣhas* balanced in her uterus. There is a special *mantra* recited by the husband, "*Ahirasi sutam*" ("O Lord, you are the procurer, you are the life, you are present everywhere, may *Dhātā* bestow on me good, may *Vidhātā* bestow the divine radiance, may *Brahman, Brihaspati, Vishnu, Soma, Sūrya, Aṣhwin*-twins, *Bhaga, Mitra*, and *Varuna* grant me a valiant son.") Male offspring were highly prized in ancient times; the prayer can be changed to replace "son" with "child."

Other *mantras* found in the *Ṛik Veda* are chanted by a priest, including, "*Viṣhṇuryāni Kalpayatu*" (May Lord *Viṣhṇu* fulfill her desire in the womb). "May Lord *Viṣhṇu* prepare the womb. May Lord *Tvastr* make the respective forms. May Lord *Prajāpati* spray the sperm. May Lord *Dhātr* protect your wife's womb." Cohabitation then occurs with affection and cheerfulness. Afterwards, the woman is sprinkled with cold water.

Lifestyle During Pregnancy

The woman is advised to take various herbs to nourish herself and the fetus, including *brāhmī, guḍūchī*, and *ghee* boiled with milk. The herbs are also worn as a talisman and held by the wife. The wife is looked at affectionately, attended to by her husband and attendants who give her all the wholesome foods she wants, especially butter, *ghee,* and milk.

Many factors may impair the pregnancy or cause abortion. Thus, she should avoid, excess sexual activities, exertion, excess sleep or staying up late, sitting on uncomfortable or seats that are too high, and walking in high heels. Grief, anger, fear, strong emotions, suppression of natural urges and desires, fasting, long walks, pungent, hot, constipating and hard to digest foods, laxative herbs, and wearing red are also avoided. Other habits to avoid include staring into deep pits, wells, or waterfalls, drinking alcohol, eating meat, sleeping on her back, and disobeying elder women. She is also advised not to undergo *pañcha karma* (until the eighth month), excessive uncomfortable travel, excessive or irritating noises.

Many activities of the parents can cause harm to their newborn child. Both husband and wife cause these troubles before conception (i.e., foods, lifestyle habits). During pregnancy, the actions of the woman mainly cause these unhealthy results through her foods and lifestyle. Of course external factors can also influence her health.

Activities Causing Diseases in the Child

Harmful Activity and the Results in the Child

1. Constantly sleeping on her back.
Result: umbilicus twists around the neck of the fetus.
2. Sleeping in the open air or traveling alone at night. Result: mental illness.
3. Verbal and physical abuse. Result: epilepsy.
4. Excessive cohabitation. Result: rudeness, lacking will.
5. Constant grief: Result: fearfulness, thinness, short-lived.
6. Thinking ill of others. Result: anti-social behavior, envious, weak-willed.
7. Stealing. Result: laziness, maliciousness.
8. Anger. Result: deceitfulness, jealousy, anger.
9. Excessive sleep. Result: dullness, lethargy, poor digestion.
10. Alcohol addiction. Result: thirst, poor memory, fickleness.
11. Eating pork. Result: red eyes, respiratory problems.
12. Eating fish. Result: eye closure problems.
13. Sweets addiction. Result: urinary disorders, diabetes, mental disorders, obesity.
14. Addiction to sour things. Result: bleeding, skin, and eye disorders.
15. Salt addiction. Result: kidney and urinary disorders, *ojas* depletion.
16. Addiction to pungent tastes. Result: weakness, reproductive problems.
17. Addiction to bitter tastes. Result: emaciation, weakness.
18. Addiction to astringent tastes. Result: gray complexion, constipation, gas, distention.

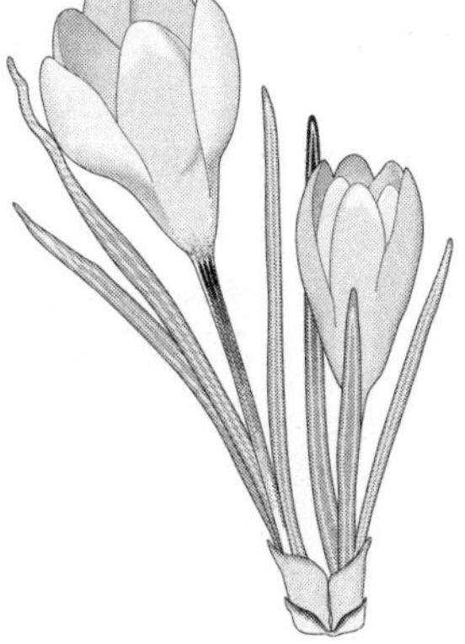

Wholesome Therapy During Pregnancy

Month	Therapy
1	cold milk
2	boiled milk with sweet tasting herbs (e.g.
3	boiled milk with honey and *ghee*
4	milk with 12 grams of butter
5	*ghee*
6	(sweet) herbal *ghee* (e.g.
7	same as 6*
8	milk, easily digested grain broth, and *ghee*
9	medicated oil enema, oleation of uterus and genital tract, daily body oil *abhyañga* **

* During the seventh month, the fetus causes pressure on the chest, leading to itching and burning sensations. Therapy: To relieve this condition, eat 12 grams of butter, boiled with sweet herbs. Breasts and abdomen are anointed with sandalwood paste (herb powder and water), *musta, mañjishṭhā,* and *triphalā*. A gentle oil *abhyañga* (massage-like) is given. Small quantities of sweet foods are to be taken every 3 to 4 hours to alleviate Vāyu. Fats and salt should be avoided.

** In the ninth month, *abhyañga* is done to soften the placenta, pelvis, waist, and the sides of the chest and back; to expel gas, for easy elimination of urine and stools; to soften skin and nails; to give strength and enhance the complexion; to create an easy delivery of a healthy child.

If the right side of a woman's abdomen is more elevated, and she first gets milk in her right breast, prefers things using her right side, longs for masculine activities, and dreams about them, it is said that she will give birth to a male child. If the opposite features are noticed, including more feminine characteristics, desires to dance, play, or sing, enjoy aromas, and flowers, she will give birth to a female.

Before the 9th month, a special room or apartment should be constructed for the woman. Pleasant aromas, colors, foods, and herbs are placed in the room. At the onset of the 9th month, female relatives and midwives attend to the pregnant women in the apartment. Auspicious days and times, favorable moon and constellation positions determine when sacred fire rites for peace and good fortune should be performed by *brāhmanas* (priests). The priests use *mantras*, grass, food, water, and cows in the ceremonies.

Impending Delivery Signs

The Āyurvedic scriptures suggest that either on the day before or on the day of delivery, the expectant mother exhibits will show signs of fatigue, looseness of the abdomen and eyes, heaviness in the lower parts of the body, loss of appetite (or taste), and increased salivation. She may feel pain or discomfort in the thighs, waist, abdomen, back, heart region, bladder, groin, and vaginal tract. Other symptoms include tearing pain, pricking, pulsating, and fluid discharge, followed by the onset of labor pains, discharge of fluid from the womb, and increased frequency of urination.

Once these signs are experienced, she observes auspicious rites, holds masculine-named fruit, is given an oil *abhyañga* and a warm bath. Following this, she drinks thin, easily digested grain soup, with *ghee*. Then she lies on a hard bed, with legs bent. Her body, especially the lower belly, is continuously rubbed with warm oil. Her female attendants console her as well. Some authorities suggest that she inhale herbal snuff, including cardamom (*elā*), *vachā* (calamus), and *chitrak*. This promotes an easy delivery by helping the fetus detach from the upper belly region and move to its lower region.

Once the fetus has detached from the heart region (upper abdomen), labor pains will increase and the fetus will have turned. The woman should lie on a bed. *Mantras* are then recited in her ears by one of her attendants. ("May the five elements, *Vishṇu* and *Prajāpati* always protect you, the pregnant one, and help the delivery of the child. O auspicious one, may the delivery take place without any distress, either to you or your child, who has the brilliance of the divine warrior [*Kartik*, or *Skandā*], and be protected by *Kartik* ."]

The attendants console her, advising her not to strain when there are no labor pains, as it causes difficult breathing, cough, enlarged spleen, and wasting diseases. When labor begins, she is advised to increase pressure slowly and gradually. When the child appears, the women announce the delivery and the gender of the baby to give the new mother relief, joy, and help her regain strength. She is then fanned, sprinkled with water, and drinks water as well.

Post-Partum Therapies For New-Born Baby (Bālopacharaṇīya Ahyāya)

Immediately after birth, the baby's skin is cleansed using rock salt and *ghee*. Then, to relieve the fatigue of its birth, the baby is anointed with (medicated) *balā* oil. Finally, two stones are hit together at the root of the baby's ears and a sacred hymn is chanted into its right ear by the father or mother:

"You have been born from every organ of the body and mind's heart (*hṛidaya*) of your parents. You are we in the form of a (son/daughter); may you live for a hundred years. May you attain long life. Let the stars, the quarters, nights, and days protect you."

After the child settles down, the umbilical cord is tied with a thread 4-finger's width above the navel, then severed. The cord is fastened around the baby's neck (without causing harm). The umbilicus is next massaged with *kuśhtā* oil and then given a bath with a decoction of tree barks with milky sap or water boiled with fragrant herbs. The water can be boiled with silver or gold in it as well.

A cloth soaked in sesame oil is placed over the baby's head while the baby is fed an herbal sweet (e.g., *brāhmī, vachā, śhaṅkh pushpī, harītakī, āmalakī, ghee*, raw honey, gold). The dose is no more than that which fits in the baby's palm. This confection will stimulate the development of intelligence, long life, and strength. Prayers for the baby to develop these qualities are chanted while the baby eats.

The baby is made to vomit the uterine fluid by eating *ghee* mixed with rock salt. Then religious rites are performed for the baby.

Breast Feeding

The milk of the mother is not considered ready for nursing for the first 3 or 4 days after delivery owing to the dilation of the milk duct orifices. Thus the child is fed the juice of *dūrva* mixed with honey and *ghee* (quantity the size of the child's handful), 3 times a day for the first 3 days. *Mantras* or prayers for the baby's protection, health, intelligence, and longevity are recited over the meals.

On the 2nd and 3rd days, the baby is given *ghee* with white *kaṇṭkārī* (or ginseng—*aralia qinquefolia*) for all three meals. On the 4th day, the child eats only two meals (morning and noon). In the evening, mother's milk is given from the right breast after squeezing a little bit of the milk out; reciting a *mantra* over the breast. A pitcher of water impregnated with *mantras* is kept near the child's head and the baby licks some fresh butter. This procedure is followed before all nursing meals. Hereafter, the baby nurses twice a day.

A *mantra* is recited over the breast as follows, "O beautiful women, may the four oceans of the earth contribute to the secretion of milk in your breasts for the purpose of improving your baby's physical strength. O you with a beautiful face, may the child, reared on your milk, attain a long life like the gods made immortal from their ambrosia drinks."

Should the mother be unable to breast-feed, two wet-nurses or women who can breast feed, substitute for the mother. These women should be affectionate, healthy, observing celibacy, of the same *doṣha* as the mother, eating foods and living a lifestyle in accordance with their *doṣha,* and have children of their own.

Breast Milk

Breast milk can become deficient as a result of grief, anger, fasting, and exertion. Happiness, love, nutrition, and rest increase breast milk. Milk, *dūrba,* and fennel, also increase breast milk. If breast milk is not available, the child can drink cow's or goat's milk boiled with the 5-herb group known as *hṛisva pañchamūl* (*bṛihatī, kaṇṭkārī, gokṣhura, śhāliparñī,* and *pṛisnaparṇī).*

Breast milk diseases occur from eating before the last meal is digested, eating unsuitable or incompatible foods, irregularity and excess of meals and habits. Other causes include regularly ingesting of salty, sour, pungent, and stale foods; mental and physical stress, staying up late, taking naps after lunch, and excess mental work. Further causes include suppressing and forcing natural urges, ingesting meat, fat, and wine; lack of exercise, injury, and anger. Other causes include weakness or wasting due to illness. The channels carrying milk cause eight forms of disorders.

Symptoms:

Vāyu causes abnormal tastes, excess froth, and roughness. Pitta causes abnormal color and malodor. Kapha causes oiliness, sliminess, and heaviness.

1. Vāyu affects the taste of milk, causing slow growth and weight loss.
2. Vāyu, churning the milk, produces excess froth that causes difficult milk flow. Upon drinking this milk, the child will develop a weak voice and will retain urine, stool, and gas. Vāyu headaches or colds with mucus (coryza) are also common.
3. Vāyu dries up the unctuous nature of the milk, causing the child who drinks it to becomes debilitated.
4. Pitta, causing abnormal coloration of milk (e.g., blue, yellow, black), will create a poor complexion, sweat, thirst, diarrhea, constant fever, and no desire to drink from the breast in the child.
5. Pitta causes the milk to spoil, giving the child who drinks it anemia and jaundice.
6. Kapha makes the milk too oily; and the child

drinking it develops vomiting, abdominal distention, salivation, sleepiness and exhaustion, difficulty breathing, cough, excessive discharge, and a pervading sense of darkness.
7. Kapha causes the milk to become slimy. The child will salivate, develop swollen face and eyes, and become dull.
8. Kapha causes heaviness of the milk, causing heart disease.

General Milk Cleansing

The mother or wet-nurse is first oiled and fomented, then undergoes emesis with a neem, calamus, and *kuṭaj* decoction. After resting, eating, and digesting her food, she is massaged with oil. Then the woman is purged with a *harītakī* and/or *triphalā* decoction with raw honey. Afterwards, she follows her Āyurvedic diet. This cleansing prepares her for nursing. Cleansing foods include rice, barley, cane sugar, vegetable soup, green legumes, lentils, made with neem, *āmalakī*, *ṭrikatu,* and rock salt. Herbs include *guḍūchī*, *aśhwagandhā*, and ginger.

General:

Vāyu: *Daśhmūl* decoction is drunk for three days. Thereafter one drinks Vāyu-reducing medicated *ghee*, followed by beer foam to lubricate the body. A mild purgative is then given, followed by enema and sweat therapy. The woman then eats cedar, cardamom, *ajamodā* mixed with *ghee* and rock candy.

Pitta: Mother and child both drink a decoction of *guḍūchī, śhatāvarī,* neem, sandalwood and cedar. Alternatively, they can take a decoction of *triphalā, mustā, bhūmīāmalakī,* and *kaṭukā. Ghee* can be taken with these herbs. Pitta-reducing purgatives, *abhyañga* (massage-like), and *lepa* (body pastes) are also required.

Kapha: The child licks *ghee* mixed with powder of licorice and myrrh, or myrrh and *pippalī. Madanaphal* is made into a paste with honey and applied to the mother's breasts and baby's lips. This will easily cause the baby to vomit (thereby removing excess Kapha). The mother should follow emetic therapies discussed in Chapter 7. After emesis, mother and child drink a decoction of cedar, *kuṭaj,* and *tagara* and follow a Kapha-reducing food plan. The mother follows the post-*vamana* food plan in Chapter 7.

Tridoṣha: This is a difficult disorder to heal. First mother and child practice emesis described above for Kapha. Herbs include *vachā,* licorice, turmeric, ginger, cedar, myrrh, *mustā*, and *guḍūchī.*

Children are by nature more Kapha from drinking milk and *ghee*. Thus, if emetics (for vomiting) are needed, mild herbs and doses are given without oleation (oil) therapy (normally required for adults). Children that only nurse or those that nurse and eat solid food are made to vomit after they are content from drinking breast milk. Children who no longer breast feed, first drink *peyā* (thin gruel—see Chapter 7) with *ghee* until sated, before making them vomit.

Enemas are given to children when purgative therapy is required (for adults) to heal a disorder. Nasal therapies (*pratimarṣhā*), purgation and other required therapies are given only to the mother.

A paste of *pippalī* and raw honey or paste of *dhātakī* and *āmalakī* are applied to the ear lobes of the child.

<u>Specific Milk Therapies</u>

<u>1. Abnormal taste</u>: One drinks *Kaṇchanar*, licorice, *vachā* (calamus) and *khadir* mixed in warm water. Paste of *śhatāvarī, triphalā*, and *kūt* is applied locally on the breasts, allowed to dry and then washed off. This purifies the milk.

<u>2. Frothy</u>: A paste of ginger, *bilwa, daśhmūl*, and *śhatāvarī* with warm water is drunk. The mother or wet nurse takes a decoction of ginger, *guḍūchī*, *nāgkeśhar*, *dhātakī*, lotus seed, and *vachā* to alleviate milk defects and apply barley, wheat, and mustard paste to the breasts.

<u>3. Rough/Dry</u>: One drinks milk or *ghee* with *śhatāvarī*, wild yam, *vidārī kand*, *aśhwagandhā,* and *balā*. Paste of *ṭrikatu, prīyañgu*, and *āmalakī* is applied to the breasts for purification.

<u>4. Abnormal Color</u>: A paste of *mañjiṣhṭhā*, *āmalakī*, *śhatāvarī*, neem, and *kulattha*

(horsegram) is taken with cold water. Apply a paste of hibiscus petals on the breasts. When it dries, milk is taken out.

5. Foul Odor: One takes a paste of *triphalā*, turmeric, and calamus with cold water. Alternately, the mother or wet nurse takes *harītakī* and *tṛikatu* with honey to remove malodor from the milk. Other therapies include eating a wholesome diet. A paste of *mañjiṣhṭhā*, sandalwood, neem, *bibhītakī*, and sarsaparilla are applied to the breasts.

6. Oily: One eats a paste of *musta*, *tṛikatu*, *daśhmūl*, *nāgkeśhar*, and *prīyaṅgu.* Rock salt with warm water is used to purify the milk.

7. Slimy: Persons drink a decoction of *harītakī*, *musta*, ginger, *vachā*, and *karañj* to purify breast milk.

8. Heavy: One drinks a decoction of *guḍūchī*, neem, *triphalā*, *motha (fenugreek)*, *patha* (cissampelos pareira, linn.), and ginger, or a paste of *pippalī*, *balā*, ginger, *chitrak*, ginger is applied to the breasts for purification.

All diseases require mild doses. Except for emergencies. Purgatives are strictly avoided.

Additional Ceremonies

On the sixth night rites are offered to protect the child from evil spirits. Parents and relatives of the child stay awake all night making sure the baby remains in a pleasant frame of mind. Certain herbs are placed around the birth room to protect the baby, and broken rice and mustard grains are spread throughout the house. For the next 10 days, a fire ceremony (*yagña*) is performed throughout the day.

At the end of the 10th day, other ceremonies are performed. The baby is anointed with sandalwood. The baby is also given two names by a priest, after proper ceremonies. The names are chosen, based on the constellation (*nākṣhatra*) the child is born under, and the family name. If the family name starts with a "g, gh, j, jh, dr, drh, d, dh, b, and bh", and ends with a "ya, ra, la, va, sha, sa or ha," the name relates to the past three generations and is a famous name. A name with an even number of letters may also be given.

In the first 10 to 12 days after childbirth, the women attend to the wife, and kind and pious people are entertained in the house. Music, food, and drinks are provided for all to enjoy.

The baby always wears auspicious amulets and herbs, such as *brāhmī* and *vachā,* on its hands, neck, and head. These bestow long life, intelligence, memory, health, and protection. During the sixth to eighth month, a ceremony is conducted to for the punching of the earlobes.

A baby should not be frightened or threatened, even if disobedient, because spirits can take possession of a frightened baby. Medicated *ghee* made with *brāhmī, vachā, kuśhtā,* and myrrh bestow voice, intelligence, memory, and long life and protect against sins, evil spirits, and cures insanity from possession by spirits.

Weaning (Stanyāparaṇa)

Once the baby's teeth begin to appear, a gradual weaning from breast milk begins. Cow's or goat's milk are easily digestible foods and are gradually begun.

Sweet balls made with raw honey, parched rice paddy and sugar candy develop a content baby. *Bilwa* and *elā* are given to kindle digestion. A nutritive drink (*tarpaṇa*) is made with *dhātakī*, parched rice paddy and cane sugar stops diarrhea.

Healing Childhood Diseases (Bālāmaya Pratihedha)

Nonverbal Communication

A child may constantly touch (sometimes press hard) on its diseased parts or organs when ill. When another person touches that area (even gently), the child will cry.

Head Disorders: If any head disease occurs, the child cannot raise or move its head and its eyes will remain closed.

Heart: Biting the tongue and lips, difficult breathing, and clenching fists.

Abdomen/Colon: Constipation vomiting, biting mother's breast, intestinal gurgling, gas, bending the back, urine and stool retention, dis-

colored complexion, and abdominal distention.
Bladder/Genitals: Urine retention, thirst, pain, frightened look, and occasional fainting.

Systemic Disease (i.e., throughout the body): The child will cry constantly and cannot be consoled.

Therapies

Herbs used for specific disorders (discussed throughout the book) are taken in small quantities by the nursing mother. The child will receive the herbs through the milk. After the first month of the child's life, a pinch of herbs is also given along with *ghee.*

For children nursing and also eating foods, herbs are taken with food as well as given to the mother (dose: several pinches of herbs). When children are only eating food (and no longer nursing), herbs are given as decoctions, but not given to the mother (dose = 1/16 teaspoon).

Dosing Details: From birth to one month, herbs should be taken with milk, honey, syrup or *ghee*, the amount of two rice grains. Then each month the size is gradually increased by two grains in size until the child is one-year-old. Thereafter the child takes about 20 grains or 1/16 of a teaspoon until age 15.

<u>Elixirs</u>: These herbs improve the health, strength, intellect and longevity of the child.

Nursing: *Ghee* cooked with a decoction of white mustard seeds, *vachā, apāmārga, śhatāvarī, brāhmī, pippalī, kuśhtā,* myrrh, and rock salt.

Nursing and Food: *Ghee* cooked with a decoction of licorice, *vachā, chitrak, pippalī,* and *triphalā*.

Food (no nursing): *Ghee* cooked with a decoction of *brāhmī, daśhmūl*, milk, *tagara,* black pepper, *viḍaṅga,* honey, and *drākṣhā* (medicated grape wine).

[Cow's or goat's milk is important for the child.]

Diseases of Growing Teeth (Dañtobheda Roga)

Āyurveda notes that all diseases can be caused by the eruption of new teeth, but especially fever, diarrhea, cough, vomiting, headache, conjunctivitis, herpes, and styes. The whole body can experience pain. Therapies are followed according to the *doṣha(s)* involved. Therapies are the same as adults, only doses are much less.

Medicated *ghee* with *vachā, bṛihatī, laghu-pāṭhā, kaṭukā*, cane sugar, milk, and raw honey are excellent promoters of healthy growth of teeth.

For all diseases arising from newly growing teeth, *balā, atibalā, bilwa, dhātakī*, milk, and the watery portion of yogurt are used. For fever, diarrhea, difficult breathing, jaundice, anemia, and cough, cedar, *pippalī, bṛihatī,* and dill are used; these herbs also promote strength and a healthy complexion. Once teeth have completely grown in, all associated diseases subside.

If the child is born with teeth or develops the upper teeth first (*sadañta janma*), a propitiatory rite is performed, money is donated to priests and prayers are offered to *Naigameṣha* (the protector of children).

Oversleeping During the Day (Bāla Śhoṣha)

Excessive napping, drinking cold water or drinking Kapha-excessed breast milk causes the child's plasma tissues (*rasa dhātu*) to become blocked by Kapha. This results in loss of appetite, excess nasal mucus, fever, cough, emaciation; greasy and white face and eyes develop.

Herbs to heal this condition include myrrh, *vachā, pippalī, bṛihatī, kākolī, musta, vāsāk, dhātakī*, and *āmalakī* mixed with honey and *ghee*. Licorice, *pippalī, tālispatra,* sandalwood, and myrrh eliminate emaciation. *Abhyañga* (massage-like) and bath include medicated oil of *vachā, tagara,* and sesame oil.

Vomiting

General: *Kadira, arjuna, tālispatra, kuśhtā*, and sandalwood mixed with *ghee* and boiled in milk.

After Nursing: Herbs include *kaṇṭkārī,* ginger, and raspberry.

Tālukaṇṭaka

Kapha becomes increased in the palate muscles, and the skull becomes depressed at the palate region. The baby develops an aversion to food, has difficulty suckling, and passes watery stool. Babies become thirsty, develop irritations in the mouth, eye pain, vomiting, and have difficulty holding their necks straight.

Therapies call for pressing a paste of ginger, myrrh, and honey onto the palate. The paste of *harītakī, vachā, kuśhtā* , and honey are taken with breast milk to heal this disorder.

Rectal Ulcer (Guda Vraṇa)

Sweat or the sticking of feces causes an excess of blood and Kapha that gives rise to an ulcer. The ulcer is copper-colored with itching and is associated with secondary complications in the rectum. It is also called *Mātṛika doṣha, Ahipūtana, Pṛiṣhṭāru, Gudakuṭṭa,* and *Anāmaka.*

The mother's breast milk needs to be purified with Pitta- and Kapha-reducing herbs. Herbs used for Pitta ulcers (Chapter 16) are boiled and then cooled, mixed with honey, and used as a drink. The rectum is bathed by sprinkling of *triphalā* decoction and by the application of dry *triphalā* powder. If redness and itching are severe, blood-letting is used.

Mud-Caused Disorder (Mṛit Bhaksaṇaja Roga)

If the child has eaten mud, medicated *ghee* with *musta, punarnavā*, and *bilwa* are licked by the child.

Therapies for the New Mother

Some authorities suggest the first two days after giving birth, herbs of safflower, myrrh, and saffron should be taken to cleanse the uterus. Both the *Aṣhṭāñga Hṛidaya* and *Charak Saṃhitā* advise the woman to take *ghee* and oil (to promote fat) and various herbs including, *pippalī* and *chitrak.* Sprinkling her with warm water is advised before eating easily digested meals (when she is hungry). She also receives an almond oil *abhyañga* (massage-like) and is then tightly wrapped in cloth and given Vāyu-reducing herbs. This helps to prevent an imbalance of Vāyu in her abdomen, stretch marks, and to help return the belly to its normal size. These therapies continue for 5 to 7 nights, then a nourishing therapy begins. She is served various herbs and foods to build her immune system and increase the flow of breast milk. Herbs include white musali, *śhatāvarī, brāhmī, āmalakī,* saffron, milk, *ghee,* and sesame oil. She remains under care for 1 1/2 months, until she begins her next menstrual cycle.

Nursery

The child's room should be clean, beautiful, light, without drafts (air entering only on one side), and without pets. It should be comfortable and properly prepared for the season (i.e., blankets in the winter, air cooling in the summer). Antiseptic aromas like *guggul*, frankincense, and cedar are burnt to fumigate the room and fabrics. The child is given talismans of jewels, and herbs to wear. There should be a variety of toys of many colors and sounds. The child should not be frightened or disciplined.

Miscarriage

Traditionally it was believed that girls under age 16 and boys under age 25 involved in conceiving a child were more likely to have a miscarriage or have a child with weak organs. The signs of impending miscarriage are pain in the uterus, bladder, waist, groin; and bleeding.

To prevent miscarriage, the person immediately receives cold baths, cold water spraying, and medicated plaster, followed by drinking boiled milk with licorice and *aśhwagandhā.* If there are unusual movements of the fetus in the womb, one drinks milk boiled with white lotus (*puṇḍarīka*), white water lily (*kumuda*), and licorice.

Fetus displacement causes pain or spasms, burning, excessive discharge of blood or reten-

tion of urine and stool. When the fetus shifts from place to place it causes abdominal swelling. In both cases cooling and soothing therapies are required.
For pain: Boiled milk with licorice flower and *kaṇtakārī* mixed with cane sugar and honey is drunk.
For stool retention or distention: Boiled milk with *asafoetida*, salt, garlic, *vachā* is mixed with raw honey and cane sugar and drunk.
Other conditions follow therapies discussed in their respective chapters.

In the event of a miscarriage, herbal emmenagogues are used to cleanse the uterus, including aloe vera gel, myrrh, turmeric, and *mañjiṣhṭhā*. This therapy continues for 1 to 2 weeks. Rest is essential to recover from the loss.

Childhood Planetary Influences (Grahākriti-Vijñānan)

There are 9 diseases of infancy exist related to the 9 planets (*graha*), *Skandā-graha, Skandā-pasmarā, śhakuni, Revati, Putanā, Andha-putanā, śhita-putanā, Mukhamandikā, Naigameṣha (priti-graha).*

Causes: These diseases result from improper breast feeding, poor hygiene, cruel treatment, and a poor spiritual environment. During these times the planetary (evil) spirits enter the child.

Symptoms:
Skandā graha: Swollen eyes, distorted facial features, aversion to breast milk.
Skandā-pasmarā-graha: The child's body emits a bloody smell, one eyelid becomes motionless. It has a frightened look, clenches fists with slight moans, rolls the eyes, is constipated and subject to fainting fits, convulsive leg and hand jerks, foaming mouth, yawning, passing gas while excreting stool and urine.
Śhakuni: Loose limbs, body odor.
Revati: The child is filled with terror, secreting ulcers or vessel eruption with burning sensation all over the body (which eventually develop pus and burst of their own nature). The child will have a reddish face, green stool and urine, deep yellow or dark brown complexion, fever with an inflamed mouth, bruising pain all over the body, and will frequently rub the nose and ears.
Putanā: Loose limbs, troubled day or night sleep, loose stools, body odor, vomiting, goose bumps, thirst.
Andha-putanā: Aversion to breast milk, develop dysentery, cough, hiccups, vomiting, fever, a discolored complexion, swollen skin, and will always lie face down.
Śhita-putanā: Constantly frightened and startled, excess shivering, comatose sleep, constant diarrhea, body odor.
Mukha-mandikā: Incessant crying, intestinal rumbling, emaciation, shiny, swollen lines of the face and body, fearful, large appetite, net-like abdominal veins, a urine-like odor.
Naigameṣha-graha: Frothy vomit, bent over, anxious, crying loudly, gazing upwards, emaciation or fever, body odor, fainting.

If a child appears stupefied, with aversion to breast milk, constant fainting spells, and full development of all symptoms, the situation is grave and not healable. When symptoms are milder or of more recent origin, healing is possible.

Origins of the Nine Planets (Grahas) [Grahotpatti-Adhyāya]

The nine presiding deities (of the nine infant diseases) are ethereal. They were created by the gods *Agni*, *Mahādeva* (*Śhiva*), the goddess *Krittikā* and *Umā*, for guarding the newborn god, *Guha*. Newborns need to be guarded for approximately 40 days. The female deities were created from the essence of the goddess *Gangā*, *Umā,* and *Krittikā*.

The *Naigameṣha graha* has the face of a sheep and was created by the goddess *Pārvati* as the friend and protector of the child *Guha*. *Skandāpasmāra* was created by *Agni* (the fire god). He is as bright as fire, and a constant companion of the god *Skandā*. He is also known as *Kartik* and *Viṣhakha*. *Skandā*, born of *Śhiva* and *Pārvati*, is also known as *Kumāra* (lit. a child, viz., of *Śhivaji*). *Skandā* is known as the Divine Warrior, the ensurer of Divine love.

The deities of the nine childhood diseases asked *Skanka* how they will survive. *Skandā* looked to his father, *Śhiva* for the answer. *Mahādeva* answered, 'Gods, men, and animals live under the principle of give and take; they are linked by the bonds of service to one another. The gods minister to the needs of humans and animals by ruling the seasons of the year and by controlling the rain and air.

'Humans return the favor by propitiating the gods through meditation, prayer, offerings. All services and their compensation between the gods and humans are complete, so there is nothing left for you. Therefore, your means of sustenance will be in the life of an infant. It is true that this form of compensation will be tainted with the tears of the anxious and haggard parents.'

'Thus, the children of the families in which the gods, ancestors (*Pitris*), the *Brāhmans*, pious, preceptors, elders, and guests are not properly worshipped, respected and served, where the rules of cleanliness and virtues are not observed, when the family members do not make daily offerings to the gods and donate money and food to the less fortunate, and those who eat food that belongs to others, are the proper persons whom you can strike with impunity, and by your malefic influence, cause them these childhood diseases.

'It is your duty to see that the payment of the parents' iniquities appears in their children. The parents will be forced to worship you and give you offerings, to return the childrens' health. Thus, you will have ample sustenance.'

The nine *grahas* (planetary deities) accepted these words. These childhood diseases are difficult to heal. When disease is caused by *Skandā*, the most dreadful of all the planets, there may be permanent damage, even if the child is healed,. If a fully developed disorder occurs from any of the other planets, the disease will be incurable.

This planetary section may sound less scientific and more mythological. For this reason, it may be more difficult to believe, or at least, harder to understand. Simply put, to prevent childhood diseases (and all diseases), live ethically, virtuously, cleanly, and spiritually according to your own path. Be kind, generous, charitable, gentle, and always make time to meditate or pray according to your own spiritual beliefs.

Therapies

General: The child should be kept in a clean and purified room, and massaged with *ghee*. Mustard seeds are spread on the floor and a mustard oil lamp is constantly lit. Cardamom, sesame and barley, and sandalwood are constantly placed in the fire with garlands of flowers. *Mantras* are also constantly recited, "Reverence to thee, lord of the fire, honor to thee, goddess *Krittikā*, obeisance to thee, lord *Skandā*, reverence to thee, lord who has cast this malefic effect. In deep respect and humility, I beseech your favor. May my child be rid of this disease, make (him/her) strong and healthy again."

Skandā-graha:

Herbs: Decoctions of *bilwa, aśhwagandhā, balā*, cardamom, *yogaraj guggul*, and other Vāyu-reducing herbs are sprinkled on the child's body. The same herbs, along with sesame oil, *guḍūchī* are used to massage the body. *Ghee* cooked with cedar and frankincense is mixed with milk and ingested.

Offerings: Mustard seeds, *vachā*, frankincense, cedar, *ghee* are burnt and the smoke is used to cover the child's body. *Bilwa, guḍūchī*, and *anantmūl* are strung together and worn as a necklace. The person taking care of the child bathes in the night (chanting the *gāyatri mantra*). They pray to lord *Skandā* for three consecutive nights, offering red flower garlands, saffron or rose incense, grains, and rice. Bells are rung.

Mantras: Daily prayers to *Skandā* (the Divine warrior) are said, "May the eternal, changeless *Skandā*, the receptacle of all energies gained by austerities, fame, valor, or vital energy be favorable to thee (the child). May almighty *Guha*, head of the army of the gods, planetary lords, and destroyer of their enemies, protect thee from all evils. May he who is the son of the supreme, whose mothers are *Gangā, Umā,* and the *Krittikās* give thee health and comfort. May the beautiful god who with a single shaft, pierced the heart of mountain *Krouncha* and who is resplendent with red rays of his own divine person, smeared with red sandalwood paste and wearing red flower garlands, protect thee from all dangers."

Skandā-pasmarā Pratiṣhedha:

A bilwa leaf decoction subdues Vāyu. Sprinkling with this decoction is useful. An oil decoction of *bilwa* root with herbs from the *sarvagandha* group (i.e., aromatic herbs like *sandalwood, tulsī, guggul, frankincense)* neem, and *guḍūchī* is pasted on the child's body.

Fumigation: Mustard seed, *vachā*, and *ghee* are burned around the body of the child. Twigs of *guḍūchī* and *bilwa* thorns are strung on a necklace and put around the child's neck. *Anantmūl*, sandalwood, *guggulu,* and *tulsī* aromas are used. Whoever is caring for the child should bathe nightly and meditate to *Skandā*, the ruler of Mars, for three successive nights in the inner area of the child's house. The bath water should be purified by reciting the *Gāyatri Mantra* (*Aum bhūr bhuvah swaha; Tat savitur warenyam; Bhargo devasya dhī mahi; Dhiyo yo nah prachidayāt*). Red-flower garlands, red flags, and red oils (e.g., *kumkum*) are offered in prayer. Fresh barley and rice are also offered. Bells are rung and sacred fires are lit with 3, 7, or 10 pourings of *ghee*.

Mantra*:* Daily recitation protects the body from this malefic planet. "May *Skandā*, the eternal and changeless deity who is the receptacle of all sorts of energies produced by austerities, fame, valor or vital energy be propitious to thee. May almighty *Guha* (the commander-in-chief of gods and planets) protect thee from all evils. He is the destroyer of the enemy of the gods. May he who is the son of the supreme deity, the god of the gods, and who acknowledges the exalted motherhood of *Gangā*, *Umā,* and the *Krittikās*, give thee health and comfort. May the beautiful god who pierced with a single shaft right through the heart of the mountain *Krouncha* and who is effulgent with red rays of his own divine person smeared with the paste of red sandalwood and decked with the garland of red flowers protect thee from all perils."

Skandāpasmāra-Pratiṣhedha:

A decoction of *bilwa* is sprinkled over the body. Medicated oils of the *sarvagandhā* herb group (i.e., aromatics) are smeared on the body. *Ghee* cooked with milk and a decoction of the barks of *kṣhīrī* trees, and herbs from the *śhatāvarī, aśhwagandhā,* and licorice are made into a paste and are eaten.

The child's body is rubbed with *vachā* and *hiṅg* paste. Fumigation with the aromatic herbs (i.e., *bilwa*, sandalwood, *guggul*). A bracelet of sandalwood, *tulsī, rudrakṣha,* or *anantmūl* is worn by the child. The child's caretaker, observing a fast, sits in a ditch and offers milk and grains (food stuff). The child is bathed at a crossroads while a *mantra* is recited: "O thou, the trusted and beloved friend of god *Skandā*, O *Skandāpasmāra*, O thou ugly-faced one whom the world knows by the epithet of *Visākha*, may good befall this child in distress."

Shakuni-Pratiṣhedha:

The child's body is sprinkled with a decoction of *kapittha* and *āmra* (mango). An oil decoction, using sweet and astringent herbs, is used to anoint the body. Plasters of *madhuka, utpala, prīyaṅgu, mañjiṣhṭhā,* and sarsaparilla are pasted on the child.

Herbs and foods discussed in the ulcers section and the fumigation described above for *Skan-dāgraha* are also used here. *Śhatāvarī*, *nāga-danti* (heliotrope), *kaṇṭkārī, lakṣhmana,* and *vrihati* (Indian nightshade) are worn as a charm by the child.

Skandā, the ruler of Mars is meditated on by the practitioner in a beech arbor. He is offered huskless sesame seeds and flower garlands. The child is bathed in the arbor as discussed under *Skandā Graha*. Medicated *ghee* used for *Skandā Graha* is also used.

Flowers are offered to *Skandā*, and *a mantra* is recited, "May the ever down-looking sharp-beaked, keen and farseeing-eyed goddess (*Śhakuni* is decked with a variety of ornaments) and who traverses the ethereal sky in her flight, be propitious to thee. May the brown-eyed, fierce-looking, huge-bodied, large-bellied and spike-eared *Śhakuni*, who strikes terror into the hearts of people with her terrible voice, be pleased with thee."

Revati-Pratiṣhedha:

A decoction of *aśhwagandhā*, *sarsaparilla, punarnavā,* and both *sahā* and *vidārī kand* are sprinkled on the child's body. Medicated oil of *kuśhtā, guggul***,** and khus-khus are anointed on the body. Medicated *ghee* cooked with lotus, *dhātakī,* and *aśhwagandhā, śhatāvarī,* and *licorice* herbs are taken internally.

Burnt *kulattha* (horse gram), powdered conch shell (*śhank bhasma*), and herbs from the *sarvagandha* group (aromatic herbs) are applied as a plaster. The child's body is fumigated morning and evening with barley, *yava-phala* (barley). A necklace is made for the child from *varuna,* neem, or *nirguṇḍī.*

The planetary ruler of this disease is *Revati*, who is meditated on in a cow barn by the practitioner. White flowers, milk, and boiled rice should be offered. The nurse and child are both bathed in the junction of rivers. A *mantra* is recited: "May the goddess *Revati*, of dark complexion, who is clad in brightly colored clothes, with garlands of multicolored flowers, and is anointed with various aromas and with oscillating earrings, be pleased with thee. May the goddess *Revati*, who is tall, drooping and terrible looking, and who is the mother of many sons be always propitious to thee."

Putanā-Pratiṣhedha:

The child is washed with a decoction of the barks of *varuna*, *pāribhadraka,* and *āsphotā* Medicated oil made with a decoction of *vachā*, *brāhmī,* and *kuśhtā* is used to anoint the child's body.

Ghee is cooked with *kuśhtā, khadira,* sandalwood, licorice, *śhatāvarī*, and *aśhwagandhā.* Cedar, *vachā, kuśhtā, hiṅg,* and aromatic herbs are used to fumigate the child's body. A bracelet made of wild licorice other aromatic herbs is worn by the child.

The ruler of this planetary disease, *Putanā*, is meditated on in a lonely room. Offerings include boiled rice and sesame butter. They are placed on a saucer and covered. The child is bathed with the water used with the offerings.

The *mantra* recited is, "May the slovenly shag-haired goddess, *Putanā*, who is dressed in dirty clothes and who loves to haunt lonely places, preserve this child. May the fierce-looking frightful goddess, who is as black as a dark rain cloud, who loves to haunt lonely and dilapidated human dwellings, and whose body gives off filthy odors, protect the child from all evils."

Andha-putanā-Pratiṣhedha:

A decoction of bitter trees (i.e., neem or *chirāyatā)* is used to sprinkle on the child's body. Wine, rice vinegar**,** *kuṣhā,* and *haritāla* should be used with medicated oil. Medicated *ghee* is made from a decoction of *pippalī*, *aśhwagandhā, śhatāvarī, vidārī kand,* licorice, and raw honey (added after cooking).

A plaster of aromatic herbs is applied to the child's body. The eyes are soothed with cold water. Fumigation is conducted with aromatic herbs**.** The child wears a necklace of *śhimbi, anatāmūl, mango,* neem, and other aromatic herbs.

The practitioner makes an offering of food at the cross roads or inside the house. The child and nurse are bathed with a decoction of aromatic herbs. The following *mantra* used chanted: "May the dreadful, brown-colored, bald-headed goddess *Andha-putanā*, wearing red-colored clothes, be pleased to save this child."

<u>*Śhita-putanā-Pratiṣhedha*</u>:

A decoction of *kapittha, bilwa,* and *bhallātaka* are used to sprinkle on the child's body. *Musta,* cedar, *kuśhtā*, and aromatic herbs are used as a medicated oil. Medicated *ghee* is made with three parts of a decoction of the herbs *rohini, khadira, palāsā, arjuna* bark, and one part milk. Neem, licorice *bilwa,* and mango are used for fumigating the child. *Gunja* (wild licorice), *tulsī*, sandalwood, and other aromatic herbs are worn as a bracelet by the child.

The ruler *Shitaputanā*, is meditated on, and offered rice and *mudga* (*mūngdal*) (cooked together). Wine is also offered. The child is bathed near a river, pond, or pool. The *mantra* recited is, "May the goddess *Śhita-putanā*, who is fond of rice and *mūng (mudga)*, who delights in drinking wine, and who resides by the side of rivers, preserve thee."

<u>*Mukha-mandikā-Pratiṣhedha*</u>:

A decoction of *kapittha, bilwa, vaṃśha lochana, jayanti, erand,* and *pātalā* are used to sprinkle on the child. Oil and *ghee* (in equal parts) is cooked with the juice of *bhṛiṅgarāj, aśhwagandhā*, and *śhatāvarī* and anointed on the child's body. Medicated *ghee* is made with *daśhmūl* and milk.

Fumigation with *vachā, kuśhtā*, and other aromatic herbs and mixed with *ghee* is ingested by the child. A bracelet of sandalwood, *tulsī, rūdrakṣha,* or *anantmūl* is also worn. The ruler is offered food in a cow barn. The child is bathed with water that the *mantra* was recited over. The *mantra* is, "May the beautiful and blessed goddess *Mukhamandikā*, who wears ornaments, who can assume different forms at will and who resides in cow barns, preserve thee."

<u>*Naigameṣha-Pratiṣhedha*</u>:

A decoction of *bilwa*, *agnimantha* (clerodendron p. or premna integrifolia), *sarvira* (sarsaparilla), and whey are sprinkled on the child's body. A medicated oil is made with *prīyaṅgu, anantamūl,* and *śhata-puṣhpa* (fennel) with yogurt whey and anointed on the child. Medicated *ghee* is made with *madhura* herbs, *daśhmūl* decoction, and milk.

The child wears the same bracelet advised for *Skandāpasmāra*. White mustard seed, *vachā, hiṅg, kuśhtā*, parched rice, *bhallātaka,* and *ajamodā* are used for fumigating the child's body. Huskies sesame seeds, garlands of flowers, and various foods are offered to *Naigameṣha*, the preserver of the child, at the base of a *banyan* tree on the sixth day of the fortnight. The child is bathed there also.

The *mantra* recited is, "May the far-famed god, *Naigameṣha*, the preserver of children, who has a goat's face with moving brow and rolling eyes and who can assume different forms at will, preserve the child."

Male Reproductive System (Punster)

Defective Semen

<u>Cause</u>: Excess sex or sex at the wrong times, masturbation, exercise, unsuitable foods, eating an excess of rough, bitter, astringent, salty, sour and hot foods, old age, anxiety, grief, suspicion, fear, anger, exorcism, emaciation from disease, suppression of natural urges, and wounds can lead to the derangement of *doṣhas* and tissues. This can reach the semen-carrying channels, causing semen defects.

Semen is considered normal when it is oily, viscous, non-slimy, sweet, non-burning, and white.

<u>Symptoms</u>: Defective semen is frothy, thin, rough, discolored, slimy, malodorous, combined with other tissues and premature.

<u>*Vāyu*</u>: Air afflicts the semen causing frothy, thin and rough, semen that is difficult to ejaculate (impotence).

<u>*Pitta*</u>: Fire affecting the semen is blue or yel-

lowish, very hot, malodorous, and burns when ejaculated.
Kapha: Water obstructs the passage of semen making it slimy.
Excessive Coitus, Injury, Wound: Bloody semen develops.
Suppression of Urges: This causes Vāyu to obstruct the passage of semen, making it difficult to ejaculate, feel knotted, or ejaculate prematurely.

Therapies: Herbs with the properties of aphrodisiacs are used, such as *śhilājit*, *śhatāvarī*, *aśhwagandhā*, *kapikachhū,* and *vidārī-kand.* For bleeding, red raspberry, *śhatāvarī*, *musta*, *mañjiṣhṭhā*, gotu kola, aloe vera gel, and *bhṛiṅgarāj* are used. Pitta-reducing foods, drinks and lifestyle are advised.
Vāyu: Herbs include *śhatāvarī*, *aśhwagandhā*, *kapikachhū*, *vidārī-kand*, sesame seeds, and almonds. Non-oily enemas are also used.
Pitta: *Śhatāvarī* and *balā* are used.
Kapha: *Pippalī*, *arjuna,* and *triphalā* are suggested.
Foods: *Ghee*, milk, barley, rice, and wheat are advised.

Impotency (Vīryalpata)

Causes: Loss or deficiency of semen and penile strength and senility.

Defective Seed: This results from ingesting cold, rough, mixed, incompatible, uncooked or insufficient food, fasting, grief, anxiety, fear, terror, and sexual intercourse. Other causes include exorcism, suspicion, deficient plasma, *doṣha* excesses, exertion, faulty application of *pañcha karma*, and impaired semen. These conditions are associated with pale complexion, weakness, low vitality, erection difficulty, heart problems, anemia, bronchial asthma, jaundice, exhaustion, vomiting, diarrhea, colic, fever, and cough.
Penile Weakness: This results from ingesting excess sour, salty, heavy, incompatible and unsuitable foods, drinking excess water, or overeating pastries. Other causes are irregular meals, meats, excess yogurt or milk, weakness from illness, coitus with a female child, not in vagina, with lust, during menses, or female tract malodor. Further causes include a defective tract, excessive discharge, chronic illness in women, with animals, not washing the penis, and injured genitals.
Senility: Old age often causes diminished semen related to a deficiency of the seven tissues, not using aphrodisiacs, gradual loss of strength, energy, motor and sensory organs; poor nutrition, physical exertion, and mental exhaustion. This results in depleted tissues, debilitation, poor complexion, and poor resistance to disease.
Deficiency: From excess mental work, grief, fear, anxiety, envy, curiosity, intoxication, agitation, habitual rough and emaciating diet and herbs, fasting, or insufficient amounts of plasma-foods by weak persons. The diminished *rasa* causes deficiency in other tissues (*dhātus*). This results in low resistance to disease and can be life-threatening.

Therapies: General
Excess Sex, Doṣha Imbalance: Enemas, *ghee*, semen-promoting herbs, such as *śhatāvarī*, *aśhwagandhā*, *balā*, and *kapikachhū* are suggested.
Exorcism: Spiritual measures are used.
Impotence: Therapies should be administered in this order: unction, fomentation, and oil purgative (e.g., castor oil). Next, a proper meal should be eaten. Later non-oil enemas and oil enemas are used. Non-oil enemas include the herbs, *musta*, *patha*, *guḍūchī*, *balā*, *punarnavā*, *mañjiṣhṭhā*, *pṛiśhinderṇī*, and *kaṇṭkārī.* The best oil enema to use is *śhi goal* oil. The ingredients of *śhi goal* oil are black pepper, *hiṅgu*, saffron, and *viola* (cotton plant seed) herbs with Spanish jasmine oil. A sustained enema containing mastoid herbs is also suggested. Lastly, semen-promoting herbs such as *śhatāvarī*, *aśhwagandhā*, *balā*, and *kapikachhū* are taken. The oil enema promotes strength. Eating proper foods gives

strength and energy. In the same way, oil enemas restore strength and energy to the local area and to the whole body through colon absorption.

Loss of penile strength: Anointing the genitals with oil, sprinkling or blood-letting is used. Persons take sesame oil, *ghee*, castor oil purgatives and enemas, then non-oil enemas. Lastly, semen-promoting herbs, such as *śhatāvarī*, *aśhwagandhā*, *balā*, *kapikachhū*, and *āmalakī* are ingested.

Senility & Semen Deficiency: Therapies include unction and fomentation, oil purgatives and enemas. This is followed with *ghee* and semen promoting herbs, such as *śhatāvarī*, *aśhwagandhā*, *balā*, *kapikachhū*, *guggul*, *śhilājit*, and sesame or castor oil enemas.

Vāyu: Deficient semen. Therapies include *ghee*, sesame seeds, almonds, cooked garlic and onions; semen-promoting herbs, such as *śhatāvarī*, *aśhwagandhā*, *balā*, *kapikachhū*, *āmalakī*, *guggul*, and *śhilājit*.

Pitta: Burning semen. Herbs include aloe vera gel, *śhatāvarī*, *āmalakī*, milk, sugar, and *ghee*.

Kapha: Loss of interest in sex, obesity, excess mucus, desiring sugar as a substitute for sex. Herbs include *pippalī*, garlic, cloves, *trikatu*, *guggul*, and *śhilājit*.

Enlarged Prostate (Vātāṣhṭhīlā)

(see also Chapter 18)

Causes: This results from aging, excessive sexual intercourse, and suppression of ejaculation.

Symptoms and Therapies:

General: *Gokṣhura*, *aśhwagandhā*, and *śhilājit* are advised.

Vāyu: Symptoms include low back pain, low energy, and constipation. Therapies include Vāyu-reducing foods, cooked garlic and onions, *balā*, *kapikachhū*, *guggul*, *gokṣhura*, and *aśhwagandhā*.

Pitta: Symptoms include infection, swelling, fever, and dark yellow or red urine. Therapies include Pitta-reducing foods, *gokṣhura*, *punarnavā*, *aśhwagandhā*, lemon grass, and *chyavan prāśh*.

Kapha: This results from water retention and excess phlegm. Kapha-reducing foods, ginger, cinnamon, *śhilājit*, and *guggul* are advised.

Venereal Diseases (Upadamśha)

Genital Herpes, Syphilis , Gonorrhea

Causes: External injury, lack of cleanliness, excessive sexual intercourse, or contact with a diseased vagina. Generally this is a Pitta-excess disease, involving heat in the liver. Pitta moves through the liver channels to the urogenital region. Impure blood and excess bile may clog the area, causing an accumulation of stress, anger, and anxiety.

Symptoms:

Vāyu: Dry skin, constipation, small, blackish painful and hard pimples; low energy, and insomnia.

Pitta: Fever, thirst, red or black, swollen or painful pimples that exude yellowish fluid; burning sensation, pimples that discharge blood, and irritability.

Kapha: Pimples that exude white fluid, swelling, itching, slight redness and pain, phlegm accumulates in the body.

Tridoṣha: Muscular tissue sprouts (resembling a rooster's crown), developing inside the foreskin, at the junction of the glands or nearby; accompanied with pain and exudation. This is difficult to heal.

Therapies:

General: Sarsaparilla, gotu kola.

Vāyu: Vāyu-reducing foods, milk, *ghee*, aloe vera gel, turmeric, barberry, sandalwood, gotu kola, *aśhwagandhā*, *śhatāvarī*, and *balā*.

Pitta: Pitta-reducing foods, raw vegetables, *mūngdal*, *basmati* rice, milk, *ghee*; avoiding hot spices, alcohol, sour, salty foods, sugar, and avoiding stress. Herbs to cleanse the blood and liver include coriander or cilantro, parsley, *mañjiṣhṭhā*, *musta*, *bhūmīāmalakī*, *gokṣhura*, aloe vera gel, *punarnavā*, *śhatāvarī*, *kaṭukā*, and sandalwood. Sex should be reduced, and rest is required. Sandalwood and coconut oil body *abhyañga* (massage-like) is important. Purgation is also useful. Sores are washed with *chitrak*, turmeric, and sarsaparilla.

Kapha: Liver-cleansing herbs, such as aloe vera gel, *chitrak*, turmeric, with hot spices like ginger, *pippalī*, cloves, and *tṛikatu*.

Females: Aloe gel, myrrh, saffron, safflower, and other menstrual herbs (see female genital tract section).

Tridoṣha: Therapies for all three *doṣhas*.

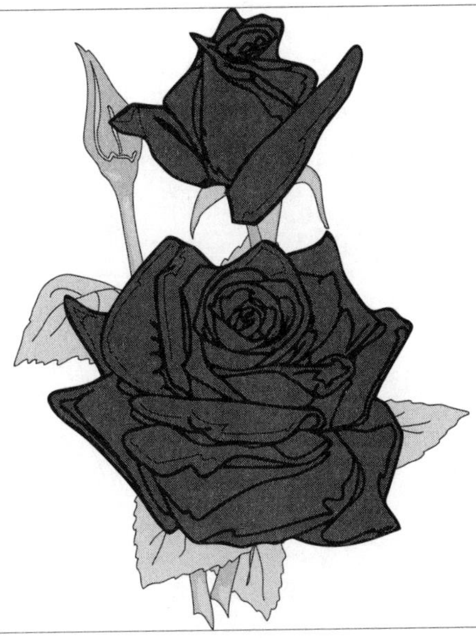

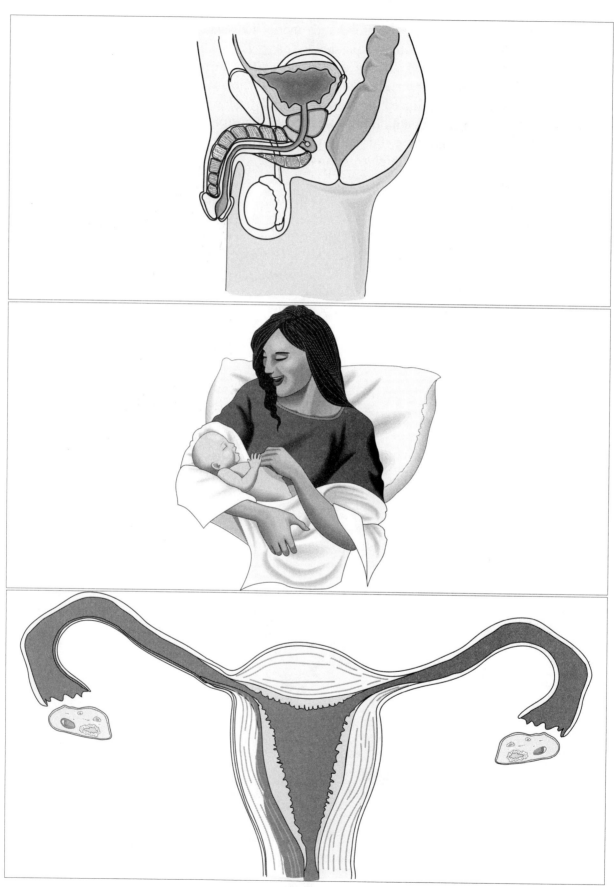

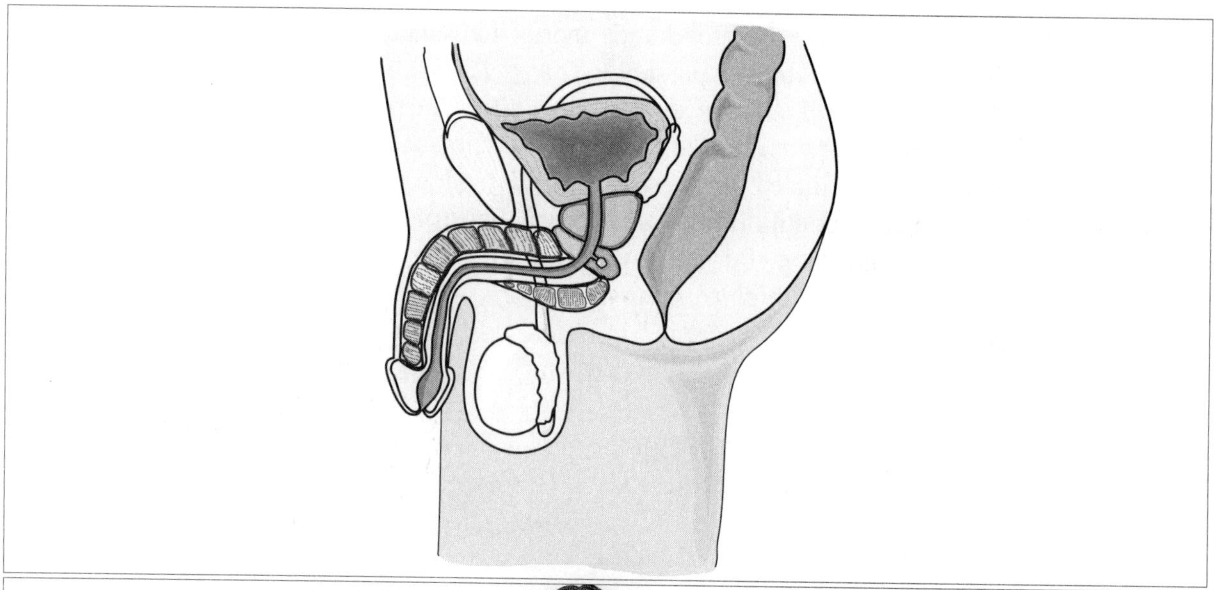

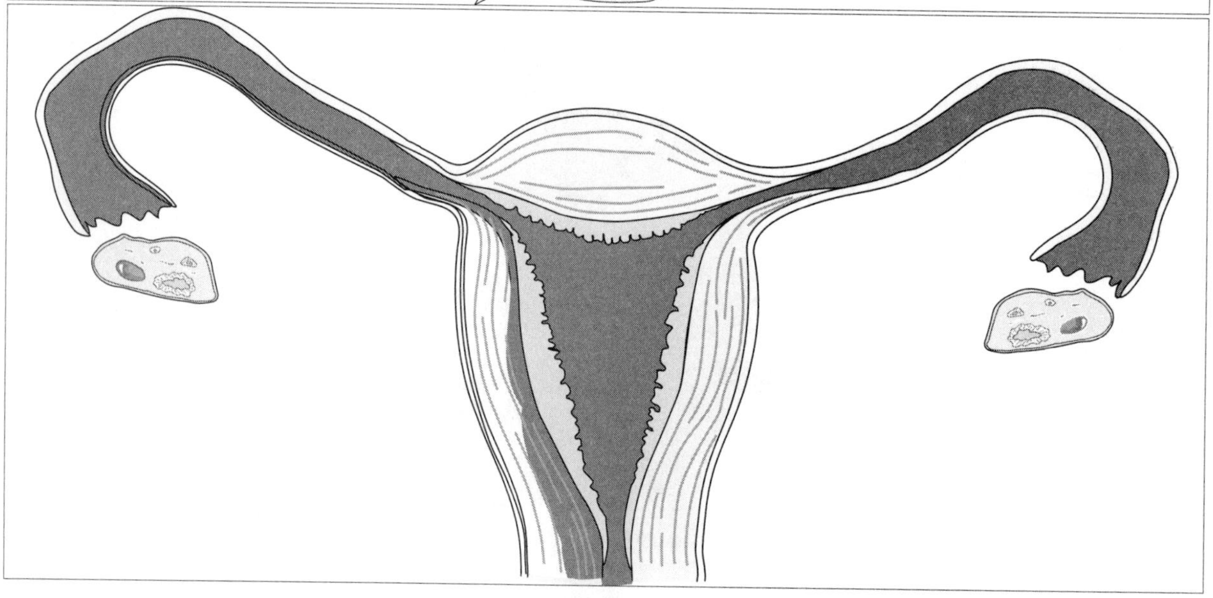

Persons should not engage in occupations that are lacking, or going contrary to the three pursuits; righteousness, wealth and pleasure...one should be moderate and avoid extremes.
Aṣhṭāñga Hṛidayam Sū. Ch. 2: ver. 30

Chapter 24
Immune System
HIV/AIDS, Epstein Barr

Immune system disorders are becoming more prevalent as modern society becomes faster paced, orients itself more toward high technology, and departs from nature's rhythms and nutritional living. Technology itself is not an inherent evil. Rather, it is the imbalance, the overreliance or the idea of conquering nature, rather than learning to live in harmony with it, that tips the scales toward an artificial or destructive lifestyle.

Āyurveda is aware of an immune system essence or life-sap. This life-sap is called *ojas*, and has been discussed throughout this book. It is this sap that covers and protects the immune system from harm. *Ojas* can be likened to the sap of a tree. When the bark of a healthy tree is cut, the sap oozes over the cut and slowly hardens. Eventually the cut is healed and the bark grows once again. Analogously, when some foreign body attacks the immune system, the *ojas* or life-sap covers, protects, and eventually repairs the damage. Healthy immune systems having an ample supply of *ojas* can even protect the system, keeping it healthy at all times.

Many of today's habits quickly deplete the immune system's *ojas*. Excess travel, overworking to the point of burnout, eating junk food, and excess sexual intercourse—to cite a few noxious influences—all overtax the system and deplete the supply of *ojas*. Mental stress can also overtax the nervous system, and cause a depletion of *ojas*. Excess worry, fear, anger, and impatience can dry or burn up *ojas*. Thus, immune system disorders are caused by both mental and physical lifestyle factors.

In contrast to these *ojas*-depleting lifestyles, Mother Nature, being all-providing, has provided various foods, herbs, colors, gems, and *mantras* that have *ojas*-building properties: organic milk and yogurt, *ghee*, whole cane sugar, maple syrup and raw honey, almonds and sesame seeds are all natural foods that are known to build *ojas*.

The gold ash formula, *Survana Vasant Malti* is excellent for all immune disorders—1 pill in the morning with 1/2 tsp. honey. For extreme immune weakness (e.g., AIDS) a second pill can be taken in the evening. In rare cases, some heartburn may occur. For this, *avipattikar chūrṇa* is used as needed.

Dairy: Milk is drunk after it is boiled and cooled. Whole sugars and *ghee* are added to the milk. The milk is drunk early in the morning or just before bed (without other foods). Yogurt water (*lassi*) is drunk with meals or between meals.

Nuts/Seeds: After a few almonds are soaked overnight, the skin should be peeled before the nuts are eaten. Sesame seeds, in the form of tahini (sesame butter), are easy to digest.

Herbs: *Aśhwagandhā* and *śhatāvarī* are two common *ojas*-boosting herbs. Cardamom or cinnamon may be added to aid digestion of these heavier herbs.

Gems: Diamonds and yellow stones such as citrine boost *ojas* in the body.

Colors: These balance physical health by balancing mental health. Gold strengthens the immune system and *ojas*.

Aromatherapy: Aromas like lotus, rose, frankin-

cense, and sandalwood help to boost *ojas* while calming the mind.
Mantras: The best *mantra* is the one given by one's personal spiritual *guru* (guide). Since many people do not have such an opportunity, Āyurveda offers *mantras* that heal the mind and body. *Aum, Ram,* and *Klīm* increase *ojas.*
Mental Peace: The health of the mind affects the health of the body: *śhiro dhārā* (warm oil flow on the head) relaxes the mind, nerves, and immune system, providing individuals with a profound state of rest. In this state, deep-seated stresses and diseases may be released.
Spiritual Lifestyle: Reading scriptures, listening to spiritual music, helping others, meditating, eating properly, and working at a job one loves are examples of lifestyles that heal the mind and body and boost *ojas*.

HIV/AIDS

In an ancient Āyurvedic text, *Mādhana Nidān*, written around 700 A.D., the author, *Mādhavakara* foretells a disease that will come to India. From its description, we know it as HIV/AIDS. Its cure was said to be *śhilājit*.

Causes: The main cause is deficient life-sap (*ojas*), which causes an extremely weakened immune system. When one has sufficient *ojas,* the HIV virus cannot develop. *Ojas* is lost or diminished by excess sex, improper diet, junk food, drugs, excess worry, thinking, and insomnia.

Symptoms: Vāyu and Pitta are primary factors, but Kapha may present symptoms of congestion and lung disorders.
Vāyu: Weakness, low energy, nerve disorders, constipation, anxiety, worry, fear, dry skin, vertigo, palpitations, and nervous system disorders, such as neuropathy.
Pitta: Blood, skin, and liver problems; nervous system disorders caused by heating, burning, diarrhea, fever, anger, impatience, and low energy-burnout. An inflamed tongue (oral candida/yeast).
Kapha: (complications—not a primary cause of HIV/AIDS) Congestion, mucus, and lung disorders. A white-coated tongue (oral candida/yeast).

Therapies:

1) The main herb suggested in *Mādan Nidān* is *śhilājit* (tridoṣhic—for all *doṣhas*). It boosts the immune system (*ojas*) and is antiviral.
2) Vāyu/Immune boosting herbs. *Śhatāvarī, aśhwagandhā, kapikachhū* and *chyavan prāśh* build the *ojas* and balance Vāyu.
3) Pitta reducing herbs.

A) Blood purifiers—gotu kola, *mañjiṣhṭhā*, turmeric.

B) Liver cleansers—gentle herbs are used if Vāyu is also high (i.e., weak or emaciated). They include gotu kola, *bhṛiṅgarāj, musta* ,and sandalwood (antibacterial/antiseptic). When persons are strong but still have infections, purpura (or other skin disorders), then stronger liver herbs, such as *bhūmīāmalakī* and *kaṭukā,* may be administered.

C) Gokṣhura may be used to treat burning or infections of the urinary tract. It is also good for seminal debility and nerve disorders.

D) Herbal antibiotics like *guḍūchī* and turmeric can also be used to treat infections.

4) Kapha-reducing herbs. Hot spices are used to treat congestion.
5) Antiviral herbs. In small doses, or when mixed with Vāyu-reducing herbs, jasmine is a gentle antiviral herb. *Śhilājit* also has antiviral properties, but is not used if the uric acid count is high.

A Vāyu- or Pitta-reducing diet and lifestyle are required; spicy, sour, bitter, and astringent tastes are not recommended. Foods that are wholesome, pure (*sattwic*), and *ojas*-building are used (e.g., sesame oil and seeds, almonds, chickpeas, boiled milk, yogurt/water, and *ghee*). Sesame oil should be applied externally. *Brāhmī* and sandalwood oil should be applied on the head. *Śhiro dhārā* is efficacious in relaxing the nervous system and boosting the immune system. Sex is also to be avoided because it drains the body of *ojas*.

Ojas-boosting *mantras* include *Aum*, *Śhum,* and *Śhrīm*. Yellow stones, moonstone, and pearl all increase *ojas*.

Thrush: Coriander or fennel (1/8 tsp.) between meals.

Epstein-Barr Virus/ Chronic Fatigue Syndrome

Western medicine describes Epstein-Barr Virus (EBV) (Chronic Fatigue Syndrome) as a ubiquitous herpes virus related to B-lymphocytes and the nasal and pharynx cells. Āyurveda suggests that this low-grade infection is caused by a depleted immune system, as discussed earlier in the introduction to this chapter. Western medicine suggests that primary EBV infection occurs in people of all ages. Fifty percent of children under the age of five may possibly carry EBV, but it is almost always in a dormant stage.

In the past decade or so a pattern of EBV has been seen in adults, ages 20 - 40. The symptoms include fatigue, low-grade fever, mild thinking dysfunction, and lymphadenopathy (lymph node inflammation that can lead to diseases related to the lymphoid system).

Although EBV is sometimes called Chronic Fatigue Syndrome, the symptoms are not always the same.

Therapies: Generally, this is viewed as a Pitta excess, often caused by burn-out and overwork. Āyurveda recommends a two-fold therapeutic approach.

1) Immune-boosting herbs that do not aggravate Pitta (e.g., *śhatāvarī*, *śhilājit*).

2) Pitta-reducing herbs to reduce infection and virus, and cleanse the blood, liver, gall bladder, spleen, and lymphoid system (e.g., *mañjiṣhṭhā*, turmeric, *bhūmīāmalakī, kaṭukā,* yellow dock, and *bhṛiṅgarāj*).

A Pitta-reducing diet and lifestyle are also essential for healing and rejuvenation.

Fibromyalgia

This is another condition that has become prevalent in more recent years. Therapies include yoga postures, *śhiro dhārā, abhyañga, mahānārāyan* oil for pain, and *survana vasant malti* (gold) pills as an immune booster. Other herbs include *śhatāvarī* and *aṣhwagandhā*. This condition takes a long time to heal.

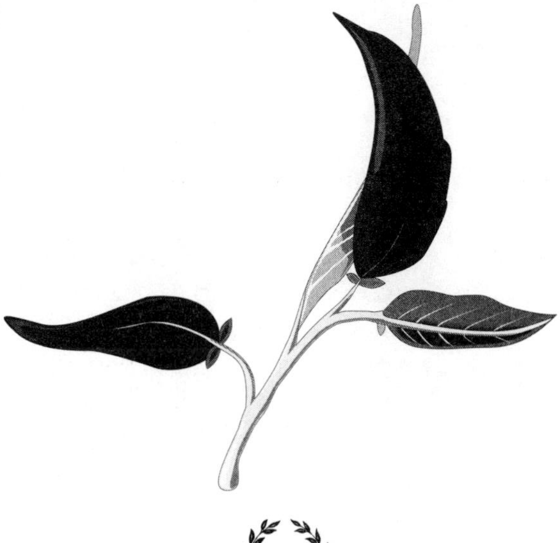

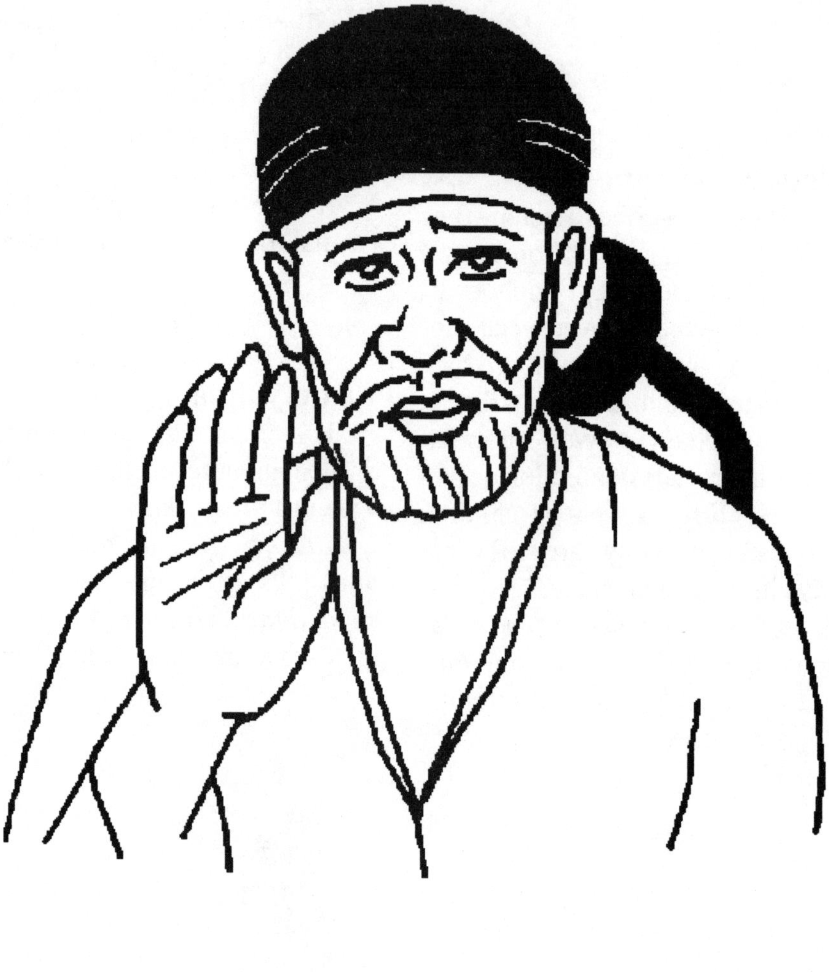

Being mindful of the nature of people,
deal with them in a way that best pleases them.
Become well versed in the art of adoring others.
Aṣhṭāñga Hṛidayam Sū. Ch. 2: ver. 26-28

Chapter 25
Metabolic System
(Edema, Tonsillitis, Gingivitis, Dental Abscess Goiter, Hypo/Hyperthyroid, Gout, Thirst)

Edema (Śhopha or Śhotha)
Non-Inflammatory

Causes: General causes occur from increased *doṣhas*. All three *doṣhas* are involved in the development of all three types of edema (Vāyu, Pitta, and Kapha), yet the predominating *doṣha* determines what *doṣha* should be balanced. Specific causes result from debilitating diseases, fasting, sudden overeating, or unhealthy foods. Other causes include eating foods that are hard to digest, fatty, heavy, hot, sharp, cold, salty, or from excessive use of diuretics or elimination therapies, leafy vegetables that are penetrating or too hot. Drinking water to excess, oversleeping, lack of sleep, eating mud, excess yogurt, dry meats, and uncooked foods also cause edema. Further causes include overexertion, long distance walking, excessive travel, and eating mutually contradictory foods (e.g., fish and milk).

It may also develop from difficult breathing, cough, diarrhea, hemorrhoids, enlarged abdomen, menorrhagia, and fever. Other causes include simultaneous vomiting and diarrhea resulting from indigestion, undigested food remaining in the stomach, vomiting, pregnancy, herpes, and anemia. This can also be caused by other diseases improperly tended to, lack of exercise, irregular delivery, abortion, or miscarriage.

External causes result only when the superficial skin layer is afflicted by injury.

Development: Edema is either organic or traumatic and may pervade the body or remain localized. It may be hard and wide, raised, or knotted/glandular.

These conditions will cause Pitta, blood, and Kapha to enter the outer channels and obstruct the circulation channels (*Vyān* Vāyu). This causes localized swelling in the skin and muscles. There are 9 types of edema: Vāyu, Pitta, Kapha, Vāyu/Pitta, Vāyu/Kapha, Pitta/Kapha, Tridoṣha, external (two causes: trauma/injury, and poison).

When the *doṣhas* are in the chest, they produce upper body swelling. When they are found in the urinary bladder, the lower body swells; in the middle of the body, the middle swells. *Doṣhas* found throughout the body cause the whole body to swell. When it occurs in the throat or palate, edema remains localized.

Premonitory Signs:

Fevers, burning sensations, dilated veins at the site of edema, heaviness.

Symptoms:

General: Heaviness, appearing and disappearing (i.e., unstable or variable); swelling, rising temperature, thinning vessels, hair standing on end, discoloration of skin on the extremities.

Vāyu: Swelling moves from place to place, is dry with rough hair; reddish or black; thin, constricting, pulsating, tingling, pricking, puncturing or cutting pains, or a lack of sensation. Swelling quickly rises and subsides and spreads to other parts. Can subside by massage with fatty and hot materials. Will be mild at night and severe during the day. May also be mildly burning or tingling. There may be numbness. When the skin is pressed the swelling disappears, but when the finger releases from the skin, the swelling rises again.

Pitta: Black, pink, yellow, or reddish white swelling with copper-red hair, malodorous, quick swelling, and subsiding. First appears in the middle of the body with thirst, burning fever, perspiration, sweating, thirst, giddiness, toxicity, and dizziness. Persons wanting cold things have painful diarrhea.

Kapha: Itchy swelling, yellowish-white hair and skin, hard, cold, oily, smooth, firm, and thick. It is associated with excessive sleep, vomiting, and weak digestion. Pressing and releasing fingers from the swelling leaves an indentation (i.e., the skin does not rise). This is known as "pitting edema." Edema is slow to appear and heal and swells more at night. When pricked, it exudes slimy fluid. Other symptoms include heavy limbs, localization of the edema. Touch and warmth are pleasing to the person.

Tridoṣha: Symptoms of all three *doṣhas* appear simultaneously.

Trauma: Results from cutting, splitting, hitting, banging, being in a cold breeze or sea breeze. It spreads from place to place, is hot to touch, blood-red color. Other Pitta symptoms pertain.

Poisons: Causes include bites, claws, contaminated things, feces, urine, semen, poisonous trees, wind, gas, and smoke. It is soft, moveable, drooping, quickly rising, burning, and painful.

Recently occurring edema without secondary complications can be healed.

Therapies:

If undigested food toxins (*āma*) have caused the edema, then fasting and laxatives are first suggested. When food is taken, it should only be fresh and wholesome. It is important to avoid dried vegetables, heavy and burning foods and drinks, naps, sexual intercourse, sweets, alcohol, and fried foods. Take cane sugar and fresh ginger (equal quantities—totaling 125 mg.) on the first day. Increase the dose by 125 mg. daily for 10 days. Continue to take this amount for 1 month. When this recipe is digested, take boiled milk, and when it can be easily digested take vegetable and *ghee* soup. Thick barley (powder) gruel with *śhatāvarī*, *āmalakī*, *vidārī kand*, *arjuna*, coriander, *chitrak*, and *bilwa* are fried in *ghee* (1 part herbs to 2 parts *ghee*) and eaten.

Vāyu: *Daśhmūl*, *punarnavā*, *harītakī*, *pippalī* with boiled milk.

External therapies: This includes 2 or 3 drops of *daśhmūl* and *mahānārāyan* oils ingested and/or applied externally to the edema. The oils may also be cooked with cardamom, *musta*, *pippalī*, and coriander. They may also be applied as a paste (*lepa*) and massaged into the skin. Afterwards, a warm bath with *vāsāk*, *musta,* and sandalwood is useful.

Burning and pain- *daśhmūl* oil and paste.

Pimples and burning- licorice, *musta*, sandalwood, *viḍaṅga*, neem, *chitrak*, *triphalā*, and *daśhmūl* as oil and paste.

Vāyu and constipation: *Nirūha* enema and castor oil, *ghee,* and cane sugar before meals. If circulatory blocks, poor digestion, or anorexia exist, fermented barley drinks are essential.

Vāyu/Pitta: *Triphalā*, *musta*, sandalwood, *arjuna*, licorice, ginger, black pepper, turmeric, *guḍūchī*, and castor oil.

Pitta and diarrhea: Drink 1/2 cup yogurt with 1/2 cup water; mixed with ginger, *chitrak*, black pepper, and *pippalī* with raw honey.

Pitta external therapies: Sandalwood, *guḍūchī* and *gokṣhura* are made into a paste and applied to the body. The same herbs may be cooked with oil and used for *abhyañga* (massage-like). Afterwards, a bath in warm water with sandalwood and *musta* is recommended.

Kapha: *Triphalā*, rhubarb, black pepper, *pippalī*, ginger, *ṭrikatu*, *punarnavā*, and *daśhmūl* are ingested.

Kapha external therapies: *Pippalī* paste or sand massages are useful. Water mixed with ginger may be poured on the body (or bathed in). Afterwards, one applies sandalwood oil to the body.

When edema is located in the lower part of the

body, purgation is advised. If the edema is found in the upper part of the body, emetics are used.

Should edema be caused by improper oleation therapy, then dry herbs and foods are used to counterbalance this effect. For symptoms of fainting, disliking everything, burning, and thirst, boiled milk is given.

Meningitis

This results from external factors. A meningococcal virus infects the brain and membranous sheath of the spinal cord. This disease was not present during ancient *Vedic* times. It is difficult to heal. It is called "brain edema" and is caused by Vāyu and Kapha. All three *doṣhas* become deranged. This is a very serious condition.

Therapies: The best herbs include *jaṭāmāṇśhī*, gotu kola, *vachā*, *chitrak*, *tṛikatu*, small cardamom, *pippalī*, and *punarnavā*. They are ingested, used as aromatherapy, and nasal oils, to evacuate the head from the excess *doṣhas*. Also useful are *śhiro dhārā* and *śhiro basti*.

Quinsy or Throat Edema (a Vāyu/Kapha disorder); may develop into meningitis.

Therapies: Herbs to heal this condition include *tṛikatu*, *daśhmūl*, *jaṭāmāṇśhī*, and *guggul*.

Tonsillitis (Bidālikā)

When edema occurs in the throat it is called *bidālikā* or tonsillitis. The swelling causes redness and burning, impairs the breathing, and causes great pain. This is a Pitta/Kapha condition. If the swelling surrounds the entire neck, it is very serious.

Therapies: The same therapies as quinsy are used. Other herbs include *kañchanar*, *triphalā*, and *tṛikatu*.

Palatal abscesses (Tālu vidradhi)

This is an abscess with burning, redness, and oozing in the throat. It is caused by all three *doṣhas*.

Therapies: Herbs include *sitopaladi, kañchanar guggul*, and also general treatment of *Vidradhi* is followed (see Chapter 16 on abscess and sinus).

Acute superficial glossitis (Upajihvikā)

This condition is located in the back of the tongue (Kapha/Vāyu), whereas sublingual abscesses or *adhijivikā* (caused by Kapha) are found on the bottom of the tongue.

Therapies: Herbs used include *tṛikatu*, *guggul*, licorice, *kūt*, and *vachā*.

Gingivitis (Puakuṣha)

This is caused by excess blood and Pitta. The condition is an inflammation of the gum muscles.

Therapies: Herbs used include sesame oil, *elā* (cardamom), licorice, and cane sugar.

Dental abscesses (Danta-Vidradhi)

This is an inflammation in the muscles around the teeth. It is caused by excess Kapha and blood in that area.

Therapies: Herbs include turmeric, small cardamom, chestnuts, *kayaphal*. The best herb is *badradanti*.

Goiter (Galaganda)

This is a single swelling (cyst) in the throat. When a chain of swellings around the lower neck (i.e., necklace-shaped) develops it is called cervical adenitis or *gandamālā*. Both diseases can be healed. However, if they are associated with chronic rhinitis (*pīnasa*), chest pain (*pārṣhva shūla*), bronchitis, vomiting, and fever, then they are incurable.

Therapies: Herbs include *kañchanar, guggul, sitopaladi, tṛikatu,* and *vachā* (calamus). Other therapies include emesis and purgation to eliminate the *doṣhas* from the body; therapeutic smoke inhalation, and fasting. If the swelling is in the mouth, then the herbs are made into a paste and rubbed onto the swelling from inside the mouth.

Hyperthyroidism

(Graves' Disease falls under this category.)

Symptoms of hyperthyroidism include enlarged thyroid, nervousness, hypersensitivity to heat, palpitations, fatigue, increased appetite, weightloss, tachycardia, insomnia, weakness, diarrhea or frequent stools; and difficult breathing. It is caused by all three *doṣhas*, but mainly Pitta.

Therapies: *Kañchanar guggul* is the main herb used. Other herbs include *triphalā* and *tṛikatu*.

Endemic Goiter: Symptoms include an enlarged thyroid gland with almost no function. It begins subtly. Persons can develop dull facial expression, hoarseness, slow speech, puffiness, intolerance to cold, drooping eyelids, sparse, coarse, and dry hair. Other indications are dry, scaly skin, weight gain, poor memory, psychosis, constipation, carpal tunnel syndrome in wrists and ankles. Further symptoms include slow reflexes, menorrhagia, mild anemia, difficult breathing, umbilical hernia, slow bone growth. This is a Vāyu disorder, usually found in iodine-deficient areas as endemic goiter. It is often found in persons living in land-locked, mountain areas, where there is no iodine from the sea salt and fish. iodised salt is used as preventive therapy. Hot spices, such as *tṛikatu*, *pippalī*, and ginger, are useful.

Hypothyroid

Herbs include *tṛikatu, shilājit,* and iron and mineral ashes (*abhrak* and *mūkta bhasmas*)

Thyroid Therapies

For all thyroid conditions: Irish moss (insufficient hormones), *tṛikatu, yogarāj guggul* (Vāyu), *kaiṣhore guggul* (Pitta) or pure *guggul* (Kapha). Mustard oil can be applied externally on the throat.

Granthi (hard, small, benign tumors)

These tumors are caused by excesses of any of the *doṣhas*. If they occur in the muscle tissues, they are large swellings. If they occur in the fat (*medas*), they are painless, oily, and movable. If surrounded by bleed vessels, they pulsate.

Therapies: Surgery is recommended. If very young or very old persons have large and rough tumors in the pelvic area, abdomen throat, or in any vital organ, surgery is not advised. Cancer and (large) tumors are treated like hard (small) tumors (see Chapter 22).

Alajī

This is a painful eruption that is copper-colored and emits a discharge from the mouth.

Therapies: Include *āmalakī*, *shatāvarī*, and turmeric.

Edema between the skin and nails (without ulceration)

This form of edema is caused by excess muscle tissue (*māṃsa*) and blood. It is called whitlow or *charmanak-hāntara shotha*.

Therapies: Herbs used include *guggul*, *triphalā*, *viḍaṅga*, ginger, and black pepper.

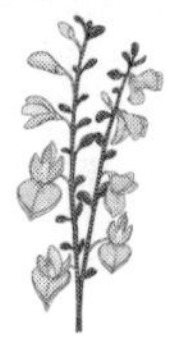

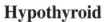

Cysts in the armpit after fever

These are painless, difficult to touch and are expansive (called *vidārikā*). It is caused by vitiated Vāyu and Kapha.
Therapies: Include *daśhmūl, guggul,* and *trikatu.*

Therapies for *Alajī*, *charmanak-hāntara,* and *vidārikā* suggest blood-letting through surgical measures.

Skin abscesses (reddish pus eruptions-*viṣhpa-take*)

These appear all over the body, along with fever and thirst. This is a Kapha/Pitta derangement.
Therapies: Herbs include *punarnavā*, neem, and *mañjiṣhṭhā.*

Gout (Vāta-ṣhonita or Vāta-rakta)

Causes: Eating foods that cause burning during digestion, incompatible foods, excess sleep, not sleeping, improper sexual intercourse, trauma, not undergoing purificatory therapies, and cold breezes, all weaken Vāyu and blood. Aggravated Vāyu, prevented from moving in its normal path, moves in the wrong directions owing to the excessed blood. Vāyu first vitiates the blood, then causes Vāyu excessed blood diseases. This generally occurs in weak-constitution people who do not walk much. It first affects legs from prolonged sitting. Eight types of gout exist: Vāyu, Blood, Pitta, Kapha, Vāyu/Pitta, Vāyu/ Kapha, Pitta/Kapha, and Tridoṣha.

Premonitory Signs: Skin is very smooth, hard to the touch, discolored, burning, itching, debilitated, looseness of the body, throbbing, pricking, intermittent, and splitting joint pain. There is heaviness and loss of sensation. Symptoms may subside and reappear intermittently.

Symptoms: Beginning in the feet (sometimes in the hands), symptoms slowly and steadily spread throughout the body. Gout occurs in the skin and muscles, with symptoms of itching, various pains, and colors, stretching, severe burning, and heat. Later, swelling, hardness, and ulcers may occur. If not tended to, Vāyu quickly moves into the joints, bones, and marrow, causing sharp pain and curvatures of the bones and joints. Eventually, it can make persons lame in one or both legs.
Vāyu: Throbbing and pricking pain, dry swelling, black or blue color, increasing during Vāyu times and decreasing at other times. Constriction of arteries and tendons in the finger or toe joints can occur along with sharp body pain, severe joint pain, aversion to cold, stiffness, tremors, and loss of feeling.
Blood: Swelling with great pain, pricking, coppery color, tingling sensation, itching, and oozing. It does not subside with either oily or dry things such as nuts and granola respectively.
Pitta: Burning, delusion, perspiration, fainting, toxicity, thirst, sensitivity to touch, pain, redness, swelling, ulceration, and severe heat.
Kapha: Inactivity, heaviness, loss of feeling, oily and cold skin, mild itching, and pain.
Dual/Tridoṣha: Symptoms of the related *doṣhas* appear simultaneously.

Healing Outlook: Gout recently caused by one *doṣha* can be healed. When caused by two *doṣhas,* it is containable. Gout caused by *tridoṣha*, that is oozing, immovable or leading to malignant nodules, cannot be healed.

Āvarana Vāyu: When Vāyu quickly spreads into the channels of the blood in the joints of the extremities, it cannot function normally. Vāyu and blood produce different kinds of pain and become life threatening.
Prāṇa Vāyu: Dryness occurs as a result of a lack of fat, over-exercise, fasting, eating, trauma, long-distance walking, forcing the elimination of or suppression of natural urges. It causes many diseases or symptoms including sensory organ disorders, nasal mucus, facial palsy, thirst,

cough, and labored breathing.

Udāna Vāyu: Excesses occur by suppressing sneezing, belching, vomiting, and not sleeping; carrying heavy loads on the head, overindulging in emotions (e.g., crying, laughing). This results in diseases of the neck and head, including throat obstructions, mental disorders, vomiting, loss of taste and appetite, nasal mucus, and enlarged neck glands.

Vyāna Vāyu: *Vyāna* becomes aggravated from excesses of walking, sexual intercourse, worry, or exercise. Other Vāyu aggravations include improper exercise, eating incompatible and dry foods. Emotional causes include fear, joy, and sorrow. This causes loss of virility, enthusiasm, strength, swelling, mental disorders, fever, and paralysis of the entire body. Other developments include intermittent pain, hair standing on end, loss of sensation, skin diseases, herpes, and other systemic diseases.

Samāna Vāyu: It becomes excessed by eating improper or uncooked foods; foods causing indigestion; cold, too much sleep or too little sleep. This causes abdominal pains or tumors, duodenal diseases, and other intestinal or alimentary tract diseases.

(Air with toxins) causes stupor, inactivity, heaviness, oily body, poor digestion, loss of taste or appetite, lassitude, cold, swelling, and a desire for pungent, dry foods.

Apāna Vāyu: This is vitiated by eating dry, heavy foods, suppressing or forcing the elimination of urges, excess travel, sitting, and walking. This causes diseases of the colon, urinary or semen disorders, hemorrhoids, rectal prolapse.

Tissues (*Dhātus*) Obstructing Vāyu:

Blood (Rakta) Obstructions: Symptoms include burning, severe skin and muscle pain, red swelling, and skin patches.

Muscle (Māmsa) Obstructions: Hard swellings, oozing, hair standing on end, feeling as though ants are crawling on the body.

Fat (Medas) Obstructions: Soft, oily, moveable body swellings. Healing is difficult.

Bone (Asthi) Obstructions: The body is overheated, severe pricking pain, weakness. It is relieved by massage.

Marrow/Nerves (Majjā): The body parts bend, excess yawning, wanting to wrap the body with clothes, pain (relieved by massage).

Reproductive (Śhukra) Obstructions: Semen is ejaculated with great force or not at all, or it may not result in fertility.

Food Obstructions: Abdominal pain shortly after eating that disappears after digestion.

Urine Obstructions: Nonelimination with urinary bladder distention.

Feces Obstructions: Constipation causes sharp colon and rectum pains. Ingested oil or *ghee* is quickly digested causing gas and dry feces.

All Seven Tissue Obstructions: When Vāyu is obstructed by all the tissues, there is pain in the pelvis, groin, and back. Vāyu moving in the wrong direction, causes poor health and severe heart pain.

Pitta Obstructing *Prāṇa Vāyu*: Occurs during digestion and causes dizziness, fainting, vomiting, burning, thirst, pain, diarrhea, momentary blindness, burning in the alimentary tract from pungent, hot, sour, and salty foods, and a desire for cold things.

Pitta Obstructing Udāna Vāyu: Internal burning, loss of strength.

Pitta Obstructing Vyāna Vāyu: Burning everywhere, exhaustion, hindered movement with fatigue and pain.

Pitta Obstructing Samāna Vāyu: This causes profuse perspiration, restlessness, thirst, burning.

Pitta Obstructing Vyāna Vāyu: Yellowish feces and urine, excess menstrual bleeding or heat discomfort from increased temperature in the female and male genitalia and the rectum.

Kapha Obstructing Vāyu: Debility, stupor, loss of appetite and taste, vomiting, expectoration of mucus or saliva, excess sneezing and belching, labored breathing, heaviness, cold, pain. It can be comforted by pungent, hot, sour, and salty things; fasting, exercise, dry or hot foods.

Kapha Obstructing Udāna Vāyu: Heaviness, loss

of taste or appetite, difficulty speaking, weakness, and a pallid complexion can develop.
Kapha Obstructing Vyāna Vāyu: Sharp throat, joint and bone pain, heaviness, impaired walking.
Kapha Obstructing Samāna Vāyu: Physical coldness, lack of sweating, poor digestion.
Kapha Obstructing Apāna Vāyu: Kapha in the urine and feces.

The five Vāyus become mutually obstructed or in various combinations.
Prāṇa Obstructing Udāna: Labored breathing, mucus, sharp head pain, heart pain, dry mouth.
Prāṇa Obstructing Udāna: Loss of complexion, enthusiasm, and strength.

The imbalances of *prāṇa*, Vāyu, Pitta, and Kapha may occur alone or together, creating an almost infinite number of diseases. Therefore, one needs to note: 1) onset of the symptoms, 2) location of symptoms, and 3) increases or decreases of bodily functions to determine causality.

Prāṇa Vāyu is the main source of life, although *Udāna* Vāyu is the main source of strength. When one of these symptoms is not clearly detectable or has lasted for over a year, they are difficult to heal. Therapies should begin as soon as possible to avoid secondary complications, such as abscesses, enlarged spleen, heart disease, abdominal tumors, or poor digestion.

Therapies:
General: Blood-letting is useful for burning, piercing pain and redness, numbness, itching, prickly sensation. If the disorder moves around, it is eliminated by venesection or scarifying. Vāyu *doṣhas* should not undergo blood-letting.

First, persons take oil (internally and externally), and a rough or mild purgative. Enemas are used frequently as well. Sprinkling, pastes, *abyañga* (massage-like), poultice, and Pitta-reducing foods are advised.
Vāyu: Sesame oil, *abyañga,* milk enemas with *ghee*, warm poultices, Vāyu-reducing lifestyle and foods, *ghee*, *śhatāvarī*, *balā*, *kapikachhū*, sugar cane, *punarnavā*, *guḍūchī*, *daśhmūl*, and boiled milk are used. Purgatives include *triphalā* and castor oil. *Gokṣhura* and *pippalī* are also useful. (Deep-seated diseases with affected blood are treated as Vāyu excesses.)
Vāyu With Pain: Boiled milk with *daśhmūl* or sprinkling warm *ghee* removes pain. Pastes made of green lentils, rice, boiled milk, *ghee,* and sesame oil are applied to the body. Alternatively, sesame and mustard are applied as a poultice.
Convulsion, Stiffness, Pain: Sprinkled with *ghee* or grape juice and cane sugar.
Pitta and Blood: Purgatives, *ghee*, boiled milk, sprinkling, enema; cooling herbs—*āmalakī, guḍūchī*, *gokṣhura, śhatāvarī*, *pittapapra*. Pitta-reducing foods and lifestyle are recommended. Purgatives include *triphalā* and castor oil.
Burning: Sandalwood and floral essential oils mixed in water and sponged on body parts; wearing a moonstone, pearl, red coral, or a sandalwood necklace.
Burning and Pain: Barley flour and licorice or milk and *ghee*.
Burning With Redness and Pain: blood-letting, followed by an application of paste of *dūrbā*, aloe vera gel, and *mañjiṣhṭhā*.
Bleeding or Pus: Incision, cleansed then healed with the above Pitta/Blood measures.

Kapha: Mild emesis, mild external oil application, sprinkling, and warm pastes, Kapha-reducing diet and habits. Herbs for all these therapies include *guggul*, *śhilājit*, *pippalī*, *gokṣhura*, *guḍūchī*, ginger, *triphalā*, calamus, cardamom, *musta*, *chitrak*, *viḍaṅga*, *vāsāk*, with *ghee* and boiled milk.
Tridoṣha: *Triphalā*, *guḍūchī*, *pippalī*, *śhilājit*, *gokṣhura*, and *punarnavā*.

Kaiṣhore guggul is the best for all types of gout. It helps to purify the blood of cholesterol and uric acid.

Thirst (Triṣhnā)

Causes: There are 6 causes of thirst: Vāyu, Pitta, Kapha, Tridoṣha, a type resulting from loss of plasma, and those resulting from other diseases, such as TB, diabetes, fevers, and wasting. Thirst may develop from dryness at the root of the tongue, throat, palate, channels supplying water, or the pancreas.

Symptoms: General experiences include dry mouth, unquenchable thirst, aversion to food, weak voice, rough throat, lips and tongue, swollen tongue, exhaustion, nonsensical conversation, mental wandering, emaciation, debility, deafness, delusion, giddiness, or heart disease.

Vāyu: Emaciation, helplessness, pain in temples, dizziness, loss of smell, bad taste in the mouth, teary eyes, insomnia, physical weakness, thirst that is increased when drinking cold water.

Pitta: Fainting, bitter taste in the mouth, reddish eyes, constant dryness in the mouth, burning sensation, hot fumes.

Kapha: As aggravated Kapha overflows and obstructs Vāyu in the channels providing water, Kapha dries up. This results in a thorny feeling in the throat, oversleeping, sweet taste in the mouth, gas, dull headache, lethargy, vomiting, loss of taste and appetite, lassitude, and indigestion.

Tridoṣha: Symptoms of all three *doṣhas* occur.

Toxins (āma): Caused by Vāyu/Pitta. Results from fasting or starvation.

Heat Exhaustion/Cold: Thirst occurs when one contracts heat exhaustion from fire or sun, then suddenly plunges into cold water. This prevents heat from leaving the body—forcing it into the abdomen—causing Pitta thirst problems.

Food/Drink: Excess alcohol or wine or eating too much fatty foods by persons with very strong digestive fires, produces Pitta-thirst problems. Excess oily, indigestible, sour, or salty foods causes Kapha thirst.

Plasma: When plasma is reduced, one experiences dryness, fatigue, emaciation, exhaustion without exertion, and a distaste for noise.

Therapies: All types of thirst relate to the predominance of Vāyu and Pitta and plasma loss (dehydration).

Plasma Loss: Cool honey water relieves thirst as does boiled water with rock candy, barley flour, cane sugar, and honey. Soothing foods include barley sweets with honey and cane sugar, *basmati* rice; for all foods, add honey and cane sugar, boiled milk, *ghee*, avoid sour and salty foods and liquids; green lentils, and other types of lentils.

Ghee is massaged on the body. Short baths in cold water are taken, followed by drinking boiled milk with bitter herbs (e.g., *chitrak*, *kaṭukā*, neem, aloe vera) honey, and cane sugar. This milk concoction may also be sprinkled over the body. *Ghee* may also be used as *nasya* (nasal massage). Paste made with *āmalakī* ginger, sandalwood, licorice and *ghee* may be applied to the heart, face, and head to alleviate thirst, fainting, and giddiness. Pastes of these herbs can also be applied to the head.

One may also gargle with milk, sugar cane, honey, and water to heal a dry palate. Drinking yogurt/water, barley with *āmalakī* is recommended. External thirst-relieving therapies include wet cloth wraps, gentle massage, cool baths, and wearing wet clothes. Wearing moonstones or pearls, visiting or visualizing beautiful, cool oceans, rivers or streams, imagining cool breezes, and moon bathing may also relieve thirst..

Vāyu: Soft, light cold, Vāyu-reducing herbs (e.g., *śhatāvarī, aśhwagandhā, and āmalakī*), foods and drinks, with *ghee*.

Vāyu/Pitta: Soft, light, cold, Vāyu- and Pitta-reducing herbs, foods, and drinks, with *ghee*, and rejuvenatives (e.g., *śhatāvarī*).

Pitta: Water with sandalwood, *guḍūchī*, cane sugar and honey, *basmati* rice.

Kapha: *Tṛikatu*, calamus, bitters, such as *chitrak*, *kaṭukā*, neem and aloe vera, astringents, such as raspberry, and *āmalakī* (sours) are ingested. If thirst is related to stiffness, anorexia, indigestion, lassitude, or vomiting, emesis with yogurt, honey, salt, and hot water are used.

Triphalā: Boiled in water and allowed to cool before drinking.

Astringents, such as red raspberry, turmeric,

āmalakī, śhatāvarī, aśhwagandhā, brāhmī, vāsāk, aṣhoka, with *ghee*, cane sugar, honey in boiled milk, or barley may be taken.

Alcoholism Thirst: Cold baths, then alcohol with 1/2 water, *āmalakī*, rock salt, aromatics, wine with 1/2 water, cane sugar and water with gotu kola.

Anorexia Thirst: Thin gruel, *ghee*, boiled milk.

Excess Intake of Fat: Thin gruel, *guggul, ghee*, boiled milk, cane sugar.

Thirst resulting from eating heavy foods: Emesis, *ghee*, milk

Fainting complications: *Mañjiṣhṭhā*, gotu kola, *chitrak, kaṭukā*.

Thirst after severe disease: Plain water is dangerous. Coriander water with cane sugar and raw honey is useful.

Although improper use of foods can lead to disease or even death, drinking alcohol additionally leads to loss of self-worth, life path, wealth, true pleasure, intelligence, and courage.

Aṣhṭāñga Hṛidayam; Nidānasthāna Ch. 6; ver. 11

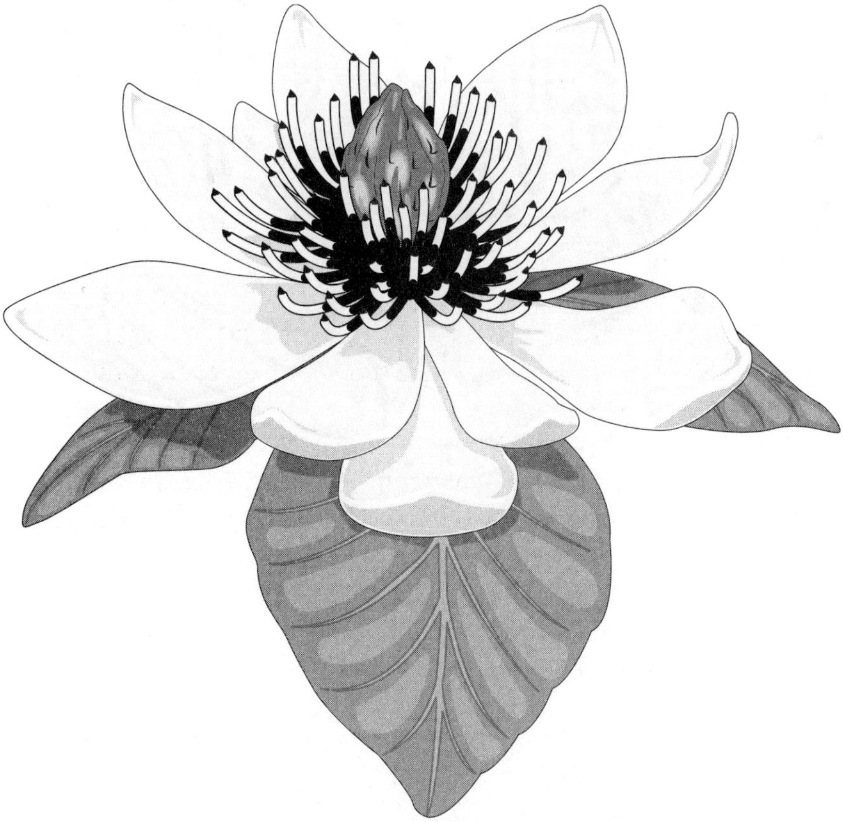

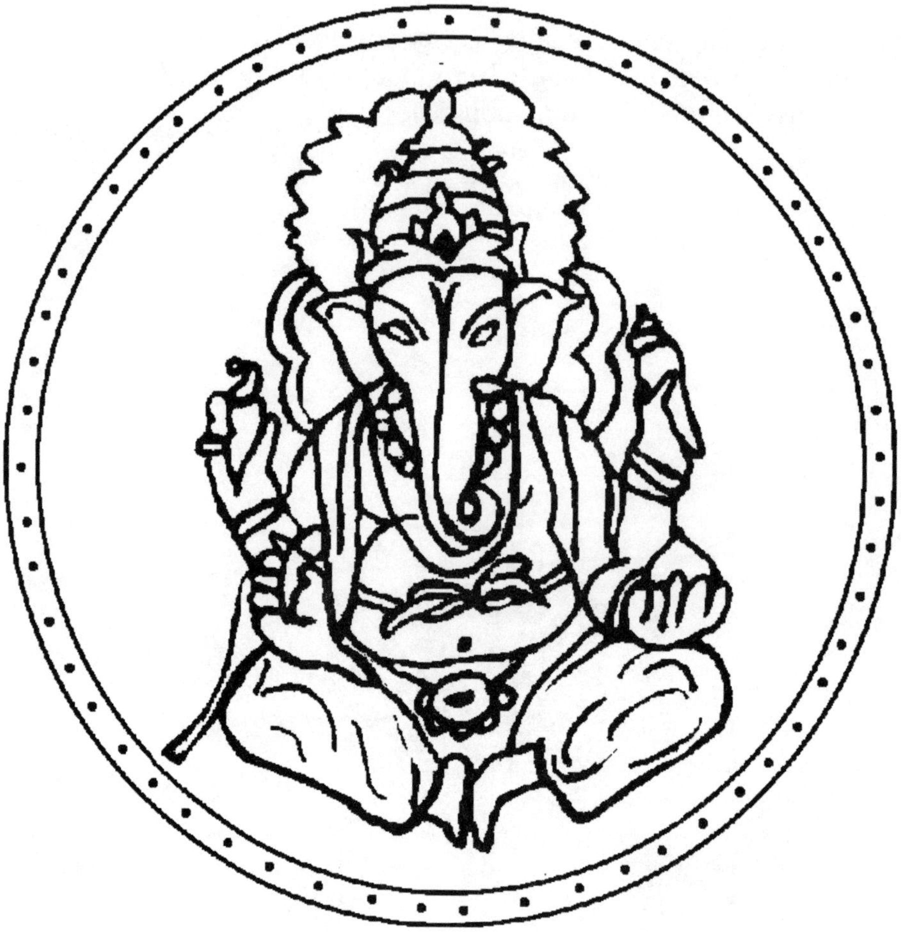

Education is not a matter of always seeing new things;
education means seeing the same things in a new light
Unknown

Chapter 26
Miscellaneous
3 Vital Organs, Dangerous Spiritual Practices, Herbs for Tissues and Organs, Definitions of Glands, Organs and Doṣhas, When to Take Herbs, Herbal Recipes, Acupuncture

3 Vital Organs (Mahā Marmas)

Definition: There are 107 vital body parts. Of these, three organs are paramount: the urinary bladder, heart, and head. They are considered the main sites because they are the seats of the vital breath (*prāṇa*) and Vāyu that can cause immediate death if wounded.

Cause & Development: Downward moving air (*Apāna Vāyu*) in the colon becomes excessed from eating and drinking pungent, bitter, astringent, and rough foods, suppressing natural urges, fasting, and sexual intercourse. These actions bring about obstructions and retention of stool, gas, and urine, and ultimately cause air to move in the reverse direction.

This results in frequent and intense pain in the pelvic and heart area, abdomen, ribs, and back. Obstructions cause abdominal distention, nausea, cutting and piercing pain, indigestion, cystitis, stool retention, enlarged organ membranes, and upward-moving Vāyu (*Udāna Vāyu*). The stool is dry and difficult to pass. The body is rough, coarse, and cold with fever, difficult urination, dysentery, heart, and digestive disorders. Persons may experience vomiting, blindness, deafness, headache, mental disorders, thirst, internal bleeding, anorexia, and tumors. Other experiences include cough, labored breathing, facial paralysis, chest pain, cold, Vāyu mental disorders, *vāta śhthīlā* (prostate disorders), and many other serious disorders.

Therapies: Oil *abhyañga* (massage-like) with sesame, *mahānārāyan* and *pañchaguṇa* oils. Fomentation (moist heat) should be applied to the troubled area. Once the illness is balanced, oil and dry enemas, suppositories, purgatives, carminatives, and other Vāyu-reducing herbs are used. Suppositories are made with oil, *tṛikatu*, *viḍaṅga*, *pippalī,* and cane sugar. Foods include barley, Vāyu-reducing (steamed) vegetables, fresh ginger, sesame oil, and *ghee*. Should the condition resolve, but gas and stool retention continue to exist, an oil enema is used. For hard bowels, colic, heart disease, tumor, indigestion, weak spleen, and upward-moving air; *vachā*, *harītakī*, *pippalī*, *chitrak*, and *viḍaṅga* are used.

Hard bowels are caused by *āma*, arising from stiffness, heaviness in the head and abdomen, retaining belches, and mucus. It is healed through emesis, reduction therapies, and digestive herbs.

Vital organ diseases include dysuria, diseases of the heart and head (including mouth, hair, eyes, ears, nose, and throat), and anorexia. These are discussed in detail in their respective chapters.

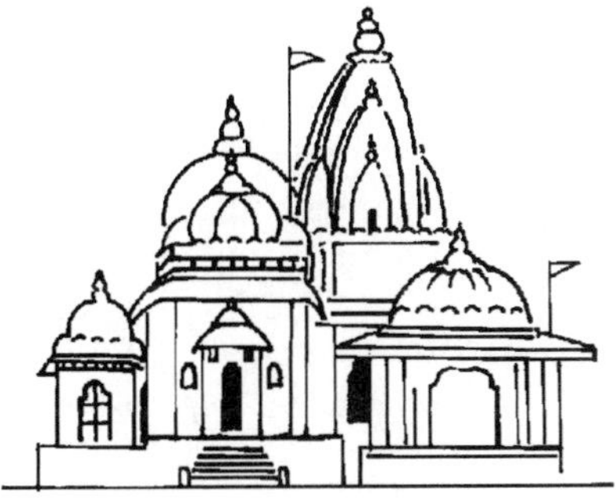

Organ	Governs
Heart	*prāṇa, apāna*, mind, intellect, consciousness, *mahābhūtas*
Head	senses
Bladder (*Basti*)	scrotum, raphe, vas deferens, middle of the rectum, and uterus: governs urine, and is the stabilizer of all fluid channels.

When each of these three sites is afflicted, various diseases occur.

Organ	Diseases
Heart	cough, labored breathing, debility, dry mouth and throat; contraction of the stomach, protracted tongue, epilepsy, insanity, delirium, vacant-mindedness
Head	stiff neck, facial paralysis, rolling eyeballs, confusion, cramps, loss of coordination and movement; labored breathing, lockjaw, loss of voice, muteness, stuttering, ptosis, quivering cheeks, yawning, salivation, crooked face
Basti	retention of gas, urine and stool; pain in groin, penis, and urinary bladder; stiffness, spasm in the navel, lower abdomen, anus, hip; *udvarta*, phantom tumors. These three vital spots are to be especially protected from Vāyu disorders as Vāyu is the cause of the other *doṣhas*, and the root cause of the vital breath. The best therapy for this is *basti*.

No other therapy equals (unctuous) enema for protecting the vital parts
Charak; Si., Ch. 9 v7

Vāyu-Reducing Therapies

Organ	Therapeutics
Heart	*asafoetida*, rock salt, sour liquid, sugar
Head	*abhyañga*, sweating, poultices, ingesting unctuous items, snuff, juice pressing (in nostrils), smoke (*dhūma*)
Basti	moist heat, suppositories, nonunctuous enema, urethra douche, *bilwa, dūrbā, gokṣhura,* barley, turmeric, *ghee, śhatāvarī, guḍūchī, lodhra, balā, vāsāk, vachā, pāṣhāṇa bheda*

Heart Disorder (Hṛidaya)

Therapies: *Arjuna*, ginger, pomegranate, rhubarb, *harītakī, asafoetida*, black salt, barley, Vāyu- and Kapha-reducing foods and lifestyles.

Urinary Bladder (Basti)

Vāyu: Becomes excessed from suppressing urine. This causes retention, distress, and itching. This is called *vātabasti*. Retention results in excess *Udāna* Vāyu in the urethra. A feeling of pierced, torn, and stiffening of the urethra occurs during urination. Other symptoms include breaking pain, heaviness, cramps, extreme pain, and retention of urine and feces.

In persons who are debilitated and have roughness, Vāyu may cause the stool to be reversed in its passage and enter the urinary canal. Thus, urine is passed with feces accompanied with malodor and straining. This is called *vidvighāta*.

Vāyu with Pitta: Drying up the urine causes the passing of red or yellow urine, with difficulty, and burning in the pelvis and perineum.

Vāyu with Kapha: This affects the blood and produces a hard nodular mass in the opening of the urinary bladder, resulting in difficult urination. This condition is called *mūtragranthi*.

Pitta: When Pitta afflicts the bladder, symptoms include burning sensation, pain, and abnormal

color.
Kapha: When Kapha afflicts the bladder, symptoms include heaviness, swelling, unctuous, and white and rushing urine.
Pitta and Kapha: When both these *doṣhas* obstruct the urethra, the condition cannot be healed.
External: Fast traveling, jumping, exertion, injury, and pressure may cause the bladder to bulge and remain extended, making one look pregnant. The bladder is painful, quivering, and burns. Urine passes in drops; however, if the bladder is pressed, urine passes in a stream. The bladder feels stiff with cramping. This severe condition is called *bastikundala*.

Depending on the *doṣha* causing these disorders, diuretics, enemas, and urethral douches (see Chapter 7 on *pañcha karma/basti* section) can be used.

Head Disorders (Śhiro-roga-Vijnāñiya)

There are 11 head diseases: Vāyu, Pitta, Kapha, Tridoṣha, blood, wastes, parasites, *suryāvarta*, *anantavāta*, *ardhāvabhedaka*, *śhamkhaka*.

Symptoms:
Vāyu: Violent headaches occur without cause. Symptoms worsen at night and are relieved by pressure or head fomentation (moist heat).
Pitta: Violent burning and aching head pain; a feeling of hot coals on the scalp; burning vapor from nostrils (diminishes at night or when applying cold packs to the head).
Kapha: Headaches; a sticky mucus-coated palate and throat that feel cold and heavy; swollen face and eyes.
Tridoṣha: Symptoms of all three *doṣhas*.
Blood: The same symptoms as Pitta; and head pain is unbearable even when touched lightly.
Wastes (Kṣhayaja): Waste in the fatty substances in the body tissues (e.g., *māṃsa, medas, majjā*), brain areas, and semen causes unbearable head pain. This condition is aggravated by fomentation, fumigation, nasal therapies, emetics, and blood-letting.
Parasites (Krimija): Pricking, tingling head pain; with liquid secretions mixed with blood and pus from the nose occur from parasites in the nose.
Suryāvarta: Tridoṣhic excesses, suppression of urine with indigestion, vitiation of blood, and brain involvement from Vāyu can cause severe eye and eyebrow pain at sunrise. This condition worsens as the day progresses, and subsides in the evening. It may be reduced from cold things (and sometimes warm things). The morning sun liquefies the excesses in the brain causing headache. Resolidification occurs after sunset.
Ananta-Vāyu (trigeminal neuralgia): Severe pain in the two nerves at the back of the neck and in the carotid arteries. This then spreads to the eyes, eyebrows, and temples, causing throbbing in the cheeks, and paralysis of the jaw bone and eye. It is associated with excesses of all three *doṣhas*. This condition develops from excess fasting (or insufficient food), grief, or cold. All three *doṣhas* become excessed. Symptoms also include twitching near the cheeks, lock jaw, and eye disorders.
Ardhāvabhedaka: Excruciating piercing, or aching pain in one half of the skull; causing giddiness when Vāyu becomes excessed from ingesting rough food, overeating, eating with indigestion, or from exposure to easterly winds and dew. Excessive coitus, suppressing natural urges, overexertion and exercise, or Kapha excesses also upset half of the head. It may recur at intervals of 10 to 14 days or at random. Some authorities say it is caused by all three *doṣhas*. Symptoms include severe, cutting, head pain; churning in one carotid artery, eyebrow, temple, ear, eye, and forehead; trembling. Severe cases may result in loss of sight and hearing.
Śhankaka: Severe head and temple pain due to local Vāyu combined with Pitta, Kapha, and blood. Pain may spread to the temples, causing severe swelling, great pain, burning, and redness. This can be fatal. Healing it is difficult. After three days, therapies may be given, including head evacuation, sprinkling, and other anti-ery-

sipelas therapies.

Apatantraka: *Udāna* Vāyu, moving upwards in excess, reaches the heart, head, and temples. This causes convulsions and confusion, labored breathing, stiff/closed eyes, unconsciousness, and groaning.

Therapies:

Vāyu: Head diseases caused only by Vāyu *doṣha* are relieved by the same measures for the nervous system (*Vāyu-Vyādhi*—Chapter 20). Sesame oil, *ghee*, boiled milk (taken tepid), and pungent and hot herbs are taken before bed. Milk cooked with *śhatāvarī, aśhwagandhā,* and *balā* is used to wash the diseased area. A lukewarm plaster of the same is applied to the scalp. Afterwards, oil, *ghee,* and Vāyu-reducing herbs are cooked together and used as a nasal oil.

Vāyu-reducing foods and lifestyle, aromatherapy (sandalwood oil on the forehead), hot-oil head *abhyañgas* (*śhiro dhārā/śhiro basti*), and gotu kola oil (3 drops in the nose followed by gentle massage) are useful therapies. Poultices made from the herbs and foods listed below may be wrapped around the head.

Herbs: *Vaṃśhā lochana, guggul, harītakī,* gotu kola, *gokṣhura, aśhwagandhā, bibhītakī, bhṛiṅgarāj, balā, daśhmūl, tṛikatu, brāhmī ghee.*

Foods: Almonds (soaked and peeled), sesame tahini, *ghee*, sesame oil, boiled milk, *basmati* rice, whole wheat, barley. Yogurt/water (*lassi*) is also useful for soothing nerves. If excess impurities develop, and the disorder is not healed from the preceding therapies, one takes mild oil purgatives (e.g., castor oil) to help the evacuation process. Warm carminative herbs such as cardamom, ginger, cinnamon, cloves, and turmeric help dispel gas, improve digestion, and assist absorption of undigested foods that cause impurities. Weak persons should use non-oil enemas and digestive herbs and foods instead of purgatives.

Pitta and Blood: Plasters of cool herbs (*vetasa*, sandalwood, licorice, *musta*) and *ghee* are pasted on the scalp and used as cooling head washes. Pitta and blood *visarpa* (erysipelas) therapies are also used: *chirāyatā, kaṭukā,* neem, aloe vera, gentian, *mañjiṣhṭhā*, barberry; first purgation then blood-letting is used. *Aśhwagandhā, vidārī kand, śhatāvarī,* licorice, and *maṣhparni* are used. Oil or *ghee* is used as nasal therapy *nasya*. Dry and oily enemas (*basti*) are also employed. *Basti* herbs include *madanphal, prīyañgu,* licorice, *bilwa,* and *dantī (baliospermum a.)* root.

Kapha: Emetics, head purgatives, inhaling aromas, and gargles are useful. The clear upper part of *ghee* is ingested and frequently used as fomentation to the head. Herbs include frankincense, myrrh, cedar, calamus, and *kuśhtā*. Meals include barley or *basmati* rice taken with hot spices like *tṛikatu* (mixture).

Tridoṣha: Therapies related to the imbalances of the three *doṣhas* are used.

Wastes (Kṣhayaja): *Bṛiṃhaṇa* enema (nourishing—honey, sesame oil, dry ginger, rock salt in hot water). *Ghee* is mixed with *śhatāvarī, aśhwagandhā,* and licorice. Vāyu-reducing herbs are used as nasal therapy and as drinks (*brāhmī ghee*).

Parasites (Krimija): Inhaling powder and smoke of *viḍaṅga* and *musta*.

Suryāvarta: Nasal oils, plaster, gargles, eating boiled rice, drinking milk with *ghee*, *vaṃśhā lochana, vachā*, licorice, sandalwood, honey; ingesting *ghee* after meals. Then, snuffs of *ghee* and *śhatāvarī, aśhwagandhā,* and licorice are used.

Other therapies include plasters of licorice, *kuśhtā,* sarsaparilla, *ghee,* and sesame oil; purgation, milk, and sprinkling with *ghee* .

Ananta-vāyu: The same therapies as *suryāvarta* are used. Blood-letting, Vāyu- and Pitta-reducing foods; and sweets made with wheat, cane sugar, milk, and *ghee* are also suggested. Other therapies include ingesting *ghee* after meals, head evacuation, purgation, milk and *ghee* sprinkling, ingesting vitalizing herbs mixed with 8 times as much milk as snuff.

Samkhaka: *Ghee* taken internally and as a snuff. Boiled rice with *ghee* is recommended. Plasters may be made of *śhatāvarī*, black sesame seeds, licorice, *dūrvā*, *punarnavā*. Cooling washes and herb powder nasal therapies are also soothing.

Apatantraka (a form of epilepsy): Cleanse channels obstructed by Vāyu and Kapha by blowing irritating powders such as black powder, *viḍaṅga, harītakī, asafoetida*, black salt, and barley powder into the nasal passages. *Brāhmī* has been found to control epilepsy.

Note: Heart, bladder, and head disorders deal with physiological diseases. *Mahā marma* is important for surgery and for wartime injuries. The surgeon must be aware of the *mahā marmas* when surgery is conducted on the head. Knowledge of *mahā marma* is contained within the martial arts. Soldiers are trained to aim at these three vital points (heart, bladder, head) to kill an enemy.

Headache/Migraine

Causes: Many situations can cause headaches: indigestion, constipation, colds, flus, poor posture, suppression of urges to urinate or pass stool, muscle tension, mental conditions such as nervousness, worry, anxiety, anger, and high blood pressure. Migraines can be caused by heartburn, congenital factors and other conditions. The climate can further aggravate migraines.

Symptoms:

Vāyu: Anxiety, depression, dry skin, constipation, and extreme pain.

Pitta: Red complexion and eyes, light sensitivity, burning sensation, anger, irritability, and nose bleeds. Liver and blood toxicity are often associated with these symptoms.

Kapha: Dull headache, heaviness, fatigue, nausea, white or clear phlegm, vomiting, and excess salivation. Respiratory disorders are often associated with these symptoms.

Therapies:

Vāyu: *Triphalā* as a purgative, *jaṭāmāṇśhī, brāhmī,* and rest. *Śhiro dhārā* (hot oil head massage) is very beneficial.

Pitta: Purgatives (e.g., aloe vera gel, rhubarb, and fennel), liver cleansers (e.g., *bhūāmalakī* and *brāhmī*), sandalwood oil on the third eye, temples, heart, and under the nose, walks in the full moon and by water; and flower gardening reduce Pitta causes of migraines. Overexertion, heat and sun should be avoided. *Śhiro dhārā* (hot oil head massage) is also highly beneficial.

Kapha: *Tṛikatu, brāhmī, tulsī* tea, inhaling eucalyptus oil, vomiting, exercise, nasal snuff of ginger or pepper. *Śhiro dhārā* (hot oil head massage) is also very helpful.

Cough, Cold, Flu, Allergy-Caused: Decongestant/expectorant herbs—Vāyu and Kapha excesses (ginger, black pepper, licorice, *viḍaṅga,* etc.) are ingested or used as nasal snuff. *Tulsī* tea and inhaling eucalyptus oil are also very helpful. Ginger paste can be applied under the nose,and on the temples and forehead. Vomiting (if the person is strong) will help rid the head of congestion and pain arising from it.

Migraines (Ardhāvabhedaka): The same therapies as *suryāvarta* (above). Medicated oils or *ghee*, using *guḍūchī, balā,* and *aśhwagandhā*; fomentation, and saturating snuff are also advised. Long-term healing includes *chyavan prāśh, brāhmī,* and *aśhwagandhā*. *Śhiro dhārā* (hot oil head massage) is also beneficial. This is usually a Vāyu and Pitta excess, caused by lack of sleep, overwork, stress, worry, poor digestion, muscular tension, heartburn, or high blood pressure.

Arthritis/Rheumatism (Āmavāta)

Modern medicine recognizes more than 100 types of rheumatic diseases. Causes are attributed to injury, infection, metabolic conditions, or tumors. In many cases the causes remain unknown to western medicine. Some disorders are related to age, gender, and climactic conditions (i.e., cold or dampness). Āyurveda also cites causes related to digestive disorders. See Chapter 15.

Causes and Development:

Eating incompatible food combinations and following incompatible lifestyles, lack of exercise or exercising after eating fatty foods—or with poor digestion, produces *āma* (undigested food toxins). *Āma* associated with Vāyu quickly moves to different seats of Kapha in the body, filling them (and blood vessels) with waxy material. Thus, *āma* associated with all three *doṣhas* blocks tissue pores and passages. This causes weakness and heaviness in the heart, which becomes the seat of the disease. Joints are simultaneously affected, causing stiffness and many other disorders. It can also be considered an autoimmune disorder.

Symptoms:

Joint pain, loss of taste, thirst, lack of enthusiasm, heaviness, fever, indigestion, swelling (inflammation).

Vāyu: Severe, throbbing, cutting pain that is variable and migrating in nature; becomes worse in cold weather or when cold water comes in contact with the affected joint(s). Other symptoms include dry or scaly skin, stiff or cracking joints, bone deformities, constipation, gas, abdominal distention, low back pain, nervousness, fear, and insomnia.

Pitta: Burning sensation, redness, swelling, inflammation; becomes worse in hot weather or when hot water comes in contact with the affected joints. Other symptoms include diarrhea, anger, irritability, and sweating.

Kapha: Loss of movement, itching, joint swelling, and edema (without inflammation); becomes worse in cold and damp or humid weather. Other symptoms include dullness, heaviness, aches, oily skin, congestion, or mucus in the stool.

Therapies:

General: If only one *doṣha* is involved, the condition is easy to heal. When two *doṣhas* are implicated, it becomes difficult to heal. When all three *doṣhas* are involved, and if swelling involves every joint in the body, healed will not be possible.

First toxins should be digested by balancing the digestive fire. Eating animal products will aggravate the condition, especially pork, red meat, and dark poultry. Heavy, *āma*-increasing foods will also increase arthritic symptoms. Many people report improvements by following these dietary suggestions.

Mahānārāyan oil improves flexibility, stiffness, muscle fatigue, and removes pain. It is mixed with sesame oil (1:1) and applied to the painful areas. This oil also breaks up blockages and begins to heal locally. After oil application, warm heat, *yoga*, bath, or mild exercise further improves this situation. *Nāḍī sweda* (local steam application; see Chapter 4) with *daśhmūl* can be applied locally.

Nārāyan oil is good for muscle and joint pain, lower body circulation, and reversing imbalances caused by aging. *Brāhmī* and sandalwood oils (mixed together) are very beneficial for Pitta types of arthritis. *Avipattikar chūrṇa* is good to ingest for rheumatism.

Vāyu: Hot spices like cinnamon and fresh ginger. *Yogaraj guggul* is the best herb for this condition; it cleanses bone tissue, strengthens bones, and improves flexibility. Castor oil or *triphalā* help keep the colon cleansed.

Pitta: *Kaiṣhore guggul,* sandalwood, *guḍūchī,* aloe, turmeric, saffron. *Musta* and *nirguṇḍī* relieve pain.

Kapha: Pure *guggul* is best for this condition. Hot herbs are also helpful, such as cinnamon, dry ginger, turmeric, *tṛikatu*. *Musta* and *nirguṇḍī* relieve pain.

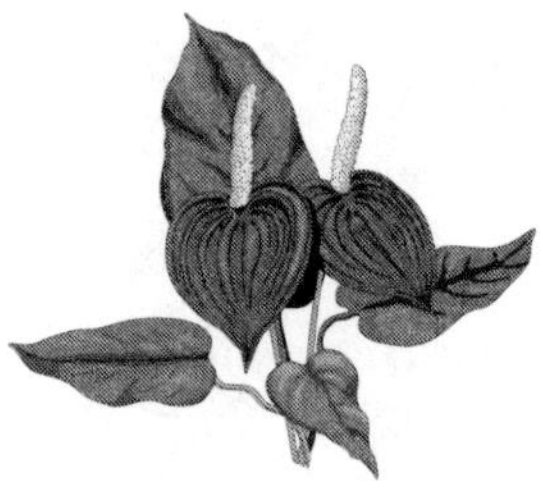

Dangerous Spiritual Practices

Channeling, especially for Vāyu persons (or Vāyu-minded persons), may render them too ungrounded. Allowing another entity to enter your being can be very dangerous.

Kuṇḍalinī (spiritual energy)—*yoga* and other techniques artificially open *chakras* (spiritual energy centers) before a person may be prepared. This can lead to numerous and serious physical and mental disorders. [This does not apply to persons naturally raising their *kuṇḍalinī* through meditation and *yoga*, but to those who target specific *chakras* for their manual opening.] Practicing a natural form of meditation that allows for the gradual and holistic opening balances the entire person.

Hypnosis is a psychically induced state in which a subject responds to suggestions from the hypnotist (within certain limitations). If the subject is not naturally ready to respond, even though they may want to, hypnosis may cause subtle anxiety and weakening of the mind-body coordination. Some modern hypnotherapists however, utilize a method whereby the client is in complete control of their choices. This may be a more natural approach to this practice.

Prāṇāyāma (breathing practices) can also be harmful if done with force, breath retention, or in excess without a proper teacher for guidance.

Tissue (Dhātu) Building Herbs

Plasma (*rasa*): *Śhilājit, punarnavā, vidārī kand, kṣhīr kākolī*

Blood (*rakta*): Green leafy vegetables, radish, *punarnavā*

Muscle (*māṃsa*): *Aśhwagandhā, śhatāvarī, mahā medha, ghee.*

Fat (*medas*): The same

Marrow (*majjā*): The same

Bone (*asthi*): *Pravāl piṣhti, vaṃśhā lochana, śhatāvarī*, sesame, black *dal*, milk.

Semen (*śhukra*): *Śhatāvarī, aśhwagandhā.*

Organs and Herbs

Kidney problems: Pitta/(Vāyu secondary). Best herb—*śhilājit.*

Pancreas: Kapha/Pitta: Glyceric acid (Pitta), insulin (sweet/Kapha). Best herb—*gurmar.*

Ojas: This means life sap, metabolism, and will power. It is not actually something that is found in the body. *Śhatāvarī, aśhwagandhā, guḍūchī,* saffron.

Brain: Vāyu/Kapha secretions, cerebral spinal fluid. *Brāhmī, jaṭāmāṇśhī, aśhwagandhā, śhaṅkh puṣhpī, tulsī, bhṛiṅgarāj.*

Nerves: Vāyu/Pitta- *prāṇavaha, raktavaha* and *majjā srotas.* Reduce Pitta to purify the nerves. Reduce Vāyu to tone the nerves. *Brāhmī, jaṭāmāṇśhī, aśhwagandhā, śhaṅkh puṣhpī, tulsī, bhṛiṅgarāj.*

Gall Bladder: *Paṣhana bedha,* dandelion

Liver: *Punarnavā, bhūāmalakī*

Blood purification: *Mañjiṣhṭhā*

Lymph: *Kaiṣhore guggul*, yellow dock, jasmine for Pitta and Kapha; bayberry for Vāyu.

Adrenals: Kapha/Pitta—*brāhmī.* Secretes adrenaline. Develops the mind and affects spiritual development.

Spleen: Pitta—*Punarnavā, kaṭukā*

Tendons, ligaments: Kapha—turmeric

Veins: Pitta - *mañjiṣhṭhā* (cleanse/circulate)

Marrow: Fluid—Kapha; Vāyu—space and pushing effect; color—Pitta (due to gall bladder). Herbs according to *doṣha. Āśhwagandhā, balā, bhṛiṅgarāj, gokṣhura, musta, pippalī, vaṃśh lochana*

Lungs: Vāyu brings Pitta (from peritoneum secretion of the heart) [carbonic acid] to the respiratory system, hemoglobin, red blood cells, and supplies oxygen in the body parts (Vāyu). Kapha relates to fluids. *Vāsāk, balā, harītakī, bibhītakī, pippalī.*

Gland Definitions

Exocrine: Channels that open into the organs, gastrointestinal tract, bloodstream, etc. (e.g., salivary glands, intestinal or digestive glands, mammary glands).

Endocrine: Secrete directly into the bloodstream or the surrounding tissues. They do not have any channel, such as the exocrine glands. Examples are hormones.

Thyroid: Responsible for the growth, calcium, and metabolism in the body. Thyroxin discharge (Kapha) digests the seven tissues (*dhātus*) and develops the mind and body.

Hyperthyroid: Disturbs the mind and body, increases the reflex action, causes fine tremors and palpitations, exophthalmic goiter, and neurosis.

Hypothyroid: Causes slowed thyroid functioning. Symptoms include anemia and Vāyu obesity; low heart rate, infertility, neuritis, goiter, exophthalmia (protrusion of the eyeball), photophobia (fear of light), and sweating.

Parathyroid: Regulates the calcium metabolism level in the body.

Pineal: (Kapha) Controls the brain.

Thalamus: Responsible for the early childhood growth until approximately age 15.

Hypothalamus: (Vāyu) Located in the brain, controlling the pituitary gland and other hormones.

Pituitary: (Pitta/Kapha) Controls all other hormone functions and levels in the body. It sits on top of the *sușhumnā* (the spiritual tube inside the spine), anterior, and posterior lobes. It is in the spinal column

Suprarenal: This secretes the hormone that controls the fight or flight response. Thus, muscular activity and glucose in the blood are increased.

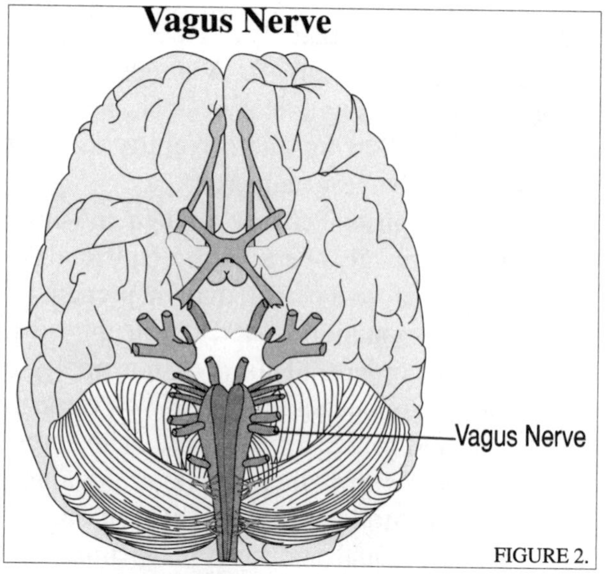

FIGURE 2.

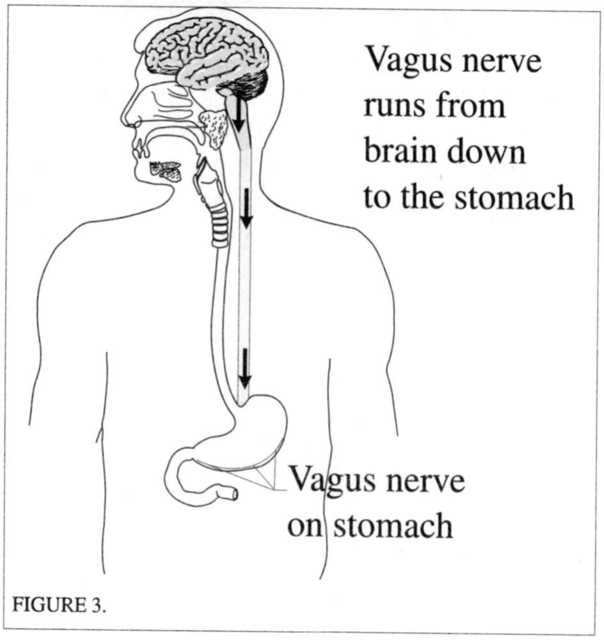

FIGURE 3.

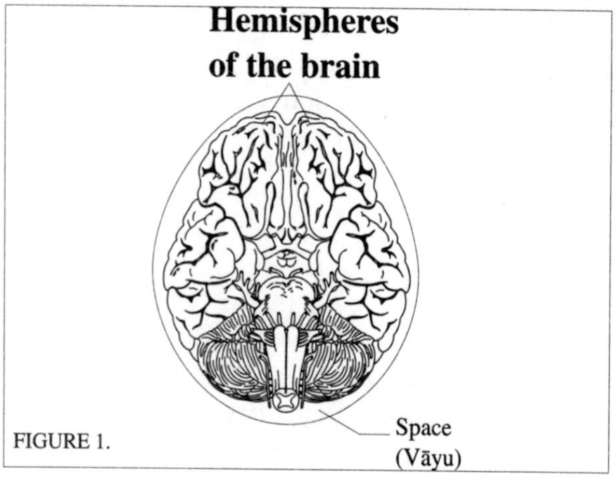

FIGURE 1.

The vagus nerve is controlled by the thalamus. It runs from the brain to the stomach. Vagus is the 10th cranial nerve supplying the heart, stomach, diaphragm, sensory-motor skills, voice, breathing, pharynx, and esophagus. These areas are affected by all three *doșhas*. When there is any reflex or response from any of these organs, it signals the brain. The response from the brain is transmitted back to all the organs (not just the one signaling trouble). In this way, if one organ is ill, it affects the functioning of all the other related organs.

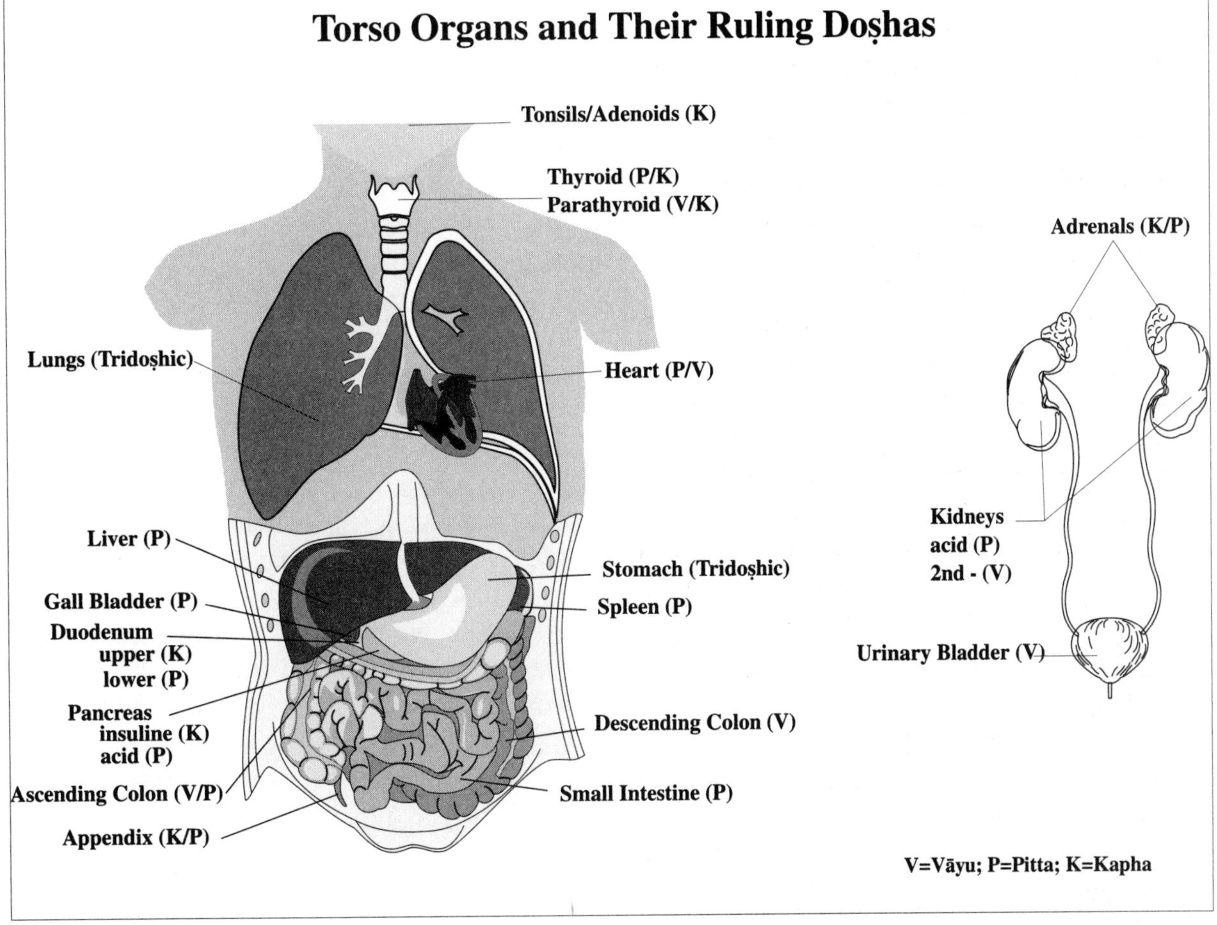

FIGURE 4: THE TORSO ORGANS AND THEIR RULING DOṢHAS

Peritoneal Layer: This is a membranous sheath covering all the visceral organs, and protecting them against friction, separating them, etc.

Sub-Doṣhas Organs: All five Pitta sub-*doṣhas* disturb one's spiritual life. *Sadhaka* Pitta and *Avalmbaka* Kapha create the most energy disturbances on one's spiritual path.

The combination of the two is called *Sam Awostha* (balance period). *Bodhak Kapha* relates to the taylin (mucus gland).

Times And Methods To Take Herbs

Stomach disorders are healed by ingesting herbs

Head disorders are removed through the nose.

Colon diseases are healed through enemas.

Strong persons take herbs in the morning on an empty stomach.

Weak persons mix herbs with a light meal or snack.

Stool, urine, gas, semen, menstrual, and pregnancy herbs (*apāna*) Herbs are taken before meals (i.e., disorders related to the lower body).

Pervasive ills (*samān*) Herbs are taken during lunch.

Vyān disorders Herbs are taken after breakfast and lunch.

Udān diseases Herbs are taken after dinner.

Prāṇa ills Herbs are taken between bites of food.

Cough, thirst and difficult breathing Herbs are used frequently.

Hiccup: Herbs are taken with delicious foods.

Some practitioners say for Vāyu conditions, herbs are taken before meals to quickly reach these lower areas; Pitta conditions require herbs with meals to affect the middle portion of the body (Pitta organs); herbs are used immediately following meals for Kapha conditions to help with upper torso conditions.

Herbal Recipes

Arteriosclerosis: *Yogaraj guggul*, turmeric, aloe, safflower, myrrh.
Athletes foot: Pitta (infections), Kapha (white). Turmeric and *guḍūchī* for infections; Tea-tree oil for Kapha (internally and externally).
Broken bones: *Mañjiṣhṭhā, arjuna,* comfrey, Solomon's seal, horsetail (internally and externally); *yogarāj* or pure *guggul*).
Cholesterol: Purified *guggul.*
Circulation (poor): Saffron, turmeric, cinnamon, black pepper, *ajwan,* cloves; *tṛikatu* for Vāyu or Kapha (*yogarāj guggul* for Vāyu; pure *guggul* for Kapha); *Kaiṣhore guggul*, turmeric, *mañjiṣhṭhā,* saffron, coriander for Pitta. Other herbs that help circulation include *brāhmī*, *āmalakī*, and *balā*.
Colic: Fennel, chamomile.
Dandruff: *Multani mitti* or curd and sesame oil
Depression: Saffron, jasmine, patchouli, and ylang ylang aromas.
Ear disorders: *Nirguṇḍī*, *ghee* ear baths.
Eczema: *Brāhmī, bhṛiṅgarāj.*
Encephalitis (brain inflammation): *Jaṭāmāṇśhī, brāhmī,* sandalwood; 2 to 6 drops of *śhadbindu* oil.
Eye disorders: *Nirguṇḍī, triphalā, guḍūchī, śhweta punarnavā.*
Food allergies: Foods that increase one's *doṣha* often cause allergic reactions. Allergies are also related to a weak immune system. Therefore, eating foods and taking immune boosting herbs according to one's *doṣha* is advised.
Gangrene: Echinacea.
Gums (bleeding): Massage gums with coconut oil or drink juice of 1/2 lemon in a cup of water.
Hang nail: A Vāyu excess (Vāyu-reducing herbs)
Hemorrhoids: 1/2 cup aloe vera juice 3 times daily. *Triphalā* is also useful.
Hodgkin's: Jasmine.
Immune: *Brāhmī, guḍūchī.*
Incontinence: Skullcap (V+), nutmeg (P+).
Liver: *Bhūāmalkī*, aloe vera gel, *kaṭukā, guḍūchī, brāhmī, bhṛiṅgarāj, chirāyatā.*
Mastitis: Marshmallow, *balā.*
Meningitis (brain edema): *Jaṭāmāṇśhī, yogaraj guggul, brāhmī*, musk, *vadam* (almonds) .
Menstrual Cramps: 1 tablespoon aloe vera gel with 1/4 teaspoon black pepper 3 times daily.
Mononucleosis: *Chyavan prāśh* and *jaṭāmāṇśhī.*
Mouth disorders: *Triphalā.*
Nail deposits (under nail): Vāyu and Kapha (local mucus). Vāyu/Kapha-reducing herbs.
Pain, aches, arthritis, back pain, strains, etc.: Ginger and water paste compress; or *mahānārāyan* oil equally mixed with sesame oil; saffron, turmeric.
P/K *Āma*: Six cloves of garlic well chopped, boiled in a cup of milk until it is reduced by half. Add cane sugar. Taken once daily for 1st week; every other day for the following week. After that, once or twice a week until *āma* is cleared.
Pleurisy: Licorice and honey to prevent Kapha excess.
Psoriasis: *Brāhmī, mañjiṣhṭhā,* barberry.
Shock: Sinus congestion—inhale one pinch of *vachā* powder.
Sore throat: Gargle with hot water mixed with turmeric, *guggul, pippalī*, ginger, *triphalā,* and black pepper.
Sprue (*grahinī*): [*āma* causes constipation or diarrhea]. Herbs include *kuṭaj, bilwa*, ginger.
Stings & Bites: Drink cilantro juice and apply sandalwood paste externally.
Swollen knees/ankles: 2 lb-salt bag heated in a pan and kept on the swelling for 5 minutes a day.
Swollen legs: Castor oil and half cooked rice mixed into a paste and massaged on the swelling.
TB: *Vāsāk, vaṃśha lochana.*
Toothache: Apply 3 drops of clove oil to tooth.
Varicose Veins: (Vāyu) Shoulder stands (10 minutes daily).

Mutually Contradictory Foods

Milk and Fish (hot and cold, respectively) vitiate the blood and obstruct circulatory channels.

Meat with honey, sesame seeds, sugar, milk, lotus stalk, or grains, causes deafness, blindness, trembling, loss of intelligence, causes voice to sound nasal, may cause death.

Milk after radish or garlic may cause obstinate skin diseases.

Milk with sour foods and drinks

Honey and *ghee* in equal quantities or honey, *ghee* and water in equal quantities, causes a subtle toxic reaction.

Drinking hot water after taking honey is contraindicated.

With very few exceptions, mutually contradictory foods cause sterility, blindness, skin diseases, ascites, eruptions, insanity, fistula, fainting, and intoxication. They can also cause tympanitis, throat spasms, anemia, *āma* poisoning, sprue, edema, acid indigestion, fever, rhinitis, fetal diseases, and death. These diseases are healed through emesis, purgation, antidotes, and can be prevented by protective measures.

The exceptions to mutually contradictory foods include, milk with garlic, and hot water after honey for emesis.

Herbal Preparation and Use

Fresh Juice (Swarasa)

Extracting the juice from fresh herbs (by crushing or pounding) has the most potent healing effect. With few exceptions (e.g., ginger and cilantro), it is difficult to obtain fresh Āyurvedic herbs for juicing. Each of the remaining preparations have slightly less potency than the previous, with confections containing the least degree of potency.

Decoctions (Kwātha)

Decoctions are made by boiling herbs in water over a low flame until 1/2 the amount of water remains. Decoctions are best suited for roots, stems, bark, and fruit, because it takes longer to transfer the energies from these parts of the plant to the decoction liquid (flower and leaf energy is quickly transferred).

Decoction Recipe: 1 part dry herbs to 16 parts water or 1/2 ounce of herbs to 8 ounces of water. The 8 cups of water are boiled over a low flame until half the amount (2 ounces) remains. The herb's energies are now transferred to the liquid from the dry herb. Herbs are then strained and the decoction is taken.

Sometimes milk decoctions are especially useful for enhancing herbal properties as for *aśhwagandhā* and *śhatāvarī.* A traditional recipe for *aśhwagandhā* milk decoction is 1/4 ounce *aśhwagandhā* to 1/4 cup milk to 1 cup water. This mixture is boiled over a low flame until the water evaporates. Less water can be used when using herbs in powdered form.

Hot Infusions (Phāṇṭa)

One ounce of herbs is mixed with 8 ounces of water (1:8 ratio) for hot infusions. After the water has boiled, the flame is turned off, and herbs are added to the water. The herbs are allowed to steep up between 1/2 hour to 12 hours, during which time their energies are transferred to the water. Then, herbs are strained before drinking the infusion.

Aromatic herbs, nonwoody plants, leaves, and flowers are best suited to hot infusion because their energies are easily transferred and would be destroyed through boiling. When a formula requires a mixture of herbs (e.g., roots and flowers), the roots are boiled and the flowers are added and steeped.

Cold Infusions (Hima)

Herbal powders release their energies more quickly than raw herbs, so they are left to steep in cold water from 1 hour to overnight (overnight is the preferred time). As with hot infusions, cold infusions are best for delicate parts of the herbs. This method offers the further advantage of preserving herbs which have cooling or refrigerant properties. Pitta-reducing therapies are best suited to this method of preparation. Herbs include jasmine, sandalwood, mint, etc.

Wet Pill, Paste, Bolus (Kalka)

Fresh or dried herbs are rubbed on a stone and mixed with a small quantity of water until they become a soft paste. This preparation is applied externally as a paste to heal wounds, sores, etc. It can also be taken internally. Some recipes call for the addition of sweets or liquids. Twice the amount of raw honey, *ghee,* or oil may be added to the paste; an equal amount of *jaggery* may be added, and 4 times the amount of any other liquid is added.

Powders (Chūrṇas)

Dried herbs are ground in a mortar and pestle or with an herb grinding machine; and strained into a fine powder. They are easily mixed with other herbs and have quick acting properties in the body. However, they stay in the body for only a few hours, and their shelf life is not as long as that of pills and other compounds.

Traditionally powdered mixtures used 20 or more different herbs per formula. Powders are best taken with *ghee,* raw sugar, or raw honey; which transport the herb's energies to all seven tissue layers. The ratio of herbs to vehicle is 1:2. If milk or water is used as a vehicle, they are used in a ratio of 4:1 to herbs.

Powders work best for the gastrointestinal tract and on the plasma tissue (*rasa dhātu*); with the exception of rejuvenative herbs like *aśhwagandhā, triphalā, śhatāvarī,* etc., that work on all seven tissues. Traditional powdered (*chūrṇa*) formulas include *lavaṇ bhāskar, triphalā, sitpaladi, hiṅgwastock*, and *sudarṣhan chūrṇas.*

Pills (Guṭi and Vaṭi)

Pills not only include herbs, but also powdered herbal extracts and burnt minerals and metals. These make the pill more potent, offering a quicker and more effective healing process. Pills also remain in the body longer than powders and have a longer shelf life. When pills are made with burnt metals and minerals (*bhasmas*), the longer the pills are stored the more potent they become.

Traditional pills include *laṣhunadi vaṭi, chandraprabhā vaṭi, kuṭajghan vaṭi, yogarāj guggul,* and *kaiṣhore guggul.*

Confections (Avaleha)

This is the solid mass obtained from boiling a decoction. Sugar or liquid is added in 4 times the quantity, while *jaggery* is only double the quantity of the mass. This makes a confection. They are best taken with boiled milk, cane juice, or decoction. *Chyavan prāśh* is perhaps the most well known confection. Being sweet in nature, children like to eat the confection. Often *avalahas* are used as tonics and rejuvenatives. Different confections help different disorders.

Medicated Ghee and Oil (Sneha)

Oils work primarily on the skin, blood, lungs, and colon; they cannot reach the deeper tissue layers because their heavy nature is difficult for the liver to digest (the colon will have some effect on the nerves, however).

The recipe for *sneha* is 1 part herb paste to 4 parts *ghee* or oil to 4 parts of any decoction (or 16 parts water). They are cooked over a low flame for 4 to 8 hours until the water evaporates. When water is sprinkled into the oil or *ghee,* it will crackle; the preparation is now ready.

When the delicate parts of the plant (i.e., leaf or flower) or aromatic herbs are used they may be directly added to the pre-cooked oil or *ghee* and left to sit for 24 to 48 hours before they are strained.

Herbs are empowered by this process, providing quick and strong healing or rejuvenation. *Snehas* are used internally, in the nose, eyes, head, as enemas, and elsewhere. Traditional formulas include *brāhmī* oil, *brāhmī ghee, mahānārāyan* oil, *daśhmūl* oil, *anu* oil, *mahābhṛiṅgarāj* oil, *triphalā ghee, piṇḍa* oil.

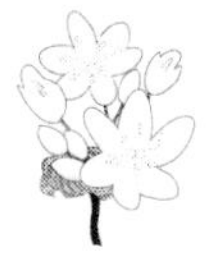

Medicated or Fermented Wines (Āsavas, Ārishṭhas)

Āsavas are prepared in cold water without boiling the herbs. *Ārishṭhas* involve boiling the herbs. Fermenting agents are added to these mixtures (e.g., *jaggery, dhātkī*) which are then stored at specific temperatures for a number of days, weeks, or months. This form of herbology is the Āyurvedic version of western liquid extracts, only more potent. These wines are easily and instantly absorbed into the blood stream (even if one has trouble digesting herbal pills or powders); improve digestive fire, and contain no alcohol. Traditional wines include *balāsava, kuṭajārishṭha, drākshāsav, arjunārishṭha, pañchāsav*.

Extracts

Herbal powdered extracts along with or instead of plain herb powders have become the industry standard. Extracts can offer a guaranteed potency of more than 3 to 6 times the power of plain herbs. *Giloy Sattwa* is a traditional Āyurveda powdered of extract of *guḍūchī*. Purified *guggul* is another common extract. In the U.S., many extracts are now offered including *garcinia* (tamarind) and turmeric.

There are 2 approaches to extraction. The common method is to take the active ingredients out of the whole herb. Newer methods to extract the whole plant yet guaranteed potency levels have been developed by Zandu Pharmacies of Bombay, and Sabinsa in New Jersey. This approach is more in line with Āyurvedic thinking because it uses the entire herb. In this method, one receives the properties of whole herb as mother nature has intended. By only using so-called "active ingredients," we are assuming that the other ingredients play no role in the healing process when they may actually prevent side effects or direct the healing effects of the herb to its appropriate site. Thus, the whole plant extract retains the integrity of the herb, ensuring safety and efficacy.

Minerals and Metals (Rasas)

Seven metals are used along with herbs in certain powerful preparations. The 7 metals (gold, silver, brass, copper, lead, tin, and magnetic iron-ore) relate to the 7 *dhātus* (tissue layers). These 7 plus 2 additional metals relate to the nine planets: copper/Sun, silver/Moon, brass/Mars, lead/Mercury, gold/Jupiter, tin/Venus, steel/Saturn, bronze/*Rahu*, magnetic iron-ore/*Ketu*. These metals undergo precise purification processes to remove toxins and make them digestible.

When the metals undergo these alchemical processes they are used for rejuvenation (*rasāyanas*) therapy. For example, therapies for healing amebic parasites include antiparasitical herbs and immune-boosting herbs. Formulas sold in India include *kuṭaj* (antiparasitical) and mercury *bhasma* (immune-boosting ash). *Bhasmas* (metal, mineral, and gem ash) are common to many Āyurvedic products in India. Some of the *bhasmas* have not yet been approved for use in the U.S. by the FDA. Many European countries, however, allow importation of these *bhasmas*.

Metals, gems, minerals (mica, red coral, sea shells) are burnt into ash (*bhasma*) in a very specific process, thereby removing all toxic properties. If these items are improperly prepared, ingesting them can be life-threatening. Even in India, only a few Āyurvedic companies are viewed as reliable manufacturers of *bhasmas*. So caution is strongly advised when considering the use of certain *bhasmas*.

Mercury conquers all diseases
and confers strength.
Shārṅgadhara Saṃhitā: Ch. 12; verse 1

Herb Mixing

Dose: The herbal dose depends on many factors, e.g., the strength of the person, the herb, the disease or disorder, the season, and geographic location. For example, doses given to person in India are generally 2 to 4 times higher than those required or tolerated by persons in the U.S. For mild conditions found in the U.S., 1/4 to 1/2 tsp. of powdered herbs; 3 times daily is adequate to produce desired healing results. For more chronic mental or physical problems, 1/2 to 1 teaspoon, 3 times daily is needed. Yet even in these cases, it is wise to allow gradual build-up from smaller doses to the full dose so that the system can adjust to the herbs. In extreme conditions (e.g., cancer), 1 to 3 ounces daily are required for certain tissue layer *(dhātus)* healing.

Children's doses have been discussed in Chapter 23. From birth to one month, herbs are given in quantities of approximating 2 rice grains, with raw honey, milk, *ghee,* or syrup (herbs may also be received through breast milk). This quantity is augmented by 2 grains each month until age 15 to a maximum dose of 1/16 teaspoon.

Pet Care: Pets (horses, cats, dogs) respond extremely well to herbs. Animals are so intuitive they often attack the bag or bottle of herbs before their owner can even give them the product. At our U.S. center, we have found that pets only require 1/16 to 1/8 teaspoon of herbs for most disorders; even chronic ones. Since it is difficult to take the pulse of a pet, deciding on appropriate therapies is achieved through observing symptoms and medical reports prepared by the vet.

Mixing**:** Mixing herb powders is a fairly simple process so long as the tridoṣhic theory is followed. Keep in mind the effects each herb has on a particular *doṣha*, disorder, organ, and tissue layer. For example, if a Vāyu *doṣha* person needs a brain tonic, Vāyu-reducing or tridoṣhic brain tonic herbs are used, such as *aśhwagandhā, jaṭāmāṇśhī,* or *brāhmī*. An herb like skullcap, although useful for insomnia and nervousness, will aggravate the Vāyu *doṣha* if used in excess. Thus, skullcap can be completely avoided or mixed with warming herbs such as cinnamon to balance out its cooling effect. Another example of herb personalization is high blood pressure. Although garlic is a well-known herb for hypertension, in Āyurveda it is helpful for Vāyu- and Kapha-caused hypertension; it will aggravate Pitta-related high blood pressure.

If a person is a dual *doṣha,* herbs that increase the third *doṣha* are used. For example if a person is a Pitta-Kapha *doṣha* and has a Pitta-Kapha health concern, such as bronchitis (Kapha symptoms) with an infection (yellow or green mucus/Pitta secondary symptoms), then Vāyu-increasing lung herbs are used (e.g., *vāsāk*). The Vāyu energies cool the excess Pitta (infection), dry the excess Kapha (phlegm), and the herb directs these energies directly to the lungs. When looking at this balancing effect from the view of the six tastes, the bitter taste is responsible for healing. Bitter herbs often have antibiotic properties (e.g., goldenseal).

When tridoṣhic disorders are involved (all three *doṣhas* are present), tridoṣhic herbs are required. If these herbs are not specific enough to affect healing then herbs are used to heal (reduce) the *doṣha* causing the most problems. As this condition improves, should another *doṣha* become aggravated due to ingesting the herbs being used, then herbs should be changed to balance this newly developed condition. Unquestionably, tridoṣhic cases are the most difficult situations to deal with.

Sometimes subtle uses of the herbs come into play. If one has an opportunity to effect healing using *sattwic* (holy) herbs (e.g., brāhmī or *tulsī,*) instead of *tamasic* or *rajasic* herbs (e.g., garlic, onions, valerian), then subtler spiritual benefits can develop as well. However, if needed for physical healing, *tamasic* and *rajasic* herbs must be used for some time.

Directing herbs to the proper organ should also be considered. Certain herbs, such as *gokṣhura* break up urinary stones. Coriander is mixed with *gokṣhura* to direct its healing effect to break up gallstones.

To summarize the rules discussed:

1) Use tridoṣhic herbs.

2) Use herbs that reduce one's *doṣha.*

3) If using herbs that increase one's *doṣha,* add other herbs that balance the herb's effects (i.e.,

add secondary herbs that will reduce the *doṣha).* Even if these herbs are not specifically used for that condition, they will balance the effects of the primary herb.

4) Dual-*doṣha* disorders require herbs that increase the third *doṣha* (i.e., reduce both *doṣhas*)

5) When tridoṣhic conditions require non-tridoṣhic herbs, constant switching of herbs is needed for balance depending upon the predominant *doṣha*.

6) Antibiotic or other specific concern herbs can be used.

7) *Sattwic* herbs are preferred over *tamasic* or *rajasic* herbs as long as they affect healing.

8) Secondary herbs may need to be used to direct the main herb to a specific organ or tissue.

Pitta/Kapha Balancing

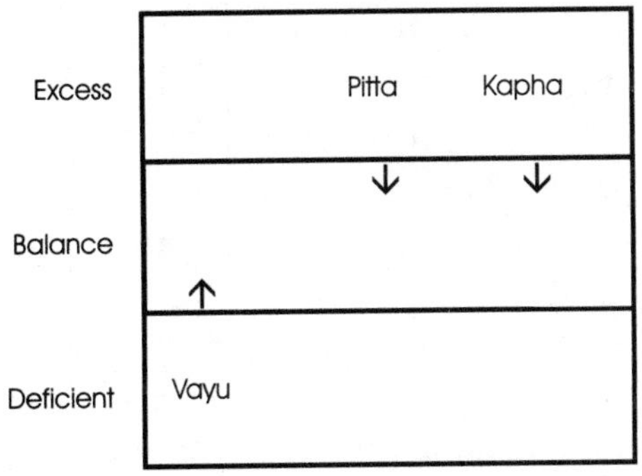

The above chart explains how a Pitta/Kapha *doṣha* excess is balanced. Pitta and Kapha are in excess, and Vāyu is deficient. Herbs and foods that increase Vāyu and reduce Pitta and Kapha, are incorporated into one's life; whereas items that increase Pitta and Kapha are avoided or reduced. Thus, the energies of Vāyu (e.g., cool, dry) will reduce the effects of Pitta (hot) and Kapha (dampness, phlegm). This tridoṣha theory is discussed in detail in Chapters 3 and 6. Below is a review of this theory.

If Pitta is in excess, heat is the main experience. Herbs that are cooling (sweet, bitter, and astringent) will balance the heat (i.e., reduce the heat). If Kapha is excessed, moistness (phlegm) is predominant or imbalanced in the individual. Herbs that are hot, pungent, and bitter will balance or reduce the moisture by their drying nature. When Pitta and Kapha are in excess, heat and moistness are the predominant symptoms. Bitter-tasting herbs will reduce both Pitta and Kapha *doṣhas* (astringent tastes may aggravate the earth element of Kapha, and pungent or hot tastes will aggravate or increase the Pitta element). Thus, bitter tastes will reduce Pitta and Kapha. See the tables below.

Taste	**Quality**	***Doṣha* Reduced**
Sweet	moist, cool	Vāyu/Pitta
Sour	hot	Vāyu/Kapha
Salty	hot	Vāyu
Pungent	hot	Kapha
Bitter	cold, light	Pitta/Kapha
Astringent	cold	Pitta/Kapha*

Doṣha	**Element**	**Qualities**
Vāyu	ether, air	cold, dry
Pitta	fire, water	hot, moist
Kapha	water, earth	wet, cold, heavy

** Sometimes astringent tastes will aggravate Kapha.*

When choosing herbs for a specific health concern, it is advisable to find an herb that works best for the situation. For example *mañjiṣhṭhā* is the best blood purifier. Other blood-cleansing herbs can then be added to the mixture, such as *brāhmī* and turmeric. Two to 4 times as much of the main herb (*mañjiṣhṭhā*) is used with the secondary herbs (2:1:1). Conditions associated with the main problem are also addressed. Should the liver also need detoxifying, liver-cleansing herbs are added to the mixture. *Brāhmī* also cleanses the liver, so it helps both conditions. However, if the liver requires serious attention, *bhūāmalakī,* the best liver cleanser, may be necessary to add to the formula. If blood purification is the predominating concern, then less *bhūāmalakī* is used (one or two parts). If the liver needs as much attention as the blood, then equal amounts of *bhūāmalakī* and *mañjiṣhṭhā* are used (2:2). One part coriander can be added to the formula to help digest the herbs, making them more effective and quick acting. If mental stress has caused the disorder, then *brāhmī* would also be added to the formula to balance the mind.

If the person with this Pitta condition is a pure Pitta *dosha,* this would be an acceptable formula. If they are a Pitta/Vāyu *doṣha,* then *bhūāmalakī* may be too aggravating for Vāyu. *Brāhmī* or *bhṛiṅgarāj* can be used instead of *bhūāmalakī.* When herbs cannot be found to heal a condition without aggravating one's *doṣha* (in this example, Vāyu) the rule is to choose herbs that will heal the excessed condition (in this case the blood and liver) and watch for any Vāyu-excess symptoms.

To summarize

1) The best herb for a condition should dominate the formula.

2) Other herbs can be used in smaller amounts.

3) Herbs used for secondary conditions are added in lesser amounts.

4) If two conditions are equally predominant, use the one herb that will help both conditions, or separate herbs for both conditions and use them in equal quantities.

5) Include herbs that digest the other herbs, thereby saving digestive energy and improving the absorption of the herbs.

Vessels and Cooking

The nature of the pot used to cook herbs (and foods) affects the final preparation. Aluminum, for example, is absorbed into the body as a poison. The best cooking materials are:

Kapha-reducing: Clay and copper (scraping and reducing properties)

Pitta-reducing: Brass or silver (cooling properties)

Vāyu-reducing: Iron (grounding properties)

Cooking over a flame (gas or wood) is better than using electric heat because it empowers the herbs and foods, making them more easily digestible. Wood fires are best, microwaves are not recommended.

Āyurvedic Acupuncture (Bhedan Karma)

In the three major Āyurvedic texts, discussions of surgery and *marma* points also involved Āyurvedic acupuncture or "needling," and *moxibustion*. The use of needles was used for both surgical and non-surgical healing. According to Dr. Frank Ross, author of *The Lost Secrets of Āyurvedic Acupuncture*; acupuncture was taught in Indian schools at least as early as 100 B.C. Students included Chinese visitors.

Very little information about Āyurvedic acupuncture is available in India today. It was first recorded in the *Suchi Veda* (science of needling) about 3,000 years ago. Since this is a very detailed science, the topic is merely mentioned here. For a more detailed explanation of the subject, please read Dr. Ros' book.

All human activities are meant for happiness of all living beings.
Such happiness is based on dharma (righteousness, right moral conduct).
Hence, every person should always adopt righteousness.
Aṣhṭāñga Hṛidayam Sū. Ch. 2: ver. 20

Chapter 27
Outer Healing
Beauty Care, Environmental Balancing Jyotiṣh, (Vāstu Śhāstra and Feng Shui), Scientific Research

Facial Doṣha-Beauty Care

Everyone has heard the sayings, 'beauty is only skin deep', and 'beauty is in the eyes of the beholder.' It is also commonly said that people in love always look beautiful. Āyurveda suggests that when persons have high self-worth or see the Divine within, they radiate true beauty. Thus, outer beauty is a reflection of inner beauty.

In Western cultures, the aging process of men has always been seen as beauty (handsome). However, the value and beauty of women more than 40-years-old seem to be ignored. Beauty has a much different definition in the ancient cultures, where, as both males and females grow older (and look older), beauty is said to grow. In other words, wisdom that comes with age is valued as a deeper beauty. This is a striking contrast to modern hi-tech cultures that see superficial, youthful faces as a sign of true beauty. Still, if persons take care of their health and cultivate their ethics, health and inner beauty radiates even through the skin. Āyurveda adds a spiritual dimension to the definition of beauty by saying:

Inner peace brings outer beauty

It is Divinity that is true beauty, that is, eternal and Divine love. Mental peace is the source of Divine beauty and develops as one realizes their Divinity. As each person sees their inner Self as Divine, they grow in beauty, both internally and externally. There are 3 aspect to beauty: inner, outer, and genetic or *karmic* beauty.

Outer beauty relates to bone structure, skin tone, muscle development, intelligence, hair quality, youthfulness, and weight. The *Vedic* sciences, such as Āyurveda and *Vedic* Astrology, discuss outer beauty as an integrated byproduct of inner beauty and virtue.

Karmic beauty results from genetic traits. Also, each person has varying degrees of grace, which enhance beauty. These *karmic* traits are enhanced through being raised to develop compassion, understanding, love, patience, sharing, and nurturing that which is in harmony with nature. This is a more fundamental aspect of beauty.

Inner beauty mainly requires development of virtue. One of the main Āyurvedic texts, the *Charak Saṃhitā*, specifically notes that longevity can be achieved through being ethical and virtuous. This aspect of character is a part of the process of developing and maintaining beauty. It, too, is more essential than mere outer beauty.

Besides ethics and virtue, healthy eating habits and life style are also necessary for inner beauty to radiate into outer beauty. Cleanliness is next to Godliness, and keeping the body clean is a twofold process: Externally, one should wash and apply healthy and nurturing cosmetics. Internal cleansing is developed through eating foods according to one's Āyurvedic constitution, virtue, and prayer or meditation. This helps develop a positive self-image or healthy self-love. Further, one's life habits must be considered.

Avoiding staying up late, excessive work, and overexposure to elements like sun, cold, and dryness is essential. In short, one should take control of or balance their outer and inner lives.

The four areas of life have already been discussed (health, harmonious career, spiritual relationships, and direct spiritual development). The truly beautiful person is then defined as one who is healthy, loves their career, and has a relationship that helps them grow spiritually. These persons also find adequate time to develop their inner spiritual Self.

Thus, outer beauty cannot by itself bring true and lasting beauty. Even those who are physically beautiful must feel some inner connection—some purpose to life to feel truly beautiful. Looking and feeling beautiful are two separate aspects. An ancient *Vedic* story tells of inner, spiritual beauty being stronger than superficial beauty:

Parvati was the loveliest goddess in all the world. She wanted to marry *Śhiva*, the Divine God. Yet even with all her beauty, *Śhiva's* meditations could not be disturbed. Seeing that mere physical attraction was insufficient, *Parvati* underwent developing her ethics, virtue, and health, and spent many long years enhancing her own spirituality through meditation. One day, by the mere purity of her soul, *Śhiva* was aroused from His meditations to see who it was who was so devoted to God. When He saw the radiance of her Divine beauty, He accepted her wish to be married.

Throughout this book, it is explained how to develop inner beauty through meditation, proper diet, ethics, a positive self-image, and various therapies, such as aroma therapy, yoga, and *abhyañga* (a massage-like therapy). These are the essential ingredients for developing a true and lasting aura of beauty.

We will now spend some time discussing how to develop and maintain outer beauty through natural methods. For example, using makeup that removes symptomatic signs of aging can harm the skin and poison the body with chemicals. It will eventually destroy one's outer looks and undermine one's inner health and spiritual beauty as well. Just as we have discussed foods that enhance and balance a person, according to their constitution, natural makeup, shampoo, and facials are also available for each person's constitution.

Skin: Sensitivity & Healing

Besides the seven *doṣhas* (Vāyu-Air, Pitta-Fire, Kapha-Water, Vāyu/Pitta, Vāyu/Kapha, Pitta/ Kapha, Tridoṣhic (all three *doṣhas*)), a special category exists known as changing skin conditions. Despite one's *doṣha*, skin conditions change depending upon one's diet, exercise, and the climate. Sensitivity towards cold, dryness, and the sun may exist. It is important to remember that it takes the body between 3 and 5 years to adjust to good or bad eating habits and climate. This is one reason that Āyurveda suggests gradual changes towards building a healthier lifestyle. It takes time for a toxic body to be cleanses; new cells and tissues built; and a new way of life and health to develop. Below are some Āyurvedic beauty care tips.

<u>Post-Surgery</u>: When the skin becomes scarred from surgery, herbs help heal the tissues. Aloe vera gel and *mañjiṣhṭhā* are the main recommendations.

<u>Acne</u>: Not only do teenagers get acne, but also many adults suffer from this condition. Acne is generally an excess of Pitta (fire). Therefore, Āyurveda approaches acne from both symptomatic and causal levels. To remove symptoms, turmeric creme and sandalwood soap, found in most Indian grocery store, work very quickly. Simultaneously, one also should reduce the causes—the excess fire and toxins inside the body. If neglected, Pitta and toxins will cause acne to reappear, or manifest as illness in another part of the body (e.g., eyes, liver, spleen, gall bladder, heat, blood, and infections). For causal balancing or healing, persons should follow a fire- (Pitta) reduction diet (discussed in Chapter

6 and appendix 1).
Seasonal Conditions: Each season (see Chapter 12) has a predominance of Vāyu (air), Pitta (fire), or Kapha (water). Āyurveda recommends that persons protect themselves from these environmental changes.

Season	Excess Doṣha/ Symptoms	Balance With
Winter	Vāyu/Kapha cold, damp, poor circulation	Pitta/Warmth warm oils, herbs, foods
Spring	Kapha/Water congestion/excess toxins, overweight	Vāyu/Pitta warm, dry oils, foods, herbs, steam
Summer	Pitta/Vāyu hot/dry, acne, rashes	Kapha/moist, cool powders, foods, herbs, creams
Fall	Vāyu/cold, windy, dry skin, wrinkles—signs of aging	Pitta/Kapha/ warm and moist oils, herbs, creams, foods

Facial Cleansing
Tridoṣhic Year-Round Cleansers

Chandrika Āyurvedic Soap	Sandalwood Soaps Kaphause only in Summer/Fall

Vāyu Cleansing Formulas
- early evening/year-round cleansers -

Sandalwood/Almond (gentle astringent)
6 drops sandalwood oil
2 oz. almond oil
4 oz. harītakī
14 oz. water
Put 4 oz. *harītakī* powder in 14 oz. of water until boiled. Strain herbs once water becomes tepid. Add sandalwood and almond oils.

Vāyu/Pitta Cleansing Formulas
- early afternoon and early evening/ year-round cleansers -

Sandalwood/Sesame (gentle astringent)
6 drops sandalwood oil
2 oz. sesame oil
4 oz. *triphalā*
14 oz. water
Steep 4 oz. of *triphalā* powder in 14 oz. of water until it boils. Strain the herbs when the water becomes tepid. Add sandalwood and sesame oils; pour into a glass jar; and store in a cool place.

Pitta Cleansing Formulas
- early afternoon/year-round cleansers -

Silver Sandalwood (astringent)
1 tsp. sandalwood oil
6 oz. vegetable glycerine
4 tbs. *mañjiṣhṭhā*
10 oz. silver water
Use 1 oz. of pure silver, or new silver quarters in 20 oz. spring water. Boil until half the water remains. Remove the silver and use the water for the cleansing formula. Boil silver water, *mañjiṣhṭhā*, and glycerine. Remove and cool until tepid. Strain *mañjiṣhṭhā*. Add warm sandalwood oil. Pour into a glass jar, cover, and shake thoroughly. Keep in a cool place.

Kapha Cleansing Formulas
- late morning/year-round cleansers -

Copper Eucalyptus
6 drops eucalyptus oil
6 oz. vegetable glycerine
2 tbs. *triphalā*
10 oz. copper water
1 oz. of copper or copper pennies can be cleaned by soaking in them lime juice for a few hours. Rinse the copper and add them to 20 oz. of spring water. Boil until half the water remains. Remove the copper and use the water for the cleansing formula. Boil copper water, *triphalā,* and glycerine. Remove and set until tepid. Strain the *triphalā*. Add eucalyptus oil. Pour it into a glass jar, cover, and shake thoroughly. Keep in a cool place.

Vāyu/Kapha Cleansing Formulas
- late morning & early evening/ year-round cleansers -

Sandalwood/Eucalyptus
3 drops sandalwood oil
3 drops eucalyptus
6 oz. vegetable glycerine
4 oz. *triphalā*
14 oz. water
Steep 4 oz. of *triphalā* powder in 14 oz. of water until it boils. Strain the herbs when the water becomes tepid. Add glycerine and bring to a boil. Add sandalwood and eucalyptus oils, and set until tepid. Pour into a glass jar, cover, and shake well. Store in a cool place.

Pitta/Kapha Cleansing Formulas
- late morning & early afternoon/ year-round cleansers -

Ylang-Ylang
6 drops ylang-ylang
6 oz. sunflower oil
4 oz. *triphalā*
10 oz. water
Bring *triphalā* and water to a boil. When tepid, strain the herbs and add the oils. Pour into a glass jar and store in a cool place.

Press a warm (organic) cotton towel on the face for several minutes

Eye Care

Triphalā and rose water may be used internally; and externally as eye washes. Boil one cup of water; add one teaspoon of *triphalā* powder. Let it sit for at least 3 minutes. Pour the *triphalā* tea through a coffee filter into another cup. Let the tea cool to room temperature before washing the eyes. Rose water may be used as an eye wash without boiling or straining.

Kajal is a black cosmetic creme that is placed on the edges of the eyelids. This Āyurvedic preparation keeps dust and pollution out of the eyes, while enhancing their beauty.

For more details on skin care and skin disorders, see Chapter 21.

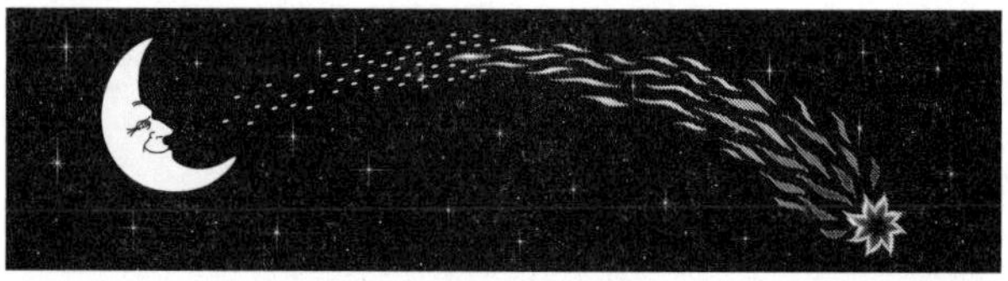

Jyotiṣh - Vedic Astrology

Jyotiṣh means inner light. This science helps reveal one's inner Divine light. Āyurveda and

Jyotiṣh were once a part of the same science, but later developed into two separate forms of healing. Although some may be skeptical towards astrology, when practiced correctly, *Jyotiṣh* is an excellent tool for uncovering planetary-caused illnesses.

This science follows the basic *Vedic* belief that four areas of life require attention: health, life-purpose or meaningful career (*dharma*), spiritual relationships, and personal spiritual path.

By looking at the planets, the 12 houses and their relationship in the astrology chart, one can determine health tendencies, planetary causes of disease, *dharma*, necessities for spiritual relationships, and tools for one's spiritual path.

Every person has some strong and weak planets. Each planet, when weak and influencing health-related houses, can cause specific disease. Instead of merely informing a person of what the chart says through *Vedic* astrology; *Jyotiṣh* additionally offers simple therapies to remove the troubling effects of planets. Therapies include *mantras, yantras* (talismans), meditations and rituals, herbs, aromas, gems, lifestyle, and spiritual suggestions. Therefore, like Āyurveda, *Jyotiṣh* offers therapies so people can take control of their lives and effect healing.

Planets

Below are the nine traditional planets used in *Jyotiṣh*, what they affect, and the corresponding mental and physical disorders that each planet can cause.

Sun: Father, ego, Soul, honor

Physical; arthritis or weak bones; low energy or resistance; pallor or anemia; cold limbs, poor appetite or digestion; weak pulse or heart; poor circulation or eyesight; edema or other disorders of water accumulation.

Mental; low self-esteem or confidence; lack of motivation, emotional or material dependency; sluggishness or dull mindedness; difficulty with independence.

Moon: Mother, emotions, personality, socializing, happiness, home, nurturing

Physical; anemia, constipation, dry skin, weak lungs or kidneys; female reproductive disorders.

Mental; depression, moodiness, ungroundedness, fear of intimacy or difficulty dealing with others.

Mars: Brothers, friends/enemies, courage, injury, energy, logic, law

Physical; lack of motivation or energy; unable to defend oneself or dominated by others; unable to express anger, unable to see through people's motivations, overly passive, easily controlled or abused (emotionally or physically).

Mental; weak immune system; appetite or absorption of nutrients; liver or small intestine disorders; anemia, injuries or slow healing of injuries; low male vitality.

Mercury: Healing, communication (writing, computers, speaking), intelligence, childhood, commerce

Physical; weak nervous system, anxiety, insomnia, dry skin, palpitations or other nerve conditions; allergies, weak lungs or heart.

Mental; difficulty communicating, immaturity or childishness; low intelligence, dependencies or addictions; dullness or daydreaming.

Jupiter: Spirituality, guru, dharma, wealth, health, creativity, music, husband (for women)

Physical; weak immune system or vitality; overly thin, liver or pancreas disorders; poor absorption of nutrients.

Mental; lack of faith, enthusiasm, meaning, or will; feeling constricted, pessimism or depression; moodiness or melancholy; anxiety, unfriendliness, financial difficulties, low creativity.

Venus: The arts, love, vehicles, beauty, comfort, the wife (for husbands)

Physical; weak kidneys, bones, or reproductive system; weak immune system or low energy; chronic urinary tract disorders, bleeding tendencies.

Mental; lack of grace, charm, beauty, taste, or

refinement; insensitivity or coarseness; feeling unloved or romantic difficulties; low feminine qualities.

Saturn: Obstacles, delays, separation, longevity, spiritual discipline, spiritual one-ness

Physical; weak bones or nerves; constipation, poor resistance or healing; mysterious diseases (e.g., cancer and epilepsy).

Mental; agitation, stress, insomnia or ungroundedness; weak or easily intimidated; impractical, poor endurance or no long-term drive; troubles making money or with government or institutions.

Rahu (North node of the Moon): Disease, psyche, illusion, mass trends, higher visions, new *karma*

Physical; weak immune or nervous system; insomnia, pallor, poor mind-body coordination; easily contracts diseases.

Mental; disillusionment or poor perception; anxiety, moodiness, no self-identity, easily influenced, spreads oneself too thin.

Ketu (South node of the Moon): Liberation, constriction, loss, past *karma*

Physical; poor digestion or circulation; ulcers, muscular or nervous system disorders; anemia or bleeding problems; mysterious diseases (e.g., cancer and paralysis).

Mental; feeling constricted, attached to the past or lost causes; poor perception, self-destructive, injuries or violence; poor eyesight, low self-esteem.

Houses

Just as Western astrology, *Jyotiṣh* uses the same 12 houses and signs. Each house relates to another domain of life. Different astrologers (*Jyotiṣhis*) have slightly different house interpretations. Below is a brief summary of the houses and areas of influence:

1. Personality, health
2. Education, livelihood potential, communication, childhood
3. Courage, socializing, siblings
4. Home, mother, material possessions, faith, travel
5. Creativity, children, speculations, devotion
6. Physical health, injury, litigation, enemies
7. Long-term partner (e.g., spouse or business partner)
8. Mental health, longevity, travel
9. *Dharma* (life purpose), religion, fortune, father, honor
10. Profession, achievement, recognition
11. Material and spiritual gains
12. Loss, liberation

Charts

Two main chart styles can be used, Northern and Southern, depending on one's preference. Examples follow.

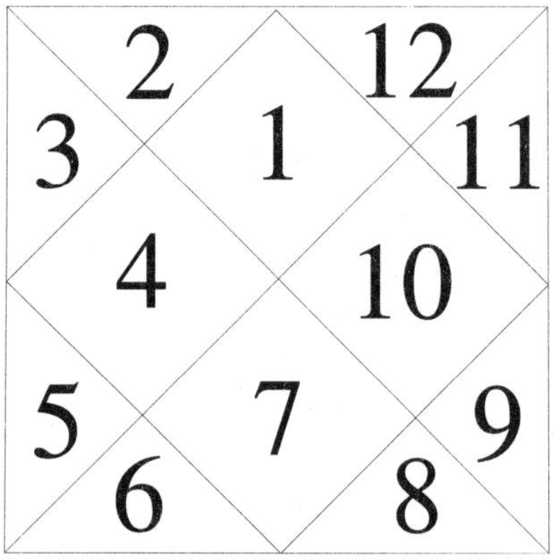

NORTH INDIAN JYOTIṢH CHART

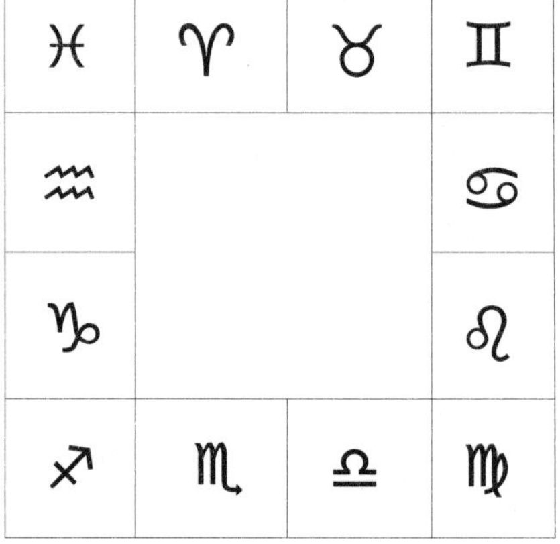

SOUTH INDIAN JYOTIṢH CHART

This science delves deeply into life and fully

compliments Āyurveda. Read Astrology of the Seers by David Frawley for more information on this subject.

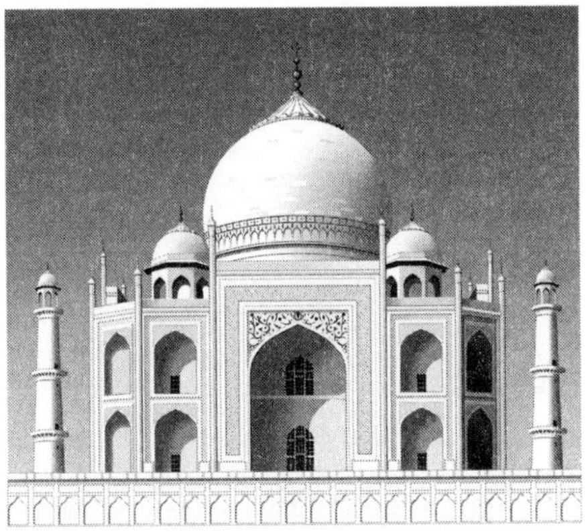

Architectural Harmony: (External Kuṇḍalinī) Vāstu Śhāstra

The focus of this book has been on healing, prevention, and rejuvenation through Āyurvedic balance. This balance is achieved by living in accordance with nature's laws. We have also discussed how meditation raises one's inner life force or *kuṇḍalinī śhakti*. The raising of one's *kuṇḍalinī* is essential for Self-Realization. We briefly discussed Vedic astrology (*Jyotiṣh*) as another influence upon health, career, lifestyle, and spiritual development.

The Vedic science of architecture, *Vāstu Śhāstra,* integrates the sciences of Āyurveda and *Jyotiṣh* by providing the link between humans and the astrological influences. *Vāstu* considers the magnetic fields of the earth, the influences of the planets and other heavenly bodies essential elements when designing commercial or residential buildings, temples, and even towns, villages, and cities. It is believed that architectural structures are alive, influenced by natural law, just as the health of humans is influenced by nature. Thus, living in a home (or working in an office) built according to natural law ensures general health and prosperity.

Vāstu's integration of astrology, earth, health, science, and spirituality or religion is wonderfully evident as one reads through the *Vāstu* texts. For example, in Hindu religion, the deity of the sun is said to ride in a chariot pulled by seven horses or deities. They are called the seven rays of the sun. It is important to have these rays enter eastern windows for health reasons. However, reading that it is useful to have these seven deities enter the home may raise the eyebrows of religious skeptics or persons of other religions. Yet these seven deities also happen to be called the seven visible colors of the spectrum of solar white light. In other words, violet, indigo, blue, green, yellow, orange, and red are merely the scientific names of these rays; whereas *Vāstu* also uses their spiritual, religious, or mythological names. Thus, Vāstu offers insights into the link between modern science and ancient universal religion or spirituality. It is only a matter of semantics whether to call the sun's rays by the names of deities or colors of the spectrum. This semantic interchangeability of scientific and religious names is found in Āyurveda and the other *Vedic* sciences, as well as in most (if not all) ancient religions.

Vāstu describes other deities (light wavelengths) associated with the sun that cannot be detected by modern scientific instruments. Thus, the rules of *Vāstu* offer deeper insights into the laws of nature that modern science has yet to discover.

Since the focus of Āyurveda is holistic (i.e., all-inclusive), it is useful to consider harmonizing or balancing the external influences involving architectural structures.

Vāstu Śhāstra considers the quality of the soil, the shape and elevations of the land, the direction placement and the number of windows and doors; the thickness and height of walls and doors. In short, the minutest details of building are considered.

Like *Āyurveda* and *Jyotiṣh*, *Vāstu* is also a spiritual science. The house is divided into a certain number of squares (e.g., 81 squares), and each square is ruled by different a deity. Windows are determined according to the path of the sun to allow the seven solar rays (or deities) to bless (enter) the house.

Persons living or working in a *Vāstu*-built structure experience the enhancement of health, general well being, and prosperity. This is due to the external influences of natural law provided through the structure.

The diagram below is one version of the blueprint that is overlaid on a building site. The rectangle represents the building. Each box inside the rectangle is ruled by a different deity. The four dark rectangles (made up of six smaller boxes) are ruled by one deity per dark box. Finally, the nine small boxes in the middle of the house are ruled by the main deity, *Brahma*. Traditionally, one does not have walls or pillars in the center of the house so as to leave room for *Brahma*. Thus, the building is seen as a very holy place.

Further, the building is seen as a body. The head is in the upper right boxes. The arms run along the top and right outer boxes. The legs extend along the left and lower outer boxes. The heart resides in *Brahma's* box. If one has a health problem, it is believed that part of the structure pertaining to that area of the house was not built in accordance with *Vāstu* natural law.

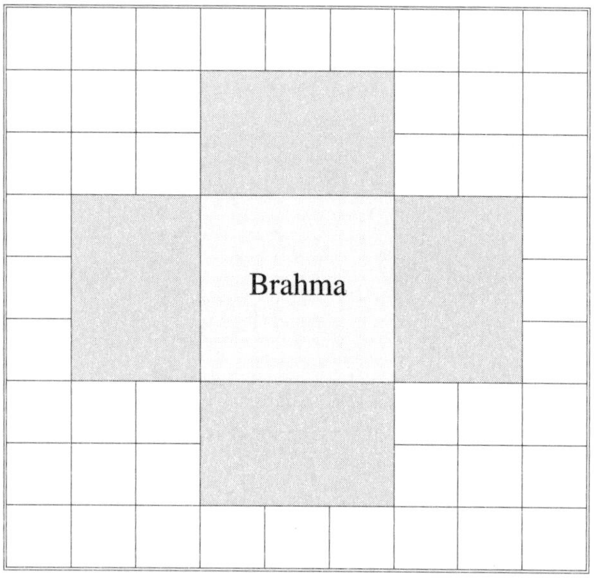

DIAGRAM: A 9 x 9 VĀSTU BUILDING BLUEPRINT

Determining the size and shape of the house is based on one's *Jyotiṣh* (*Vedic* astrology) birth chart. In this way, Āyurveda and *Jyotiṣh* are linked with the home, earth, and the natural laws that govern all things.

It is difficult to discuss the details of *Vāstu* for two reasons. First, it is a subject requiring more space than can be provided in a book on Āyurveda. Second, there are several schools of *Vāstu* . To date, there is no clear, simple book that outlines one consistent approach from start to finish. Most *Vāstu* architects live in India, but a few of them live in or visit other countries.

The lack of information on *Vāstu* creates a second practical drawback. Information to remedy existing buildings inexpensively (without changing the structure) is all but nonexistent.

Interest in Vāstu has dramatically increased in India. Perhaps the growing interest in Āyurveda and *Jyotiṣh* will awaken desires to learn more about *Vāstu Śhāstra* in Western countries. Then these spiritual architects can be inspired to write, teach, and lecture on the subject.

Throughout India and other Asian countries *Vāstu*-built temples abound. Some Hindu temples in the U.S. have also been built according to traditional *Vāstu* guidelines. *Vāstu* guidelines have been applied to some modern homes, apartments, offices, and factories in India and the U.S. Several books provide photographs of both traditional and modern *Vāstu* structures to give readers a better idea of these buildings.

Feng Shui

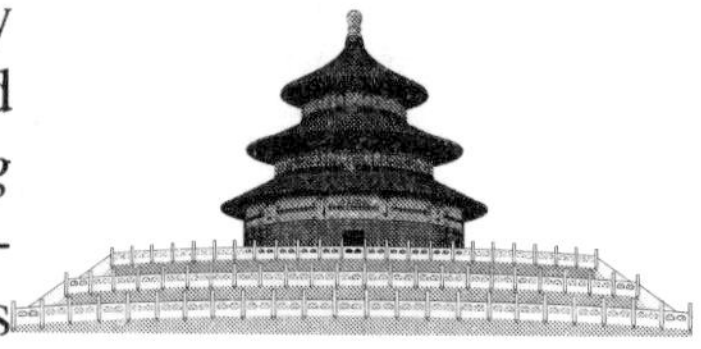

The Chinese version of natural-home living (i.e., harmony with nature) is called *Feng Shui* ("*fung shway*"). Its principles and goals are as universal and as natural as Āyurveda and *Vāstu Ṣhāstra*. In fact, *Feng Shui* practitioners believe that this science was adapted from

India's *Vāstu Śhāstra*.

Much more information is currently available about *Feng Shui*. Further, there are many *Feng Shui* practitioners in the U.S. and throughout the world. It is reported that in Hong Kong today, people will not work for a company if the building is not built or adjusted according to *Feng Shui*; so strong is their belief in the science. Even U.S. companies, such as Chase Manhattan Bank and Citibank, with branches in Hong Kong, Singapore, and Taiwan, have had to build their offices according to these principles before local employees would agree to work in the buildings. In the U.S. as well, many companies use *Feng Shui* in their offices. Even television shows and newspaper cover this science (including Donald Trump's use of *Feng Shui*).

In addition to providing guidelines on building structures, *Feng Shui* also offers very practical and inexpensive methods to correct architectural problems in a building without having to remodel or rebuild. Extensive knowledge of *Feng Shui* and the ability to remedy without expensive remodeling make *Feng Shui* a very appealing alternative to *Vāstu Śhāstra*.

The basic premise of *Feng Shui* is that the structure (e.g., the home) has a life force of its own. This external life force or *chi* (pronounced *chee*) is the same as *kuṇḍalinī*. Although it is most important to have one's inner *kuṇḍalinī* raised for Self-Realization, there is no harm (and it is helpful) to ensure that the outer *kuṇḍalinī* or *chi* also flows properly. To this end, a brief discussion of *Feng Shui* follows.

Various schools of *Feng Shui* exist. One school works with a compass, using precise measurements and calculations. Other schools rely on some basic guidelines and then infuse intuition into the decision making process. Still other schools have more modern integrative interpretations. One popular school of thought will be discussed here. Its basic theory is simple and straight forward, and has become a very popular practice over the last decade.

This intuitive form of *Feng Shui* was popularized by author Sarah Rossbach. She is a student of Lin Yun of the *Tantric* Black Hat branch of Tibetan Buddhism, who is credited with making this approach widely available in the West.

Although it is always better to hire a trained practitioner of *Feng Shui*, many simple therapies can be done by reading Rossbach's book, *Interior Design with Feng Shui*. The do-it-yourself approach to *Feng Shui* is simple and inexpensive.

Simple remedies include rearrangement of desks, couches, chairs, and beds. Structural considerations, such as placement of stairs by the front door, hallways, angled ceilings, and ceiling beams require minor remedies. Three inexpensive methods to remedy structural problems in the home or office include mirrors, wind chimes, and small crystal balls.

One use of mirrors will be explained to provide a basic understanding of the science. A structure (e.g., a home) is divided into nine equal rectangles (or squares) by applying a tic-tac-toe-like grid over a drawing of the building. Each rectangle relates to a specific area of one's life (except for the center rectangle—similar to *Vāstu*). The placement of the front door determines the personality of each rectangle.

Feng Shui building blueprint

Wealth	Fame	Marriage/ Relationship
Family/ Health		Children
Knowledge	Career	Helpful People

The front door is somewhere on this wall of the house.

The diagram above shows a floor plan of a building with nine equal rectangles. Eight of the areas relate to eight different aspect of life. In this drawing the front door is placed along the bottom of the chart. Thus, areas of knowledge, career, and helpful people will reside on the wall wherever the front door is.

To enhance any of these areas, a mirror can be placed on the wall to symbolically reflect the positive flow of life force of that domain of life. Some companies sell inexpensive 3-inch hexagonal or octagonal mirrors with the names of each domain written on them both in English and in Chinese.

For example, if a person has an unusual or severe health problem, a health mirror is placed on a wall in the family/health area. It does not matter what room of the house it is (i.e., bedroom or kitchen) The focus is on the area itself as the domain of health (in relationship to the front door). Thus, in addition to herbs, foods, and other Āyurvedic therapies for healing, the placement of the mirror will help harmonize any external causes related to health.

Career mirrors are used for healing certain health problems. Career troubles (such as job dissatisfaction, fearing loss of job) can lead to anxiety and worry. This mental tension can cause mental and/or physical health disorders. In addition to brain tonic herbs like *brāhmī*, to calm the mind, a career mirror can be placed in this sector of the home to bring positive changes in one's career. Thus, *Feng Shui* offers an additional healing therapy option.

The layout of a building is also said to influence each area of life. As an example, the diagram below gives an example of a second-floor apartment.

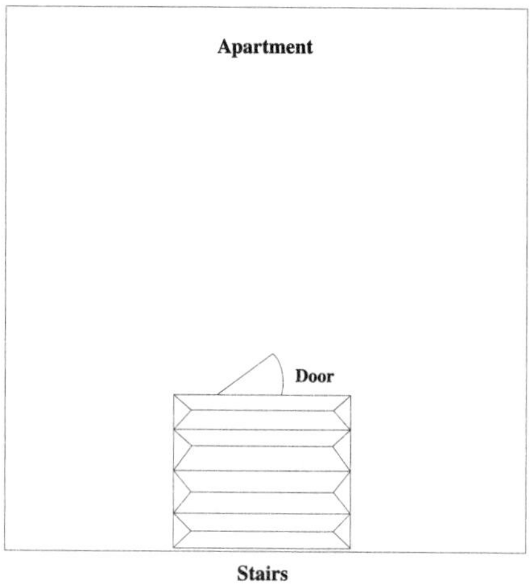

If the stairway rises up into the career area of the apartment, it will cut out a large section of the space. This can indicate trouble with career because that part of the apartment is missing. It is likely that the resident will have trouble keeping a job or finding a good job. Placing a career mirror on the wall in this area would help rectify this situation.

Changes can occur in one of two ways. Sometimes the change is very noticeable, such as finding a job. In other cases, changes occur on the level of thinking. For example if a person had previously been resigned to the belief that they were stuck in their job and there was no way out; they may never have given a thought to changing jobs or careers. After placing a career mirror in the career area of their home, they may begin to consider job improvement. In other words, before a job change can occur, one must be ready for it; one should consider the topic or be aware of it.

Positive change means leading one a step further from where one began when the mirror was placed. Some people may be ready for a job or healing to occur. Others may need further information before making such choices or and allowing such developments.

Healing Structural Problems

Sometimes the actual structure of the home, apartment or office blocks the proper flow life force. Through the use of simple and inexpensive therapies, such as mirrors and crystal balls, the flow of proper life force can be restored. Three examples are listed below.

If the front door opens to face a wall, the life force is blocked. It is psychologically cramping or inhibiting to always feel one is walking into a wall and leads to a life of struggle. To resolve this a mirror is placed on the wall (see diagram a).

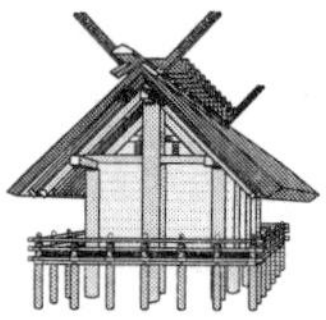

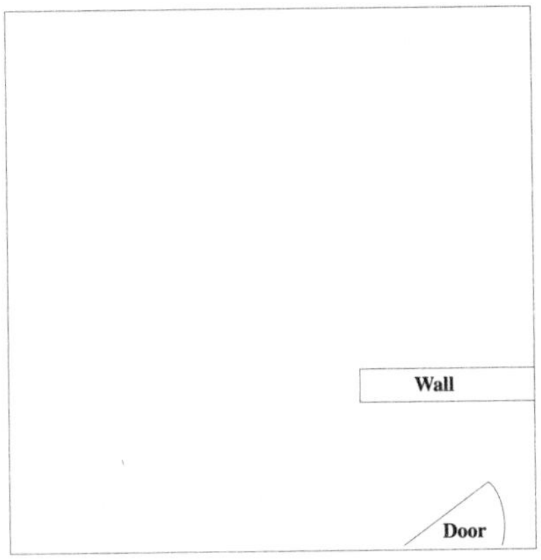

DIAGRAM A—WALL OBSTRUCTION AT FRONT DOOR

Another structural problem involves having a stairway facing the front door. This allows the life force and money to flow out the door. The remedy is to hang a crystal ball or wind chime between the bottom stair and the front door. This improves the life force.

The entranceway or foyer should be well lit and spacious; dark spaces are psychologically depressing; narrow spaces evoke oppressive feelings that choke the home owner's luck and health, leading to breathing problems. Placing a large mirror on the wall gives a sense of depth to the foyer.

Stairways should be well lit and wide, with high ceilings. Hanging a mirror on the ceiling gives a sense of spaciousness and brightens the stairs, thereby preventing the feeling of constriction.

Many other simple and inexpensive therapies are available for slanted ceilings, long corridors, aligned doors and windows, and more.

Furniture Placement

The arrangement of furniture can also enhance or hamper the life force. It is possible to set up living room and office chairs that empower everyone. Placement of the bed is crucial for health, strength, and mental peace. A person's head should be able to see anyone entering through the bedroom door. If a person doesn't see someone entering the room it may startle them. This shocks the life force, causing nervousness and anxiety. The best bed placement is to have the bed at an angle to the door. Other helpful placements are shown below. Should the room not allow for proper bed placement, mirrors can be hung on the walls to reflect the door.

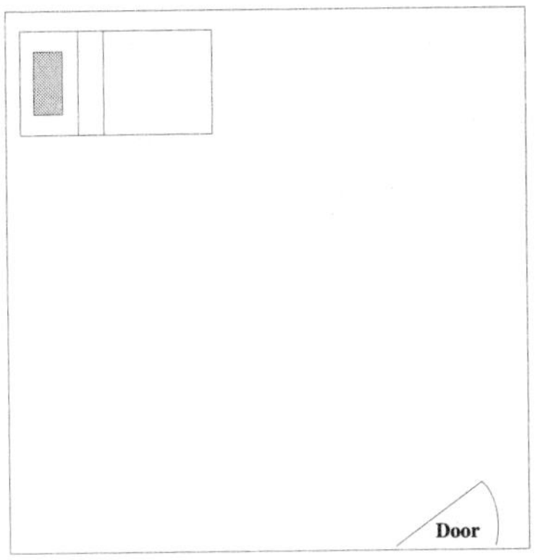

CATER CORNERED BED

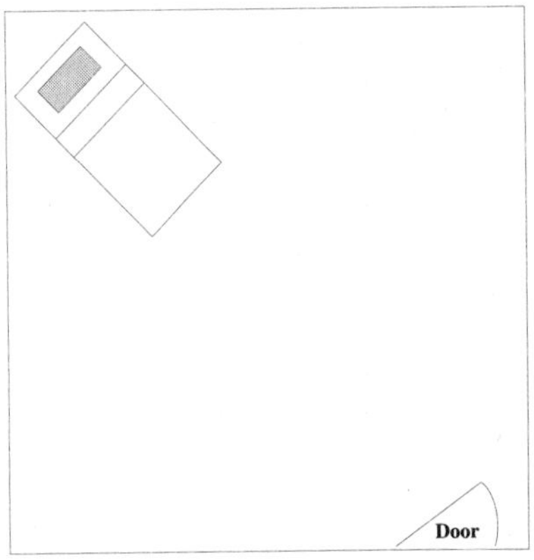

HELPFUL BED PLACEMENT OPTION

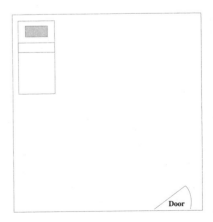

HELPFUL BED PLACEMENT OPTION

Feng Shui balances or harmonizes the outer life force, enabling life to flow according to natural law. Thus, it follows the same principles as Āyurveda. Thus, it can be considered a useful Āyurvedic therapy for external influences on health.

Herbs and Their Effects
A New Paradigm of Healing

In the light of modern science, persons may wonder how such an ancient science compares with the technological advantages of today's medicine. In fact, it is astonishing to see just how specific and comprehensive Āyurvedic insights are.

In addition to understanding herbal application for *doṣhas* and specific disorders, it is interesting to know that herbs send their healing energy to specific organs. *Pippalī*, for example, has an affinity for the liver. *Guḍūchī* has a predisposition for the blood tissue (*rakta dhātu*). Thus, herbs can target specific sites for precise therapy.

Further, if a preliminary site is blocked along with a secondary site, an additional herb can be used to remove the primary block so that the second herb can travel to the latter site. For example, if the blood tissue needs repairing, but the blood cell receptors are unable to receive *guḍūchī, kaṇṭkārī* is first used to correct the blood cell receptors. In this way, *guḍūchī* will be received by the cells and will reach the blood tissue. This aspect of Āyurveda falls under pharmacokinetics (the study of absorption, distribution, metabolism, and excretion).

Another branch of Āyurvedic knowledge is pharmacodynamics, or the study of the action and effect of herbs on *doṣhas, dhātus*, wastes (*malas*), and channels (*srotas*).

Pharmacotherapeutics is the study of matching herbs to people. Specific conditions must be taken into consideration: the size of the dose, the age of the person, their level of strength and tolerance, mental condition, and digestive functioning. Other factors include the season, time of day, time of collection, method of herb storage, the potency of the herbs, the client's diet, and whether the herbs are fresh or dry.

One herb can have many different applications; seemingly unrelated disorders can be healed from the same herb. For example, *kuṭkī* can be used for heart disease, colic, painful urination, respiratory conditions, convulsions, and insomnia.

Medicine should be considered to perform diverse functions.
Charak Saṃhitā: Sū. 4; verse 22

This is very different from the modern idea that one drug can be used for one disease; although this idea is not entirely foreign to Western practitioners. Sometimes, when studying many patients who are taking a drug for one condition, it is found that the drug also helps another condition. The reverse of this finding is also true; various adverse side effects can unknowingly develop from taking a drug. Here, too, Āyurveda reveals the possible side effects of herbs (if any), so there are no surprises. The main principle of Āyurveda is to cause no harm. Armed with knowledge of uses and side effects, Āyurvedic practitioners can avoid such mistakes.

A therapy that helps some symptoms but causes other symptoms is not a pure therapy.
- Aṣhṭāñga Hṛidayam: Sū. 12; verse 16

Holistic Interrelation

Western thinking seems to focus on pieces, remaining unaffected by the whole picture. For example, illness and unhealthy organs are viewed independently. Other symptoms, such as nutrition, lifestyle, and career, are too often not taken into account. Āyurveda, on the other hand, is founded on the principle that all aspects of one's life are interrelated. The whole is greater than the sum of its parts. This is clearly seen in the way drugs are made, versus how herbs are prepared. Western medicine isolates active ingredients from known herbs to guarantee certain levels of active ingredients in their drugs, ignoring the possibility that other unknown active ingredients may also play a part in the process; directing the ingredient to a specific site or preventing side effects. Some holistic practitioners have also fallen into this piecemeal frame of thinking. Āyurveda encourages persons to look at healing from the truly holistic vantage.

Certain herbs perform unique actions and do not follow the general rules. For example, many herbs have been found helpful in reducing hypoglycemia (mostly bitter and astringent taste). Yet, why these herbs perform this action cannot be explained phytochemically, or taxonomically. In other words, no one active ingredient can be said to effect healing. This example lends more credence to the idea that much can be lost through the extraction and use of only extracted parts of a plant.

The aim of the herb's action is the whole plant, thus, examine the whole patient.
Charak Saṃhitā: Vi. 8; verse 94

Healing the Unhealable

Some diseases are considered incurable, and in some cases untreatable. These include psoriasis, certain liver disorders, obesity, malabsorption, rheumatoid arthritis, osteoarthritis, asthma, skin allergies, diabetes, epilepsy, MS, certain cancers, and some mental disorders, to name a few. Patients may be told by their doctors that not much can be done other than live with the condition. In some cases, drugs can lessen the symptoms, but healing is not available.

Āyurveda has found that many of these conditions can be healed, so long as the conditions are not genetic in origin. Even when heredity is a factor, Āyurveda can at least contain, lessen, and sometimes remove the symptoms; however, persons may be required to remain on the herbal and nutritional therapies for the rest of their lives.

These statements are not being made to discredit Western medicine; it has its place. The point here is that Āyurveda offers valid complimentary therapies that can help in many cases where Western medicine presently has no answers.

Healing vs Curing

It is useful to review the concept of curing versus healing. Western terminology centers on the notion of curing, as if one can achieve a permanent state of health. Āyurveda suggests that health does not necessarily mean the absence of disease or even the absence of symptoms. Rather, if one achieves a state of homeostasis or balance (i.e., a harmonious integration of all mental and physical systems), a person will feel healthy. The Āyurvedic view makes sense because we know there are such things as viruses and parasites within our system. When the immune system is weak these elements cannot take hold and cause disease.

The mind and body continually undergo rhythmic changes as a result of age, season, time of day, and metabolism. Consequently, persons must adjust to these internal and external influences to maintain their balance. It does not make sense that once a medicine is taken and the symptoms are 'cured' that the body will no longer be challenged.

An example of how rhythms affect the physiology is given in a study discussed in the *Principles of Āyurvedic Therapeutics* by A.V. Kumar. The chemicals acetylcholine, catecholamine, and histamine were more predominant in the blood of the subjects during summer, rainy, and winter seasons. Thus, these three chemicals, also related to Vāyu, Pitta, and Kapha respectively, increase and decrease in the human body according to seasonal rhythms. This is why Āyurveda suggests subtle changes in diet and lifestyle according to the season.

Working With Natural Rhythms

Āyurveda also delineates the best time of year to collect herbs to ensure their maximum potency, and also the best time of day to take the herbs depending upon it's properties. Below are two tables discussing these rhythmic schedules.

Plant Part	Time to Collect
rhizomes, roots, bark	late autumn, early spring
leaves	at the time the flower develops and before the maturing of the fruits and seeds
flowers	just before pollination
fruit	when ripe
seeds	when fully matured
juicy parts	winter
emetics and purgatives	at the end of spring

Further, when collecting thick roots, only the root bark is collected. When roots are thin, the whole root is collected.

Herb Property	Time To Take Herb
gastric sedatives	on an empty stomach
stomachics, bitter tonics	1/2 hour before bed
emetics	morning (to remove undigested food from the previous night)
purgatives	morning or evening
diuretics	daytime (when skin is kept cool)
diaphoretics	during fever

Rejuvenation

Other areas unique to Āyurveda include rejuvenation, longevity, or age reversal (*rasāyanas*). The concept of *rasāyanas* takes healing to another level. Beyond healing and prevention, Āyurveda says that through special herbs, diet, lifestyle, ethics, and spirituality, the mind and body can actually rebuild new healthy cells and tissues, thus slowing or reversing the aging process. Brain tonics like *aśhwagandhā*, *śhaṅkh puṣhpī*, and *brāhmī* have been found to prevent senility and memory loss. Physically, the essential life sap in the body that protects the immune system can actually continue to develop through eating herbs like *śhatāvarī* and *aśhwagandhā.*

Rejuvenation is new to Western medicine. Rejuvenation views the psychological, neurological, endocrinological, and immunological systems as an integrated whole. The key organ studied in rejuvenation is the brain. The brain influences its peripheral systems, the immune system, and harmonizes body functions. Through the use of special herbs, foods, and *pañcha karma* practices, the chemical age of individuals can be reversed.

Herbal Catalytic Agents (Anupans)

In addition to the advanced knowledge of herb usage, Āyurveda offers various herbs, liquids, and foods to empower the main herb, thereby healing even more quickly. For many conditions, mercury ash is suggested. Presently it is not allowed in some Western countries in this form because it is erroneously believed to be harmful. Mercuric oxide, however, is used for healing styes in the U.S. Although it is true that mercury in its natural state is toxic, it becomes a powerful healing agent after undergoing a specific burning process. Other catalysts include:

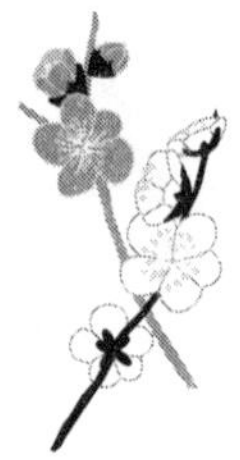

Disease	Catalyst (*Anupana*)
Acidity	*ghee* and sugar
Anemia	butter and rock candy
Anorexia	ginger juice and honey
Bronchitis	honey, *ghee*
Epilepsy	buttermilk
Facial Palsy	honey
Leukoderma	castor oil
Renal Calculus	honey and hot water
Rheumatism	*śhilājit* and *gokṣhura*
Tumors	castor oil, lemon juice

Knowledge vs Experience

In the West, knowledge is most highly revered. Experience and knowledge are equally important in the East, but experience is seen as the crucial validating factor.

The essence of Āyurveda is to remove the obstacles to health on one's spiritual path. Thus, the most important aspect of learning Āyurveda is to learn to follow one's personal Āyurvedic regimen to achieve balance.

Too often, in the name of helping others, compassionate healers will ignore their own health and lifestyle. Developing and maintaining balance deepens one's intuition, compassion, ethics, and overall spiritual life; thereby ever improving one's abilities as a healer. In contrast, many Westerners will absorb themselves in the intellectual study of a subject (even Āyurveda), forgetting to include themselves in the holistic picture.

Parallels: East and West

Although we have discussed at some length the unique aspects of Āyurveda, many parallels do remain between East and West. In fact, one can more readily accept the validity of the Āyurvedic system when the anatomical, physiological, endocrinal, systems discussed are found to be identical to those known through modern science.

One such example is the discussion of *srota*: *srotasmi, siras, rakta,* and *hṛidaya*. Although these words may seem foreign, they are merely the *Sanskrit* words for channels, arteries and arterioles, capillaries, veins and venules. The blood flow process (from the heart through the arteries and arterioles, branching into the capillaries and supplying nutrients to the body) is identical in both Āyurvedic and modern medical descriptions. Thus, as the Āyurvedic system is examined more thoroughly, it will reveal many similarities to modern medicine.

Āyurvedic Research
Modern Scientific Validation

This book has been dedicated to the compilation and presentation of Āyurveda, the holistic healing alternative from India. Throughout the chapters, modern terminology has been added to reveal the parallels between the ancient and modern sciences. These similarities suggest just how credible this ancient science is. Still, one may wonder whether Āyurveda would be applicable in today's society, or in other cultures other than Indian. In short, can holistic healing alternatives (e.g., herbs, meditation, proper nutrition, *yoga*) offer solutions to diseases in our time?

Over the past decade, many studies focused on just this question. This section offers a brief look into the extensive research being done on Āyurvedic herbs over the past 10 years. Summations of the research from books and journals, including studies listed for those who wish to take a more scientific approach, are given here.

There are different forms of Āyurvedic research: studying of the effect of herbs on humans, on animals, and in vitro (isolated tissue cell or organ preparation). Another group of herbal research involves whole-plant versus isolated-active ingredients; and whole plant versus herbal extracts. In order to keep the integrity and spirit of Āyurvedic holistic healing, it is important to emphasize human research, whole plant research, and whole-plant extracts. Human studies do not inflict unnecessary cruelty on animals. Whole plant and whole plant extracts offer the entire preparation made by mother nature. Anything less can potentially cause harm.

First, these herbs have been safely and successfully used for thousands of years, and their effects are fully documented in Āyurvedic texts. To inflict illness, suffering and pain on animals just to study these results seems cruel and unnecessary. Further, effects on animals does not automatically assume the same results will be found in humans—it is a jump in logic. So research on animals is not advocated.

Second, in trying to prove the efficacy of Āyurvedic herbs, some people try to make it fit into the western allopathic paradigm of drugs. In other words, find the active ingredient, isolate it, and boost its strength—if something is good, more of it must be better. It is this very process that has led to the harmfulness of drugs. Isolated ingredients—even from herbs—can cause side effects. Mother nature has added to each whole plant part not only active ingredients, but also protective ingredients. This is the value of holistic vision. These days pharmacies and health food stores are selling herbal products containing only active isolated ingredients. This is just what drugs are. This will be equally harmful. Further, making a man-made version of an herb, it is now enhanced by using only the extracted version—a more potent version of this isolated herb. Thus, if there is potential harm from the herb, the danger is not increased exponentially.

In short, it is hoped that future researcher will consider keeping the integrity of Āyurveda in mind when they design their tests. It is further hoped that herbal and pharmaceutical companies will not try to mold the integrity and value of Āyurvedic medicine into the less effective and more dangerous mindset of allopathic drugs. In an April 15, 1988 JAMA article (pages 1200-1205), it was reported that death due to allopathic drugs was the fourth leading cause of death in the US for 1997. This is 21/2 times more deaths than from AIDS. If AIDS is an epidemic, what do we call death due to prescription drugs. One person figured out these deaths are equivalent to a plane crash a day. Why do we insist on molding herbal research to become like allopathic drug research? Simple double-blind studies on humans using whole plant herbs will be safe, effective, and still produce acceptable and reliable research. It is hoped that this information is heeded before herbs are used in a way that makes them as harmful as prescription drugs.

Discussed below are some research studies. The Āyurvedic herbal section includes studies using various forms of research from human-whole plant, to animal-active ingredient extracts. This small sample of more than 2,000 Āyurvedic studies are presented to show the efficacy of Āyurvedic herbs; it is not meant to condone the various forms of research that have potentially harmful outcomes as discussed above.

Another notion to keep in mind when maintaining the integrity of the Āyurvedic system is that Āyurveda uses herbs to heal the root-cause of illness, not merely treating the symtoms. Also, Āyurveda considers the whole person and their lifestyle. To ignore this would be to weaken the healing power of Āyurveda, as well as destroy its spiritual link. Therefore, for all the above reasons, researchers, herbal and pharmaceutical companies, doctors, and practitioners are respectfully urged to avoid attempting to fit Āyurveda into the mold of modern medicine.

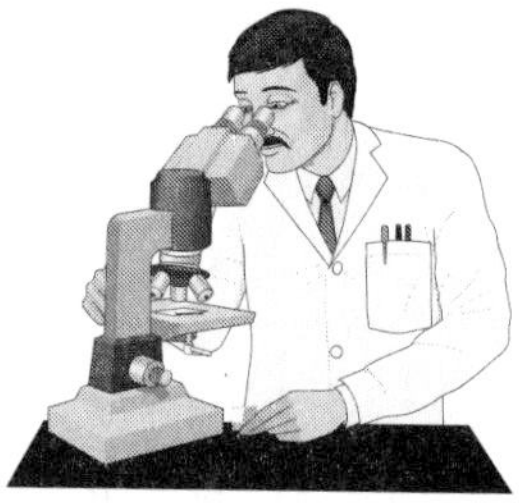

Research

Modern research has begun to investigate the power of prayer and meditation, low-fat vegetarian diets, and *haṭha yoga* exercises. The results of the research suggest that meditation or prayer, *yoga*, diet, and lifestyle changes play an effective role in the healing and prevention process. Further, scientific studies are underway on various Āyurvedic herbs to determine if the suggestions of the Āyurvedic texts are valid for people of this era. Diseases presently be researched using Āyurvedic herbs include the heart, liver, cholesterol, asthma, osteoarthritis, and AIDS.

Alternative Healing and Arteriosclerosis

Dr. Dean Ornish, in his book, *Reversing Heart Disease*, has discussed scientific studies he had conducted on reversing heart disease, specifically, coronary artery disease (CAD) or coronary arteriosclerosis. Because of his studies, the Mutual of Omaha Insurance Company and Oxford Health Insurance have begun to offer compensation for coronary heart patients who enroll in Dr. Ornish's heart therapy program.

In a 1-year, randomized, single-blind study, 28 patients were placed in an experimental group. They were given a low-fat vegetarian diet and stopped smoking cigarettes and drinking coffee. They also began various "stress management" routines (i.e., exercises of *haṭha yoga* stretching, *prāṇāyāma* breathing, moderate walking, relaxation and visualizations, and group support sessions). Another group of 20 patients comprised the control group. This latter group followed the currently recommended 30% fat reduction diet.

The experimental group improved significantly, whereas the control group actually grew worse. Specifically, in the experimental group there was a significant decrease in cholesterol. Other reductions include the frequency of angina, lesion size, and apolipoprotein B. The control group had increases in these areas.

Stress management measures may have proved effective owing to their ability to reduce emotional stress that stimulates the sympathetic nervous system. This increased stimulation may lead to chemical reactions that cause coronary problems and blood clots.

It may also be that a holistic healing approach (i.e., mediation, *haṭha yoga*, breathing, diet, group support) is a more effective way to recover and prevent coronary heart disease. This is because holistic health considers persons as a whole, beyond an isolated physical organ. For example, all the patients in the experimental group had a common feeling of isolation or emotional loneliness. Thus, a correlation may exist between emotional (e.g., a breaking heart) and physical health. Group support sessions helped remove the barriers causing emotional isolation.

Group support and the educationally motivating aspects of the holistic approach worked to inspire the experimental group to comply with the program.

Prayer, Meditation, and Healing

In Dr. Dossey's new book, *Healing Words*, he discusses various studies on the use of prayer and meditation by people to heal and prevent illness from occurring, or becoming worse.

In a randomized, double-blind study by Dr. Randolph Byrd, an experimental group of 192 coronary patients (versus 201 control coronary patients) arranged to have between 5 and 7 people praying for them daily over a 10-month period. No one prayed for the control group. The experimental group was five times less likely to require antibiotics and three times less likely to develop pulmonary edema. None of the experimental group needed artificial air tubes, whereas 12 people in the "unremembered" group had this need; and fewer people died in the experimental group (but this was not statistically significant). The study was widely respected, but inconclusive and requiring further research and a larger study group.

In another study by Braud and Schlitz, 62 people (influencers) were asked to perform healing on 271 subjects, whose health concerns ranged from overly emotional, hyperactivity, tension headaches, high blood pressure, and ulcers. The influencers were asked to perform mental imagery and self-calming techniques; depending upon the needs of the subjects. Influencers and subjects were located in different rooms in the same building (20 meters away). Thirteen experiments were performed. Results were strong, consistent, and replicable.

Dossey also mentioned the Spindrift group, who for more than 10 years has performed laboratory experiments suggesting that prayer helps healing. Two types of prayer were measured: directed (goal-oriented or image, i.e., praying for cancer to be cured) and nondirected (whatever is best for the patient, or 'let God's will be done'). They found that both methods work, but the nondirected approach was determined to be more powerful. These findings suggest that a person need not know how the healing process occurs, but pray for healing to occur, however it is best for the patient.

Dr. Dossey cites a study by Dr. Daniel Benor who investigated 131 studies on spiritual healing done before 1990 (mostly nonhuman studies). In 56 of the studies, the positive findings were said to be 1 in 100 to result from chance. In another 56 studies, between 2 and 5 in 100 were said to result from chance.

Benor found in 151 out of 194 fungus cultures that growth was inhibited or retarded after 15 minutes of concentration. This took place from about 1.5 yards distance away from the fungus. This study was replicated when distances increased from 1e to 15 miles away from the fungus cultures. Results were replicated in 16 experiments. Another study found people with no known healing abilities to retard and stimulate significant bacterial culture. Other studies demonstrated the ability to inhibit cancer cells in simple organisms (e.g., one-celled algae, paramecia, moth larvae), plants, and animals.

In light of this research, the relevance and effectiveness of Āyurvedic therapies of meditation, nutrition, *haṭha yoga*, *prāṇāyāma* in healing and preventing modern-day illness is most encouraging. It suggests that medical technological developments do not imply a more advanced culture in terms of healing. Rather, it suggests that the ancient healers were as adept (or more so) in healing and preventing illness. This wisdom was lost or overlooked for some time.

In the coming decade, much scientific research should validate the use and need for a more spiritual and holistic approach to true healing. It is more than likely that Āyurvedic wisdom will play a significant role in this regard.

Āyurveda, Allopathy, and Health Care

As discussed earlier, not only might alternative, natural, Āyurvedic care be a useful complement to Western medicine in terms of healing, but it can also be financially practical. In a recent Yoga Journal article about Dr. Ornish's "reversing heart disease" program, the difference in cost between traditional heart care and a holistic approach, such as Dr. Ornish's, was staggering. Heart bypass operations cost about $43,000, and the process of opening the arteries through surgery (angioplasty) costs around $18,000. Cholesterol lowering medicine alone, such as Lovastatin, can cost up to $1,500 a year per person. When compared with the $3,500 cost of Ornish's 12-week program, it is enough to make any hospital administrator think twice, and in fact, it has. David M. Liff, the Program Development Consultant for Dean Ornish's program said that they are inundated with requests from clinics around the United States to set up the heart disease reversal programs. It is interesting to note that the main Āyurvedic herb for cholesterol, *guggul*, may only cost $150 for an entire year; making this the most cost-effective cholesterol program.

As more favorable research emerges on holistic healing alternatives for modern diseases, hospital administrators will want to expand their alternative healing programs to include other diseases as well.

Āyurvedic Research

In the Garden of Life, by Naveen Patnaik, several studies on Āyurvedic herbs are discussed.

Brāhmī (gotu kola) was used in a double-blind clinical test on 30 mentally retarded children (free from epilepsy and other neurological conditions). The study attempted to see if there was an effect on their mental abilities. The results suggested that there was a significant improvement in both general mental ability and behavioral patterns after only 12 weeks.

Punarnavā (hogweed) was found to be an effective therapy for nephritic syndrome (kidney) in 22 patients, producing an increased flow of urine, reducing edema, and in an overall improvement of albumin urea, serum protein rise, and decreases in serum cholesterol levels.

Guggul (Indian bedellium) was used in preliminary tests on 22 patients having hypercholesterolemia, associated with obesity, ischemic heart disease, hypertension, and diabetes. In all cases, the total serum cholesterol and serum lipid phosphorus levels diminished. A significant decrease in weight was found in 10 of the patients. In later studies involving 12 cases, *guggul* was found to reduce serum turbidity and prolong coagulation in all instances.

Other Āyurvedic Research

Brāhmi (gotu kola; Centella asiatica or hydrocotyle asiatica)

This herb was found to be useful for cirrhosis of the liver, periodontal disease, peripheral vascular disease, scleroderma, vascular fragility, enhanced wound healing, enhanced connective tissue structure of the vascular sheath, and reduced sclerosis or hardening. It was found to reduce feelings of heaviness in the lower legs, numbness, nighttime cramps, swellings, spider veins and skin ulcers, vein distensibility, and improve blood flow through affected limbs in 80% of patients in clinical trials.

Brāhmī has been found to relieve depression, anxiety, mental fatigue, and enhance memory. [Journal of Research in Āyurveda and Saddai: 1980]

It has also been helping mentally handicapped and emotionally disturbed children. [Indian Journal of Psychiatry: 1977]

It has been found helpful in treating cirrhosis. [Sem. Hop. Paris 55(37-8):1749-50, 1979]

Brāhmī has been reported to heal brain tumors as well. [Herbal Gram No. 36]

Harītakī (Terminalia chebula), *Keṣharāja* (Eclipta alba), *Tulsī* (Ocimum sanctum) were found to be useful antibacterial herbs. *Harītakī* was the strongest and had the widest spectrum of antibacterial activity. *Keṣharāja* had the second widest spectrum of effect. Additionally, salmonella was treated by *harītakī*. Shigella was treated by *harītakī* and *keṣharaja*. [Indian Journal of Medical Sciences. 43 (5):113-7, 1988 May]

Āmalakī (Emblica officinalis, Gaertn.) was studied in normal and hyper-cholesterololemic men. The herb was taken for 28 days. Both normal and hypercholesterolemic subjects showed a decrease in cholesterol levels. Two weeks after stopping the therapy, the total serum cholesterol levels of the hypercholersterolemic subjects rose significantly, almost to initial levels. [European Journal of Clinical Nutrition. 42 (11): 939-44, 1988 Nov.]

Neem (Azadirachta indica ADR) and Turmeric (Curcuma longa) were tested to heal chronic ulcers (external) and scabies. They were used as a paste in 814 persons. 97% of the people were cured within 3-15 days. There were no toxic or adverse reactions. [Tropical and Geographical Medicine 44 (1-2): 178-81, 1992 Jan.]

Śhatāvarī (Asparagus racemosus) was used to test dyspepsia and as a galactogogue. It was compared with a modern drug (metoclopramide) which is used in dyspepsia to reduce gastric emptying time. The gastric emptying half-time was studied in 8 healthy males. *Śhatāvarī* was found to work as effectively as the allopathic drug. [Postgraduate Medicine 36(2): 91-4, 1990 April]

Aśhwagandhā (Withania somnifera, stem of *Shallaki* (Boswellia serrata, rhizomes of Turmeric (Curcuma longa) and a zinc complex (Articulin-F) were studied in a randomized, double-blind, placebo-controlled, crossover study in persons with osteoarthritis. First, a 1-month single blind study on 42 persons with osteoarthritis was conducted. Persons were randomly allocated to receive either the herbs or a placebo for a period of 3 months. After a 15-day "wash out" period, the two groups switched therapies for another 3 months. Evaluations were given every 14 days based on pain severity, morning stiffness, Ritchie articular index, joint score, disability score, and grip strength. Erythrocyte (red blood cell) sedimentation rate was monitored and radiological examinations were compared. The herbs were found to cause a significant drop in the severity of pain ($P = .001$) and a disability score ($P = .05$). No significant changes were noted in either group from the radiological assessment. [Journal of Ethnopharmacology. 33 (1-2) 91-5, 1991 May-June]

In another study, the adaptogenic mechanism of *aśhwagandhā* was compared to ginseng. A 40-day double-blind study found *aśhwagandhā* equal or better than ginseng in the areas of improved problem solving, physical performance, and reaction time in healthy volunteers. [Indian Medicine: 3 (2,3): 1-5, 1991 April-July]

The effects of *aśhwagandhā* were again measured in a double-blind study on 101 healthy persons, aged 50 to 59 years old. After taking *aśhwagandhā* for 1 year the volunteers showed significantly reduced signs of aging compared with the placebo group. Anti-aging was found in areas of increased melanin (hair pigment that declines with age that is responsible for graying) and significantly lower levels of calcium loss (measured in the nails) than the control group. [Journal of Research in Āyurveda and Saddai: 247-258, 1980 - Kuppurajan, K., et al.]

Aśhwagandhā has also been found to relieve a reactive form of depression. [Journal of Research in Āyurveda and Saddai, 1989]

Guḍūchī (Tinospora cordifolia) was tested for its immunosuppression activity associated with deranged hepatic function and sepsis resulting from poor surgical outcomes. Preliminary studies suggested *guḍūchī* contains hepatoprotective and immunomodulatory properties in surgical outcomes in patients with malignant obstructive jaundice. This follow-up study tested 30 patients, randomly divided into two groups (matched with respect to clinical features, impairment of hepatic function, as judged by liver function testes including antipyrine elimination, and immunosuppression/phagocytic capacities of neutrophils). The first group received conventional treatment, namely, vitamin K, antibiotics, and biliary drainage. Group two also received *guḍūchī* (16 mg/kg/day orally) during their biliary drainage. Hepatic function was comparable in the two groups after drainage, but the phagocytic and killing capacities of neutrophils were normalized only in persons receiving *guḍūchī*. Clinical evidence of septicemia was observed in 50% of patients in group one, whereas none was found in the second group ($P = .05$). Postoperative survival in groups one and two were 40% and 92.4%, respectively ($P = .01$). The conclusion drawn was that *gudūchī* appears to improve surgical outcomes by strengthening host defenses. [Indian Journal of Gastroenterology. 12(1) :5-8, 1993 Jan.]

Turmeric (Curcuma longa) has been found to be a strong antioxidant, anti-inflammatory, antiviral, antibacterial, antifungal, anticancer, and a detoxifying herb. [Planta Med., 57: 1-7, 1991]

Other research has found that turmeric's active ingredient, circuminoids, have significant antioxidant activities in both prevention and intervention. [Nutracon 95; Majeed, M., and Badmaev, V.]. It was also found useful for the treatment of rheumatoid arthritis minus side effects. [Ind. J Med Res 71:632-4, 1980)]

Triphalā (*Āmalakī* (Emblica Offic.), *Harītakī* (Terminalia chebula), *Bibhītakī* (Terminalia bellerica) have been found to improve digestion, absorb nutrients, and assist the body's metabolism. It is also useful for psychosomatic conditions that affect the gastrointestinal tract. [Journal of Ethnopharmacology, 1990]

Bhūmiāmalakī (Phyllanthus amarus) was tested in persons with chronic active hepatitis resulting from the chronic hepatitis B virus. In a 30-day study, a significant number of persons using *bhūmiāmalakī* were rid of the viral antigen compared with the placebo group. [Lancet, 1988]

Arjuna (Terminalia arjuna), *Bibhītakī*, and *Harītakī* helps protect the heart muscle. [Indian Drugs: 1990]

Pippalī (Piper longum), alone or in *tṛikatu*, has been found to relieve asthma and chronic bronchitis. One study measured 240 children of various ages who frequently had bronchial asthma. *Pippalī* was found to reduce the frequency and severity of attacks. [Indian Drugs: 1984]

Balā (Sida cordifolia) has also been found to effectively relieve bronchitis and asthma. [Lancet: 1984]

Guggul (Gugulipid- Commiphora mukul), was found useful in healing acne vulgaris [Indian Journal of Dermatology Leprol 56(1):381-3, 1990] and atherosclerosis (cholesterol reduction). HDL cholesterol gradually increased, whereas VLDL and LDL cholesterol significantly decreased [J Assoc Phys India 37(5):323-8, 1989; Indian J Med Res 87:356-60, 1988]

The active components of gugulipid is Z-guggulesterone and E-guggulesterone. This active ingredient has been found to prevent Pitta- (heat) related side effects, caused by using the pure, whole resin. If Pitta conditions develop, it is useful to research *kaiṣhore guggul*—Pitta-reducing *guggul*. In this way, the benefits of avoiding side effects as well as using the whole resin may be simultaneously accomplished.

Licorice (Glycyrrhiza glabra), has been found to be effective in healing eczema [Br. J Clin. Pract. 12:269-79, 1958], peptic ulcer [Hepatogastroenterol 32(6):293-5, 1985], duodenal and gastric ulcer [Scand J Gasterenterol suppl. 65:85-91, 1980], and dental plaque [Isr J Dent Sci 2(3):153-7, 1989].

Licorice may cause some side effects when taken alone for more than 6 weeks. It may increase sodium and water retention, hypertension, hypokalemia, and suppress the renin-aldosterone system. Monitoring blood pressure and electrolytes and increasing potassium intake is suggested. However, in Āyurveda these side effects can be avoided by mixing licorice in warm milk. To date, we have not found any studies measuring this formula.

Cranberry (Vaccinium macrocarpon)- Drinking cranberry juice has been found to effectively treat urinary tract infections [JAMA 271:751-4, 1994; J. Naturopathic Med 2(1):45-7, 1991; Southwest Med. 47(1):17-20, 1966; Wisconsin Med. J. 61:282, 1962]

It has also been found helpful in kidney stone conditions, reducing the amount of ionized calcium in the urine [Urology 1(1):67-70, 1973]

Īśhabgol (Plantago ovata) was found to help irritable bowel syndrome—diarrhea: [Acta Gastroenterol Latinoam 17(4):317-23, 1987; Ir Med J 76(5):253, 1983]. It has also been helpful for constipation. [Gut 28(11):1510-13, 1987]

Īśhabgol was found to be useful for treatment of anal fissure (except in cases of advanced anal stenosis). [Dis. Colon Rectum, 21: 8, 1978 Nov-Dec, 582-3]

When mixed with food, *īśhabgol* was found to reduce blood glucose responses. [J Am Coll Nutr, 10: 4, 1991 Aug, 364-71]

Ginger (Zingiber officinale) has been found to reduce gastrointestinal complaints, atherosclerosis, headache, nausea, vomiting, and vertigo (numerous studies, including [Anaesthesia 45(8):669-71, 1990; Acta Otolaryngol 105(1-2):45-9, 1988], osteoarthritis [Med Hypothesis 39:342-8, 1992], rheumatic pain, and rheumatoid arthritis [Med Hypothesis 39:342-8, 1992; Med

Hypothesis 29:25-8, 1989; ORL J Otorhinolaryngol Relat Spec, 48: 5, 1986, 282-6]. It was also found to contain high levels of anti-oxidants. [Chung Kuo Chung Yao Tsa Chih, 17: 6, 1997 Jun, 36809, 373 backcover]

Garcinia Spp. (Malabar Tamarind) may help reduce obesity. The dried fruit contains 20-30% of the active ingredient (-)Hydroxycitric acid (HCA). [Arch Biochem Biophys 135:209-17, 1969; J Biol Chem 245:599, 1970]. HCA has been found to divert glucose from being used as building blocks of fatty tissue and increase the body's supply of stored glucose, called glycogen. Glycogen also turns off food cravings. [Alt. Comp. Ther. 1(4) 212-215, 1995]. In another study, insulin requirements for persons with diabetes mellitis decreased along with fasting blood glucose and glycosylated hemoglobin (HbA1c), and glycosylated plasma protein levels. Serum lipids returned to near normal levels with GS water soluble extract, glycosylated hemoglobin, and glycosylated plasma protein levels remained higher than control group. Enhances indogenous insulin. [J Ethnopharmacol, 30: 3, 1990 Oct, 281-94]

Gurmar (Gymnema sylvestre) was found to remove sweetness from bittersweet mixtures, increasing bitterness. [J Comp Physiol Psychol, 93: 3, 1979 June, 538-47]. In another study *gurmar* reduced sweet cravings. [Physiol Behav, 30: 1, 1983 Jan, 1-9]

Research by Disease

In the book, *Botanical Influences on Illness* by Werbach and Murray, research is cited on foods and herbs that help various disorders. Some of the following were described earlier in this book.

Atherosclerosis: (including coronary heart disease) Foods and herbs found to help these conditions (in scientific research) include alfalfa, artichoke, eggplant, berberine (from barberry), curcumin (from turmeric), fenugreek, garlic, onion, ginger, gugulipid, and garcinia camboga (Malabar Tamarind).

Bronchial Asthma: Numerous studies have found herbs that help ease this condition including, aloe vera, coleus forskohlii (containing forskolin), licorice, onion, picrorrhiza kurroa (*kaṭukā*)

Cancer: Research has found many useful herbs for healing cancer, including barberry root (berberine), garlic, onions, and turmeric.

Diabetes: Herbs and foods found to be helpful in diabetes include aloe vera, bitter melon (momordica charantia/*Kerala*), fenugreek (Trigonella foenum graecum/methi), *Gurmar*, (gymnema sylvestre/*Śharkunikha*)

Psoriasis: Two herbs found useful in treating this condition are *Bākuchī* (psoralea corylifolia) [Pharmac Ther 34:75-97, 1987] and sarsaparilla (Smilax sarsaparilla) [Br J dermatol 108:33-7, 1983; N Engl J Med 227:128-33, 1942]. *Bākuchī* has also been found effective in treating vitiligo [Pharmac Ther 34:75-97, 1987].

Collaborative Research

Several cooperative studies between Zandu Pharmaceutical Works, Bombay India and various research institutions are discussed below. The herbs contained in the following formulas are readily available from many sources. This author is grateful for Zandu for making these studies available.

Diabetes: One formula that includes *gurmar*, neem, and *śhilājit* was tested on 20 persons with proved maturity onset of diabetes over an 8-week period. Eighteen persons had hereditary histories of diabetes. Ten people were randomly chosen as a control group. Both groups followed certain dietary restrictions.

All 10 people taking the herbal formula reported subjective, as well as objective improvement of all symptoms (polyphagia, polyuria, polydypsia, excessive sweating, dryness of throat, numbness, fatigue, weakness, and constipation). Objective and subjective symptoms of the control group remained the same or increased.

The group taking the herbal product) experienced decreased mean blood sugar values, dropping from 204.1 mg/dL before the study to 119.65 mg/dL at the end of the study. The mean blood sugar levels levels in the control group rose from 189 mg/dL before the study to 205 mg/dL at the end of the study.

Effects of a Herbomineral Compound on Diabitis by K. N. C. Pal. Ayurved Samachar: Issue 8; vol 10 2 Feb. 1988

Indigestion: A group of 20 general practitioners tested a digestive herbal in their private practices for 15 days on patients with anorexia, nausea, vomiting, heaviness in the chest, heaviness in the body, burning sensation, and constipation. Patients were clinically assessed after the 4th, 7th, 11th, and 15th days of treatment. The herbal product included cumin, *asafoetida*, cinnamon, cardamom, ginger, *pippalī*, coriander (*dhanyāka*), *musta*, and *triphalā*.

Significant improvement ($p < 0.001$) was seen in all clinical symptoms and signs.

Effects of Ayurvedic Drug (AB + R) in Indigestion. Thakur, M. Bhatt, N.S. Mishra S. et. al. Medicine & Surgery. May - August '96/23

Schizophrenia: A herbal product including *śhankapuṣhpī, brāhmī, aśhwagandhā, yaṣhtī madhu, vachā*, and *sarpagandha* was administered to 17 schizophrenia patients taking medication and 22 patients not taking any medication for six weeks. Approximately 50% of both groups showed more than 50% improvement on the Brief Psychiatric Rating Scale. The herbs were relatively free from side effects.

Evaluation of Indigenous Psychotoropic Drugs - A Preliminary Study. Parikh, M.D., Pradhan, P.V., Shah, L.P., Bagadia, V.N. Journ. Res. Ay. Sid. Vol 5; no. 1-4 pp. 12-17

Urinary Tract Infections: A total of 51 inpatients and outpatients with various urinary tract symptoms (pain, burning, fever, frequency, blood in urine) was tested for 45 days using an herbal product that included *guḍūchī, haridrā, bilwa*, and *karella* (bitter melon). Patients were monitored every 15 days.

After 15 days, 50% of the patients began to show reduction of symptoms. At the end of 30 days more than 75% of the patients were symptom-free. By the end of the study only 3 patients (6%) had painful or burning urination. Since modern antibiotic therapy cannot always guarantee long-term benefits, these herbs offer encouraging options to healing urinary tract infections. Further, these herbs did not cause any side effects, even after 2 months of use.

Clinical Trial of Ayurvedic Drug U-144 (K-4 Tablets) in Urinary Tract Infections. Deshpande, P.J., Singh Raman, Bhatt, N.S. The Medicine & Surgery. Vol. 32; no. 10/11. Oct. - Nov. 1944

Liver/Bile Disorders: Forty-five persons who developed liver- and bile-related disorders following surgery were given an herbal product containing *punarnavā, bhṛingarāj, chirāyatā, arogyavardhini* ,and *mandur bhasma* (iron ash) for 45 days. Seven patients had cholecystectomy, 21 previous gall bladder operations, 12 hepatitis, and 5 T-tube biliary drainage following cholecystectomy. Subjects were monitored every 15 days.

Measurements after herbal therapy revealed increased liver function and control of hepatitis. Biliary flow was restored. Associated symptoms of nausea, dyspepsia, pain, tenderness, vomiting, belching, anorexia, vertigo, fever, swelling, constipation, weakness, and flatulence were alleviated in all subjects except for 1 symptom of jaundice and 3 signs of weakness. Four of the five biliary T-tube drainage cases showed definite increase in the biliary flow.

Clinical Effect of an Ayurvedic Drug L 2002 on Hepatobiliary Disorders. Deshpande, P.J., Singh, R., Bhatt, N.S. Journal of NIMA, December 1994.

Music Research

The India Currents Magazine reports of scientific research involving music to heal heart disease and high blood pressure. Researchers in Berlin played music by Ravi Śhankar, Strauss, and modernist H. W. Henze for 40 heart patients. Blood samples and stress levels of patients were measured before and after listening to the music.

The results were reported at the European Society of Cardiology in Amsterdam. Strauss' music lowered stress hormones in the patients. However, levels were even lower after listening to the *sitar* music of Ravi Śhankar. Blood pressure also reduced after listening to his music. By contrast, the modern music raised stress levels.

Pañcha Karma Research

Rheumatoid arthritis: During the 1970s at Benares Hindu University, *piṇḍa sveda* was found to relieve pain, swelling, stiffness, and swollen joints caused by rheumatoid arthritis within 1 week of treatment. Patients' body weight (formally underweight) was also increased to healthier levels. Measurements involved ease of walking, gripping, pressing power with both hands and body weight.

Chronic rheumatoid arthritis and bronchial asthma: Two groups of patients were administered *vamana* and *virechana*, followed by *saṃsarjana* diet. One group suffered from chronic rheumatoid arthritis. The other group had bronchial asthma.

Both groups of patients received 3 days of *snehapāna* (ingesting oil or *ghee*),whole body *sveda* for the next 3 days, *vamana,* and *virechana*, followed by the *saṃsarjana* diet. Within 1 week post therapy measurements of physical, physiological, and biochemical parameters of the patients were taken.

All rheumatoid arthritis patients showed statistically significant improvements in ease of walking, and gripping power and pressing power (in both hands) ($P < 0.05$). Asthmatic patients showed a statistically significant increase in vital capacity and length of time to hold the breath ($P < 0.05$). Biochemically, a statistically significant reduction in D-xylose ($P < 0.001$) caused improved gastrointestinal absorption capacity.

Current OAM-NIH Studies

The Office of Alternative Medicine, a part of the National Institutes of Health has funded several currently ongoing Āyurveda and yoga studies. Topics include Parkinsonism, general promotion of health, and yoga therapy for heroin addiction.

Āyurveda at Columbia University

In November 1994, the *Dharma Hinduja Indic Research Center* held its first 2-day conference in New York at Columbia University. It was entitled *Health, Science and the Spirit: Veda and Āyurveda in the Western World.* Āyurvedic Doctors from India and the U.S. met and spoke with Western allopathic doctors, professors, and students from universities across the country including Harvard, Columbia, New York University.

One aim of the conference was to have Āyurvedic and allopathic medical professionals work together to develop valid scientific research on healing through Āyurvedic herbs and *pañcha karma*. The scientific validation of the ancient Āyurvedic practices appears imminent.

Since this conference, Columbia has begun offering weekend symposia with Āyurvedic doctors several times a year. They have also embarked on scientific research projects.

The scientific community is beginning to study the effects of Āyurvedic therapies. It would also be interesting to test Āyurvedic therapies on diseases that are presently considered unhealable. The advantages to healing through Āyurveda include no side effects, inexpensive treatment, and dramatically lower health care costs. Already, several health insurance companies across the U.S. are covering customers for Āyurvedic consultations.

Modern-Day Challenges for Future Generations

One reason Āyurveda is so effective is that it is a living science; it addresses new diseases and provides appropriate therapies continually. The use of mercury as a powerful rejuvenative was introduced in the 14th century. Minerals were first used in Āyurveda in the 16th century. To accommodate new developments and discoveries, Āyurveda also adapts and adjusts.

In the early 20th century, the effects of the industrial revolution's such as water and air pollution had a significant impact on the health of the wildlife, nature and humans-including infants and fetuses. In time, a growing body of research would show that the development and use of chemicals (e.g., those used for pesticides and plastics) and drugs had also added to the poisoning of the planet and its creatures, manifesting as a sharp increase in the incidence of cancer, asthma, neurologic and immune disorders, and physical deformities in children. Research suggests that there is a link between chemicals, environmental pollutants, and certain diseases. Today depletion of soil nutrients and erosion of soil, air and water pollution due to unnatural farming methods and deforestation continues.

Modern Āyurveda must address these trends and their consequences. Although Āyurveda can address the symptoms, such as using herbs to remove toxins from the body, the scope of healing must be expanded to address issues that currently are being overlooked, such as the poor nutrient quality of food, air, and water. Today, disease prevention includes eating organic foods to avoid harmful preservatives and insecticides.

In the book, Our Stolen Future, the authors suggested that the use of man-made products has contributed to the ill health of wildlife and humans. Detergents, drugs (i.e., synthetic estrogen), industrial chemical waste, agricultural pesticides and runoff, pesticides, and cooking vessels and containers made of plastics or other unnatural products may also be poisoning our children, unbalancing their hormones, and interfering on the genetic and neuronal levels.

Therefore, the substances that contaminate our food bear examination. The authors report that damage from these hormone-disrupting chemicals is most clearly seen in the offspring of women exposed to the pollutants during the first months of pregnancy.

Āyurvedic Healing of Environmental Toxins

If we address the three areas of the body that are most critically affected by environmental pollutants-the brain and the reproductive and immune systems-we can apply Āyurvedic therapies discussed earlier. The following therapies are listed according to condition-not according to one's *doṣha*. Therefore, doṣha must also be considered before choosing these suggestions.

Herbs

Hormonal/Reproductive: *Aṣhwagandhā*, yam (*vārāhīkānd*), *śhatāvarī* and *yogaraj guggul*
Liver detox: *Bhūāmalakī* (main herb), *kuṭki* (for chemical and biological poisoning), barberry, *chirāyatā*, *triphalā*, *mahāsudarṣhan*, neem, *musta* and *mañjiṣhṭhā*.
Toning: *Āmalakī, bākuchī* and *bhṛiṅgarāj*

Massage

Hormones: Releases growth hormones; massage (especially between eyebrows, neck and top of head; just below navel [*basti*], reproductive organ area [*guda*])
Liver: Elbow and knee joints, throat, heart and navel

Foods

Hormones: Organic foods (has no hormones added)-B6 vitamin (found in buckwheat, beans, carrots, brown rice); tofu (female hormones); thyroid: sea vegetables, watercress oats, green foods such as wheatgrass juice or powder.
Liver: Organic foods-cherries, figs, grapes, melons, papayas, pears, pineapples, raspberries, artichokes, beets, bitter melon, avocado, beans, Brussels sprouts, mung sprouts, celery, watercress, barley, corn, mung beans, ghee, fenugreek,

B2 vitamin (found in millet, soy, whole wheat, wheat germ, beans, milk, nuts, dark greens, molasses), green foods such as wheatgrass juice or powder.

Yoga Poses
Hormones: Siddhāyogāsana/siddha yoni āsana, cow pose, any of the spinal twist poses, shoulder stand, fish pose and tortoise
Liver: *Siddhāyogāsana/siddha yoni āsana,* lotus pose, any bow pose, spinal twist, tortoise and fish

Breathing Exercises (prāṇāyāma)
Hormones: *Śhītkarī kumbhaka* (hissing breath exercise) and solar *prāṇāyāma*
Liver: *Śhītkarī kumbhaka,* frontal brain cleanse

Bandhas & Mūdras
Jālandhara bandha (throat lock), *mūla bandha, mahā bheda mūdra*

Miscellaneous
Purgation for liver cleansing. Aromatherapy—iris and gardenia for the liver.

Āyurveda and Environmental Food Considerations

Why buy Organic?

Organic foods are preferred for two reasons: personal and environmental health. In both cases, the concern is not so much for adults, but for children and parents who plan to have children-the concern is for future generations of people and the future of the planet.

The Organic Trade Association offer the following reasons one should buy organic foods:

1. Organic products meet stringent standards.
2. Organic certification is the public's assurance that products have been grown and handled according to strict procedures without persistent toxic chemicals.
3. Organic food has more flavor.
4. Well-balanced soils nourish strong healthy plants. Many chefs use organic foods in their recipes because they taste better.
5. Organic production reduces health risks.
6. Many Environmental Protection Agency (EPA)-approved pesticides were registered long before extensive research linked these chemicals to cancer and other diseases. Organic agriculture does not release additional chemicals into the air, earth, and water.
7. Organic farms protect water resources.
8. Eliminating polluting chemicals and nitrogen leaching in combination with soil building protects and conserves water resources. Water makes up two-thirds of our body mass and covers three-fourths of the planet. In the US, the EPA estimates that pesticides (including cancer-causing pesticides) have contaminated groundwater in 38 states, thus polluting the primary drinking water source for more than half the country's population.
9. Organic farmers build soil rather than deplete it.
10. Soil is the main focus of organic farming. We are facing the worst topsoil erosion in history owing to chemical intensive, mono-crop farming. The Soil Conservation Service estimates that more than 3 billion tons of topsoil are eroded from US croplands each year. This means that soil is eroding seven times faster than it is being replaced.
11. Organic farmers work in harmony with naature, respecting the balance required of a healthy ecosystem: wildlife is encouraged by including forage crops in rotation and by retaining fence rows, wetlands, and other natural areas.
12. Organic farmers have led the way, largely at their own expense, with innovative on-farm research aimed at minimizing the impact that agriculture has on the environment.
13. Organic producers strive to preserve diver sity. The loss of a large variety of species (biodiversity) is one of our most pressing environmental concerns. Organic farmers and gardeners have been collecting and preserving

seeds, and growing unusual varieties for decades.

14. Organic farming helps keep rural communities healthy.
15. The USDA predicts that by the year 2,000, half of the US farm production will come from 1% of farms. Organic farming may be one of the few survival tactics left for the family farm and the rural community.
16. Every food category has an organic alternative. Even non-food crops are also being grown organically, including cotton.

For further information contact:
The Organic Trade Association
PO Box 1078
Greenfield, MA 01302 USA
Phone 413-774-7511
Web: http://www.ota.com

Āyurveda and Environmental Home Safety An Ounce of Prevention

In addition to buying and eating organic foods, we can further avoid polluting our home environment. Below is a list of household and office products that should be avoided and possible substitutes for them. For further information, read Debra Dadd's book, *Home, Safe Home*. The book also gives many homemade ingredients for most healthy product substitutes.

Suburban homeowners use more pesticides per acre on their lawns than farmers use on their fields

Instead of using toxic pesticides, many pests can be eliminated using natural products, such as cayenne pepper, strong mint tea, vacuuming, and

Harmful Products	Helpful Substitutes
Nonorganic fertilizer	Organic fertilizer, home compost, organic seeds. Flower, vegetable, fruit, lawn & tree pesticide sprays Neem and other natural pesticides, traps, noise repellants, ladybugs. Certain flowers and plants can be used to repel insects.
Toxic weed killers	Grow and eat your own dandelions (provided they have not been sprayed with harmful substances).
Genetically engineered foods	Naturally grown foods
Cleaning products, such as ammonia, aerosol propellants, detergents, ethanol, synthetic fragrances, lye, chlorine, artificial dyes, detergents, fluorescent brighteners, cresol, phenol, formaldehyde, petroleum distillates, sulfur compounds; ammonia (and all purpose cleansers), basin, tub, tile cleaners; bleach, dishwasher detergents & liquids; disinfectants, drain cleaners, fabric softeners, glass cleaners, laundry detergent & starch; mold & mildew cleaners, rug, carpet & upholstery shampoo; scouring powder, shoe polish, silver/metal polishes, spot remover, water softeners	Homemade ingredients (see *Home Safe Home* by Dadd) or buy all these products in natural forms at health food stores

keeping a clean home. Check your health food store for safe products, including termite, rat and mouse prevention products.

Problem	Natural Solutions
Ants	patchouli, chili pepper, paprika, dried peppermint, lemon juice; grow mint near entrances
Cockroaches	borax, bay leaves, eucalyptus oil
Flies	cloves, lavender, patchouli, *vāsāka* (Āyurvedic herb)
Beetles/ weevils	add bay leaf to food products; use black pepper sacks in food bins
Mosquitoes	*vāsāka*, lavender, patchouli
Miscellaneos bugs and insects	lavender, eucalyptus, *vāsāka*
Moths	patchouli
Gnats	patchouli
Fleas	*vāsāka*

Personal Care

Use natural deodorants, cosmetics, bath products, body oils and powders, toothpastes, mouthwash, soaps, air fresheners, hair sprays, shampoos, hair coloring, hairspray, skin moisturizers, shaving cream.

Nonorganic personal care products have numerous toxic chemicals, including aerosol propellants, benzyl alcohol, artificial colors, synthetic fragrance, formaldehyde, ammonia, ethanol, glycerin, detergents, plastics, paraffin, saccharin, BHA-BHT. Substitutes found in health food stores contain none of these chemical toxins.

Miscellaneous

Air purifiers: Basil or tulsī (natural negative ion machines), cedar, frankincense, sandalwood, *agnihotra (Vedic* fire rituals).
Plastic containers: Leach chemicals into the liquids. Use glass, stainless steel or ceramic containers instead.
Cooking utensils: Cast iron, stainless steel, copper are best; non-stick and aluminum pans leech toxic chemicals into the food (aluminum foil is also not advised).
Fabrics: Use natural fibers like cotton, linen and wool. Ideally organic, dye-free fabric is best for the skin, and for the earth. Products include clothing, towels, sheets, bedding, blankets, pillows,
Paper products: computer, typing, note and bathroom paper, and paper towels that are recycled and acid-free is safest for the environment. The dyes used to whiten paper also pollute the environment.
Shopping: Carry cotton bags to the store to use instead of paper and plastic (or at least reuse the paper and plastic bags). Some health food stores also sell re-useable bags to carry fruit and vegetables in.
Other Products: Baby products, office, art and computer supplies; building & furnishing products, pet care, recycling garbage.

Conclusion

In summary, the underlying notion of Āyurveda is to cause no harm to oneself, others, animals, or to nature. This basic *Vedic* tenet of nonviolence is followed in action, word and thought. This is accomplished by accepting all people and paths in life and quickly leads to peace, self-worth, appreciation and respect for all things. May you, dear readers, find and live in growing health and divinity, seeing the Divine in all.

ॐ शान्तिः शान्तिः शान्तिः

Aum śhānti, śhānti, śhānti
Peace in the body, mind and soul.
Peace on earth.

Appendix 1: Sanskrit Alphabet

Vowels

अ	आ	इ	ई	उ	ऊ
A	Ā	I	Ī	U	Ū

ए	ए	ओ	औ	अ	अः
E	AI	O	AU	AṄ	AḤ

ऋ	ॠ	ऌ
Ṛ	Ṝ	ḶṚ

Pronunciation

A as in rural; Ā as in father
I as in lily; Ī as in police
U as in push; Ū as in rude
E as in they; AI as in aisle
O as in home; AU as in house
AṆ as in thong
AḤ as in aha (accent the 'h')
Ṛ as in merrily; Ṝ as in marine (harder 'r')
ḶṚ as in revelry

Consonants

Gutterals (back of throat)	क Ka	ख Kha	ग Ga	घ Gha	ङ Ṅa
Palatals (back or soft palate)	च Cha	छ Chha	ज Ja	झ Jha	ञ Ñya
Cerebrals (tongue on top palate)	ट Ṭa	ठ Ṭha	ड Ḍa	ढ Ḍha	ण Ṇa
Dentals (tongue on teeth)	त Ta	थ Tha	द Da	ध Dha	न Na
Labials (Lips)	प Pa	फ Pha	ब Ba	भ Bha	म Ma

Consonant Pronunciation

Ka as in kite; Kha as in inkhole
Ga as in go; Gha as in loghouse
Ṅ as in pink (nasal sound)

Cha as in charge; Chha as in Curchill (hard 'h')
Ja as in joy; Jha as in hejhog (hedgehog)
Ñ as in hinge

Ṭa as in trust; Ṭha as in anthill
Ḍa as in drum; Ḍha as in redhorn
Ṇ as in one

Ta as in top; Tha as in hothouse (tongue/teeth)
Da as in dye; Dha as in adhere
Na as in nine

Pa as in poet; Pha as in uphill
Ba as in boat; Bha as in abhor
Ma as in mother

Semivowels

य	र	ल	व
Ya	Ra	La	Va

Sibilants (Hard) and Aspirate (Soft)

श	ष	स	ह
Śha	Ṣha	Sa	Ha

Miscellaneous Combinations

कि	की	कु	कू	के	कै	कौ	को
Ki	Kī	Ku	Kū	Ke	Kai	Kau	Ko

When vowels are written with consonants they look as above (using K as an example, such as kit, kola, etc.)

क + य = क्य (right side of ka is shortened)
क + ष = क्ष (kṣha)

ग + द = ग्द (gda - the vertical bar is removed. This is true for all consonants with bars cha (घ) ñya (ञ), 'a (ख), ta (त), tha (थ), dha (ध), na (न), प त्रप), ba (ब), bha (भ), ma (म), and semi vowels ya (य) la (ल), and va (व).

Other common combinations are

त + र = त्र Ta + Ra = Tra	र + उ = रु Ra + U = Ru
ज + ञ = ज्ञ	क + त = क्त
Ja + Ña = Jña *(pronounced gña)*	Ka + Ta = Kta
द + य = द्य Da + Ya = Dya	द + ध = द्ध Da + Dha = Ddha

Many more combinations exist, but this book is about Āyurveda, not Sanskrit. This brief introduction is merely to offer some basic guidance to those wishing to understand the Sanskrit in this text.

Appendix 2: Client Forms

On the following page is a sample self-test to determine one's mental and physical constitution or *doṣha*. Read the topics in bold in the left column and circle the choice that best describes you (from the right three columns). Circle all columns that are applicable. Choose answers according to your total life experience, not based solely on how you feel the past few weeks or years. Add up the columns under the total sections.

Āyurveda Doṣha Self-Test

BODY	Vāyu	Pitta	Kapha
Body Frame	thin	medium	large
Fingernails	thin or cracking	medium, pink, soft	thick or white
Pulse	80 - 100	70 - 80	60 - 70
Weight	low or bony	medium, muscular	gains easily
Stool- move bowels	small, hard, gas	loose or burns	moderate or solid
Forehead size	small	medium	large
Appetite	varible	strong or sharp	constant or low
Eyes	small or unsteady	reddish or piercing	white or wide
Voice	low or weak	high or sharp	deep or tonal
Lips	thin or dry	medium or soft	large or smooth
Chest	flat or sunken	medium	round or large
Bothers you most	cold and dry	heat and sun	cold and damp
Neck	thin or tall	medium sized	big, wide, or folded
Chin	thin or angular	tapered	round or double chin
Body Totals			
MIND	ॐ	ॐ	ॐ
Memory	quick to grasp ideas- soon forgets	sharp or clear	slow to learn- but never forgets
Beliefs	radical or changing	leader, goal oriented	constant or loyal
Dreams	flying or anxious	in color or fighting	romantic or few
Speech	quick or talkative	moderate or argues	slow or silent
Sleep	light	moderate	heavy
Habits	travel or nature	sports or politics	water or flowers
Mind	quick or adaptable	penetrating or critical	slow or lethargic
Emotions	enthusiastic, worries	warm, can get angry	calm or attached
Temperament	nervous or fearful	impatient	easy going
Finances	spends on trifles	spends on luxuries	saves money
Mind Totals			

Āyurvedic Client Health Form

Name			Phone ( )
Address			Country
Town		State	Zip
Consultation Date		Practitioner	Age
List any serious childhood diseases			
Number of stools passed each day		Referred by	Marital Status
List any medicines, herbs or vitamins you are taking			
List any genetic or heredity disease in you family.	Mother	Gmother	Gfather
	Father	Gmother	Gfather
	Brother	Sister	Relatives
Do any family members have addiction problems (e.g., alcohol, drugs)?			
Did you experience any physical or emotional abuse in your life?			
Current Job		Highest grade completed	
Reason For Visit?			
List any female reproductive disorders:			
Career Satisfaction: Love the career_____ OK career_____ Unhappy with career_____			
Family/social life is: Good_____ Average_____ Not Good_____			
Is your life spiritual?		Is your life purposeful?	
Prakṛiti: Body; V__ P__ K__ Mind: V__ P__ K__			Vikṛiti: V__ P__ K__
Pulse Quality: Snake Frog Swan		Pulse Position: V_____ P_____ K_____	
Organ Pulses:	Left	Right	Comments:
Superficial	Small Intestine	Colon	
	Stomach	G. Bladder	
	Bladder	Spiritual Pulse	
Deep	Heart	Lungs	
	Spleen	Liver	
	Kidney	Spiritual Pulse	
Tongue:		Nails:	

Check Current Health Issues	✓	Check Current Health Issues	✓
Respiratory		Anemia	
Cardiovascular/heart		High Blood Pressure	
Gastrointestinal		Low Blood Pressure	
Anorexia		Arteriosclerosis	
Diabetes		Jaundice	
Diarrhea		Gall Bladder	
Constipation		Acidity	
Menopause		Overweight	
PMS		Fever	
Colic/abdominal pain		Sinus	
Abdominal distention		Food Allergies	
Mouth		Environmental Allergies	
Stomach		Asthma	
Small Intestine		Bronchitis	
Ulcers		Addiction	
Colon		Epilepsy	
Rectum		Cancer	
Blood		Tumors	
Urine		Female Reproductive	
Parasites		Male Reproductive	
Metabolic/Endocrine		Skin Disorder	
Hemorrhoids		Epstein Barr	
Hernia		Nose	
Edema		Throat	
Hyperthyroid		Eyes	
Hypothyroid		Ears	
Gout		Arthritis	
Cholesterol		Rheumatism	
Head		Headaches/Migraines	
Emotional		Worry, Fear, Anxiety, Nervous	
Anger, Impatience		Lethargy	
Immune System		Nervous System	
HIV\AIDS		Muscles	
Bones		Other: ______________	

Appendix 3: Prakṛiti Food Plans

Traditional Āyurvedic Life Health Analysis Vāyu Doṣhas

Your constitution is predominantly air. An excess of air element creates cold, light, and dryness in the body, colon, skin, and bones. When balanced, you are energetic, adaptable, and cheerful. An excess of air causes dry skin, gas, constipation, anxiety, nervousness, and worry. The aim of Āyurveda is to create a balance between the elements of air, fire, and water. To bring air into balance Vāyu *doṣhas* need to

- Consume more steamed, heavy and moist foods.
- Ingest herbs to help digest the heavy foods.
- Eat smaller meals, no more than 3 to 4 hours apart.
- Eat sour, sweet, and salty substances that reduce excessive air. Pungent herbs, such asginger, are good if combined with sweet, sour, and salty foods and herbs.
- It's better not to eat alone. Have your food cooked for you if possible.
- Avoid nightshades (potatoes, tomatoes, eggplant, peppers, chilies) as they may cause allergic reactions.
- Don't combine milk with yeasted grains.
- Eat in a calm to celestial frame of mind.

HERBOLOGY

DIGESTION Cardamom, coriander, cinnamon, ginger, rock salt are among the major herbs to use.

ELIMINATION Licorice, soaked prunes, psyllium seeds, flax seeds, bran and *triphalā* before sleep.

ENERGY Ginseng, comfrey root, marshmallow, *aśhwagandhā, balā,* and *śhatāvarī.*

MIND Calamus, *aśhwagandhā,* basil, chamomile, *brāhmī.*

ANTI-RHEUMATICS Angelica, myrrh, *yogaraj guggul.*

OIL and MASSAGE Sesame oil and almond oil are heavy and warm, and therefore good for Vāyu *doṣha*. Oil massage the feet, head, back, and lower abdomen to reduce air. Essential oils include sandalwood, cinnamon, and frankincense.

FRUIT Most fruit is purifying, though not grounding. Dry fruit, melons, uncooked apples and pears, and cranberries increase air; they are not advised (baked apples and pears, or soaked dry fruits are alright). The best fruits for Vāyu *doṣhas* are, lemons, limes, grapefruit, cherries, grapes, strawberries, raspberries, pineapples, papayas, mangos, soaked—prunes, raisins, dates, and figs; other berries, kiwi, sweet melons, and rhubarb. Second best are oranges, cooked pears, cooked apples, peaches, plums, apricots, pomegranates, and persimmons. Fruit is best eaten between meals.

VEGETABLES also are too light for air constitutions to live on. However, if steamed and prepared with oils and spiced, eating them with whole grains is fine. The cabbage family causes gas (broccoli, cauliflower, Brussels sprouts). Other air-increasing vegetables are cucumbers, sprouts, celery, asparagus, spinach, and chard. The best vegetables for Vāyu *doṣhas* are sweet potatoes, carrots, beets, cilantro, parsley, seaweed, and small amounts of avocado. Second best are fresh corn, green beans (well-cooked), fresh peas, zucchini, squash, artichoke, kira, mustard greens, watercress, bell peppers, and okra. Some practitioners recommend moderate amounts of fenugreek greens, cooked leeks, black and green olives, parsnip, pumpkin, rutabaga, and watercress.

GRAINS Cooked whole grains are best. Bread is fine if toasted (but the yeast in bread is still heavy and hard to digest). The best grains for Vāyu *doṣhas* are wheat, then other moist grains like *basmati* rice, oats, and khus khus. Whole grain pasta is good. Dry grains like granola and chips aggravate the air element.

BEANS Most beans cause gas, are drying, and promote constipation. The best bean is *mūng*. Tofu is also acceptable, but may be hard to digest.

NUTS and SEEDS Raw or lightly roasted nuts are heavy, nourishing and moistening. They are hard to digest and so they are taken in small amounts at any one time. Vāyu recommendations include almonds (peel off the skin), walnuts, pecans, pine nuts and sesame seeds (or tahini); these should be soaked overnight.

OILS The best are sesame oil and *ghee* (one teaspoon per serving). Second best include almond, olive, avocado, and butter.

DAIRY is good for air constitutions, though hard to digest. Dairy is taken with spices, and milk should be boiled then left to cool slightly. The best dairy for Vāyu *doṣhas* include *lassi* (1/2 cup yogurt to 1/2 cup water, digestive herbs, all mixed and drunk at mealtime to aid digestion). *Ghee* is also excellent. Other suggestions include yogurt, kefir, cream, sour cream, butter, and cottage cheese. A little cheese may be eaten (especially homemade *paneer*).

SWEETENERS It is best not to eat sweets during meals. Natural sugars assist air types more than any other constitution in tissue building and body fluid maintenance. The best sweeteners are *jaggery* (*guḍ*-Indian), turbinado sugar, or natural sugar cane (sold in stores as Sucanat), maple syrup, and raw sugar. Raw honey and fruit sugar are acceptable but in smaller amounts.

CONDIMENTS A little rock salt improves digestion. Other suggestions include cardamom, fennel, ginger, cloves, coriander, cumin, cinnamon, basil, and fenugreek.

ANIMAL PRODUCTS Generally it is best to avoid animal products except when needed to regain strength following illness. Animal products give strength but are inharmonious on finer levels. *(Ghee* and *lassi* are good substitutes). Next best is fish and eggs. White chicken and turkey are also acceptable.

BEVERAGES Air constitutions require fluids. The best liquids are dairy, fruit or vegetable juices, tonic teas (taken with sweetener and milk), water with lime or lemon, and sour fruit juices.

VITAMINS and MINERALS are not generally used, but if needed, the following are best for Vāyu *doṣhas*: oily A, D and E, sour C, zinc, and calcium. Spices (e.g., ginger, cardamom) are taken with vitamins to aid digestion.

Herbal Preparations: The average amount of herbs to take is between 1/4 to 1 teaspoon of an herb or of an herbal mixture 1/2 hour before meals. *Ghee*, honey, or water may be mixed herbs (until paste) (2 parts to one part herbs). It is also advisable to cook herbs in 1 teaspoon of heated *ghee* or oil, and then add them to food. Teas can be made with 1 to 2 teaspoons of herbs.

* * * * * * * * * * * * * * * *

AROMA THERAPY Sandalwood, lotus, frankincense, cinnamon, or basil can be used as oil, incense, soap, or candles to calm the mind.

COLOR THERAPY Most colors are uplifting, particularly white, yellow, gold, orange, and some red. Lighter and pastel shades are preferred. Dark grays, browns and black upset the wind element.

GEM THERAPY Emerald, jade, peridot, yellow sapphire, topaz, and citrine set in gold.

YOGA Sitting and prone positions are good. Shoulder stands and back bends are also helpful if there are no heart problems. Deep breathing promotes calming.

MANTRAS

Ram—for Divine protection, immune boosting, insomnia, anxiety, fear, mental disorders

Hoom—wards off negativity, helps digestion, removes *āma,* and clears *srotas* (channels)

Śhreem—for general health, overall health and harmony, builds reproductive tissue.

MEDITATION can be done anywhere, at any time, lying down, sitting, or walking. *Mantra*s, thoughts, feelings, looking at nature, thinking about God, love, virtually anything that doesn't cause strain or worry are acceptable forms of meditation. Practice giving up worry, fear, negativity, anxiety, and lack of faith. Knowledge and devotion are the most important aspects to practice. If the opportunity arises, consider a meditation practice with a qualified spiritual teacher.

* * * * * * * * * * * * * * * *

Please Remember Do not force anything! If your system tells you it wants or doesn't want something, countering these guidelines, by all means follow your intuition!! The Inner Self is the best healer. Āyurveda helps us take control of our health. Seasonal changes may also require some modification of these recommendations. Enjoy these suggestions and feel increasingly healthy and harmonious.

Aum Śhānti, Śhānti, Śhānti
Peace.

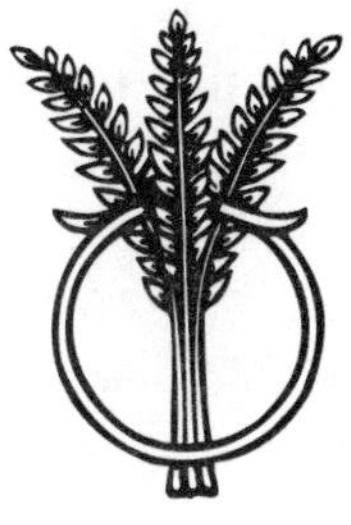

Traditional Āyurvedic Life Health Analysis Vāyu/Pitta Doṣhas

Your constitution is predominantly air and fire. An excess of air element creates cold, light, and dryness in the body, and colon, skin, and bones. When balanced, you are energetic, adaptable, and cheerful. An excess of air causes dry skin, gas, and constipation. Fire excess causes heat in the form of hot temper, impatience, rashes, infections, ulcers, etc.

When balanced, fire helps one be more goal-oriented, express leadership qualities, warmth, and gives physical strength. The aim of Āyurveda is to create a balance between the elements of air, water, fire, and earth. To bring air and fire into balance one needs to:

- Consume more cooked, moist, and somewhat heavier foods.
- Eat herbs to help digest the more grounding foods.
- Avoid hot foods (e.g., onions, garlic, red peppers), fermented or fried foods, salt.
- Eat smaller meals, no more than 3 to 4 hours apart.
- Avoid nightshades (potatoes, tomatoes, eggplant, peppers, chilies) as they may cause allergic reactions.
- Don't combine milk with yeasted grains.
- Don't combine fruit with other foods.
- Eat meals in a serene, thankful state of mind.

HERBOLOGY

DIGESTION Cardamom, cinnamon, fennel, mints, coriander.

ELIMINATION Licorice, *triphalā* (before sleep and in the morning), soaked raisins.

ENERGY Comfrey root, marshmallow, *balā,* and *śhatāvarī.*

MIND Calamus, basil, chamomile, gotu kola, *aśhwagandhā, jaṭāmāṇśhī* (insomnia).

ANTI-RHEUMATICS Angelica, myrrh, *yogaraj guggul* on occasion.

OIL and MASSAGE Sesame oil is heavy and therefore grounding. Massage the feet, head, back, and lower abdomen with oil to reduce air. Include the chest and third eye. *Brāhmī* oil in the hair is excellent. *Mahānārāyan* oil is said to help with pains, arthritis, and other pains and injuries.

AROMATHERAPY Essential oils include sandalwood, rose, geranium, lily.

FRUIT Most fruit is purifying, although it is not grounding. Soak dry fruit, and bake apples and pears. Sweet fruits of berries, cherries, coconut, fresh figs, grapes, kiwi, mangos, sweet melons, sweet oranges, peaches, pineapples, rhubarb, and plums are balancing. Avocado (small amounts), watermelon (chew and eat several of the seeds).

VEGETABLES also are too light for air constitutions to live on. If vegetables are steamed and prepared with oils—and spiced, eating them with whole grains is acceptable. Most forms of squash (acorn, butternut, scaloppini, summer, winter and yellow creek neck), artichoke, asparagus, fresh corn, cucumber, green beans, okra, sweet potatoes, rutabaga, and zucchini are excellent for balance. (The cabbage family causes gas, i.e., broccoli, cauliflower, Brussels sprouts; root vegetables like beets and carrots may cause too much heat).

GRAINS Cooked whole grains are best. Bread is acceptable if toasted, but yeast (contained in bread) is not a recommended product because it is difficult to digest. White *basmati* rice, wheat, oats, amaranth, wild rice, khus khus are good. Dry grains like granola, chips aggravate the air element. Barley is good for reducing fire, but may create gas for the air aspect of your constitution.

BEANS Most beans cause gas, are drying, and promote constipation. The best bean is *mūng*. Tofu is also acceptable, but may be hard to digest. Aduki, soy cheese, soy milk, and tepery beans may be taken in moderation.

NUTS and SEEDS Raw or lightly roasted nuts are heavy, nourishing, and moistening. They are hard to digest, thus, small amounts should be taken at any one time. Best is almonds (soaked overnight and peeled) and sesame seeds in moderation (grounds air); coconut and sunflower seeds are also good (cools fire).

OILS Best is sesame oil (for air conditions) and *ghee* (clarified butter). Sunflower is better for fire-related issues; soy and unsalted butter are also good.

DAIRY Is good very good in its organic state and/or from raw sources. It may be hard to digest. Dairy should be taken with spices; milk should be boiled, then cooled. Best is *lassi* (1/2 cup yogurt to 1/2 cup water; and digestive herbs, all mixed and drunk at mealtime to aid digestion). *Ghee* is also excellent. Other good dairy products includes yogurt, kefir, cream, unsalted butter, and cottage cheese. A little cheese is acceptable also, but only 'renetless' cheese qualifies as vegetarian.

SWEETENERS It is best not to combine sweets with other foods. Use only natural sugars which aid air types more than any other constitution in tissue and body fluid maintenance. Best is *jaggery* (*guḍ*-Indian), turbinado, maple syrup, or Sucanat. Raw honey (for air conditions) is acceptable.

CONDIMENTS Best is cardamom, fennel, coriander, cumin, cilantro, turmeric, vanilla, saffron, rose water, mint. Cinnamon, cloves, mustard seeds, *pippalī* will aggravate fire conditions.

ANIMAL PRODUCTS Generally it is better to avoid animal products except for strength when extremely ill. It gives strength, but is difficult to digest, is toxic and disharmonious on finer levels. *Ghee* and lassi are excellent substitutes. Next best is poached or boiled egg whites and white poultry because they are easily digested.

BEVERAGES Air/Fire constitutions need fluids. Suggestions include boiled milk, teas such as bansha (with milk), catnip, chamomile, elder flower, fennel, hibiscus, jasmine, lavender, lemongrass, licorice, lotus, marshmallow, oat straw, raspberry, rose, and saffron. All fruits, vegetables, and herbs listed above are good as juice.

VITAMINS and MINERALS For air conditions, oily A, D, and E, sour C, minerals—particularly zinc and calcium. However, vitamins and minerals should be taken with spices to help digest them. For excess fire, B vitamins, K, calcium, and iron may be needed, but it is better to get them from steamed vegetables.

Herbal Preparations: Take an average of between 1/4 and 1 teaspoon of an herb or of an herbal mixture, 1/2 hour before meals. You may mix them with twice as much *ghee* or water (until paste). It is also advisable to cook herbs in heated *ghee* or oil, and then add to your food. Teas can be made with 1 to 2 teaspoons of herbs.

* * * * * * * * * * * * * * * *

AROMA THERAPY Sandalwood, rose, gardenia, jasmine (white flowers). Basil, frankincense, cedar, myrrh (warming). Aromas can be used as oil, incense, soap, candles, etc., to calm and refresh the mind.

COLOR THERAPY Most colors are uplifting, particularly white, lighter, and pastel shades. Dark grays, browns, and black upset air and fire elements. White shades of green, pink, and blue (i.e., emerald, sky blue) are also very good colors for balance. For air, warmer colors like gold, yellow, and a bit of red are suggested. For fire, bright, cheery greens, such as emerald, are suggested.

GEM THERAPY White stones, such as pearl and moonstone set in silver, are recommended for both air and fire. For air, red, yellow, or orange stones set in gold. For fire, green stones set in silver.

YOGA Sitting and prone positions are good; shoulder stands (so long as there are no heart problems) and back bends are also good. Deep breathing is calming.

MANTRAS

Śhānti—for mental peace.

Ram—for Divine protection, immune boosting, insomnia, anxiety, fear, mental disorders

Hoom—wards off negativity, helps digestion, removes *āma,* and clears *srotas* (channels)

Śhreem—for general health, overall health and harmony, builds reproductive tissue.

MEDITATION can be done anywhere, at any time; lying down, sitting, walking. It can be with a *mantra,* with a thought, a feeling; looking at nature, thinking about God, love; virtually anything that doesn't cause strain, anger; or worry that you are not meditating properly. Practice giving up worry, fear, negativity, anxiety, impatience, anger, harsh speech, a critical mind, and lack of faith. Knowledge and devotion are the most important aspects to practice.

EXERCISE Moderate; walking, swimming, trampoline, cross-country or downhill skiing.

OIL MASSAGE Apply oils to heart, forehead (third eye), feet, lower back and belly, neck, and shoulders. *Brāhmī* oil for the head is excellent. Sesame or Sunflower is acceptable for the body. *Mahānārāyan* oil is used for pains and arthritis.

* * * * * * * * * * * * * * * *

Please Remember Do not force anything! Listen to what your system tells you. One's intuition is, in the final analysis, the best doctor. Enjoy these suggestions and feel an increasingly healthy and harmonious life.

Aum Śhānti, Śhānti, Śhānti—Peace

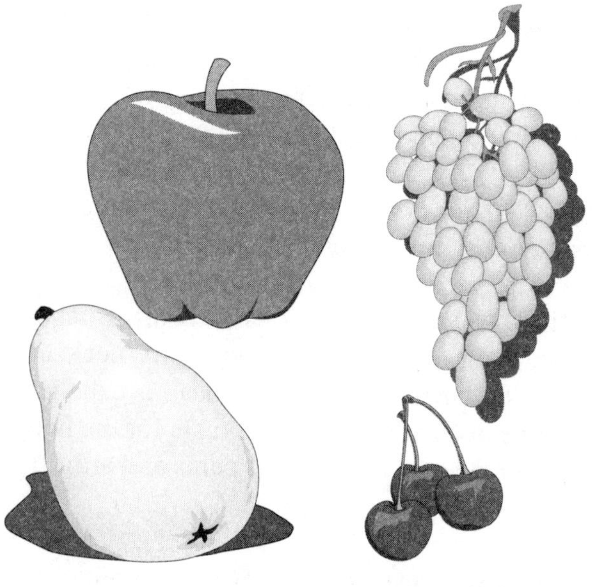

Traditional Āyurvedic Life Health Analysis Vāyu/Kapha Doṣhas

Your constitution is predominantly air and water. An excess of air element creates cold, light, and dryness in the body—colon, skin, and bones, causing dry skin, gas, and constipation. When balanced, air makes one energetic, adaptable, and cheerful. An excess of water creates moistness, coldness, and heaviness, leading to congestion, excess weight, and mental lethargy. When balanced, water creates loyalty, consistency, and comfort. The aim of Āyurveda is to create a balance between the elements of air, water, fire, and earth. To bring air into balance one needs to:

· Consume more cooked foods.

· Take herbs that help digest food

· Eat smaller meals, 3 to 4 hours apart. Breakfast may be skipped if so desired.

· Eat mainly pungent, hot substances that reduce excessive air and water. Bitter foods are useful to reduce water, but increase air. Sweet foods reduce air but increase water. So, one must monitor the effects of the foods eaten.

· Avoid nightshades (potatoes, tomatoes, eggplant, peppers, chilies) as they may cause allergic reactions.

· Don't combine milk with yeasted grains.

· Eat in a calm to celestial frame of mind.

HERBOLOGY

DIGESTION Cardamom, coriander, cinnamon, and ginger help digestion.

ELIMINATION Licorice, prunes, psyllium seeds, flax seeds, bran, and *triphalā* can be taken first thing in the morning. *Triphalā* can also be taken before sleep.

MIND Calamus, *aśhwagandhā*, basil, *brāhmī,* chamomile.

ANTI-RHEUMATICS Angelica, myrrh.

OIL & MASSAGE Sesame oil is suggested. Oil massage the feet, head, back, and lower abdomen. Essential oils include sandalwood, cinnamon, musk, frankincense, myrrh.

ENERGY Ginseng, *aśhwagandhā, balā,* and *śhatāvarī.*

FRUIT The best fruits are lemons, limes, grapefruit, apricots, berries, baked apples, cherries, peaches. Because this is a dual *doṣha,* all other fruit intake should be monitored.

VEGETABLES The cabbage family causes gas (broccoli, cauliflower, Brussels sprouts). Cucumbers, sprouts, celery, asparagus, spinach, and chard also increase air. Best are sweet potatoes, carrots, beets, cilantro, parsley, fresh corn, green beans (well cooked), fresh peas, squash, artichoke, kira, mustard greens, moderate amounts of fenugreek greens, cooked leeks, black and green olives, parsnips, and pumpkin.

GRAINS Cooked whole grains are best. Bread is acceptable if toasted, but it best avoided (it contains yeast—difficult to digest). *Basmati* rice and barley (if it doesn't cause gas) are the best grains. All other grains should be monitored owing to your dual *doṣha.*

BEANS Most beans cause gas, are drying, and promote constipation. The best bean is *mūng.* Tofu is also good, but may be hard to digest. If there is no gas or constipation problem, then any bean is good to eat.

NUTS & SEEDS Raw or lightly roasted nuts are heavy, nourishing, and moistening. They are hard to digest, thus, small amounts should be taken at any one time. The best is 3 to 5 almonds (soaked overnight and peeled), and sesame seeds.

OILS Best is 2 to 3 teaspoons sesame oil or *ghee* per meal.

DAIRY Is good for air constitutions, though hard to digest. It should be taken with spices. Milk should be boiled. *Lassi* (1/2 cup yogurt to 1/2 cup water, or 1/4 cup yogurt to 3/4 cup water if Kapha is excessed) mixed with digestive herbs and taken at mealtime, aids digestion. *Ghee* is also excellent.

SWEETENERS It is best not to combine sweets with other foods. Use only natural sugars which aid air types more than any other constitution in tissue and body fluid maintenance. Raw honey is best for Vāyu/Kapha. Turbinado sugar or Sucanat may be used if it does not cause congestion.

CONDIMENTS The best is cardamom, asafoetida, and fennel. Next best is ginger, cloves, coriander, cumin, cinnamon, basil, and fenugreek.

ANIMAL PRODUCTS Generally it is better to avoid animal products except for strength when ill. It gives strength but is difficult to digest, is toxic, and disharmonious on finer levels. *Ghee* and *lassi* are the best substitutes. Next best is eggs. Chicken and turkey (white meat) are also all right.

BEVERAGES Herbal teas and vegetable or fruit juices should be taken using the recommended fruits and vegetables.

***Herbal Preparations*:** Between 1/4 to 1 teaspoon of an herb or of an herbal mixture should be taken 1/2 hour before meals and during meals. They can be mixed with twice as much raw honey, *ghee,* or water (until paste), With meals, herbs can be sprinkled on food. They may also be cooked in heated *ghee*, then added to food. Teas can be made with 1 to 2 teaspoons of herbs.

* * * * * * * * * * * * * * * * *

OIL MASSAGE Massage the feet, lower back, shoulders, and neck before bed or exercise.

AROMA THERAPY Sandalwood, lotus, frankincense, cinnamon, basil and camphor can be used as oil, incense, soap, or candles to calm and refresh the mind.

COLOR THERAPY Most colors are uplifting, particularly yellow, gold, orange, and some red. Lighter and pastel shades are preferred. Dark grays, browns and black upset wind elements.

GEM THERAPY Emerald, jade, peridot, yellow sapphire, topaz, and citrine set in gold are warming, and thus balancing for Vāyu and Kapha. Ruby and garnet improve circulation and energy. Stones work best when set to touch the skin.

YOGA Sitting and prone positions are good. Shoulder stands and back bends are also good. Standing postures are good for Kapha. Deep breathing and alternate nostril *prāṇāyāma* are calming and balancing.

MANTRAS

Ram—for Divine protection, immune boosting, insomnia, anxiety, fear, mental disorders

Hoom—wards off negativity, helps digestion, removes *āma,* and clears *srotas* (channels)

MEDITATION Meditation can be done anywhere, at any time: lying down, sitting, or walking. It can be with a *mantra*, a thought, feeling, looking at nature, or thinking about God, or love. Virtually anything that doesn't cause strain or worry is useful. Practice giving up worry, fear, negativity, anxiety, lack of faith, attachment, or greed. Knowledge and devotion are the most important aspects.

EXERCISE Moderate to heavy; walking is best.

* * * * * * * * * * * * * * * *

Please Remember Do not force anything! Listen to what your system tells you. One's intuition is the best doctor. Please enjoy these suggestions and feel an increasingly healthy and harmonious life.

Traditional Āyurvedic Life Health Analysis Pitta Doṣhas

Your constitution is predominantly fire. An excess of the fire element creates heat in the body, specifically in the small intestines, liver, spleen gall bladder, blood, and heart. When balanced, you are warm, adaptable, cheerful, goal oriented, have leadership qualitites. An excess of fire causes heat-related behavior, such as hot temper, being overly critical and impatient, skin rashes, allergies, eye problems, ulcers, diarrhea. The aim of Āyurveda is to create a balance between the elements of air, water, and fire. To bring fire into balance one needs to:

- Consume more bitter and astringent energies in the form of food, aromas, and herbs.
- Avoid hot foods (e.g., onions, garlic, red peppers), fermented or fried foods, salt.
- Eat every 4 to 5 hours.
- Avoid nightshades (potatoes, tomatoes, eggplant, peppers, chilies) as they may cause allergic reactions.
- Don't combine milk with yeasted grains.
- Eat in a calm to celestial frame of mind.
- Increase consumption of sweet fruit juices and herbal teas
- Consume cold, heavy, moist, blander foods
- Avoid alcohol and smoking because of their heating nature
- Emotionally cultivate clarity rather than a critical nature

HERBOLOGY

DIGESTION: Coriander, mint, aloe, gentian, barberry, fennel, turmeric.

ELIMINATION: *Triphalā*, senna, boiled milk and *ghee*, rose petals, *gokṣhura, guḍūchī*.

***ENERGY*:** *Śhatāvarī, balā, āmalakī*, saffron, aloe, licorice, *guḍūchī*, comfrey, Solomon's seal, marshmallow, dandelion, burdock.

***MIND*:** Gotu kola, sandalwood, *bhṛiṅgarāj*, rose, lotus, *jaṭāmāṇśhī,* chamomile, betony, chrysanthemum, hibiscus.

***DETOXIFICATION* (blood, liver, etc.):** *Guggul, mañjiṣhṭhā*, gotu kola, *musta.*

***HEART*:** *Arjuna.*

FRUIT Most fruit is calming and cooling, harmonizing and thirst quenching. Apples, pears, pomegranates are excellent. Pineapples, cranberries, persimmons, melons, prunes, dates, figs, grapes are also very good. Mangos, plums, and raspberries are helpful. Sour and certain other fruits, such as lemons, limes, apricots, bananas, cherries, papayas, peaches, and strawberries, will aggravate heat.

VEGETABLES Most vegetables are also good for Pitta *doṣha*, especially if eaten raw or lightly steamed. The best vegetables are cauliflower, cilantro, alfalfa sprouts, sunflower sprouts, celery. Second best is broccoli, cabbage, Brussels sprouts, asparagus, lettuce, beans, peas, cucumbers, and okra. Finally, parsley, bell peppers, fresh corn, and squash are acceptable. Root vegetables (beets and carrots), nightshades (eggplant, tomato, potato), mustard greens, parsley, spinach, and sweet potatoes may cause difficulty. Hot spicy foods like chilies, garlic, onions, pickles, and radishes greatly increase the fire element.

GRAINS Most grains are cooling for Pitta. The best are cooked whole wheat, *basmati* rice, oats, barley, granola, couscous, and quinoa. Finally, long grain brown rice, blue corn, and millet. Short grain brown rice, buckwheat, corn, and rye may be too heating and create Pitta discomfort. Whole grain pastas are good. Yeast-free breads are good; bread containing yeast should be toasted.

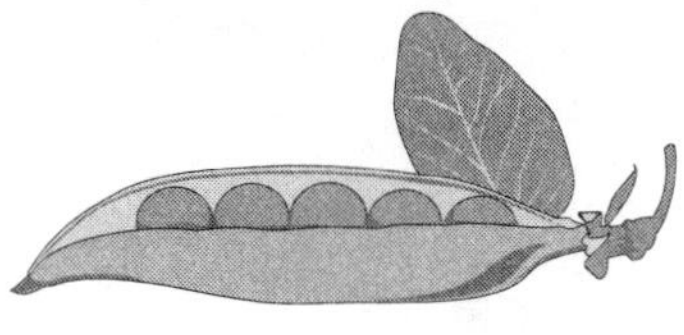

BEANS Best is *mūng,,* which does not cause gas. Most beans are acceptable for Pitta *doṣha,* though it is better to cook them with cumin or cardamom to aid in digestion. Also good are aduki, tofu, lima, kidney, soy, split, and chick peas. Lentils and peanuts may cause indigestion. (Some practitioners accept various forms of lentils).

NUTS and SEEDS The best are coconut and sunflower seeds. Seeds are a preferred source of protein over fish and poultry.

OILS *Ghee (*clarified butter), sunflower, butter (unsalted), soy.

DAIRY *Ghee*, boiled milk (then left to cool), yogurt *lassi* (1 part organic yogurt to 1 part water), cottage cheese (unsalted).

SWEETENERS Most sweeteners are good, including Sucanat. It is better to avoid white sugar, honey; and molasses in excess.

ANIMAL PRODUCTS Generally, it is better to avoid animal products except when needed for strength. Animal products give strength but are inharmonious on finer levels. Animal foods that balance Pitta include egg whites, chicken, and turkey (white meat).

BEVERAGES Juice of aloe vera, apple, pear, berry, carob, vegetables according to above section, fig shake, milk boiled, other fruit juices mentioned above. Teas include alfalfa, barley, bansha, burdock, chamomile, chicory, chrysanthemum, dandelion, hibiscus, jasmine, lavender, lemon grass, nettle, raspberry, red clover, rose, saffron, sarsaparilla, mint.

VITAMINS: *B, K, calcium, iron* Take with herbs, such as coriander, to digest vitamins.

Herbal Preparations: The average amount of herbs to take is between 1/4 to 1 teaspoon of an herb or of an herbal mixture with meals. You may mix with twice as much *ghee* or with water (until paste). It is also advisable to cook herbs in heated *ghee* or oil and then add to your food. Teas can be made with 1 to 2 teaspoons of herbs. You may also sprinkle herbs directly on meals.

* * * * * * * * * * * * * * * *

OIL MASSAGE Massage the feet, lower back, shoulders and neck before bed or exercise.

AROMA THERAPY Sandalwood, lotus, rose, jasmine, and any white flowers (cool energies) can be used as essential oil, incense, sachet, soap, or candles to calm and refresh the mind.

COLOR THERAPY Green, sky blue, or white to reduce Pitta. Reds, oranges, yellows, and brights aggravate Pitta. Apply color suggestions to home and office furnishings and clothing.

GEM THERAPY Emerald, jade, peridot, moonstone and pearl, blue sapphire and amethyst set in silver.

YOGA Sitting and prone positions are good for Pitta *doṣha*. Shoulder stands (only if there is no heart problems) and back bends are also good. Deep breathing is calming.

MEDITATION can be done anywhere, at any time; lying down, sitting, walking. It can be with a *mantra*, with a thought, a feeling, looking at nature, thinking about God, or love, or virtually anything that doesn't cause strain or worry. Practice giving up anger and impatience. Knowledge and devotion are the most important aspects.

MANTRAS Chanting, contemplation of 'Who am I?' Practice giving up hostility, anger, and criticism.

Śhanti—for peace

Śhrīm—for general health and harmony

LIFESTYLE Take walks by the water or in gardens in the full moon. Work in flower gardens and practice sweet speech, forgiveness, and contentment. Moderate exercise. Walking is best.

* * * * * * * * * * * * * * * *

Please Remember Do not force anything! Listen to what your system tells you. One's intuition is the best doctor. Please enjoy these suggestions and feel an increasingly healthy and harmonious life.

Aum Śhānti, Śhānti, Śhānti

Peace

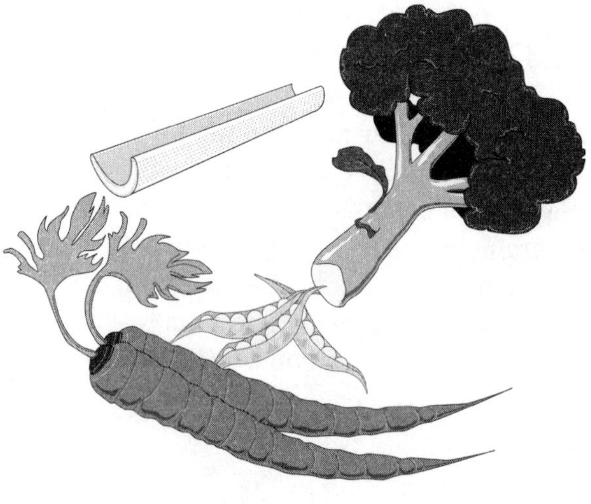

Traditional Āyurvedic Life Health Analysis Pitta/Kapha Doṣhas

Your constitution is predominantly fire and water. An excess of fire and water elements creates cold and heat, and heaviness and dampness in the body, specifically in the chest, lungs, sinuses, stomach, and small intestines. When balanced, you are adaptable and cheerful, goal-oriented, and a leader. An excess of fire causes heat-related issues like hot temper, being overly critical and impatient, skin rashes, allergies, eye problems, ulcers, and diarrhea. An excess of water creates bronchitis, overweight, and mental lethargy. The aim of Āyurveda is to create a balance between the elements of air, water, and fire. To bring fire and water into balance one needs to:

- Consume more bitter and astringent energies in the form of food, aromas, herbs.
- Avoid nightshades (potatoes, tomatoes, eggplant, peppers, chilies) because they may cause allergic reactions.
- Avoid hot foods (e.g., onions, garlic, red peppers), fermented or fried foods, salt.
- Don't combine milk with yeasted grains.
- Eat in a calm to celestial frame of mind.

HERBS Coriander, mint, rose petals, saffron, turmeric, *triphalā, guggul, gokṣhura, āmalakī, mañjiṣhṭhā, arjuna*, gotu kola, chamomile, cardamom, *guḍūchī, jaṭāmāṇśhī*, musta, raspberry, *śhilājit*.

FRUIT (between meals): Apples, mango, pears, pomegranate, prunes, quince, raisins.

VEGETABLES Asparagus, bell pepper, broccoli, Brussels sprouts, burdock root, cabbage, fresh corn, cauliflower, celery, green beans, dandelion, collards, lettuce, okra, parsley, peas, green peppers, squash (scaloppini, spaghetti, summer, yellow creekneck), sprouts, watercress. Avoid fermented foods, pickles, onions, garlic, and chilies because they will aggravate Pitta.

GRAINS Barley is best, *basmati* rice, cooked oat bran, wheat bran (moderation). Bread without yeast (or toasted) is advised.

BEANS The best is *mūng,* which does not cause gas. Aduki, black, black-eyed, chana *dal* (garbanzos), lima, navy, pinto, white, and *tūr dal* are acceptable.

NUTS and SEEDS Pumpkin and sunflower in moderation.

OILS *Ghee* (clarified butter) can be taken in moderation (2 tsp./day). Sunflower in moderation.

DAIRY *Ghee,* yogurt *lassi* (1 part organic yogurt to 3 parts water).

SWEETENERS It is better to use very little. Either raw honey or a cane sugar, such as turbinado or Sucanat, can be used sparingly.

ANIMAL PRODUCTS Generally it is better to avoid animal products except for strength when ill. It gives strength but is inharmonious on finer levels. *Ghee* and *lassi* are good substitutes. Acceptable foods include poached or boiled egg white, and white meat of chicken and turkey.

BEVERAGES Juice of aloe vera, apple, pear, berry, carob, fig shake, and fruits and vegetables mentioned above. Teas of alfalfa, barley, bansha, burdock, chamomile, chicory, chrysanthemum, dandelion, hibiscus, jasmine, lavender, lemon grass, nettle, raspberry, red clover, rose, saffron, sarsaparilla, mint.

Herbal Preparations: Between 1/4 to 1 teaspoon of an herb or of an herbal mixture should be taken 1/2 hour before meals. Twice as much *ghee* or water are mixed with herbs (until paste). It is also advisable to cook herbs in heated *ghee*, then add them to your food. Teas can be made with 1 to 2 teaspoons of herbs.

* * * * * * * * * * * * * * * *

OIL MASSAGE Massage the feet, lower back, shoulders and neck before bed or exercise.

AROMA THERAPY Sandalwood, lotus, rose, jasmine (cool energies); mixed with frankincense, cinnamon, basil, camphor (warm energies) can be used as oil, incense, soap, or candles to calm and refresh the mind.

COLOR THERAPY Reds, oranges, yellows, and brights will help Kapha, but will tend to aggravate Pitta. Green and sky blue are best. White and pink reduce Pitta but will derange Kapha. Choose colors as needed for home and office furnishings and in clothing.

GEM THERAPY Emerald, jade, peridot, moonstone, and pearls set in silver reduce Pitta.. Ruby and garnet, yellow sapphire, topaz and citrine, improve circulation and energy for Kapha.

YOGA Sitting and prone positions are good when Pitta is in excess; standing postures are best when Kapha is aggravated.. Shoulder stands (only if there are no heart problems, blood, ear, or eye pressure) and back bends are also good. Deep breathing is calming.

MANTRAS Chanting, contemplation on 'Who am I?,' practice giving up hostility, anger, and criticism; visualize meditating on specific deities of your choice, such as Christ, *Kṛiṣhṇa*.

MEDITATION can be done anywhere, at any time, either lying down, sitting, or walking. It can be with a *mantra*, with a thought, a feeling, looking at nature, thinking about God, or love; virtually anything that doesn't cause strain or worry. Practice giving up worry, fear, negativity, anxiety, and lack of faith. Knowledge and devotion are the most important aspects to practice.

EXERCISE Moderate to strong; walking is best.

* * * * * * * * * * * * * * * *

Please Remember do not force anything! Listen to what your system tells you. One's intuition is the best doctor. Please enjoy these suggestions and feel an increasingly healthy and harmonious life.

Aum Śhānti, Śhānti, Śhānti
Peace

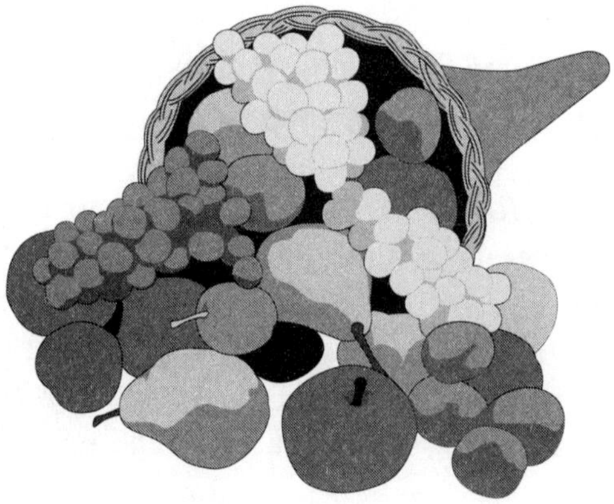

Traditional Āyurvedic Life Health Analysis Kapha Doṣhas

Your constitution is predominantly water. An excess of water element creates cold, heavy, and dampness in the body; specifically in the chest, lungs, and sinuses. When balanced, you are loyal and calm by nature. An excess of water causes water retention (e.g., edema, overweight), sinus problems, bronchitis. The aim of Āyurveda is to create a balance between the elements of air, water, and fire. To bring water into balance one needs to:

- Consume more steamed, light, hot, and dry foods.
- Take herbs to help digest the heavy foods.
- Eat smaller and fewer meals; eat more herbs. Breakfast may be skipped.
- Eat pungent, bitter, and astringent foods to reduce excessive water.
- It is better to cook for others, especially for Vāyu individuals.
- Do not use food as an emotional support.

HERBOLOGY

DIGESTION Hot spices: Dry ginger, black pepper, cloves, and cinnamon improve the metabolism.
Bitters: Aloe, turmeric, barberry, and gentian reduce the desire for sugars and fats.

ENERGY Pungent and bitter tonics: Black pepper, cinnamon, saffron, ginger, *śhilājit, guggul*, myrrh, aloe gel, or juice.

MIND Stimulants and mental clearing: musk, gotu kola (*brāhmī*), basil (*tulsī*), *guggul*, myrrh, sage, bayberry, betony.

FRUIT Generally increases water, causing mucus and depressing the digestive fire (*agni*). It is better to not combine fruits with other foods. Best are lemon, limes, and grapefruits (which dissolve mucus and reduce fat). They should be eaten without sugar. Other good fruits include cranberries, apples, and dried fruits.

VEGETABLES Most are diuretics (naturally drawing water from the system). Steamed vegetables are easiest on the digestive system. The best are chilies, broccoli, cabbage, and celery. Next best are carrots, green beans, fresh peas, beets, asparagus, lettuce, cilantro, watercress, mustard greens, alfalfa, sunflower sprouts, and chard. Third best are bell peppers, cauliflower, parsley, and spinach. Other vegetables increase water.

GRAINS are nourishing and balancing for Kapha *doṣha*. Whole grains of barley, quinoa, dry or popped grains are best. Second best are corn, millet, rye, and buckwheat. *Basmati* rice is alright in moderation. Barley is a diuretic that reduces water and weight. Avoid yeasted breads.

BEANS Most beans are good, particularly aduki, followed by soy, lima, and lentils. Other useful beans include tofu, *mūng*, kidney, peanut (but not roasted), and split peas. *Mūng* is a pure or *sattwic* bean, and will not encourage gas.

NUTS and SEEDS are eaten only in small quantities because they are heavy and hard to digest. Sunflower and pumpkin are acceptable. These are a good meat (protein) substitute.

OILS in moderation: Mustard, canola, sunflower, safflower. Corn oil is also acceptable.

DAIRY Buttermilk (*lassi*: 1/4 cup organic yogurt: 3/4 cup water) with meals; soy milk and goat's milk are acceptable when there are no congestion or digestive disorders.

SWEETENERS A little raw honey is acceptable.

CONDIMENTS Cardamom, ginger (dry), mustard horseradish, turmeric, cloves. Second best are cinnamon, coriander, basil, cilantro, and parsley. Avoid salt because it retains water in the body (if absolutely necessary, black or rock salt may be used because it is the least aggravating).

ANIMAL PRODUCTS are best avoided, except if the person is extremely weak. Animal products boost strength, but are inharmonious, toxic, increase water, and do not generate new tissue growth. White, lean poultry is the least aggravating.

BEVERAGES Astringent or pungent teas (warm or at room temperature): Alfalfa, raspberry, hibiscus, and dandelion. Boiled, organic goat's milk (without food) with cinnamon and honey. Pineapple, pomegranate, cranberry, grapefruit, lemon, and lime juices are good. Celery and other green vegetable juices are also helpful. Avoid wine, alcohol, ice, or any cold drinks.

Herbal Preparations: The average amount of herbs to take is between 1/4 to 1 teaspoon of an herb or of an herbal mixture just after meals. Twice as much raw honey, *ghee*, or water may be mixed with herbs to form a paste. It is also advisable to cook herbs in a little oil or *ghee*, then add them to your food. Teas can be made with 1 to 2 teaspoons of herbs.

* * * * * * * * * * * * * * * *

OIL and MASSAGE Warm and light oils, such as canola, mustard, flaxseed (linseed), or dry rough massage are advised. Rubbing alcohol mixed with warm herbal oils (eucalyptus, frankincense, myrrh, clove, cedar, cinnamon, mustard) is also good. These oils stimulate and clear the mind.

AROMA THERAPY Frankincense, myrrh, cedar, cloves, cinnamon, and musk stimulate and clear the mind. Use as incense, soap, sachet, or candles.

COLOR THERAPY Warm, bright colors: Yellow, orange, gold, or red. Avoid white, or pale shades of blue, green, and pink. Use black, brown, and gray in moderation, or not at all. Colors apply to clothing, office, and home furnishings.

GEM THERAPY Ruby, garnet, and cat's eye set in gold are warming, and therefore, reduce water. Weight-reducing gems: amethyst and lapis, set in gold, and worn with warmer stones. Set rings or pendants to touch the skin for the strongest effect.

YOGA Strong workouts and more standing postures, along with headstands (if there is no heart condition). Solar *Prāṇāyāma* and breath of fire (*bhastrika*) breathing are advised.

MANTRAS Stimulating and clearing *mantras:* are useful, like *Aym, Hreem, Hoom* are useful.

MEDITATION Devotion (*bhakti*) and service (*karma*) harmonize one's nature. Worship the Divine as a particular deity or incarnation you like, e.g., *Rama, Kṛiṣhṇa,* or Christ. Renounce greed, desire, attachment and sentimentality to clear the mind. Chanting is excellent.

LIFE STYLE Strong and aerobic workouts, sunbathing, warm breezes, discipline, physical hardship. Stay up at night, avoid day naps, increase mental stimulation, travel, and pilgrimage. Avoid cold and dampness.

* * * * * * * * * * * * * * * * *

Please remember do not force anything! Listen to what your system tells you. One's intuition is the best doctor. Please enjoy these suggestions and feel an increasingly healthy and harmonious life.

Aum Śhānti, Śhānti, Śhānti
Peace

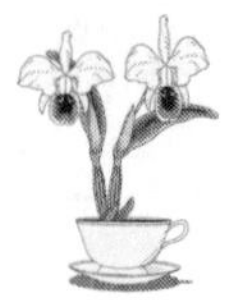

Tridoṣha Food Plan

If persons have an equal amount of all three *doṣhas*, food plans depend upon whether they are healthy or have some illness. If ill, Āyurvedic practitioners determine the *doṣha* or *doṣhas* causing the illness and suggest the food plan that reduces that excessed *doṣha* (i.e., a *vakṛiti*-reducing diet). When tridoṣhic persons have no health concerns, they are able to eat all foods in moderation.

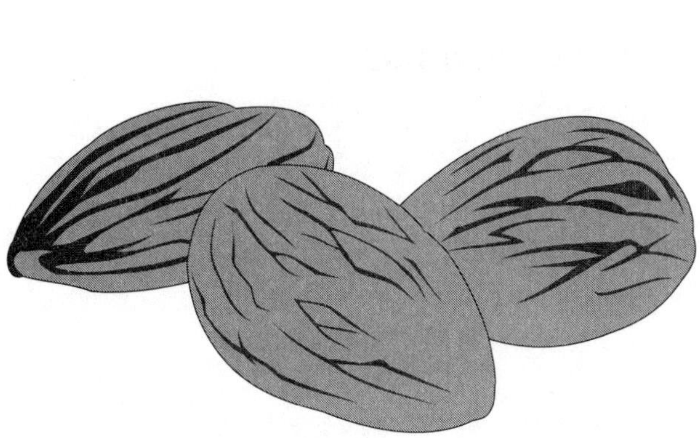

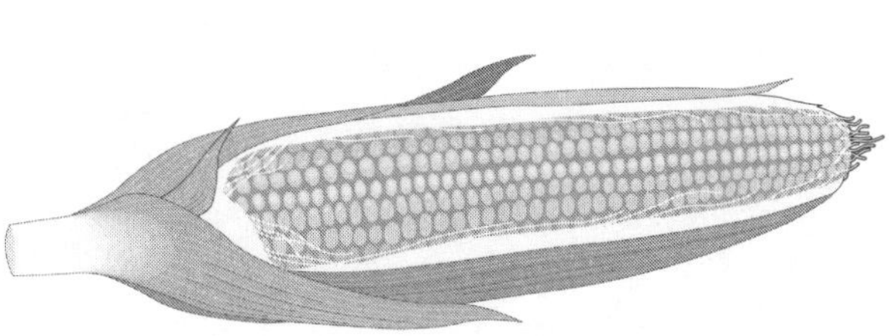

Āyurvedic Vegetarian Food Pyramid

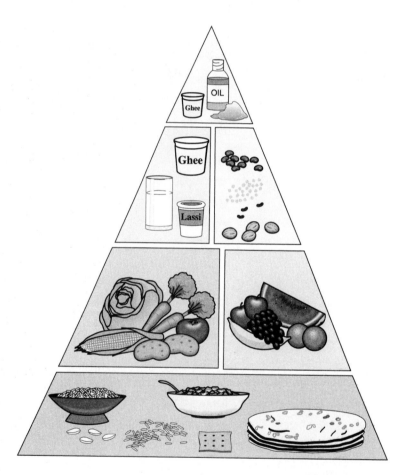

Āyurvedic Resources

Āyurveda Holistic Centers

Āyurveda Holistic Center - Distance Learning
82A Bayville Ave
Bayville, NY 11709 USA
Web brochure: http://ayurvedahc.com

Āyurveda Holistic Center - Residentail Training
460 Ridgedale Ave #2
E. Hanover, NJ 07936
Web brochure: http://www.lotusfair.com
800-452-1798
fax: 973-887-3088

Uniyal Clinic
Dr. Ram Chandra Uniyal - Director
Bhai Rava Chowk
Uttarkaṣhi, Himalayas 249193
India

Maa Parvati Memorial Clinic
Dr. J.K. Chandhok and
Dr. Archana Chandhok - Directors
Main Market
Uttarkaṣhi, Himalayas 249193
India

Āyurvedic Research

The Āyurveda Holistic Center has begun several pilot studies on cost-effectiveness, safety, holistic therapeutics, prevention and long-term results. The center is open to funding as well as working with other researchers in other parts of the country for wider geographical studies. Contact the center at the above New York number.

Āyurveda 2-Year Certification Program

A two-year certification program at our NJ center and/or through distance learning (mail & internet) for health professionals.

Program Information: The course is designed for health care professionals (i.e., MDs, RNs, pharmacists, chiropractors, psychologists, *yoga* teachers, herbalists, holistic practitioners, etc.) or for persons planning to practice Āyurveda full or part-time.

Teachers:
Residential:
Punita Desai, B.A.M.S.: Āyurveda
Dr. Patrick Conte, MD: Allopathy
Bharat Shukla: Pharmacology, Pharmacognosy

Distance Learning:
Swami Sada Shiva Tirtha: Āyurveda, Vedanta

Gentle, natural, personal. The practitioner integrates all forms of holistic healing through this unique healing system.

750 Hour Certification Program
300 classroom & internship
450 guided study program

ॐ ॐ ॐ

Syllabus

Āyurveda

101: History, tridoṣha theory, diagnosis, herbology, nutrition
102: Pañcha karma, aroma & sound therapy, cooking
201: Color & gem therapy, external influences, lifestyle therapy, Āyurvedic psychology, circulatory & digestive systems
202: Infections/wounds, respiratory, urinary & nervous systems; & ears/nose/throat/mouth/eyes
301: Skin system
302: Skin, neoplasm, reproductive systems

401: Reproductive, immune systems
402: Immune, metabolic systems, herb mixing/ preparation, miscellaneous
403: Kerala pañcha karma
404: Traditional pañcha karma

Āyurvedic-Yoga (optional local training)
101: Student training: yoga, prāṇāyām, meditation, chanting
102: Teacher training: yoga, prāṇāyām, meditation, chanting (students receive Āyurvedic-yoga teacher certification.

Vedanta
Topics: Self-realization, dharma, ethics, spiritual counseling for students & their clients. Books:
201: Bhagavad Gīta
202: Bhagavad Gīta
301: Upanishads
302: Upanishads
401: Guru Bani
402: Yoga Bani

Sanskrit (optional local training - 3rd year)
Students should have a moderate ability to read, write, and understand Āyurvedic and Vedantic Sanskrit literature at the end of the two years.
201: Introduction- read, write, & speak Sanskrit
202: Intermediate - read, write, & speak Sanskrit
301: Advanced - understanding Sanskrit
302: AdvancedII - understanding Sanskrit

Allopathy(under development)
101: Intro to Anatomy
102: Intro to Physiology
201: Intro to Pathology
202: Intro to Pharmacology
301: Intro to Pediatrics
302: Intro to OB/Gyn
401: Pharmacognosy

Research (under development)
402: Data gathering & analysis
403: Research methods

Yearly Overview
Year 1: Āyurveda, Vedanta
Year 2: Āyurveda, Vedanta
Year 3: Āyurvedic-Yoga, Sanskrit (optional)
Year 4 & 5: under development

The course is approved by the State of New York
Course focus is spiritually and practical
Email correspondence available!

ॐ ॐ ॐ

Certification is Granted When
1) Students are properly practicing and understanding their own Āyurvedic routine
2) Students display adequate knowledge in homework, exams and internships
3) Students integrate spirituality,ethics, humility and respect with classroom knowledge.

Degree Programs
Upon graduation from this training program one receives certification from the Āyurveda Holistic Center. 50 "credit hours" are transferable to a BA, MA, or Ph.D. degree in Āyurvedic Medicine through Westbrook University in Aztec, NM. Westbrook is a distance learning university. The Āyurveda Holistic Center is an affiliate member of Westbrook University.

Certification Program Options
Distance Learning Program: A video of *pañcha karma* therapies are sent to correspondence students. Students send a written outline of 50 hours of intern consultations (each consultation can last up to three hours) for grading. Exams are based on understanding principles and referencing materials. Memorization is not emphasized. Yoga training done locally through qualified centers - monitored by our center.

Center Classes: Each year lasts for 140 hours/10 months: one evening a week (2 hours) and 10 Sundays (one per month- 6 hours/day) or two 7-hour weekends a month. Final exams are based on understanding principles and referencing materials. Memorization is not emphasized. Classes held at NJ center.

Pre-requisites (for both programs)

1) For health care professionals or those who plan to practice Āyurveda full or part time.
2) Receive and follow Āyurvedic consultation suggestions for some months. If you are still eager to learn more, register.
3) Interview (in person/ phone/ email/ mail).

ॐ ॐ ॐ

Graduates Comments

'I have previously studied Western and Chinese medicine...the Āyurvedic approach is the most effective and easy to understand.'
-Dr. F. Cassis/NY

'The information was presented simply, spiritually and practically...I have already begun Āyurvedic consultations and incorporated my other holistic trainings...This course and the teacher were truly an inspiration.'
-W. Lawder/NJ

'I very much enjoy helping people, so I was searching for a healing program that will help me help others. This course has given me everything that I was looking for.'
-T. Fyssoun/Greece

ॐ ॐ ॐ

Call or write for program registration:

Āyurveda Holistic Center- Residential Program
460 Ridgedale Ave #2
E. Hanover, NJ 07936
800-452-1798 (fax: 973-887-3088)
Online Registration: http://ayurvedahc.com

Āyurveda Holistic Center- Distance Learning
82A Bayville Ave
Bayville, NY 11709
516-628-8200
Online Registration: http://ayurvedahc.com

ॐ ॐ ॐ

Web Site
Āyurveda Holistic Center

Visit our web site for articles, *doṣha* self-test, excerpts from this book, product and service links, detailed certification brochure and more. The site discusses Āyurveda, Vedic Astrology (*Jyotiṣh*), the *Swami Narayan Tirtha Math* (*ashram*), more.
Web address: *http://ayurvedahc.com.*

Other books from the Āyurveda Holistic Center Press

Yoga Bani;
Instructions for the Attainment of Siddhayoga- by the late Swami Shankar Purushottam Tirtha, founder of the *Siddhayogashram* in India. The topics discussed include *sādhanā* (meditation) experiences, how to find a *guru*, when to change *gurus*, discussions of *kuṇḍalinī śhaktipat, suṣhumna,* the 10 *chakras*, *yoga*, much more.

Guru Bani; 100 Ways To Attain Inner Peace
by Swami Shankar Purushottam Tirtha. This sequel to *Yoga Bani* offers simple guidance on how to live spiritual, ethical life outside of meditation (for families and monks)

To order books call or order online
800-452-1798 or 973-8828
http://www.lotusfair.com

ॐ ॐ ॐ

Columbia University Initiative on Āyurveda

To receive information contact Nancy Braxton at the Dharam Hinduja Indic Research Center; Columbia University; Mail code 3367; 420 West 118th St. New York, NY 10027; 1-212-854-5300; email: dhirc@columbia.edu.

ॐ ॐ ॐ

Other Āyurvedic Herb Resources

Bulk Herbs
Distributor/Wholesaler/Retailer
Fairdeal Distributors
http://www.lotusfair.com
1-800-452-1798 / Fax: 1-973-887-3088
460 Ridgedale Ave. Suite 2;
E. Hanover, NJ 07936 USA

Wholesale Herbs - sold in 1 pound orders only
Bazaar of India
1-800-261-7662 or 1-510-548-4110
1810 University Ave; Berkeley, CA 94703

Organic Ghee Retail/Wholesale
Purity Farms
1-800-568-4433 or 1-303-647-2368
Fax: 1-303-647-9875
14635 Westcreek Rd.; Sedalia, CO 80135 USA

Other Āyurveda Certification Programs
New England Institute of Āyurvedic Medicine
1815 Massachusetts Ave. Ste 318
Cambridge, MA 02140
(617) 876-2401
[Correspondence/2 week visits]

Āyurvedic Institute
P.O. Box 23445
Albuquerque, NM 87192
1-505-291-9698
http://www.ayurveda.com
[Residential]

American Institute of Vedic Studies
P.O. Box 8357
Santa Fe, NM 87504
[Correspondence]

Pañcha Karma Clinics In India

The main concern when choosing a clinic in India is to find a reputable facility. Among the reputable clinics, conditions and prices vary. Generally for basic 4-week treatments including room and board, the cost is around 5,000 rupees ($145 US). In clinics offering air conditioning and other comforts, the price can double. General treatments last from 4-6 weeks. Chronic or severe conditions (e.g., paralysis) can take longer.

Below is a select list of clinics that have been recommended to us as being reputable. Please check further before choosing a center.

Akhand Anand Āyurvedic Hospital
Ahmedabad, Gujarat

A.L. Podar Āyurvedic Hospital & College
Bombay

Dr. S. N. Srivastava
Govt. Āyurvedic College
Gurukul Kangri
Hardwar

Āyurveda College at
Benares Hindu University
Varanasi

Indian Foods & Spices

Chapatti flour, rock candy, *jaggery*, split yellow *moongdal, channa dal, tur dal,* rose water, *ghee, basmati* rice, hair oil, classical Indian music, etc. are all available wherever you find an Indian grocery. In most big cities and towns, or wherever you find a large Indian population, you will find the groceries.

Āyurveda Encyclopedia available through
Canada through Mond Trading 416-504-5755
UK: Gazelle Books 44-1524-68765
India: Sri Sat Guru Press - Delhi
Australia: Boobook Pub. 61-2-4997-0811
New Zealand: Jay Books 04-586-0226

The book is available in many other countries. Check local bookstores, holistic shops and health food stores.

About the Author

1974 Began practicing organized meditation
1975 BA-Interdisciplinary Studies
1976 Certified meditation teacher
1980 MA- Non-Verbal Communication Research
1988 Āyurveda certificate, Āyurvedic Institute, Jyotiṣh (Vedic Astrology) certification, American Institute of Vedic Studies; Began an Āyurveda practice; Visited India, initiated into science of mysticism by his *guru* (spiritual teacher) - Swami Narayan Tirtha; Advanced Āyurveda training with Benares Hindu University professors; *Varanasi,* India
1989 Āyurveda certification from American Institute of Vedic Studies, Santa Fe, NM
Founded the Swami Narayan Tirtha Math (Hindu monastery in the US)
1990 Published *Yoga Vani: Instructions for the Attainment of Siddhayoga*
Developed an Āyurvedic herbal product line
1991 Began offering Āyurveda certification training programs internationally
Received initiation as swami (monkhood) from his *guru* in India
Advanced study with Āyurvedic doctors in the Himalayas
1995 Published *Guru Bani; 100 Ways to Attain Inner Peace*
Began wholesale and distribution of herbal products
1997 Went online with an Āyurvedic website
1998 Āyurveda Encyclopedia was first published**;** completed pilot scientifc research study on Āyurveda & allopathy cost comparison for seasonal allergies
1999 PhD. Āyurvedic Medicine & Research; Westbrook University

1990-present Writing articles on Āyurveda for magazines and newspapers
1991- present Advanced spiritual training with *guru* in *Uttarkaṣhi,* India. Advanced study of Āyurveda with Āyurvedic *vaidyas* in India.

Swami Sada Shiva Tirtha is listed in Natural Living Magazine's "Best Alternative Health Practitioners in the Country" guide, and his center as been listed as respected Āyurveda resource in numerous holistic health magazine including Yoga Journal, Natural Remedies, Delicious Magazine; and in various holistic reference books including the American Holistic Health Association Complete Guide to Alternative Medicine.

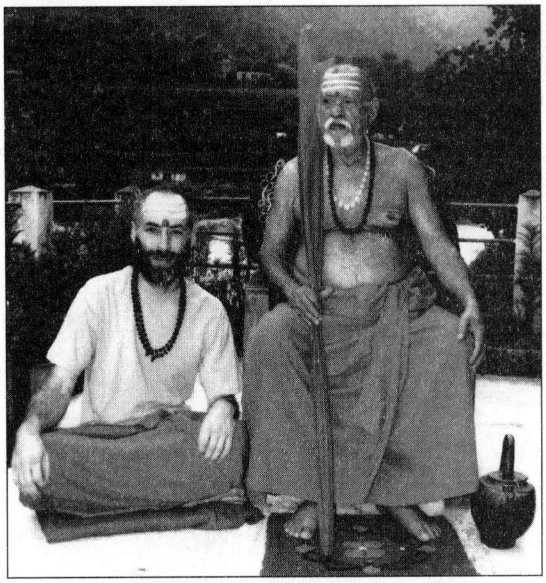

Author (left) with his Guru,
His Holiness Sri, Sri, Srimat 1008
Swami Narayan Tirthaji Maharaj

Order Form

Name____

Address____

City__________________ State ________ Zip ______ Country____________

Phone (daytime- in case we need to reach you) (_____) ____________________

Discover/Visa/MC # ______________________________ exp. date: ______________

Books	Price	Quantity	Total
Āyurveda Encyclopedia	$40.00 pp (U.S.)		
Yoga Vani	$13.50 pp		
Guru Bani	$9.75 pp		
NY State Residence add sales tax			
Total			

Email, fax or mail to:
Āyurveda Holistic Center
460 Ridgedale Ave #2
E. Hanover, NJ 07936 USA

phone/fax: (800) 452-1798
fax: 973-887-3088
email:lotusfair@aol.com
website: http://www.lotusfair.com

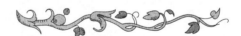

Inspiration from Tagore

God respects me when I work; but he loves me when I sing.

Those who want to help knock on the door. Those who love find the door already open.

I slept and dreamt life was joy.
I awoke and saw life was service.
I served and lo, service was joy.

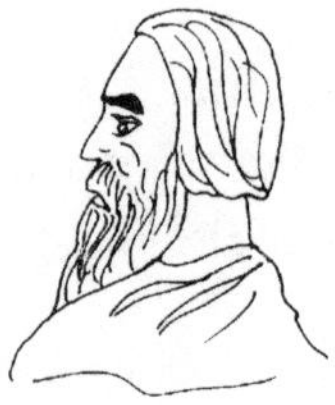

This book is also sold throughout the world

Āyurvedic Glossary

A

abaran concealment energy of the causal or essential body
abhyañga massage-like therapies
agni digestive enzymes
ahimsa non-violence
ajapa the Gāyatrī mantra that brings salvation
ajīrna indigestion
ājñā chakra third eye or intuitive eye
akaṣha space
akshe-paka convulsions
alajī a painful mouth erruption emitting discharge
alasaka a digestive disorder
alepa/ātepanam medicated pastes for ulcers
allaepauk ginger jam with additonal spices
ālochaka Pitta one of the five Pitta subdoṣhas; resides in the retina of the eyes and governs sight.
āma undigested food toxins
āmāṣhaya stomach
amla sour
amlapitta acid gastritis
anāha a digestive disorder involving āma and/or
feces accumulation in the digestive tract
anahāta chakra fourth or heart chakra
anasarca an edema-like swelling
aṅguli/aṅgula finger width measurement
ani marma energy point governing muscle tension (located just above the knees)
anjana eye salves
anjana vidhi eye therapies
anna lepa poultice used when pinḍa sweda is contraindicated or ineffective
annamaya koṣha food cell
annavaha srota digestive system channels of transport
antraja vṛiddhi inguinal hernia
anupana a food medium or vehicle that transports herbs to the tissue levels (e.g., honey)
anuvāsana basti unctuous medicated enema
ap water element
apān Vāyu one of the five Vāyu subdoṣhas; downward moving air
aparigraha not chasing after material wealth
apartarpaṇa reducing or detoxifying therapies
apasmāra epilepsy
arbuda cancer
ardha matsyendrāsana alternate spinal twist yoga pose
āriṣhṭha/āsava medicated wines
arochaka anorexia
arogya health
arṣhas hemorrhoids
artavaha srota uterus channels
āsana haṭha yoga postures
āsava, āriṣhṭha medicated wines
āṣhaya containers within the body
āṣhcotana therapy using eye drops
aṣhtabindu eight drops
Aṣhṭāñga Hṛidayam one of the three main ancient Āyurvedic texts
asṛigdara menorrhagia
asthi bone tissue
astivaha srota bone channels
atīsāra diarrhea
Ātreya author of Charak Saṃhitā
asthāpana or nirūha basti non-oily enema
aum first sound of creation
aupadravikam adhyayam eye diseases
avagāhan soaking in a tub of medicated water
avalaṃbaka Kapha one of the five Kapha subdoṣhas; found in the chest and creates cohesion, softness, moistness, and liquidity, which results in maintaining body strength.
avaleha confections
avapīda nasal therapy using fresh herb juices
Āyurveda science of life and longevity

B

bahihpragña perceiving the world through

the senses
bahya kumbhaka outer breath retention
baikhari audible sounds produced by the throat
bajra nāḍī first subtler channel in suṣhumṇā
bālāmaya pratihedha children's diseases
bandhas energy locks used during yoga poses
basmati rice a sweet, nutritious, and easily digesed rice
basti bladder or medicated enema- one of the five pañcha karma therapies
basti marma energy center below the navel; governing apāna Vāyu, Kapha, urine function
bhagandara fistula-in-ano
bhagnam fractures
bhajans singing of religous songs
bhasma burnt metals or gems (generally for ingesting)
bhastra kumbhaka bellows breath exercise
bhesan chick pea (also called garbanzo and channa)
bhrājaka Pitta one of the five Pitta subdoṣhas; resides in the skin. It regulates complexion by keeping secretions from the sweat and sebaceous glands of the skin active.
bhramarī kumbhaka humming-bee breath
bhujaṅgāsana serpent pose
bhujangini mudrā breathing exercise for stomach diseases and digestion
bhūta vidyā Āyurvedic psychiatry
bhutagnis five digestive enzimes that metabolize the five elements
bhūta Vidyā Āyurvedic psychiatry
bidālikā tonsillitis
bīj seed
bikṣhepa hallucination energy of the causal or essential body
bindū semen or ovum
bodhaka Kapha one of the five Kapha subdoṣhas; found in the tongue and is responsible for taste.
Brahmā name of God of creation
brahmacharya celibacy; one who follows a spiritual lifestyle including celibacy (certain religious married couples have their ownform of brahmacharya)
Brahman a name for eternal, unmanifest God
brahmanāḍī subtlest channel in the suṣhumṇā
brahmarandhra area in the crown chakra
brāhmī gotu kola
brāhmī ghee a rejuvenating herbal/ghee therapy with brāhmī as the main ingredient
Brihat Samhitā a Jyotiṣh astrology text
bṛiṃhaṇa nourishing therapies in pañcha karma

C

cala moving quality of food
chai tea
chaitanya consciousness
chakra spiritual energy centers in the body
chandrabheda prāṇāyāma left-nostril breathing exercise
channa dal chick peas or garbanzo beans
Charak pen name of author of Charak Saṃhitā (Lord Ātreya)
Charak Saṃhitā One of the three main ancient Āyurvedic texts
chardi vomiting
chitrini second subtlest channel in the suṣhumṇā
choti elā small cardamom seeds
chūrṇas herb powders
chyavan prāśh herbal rejuvanative jam with āmalakī and ghee as its main ingredients

D

danta roga tooth disorders
danta vidradhi dental abscess
dantamūla gums
dārdhya sturdiness
deha-manasa psychosomatic
dhamanī arteries
dhanurāsana bow pose (yoga posture)
Dhanvantari divine father of Āyurveda
dhārā drava medicated oil for the head
dhārā karma certain pañcha karma therapies
dhārā svedhana pouring warm oil on body, causing sweating
dhāraṇā God-visualization
dharma life purpose or life path; God-given talent

dhatagnis seven digestive enzymes that metabolize the seven tissue layers; it includes anabolic and catabolic activity
dhātu tissue
dhūma medicated smoke therapy
dhyāna fixed God-visualization
doṣha humors; elemental or energetics related to personal constitution or current health imbalance (Vāyu, Pitta, Kapha, Tridoṣha)
drakṣha herbal wine
drava liquid quality of food
drava svedhana see dhārā svedhana
driṣhti eye
driṣhti-gata-roga-vijnāñiya eye pupil diseases

G

galaganda goiter
Ganges famous river in India believed to believed to posess spiritual healing powers
Gangotri a holy place near the source of the
Garuda Purana ancient Vedic text that discusses gems
gāyatrī mantra mantra for salvation
ghee clarified butter
ghrita another word for ghee
grahanī duodenum
gomedha hessonite garnet used for healing in Āyurveda and Jyotiṣh astrology
gomukhāsana cow-face yoga pose
Gorakṣha Saṃhitā a major haṭha yoga treatise
grahanī digestive disorders
gṛidhrasī sciatica
grīṣhma summer
gulma abdominal tumors
guḍa (jaggery) a form of pure cane sugar
guṇas three qualities or the fundamental laws of nature (sattwa: creation, rajas: maintainance, tamas: disolution)
guru teacher; also heavy quality of foods
guṭi herbal pills

H

halāsana plough pose
haṅg saḥ mantra sound of the life-breath
haṭha yoga gentle stretching exercises that improve health, mind/body coordination and spiritual foundations
hataratnavali major haṭha yoga treatise
hemanta winter season
hikkā hiccup
hima cold infusions
hiranyagarbha Supreme God, golden egg, universal consciousness, or Supreme Self
hirchula cardiac colic
hṛidaya heart
hṛidroga heart disease

I

iḍā left or lunar channel, associated with piṅgalā;
surrounding the suṣhumṇā

J

jaggery (guḍa) a form of pure cane sugar
jālandhara bandha throat lock used with yoga postures to keep the bindū from flowing down-
out of the head
jarā aging
jatharagni digestive enzymes in the G.I. level
jathara parivartanāsana belly roll yoga pose
jatrūrdhva marma energy point group: those points on the neck and head
jihwā roga tongue disorders
jñyān mudrā finger position to keep energy from flowing out of the fingers
jwara fever
Jyotiṣh Vedic astrology

K

kaki mudrā a breathing exercise- pursing lips and inhaling; cools Pitta (heat)
kama healthy and spiritual use of the senses
kāmalā roga jaundice
kaṇṭha roga throat disorders
kapālbhāti kumbhaka frontal brain cleanse
Kapha biological phlegm; water/earth energetic, constitution, or humor
kapitthaparni a name for frankincense

kapotāsana pigeon yoga pose
karana śharīra causal or essential body
karma action
karna pūrana ear bath therapy
karnapālī roga ear lobes
karṇa-gata-roga-vijnāniya ear disorders
karpūr camphor
kāsa cough
kaṣhaya astringent
kathina hard quality of food
katti basti lower back bath therapy
katu pungent
kaumāra bhṛitya pediatrics; one of the eight branches of Āyurvedic medicine
kāya seka oil poured over the body (therapy)
kāyachikitsā internal medicine; one of the eight branches of Āyurvedic medicine
kayvala kumbhaka automatic still breath exercise
khara rough quality of food
kicharī grain/legume meal; usually basmati rice and mūngdal. Sometimes some veges are included
kledaka Kapha one of the five Kapha subdoṣhas; found in the stomach, liquefying hard food masses.
koṣṭhāgni digestive fire/enzymes
krimi parasites
Kṛiṣhṇa a name of God
krishna-gata-roga-vijñāniya chorid and iris
kriyā yoga form of yoga exercises
kṣhaya atrophy
kukkutāsana cockerel yoga pose
kukṣhi-śhūla a Vāyu digestive disorder
kumbhaka yogic breathing exercises
kuṇḍalinī śhakti spiritual life-force
kūrmāsana tortoise yoga pose
kuṣhṭha obstinate skin diseases
kwātha herbal decoction

L

laghu light quality of food
lalanā chakra energy center in the palate
laṅghana reducing therapies
lavaṇa salty
laya yoga yoga stage where breathing stops
lekhana scraping therapies
lepa herbal paste or poultice

M

madāt-yaya alcohol recovery
madhāyamañga marma energy point group: those points on the trunk of the body
madhura sweet
madhya medium (level)
madhyama sound (nāda) rising to the heart that is felt by the ears (but not heard)
mahā bandha great lock pose
mahā bheda yoga pose that brings life-breath into suṣhumṇā
mahā bheda mudrā great piercing (yoga) position
mahā marma the 3 vital organs: head, heart, urinary bladder
mahā mudrā great sealing pose
Maharishi Kanada author of Nāḍīvijñānam
Mahavīr Hanuman the Monkey-God; Lord of selfless service and devotion
majjāvaha srota marrow/joint lubrication channels
mala waste produce (i.e., urine, sweat, feces)
māṃsa muscle tissue
māṃsavaha srota muscular channels
manas chakra energy center slightly above the the 3rd eye on the forehead
manda slow quality of food; also rice water
mandāgni Kapha-produced digestive enzymes
manipūra chakra energy center located at the navel
manomaya koṣha mind cell
mantra special words or sounds for health and spiritual development
mantra yoga meditation using words or sounds
manyā marma energy points in the neck governing lymphatic and Kapha function
marga tracts in the body
marma energy points on the body
matsyāsana fish pose
matsyendrāsana spinal twist
medas fat/adipose tissue
medovaha srota adipose/fat channels
majja marrow/bones and joint tissue

majjavaha srotas marrow/bones and joint channels
mūtra urine
mūtravaha srota urinary channels
mithya āhar vihar improper lifestyle
mokṣha Self-Realization
mridu soft quality of food
mudrās body and hand positions that channel energy into the chakras and suṣhumṇā
mukha roga mouth cavity
mūla bandha perineum/cervix contraction used with yoga poses
mūlādhāra chakra energy center at the base of the spine
mūrchā fainting
mūrchha kumbhaka swooning breath exercise
mūrdha taila head oil
mūtra urine
mūtra vṛiddhi scrotum fluid
mūtrā-śharkarā urinary gravel
mūtrā-āṣhmarī urinary stones
mūtrā-ghāta urinary diseases
mūtrā-ghātādi urine retention
mūtrā-kṛichra dysuria
mūtraghāta urine obstruction
mūtravaha srota urinary channel

N

nābhi navel
nabho mudrā yoga exercise involving head extention and breathing
nāda sound
nāḍī nerve channels
nāḍī śhodhana prāṇāyāma dual-nostril breathing exercise
nāḍī sveda medicated herbal steam directed through a tube and applied to localized body areas
naḍīprakaṣham/nāḍīvijñānam pulse diagnosis
nāḍī-vraṇa sinus
nasikagra driṣhti eyes gazing at tip of nose
nasya therapies applied through the nose; one of the five pañcha karma therapies
nāsā-gata-roga-vijñāniya nose diseases
nayanā-bhighāta-pratiṣhedha externally caused eye injury
nayana-budbuda eyeball diseases
neti pot a small vessel that looks like a miniature watering can; used for nasal channel washing
netra basti medicated eye baths
nidāna diagnosis, etiology, cause of disease
niketa abodes within the body
nilā marma energy points on the neck
nirāma non-clogged (no āma) digestive system
nirbikalpa samādhi second stage of samādhi (absorption in eternal consciousness)
nirūha basti oily enema
nirvana śhakti mother of the three worlds—experienced when crown chakra opens
niyama ethical codes of conduct; purity, contentment, devotion, spiritual study, faithin God; included with Yama

O

odana soft, plain basmati rice meal
ojas life sap; essence of immune system and spiritual energy

P

pāchaka agni responsible for digestion
pāchaka Pitta one of the five Pitta subdoṣhas; the main digestive enzymes, they are foundin the small intestine, stomach, and colon as non-liquid heat, bile, or digestive fire. The fire digests and transforms food, emulsifying food fats and separating absorbable nutrients from waste, so they may be passed to lacteals by absorption.
pādābhyañga foot massage
padma lotus
padmāsana lotus yoga pose
pañcha karma five cleansing therapies; vaman, virechan, basti, nasya, rakta mokṣha
pañchang ephemeris
panīr home made Indian ricotta cheese
pantha passages within the body
pāṇḍu-roga anemia
para nāda sound evolving from kuṇḍalinī at the first chakra
pariṣheka medicated water sprinkled over localized areas of the body for therapeutic benefits

pārṣhva-śhūla a form of colic
paschimottanāsana back stretching yoga pose
pāṣhāsana chord yoga pose
pasyanti sound only heard by advanced yogis
Patañjali author of the Yoga Sutras and commentator on yama and niyama
payasam semi-solid pudding for piṇḍa sveda
peyā thin soup taken after pañcha karma therapies
phāṇṭa hot infusions
pīnasa rhinitis
piṇḍa sveda abhyañga therapy using a heated bolus
piṅgalā the right or solar nerve channel- related to iḍā; both surround the suṣhumnā
Pitta biological bile; fire energetic, a constitution, or humor
pizhichil abhyañga therapy involving the continuous pouring of warm oil over the body
prabhāva special effects of herbs
pradara menorrhagia
pradhama herbal evacuative nasal therapy using
pradhamana nasal therapy: herbs blown through a tube
pradhana karma primary pañcha karma practices
pradhena non-absorbing topical pastes for Vāyu and Kapha doṣhas
prakṛiti one's life constitution or nature
pralaya universal sound sleep
pralepa topical pastes for Pitta doṣha
prameha obstinate urinary diseases (including diabetes)
prameha piḍakā diabetic ulcer
prāṇa life force
prāṇa Vāyu one of the five Vāyu subdoṣhas; outward moving air.
prāṇavaha srota channel which prāṇa flows
prāṇāyām breathing exercises
prasad food offered to God
prasādana vision-clearing eye salves
pratimarṣha oil/uncting nasal therapy
pratiṣhyāya colds
pratyāhāra withdrawal and liberation of the mind from the senses and objcets (5th stage of yoga)
pravāhika dysentery
pṛitivi earth
puakuṣha gingivitis
pūja worship ritual
punster male reproductive system
purīṣha feces waste product
purīshavaha srota feces elimination channels
Puruṣha eternal, unmanifest consciousness
purva karma preliminary pañcha karma therapies (oleation & sudation)
pūrvarupa hidden or incubatory signs of disase
puṣhti nourishing
puta-pāka a group of eye therapies

R

rajas/rajasic law of nature that maintains life; one of the three guṇas
raja yoga final stage of yoga; one remains ever centered within their Self
rājā-yakṣhmā pulmonary TB
rakta blood
raktaja gulma blood/ovarian tumors and cysts
rakta mokṣha blood letting; one of the five pañcha karma cleansing methods
raktavaha srota blood circulatory channels
rañjaka Pitta one if the five Pitta subdoṣhas; located in the stomach, liver, and spleen, and gives color to lymph chyle when it is transformed into blood as it passes through the liver and spleen.
rasa plasma; taste; also products containing mer cury ash
rasavaha srota plasma channels
rasa dhātu plasma tissue
rasavahini capillaries
rasāyana rejuvenation
Ravi Śhankar reknown sitar musician
Ṛig Veda One of the four main Vedic scriptures
Ṛig Veda Bhasyabhumika ancient Vedic scripture
ṛishi seer or sage
roga disease
rudhrapuṣhpa rose
rūkṣhaṇa drying therapies in pañcha karma
rupa form; signs or symptoms of disease

rūṣha dry quality of food

S

sādhaka Pitta one of the five Pitta subdoṣhas; found in the heart. It helps in performing mental functions such as knowledge, intelligence, and consciousness by maintaining rhythmic cardiac contractions.
sādhanā meditation
sahasrāra chakra energy center at the crown of head
saibikalpa samādhi first stage of samādhi; sattwic mind
sālamba sarvāṅgāsana shoulder stand pose
sāma coated tongue due to āma in the digestive system
Sama Veda one of the four main Vedic scriptures
samādhi various stages of Self-Realization
samāgni normal digestion
samāna Vāyu one of the five Vāyu subdoṣhas; equalized moving air
saṃnyāsa coma
samprapti pathogenesis; disease development
samsarajana special diet after undergoing pañcha karma therapies
saṃśhamana gentle reducing therapies for mild imbalances
saṃaśhodhana strong reducing therapies for more serious imbalances
saṃtarpaṇa nourishing pañcha karma therapies
samvritāsamvrita ducts within the body
sanātana dharma fundamental Hindu philosophy that states everything has its use in its own time and place; so reject nothing and accept everything (in its time and place)
sandhi mukti fractures
sandhigata-roga-vijñaniya eyes
sapta dhātus seven tissue layers
Saraswati Goddess of wisdom, education, and music
sāndra solid quality of food
sarva-gata-roga-abhiṣhyandha conjunctivitis
sarvānga dhārā whole-body abhyañga therapies
sarvānga senchana another name for kāya seka
sattwa/sattwic purity; one of the three guṇas
sattwavajaya holistic psychotherapy
setu bandha sarvāṅgāsana bridge yoga pose
śhakti spiritual energy
śhalabhāsan locust pose
śhālākya tantra ears, nose, throat; one of the eight branches of Āyurvedic medicine
śhalyā tantra surgery; one of the eight branches of Āyurvedic medicine
śhamana palliation therapy
śhāṃbhavī mudrā staring at 3rd eye exercise
śhankha marma energy point group on the legs and feet
Śhaṅkar Sen author of Nāḍīprakaṣham
sharat autumn
śharīrachidra spaces within the body
śhastra Vedic laws
śhatapatra lotus
śhavāsana corpse pose
śheka eye sprinkling therapy
śhikṣha, dīkṣha, parīkṣha learning, dedicated practice, evaluation
śhirā veins
śhiro basti medicated oil soaking on the head
śhiro dhārā warm oil flow to the forehead
śhiro lepa medicated head pastes or poultices
śhiro-roga-vijñāniya head disorders
śhiro virechana nasya nasal evacuative therapies
shiśhira cold season
śhishya disciple/student
śhītalī cooling breath exercise
śhītkarī kumbhaka hissing breath exercise
Śhiva one name of God in Hinduism
śhlakṣhna smooth quality of food
śhlīpada elephantiasis
śhleṣhaka Kapha one of the five Kapha subdoṣhas; located in the bone joints and lubricates them.
śhodhana strong reducing therapies
śhopha/śhotha edema
śhrama fatigue
śhuklagata-roga-vijñāniya sclerotic coat
śhukra dhātu reproductive tissue
śhukra-śhmarī seminal stones
śhukravaha srota reproductive system channels

śhūla colic
śhvāsa breahing difficulty
siddha yoni āsana perfection pose (for women)
siddhāsana perfection pose (for men)
simhāsana lion yoga pose
sīta cold quality of food
sneha medicated ghee and oil
snehana oil therapy (external)
snehapāna internal oil therapy
snighda oily quality of food
soma spiritual nectar
soma chakra between third eye and crown chakras
srota channels or pores
srutis Vedic laws
stambhana astringent therapies
sthāna residence sites within the body
stanyavaha srota breast milk channel
sthira stable quality of food
sthūla large quality of food
sthula śharīra physical body
sūkṣhma subtle quality of food
sukṣhma śharīra astral body
sūrya the sun
sūryabheda prāṇāyāma solar breathing exercise
sūryāsana sun salute yoga pose
Suṣhrut author of Suṣhrut Saṃhitā
Suṣhrut Saṃhitā one of the original three main Āyurvedic texts; mainly covers surgery
suṣhumṇā spiritual tube within the spine. Life force energy rises through this tube as
sutrātma thread of the Self; Universal Consciousness
svara-bedha hoarsness
svedhana preliminary pañcha karma sweat therapy
swabhavoparama recession by nature
swādhiṣhṭhān chakra second or navel energy center
Swami Narayan Tirtha successor of Swāmī Śhaṅkar Puruṣhottam Tīrtha
Swāmī Śhaṅkar Puruṣhottam Tīrtha author of Yoga Vani & Guru Bani
swapna sleep
swarasa herb juice
swastikāsana auspicious pose (a yoga pose)
swabhavoparama health returns from recession by nature, resulting from administering therapies
swādus weet
sweda sweat
swedavaha srota sweat-transporting channels

T

tadan kriyā great piercing (yoga) position
taila seka another name for kāya seka
tālu vidradhi palatal abscesses
talugata roga palate disorders
tamas/tamasic one of the three guṇas; lethargy destruction property
tanmatras primal sensory energies before they develop into the five senses
tarpaka Kapha one of the five Kapha subdoṣhas; found in the head and nourishes the sense organs.
tāpa svedhana heated object placed on body to cause sweating
tapas a form of spiritual practice
tarpaka Kapha subdosha that nourishes the senses
tarpana soothing eye therapies
tejas mental fire
tekṣhna quick quality of food
tikṣhna strong smoke therapies
tīkṣhnāgni Pitta-produced digestive enzymes
tikta bitter
til sesame seeds
timira blindness
tridosha/tridoṣhic a physical constitution involving all three doṣhas
triṣhnā thirst
tur dal a legume high in protein

U

udakavaha srota water metabolism system
udān Vāyu one of the five Vāyu subdoṣhas; upward moving air
udara roga abdominal diseases
uḍḍīyāna bandha exercise that contracts the lower abdomen
udgharṣhana body powder rub

ugrāsana (paschimottanāsana) back stretching pose
ujjāyī kumbhaka conquering breath exercise
unmāda insanity
upajihvikā glossitis
upanāha svedhana hot poultice applied to body then wrapped in heated cloth
Upanishads a series of Vedic scriptures
upaṣhaya diagnostic tests
upaveda a secondary branch of the main Vedas
uro basti chest/heart bath
urustambha paraplegia
uṣhmā svedhana steam therapy
ūṣhnā hot quality of food
uttara karma pañcha karma follow-up therapies
uttara basti upper tract medicated enema

V

vaiswanara Consciousness in the universal ma terial body
vājikarana aphrodisiacs
vajrolī mudrā thunderbolt yoga pose
Vala a demon who when killed was cut into pieces that became various gems
vamaka vamana herbs that induce vomiting
vamana medicated emesis; one of the pañcha karma cleansing processes
vamanopaga vamana herbs that enhance vamaka herbs
varṇya lepa cosmetic plasters
varṣhā rainy season
vartmagata-roga-vijñāniya eyelids
vasant spring
Vāstu Śhastra Vedic architecture
vāta-rakta (also called vāta-ṣhonita) gout
vāta-ṣhonita (vāta-rakta) gout
vāta-vyādhi nervous system
vātāṣhṭhīlā enlarged prostate
Vāyu/Vāta biological wind; ether/air element, constitution, or humor (traditional word for Vāta)
VedasThe ancient scriptures of India
Veda Vyasa ancient sage who transcribed the Vedas
vidradhi abscess
vigñanamaya koṣha knowledge cell
vikṛiti current doṣha imbalance (as differentiated from prakṛiti or life constitution)
vilambikā digestive disorder due to excess Vāyu and Kapha
vilepī thick rice soup
vipāka post digestive taste
vīrāsana hero's yoga pose
virat consciousness in the universal physical body (also called vaiswanara)
virechana medicated purgation; one of the pañcha karma cleansing processes
vīrya potency (related to the taste of herbs,foods, etc.)
vīryalpata impotence
visāsana alternate yoga pose for vīrāsana
viṣhada non-slimy quality of food
viṣhagara-vairodh tantra toxicology; one of the eight branches of Ayurvedic medicine
viṣhamāgni Vāyu-produced digestive enzymes
Viṣhṇu maintainer of the universe (one of the triad of Brahma , Viṣhṇu, Maheṣhwara: creator, maintainer, and destroyer of the universe respectively); also One name of God in Hinduism
viṣhuddha chakra 5th or throat energy center
visūchikā gastro enteritis
viswa consciousness in the individual material body
vraṇa wounds
vṛiddhi enlarged scrotum
vyān Vāyu one of the five Vāyu subdoṣhas; air movement throughout the body
vyayama exercise

Y

Yajur Veda one of the four main Vedic texts
yakrit janya raktalplata sickle cell anemia
yama codes of ethical behavior non-envy, truth, non-stealing, continence, not desiring of material wealth (included with niyama)
yoga uniting of mind and body, and the various subtle energies within; also a form of stretching postures (see haṭha yoga)
Yoga Vani an instructional book for the attainment of siddhayoga (a guide to Selfealization)

yoni mudrā hand position to awaken raja yoga
yonivyāpat female reproductive
yuṣha rice and split yellow mūng dal soup

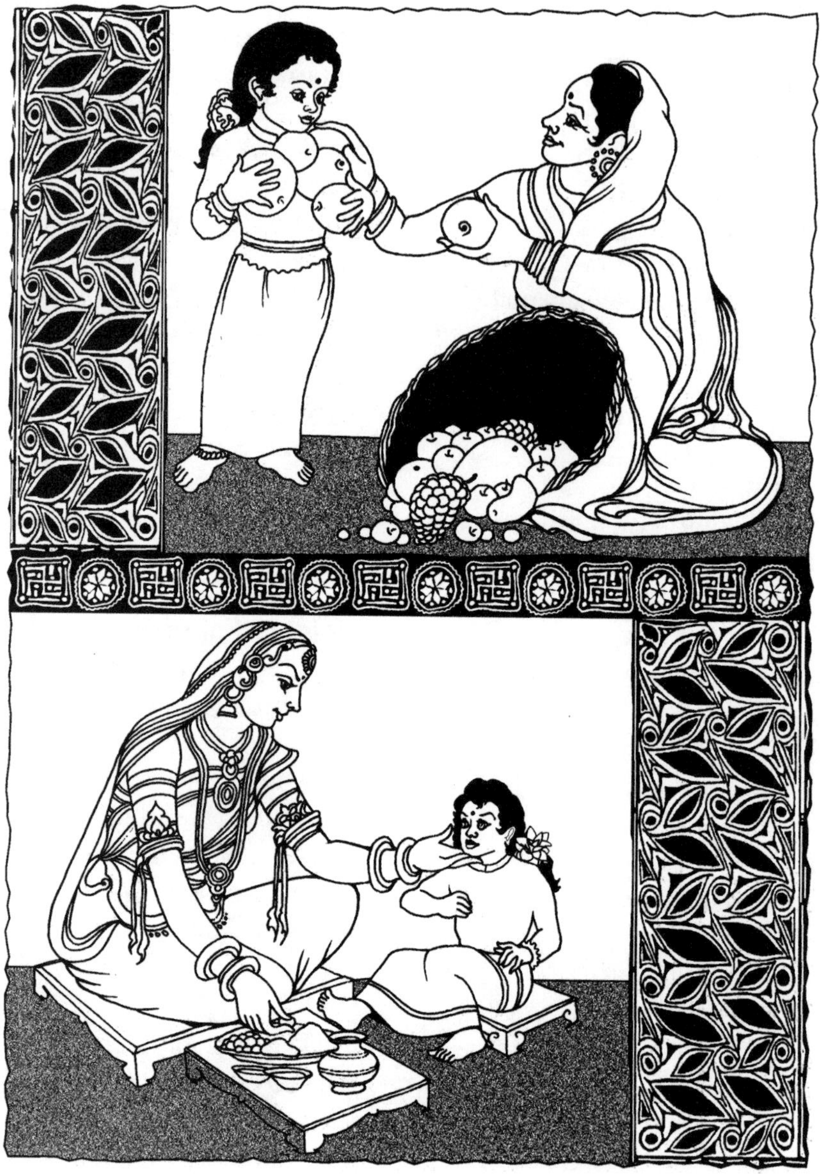

Bibliography

Acharya PK. *Encyclopedia of Hindu Architecture*. New Delhi, India: Oriental Book Reprints Co.; 1979.

Amber B. *Pulse Diagnosis*. Santa Fe, NM: Aurora Press; 1993.

Badmaev V, Majeed M. Effects of Āyurvedic Herbs. *Health Supplement Retailer Magazine*. November 1995.

Badmaev V, Majeed M.Āyurvedic Adaptogens and Bioprotectants. *Natural Food Merchandiser's Nutrition Science News Magazine*. September 1995.

Bhat MR. *Bṛihat Saṃhita*. New Delhi, India: Moltilal Banarsidass; 1986.

Bhishagratna KL. (transl.) *Suṣhrut Saṃhita*. Varanasi, India: Chowkhambha Sanskrit Series; 1991.

Brala PM, Hagen RL. Effects of Sweetness Perception and Caloric Value of a Preload on Short Term Intake. *Physiol Behav*, 30: 1, 1983 January: 1-9.

Colborn T., Dumanoski D., Myers JP. *Our Stolen Future*. New York, NY: Plume/Penguin; 1997

Collinge W. *The American Holistic Health Association Complete Guide to Alternative Medicine*. New York, NY: Warner Books; 1996.

Dadd DL. *Home Safe Home*. New York, NY: Tarcher/Putnam; 1997

Dagens B. (transl.) *Mayamatma*. New Delhi, India: Sitaram Bhartia Institute of Scientific Research; 1985.

Dash B, Kashyap L. *Diagnosis and Treatment of Diseases in Āyurveda. (vols. 2-7)* New Delhi, India: Concept Publishing; 1981-87.

Dash B. Massage *Therapy in Āyurveda*. New Delhi, India: Concept Publishing; 1992.

Dash B, Kashyap L. *Materia Medica of Āyurveda*. New Delhi, India: Concept Publishing; 1987.

Davis P. Aromatherapy A—Z. Essex, England: C.W. Daniel Ltd.; 1988.

Deshpande PJ, Singh R, Bhatt NS. Clinical Trial of Ayurvedic Drug U-144 (K4 Tablets) in Urinary Tract Infections. *Medicine & Surgery*. Vol 32, no 10/11, Oct. - Nov. 1994.

Deshpande PJ, Singh R, Bhatt NS. Clinical Effect of an Ayurvedic Drug L2002 on Hepatobiliary Disorders. *Journal of NIMA*. Dec. 1994.

Devaraj TL. *The Pañchakarma Treatment of Ayurveda*. Bangalore, India: Dhanwantari Oriental Publications; 1986.

Dossey L. *Healing Words*. San Francisco, CA: Harper; 1993

Fields D. Foods That Heal. *New Age Journal* July/August, 1993.

Frawley D. *Āyurveda Certification Course*. Santa Fe, NM: American Institute of Vedic Studies; 1992.

Frawley D. *Āyurvedic Healing*. Salt Lake City, UT: Passage Press; 1989.

Frawley D, Lad V. *The Yoga of Herbs*. Santa Fe, NM: Lotus Press; 1986.

Gould KL, Ornish D., et. al. Improved Geometry by Quantitative Coronary Arteriography After Vigorous Risk Factor Modification. *American Journal of Cardiology*. Vol 69, 10 April 1, 1992: 845 - 853

Govindan S.V. *Massage for Health and Healing*. New Delhi, India: Abhinav Publications; 1996

Gray H. *Gray's Anatomy*. Philadelphia, PA: Running Press; 1974.

Grontved A, Hentzer E. Vertigo-reducing Effect of Ginger Root. A Controlled Clinical Study. *ORL J. Otorhinolaryngol Relat. Spec.*, 48: 5, 1986: 282-6.

Gupta KRL. *Science of Sphygmica or Sage Kanad on Pulse*. Delhi, India: Sri Satguru Publications; 1987.

Guyton A. *Textbook of Medical Physiology*. Philadelphia, PA: Saunders Co.; 1981.

Heinerman J. *Encyclopedia of Nuts, Berries and Seeds*. West Nyack, NY: Parker Publishing; 1995.

India Currents Magazine. Stressed Out? Try Sitar Music. Dec '95-Jan '96: 14.

Institute for Wholistic Education. *Marma Point Therapy*. [video] Twin Lakes, WI: 1989.

Iyengar BKS. *Light On Yoga*. New York, NY: Shocken Books; 1976.

Johari H. *Ancient Indian Massage*. New Delhi, India: Munshiram Manoharlal Publishers; 1988.

Johari H. *Ayurvedic Massage*. Rochester, VT: Healing Arts Press; 1996.

Johari H. *The Healing Cuisine*. Rochester, VT: Healing Arts Press; 1994.

Jordan S. *Yoga For Pregnancy*. New York, NY: St. Martin's Press; 1987.

Joshi SV. *Āyurveda & Pañcha Karma*. Twin Lakes, WI: Lotus Press; 1997.

Kumar AV. *Principles of Ayurvedic Therapeutics*. Delhi, India: Sri Satguru Publications; 1995.

Kushi A, Esko W, Tiwari M. *Diet for Natural Beauty*. New York, NY: Japan Publications; 1991.

Lad, U & Vasant. *Āyurvedic Cooking*. Albuquerque, NM: Āyurvedic Press; 1994.

Lad, V. *Āyurveda; The Science of Self Healing*. Santa Fe, NM: Lotus Press; 1984.

Lidell N, Rabinovitch N & G. *Shivananda Companion To Yoga*. New York, NY: Fireside/Simon & Schuster; 1983.

Murthy KRS. (transl.) *Aṣhṭāñga Hṛidayam*. Varanasi, India: Kṛiṣhṇadas Academy; 1991.

Merck Manual. 16th ed. Merck Research Laboratories: Rahway, NJ; 1992.

Mindell E. *The Vitamin Bible*. New York, NY: Time Warner Books; 1991.

Murthy SK. (transl.) *Aṣhṭāñga Hṛidayam*. Varanasi, India: Kṛiṣhṇadas Academy; 1991.

Murthy SK. (transl.) *Mādhava Nidānam*. Varanasi, India: Chowkhamba Orientalia; 1993.

Murthy SK. (transl.) *Śhāngadhar Saṃhitā*. Varanasi, India: Chowkhamba Orientalia; 1984.

Nadkarni KN. *Indian Materia Medica*. Bombay, India: Popular Prakashan; 1993.

Ornish D. et. al. Can Lifestyle Changes Reverse Coronary Heart Disease? *Lancet*. Vol 336, no 8708, 21 July: 129-133. 1990.

Ornish D. Reversing Heart Disease Through Diet, Exercise, and Stress Management. *Journal of the American Dietetic Association*. Vol 91, no. 2, February, 1991: 162-165.

Pal KNC. Effect of a Herbomineral compound on Diabetes. *Ayurved Samachar* Issue 8, vol 10, February 2 1988.

Parikh, Pradhan PV, Shah LP, Bagadia VN. Evaluation of Indigenous Psychotropic Drugs - A Preliminary Study. *Journ Res Ay Sid* Vol 5, no 1-4, 1984.

Patnaik, N. *Garden of Life*. New York, NY: Doubleday; 1993.

Ranade S. *Natural Healing Through Āyurveda*. Salt Lake City, Utah: Passage Press; 1993.

Rossbach S. *Chinese Art of Placement*. New York, NY: Penguin Books; 1983.

Rossbach S. *Interior Design*. New York, NY: Penguin Books; 1987.

Rossbach S. *Living Color*. New York, NY: Kodansha, America, Inc.; 1994.

Sachs M. *Āyurvedic Beauty Care*. Twin Lakes, WI: Lotus Press; 1994.

Saraswati Swami Mūktībodhāndana (transl.) *Haṭha Yoga Pradīpikā*. Bihar, India: Bihar School of Yoga; 1985.

Savnur HV. *Ayurvedic Materia Medica*. Delhi, India: Sri Satguru Publications; 1988.

Shanmugasundaram ER, Rajeswari G, Baskaran K, Rajesh KBR, Shanmugasundaram K, Kizar AB. Use of Gymnema Sylvestre Leaf Extract in the Control of Blood Glucose in Insulin-Dependent Diabetes Mellitus. *J Ethnopharmaacol* 30: 3, 1990 Oct: 281-94 .

Sharadini U, Dahanukar T. *Ayurveda Revisited*. Bombay, India: Popular Prakashan;

1993.

Sharma RK, Dash B. (transl.) *Charaka Saṃhitā.* Varanasi, India: Chowkhamba Sanskrit Series Office; 1992.

Shastri Acharya Vaidyanath (transl.) *Atharva Veda.* New Delhi, India: Sarvadeshik Arya Pratinidhi Sabha.

Shub HA, Salvati EP, Rubin RJ. Conservative Treatment of Anal Fissure: an Unselected, Retrospective and Continuous Study. *Dis Colon Rectum* 21: 8, 1978 Nov-Dec: 582-3.

Shukla DN. *Vāstu Śhāstra.* New Delhi, India: Munshiram Manoharlal Pub.; 1993.

Sikdar JC. (transl.) *Nadivijnanam and Nadiprakasham* Jaipur, India: Prakrit Bharti Academy; 1988.

Singh RH. *Pañcha Karma Therapy.* Varanasi, India: Chowkhhamba Sanskrit Series; 1992.

Srivastava KC, Mustafa T. Ginger (Zingiber officinale) in Rheumatism and Musculoskeletal Disorders. *Med Hypotheses* 39: 4, 1992 December: 342-8.

Thakur M, Bhatt NS, Mishra S. others. Effect of Ayurvedic Drug (AB + R) in Indigestion. *Medicine & Surgery.* May - Aug. 1995: 25.

Thorne T. *Thorne's Guide to Herbal Extracts* (vol. 2). Royal Oak, MI: Wisteria Press; 1994.

Tirtha Swami Sada Shiva. *Ayurveda Certificaton Program.* Bayville, NY: Ayurveda Holistic Center Press; 1992.

Tirtha Swami Shankar Purushottam. *Guru Bani.* Bayville, NY: Āyurveda Holistic Center Press; 1995.

Tirtha Swami Shankar Purushottam. *Yoga Vani.* Bayville, NY: Āyurveda Holistic Center Press; 1990.

Tisserand M. *Aromatherapy for Women.* Rochester, VT: Healing Arts Press; 1988.

Tisserand R. *Aromatherapy to Heal and Tend the Body.* Santa Fe, NM: Lotus Press; 1988.

Vasu RBSC. (transl.) *Gheranda Saṃhitā.* New Delhi, India: Oriental Books Reprint Corp.; 1980.

Werbach M, Murray M. *Botanical Influences on Illness.* Tarzana, CA: Third Line Press; 1994.

Yoga Journal. Rx: Yoga. January/February 1994: 14

Wolever TM, Vuksan V, Eshuis H, Spadaora P, Peterson RD, Chao ES, Storey ML, Jenkins DJ. Effect of Method of Administration of Psyllium on Glycemic Response and Carbohydrate Digestibility. *J Am Coll Nutr* 10: 4, 1991 August: 364-71.

Zhou Y, Xu R. Antioxidative Effect of Chinese Drugs. *Chung Kuo Chung Yao Tsa Chih* 17: 6, 1997 June: 373, backcover.

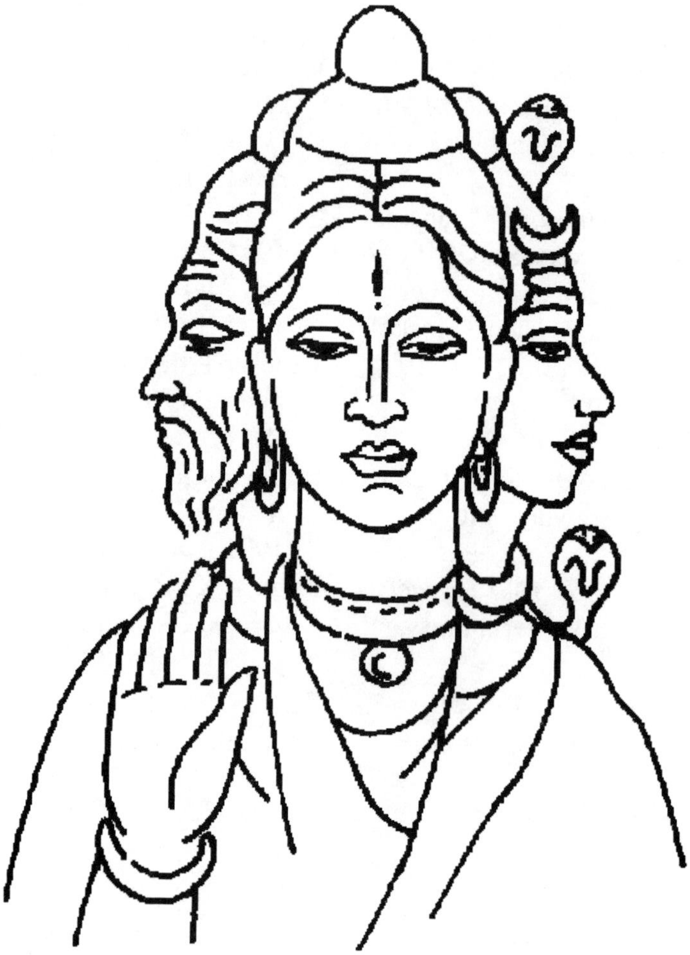

INDEX

P

T

U

W

"Oh, East is East, and West is West,
and never the twain shall meet,
Till earth and sky stand presently at
God's great Judgment Seat.

But there is neither East nor West,
border, nor breed, nor birth,
when two strong men stand face to face,
though they come from the ends of earth!"

Kipling - The Ballad of East and West